Register Now for Online Your Book!

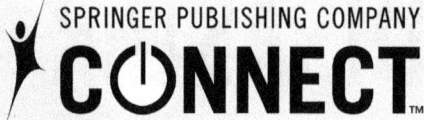
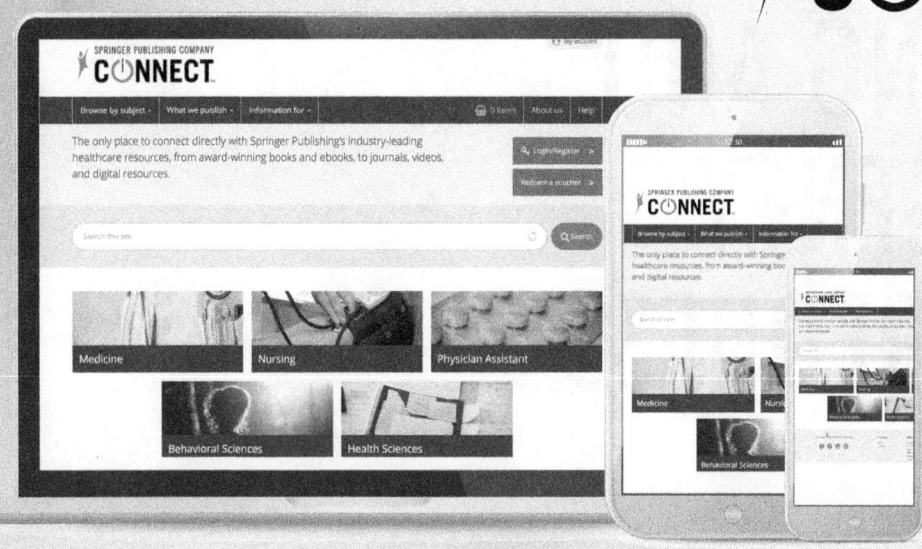

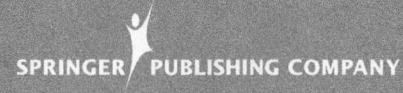

DISASTER NURSING AND EMERGENCY PREPAREDNESS

Tener Goodwin Veenema, PhD, MPH, MS, RN, FAAN, is Professor of Nursing and Public Health at the Johns Hopkins School of Nursing and the Center for Humanitarian Health at the Johns Hopkins Bloomberg School of Public Health. As an internationally recognized expert in disaster nursing and public health emergency preparedness, she has served as senior scientist to the U.S. Department of Health and Human Services (HHS) Office of Human Services Emergency Preparedness and Response (OHSEPR), Department of Homeland Security (DHS), Department of Veterans Affairs (VA), Veterans Affairs Emergency Management Evaluation Center (VEMEC), and the Federal Emergency Management Agency (FEMA). An accomplished disaster researcher, Dr. Veenema has received significant career funding and numerous awards for her work. She is a member of the American Red Cross National Scientific Advisory Board and is an elected fellow in the American Academy of Nursing, the National Academies of Practice, and the Faculty of Nursing and Midwifery at the Royal College of Surgeons, Dublin, Ireland. In 2013, Dr. Veenema was awarded the Florence Nightingale Medal of Honor (International Red Crescent), the highest international award in nursing, for her professional service in disasters and public health emergencies. She was awarded a Fulbright U.S. Scholar Award (2017) and was selected as the 2017–2018 Distinguished Nurse Scholar-in-Residence at the National Academy of Medicine (Washington, DC).

A highly successful editor and a prolific author, Dr. Veenema has published textbooks, handbooks, decision support software, and over 90 articles on emergency nursing and disaster preparedness. She has taught public health preparedness for over 25 years and has authored four highly successful national e-learning courses in disaster and public health preparedness for healthcare providers (Coursera, Elsevier, MC Strategies, American Red Cross). These interactive, e-learning programs have trained thousands of nurses and other disaster health services responders in caring for victims of disasters, terrorist events, and public health emergencies. A motivated, energetic, and self-directed leader with an impressive degree of creativity and innovation, Dr. Veenema is in high demand as a speaker and her information technology applications for disaster response have been presented at conferences around the globe. Dr. Veenema is the developer of *Disaster Nursing*, an innovative technology application ("App") for the smartphone and tablet (Unbound Medicine).

Dr. Veenema received her Bachelor of Science degree in Nursing from Columbia University in 1980, a Master of Science in Nursing Administration (1992), post-master's degree in the Care of Children and Families (1993) from the University of Rochester School of Nursing, and a Master's in Public Health (1999) and PhD in Health Services Research and Policy (2001) from the University of Rochester School of Medicine and Dentistry. A nationally certified pediatric nurse practitioner, Dr. Veenema was the recipient of the 2010 Distinguished Alumni Leadership Award from her alma mater Suffield Academy (Suffield, CT).

DISASTER NURSING AND EMERGENCY PREPAREDNESS

For Chemical, Biological, and Radiological Terrorism, and Other Hazards

Fourth Edition

TENER GOODWIN VEENEMA, PhD, MPH, MS, RN, FAAN

SPRINGER PUBLISHING COMPANY

Springer Publishing Company, LLC
11 West 42nd Street
New York, NY 10036
www.springerpub.com

Acquisitions Editor: Joseph Morita
Managing Editor: Cindy Yoo
Compositor: S4Carlisle Publishing Services

ISBN: 978-0-8261-4417-1
e-book ISBN: 978-0-8261-4422-5
Instructor's Manual ISBN: 978-0-8261-4492-8
Instructor's PowerPoints ISBN: 978-0-8261-4439-3

Instructor's Materials: Qualified instructors may request supplements by emailing textbook@springerpub.com.

18 19 20 21 22/5 4 3 2 1

The author and the publisher of this Work have made every effort to use sources believed to be reliable to provide information that is accurate and compatible with the standards generally accepted at the time of publication. Because medical science is continually advancing, our knowledge base continues to expand. Therefore, as new information becomes available, changes in procedures become necessary. We recommend that the reader always consult current research and specific institutional policies before performing any clinical procedure. The author and publisher shall not be liable for any special, consequential, or exemplary damages resulting, in whole or in part, from the readers' use of, or reliance on, the information contained in this book. The publisher has no responsibility for the persistence or accuracy of URLs for external or third-party Internet websites referred to in this publication and does not guarantee that any content on such websites is, or will remain, accurate or appropriate.

Library of Congress Cataloging-in-Publication Data

Names: Veenema, Tener Goodwin, editor.
Title: Disaster and emergency preparedness / [edited by] Tener Goodwin
  Veenema.
Other titles: Disaster nursing and emergency preparedness for chemical,
  biological, and radiological terrorism and other hazards.
Description: Fourth edition. | New York : Springer Publishing Company, [2018]
  | Preceded by Disaster nursing and emergency preparedness for chemical,
  biological, and radiological terrorism and other hazards / Tener Goodwin
  Veenema, editor. 3rd ed. c2013. | Includes bibliographical references and
  index.
Identifiers: LCCN 2018016746| ISBN 9780826144171 | ISBN 9780826144225 (e-book)
Subjects: | MESH: Emergencies--nursing | Disasters | Disaster Planning |
  Terrorism
Classification: LCC RT108 | NLM WY 154.2 | DDC 616.02/5--dc23 LC record available at https://lccn.loc.gov/2018016746

Contact us to receive discount rates on bulk purchases.
We can also customize our books to meet your needs.
For more information please contact: sales@springerpub.com

Printed in the United States of America.

Our world is not safe. Fraught with peril, it continues to be a dangerous place in which to live. And yet we know that our children and grandchildren need safe homes, safe schools, and safe communities to live in if they are to grow to be healthy, happy, and secure adults. They are counting on us to be there for them—no matter what the circumstances. They are counting on us to provide love, protection, and a safe harbor in the storm. They are counting on us to be prepared. They are counting on us to rescue them when they need rescuing. This textbook is dedicated to the children of the world—and to Kyle, Kendall, Blair, and Ryne in particular—you are everything to me. Always know how much I love you and how proud I am of you. Know that no matter how far away life takes you, home is always a safe harbor. And know that I tried to make the world a safer place.

Brief Contents

Contents

**3.   Hospital and Emergency Department
      Preparedness   51**
David Markenson and Sarah Losinski

**4.   Emergency Health Services in Disasters
      and Public Health Emergencies   67**
Jeremy T. Cushman, Manish N. Shah, and Mahshid Abir

**5.   Emergency Medical Consequence Planning
      for Special Events, Mass Gatherings, and
      Mass Casualty Incidents   81**
Tener Goodwin Veenema, Paul Arbon, and Alison Hutton

Contributors

Mahshid Abir, MD, MSc
Director, Acute Care Research Unit
Institute for Healthcare Policy & Innovation
Assistant Professor, Emergency Medicine
University of Michigan Medical School
Natural Scientist and Affiliated Adjunct,
    RAND Corporation
Ann Arbor, Michigan

Gary Ackerman, PhD
Associate Professor
College of Emergency Preparedness, Homeland Security,
    and Cybersecurity
University at Albany, State University of New York
Albany, New York

Janice B. Griffin Agazio, PhD, CRNP, RN,
    FAANP, FAAN
Assistant Dean
Professor
PhD and DNP Program Director
School of Nursing
The Catholic University of America
Washington, District of Columbia

Eileen M. Amari-Vaught, PhD, RN, MSN, FNP-BC
Clinical Assistant Professor
School of Nursing and Health Studies
University of Missouri-Kansas City
Kansas City, Missouri

Paul Arbon, RN, BSc, DipEd, Grad Dip Health Ed, MEd
    (Studies) PhD (Sydney), FACN, FAAN
Matthew Flinders Distinguished Professor
College of Nursing and Health Sciences
Director
Torrens Resilience Institute
Flinders University
Adelaide, Australia

Michael Beach, DNP, ACNP-BC, PNP, FAAN
Assistant Professor
University of Pittsburgh School of Nursing
Pittsburgh, Pennsylvania

Sue Anne Bell, PhD, FNP-BC, NDHP-BC
Clinical Associate Professor
School of Nursing
University of Michigan
Ann Arbor, Michigan

John G. Benitez, MD, MPH, FAACT, FACMT,
    FACPM, FAAEM
Medical Director
Emergency Preparedness Program
Tennessee Department of Health
Professor of Medicine and Emergency Medicine
Vanderbilt University School of Medicine
Nashville, Tennessee

Kelly J. Betts, EdD, MNSc, RN, CNE
Assistant Professor
University of Arkansas for Medical Sciences
College of Nursing
Little Rock, Arkansas

Joanne Bosanquet, MBE Queen's Nurse, RN, RHV,
    HonDUniv (Greenwich)
Deputy Chief Nurse
Public Health England
London, United Kingdom

Jody Bryant, MSN, RN
Clinical Nurse Educator
Central Arkansas Veterans Healthcare System
Little Rock, Arkansas

Frederick M. Burkle, Jr., MD, MPH, DTM,
    FAAP, FACEP
Professor (Ret.)
Senior Fellow and Scientist
Harvard Humanitarian Initiative
Harvard School of Public Health and T. C. Chan School of
    Public Health
Cambridge, Massachusetts
Senior International Public Policy Scholar
Woodrow Wilson International Center for Scholars
Washington, District of Columbia
Member, National Academy of Medicine, elected 2007

Wilma J. Calvert, PhD, MPE, MS(N), RN
Associate Professor
College of Nursing
University of Missouri–St. Louis
St. Louis, Missouri

Kathleen Leask Capitulo, PhD, RN, FAAN, IIWCC-NYU, FACCE
Chief Nurse Executive, James J. Peters VA Medical Center
Bronx, New York
Professor, Icahn School of Medicine at Mount Sinai
Faculty, Myers School of Nursing, New York University
New York, New York
Faculty, Frances Payne Bolton School of Nursing, Case
    Western Reserve University
Cleveland, Ohio

Susan M. S. Carlson, DNP
Assistant Professor
St. John Fisher College
Rochester, New York

Mary Casey-Lockyer, MHS, BSN, RN, CCRN
Senior Associate
Disaster Health Services
American Red Cross National Headquarters
Fairfax, Virginia

Thomas Chandler, PhD
Research Scientist
The National Center for Disaster Preparedness
Earth Institute, Columbia University
Adjunct Associate Professor
Teachers College, Columbia University
New York, New York

Valerie Cole, PhD
Manager
Individual Disaster Care
American Red Cross National Headquarters
Fairfax, Virginia

Andrew Corley, MSN/MPH, RN
Nurse Clinician
Johns Hopkins Hospital
Baltimore, Maryland

Mary Pat Couig, PhD, MPH, RN, FAAN
Program Manager, Emergency Management and RN
    Transition-to-Practice Residency
Office of Nursing Services
U.S. Department of Veterans Affairs
Washington, District of Columbia

Eric Croddy, MA
Astoria, Oregon

Jeremy T. Cushman, MD, MS, EMT-P, FACEP
Assistant Professor
Department of Emergency Medicine
University of Rochester
Medical Director, City of Rochester and County of Monroe
Rochester, New York

Kevin Davies, MBE, RRC, TD, DL PhD, MA, RN, PGCE
Emeritus Professor of Nursing and Disaster Healthcare
Faculty of Health and Education
University of South Wales
Glyntaff, Pontypridd
South Wales, United Kingdom

Elizabeth A. Davis, JD, EdM
Executive Director
EAD & Associates, LLC
Inclusive Emergency Management Consultants
Brooklyn, New York

Pat Deeny, RN, MSc Nursing, SFHEA
Senior Lecturer
School of Nursing
University Ulster, Magee Campus
Derry-Londonderry, Northern Ireland

Aram Dobalian, PhD, JD, MPH
Director
Veterans Emergency Management Evaluation Center
Office of Patient Care Services
Veterans Health Administration
U.S. Department of Veterans Affairs
North Hills, California

Shannon Finley, MSN, RN, CPHQ
Quality Assurance/Performance Improvement Manager
University of Arkansas for Medical Sciences Medical Center
Little Rock, Arkansas

Anne F. Fish, PhD, RN, FAHA
Associate Professor
College of Nursing
University of Missouri–St. Louis
St. Louis, Missouri

Dona M. Friend, MNSc, RN, RNP
Clinical Educator, Coordinator for Interprofessional
    Clinical Orientation
University of Arkansas for Medical Sciences
    Medical Center
Little Rock, Arkansas

Patricia Frost, RN, MS, PNP
Director
Emergency Medical Services
Contra Costa Health Services
Contra Costa County, California

Alicia R. Gable, MPH
Senior Project Director
Veterans Emergency Management Evaluation Center
Office of Patient Care Services
Veterans Health Administration
U.S. Department of Veterans Affairs
North Hills, California

Kristine M. Gebbie, DrPH, RN
Adjunct Professor, University of Adelaide and Flinders
   Universities
Associate Director, Torrens Resilience Institute
Adelaide, South Australia

Anne Griffin, MPH, BSN, RN, CNOR
Clinical Investigator and Senior Program Manager
Veterans Emergency Management Evaluation Center
Office of Patient Care Services
Veterans Health Administration
U.S. Department of Veterans Affairs
North Hills, California

Sheila R. Grigsby, PhD, MPH, RN, PHNA-BC
Assistant Professor
College of Nursing
University of Missouri–St. Louis
St. Louis, Missouri

Rebecca Hansen, MSW
Managing Director
EAD & Associates, LLC
Inclusive Emergency Management Consultants
Brooklyn, New York

Kevin D. Hart, JD, MPH, PhD

**Alison Hutton, RN, DipAppSc (Nsg), Paediatric
   Certificate, BNg, MNg, PhD, FACN**
Professor
School of Nursing and Midwifery
University of Newcastle
Newcastle, Australia

Joy Jennings, MSN, RN-BC
Clinical Assistant Professor
Arkansas State University-Beebe Campus
College of Nursing
Beebe, Arkansas

P. Andrew Karam, PhD, CHP
Karam Consulting
New York, New York

Ziad N. Kazzi, MD, FAAEM, FACEP, FACMT, FAACT
Associate Professor
Medical Toxicologist
Department of Emergency Medicine
Emory University
Assistant Medical Director
Georgia Poison Center
Atlanta, Georgia

Sean J. Kice, MS
Strategic National Stockpile Coordinator
Emergency Preparedness Program
Tennessee Department of Health
Nashville, Tennessee

Joanne C. Langan, PhD, RN, CNE
Associate Dean, Undergraduate and Pre-Licensure Education
Professor
Coordinator, Disaster Preparedness & RN Return
   to Practice
Saint Louis University School of Nursing
St. Louis, Missouri

Roberta Proffitt Lavin, PhD, FNP-BC, FAAN
Professor and Associate Dean for Academic Programs
University of Missouri-St. Louis
St. Louis, Missouri

E. Brooke Lerner, PhD, FAEMS
Professor, Departments of Emergency Medicine
   and Pediatrics
Co-Director, Comprehensive Injury Center
Medical College of Wisconsin
Milwaukee, Wisconsin

Karen Levin, RN, CCRN, CPHN, MPH, MCHES
Adjunct Associate Professor of International and Public
   Affairs
Columbia University
New York, New York

Juliana Soares Linn, MD, MPH, MSc
Deputy Director, Implementation Unit
ICAP at Columbia University
New York, New York

Justin K. Loden, PharmD, CSPI
Director of Education
Tennessee Poison Center
Nashville, Tennessee

Sarah Losinski, MPH, BSN, RN
Research Assistant
Community Public Health Nursing
Johns Hopkins School of Nursing
Baltimore, Maryland

Linda M. MacIntyre, PhD, RN
Chief Nurse, American Red Cross
Volunteer Services
American Red Cross National Headquarters
Washington, District of Columbia

Rishma Maini, BSc, MBChB, DTMH, MPH, MFPH
Senior Public Health Registrar in Global Disaster Risk
    Reduction
Public Health England
London, United Kingdom

David Markenson, MD, MBA, FAAP, FACEP, FCCM
National Chair
Scientific Advisory Council
American Red Cross

Elizabeth C. Meeker, PsyD
Director, Practice Transformation
Coordinated Care Services, Inc.
Rochester, New York

Susan Michaels-Strasser, PhD, MPH, RN, FAAN
Assistant Professor in Epidemiology
Columbia Mailman School of Public Health
Implementation Director of ICAP at Columbia University
New York, New York

Amanda Fuller Moore, PharmD
Pharmacist
Division of Public Health
North Carolina Department of Health and Human Services
Raleigh, North Carolina

Virginia Murray, FFPH, FRCP, FFOM, FRCPath
Public Health Consultant in Global Disaster Risk Reduction
Public Health England
Visiting Professor, UNU-International Institute of Global
    Health
Member of the WHO Collaborating Centre on Mass
    Gatherings and Global Health Security
London, United Kingdom

Sarah D. Nafziger, MD, FACEP, FAEMS
Professor of Emergency Medicine
University of Alabama at Birmingham
Birmingham, Alabama

Susan M. Orsega, MSN, FNP-BC, FAANP, FAAN
Chief Nurse Officer
United States Public Health Service
Washington, District of Columbia

Lori Peek, PhD
Professor, Department of Sociology
Director, Natural Hazards Center
University of Colorado
Boulder, Colorado

Marilyn M. Pesto, JD, MSN, RN
Director and Assistant Professor
Sirridge Office of Medical Humanities and Bioethics
School of Medicine
University of Missouri-Kansas City
Kansas City, Missouri

Brenda Phillips, PhD
Dean, College of Liberal Arts and Sciences
Professor of Sociology
Indiana University South Bend
South Bend, Indiana

David C. Pigott, MD, RDMS, FACEP
Professor and Vice Chair for Academic Development
Co-Director of Emergency Ultrasound
Department of Emergency Medicine
University of Alabama at Birmingham
Birmingham, Alabama

Kathleen Coyne Plum, PhD, RN, NPP
Adjunct Faculty
Wegmans School of Nursing
St. John Fisher College
Rochester, New York

Robbie Prepas, CNM, MN, NP, JD
Adjunct Professor, UCLA School of Nursing
Los Angeles, California
Co-Chairperson, Disaster Preparedness Caucus
American College of Nursing
Consultant, CDC Pandemic Flu Planning
Member, Disaster Preparedness Medical Team
Silver Spring, Maryland

Erica Rihl Pryor, PhD, RN
Associate Professor (retired)
School of Nursing
University of Alabama at Birmingham
Birmingham, Alabama

Lisa Puett, BSN, RN
Coordinator, Pediatric Trauma & Burn Programs
Division of Pediatric Surgery
John Hopkins Children's Center
Baltimore, Maryland

Kristine Qureshi, PhD, RN, FAAN, CEN, PHNA-BC
Professor
Associate Dean for Research and Global Health Nursing
School of Nursing and Dental Hygiene
University of Hawaii at Manoa
Honolulu, Hawaii

Adam B. Rains, MSc
Lead PHM Analyst
Center for Population Health Outcomes and Informatics
Department of Population Health Management
    Informatics
University of Rochester Medical Center
Rochester, New York

Richard Ricciardi, PhD, NP, FAANP, FAAN
Director, Division of Practice Improvement
Senior Advisor for Nursing
Agency for Healthcare Research and Quality
Rockville, Maryland

Susan Roettinger Ritchie, MN, RN (retired)

J. Christie Rodgers, LICSW
Senior Associate
Disaster Mental Health, Program Development
American Red Cross National Headquarters
Fairfax, Virginia

Lou E. Romig, MD, FAAP, FACEP
Medical Director
After Hours Pediatrics Urgent Care Clinics
Tampa, Florida

**Tara L. Sacco, MS, RN, CCRN-K, AGCNS-BC,
    ACCNS-AG**
Visiting Assistant Professor
Wegmans School of Nursing
St. John Fisher College
Clinical Nurse Specialist
Adult Critical Care Nursing
University of Rochester Medical Center
Rochester, New York
PhD Student & Jonas Scholar 2016–2018 Cohort
M. Louise Fitzpatrick College of Nursing
Villanova University
Villanova, Pennsylvania

Juliana Sadovich, PhD, RN
Director of Quality Management
Indian Health Service
U.S. Department of Health and Human Services
Rockville, Maryland

Cheryl K. Schmidt, PhD, RN, CNE, ANEF, FAAN
Clinical Professor
College of Nursing and Health Innovation
Arizona State University
Phoenix, Arizona

Manish N. Shah, MD, MPH
Associate Professor
The John & Tashia Morgridge Chair of Emergency
    Medicine Research
Vice Chair for Research
BerbeeWalsh Department of Emergency Medicine
University of Wisconsin School of Medicine & Public
    Health
Madison, Wisconsin

CAPT. Lynn A. Slepski, PhD, RN, PHCNS-BC, FAAN
Senior Public Health Advisor
United States Public Health Service
Office of the Secretary, U.S. Department of Transportation
Washington, District of Columbia

Janice Springer, DNP, RN, PHN
Volunteer Partner to Vice President International
    Services
Disability Integration Advisor
Disaster Health Services Manager
American Red Cross
Foley, Minnesota

Kandra Strauss-Riggs, MPH
Education Director
National Center for Disaster Medicine and Public Health
Uniformed Services University of the Health Sciences
Bethesda, Maryland

Susan Sullivan, MS, RN-BC
Public Health Nursing Consultant
Vaccine Preventable Disease Program
Communicable Disease Branch
Raleigh, North Carolina

Devin Terry, MSN, RN, ACNS-BC, CQHQ
Advanced Practice Partner for Ambulatory Services
University of Arkansas for Medical Sciences
    Medical Center
Little Rock, Arkansas

Clifton P. Thornton, MSN, RN, CNMT, CPNP
Pediatric Nurse Practitioner
Johns Hopkins University School of Medicine
Johns Hopkins Bloomberg Children's Hospital
Baltimore, Maryland

Sarah Tuneberg, MPH
Chief Executive Officer
Geospiza, Inc.
Denver, Colorado

Tener Goodwin Veenema, PhD, MPH, MS, RN, FAAN
2018 Distinguished Nurse Scholar in Residence
National Academy of Medicine
Washington, District of Columbia
Professor of Nursing and Public Health
Johns Hopkins School of Nursing
Center for Humanitarian Health
Johns Hopkins Bloomberg School of Public Health
Baltimore, Maryland

Jonathan D. White, PhD, LCSW-C, CPH (Commander, USPHS)
Chief, Domestic Policy Branch
Office of the Assistant Secretary for Preparedness and Response
U.S. Department of Health and Human Services
Washington, District of Columbia

Reviewers

Lavonne Adams, PhD, RN, CCRN
Associate Professor
Texas Christian University
Fort Worth, Texas

Mary Pat Couig, PhD, MPH, RN, FAAN
Program Manager, Emergency Management and RN
    Transition-to-Practice Residency
Office of Nursing Services
U.S. Department of Veterans Affairs
Washington, District of Columbia

Sarah Schneider-Firestone, MSW
Research Associate
Johns Hopkins School of Nursing
Baltimore, Maryland

Roberta Proffitt Lavin, PhD, FNP-BC, FAAN
Professor and Associate Dean for Academic Programs
University of Missouri-St. Louis
St. Louis, Missouri

Mary Casey-Lockyer, MHS, BSN, RN, CCRN
Senior Associate
Disaster Health Services
American Red Cross National Headquarters
Fairfax, Virginia

Zoe Rush
Medical Editor
Johns Hopkins School of Nursing
Baltimore, Maryland

Janice Springer, DNP, RN, PHN
Volunteer Partner to Vice President International Services
Disability Integration Advisor
Disaster Health Services Manager
American Red Cross
Foley, Minnesota

*With special gratitude for his review and oversight of the
    previous editions:*

Adam B. Rains, MSc
Lead PHM Analyst
Center for Population Health Outcomes and Informatics
Department of Population Health Management Informatics
University of Rochester Medical Center
Rochester, New York

Foreword

It is a humbling honor to be chosen to write this foreword for the Fourth Edition of *Disaster Nursing and Emergency Preparedness*, a scholarly compendium of the work of the most experienced practitioners and researchers involved in disaster and crisis nursing. As I write this foreword, I am fully aware that we collectively face, in this increasingly globalized world, an unprecedented number of major challenges to the preparation and protection of victims from an expanding array of threats to their safety and livelihood. While our knowledge base in the science of disasters has made great strides, especially in technical and communication innovations, this information has not always been successfully translated into improved preparedness and response capabilities. Nor has this evidence base been successfully translated into improved effectiveness and efficiency in meeting increasing healthcare challenges to the ever-changing variety of crisis events leading some humanitarian sector experts to claim that the "system is broken." Admittedly, improvements will arise first from a commitment to scale up research in improving evidence for healthcare prevention, preparedness, and response, placing a priority on identifying research gaps, and finally translating these advances into educational and training priorities. The fourth edition speaks to those advances.

Nursing is the world's largest health profession and consistently contributes 70% or more of professionals responding to local, national, regional, and global crises. Historically, nursing organizations and leadership have always considered disaster preparedness and response a vital role of nursing practice; however, it has been only in the last several decades that both professional and academic institutions have formally focused on preparing nurses with the required educational and operational competencies and courses for response and on implementing the vital roles the nursing profession has in advancing disaster research, policy, practice, and administration.

Research has shown that the nature of major crises and how the world responds to them have dramatically changed every 10 to 15 years or sooner. Whereas the first edition clearly met the challenge to be relevant to that era, subsequent editions have been remarkable in guaranteeing the most updated evidence-based information necessary to meet new educational and operational competencies—whether the crisis occurs in one's community or demands a global workforce deployment of medical teams to sudden onset natural disasters, public health emergencies of international concern such as the Ebola epidemic, war, armed conflict, and complex humanitarian emergencies. Each edition historically chronicles the unique advances across the disaster cycle from prevention, preparedness, response to recovery, and rehabilitation. The diligent work of editor Dr. Tener Goodwin Veenema, a highly respected academic nursing scholar with firsthand field experience and solid policy credentials, has consistently focused on ensuring that each volume in the series has met the operational requirements facing the individual nurse and the profession at large.

The fourth edition is unique in recognizing the rapid changes in both the causes of these crises and the latest attempts to provide timely multidisciplinary approaches to the practice of this growing specialty, as well as the inclusion of the rapidly growing influence of advances in science, technology, social sciences, international law and policy, and globalization, to name but a few. What we do as healthcare professionals in mitigating mortality and morbidity is most evident in new chapters that reflect the emerging operational vocabulary such as "public health emergencies"—one of the most crucial challenges of our time. Unfortunately, while we have embraced the fact that disasters possess the unique quality of defining the state of the public health and immediately exposing its deficiencies, collectively we have a poor history in overcoming political barriers to uncover and prevent the deficiencies in essential public health infrastructure: food, shelter, water, sanitation, access to and availability of health services, and energy that each disaster, once again, predictably reveals. Interestingly, energy was added to the list of essential infrastructure only after the 1988 Armenian earthquake resulted in an unprecedented rapid rise of preventable mortality as victims froze from the lack of heat during the following cruel winter months. Yet again, the loss of energy to posthurricane rehabilitation of Puerto Rico in 2017 was predictable and preventable and underscores societal failures in accepting that 1 U.S. dollar put to prevention can save 4 U.S. dollars in response—an economic fact rarely heeded by decision makers in the planning for disaster recovery and rehabilitation.

Additional new and timely chapters address the Sendai Agreement for Disaster Risk Reduction and the targets adopted by the United Nations (UN) Sustainable Development Goals (SDGs) designed to both prevent public health crises and protect vulnerable populations; the consequences of climate-related disasters that have increased by over 50% in the last decade with loss of essential aquifers, major droughts, and loss of viable land, leaving developing countries unable to survive or participate in adapting, further resulting in unprecedented internal migration, escalation of internal conflicts, urban warfare, and massive numbers of refugees leaving the Middle East and Northern Africa; the rapidly escalating incidence of domestic civil unrest and community violence; active shooters and mass shootings and the burden that is creating for healthcare systems; and the ever-compelling importance of preparedness for radiation emergencies and blast injuries that leave no country unprotected. In many situations, public health interventions could have prevented the acceleration of governmental mismanagement, poverty, and the mass exodus of refugees, especially those in the health professions.

A persuasive argument of Dr. Veenema's that is evident throughout this edition is the call to identify crisis leadership among the increasingly talented base of nurses who have

responsibility to move the profession to recognize and accept that they can be advocates for better planning, coordination, education, and training. Whereas nursing duties today are extremely demanding, there remain unfilled requirements for those willing to be leaders in disasters, crisis nursing, and especially public health emergencies. There is no other option but for nurses to take ownership of their responsibility to be prepared.

Frederick M. Burkle, Jr., MD, MPH, DTM, PhD(Hon.),
FAAP, FACEP
Professor (Ret.)
Senior Fellow and Scientist
Harvard Humanitarian Initiative, Harvard University and
T.C. Chan School of Public Health Boston, Massachusetts

Senior International Public Policy Scholar
Woodrow Wilson International Center for Scholars
Washington, District of Columbia
Member, National Academy of Medicine, elected 2007

Foreword

The burden upon healthcare systems that disasters create is immeasurable and stretches across all levels of society and the capacities of both official and civilian responses. Regardless of the setting, nurses play a pivotal role in disaster management. In December 2016, the Johns Hopkins School of Nursing was pleased to host *Society for the Advancement of Disaster Nursing: Nursing Administration and Leadership in an Emerging Clinical Arena*, a 2-day national conference that brought together nurse leaders, hospital administrators, and public health and emergency management specialists from across the country who are committed to the advancement of national nurse readiness. Convening thought leaders was pivotal to sustaining our U.S. National Health Security Strategy, which is "built on a foundation of community resilience—healthy individuals, families, and communities with access to health care and the knowledge and resources to know what to do to care for themselves and others in both routine and emergency situations."[1] Little did we know that this system would be further tested in the natural disasters of 2017—from hurricanes, floods, and forest fires.

While much has been accomplished over the past few years to increase awareness of nursing's many roles and responsibilities during disasters and large-scale public health emergencies, much remains to be done. Nursing as a profession represents the largest sector of the healthcare workforce and a potentially untapped resource for achieving surge capacity goals and optimizing population health outcomes following these challenging events. Ensuring that our national nursing workforce has the knowledge, skills, and abilities to respond to a disaster or public health emergency in a timely and appropriate manner must be a priority and is certainly worthy of our continued efforts.

In this Fourth Edition of *Disaster Nursing and Emergency Preparedness*, Dr. Veenema continues her mission to help our nation's nurses develop the knowledge, skills, and abilities needed to efficiently and effectively respond to disasters. In order to achieve the goal of Making Every Nurse a Prepared Nurse, it is essential to ensure that all nurses understand the implications of natural and man-made disasters, so they are prepared to respond if required. This impressive edition builds upon the solid foundation of the first three award-winning editions with an expanded focus on climate change–related disasters, globalization and its implications for emerging and reemerging infectious diseases, the accommodation of high-risk, high-vulnerability populations, and the potential for disaster arising from a world witnessing increasing community violence and civil unrest. From her work at the National Academy of Medicine in medical and public health preparedness, Dr. Veenema has woven the current state of the science throughout the book.

Internationally regarded for her expertise in workforce development for disasters, mass gatherings, and public health emergency preparedness, Dr. Veenema has maintained a laser focus on the importance of the international relevance of the book, adding new chapters that address the landmark agreements: the Sendai Framework for Disaster Risk Reduction 2015–2030, the UN Sustainable Development Goals (SDGs), and the Paris Climate Agreement. Global disaster nursing leadership has never been more important and nursing's voice across all continents can advocate for the achievement of these policies that will reduce and mitigate the impact of natural disasters and complex human emergencies.

Many times nurses assume that they are not emergency responders, so they do not need to understand how the emergency health system works. When a disaster strikes a community—whether a bus accident, an earthquake, a hurricane, terrorist attack, or riots and civil unrest—nurses will be on the front lines helping those who are in need. To protect themselves, their families, and their communities, nurses need to understand the principles and content of this comprehensive textbook. An all-hazards and whole-community approach is needed for our nation to be resilient in the face of disaster and this must include the nurses in our country and across the globe.

---

[1] Department of Health and Human Services Office of the Assistant Secretary for Preparedness and Response. Retrieved from https://www.phe.gov/Preparedness/planning/authority/nhss/Pages/default.aspx

Dr. Veenema has achieved a masterful accomplishment with the publication of this edition, and I encourage all nurses to develop the knowledge, skills, and abilities presented here, which are needed to achieve the vision of disaster preparedness locally, nationally, and internationally.

Patricia M. Davidson, PhD, MED, RN, FAAN
Professor and Dean
Johns Hopkins School of Nursing
Sigma Theta Tau International
Institute for Global Leadership Advisory Board
Counsel General International Council on
Women's Health Issues
Board Member Consortium of Universities for
Global Health
Baltimore, Maryland

Foreword

In the past, each new edition of *Disaster Nursing and Emergency Preparedness* seemed like the "best time" for the arrival of a new update. Today, more than ever before, is unquestionably the most propitious time for the fourth edition. What supports that observation? I believe it is the particular social, economic, technological, political, and environmental climate of our times. Natural and man-made disasters are not new, but the global nature, rate, type, and totality of the environments impacted are increasing. Complex human emergencies leading to population migration, violence, and infectious disease outbreaks now persist for years without resolution. These horrendous and tragic human situations are generating the urgency for a greater need for awareness, preparedness, political prowess, and leadership, and, most of all, teamwork on all levels of governments, educational institutions, human services, environmental organizations, and many others. Social media and the lightning transmission of reporting of these events and our responses make these happenings unique. Rather than separating us from the rest of the world, they may be a uniting factor with all of us sharing the same concerns, risks, threats, and consequences. They may require us to not only communicate more fully and swiftly but also plan strategies of information sharing, preventive designs, and positive promotional activities that will not only offer societies protection but also institute environments of problem solving that are more predictive, productive, and positive than we are experiencing today. Given the speed of global communications and cyberspace capacity, worldwide attention must be paid to our population's mental as well as physical health, our communities' resources and preparation, national polices and plans for prevention as well as response, and our commitment for everyone to be involved. Disasters are everyone's problem and should not be left to the professional responders alone. Each and every one of us, as citizens and as nurses, has a responsibility for preparedness, not only for ourselves, but our neighbors and communities as well. We need to think of ourselves as "first responders," not as standby observers or the last hope for survival.

This new and greatly expanded edition addresses all of these needs with an in-depth focus on the impact of climate change, the threat of growing civil unrest and community violence, the critical importance of planning for and accommodating vulnerable populations, and the design of disaster health services for those at high risk such as children, pregnant women, the elderly, and chronically ill.

The contributing authors read like a "Who's Who" of disaster leaders. They lend their special expertise and insights, which are supported and elucidated by cogent learning strategies in the use of case studies, student questions, and packed content in all areas of disaster participation, preparedness, policies, and research.

Many teachers, students, practitioners, and policymakers will find this edition a treasure trove of new information, ideas, and ideologies and will use this volume as a text, a reference, and resource for the challenging work they do in disaster preparedness and practice. For over 16 years, *Disaster Nursing and Emergency Preparedness* has been the hallmark text in its field, and this edition proves to be the best ever.

Loretta C. Ford, RN, PNP, EdD
Dean Emeritus
University of Rochester School of Nursing
Founder of the National Nurse Practitioner Program
Member, National Women's Hall of Fame
Seneca Falls, New York

Preface

Chance favors the prepared mind.

—*Louis Pasteur*

In the global community within which we live, concern for the sustainability of our environment, the health and well-being of our citizens, and the overall planetary health has rapidly accelerated. In light of recent world events and increasing geopolitical tensions, our concerns have now expanded to include the ubiquitous threat of terrorism; the potential detonation of thermonuclear weapons; acknowledgment of the devastating impact of climate change; emerging and reemerging infectious diseases such as Ebola, Zika, and coronavirus; and the increasing frequency and intensity of natural disasters such as hurricanes, floods, tsunamis, and earthquakes.

Disaster Nursing and Emergency Preparedness has always evolved to meet the unique learning needs of nurses across the globe, and the fourth edition of this hallmark text promises to be the most comprehensive ever. As the leading textbook in the field approaches 20 years, I am extremely proud and excited to present our newest edition along with its sister "e-book" and companion digital instructor's manual.

The fourth edition of this textbook holds us to our highest standards ever with an ambitious goal—to once again provide nurses, nurse midwives, nurse practitioners, and nurse executives with the most *current, valid, and reliable evidence-based* content available. The text presents a broad and comprehensive overview of existing domestic and international disaster health policy coverage. The genesis of the book was predicated on the belief that *all nurses should possess the knowledge, skills, and attitudes (KSAs) to be able and willing to respond in a timely and appropriate manner to any disaster or major public health emergency and keep themselves and their patients safe.* Our goal is simple—*to improve population health outcomes following a disaster event or public health emergency.*

Every chapter in this fourth edition has been carefully researched, fact-checked, reviewed by subject matter experts, and matched to the highest standards in disaster education. Whenever possible, we have mapped all content to published core competencies for preparing the health profession's students for response to terrorism, disaster events, and public health emergencies. As with previous editions, this edition contains a significant amount of new content and strives to expand our focus as nurses to: (a) acknowledge anthropogenic climate change, (b) deepen our understanding of the importance of global disaster risk reduction and mitigation strategies, (c) continually expand the international scope of the book to meet the needs of our global nursing colleagues, (d) address the growing threat of pandemics, and (e) increase our awareness of the health implications of urban civil unrest and community violence.

We have remained vigilant to the release of relevant major policy recommendations by international organizations, congressionally convened commissions, panels, scientific advisory boards, and organizations such as the National Academy of Medicine (Washington, DC) to inform the evolution of our discipline. In 2015, several notable UN agreements were adopted and include: the Sendai Framework for Disaster Risk Reduction, the Sustainable Development Goals (SDGs), and the Conference of the Parties 21's (COP21's) Paris Climate Agreement. The policy areas pertaining to these landmark frameworks are closely interrelated, and their importance in protecting the future of human health is incalculable. For example, climate mitigation and adaptation strategies may contribute to reducing the frequency of disasters, which in turn supports sustainable development and healthy communities. We recognize the forces of globalization and the importance of addressing "One Health."

The framework of the book relates directly to the 2015 UN agreements, the World Health Organization (WHO) Global Health Security Strategy, and the WHO and U.S. Centers for Disease Control and Prevention (CDC) Office of Emergency Preparedness and Response Guidelines for response to public health emergency events. The fourth edition aligns with the U.S. National Health Security Strategy and remains consistent with the five U.S. National Planning Frameworks and the National Incident Management System. It describes activation and deployment of the U.S. Strategic National Stockpile and the use of medical countermeasures. As with the previous editions, the overarching concepts of the book have been mapped to the Public Health Preparedness and Response Core Competency Model (www.asph.org), the Office of the Assistant Secretary for Preparedness and Response 2017–2022 Healthcare Preparedness and Response Capabilities, and the International Council of Nurses foundational competencies for disaster nursing practice. We have added several new chapters addressing critical topics such as (a) public health emergencies involving community violence and civil unrest; (b) nursing in disasters, catastrophes, and public health emergencies worldwide; (c) disaster nursing and the 2015 UN landmark agreements; and (d) national disaster nurse readiness. We have expanded our coverage of planning for and accommodating high-risk, high-vulnerability populations and have built upon our fundamental belief in a safe and clean environment as a foundational building block for health. We have updated and expanded existing chapters on natural disasters, environmental disasters, CBRNE events, and restoring public health following a disaster. We have addressed the importance of "One Health," which recognizes that the health of people is connected to the health of animals and the environment. Nurses can advance the goal of One Health by working locally, nationally, and globally—to achieve the best health for people, animals, and our environment.

We live in an increasingly complicated world where our healthcare systems are severely taxed, financially stressed, and our emergency departments are functioning in disaster mode on a daily basis. The concept of accommodating a sudden, unanticipated "surge" of patients remains overwhelming. We have reason to believe that these challenges will continue and clinical demands on staff and the need for workforce preparedness will continue to grow in the future. We will need many nurses to get involved in efforts to increase both U.S. national and global nurse readiness. Working with colleagues at the U.S. Veterans Administration Emergency Management and Evaluation Center (VEMEC) and supported by nurses from major universities and professional nursing organizations, the recently established Society for the Advancement of Disaster Nursing (2017) is working to engage more U.S. nurses in this effort. Led by a dynamic group of nurses with an unwavering commitment to disaster nursing, this group is making major inroads in advancing disaster nursing practice, education, research, and policy. Several of these amazing nurses are chapter authors in this book, which brings me to note that this textbook, like the previous editions before it, represents a major "team" effort. I gratefully acknowledge the wonderful contributions of each of my coauthors and reviewers. Many of these nurse and physician colleagues have been authors in previous editions of this book. Several authors are former graduate students of mine, now trusted colleagues. There is no way to adequately express my gratitude for the time, talent, and treasure of their work and the friendship provided by these subject matter experts. Thank you most sincerely.

This textbook represents one step in my lifelong journey to contribute to building strength and safety in emergency health services and readiness within our nursing workforce. I remain personally committed to my work in preparing a *global nursing workforce that is adequately prepared* to respond to any disaster or public health emergency and I encourage you to join me and get involved. This work involves improving and expanding programs for interdisciplinary disaster education, lobbying for the advancement of nurses in federal and other key leadership positions to develop disaster-related policies, coalition building across key stakeholders, ensuring access to appropriate and sufficient supplies of personal protective equipment, and much more. This includes working to establish functional and ongoing community partnerships that foster collaboration and mutual planning for the health of our communities and the sustainability of our environment. It includes acknowledging and aggressively addressing climate change. It means giving reflective consideration to the realities of the clinical demands placed on nurses during catastrophic events and the need for consideration of crisis standards for clinical care during disasters and public health emergencies. It includes looking at innovative applications of technology to enhance sustainable learning and disaster nursing response. Take a look at *Disaster Nursing* (Unbound Medicine, at the App store), a digital app for the smartphones that includes just-in-time information and clinical guidelines for over 400 disaster and public health emergency events, designed specifically for nurses!

This fourth edition of this textbook continues to be a reflection of my love for writing and research, as well as a *deep desire to help nurses protect themselves*, their families, and their communities. Disaster nursing is a patient safety issue. Nurses can protect their patients only if they themselves are safe first. The fourth edition represents a substantive attempt to collect, expand, update, and include the most valid and reliable information currently available about various disasters, public health emergencies, and acts of terrorism. As stated earlier, the target audience for the book is all nurses—*making every nurse a prepared nurse*—staff nurses, nurse practitioners, educators, and administrators.

This book continues to represent the foundation for *best practice in disaster nursing and emergency preparedness*, and is a stepping-stone for the discipline of disaster nursing research. There is much work to be done, and it continues to be very rewarding to witness increased interest in disaster nursing as more nurses get involved. The editor welcomes constructive comments regarding the content of this text.

Tener Goodwin Veenema

How to Use This Book

GUIDELINES FOR NURSING FACULTY AND STAFF DEVELOPMENT SPECIALISTS

Update on What Is New in the Fourth Edition

Greetings colleagues! The newest edition of this AJN Book of the Year is bigger and better than ever and continues to provide U.S. and international nurse educators with the high-quality evidence-based content needed to incorporate into both undergraduate and graduate course curricula for optimal student learning related to disaster nurse readiness. The book provides student nurses with the most comprehensive, current, and reliable information available so they can acquire the unique knowledge and develop the skills they need to efficiently and effectively respond to all types of disasters or public health emergencies. Meticulously researched and reviewed by the world's foremost experts in preparedness for terrorism, natural disasters, and other unanticipated public health emergencies, the text has been revised, expanded, and updated with significant new content, including a new chapter.

The book provides comprehensive coverage related to leadership and management in disaster and emergency health systems as well as both basic and advanced disaster clinical nursing response. This new edition has strengthened its pediatric focus with updated and expanded chapters on caring for children's physical, mental, and behavioral health following a disaster. Additional new chapters address 21st-century threats including climate change, emerging infectious diseases, global complex human emergencies, caring for patients with HIV/AIDS following a disaster, disaster information technology, and hospital and emergency department preparedness. The book provides a vast amount of evidence-based information on disaster planning and response for natural and environmental disasters and those caused by chemical, biological, and radiological elements, as well as disaster recovery. It also addresses leadership, management, and policy issues in disaster nursing and deepens our understanding of the importance of protecting mental health throughout the disaster life cycle. Each chapter is clearly formatted and includes key messages and learning objectives. Appendices present diagnosis and treatment regimens, creating personal disaster plans, a damage assessment guide, a glossary of terms, and more. Consistent with the National Response and Recovery Framework, the Centers for Disease Control and Prevention (CDC) Public Health Emergency Preparedness and Response Capabilities, and the National Health Security Strategy, the book promotes competency-based expert nursing care during disasters and positive health outcomes for small and large populations.

KEY FEATURES OF THE FOURTH EDITION

- Disseminates state-of-the-science, evidence-based information
- Provides a new chapter and new expanded content throughout the book
- Includes digital teacher's guide with exercises and critical thinking questions
- Is consistent with current U.S. federal and international guidelines for disaster response
- Empowers nurses as leaders in disaster and public health emergency preparedness planning

DIGITAL INSTRUCTOR'S GUIDE

This edition of the textbook is accompanied by a digital adjunct teacher's guide with PowerPoint presentations, student group exercises, and critical thinking questions. Faculty will find that the use of selected chapters from the text along with the digital instructor's guide and supportive materials will allow easy integration of crucial disaster content into existing courses across programs.

The goal of all nursing education programs as it relates to disaster preparedness is to ensure that all nurses possess a minimum knowledge base and skill set before graduation to ensure that they will be able to participate in a disaster response in a timely and safe manner. Both patient safety and nurse safety are critical elements in any disaster response effort. The optimization of population-based health outcomes will be achieved only if nurse responders are safe and prepared to meet the demands of a sudden surge of victims from a disaster event or major public health emergency.

In order to meet the *Essentials in Baccalaureate Education* for population-based healthcare:

Assess the health, healthcare, and emergency preparedness needs of a defined population.
Use clinical judgment and decision-making skills in appropriate, timely nursing care during disaster, mass casualty, and other emergency situations.

For the *Essentials for Master's Education* topic areas in disaster preparedness and management, **faculty** are strongly encouraged to first read the following chapter before teaching this content:

> *Chapter 36: U.S. National Disaster Nurse Readiness: Practice and Education for a Prepared Workforce*

Nurse educators may find it extremely helpful to use the following rubric in determining what components of the book and course materials they wish to integrate into their courses.

DISASTER CONTENT RUBRIC

1. Nurse educators are encouraged to include the following chapters and digital instructor's materials to present a basic CORE clinical/health systems disaster nursing overview:
   - Essentials of Disaster Planning
   - Leadership and Coordination in Disaster Healthcare Systems: The U.S. National Preparedness System
   - Hospital and Emergency Department Preparedness
   - Disaster Management
   - Disaster Triage
   - Legal and Ethical Issues in Disaster Response
   - Understanding the Psychosocial Impact of Disasters
2. Nurse educators are encouraged to include the following chapters and digital instructor's materials to present a program for ADVANCED clinical disaster nursing:
   - Decontamination and Personal Protective Equipment
   - Chemical Agents of Concern
   - Radiological Incidents and Emergencies
   - Management of Burn Casualty Incidents
   - Traumatic Injury Due to Explosives and Blast Injuries
   - Management of the Psychosocial Effects of Disasters
3. Nurse educators are encouraged to include the following chapters and digital instructor's materials to present content for Maternal & Child Health programs:
   - Identifying and Accommodating High-Risk High-Vulnerability Populations in Disasters
   - Unique Needs of Children During Disasters and Other Public Health Emergencies

- Disaster Nursing in Schools and Other Child Congregate Care Settings
- Care of the Pregnant Woman and Newborn Following a Disaster
- Human Services Needs Following Disaster Events and Disaster Case Management

4. Nurse educators are encouraged to include the following chapters and digital instructor's materials to present content related to Public Health Outbreak Management:
   - Surveillance Systems for Detection of Biological Events
   - Biological Agents of Concern
   - Infectious Disease Emergencies
   - Medical Countermeasures Dispensing
   - Role of the Public Health Nurse in Disaster Response
5. Nurse educators are encouraged to include the following chapters and digital instructor's materials to present content related to *global* disaster nursing and humanitarian response:
   - Disaster Nursing and the United Nations 2015 Landmark Agreements—A Vital Force for Change in the Field of Disaster Nursing
   - Natural Disasters
   - Complex Human Emergencies
   - Nursing in Disasters, Catastrophes and Complex Humanitarian Emergencies Worldwide
   - Restoring Public Health Under Disaster Conditions: Basic Sanitation, Water and Food Supply, and Shelter
   - Human Services in Disasters and Public Health Emergencies: Social Disruption, Individual Empowerment, and Community Resilience
   - Climate Change and Health: The Nurse's Role in Policy and Practice

My hope is that you find this information valuable, facilitating your adoption of the book and supportive materials into your educational setting. Let us work together to *Make Every Nurse a Prepared Nurse*. We owe it to our patients, our families, and our communities for they are counting on us as a profession to be there when they need us.

Most sincerely,

Tener Goodwin Veenema
Editor
2017–2018 Distinguished Scholar in Residence
National Academy of Medicine
Washington, District of Columbia

Editor's Note

The information presented in this book has been verified up to the date of submission for publication; however, this field is dynamic and the science and relevant health policies related to disasters and public health emergencies are constantly changing. References, clinical guidelines, and resources frequently change to reflect new knowledge. Readers are strongly encouraged to use this textbook as a resource and as a guide, and to frequently visit web links at the WHO and the U.S. federal websites (ASPR, CDC, FEMA, DHS, EPA, etc.) for updates. Visit the ASPR website at www.phe.gov, the CDC website at www.cdc.gov, the DHS website at www.dhs.gov/index.shtm, the FEMA website at www.fema.gov, and the preparedness page of the ASPR at www.phe.gov/preparedness/pages/default.aspx for the most current, available information.

DISASTER PREPAREDNESS

1

ESSENTIALS OF DISASTER PLANNING

Tener Goodwin Veenema

LEARNING OBJECTIVES

When this chapter is completed, readers will be able to:

1. Classify the major types of disasters based on their unique characteristics and describe their impact.
2. Identify societal factors that have contributed to increased losses (human and property) as a result of disasters.
3. Describe basic principles of disaster planning, including the agent-specific and the all-hazards approach, and the basic components of a disaster plan.
4. Discuss areas of focus in emergency and disaster planning—preparedness, mitigation, response, and recovery—and the critical importance of evaluation.
5. Describe risk assessment, hazard identification, and vulnerability analysis.
6. Assess constraints on a community's or organization's ability to respond.
7. Describe the core preparedness actions.
8. Recognize situations suggestive of an increased need for additional comprehensive planning.

KEY MESSAGES

In 2017, the United States experienced a series of devastating events such as Hurricanes Harvey, Irma, and Maria, and the California Wildfires, revealing ongoing vulnerability, inadequate level of community and organizational preparedness, and the perpetual struggle to mitigate the societal and environmental impacts of these destructive disasters.

NOTE—This chapter is mapped to the Centers for Disease Control and Prevention's (CDC) Public Health Preparedness Capabilities (Appendix I) and to the CDC Public Health Preparedness and Response Core Competency Model (www.aspph.org/teach-research/models/public-health-preparedness-response). This model states that nurses should able to

■ Contribute their expertise to a community hazard vulnerability analysis (HVA)
■ Contribute their expertise to the development of emergency plans
■ Participate in improving the organizations' capacities
■ Maintain situational awareness

The frequency and intensity of natural and man-made disasters, the individuals and families affected by them, and the economic costs associated with loss have been steadily increasing over recent years.

While disasters are often unexpected, sound disaster planning and preparedness can anticipate common problems and mitigate the consequences of an event.

Different types of disasters are associated with distinct patterns of illness and injury, and early assessment of risks and vulnerability can reduce morbidity and mortality later on.

Disasters are different from daily emergencies; most cannot be managed simply by mobilizing additional personnel and supplies. Certain commonly occurring problems can be anticipated and addressed during planning.

Effective disaster plans and preparedness activities are based on knowledge of how people behave. Key components and common tasks must be included in any disaster preparedness plan.

Nurses are well positioned to participate as full partners with the medical, public health, and emergency management community in all aspects of disaster planning, mitigation, response, and recovery.

Planning must advance the U.S. National Preparedness Goal of "A secure and resilient nation with the capabilities required across the whole community to prevent, protect against, mitigate, respond to, and recover from the threats and hazards that pose the greatest risk."

CHAPTER OVERVIEW

The foundational principles of disaster planning, preparedness, and mitigation, and the key components of a disaster preparedness plan are introduced in this chapter. Definitions of the different types of disasters are provided along with a classification system based on their common and unique features, onset, duration, effect (immediate aftermath), and recovery period. The concept of the disaster nursing timeline as an organizational framework for strategic planning is introduced. Areas of focus in emergency and disaster preparedness—preparedness, mitigation, response, and recovery—are addressed and the importance of evaluation is proposed. Risk assessment, hazard identification and mapping, and vulnerability analysis are presented as methods for decision making and planning. The concepts of disaster epidemiology and measurement of the magnitude of a disaster's impact on population health are explored. The Centers for Disease Control and Prevention (CDC) of Public Health Preparedness Core Capabilities provides a strategic framework for planning. The six domains of preparedness—community resilience, incident management, information management, countermeasures and mitigation, surge management, and biosurveillance—are discussed.

Disasters have been an integral part of the human experience since the beginning of time causing premature death, impaired quality of life, dislocation, and altered health status. The risk of a disaster is ubiquitous and on average, a disaster requiring international assistance occurs somewhere in the world every week. In 2017, the United States experienced an unprecedented year of devastating disasters. The effects of three major Atlantic and Gulf Coast hurricanes (Harvey, Irma, and Maria) on communities along the Texas gulf coast, throughout Florida, and in the U.S.

Caribbean islands were both widespread and substantial. In the Houston area, 1,500 patients from 20 different care facilities were relocated due to the storm. In Florida, 435 facilities, including 30 hospitals and over 60 nursing homes, were evacuated. At the time of publication of this book, much of Puerto Rico did not have electricity and the healthcare system in Puerto Rico was currently being supported by the deployment of the U.S. Navy's ship the USNS Comfort and other federal resources. Educational systems were similarly affected, with over 1.65 million students across the affected communities missing at least 1 day of school, and many schools in Texas and Florida closed for 2 weeks. With regard to housing, over 190,000 homes were damaged between Florida and Texas, and the extent of damage to the housing stock in Puerto Rico is still considered immeasurable. The scope of the federal response to the 2017 disasters was significant with nearly 19,000 civilian and military personnel deployed to Puerto Rico alone. Within weeks, Northern California was engulfed in flames and in December, Southern California was also in flames, making 2017 the year of the worst wildfires in the history of the state. The U.S. federal investment in response and recovery was substantial, with Congress appropriating $51.5 billion to fund disaster response and recovery efforts in the wake of these hurricanes and other disasters affecting the United States (Federal Emergency Management Agency [FEMA], 2017b).

Hurricanes Harvey, Irma, and Maria, and the California Wildfires revealed our ongoing vulnerability, inadequate level of community and organizational preparedness, and our perpetual struggle to mitigate the societal and environmental impacts of these destructive events. The recent dramatic increase in natural disasters, their intensity, the number of people affected by them, and the human and economic losses associated with these events have placed an imperative on disaster planning for emergency preparedness. Global warming, climate change, sea level rise, resource depletion, and societal factors are likely to coalesce to create future calamities. Population shifts to urban settings and the growth of "megacities" contribute to the increased risk (International Federation of Red Cross and Red Crescent Societies [IFRC], 2017; United Nations, 2016). Globalization, with increased rate of travel between continents, will continue to contribute to the international spread of lethal communicable diseases, like the Ebola outbreak of West Africa from 2014 to 2016 or the Zika outbreak in Central America and the Caribbean in 2016. Acts of aggression including events like the Orlando Nightclub shooting (2016), the Las Vegas concert shooting (2017), or international conflicts like the Syrian civil war and the resultant mass refugee crisis, along with the ongoing incidence of global terrorist attacks are reminders of the potentially deadly consequences of our inhumanity toward each other.

An extensive review of the past two decades of disasters, including significant political strife and conflicts in the Middle East, Africa, Asia and elsewhere, indicates that few disasters are the result of a single cause and effect. More frequently, they are complex human emergencies associated with global instability, economic decay, political upheaval and collapse of government structures, violence and civil conflicts, famine, and mass population displacements (IFRC, 2017). Current humanitarian crises are near the "tipping point" of being beyond recovery and represent ongoing and profound public health emergencies with a preponderance of excess or indirect mortality and morbidity. Risks to health posed by humanitarian emergencies continue to be at an all-time high and will require global solutions for resolution in the future (World Health Organization [WHO], 2016). Finally, epidemics, famine, as well as the effects of Hurricanes Katrina (2005), Sandy (2012), Harvey, Irma, and Maria (2017); the Indonesian (2004), Haitian (2010), and Iran-Iraq (2017) earthquakes; and the Japanese (2011) tsunami and nuclear event point to the complexities of managing disasters within a broader sociopolitical context. While our understanding of the environment and its associated hazards has improved significantly over the past decade, and while we now possess increasingly sophisticated tools for hazard monitoring and risk communication, the political willingness and financial resources required to successfully confront these hazards is often lacking (Burkle, 2010; Smith & Petley, 2009; Tierney, 2012). Furthermore, individual nursing and medical willingness to respond to disasters is variable and research suggests that many nurses and other healthcare providers feel unequipped to respond (Connor, 2014; Veenema, 2008) or to keep themselves safe (Subbotina & Agrawal, 2018).

In the United States, as in many countries across the globe, nurses constitute the largest sector of the healthcare workforce and will certainly be on the frontlines of any emergency response (American Nurses Association [ANA], 2018; U.S. Department of Labor, Bureau of Labor Statistics [DOL], 2018). As part of a country's overall plan for disaster preparedness, all nurses must have a basic understanding of disaster science and the key components of disaster preparedness, including the following:

1. The definition and classification system for disasters and major incidents based on common and unique features of disasters (onset, duration, effect, and recovery period)

2. Disaster epidemiology and measurement of the health consequences of a disaster

3. The areas of focus in emergency and disaster preparedness: preparedness, mitigation, response, recovery, and evaluation

4. Methods that serve as a base for strategic planning including risk assessment, hazard identification and mapping, and vulnerability analysis

5. The six domains of preparedness—community resilience, incident management, information management, countermeasures and mitigation, surge management, and biosurveillance

6. The 15 public health core capabilities as defined by the CDC as a framework for planning and preparedness (Appendix I)

7. Awareness of the roles and responsibilities of the nurse in a much larger response system

This chapter introduces the reader to the principles of disaster planning, the common tasks consistent across all disaster responses, and the key components of disaster planning and preparedness.

DEFINITION AND CLASSIFICATION OF DISASTERS

How do we define a "disaster"? A disaster is defined as: "a serious disruption of the functioning of a community or a society at any scale due to hazardous events interacting with conditions of exposure, vulnerability and capacity, leading to one or more of the following: human, material, economic and environmental losses and impacts" (United Nations International Strategy for Disaster Reduction [UNISDR], 2017). It may be viewed as an ecological disruption, or emergency, of a severity and magnitude that result in deaths, injuries, illness, and property damage that cannot be effectively managed using routine procedures or resources and that require outside assistance. Healthcare providers characterize disasters by what they do to people—the consequences on health and healthcare and human services. A "health disaster" is a catastrophic event that results in casualties that overwhelm the healthcare resources in that community (Al-Madhari & Keller, 1997) and may result in a sudden unanticipated surge of patients (Institute of Medicine [IOM], 2015b), a change in standards of care (IOM, 2009), and a need to allocate scarce resources (IOM, 2012; Timbie et al., 2012). Disasters may be classified into two broad categories: *natural* (those caused by natural or environmental forces) and *man-made* or *anthropogenic* (human generated). The WHO defines "natural disaster" as the "result of an ecological disruption or threat that exceeds the adjustment capacity of the affected community" (Lechat, 1979). Natural disasters include earthquakes, floods, tornadoes, hurricanes, volcanic eruptions, ice storms, tsunamis, and other geological or meteorological phenomena. Natural disasters are the consequence of the intersection of a natural hazard and human activity. Anthropogenic disasters are those in which the principal direct causes are identifiable human actions, deliberate or otherwise (Jha, 2010). Anthropogenic disasters include biological and biochemical terrorism, chemical spills, radiological (nuclear) events, fire, explosions, transportation accidents, armed conflicts, and acts of war.

Human-generated disasters can be further divided into three broad categories: complex emergencies, technological disasters, and disasters that are not caused by natural hazards but occur in human settlements. *Complex human emergencies* involve situations where populations suffer significant casualties as a result of war, civil strife, or other political conflict. Some disasters are the result of a combination of forces such as drought, famine, disease, and political unrest that displace millions of people from their homes. These humanitarian disasters can be epic in proportion such as civilians fleeing the genocide in Darfur (2003–2010), Rohingyas in Myanmar, or refugees displaced by the conflict in Syria. With *technological disasters*, large numbers of people, property, community infrastructure, and economic welfare are directly and adversely affected by major industrial accidents, unplanned release of nuclear energy, and fires or explosions from hazardous substances such as fuel, chemicals, or nuclear materials. Frequently, natural and human-made disasters trigger each other and the distinctions between the two disaster types may be blurred. A natural and human-generated disaster may trigger a secondary disaster, the result of weaknesses in the human environment. An example of this is a chemical plant explosion following an earthquake. Such combinations, or *synergistic disasters*, are commonly referred to as NA-TECHs (natural and technological disasters; Subbotina & Agrawal, 2018). A NA-TECH disaster occurred in Japan (March, 2011) when an earthquake and tsunami caused damage to the Fukushima Daiichi nuclear reactor, resulting in wide-scale evacuation, illness, and long-term population displacement (referred to as an indirect causality event). Disasters can and do occur simultaneously (e.g., a chemical attack along with a nuclear assault), potentiating the death and devastation created by each indirect casualty event (Subbotina & Agrawal, 2018).

Disasters are frequently categorized based on their *onset*, *impact*, and *duration*. For example, earthquakes and tornadoes are rapid-onset events—short durations but with a sudden impact on communities. Hurricanes and volcanic eruptions have a sudden impact on a community; however, advanced warnings are issued enabling planners to implement evacuation and early response plans. A bioterrorism attack may be sudden and unanticipated and have a rapid and prolonged impact on a community.

In contrast, droughts and famines have a more gradual onset or chronic genesis (the so-called creeping disasters) and generally have a prolonged impact. Factors that influence the impact of a disaster on a community include the nature of the event, time of day or year, health and age characteristics of the population affected, and the availability of resources (Burstein, 2014). Further classification of terms in the field of disaster science distinguishes between hazards, disasters, and risk. A *hazard* (cause) is a potential threat to humans and their welfare (Smith & Petley, 2009). *Risk* is the actual exposure of something of human value and is often measured as the product of probability and loss (Smith & Petley, 2009). *Hazards* present the possibility of the occurrence of a disaster caused by natural phenomena (e.g., hurricane, earthquake), failure of man-made sources of energy (e.g., nuclear power plant), or human activity (e.g., war).

Defining an event as a disaster also depends on the *location* in which it occurs, particularly the population density of that location. For example, an earthquake occurring in a sparsely populated area would not be considered a disaster if no people were injured or affected by loss of housing or essential services. However, the occurrence of even a small earthquake could produce extensive loss of life and property in a densely populated region (e.g., San Francisco or Los Angeles) or a region with inadequate construction or limited medical resources. Similarly, numbers and types of casualties that might be handled routinely by a large university hospital or metropolitan medical center could overwhelm a small community hospital.

Hospitals and other healthcare facilities may further classify disasters as either *internal* or *external*. *External* disasters are those that do not affect the hospital infrastructure but tax hospital resources due to numbers of patients or types of injuries (Burstein, 2014). For example, a tornado that produced numerous injuries and deaths in a community would be considered an external disaster. *Internal* disasters cause disruption of normal hospital function due to injuries or deaths of hospital personnel or damage to the facility itself, as with a hospital fire, power failure, or chemical spill (Hendrickson & Horowitz, 2016). Unfortunately, one type of hospital disaster does not necessarily preclude the other, and features of both internal and external disasters may be present if a natural phenomenon affects both the community and the hospital. This was the case with Hurricanes Andrew (1992), which caused significant destruction in hospitals, clinics, and the surrounding community when it struck south Florida (Sabatino, 1992); Katrina (2005) when it impacted the Gulf Coast, rupturing the levee in New Orleans (Berggren, 2005; Danna, Bernard, Schaubhut, & Matthews, 2009; Rodriguez & Aguirre, 2006); and Sandy (2012) when it impacted the East Coast resulting in flooding and the forced evacuation of two of New York City's flagship hospitals. Hurricanes Harvey, Irma, and Maria (September and October 2017) resulted in major interruptions and closures in hospital and healthcare organizations across Texas, Florida, and Puerto Rico.

DECLARATION OF A DISASTER

In the United States, the Robert T. Stafford Disaster Relief and Emergency Assistance Act,[1] passed by Congress in 1988 and amended most recently in August 2016, provides for federal government assistance to state and local governments to help them manage major disasters and emergencies. Under the Stafford Act, a "major disaster" means any natural catastrophe (including any hurricane, tornado, storm, high water, wind-driven water, tidal wave, tsunami, earthquake, volcanic eruption, landslide, mudslide, snowstorm, or drought), or, regardless of cause, any fire, flood, or explosion, in any part of the United

---

[1] Robert T. Stafford Disaster Relief and Emergency Management-related Provisions of the Homeland Security Act, as amended FEMA 592, August 2016. The Robert T. Stafford Disaster Relief and Emergency Assistance Act (Public Law 100–707), signed into law on November 23, 1988, amended the Disaster Relief Act of 1974 (Public Law 93–288). The Stafford Act constitutes the statutory authority for most federal disaster-response activities, especially as they pertain to the Federal Emergency Management Agency (FEMA) and FEMA programs.

States, which in the determination of the President causes damage of sufficient severity and magnitude to warrant major disaster assistance under this Act to supplement the efforts and available resources of states, local governments, and disaster relief organizations in alleviating the damage, loss, hardship, or suffering caused thereby (The Stafford Act, as amended and Emergency Management-related Provisions of the Homeland Security Act, as amended FEMA 592, August 2016). Through this amended act, the President may provide federal resources, medicine, food and other consumables, work assistance, and financial relief. These federal resources may now be prepositioned prior to the disaster event in order to facilitate more timely and effective response. Review of recent years' data suggests that the number of presidential disaster declarations is increasing (see Table 1.1; FEMA, 2017a; Lindsay & McCarthy, 2011, 2015). In 2011, there were 242 disasters declared by the President, the highest on record in the United States (FEMA, 2017a). If the consequences of a disaster are clear and imminent and warrant redeployment actions to lessen or avert the intensity of the threat, a state's governor may request assistance even before the disaster has occurred. A library of all past and current federally declared disasters in the United States can be located at the FEMA website (www.fema.gov/news/disasters.fema).

TABLE 1.1 Disaster Declaration by Year

Year	Total
2001	112
2002	119
2003	123
2004	118
2005	155
2006	143
2007	136
2008	143
2009	114
2010	108
2011	242
2012	112
2013	95
2014	84
2015	79
2016	102
2017	136

Source: Federal Emergency Management Agency. (2017a). *Disaster declarations by year.* Retrieved from https://www.fema.gov/disasters/year

A current list of international declared disasters and emergencies and links to disease outbreaks can be located on the WHO's website (www.who.int/topics/disasters/en).

HEALTH EFFECTS OF DISASTERS

Disasters affect communities and their populations in different ways. Damaged and collapsed buildings are evidence of physical destruction. Roads, bridges, tunnels, rail lines, telephone and cable lines, and other transportation and communication links are often destroyed; public utilities (e.g., water, gas, electricity, and sewage disposal) may be disrupted and a substantial percentage of the population may be rendered homeless and forced to relocate temporarily or permanently. Disasters damage and destroy businesses and industry, agriculture, and the economic livelihood of the community. The impact of disasters caused by weather in 2017 alone has generated a huge impact (Figure 1.1). By fall 2017, the United States had already experienced 11 weather and climate disasters that each exceeded a cost of $1 billion in response efforts (National Oceanic and Atmospheric Administration [NOAA], 2017). Hurricane Harvey, which devastated Texas in late August 2017, dumped over 50 inches of rain in Houston and neighboring counties and resulted in the largest storm-related economic losses in U.S. history (NOAA, 2017). Hurricane Maria (2017) caused widespread devastation in Puerto Rico, rendering the island without power or fresh water for months and caused billions of dollars in damages. In 2017, northern California wildfires raged across Napa, Sonoma, and Yuba counties and the southern California wildfires around San Diego and Los Angeles killed many people and caused billions of dollars in property damage.

The health effects of disasters may be extensive and broad in their distribution across populations. In addition to causing illness and injury, disasters disrupt access to primary care, preventive services, and exacerbate underlying psychiatric illness (Potash, 2008; Rabins, Kass, Rutkow, Vernick, & Hodge, 2011). Depending on the nature and location of the disaster, its effects on the short- and long-term health and mental health of a population may be difficult to measure (Lillibridge, Noji, & Burkle, 1993).

"Epidemiology," as classically defined, is the quantitative study of the distributions and determinants of health-related events in human populations (Gordis, 2013). "Disaster epidemiology" is the measurement of the adverse health effects of natural and human-generated disasters and the factors that contribute to those effects, with the overall objective of assessing the needs of disaster-affected populations, matching available resources to needs, preventing further adverse health effects, evaluating program effectiveness, and planning for contingencies (Kano, Wood, Siegel, & Bourque, 2017; Lechat, 1990). Disasters affect the health status of a community in the following ways:

- Disasters may cause premature deaths, illnesses, and injuries in the affected community, generally exceeding the capacity of the local healthcare system.
- Disasters may destroy the local healthcare infrastructure, which therefore will be unable to respond to the emergency. Disruption of routine health and mental healthcare

services and prevention initiatives may lead to long-term consequences in health outcomes in terms of increased morbidity and mortality.

- Disasters may create environmental imbalances, increasing the risk of communicable diseases and environmental air, soil, and water hazards.
- Disasters may affect the psychological, emotional, and social well-being of the population in the affected community. Depending on the specific nature of the disaster, responses may be fear, anxiety, depression, widespread panic, terror, and exacerbation of preexisting mental health problems. Children, in particular, may be deeply affected by the impact of a disaster (Save the Children, 2017).
- Disasters may cause shortages of food and cause severe nutritional deficiencies.
- Disasters may cause large population movements (refugees) creating a burden on other healthcare systems and communities. Displaced populations and their host communities are at increased risk of communicable diseases and the health consequences of crowded living conditions (Lam, McCarthy, & Brennan, 2015).
- Disaster frameworks for response are increasingly shaped by globalization, changing world dynamics, social inequality, and sociodemographic trends (Tierney, 2012; WHO, 2016).

THE DISASTER CONTINUUM

The life cycle of a disaster is generally referred to as the "disaster continuum," or "emergency management cycle." This life cycle is characterized by three major phases—*preimpact* (before), *impact* (during), and *postimpact* (after)—and provide the foundation for the disaster time line (Figure 1.2). Specific actions taken during these three phases, along with the nature and scope of the planning, will affect the extent of the illness, injury, and death that occurs.

The basic phases or "life cycle" of a disaster management program include *preparedness, mitigation, response, recovery, and evaluation* (Kim, Proctor, & Amos, 2002; Landesman, 2011; Landesman & Morrow, 2013). There is a degree of overlap across phases, but each phase has distinct activities associated with it.

Preparedness refers to the proactive planning efforts designed to structure the disaster response prior to its occurrence. Disaster planning encompasses evaluating potential vulnerabilities (assessment of risk) and the propensity for a disaster to occur. "Warning" (also known as "forecasting") refers to monitoring events to look for indicators that predict the location, timing, and magnitude of future disasters.

Mitigation includes measures taken to reduce the harmful effects of a disaster by attempting to limit its impact on human health, community function, and economic infrastructure. These

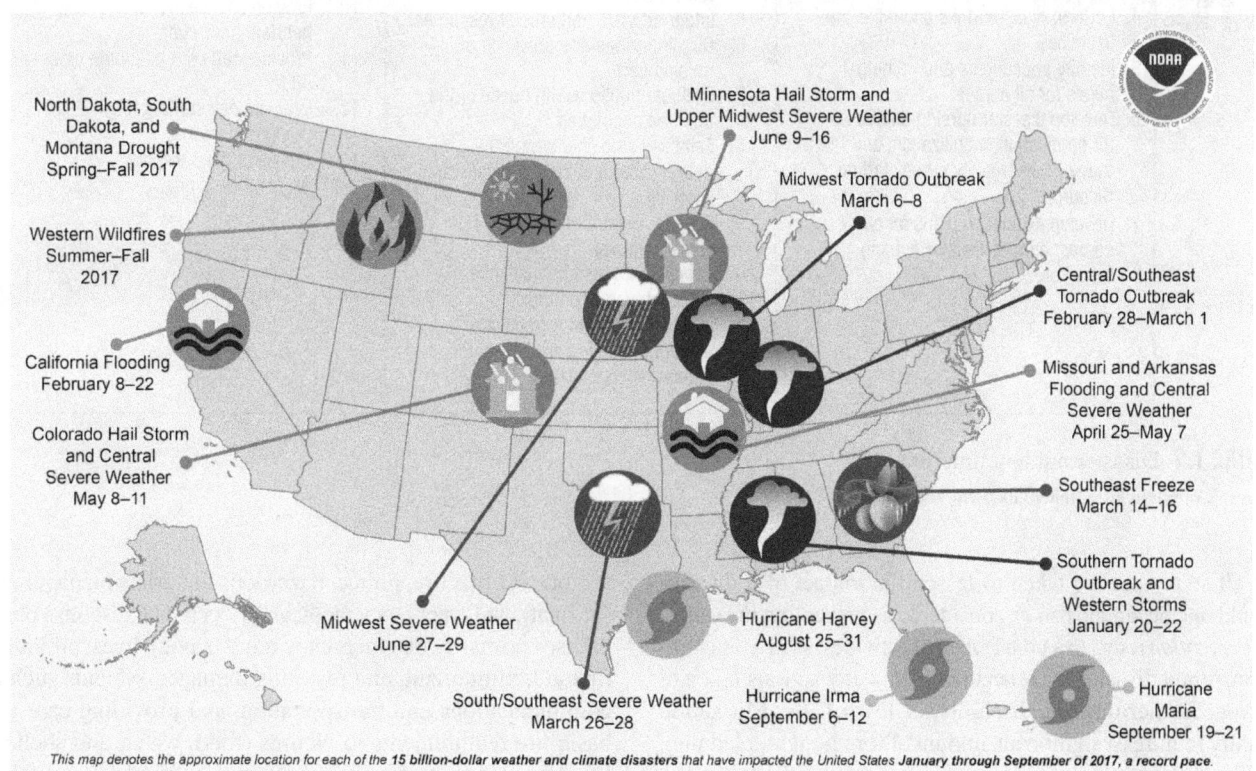

FIGURE 1.1 U.S. 2017 billion-dollar weather and climate disasters.

Source: National Oceanic and Atmospheric Administration. (2017). Billion-dollar weather and climate disasters: Overview. Retrieved from https://www.ncdc.noaa.gov/billions

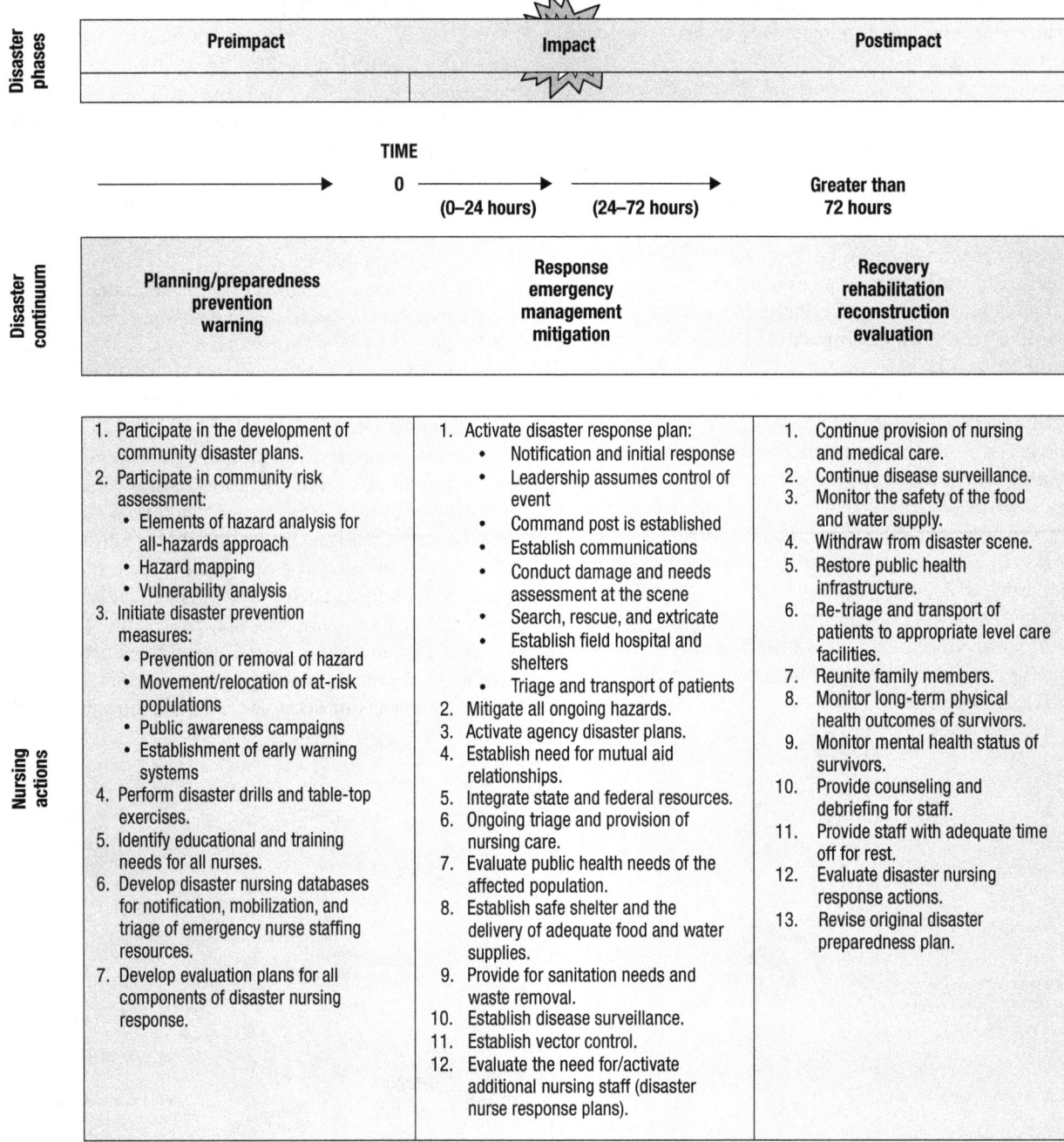

FIGURE 1.2 Disaster nursing timeline.

Source: Copyright 2018 Tener Goodwin Veenema.

are all steps that are taken to lessen the impact of a disaster should one occur and can be considered as prevention measures.

Prevention refers to a broad range of activities, such as attempts to prevent a disaster from occurring, and any actions taken to prevent further disease, disability, or loss of life. Mitigation usually requires a significant amount of forethought, planning, and implementation of measures *before* the incident occurs.

Response phase is the actual implementation of the disaster plan. Disaster response, or emergency management, is the organization of activities used to address the event. Traditionally, the emergency management field has organized its activities in

sectors, such as fire, police, hazardous materials management (hazmat), and emergency medical services. The response phase focuses primarily on emergency relief: saving lives, providing first aid, minimizing and restoring damaged systems such as communications and transportation, and providing care and basic life requirements to victims (food, water, and shelter). Disaster response plans are most successful if they are clear and specific, simple to understand, use an incident command system (ICS), are routinely practiced, and updated as needed. Response activities need to be continually evaluated and adjusted to the changing situation.

Recovery actions focus on stabilizing and returning the community (or an organization) to normal (its preimpact or improved status). This can range from rebuilding damaged buildings and repairing infrastructure to relocating populations and instituting physical, behavioral, and mental health interventions. Rehabilitation and reconstruction involve numerous activities to counter the long-term effects of the disaster on the community, its economy, and future development. "Build Back Better" should be the goal of all recovery actions with a focus upon resilient and sustainable communities.

Evaluation is the phase of disaster planning and response that often receives the least attention. FEMA recognizes the previously mentioned phases of the disaster life cycle; however, the importance of response and recovery evaluation cannot be underestimated. After a disaster, it is essential that evaluations be conducted to determine what worked, what did not work, and what specific problems, issues, and challenges were identified. Future disaster planning needs to be based on empirical evidence derived from previous disasters (Auf der Heide, 2006, 2007).

DISASTER PLANNING

The U.S. National Preparedness Goal is "A secure and resilient nation with the capabilities required across the whole community to prevent, protect against, mitigate, respond to, and recover from the threats and hazards that pose the greatest risk" (U.S. Department of Homeland Security, 2015, p. 1). Effective disaster planning addresses the problems posed by various potential events, ranging in scale from mass casualty incidents, such as motor vehicle collisions with multiple victims, to extensive flooding or earthquake damage, to armed conflicts and acts of terrorism (Burstein, 2014). The disaster planning continuum is broad in scope and must address collaboration across agencies and organizations, advanced preparations, as well as needs assessments, event management, and recovery efforts. Although public attention frequently focuses on medical casualties, it is imperative to consider numerous other factors when disaster plans and responses are being designed and developed. Participation by nurses in all phases of disaster planning is critical to ensure that nurses are aware of and prepared to deal with whatever these numerous other factors may turn out to be. Individuals and organizations responsible for disaster planning or implementation of the disaster plan should consider all possible eventualities—from the sanitation needs of crowds at mass gatherings, to the psychosocial needs of vulnerable populations, to evacuation procedures for buildings and geographic areas—when designing a detailed response (Parillo, 1995). Completion of the disaster planning process should result in the production of a comprehensive disaster or "emergency management operations plan."

ALL HAZARDS DISASTER PLANNING

The two major types of disaster plans are those that take the *agent-specific approach* and those that use the *all-hazards approach*. Historically, communities that embraced the

agent-specific approach focused their preparedness activities on the most likely threats to occur based on their geographic location (e.g., hurricanes in Florida). The all-hazards approach is a conceptual model for disaster preparedness recommended by FEMA that incorporates disaster management components that are consistent across all major types of disaster events to maximize resources, expenditures, and planning efforts. Despite their differences, many disasters share similarities because certain challenges and similar tasks occur repeatedly and predictably. The Department of Homeland Security's National Response Framework (NRF) encourages all communities to prepare for disasters using the all-hazards approach instead of stand-alone plans. FEMA has published its guidelines for all-hazards preparedness and planning titled *Comprehensive Preparedness Guide 101: Developing and Maintaining Emergency Operations Plans*, Version 2.0 (FEMA, 2010). This edition of guidelines places greater emphasis on representing and engaging the whole community—to include those with access and functional needs, children, and those with household pets and service animals—in developing community emergency operations plans.

Problems, issues, and challenges are commonly encountered across several types of disasters (Auf der Heide, 2006). Frequently, these issues and challenges can be effectively addressed in core preparedness activities through enhanced cooperation, collaboration, and communication. Attention should be addressed in disaster planning to the following:

1. Anticipate communication problems
2. Address operational issues related to effective triage, transportation, and evacuation
3. Accommodate the management, security of, and distribution of resources at the disaster site
4. Implement advanced warning systems and increase the effectiveness of warning messages
5. Enhance coordination of search and rescue efforts
6. Effective triage of patients (prioritization for care and transport of patients)
7. Establish plans for the distribution of patients to hospitals in an equitable fashion
8. Patient identification and tracking
9. Damage or destruction of the healthcare infrastructure
10. Management of volunteers, donations, and other large numbers of resources
11. Organized improvisational response to the disruption of major systems
12. Encountering overall resistance (apathy) to planning efforts

In a sentinel article, Auf der Heide (1989) stated, "Interest in disaster preparedness is proportional to the recency and magnitude of the last disaster."

DISASTER PLANNING AND PUBLIC HEALTH PREPAREDNESS

According to the CDC, the six domains of preparedness are as follows: community resilience, incident management, information management, countermeasures and mitigation, surge management, and biosurveillance (Figure 1.3).

SIX DOMAINS OF PREPAREDNESS

The **Public Health Emergency Preparedness Program** works to advance six main areas of preparedness so state and local public health systems are better prepared for emergencies that impact the public's health.

Community Resilience:
Preparing for and recovering from emergencies

Incident Management:
Coordinating an effective response

Information Management:
Making sure people have information to take action

Countermeasures and Mitigation:
Getting medicines and supplies where they are needed

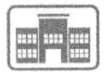

Surge Management:
Expanding medical services to handle large events

Biosurveillance:
Investigating and identifying health threats

www.cdc.gov/phpr/readiness

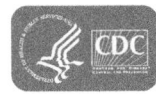

FIGURE 1.3 Six domains of preparedness.

Source: Centers for Disease Control and Prevention. (n.d.). State and local readiness. Retrieved from https://www.cdc.gov/phpr/readiness/sixdomains.htm

Adequate planning should address each of these domains in advance in order to eliminate common challenges associated with disaster situations. Common challenges to address proactively are discussed next.

Communication. Communication among organizations and across many people is a major priority in any disaster-planning initiative and is particularly difficult in today's changing communication environment (Haddow & Haddow, 2014). Communication and coordination are crucial aspects of emergency management. Information communication technology may be underused in emergency response networks (Hu & Kapucu, 2016). Failure of the communication system may occur in the event of a disaster as a result of damage to the infrastructure caused by the disaster, as well as lack of operator familiarity, excessive demands, inadequate supplies, and lack of integration with other communications providers and technologies. Backup communications systems, such as wireless, hardwire, and cellular telephones, may reduce the impact of disrupted standard communications, but, frequently, even advanced technology has been ineffectual during disasters (Garshnek & Burkle, 1999). Alternative communication tools such as texting and the use of social media for the public, as well as health providers, to get accurate information are critically important.

Information Management. Planning activities should ensure the necessary leadership and accountability to support the establishment of the interconnected data systems and analytic capacity that are essential to the continuity of healthcare and social services delivery across the continuum of disaster response and recovery. Coordination of efforts will be required among local and regional public health, healthcare, health insurance plans, private sector information technology innovators and vendors, and regulatory and governmental stakeholders at all levels. Disaster plans should be designed to facilitate data sharing and portability of individual health records across healthcare settings in support of pre- and post-disaster recovery healthcare planning and optimal recovery of essential infrastructure for medical and behavioral healthcare, public health, and social services (IOM, 2015a).

Coordination. When a disaster strikes, it rarely impacts just one isolated geographical area or jurisdiction. It is important for jurisdictions to consider how they will respond to a scenario in which the entire region is impacted. Planning activities should include identification of opportunities to strengthen the regional coordination required to ensure effective medical and public health response to a large-scale multijurisdictional disaster (IOM, 2015b). A detailed process for the efficient and effective large-scale *distribution of all types of resources*, including supplemental personnel, equipment, and supplies across multiple organizations, should be included in the plan. Leadership responsibilities and coordination of all rescue efforts (across territories and jurisdictions) should be worked out in advance of any event.

Advanced warning systems and the use of evacuation from areas of danger save lives and should be included in community disaster response plans whenever appropriate (Basher, 2006; Zschau & Kuppers, 2003). Warnings can now be made months in advance, as in the case of El Niño, to seconds in advance of the arrival of an earthquake and tsunami waves at some distance from the earthquake. Computers are programmed to respond to warnings automatically, shutting down or appropriately modifying transportation systems, lifelines, and manufacturing processes. Warnings are becoming much more useful to society as lead time and reliability are improved and as people devise ways to respond successfully. Effective dissemination of warnings provides a way to reduce disaster losses that have been increasing in the United States as citizens move into at-risk areas (FEMA, n.d.). The emergency alert system (EAS) and integrated public alert warning system (IPAWS) are examples of coordinated efforts across federal agencies (FEMA, NOAA) to provide timely and accurate emergency warnings as "an effective, reliable, integrated, flexible, and comprehensive system to alert and warn the American people … and to ensure under all conditions the President can communicate with the American people" (Executive Order 13457 [Executive Office of the President, 2006]; for more detailed information regarding the development and operation of this emergency early warning system, see www.fema.gov/emergency/ipaws).

Surge Management. A comprehensive disaster plan will account for a sudden unanticipated "surge" of patients, the effective *triage* of patients (prioritization for care and transport of patients), and *distribution* of patients to hospitals (a coordinated, even distribution of patients to several hospitals as opposed to delivering most of the patients to the closest hospital). Review of previous disaster response efforts reveals that patients are frequently transferred without adequate triage and that patient distribution to existing healthcare facilities is often grossly unequal and uncoordinated (Auf der Heide, 1996, 2002, 2006).

Disaster planning must include a community mutual aid plan in the event that the hospital(s), nursing home(s), or other residential healthcare facilities need to be evacuated. Plans for evacuation of healthcare facilities must be realistic and achievable, and contain sufficient specific detail about where patients will be relocated and who will be there to care for them. Evacuation of patients was a major challenge to disaster response efforts following Hurricane Katrina, and it was hampered by the destruction of all major transportation routes in and out of the city (Burkle, 2009). Twelve people died after a Florida nursing home failed to evacuate its residents, who suffered for days in oppressive heat with no air-conditioning after Hurricane Irma (Nedelman, 2017). Preplanning for the possibility of evacuation of entire healthcare facilities must address alternative modes of transportation and include adequate security measures (see Figure 1.4).

Nuclear events, highlighted by the Fukushima and the Chernobyl experiences and the inherent threat posed by North Korea for nuclear warfare, present serious challenges for disaster planning. Considering that over one-third of the U.S. population lives within 50 miles of a nuclear reactor (Physicians for Social Responsibility, 2011), determining appropriate evacuation zones is crucial. The correct evacuation distance from a nuclear event depends on the style of the nuclear device, type of radiation released, building structures, prevailing wind patterns, river/ocean currents, and populations living in the fallout area (Fong, 2007; U.S. Department of Health and Human Services, 2017a, 2017b). Disaster planners need to evaluate all of these elements when planning and establishing evacuation zones in nuclear events (see Figures 1.5 and 1.6).

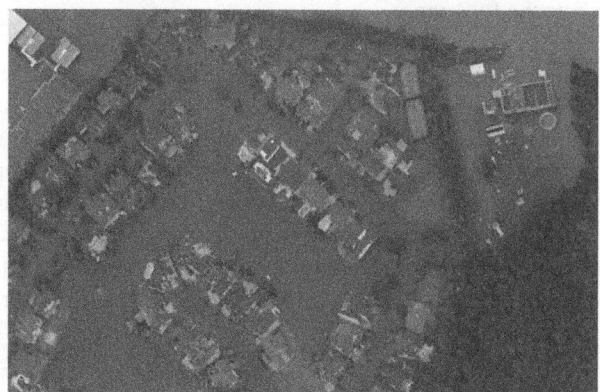

FIGURE 1.4 Floodwaters in Houston, Texas after Hurricane Harvey.

Source: National Ocean Service, National Oceanic and Atmospheric Administration. Retrieved from https://oceanservice.noaa.gov/news/sep17/hurricane-harvey.html

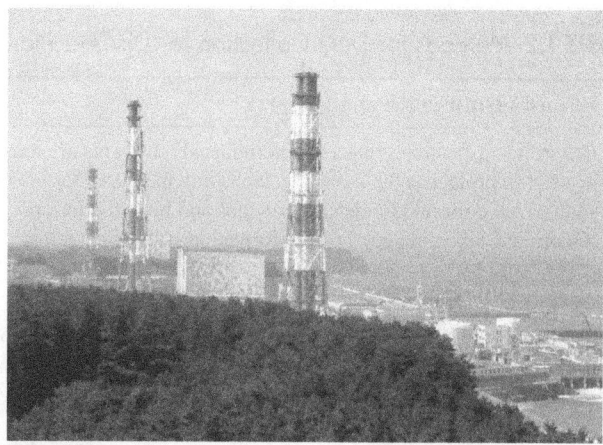

FIGURE 1.5 Fukushima I nuclear power plant before the 2011 explosion.

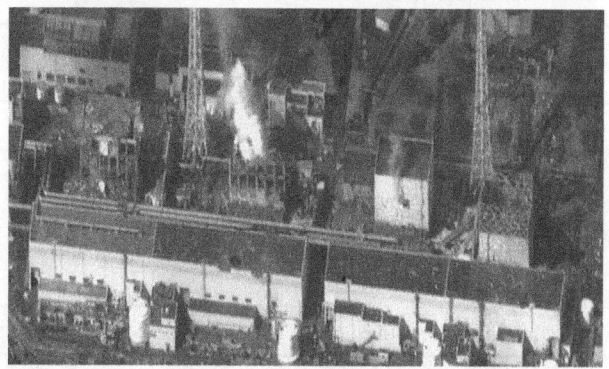

FIGURE 1.6 Fukushima Power Plant after the March 24, 2011 meltdown. The composition of the gas escape cloud is a key determinant for the safe evacuation distance from the nuclear plant.

Source: Digital Globe (2011) released under Creative Commons Attribution-Share Alike 3.0 license.

Information systems need to be identified or developed that will track patients across multiple (and perhaps temporary) settings. *Patient evacuation and tracking* during disasters is a major challenge because of lack of interoperable registration systems at shelters, and hospital communication systems that do not interface with other hospitals or county health departments. Family reunification has persisted as a major challenge to meaningful recovery initiatives.

HAZARD IDENTIFICATION, VULNERABILITY ANALYSIS, AND RISK ASSESSMENT

Hazard identification and mapping, vulnerability analysis, and risk assessment are the three cornerstone methods of data collection for disaster planning (see Table 1.2). The first step in effective disaster planning requires *advanced identification of potential problems* for the institution or community involved. Different types of disasters are associated with

TABLE 1.2 Methods for Data Collection for Disaster Planning

Hazard Identification and Mapping
Hazard identification is used to determine which events are most likely to affect a community and to make decisions about whom or what to protect as the basis of establishing measures for prevention, mitigation, and response. Historical data and data from other sources are collected to identify previous and potential hazards. Data are then mapped using aerial photography, satellite imagery, remote sensing, and geographic information systems.
Vulnerability Analysis
Vulnerability analysis is used to determine who is most likely to be affected, the property most likely to be damaged or destroyed, and the capacity of the community to deal with the effects of the disaster. Data are collected regarding the susceptibility of individuals, property, and the environment to potential hazards in order to develop prevention strategies. A separate vulnerability analysis should be conducted for each identified hazard.
Risk Assessment
Risk assessment uses the results of the hazard identification and vulnerability analysis to determine the probability of a specified outcome from a given hazard that affects a community with known vulnerabilities and coping mechanisms (risk equals hazard times vulnerability). The probability may be presented as a numerical range (i.e., 30%–40% probability) or in relative terms (i.e., low, moderate, or high risk). Major objectives of risk assessment include the following:
• Determining a community's risk of adverse health effects due to a specified disaster (i.e., traumatic deaths and injuries following an earthquake)
• Identifying the major hazards facing the community and their sources (i.e., earthquakes, floods, industrial accidents)
• Identifying those sections of the community most likely to be affected by a particular hazard (i.e., individuals living in or near floodplains)
• Determining existing measures and resources that reduce the impact of a given hazard (i.e., building codes and regulations for earthquake mitigation)
• Determining areas that require strengthening to prevent or mitigate the effects of the hazard

Source: Information obtained from Landesman, L. Y. (2011). *Public health management of disasters: The practice guide* (3rd ed.). Washington, DC: American Public Health Association. The author gratefully acknowledges Dr. Linda Landesman and the American Public Health Association for permission to reproduce this work.

distinct patterns of illness and injuries, and limited predictions of these health outcomes can sometimes be made in advance, with appropriate and adequate data. Hazards are situations or items that create risk and the potential for the disaster to occur. Hazard identification and analysis is the method by which planners identify which events are most likely to affect a community and serves as the foundation for decision making for prevention, mitigation, and response. Hazards may include items such as chemicals used by local industry; transportation elements, such as subways, airports, and railroad stations; or collections of large groups of people in areas with limited access, such as skyscrapers, nursing homes, or sports stadiums (see Box 1.1). Environmental and meteorological hazards must also be considered, such as the presence of fault lines and seismic zones and the seasonal risks posed by blizzards, ice storms, tornadoes, hurricanes, wildfires, and heat waves. The National Fire Protection Association's (NFPA) Technical Committee on Disaster Management issued international codes and standards that require a community's hazard identification to include *all* natural, technological, and human hazards (National Fire Protection Administration [NFPA], 2017).

In the United States, planners leverage the findings from the Strategic National Risk Assessment (SNRA) to build

and describe the response core capabilities within our NRF for disaster response. The SNRA identifies the threats and hazards that pose the greatest risk to the United States. These findings affirm the need for an all-hazards, capability-based approach to preparedness to ensure that all types of scenarios are accounted for. The risks and threats identified by SNRA include the following:

- Natural hazards—including hurricanes, earthquakes, wildfires, and floods—present a significant and varied risk across the country.
- A virulent strain of pandemic influenza could infect thousands of Americans, affect millions more, and result in considerable morbidity and mortality and economic loss.
- Additional human and animal infectious diseases, including those previously undiscovered, may also present significant risks.
- Technological and accidental hazards, such as dam failures or chemical substance spills or releases, have the potential to cause extensive fatalities and severe economic impacts, and the likelihood of occurrence may increase due to aging infrastructure.
- Terrorist organizations or affiliates may seek to acquire, build, and use weapons of mass destruction. Conventional

terrorist attacks, including those by lone actors employing explosives and armed attacks, present a continued risk to the nation.
- Cyberattacks can have catastrophic consequences and may also have cascading effects such as power grid or financial system failures.
- No single threat or hazard exists in isolation. As an example, a hurricane can lead to flooding, dam failures, and hazardous materials spills (FEMA, 2013, p. 7).

Those who are vulnerable are "capable of being physically or emotionally wounded, open to attack or damage" (*Merriam Webster's Collegiate Dictionary*, 2017). The disaster-planning team must identify vulnerable groups of people—those at particular risk of injury, death, or loss of property from each hazard. Vulnerability analysis can provide predictions of what individuals or groups of individuals are most likely to be affected, what property is most likely to sustain damage or be destroyed, and what resources will be available to mitigate

the effects of the disaster. Vulnerability analysis should be conducted for each hazard identified and regularly updated to accommodate population shifts and changes in the environment (Landesman, 2011).

Risk assessment is an essential feature of disaster planning and is, in essence, a calculation or model of risk, in which a comprehensive inventory is created, including all existing and potential dangers, the population most likely to be affected by each danger, and a prediction of the health consequences. Risk analysis uses the elements of hazard analysis and vulnerability analysis to identify groups of people at particular risk of injury or death from each individual hazard. The calculation of estimated risk (probability estimate) may be constant over time, or it may vary by time of day, season, or location relative to the community (Burstein, 2014). Risk assessment necessitates the cooperation of corporate, governmental, and community groups to produce a comprehensive listing of all potential hazards (Leonard, 1991; Waeckerle, 1991).

BOX 1.1 Hazard Analysis

NATURAL EVENTS

Drought
Wildfire (e.g., forest, range)
Avalanche
Winter storm/blizzard; snow, ice, hail
Tsunami
Hurricane/windstorm/typhoon/cyclone
Biological event
Heat wave
Extreme cold
Flood or wind-driven water
Earthquake
Volcanic eruption
Tornado
Landslide or mudslide
Dust storm or sandstorm
Lightning storm

TECHNOLOGICAL EVENTS

Hazardous material release
Explosion or fire
Transportation accident (rail, subway, bridge, airplane)
Building or structure collapse
Power or utility failure
Extreme air pollution
Radiological accident (industry, medical, nuclear power plant)
Dam or levee failure

Fuel or resource shortage
Industrial collapse
Communication disruption

HUMAN EVENTS

Economic failures
General strikes
Terrorism (e.g., ecological, cyber, nuclear, biological, chemical)
Sabotage, bombs
Hostage situation
Civil unrest
Enemy attack
Arson
Mass hysteria/panic

SPECIAL EVENTS

Mass gatherings, concerts, sporting events, political gatherings

CONTEXT HAZARDS

Climate change
Sea level rise
Deforestation
Loss of natural resources
Intensive urbanization
Catastrophic earth changes

Source: From Smith, K., & Petley, D. N. (2009). *Environmental hazards: Assessing risk and reducing disaster* (5th ed.). New York, NY: Routledge.

The following disaster-prevention measures can be implemented following the analysis of hazards, vulnerability, and risk:

- Prevention or removal of hazard (e.g., closing down an aging industrial facility that cannot implement safety regulations)
- Containment of the hazard or implementation of mitigation strategies (e.g., enforcing strict building regulations in an earthquake-prone zone, increased engineering codes for buildings in coastal areas)
- Removal of at-risk populations from the hazard (e.g., evacuating populations prior to the impact of a hurricane; resettling communities away from flood-prone areas)
- Provision of public information and education (e.g., providing information concerning measures that the public can take to protect themselves during a tornado)
- Establishment of early warning systems (e.g., using satellite data about an approaching hurricane for public service announcements)
- Mitigation of vulnerabilities (e.g., sensors for ventilation systems capable of detecting deviations from normal conditions; sensors to check food, water, currency, and mail for contamination)
- Reduction of risk posed by some hazards (e.g., relocating a chemical depot farther away from a school to reduce the risk that children would be exposed to hazardous materials)
- Enhancement of a local community's capacity to respond (e.g., healthcare coordination across the entire health community, including health departments, hospitals, clinics, and home care agencies)

Regardless of the type of approach used by planners, all hazards and potential dangers should be identified before an effective disaster response can be planned.

EVALUATING CAPACITY TO RESPOND

Resource identification is an essential feature of disaster planning. A community's capacity to withstand a disaster is directly related to the type and scope of resources available, the presence of adequate communication systems, the structural integrity of its buildings and utilities (e.g., water, electricity), and the size and sophistication of its healthcare system (Burstein, 2014; Cuny, 1998). Resources include both human and physical elements, such as organizations with specialized personnel and equipment. Disaster preparedness includes assembling lists of healthcare facilities; medical, nursing, and emergency responder groups; public works and other civic departments; and volunteer agencies, along with phone numbers and key contact personnel for each. Hospitals, clinics, physician offices, mental health facilities, nursing homes, and home care agencies must all have the capacity to ensure continuity of patient care despite damage to utilities, communication systems, or their physical plant. Redundant communication systems must be put in place so that hospitals, health departments, and other agencies, both locally and regionally, can effectively communicate with each other and share information about patients in the event of a disaster. Within hospitals, departments should

have a readily available, complete record of all personnel, including cellular phone numbers to ensure access 24 hours a day. Resource availability will vary with factors such as time of day, season, and reductions in the workforce. Creativity may be needed in identifying and mobilizing human resources to ensure an adequate workforce. Disaster plans must also include alternative treatment sites in the event of damage to existing healthcare facilities or in order to expand the surge capacity of the present healthcare system.

Coordination *between agencies* is also necessary to avoid chaos if multiple spontaneous volunteers respond to the disaster and are not directed and adequately supervised. As with the September 11 (9/11) disaster, many national healthcare workers and emergency medical services responders who came to New York to help returned home because the numbers of volunteer responders overwhelmed the local response effort.

CORE PREPAREDNESS ACTIVITIES

1. *Prepare a theoretical foundation for disaster planning.* Disaster plans are "constructed" in much the same way as one builds a house. Conceptually, they must have a firm foundation grounded in an understanding of human behavior. Effective disaster plans are based on empirical knowledge of how people normally behave in disasters (Landesman, 2011; Lasker, 2003). Any disaster plan must focus first on the local response and best estimates of what people are *likely to do* as opposed to what planners *want people to do*. Realistic predictions of population behaviors accompanied by disaster plans that are flexible in design and easy to change will be of greater value to all personnel involved in a disaster response.

2. *Disaster planning is only as effective as the assumptions upon which it is based.* The effectiveness of planning is enhanced when it is based on information that has been empirically verified by systematic field disaster research studies (Auf der Heide, 2002, 2006). Sound disaster preparedness includes a comprehensive review of the existing disaster preparedness literature.

3. *Core preparedness activities must go beyond the routine.* Most disasters cannot be managed merely by mobilizing more equipment, personnel, and supplies. Disasters differ from routine daily emergencies, and they pose significant problems that have no counterpart in routine emergency responses. Many disaster-related issues and challenges have been identified in the disaster literature, and they can be anticipated and planned for (Auf der Heide, 2007).

4. *Have a community needs assessment.* A community needs assessment must be conducted and routinely updated to identify the preexisting prevalence of disease and to identify those high-risk, high-need patients who may require transport in the event of an evacuation or whose condition may necessitate the provision of care in nontraditional sites. This needs assessment provides a foundation for planning along with baseline data for establishing the extent of the impact of the disaster.

5. *Identify leadership and command post.* ICS is the mandated leadership form for leading an emergency response (FEMA, 2015). The issue of "who's in charge" is critical to all components of the disaster response and must be determined

before the event occurs. The process of disaster planning is important for establishing relationships, identifying leaders, and laying the groundwork for smooth responses. ICS is an excellent management structure for the immediate post event response. The planning process, often more important than the final written plan, benefits from a participatory process. Those who take part in planning are more likely to agree to and abide by the final product resulting in plans with a higher likelihood of acceptance and compliance (Lasker, 2003). Identification of the command post must also be decided in advance and communicated to all members of the organization or community.

6. *Design a local response for the first 72 hours.* "All disasters are local" and the plan for the mobilization of local authorities, personnel, facilities, equipment, and supplies for the initial postimpact, 72-hour period is the next level of foundation of the disaster response. Most disaster casualties will arrive at the hospital within 1 hour of impact, and very few trapped casualties are rescued alive after the first day. Thus, the effectiveness of the local response is a key determinant in preventing death and disability (Auf der Heide, 2007). Communities must be prepared to handle the immediate postimpact phase in the event that they are also isolated from outside resources or supplies (as happened in the immediate aftermath of 9/11 when all planes were grounded for the first time in U.S. aviation history). This stage of the disaster planning will involve many organizations and disciplines, from local institutions to municipal, state, and federal governments, including private, volunteer, and international agencies. Local organizational leaders and executives from each agency must come together and work as a planning group to conduct the initial assessments (risk, hazard, and vulnerability), establish a coordinated process for response, design effective and complementary communication systems, and create standard criteria for the assessment of the scope of damage to the community.

7. *Identify and acccommodate vulnerable populations.* A community disaster plan must accommodate the needs of all people, including patients residing in hospitals, long-term care facilities such as nursing homes, assisted living, psychiatric care facilities, and rehabilitation centers. Children in the child welfare system or living in residential living centers, homeless individuals, and people detained in the criminal justice system must all be accommodated within the plan. "Invisible populations" such as the undocumented and migrant workers must be considered. Poison control and suicide hotlines need to be maintained, and the continuity of home healthcare services must be safeguarded as well. School districts, day-care centers, and employers must be kept aware and up to date regarding the community's disaster plan.

8. *Know about state and federal assistance.* Finally, state and federal assistance programs are added to the plan, and consideration of the need for mutual aid agreements (between communities or regions) is begun. Groups and organizations are most helpful when they understand their own capabilities and limitations, as well as those of the organizations with which interactions are anticipated or intended. Disaster plans should be designed to be both structured and flexible, with provisions made for plan activation and decision making by first-line emergency responders or field-level personnel, if necessary.

9. *Identify training and educational needs, resources, and personal protective equipment (PPE).* The disaster plan provides direction for identifying training needs including mock drills, acquiring additional resources, and PPE.

10. *Plan for the early conduction of damage assessment.* In emergency medical care, response time is critical (Schultz, Koenig, & Noji, 1996). A crucial component to any disaster response is the early conduction of a proper damage assessment to identify urgent needs and to determine relief priorities for an affected population (Lillibridge, Noji, & Burkle, 1993). Disaster assessment provides managers with objective information about the effects of the disaster on a community and can be used to match available resources to the population's needs. The early completion of this task and the subsequent mobilization of resources to areas of greatest need can significantly reduce the adverse effects of a disaster. Identification of *who* will be responsible for this rapid assessment and *what* variables the assessment will contain needs to occur in advance as part of the disaster-planning process. Ongoing assessment of the affected population's burden of chronic disease is an element of evaluation often overlooked in disaster preparedness planning. As a result, many disaster victims may experience untimely death simply because they do not receive treatment for these preexisting conditions (Burkle, 2007).

EVALUATION OF A DISASTER PLAN

An essential step in disaster planning and preparedness is the evaluation of the disaster response plan for its effectiveness and completeness by key personnel involved in the response. The comprehension of people expected to execute the plan and their ability to perform duties must be assessed. The availability and functioning of any equipment called for by the disaster plan needs to be evaluated and reviewed on a systematic basis. Several methods may be used to exercise the disaster plan, the most comprehensive of which would be its full implementation in an actual disaster. Disaster drills may also provide an excellent means of testing plans for their completeness and effectiveness. Drills can be staged as large, full-scale exercises, using triaged victims and requiring vast resources of supplies and personnel, or they may be limited to a small segment of the disaster response, such as drills that assess the effectiveness of communications protocols or notification procedures. The disaster plan may also be assessed by using "table-top" academic exercises, mock patients, computer simulations, or seminar sessions focusing on key personnel or limited aspects of the disaster response.

Improved performance during the drill, with enhanced understanding of disaster planning and response, is more likely when personnel are notified in advance that a drill is scheduled. The specific goal of any drill should be clearly communicated. If drills are to be used as training sessions as well as evaluations of preparations and response plans, personnel are more likely to make the correct or most appropriate response choices during the drill if they are prepared. Frequent drills will ensure that knowledge and skills are current. Consequently, they will be more likely to take appropriate actions when faced with an unexpected disaster situation in the future. The more realistic the exercise, the more likely it is that useful information about the strengths and weaknesses of both the disaster plan and the responders will be acquired. A shortage of available resources is a common factor in many disasters; without experiencing at least some of the stress that accompanies that situation, it is unlikely that the disaster plan and response will be taxed at a level that realistically simulates the circumstances of an actual disaster.

Essential features of all effective disaster drills are the inclusion of all individuals and agencies likely to be involved in the disaster response and a critique, with debriefing, of all participants following the exercise. The drill should include representation from all sectors of the emergency management field, all healthcare disciplines, governmental officials, school officials, and the media. The news media has a vital role in disasters, and failure to include the media in planning activities can lead to a dysfunctional response (Haddow & Haddow, 2014). Regardless of the format used, the critique should consider comments from everyone involved in the drill. Disaster planners should review all observations and comments and respond with modifications of the disaster plan, if necessary. Any modifications made to disaster plans or response procedures must be communicated to all groups involved or affected. Periodic evaluations of disaster plans are essential to ensure that personnel are adequately familiar with their roles in disaster situations, as well as to accommodate changes in population demographics, regional emergency response operations, hospital renovations and closings, and other variables. At a minimum, disaster drills should take place once every 12 months in the community, and more frequently in hospitals and other long-term care facilities.

SITUATIONS SUGGESTIVE OF AN INCREASED NEED FOR PLANNING

Megacities

Globally, the intensity and frequency of disasters are escalating and urban areas, where half of the world population lives, have been exposed to numerous disasters. In 2016, an estimated 54.5% of the world's population lived in urban settlements. By 2030, urban areas are projected to house 60% of people globally and one in every three people will live in cities with at least half a million inhabitants (United Nations, 2016). Megacities—those in which the population exceeds 10 million—present unique challenges in disaster. Of the world's 31 megacities in 2016, 24 are located in the less developed regions or the "global South." China alone was home to six megacities in 2016, while India had five. The 10 cities that are projected to become megacities between 2017 and 2030 are all located in developing countries. They include: Lahore, Pakistan; Hyderabad, India; Bogotá, Colombia; Johannesburg, South Africa; Bangkok, Thailand; Dar es Salaam, Tanzania; Ahmedabad, India; Luanda, Angola; Ho Chi Minh City, Vietnam; and Chengdu, China (United Nations, 2016). Cities in the developing world are growing at an alarming rate and, as a consequence, increase their vulnerability to disasters. In these cities, over 37% of residents are living in slums and squatter settlements. As a consequence, the intensity and occurrences of urban disasters have increased, and authorities have been hard-pressed to cope with and build urban resilience to such events (Atta-ur-Rahman, Shaw, Surjan, & Parvin, 2016). These cities are at increased risk of environmental and occupational hazards and infectious disease outbreaks. The concentration of people, the lack of urban planning, unavailability of quality building materials, and substandard construction practices result in crowding (Kapadia & Badhuri, 2009; Khan & Pappas, 2011). Extreme disasters have hit urban areas in both developing and developed locations, but cities in the developing world have extremely high vulnerability and low resilience. Whenever a disaster hits an urban area, it creates widespread damage and redirects budget allocation from development to immediate emergency response. These cities present extremely difficult challenges to planning for an effective disaster response. Limited access (ingress and egress), potentially widespread shortages of technical equipment and supplies, and the underlying existing urban ecology combine to create seemingly overwhelming obstacles to disaster planning. Existing megacities have severely taxed public health's capacity in many parts of the world (Khan & Pappas, 2011) and disaster events will serve to intensify these challenges.

Disasters Within Hospitals and Healthcare Settings

"Internal" disasters refer to incidents that disrupt the everyday, routine services of a medical facility and may or may not occur simultaneously with an external event. Although these concurrent events are rare, experiences such as the Haitian and Japanese earthquakes, and Hurricanes Katrina and Rita are evidence that they can happen with devastating consequences (Quarantelli, 1983; Rudowitz, Rowland, & Shartzer, 2006; Wolfson & Walker, 1993). Before Hurricane Katrina's impact, there were 22 hospitals in New Orleans. Following the rupture of the city's levee system, all 22 hospitals had to be evacuated. Healthcare facilities need to define what constitutes an internal disaster. In general, an internal event can be defined as any event that threatens the smooth functioning of the hospital, medical center, or healthcare facility, or that presents a potential danger to patients or hospital personnel. In the United States, the Joint Commission on Accreditation of Healthcare Organizations (JCAHO) requires that all hospitals have comprehensive plans for both internal and external disasters. Nurses should be aware of the current JCAHO standards for hospital disaster preparedness (JCAHO, 2017). These standards provide guidance for developing an emergency management program that identifies six critical functions, regardless of the cause or causes of an emergency. It is important that organizations have an understanding of their capabilities in meeting these six critical functions when a facility's infrastructure, the community's infrastructure, or both are compromised. These functions are:

- Communicating during emergency conditions
- Managing resources and assets during emergency conditions
- Managing safety and security during emergency conditions
- Defining and managing staff roles and responsibilities during emergency conditions

- Managing utilities during emergency conditions
- Managing clinical activities during emergency conditions

Hospitals are dependent upon the infrastructure of the community where they are located and must be able to survive and sustain operations in the event of a loss of this essential infrastructure. Unplanned (unanticipated) and planned (scheduled maintenance) disruptions to infrastructure can disrupt the ability of the hospital to remain functional and create a dangerous environment for patients and staff. *Any event* that may result in the disruption of electrical power, water, steam, cooling, sewer, oxygen, and suction systems must be accounted for in the hospital's internal disaster plan. Internal disasters or system support failures can result in a myriad of responses, such as evacuation of patients and staff; decreased levels of service provision; diversion of ambulances, helicopter transport, and other patients; and relocation of patient care areas. Sources of internal events include power failures, flood, water loss, chemical accidents and fumes, radiation accidents, fire, explosion, violence, bomb threats, loss of telecommunications (inability to communicate with staff), and elevator emergencies. The hospital setting is full of flammable and toxic materials. The use of lasers near flammable gases, multiple sources of radiation, storage of toxic chemicals, and potentially explosive materials in hospitals and medical centers magnifies the potential for a catastrophic event. Internal disaster plans are based on a "Hospital Incident Management System" and address the institution's response to any potential incident that would disrupt hospital functioning. Similar to the disaster continuum, the phases of a hospital's internal disaster response plan generally include the identification of a command post and the following three phases:

1. *Alert phase*, during which staff remain at their regular positions, service provision is uninterrupted, and faculty and staff await further instructions from their supervisors
2. *Response phase*, during which designated staff report to supervisors or the command post for instructions, the response plan is activated, and nonessential services are suspended
3. *Expanded response phase*, when additional personnel are required, off-duty staff are called in, and existing staff may be reassigned based on patient needs.

Internal disaster plans must address all potential scenarios, including:

- Loss of power, including auxiliary power
- Loss of oxygen and other medical gases
- Loss of water, steam, and/or water pressure
- Loss of compressed air and vacuum (suction)
- Loss of telecommunications systems
- Loss of information technology systems
- Threats to the safety of patients and staff (violence, terrorism, and bombs)
- Toxic exposures (fumes, chemicals, or radiation)
- Immediate evacuation of all patients and personnel

Internal disaster plans should be integrated with the hospital's overall disaster preparedness protocol. Training should be mandatory for all personnel. Disaster drills and table top exercises should be designed and routinely performed to ensure that staff are adequately prepared. Emergency or preventive evacuations of patients and staff are also key components of an effective hospital disaster plan.

Pandemics

The lessons learned from the recent Ebola (2014), Middle East respiratory syndrome (2015), Zika (2016), and cholera (2017) outbreaks provided evidence that infectious disease outbreaks create unique challenges to planners both in the United States and internationally. The investigation and management of any communicable disease outbreak requires three steps: (a) recognition that a potential outbreak is occurring; (b) investigation of the source, mode of transmission, and risk factors for infection; and (c) implementation of appropriate control measures. If outbreak management exceeds or threatens to exceed the capability and resources available, then a population-based triage management model may be needed (Burkle, 2006).

Institutional outbreaks of communicable disease are common. Most institutional outbreaks involve relatively few cases with minimum effect on the hospital and external community. However, large outbreaks, outbreaks of rare diseases, smaller outbreaks in institutions lacking infection control departments, or outbreaks in those with inadequate infection control personnel may exceed an institution's or a community's coping capacities. The need for widespread quarantine for the purposes of disease control (e.g., smallpox epidemic) would rapidly overwhelm the existing healthcare system and create significant staffing issues. Staff may refuse to come to work fearing exposure of themselves and their families to the disease. Healthcare facilities play a vital role in the detection and response to biological emergencies, including emerging infections, influenza outbreaks, and use of biological weapons by terrorists. Assessment of the preparedness and capacity of each hospital to respond to and treat victims of an infectious disease outbreak or biological incident must be conducted as part of disaster planning.

Hazardous Materials Disaster Planning

Every industrialized nation is heavily reliant on chemicals. The United States is no exception; it produces, stores, and transports large quantities of toxic industrial agents. In fact, hazardous materials are present in every sector of American society and represent a unique and significant threat to civilians, military, and healthcare workers both in the field and in the hospital emergency department. Situations involving hazardous materials will require additional planning efforts. In the United States, the Superfund Amendment and Reauthorization Act requires that all hazardous materials manufactured, stored, or transported by local industry that could affect the surrounding community be identified and reported to health officials. Gasoline and liquid petroleum gas are the most common hazardous materials, but other potential hazards include chlorine, ammonia, and explosives. Situations involving relocation of nuclear waste materials also pose a considerable risk to the communities involved. Material safety data sheets standardize the method of communicating relevant information about each material—including its toxicity, flammability, and known acute and chronic health effects—and can be used as part of the hazard identification process.

Clinically, the removal of solid or liquid chemical agents from exposed individuals is the first step in preventing serious injury or death. Hospitals need to be prepared to decontaminate patients, despite plans that call for field decontamination of patients prior to transport. During a hazardous materials (HAZMAT) accident, the victims often ignore the rules of the disaster plan by seeking out the nearest hospital for medical care, regardless of that institution's capabilities. If first receivers rush to the aid of contaminated individuals arriving in the emergency department without taking proper precautions (e.g., donning PPE), they may become contaminated and risk becoming victims themselves (Levitin & Siegelson, 1996, 2007). Because mismanagement of a hazmat incident can turn a contained accident into a disaster involving the entire community, disaster-planning initiatives must incorporate victim decontamination and PPE into the planning process (Levitin & Siegelson, 1996, 2007).

PROFESSIONAL NURSING MANDATE

Caring for patients and the opportunity to save lives are what professional nursing is all about, and disaster events provide nurses with an opportunity to do both. According to the ANA (2010, pp. 1–3), "the aim of nursing actions is to assist patients, families and communities to improve, correct or adjust to physical, emotional, psychosocial, spiritual, cultural, and environmental conditions for which they seek help." Definitions of nursing have evolved to acknowledge six essential features of professional nursing:

- Provision of a caring relationship that facilitates health and healing
- Attention to the range of human experiences and responses to health and illness within the physical and social environments
- Integration of objective data with knowledge gained from an appreciation of the patient or group's subjective experience
- Application of scientific knowledge to the processes of diagnosis and treatment through the use of judgment and critical thinking
- Advancement of professional nursing knowledge through scholarly inquiry
- Influence on social and public policy to promote social justice (ANA, 2010, p. 12)

All nurses should have an awareness of the basic life cycle of disasters, the distinct patterns of illness and injury associated with the major events, and a framework to support the necessary assessment and response efforts. Both national and international nursing organizations have focused on the need for improved disaster nursing preparation. The ANA, the Emergency Nurses Association, and the Society for the Advancement of Disaster Nursing, to name a few, have each issued position statements regarding the need for nurses to advance their disaster knowledge and preparedness skills. Multiple sets of disaster nursing competencies have been proposed along with a variety of educational programs.

As every nurse has the potential to be involved in a disaster at some point in his or her personal or professional life, disaster nursing is "everyone's subspecialty." It is imperative that all nurses acquire a minimum knowledge base and set of skills to enable them to plan for and respond to a disaster in a timely and appropriate manner. In doing so, nurses are better prepared to keep themselves, their colleagues, their patients and families, and ultimately their communities safe.

SUMMARY

Disasters are highly complex events that bring significant destruction and devastation to the communities they strike. A disaster's immediate effects may be seen in injuries and deaths, disruption of the existing healthcare system and public health infrastructure, and social chaos. The recent dramatic increase in natural disasters, their intensity, the number of people affected by them, and the human and economic losses associated with these events has placed an imperative on effective disaster planning and preparedness. Sound community disaster planning must be based on a rigorously conducted hazard vulnerability assessment and an understanding of how people behave during a disaster. Disasters often share a common set of challenges that can be addressed during the planning process. Ideally, all disaster plans should be consistent with the CDC public health emergency capabilities and will advance the U.S. National Preparedness Goal of "a secure and resilient nation with the capabilities required across the whole community to prevent, protect against, mitigate, respond to, and recover from the threats and hazards that pose the greatest risk" (U.S. Department of Homeland Security, 2015, p. 1). Nurses who possess an awareness and understanding of the concepts of disaster planning and preparedness are better able to keep themselves and their patients safe.

STUDY QUESTIONS

1. Differentiate "disaster," "hazard," and "complex human emergency." What are the criteria used to classify the different types of disasters into categories? Explain how these unique features provide a structure for strategic planning.

2. What are the phases of the disaster life cycle?

3. Compare and contrast risk assessment, hazard identification, and vulnerability analysis.

4. What are common problems, issues, and challenges associated with disaster response? How can these problems and issues be addressed during the preparedness phase?

5. The Puerto Rico Department of Health is holding an After Action planning meeting with key public health officials and healthcare clinicians to address the 2017 hurricanes and responses. Building upon your answer to question #4, and using the focus areas of disaster planning, construct a new

and improved comprehensive disaster response plan for this island community.

6. What types of activities must a community be prepared for during the first 72 hours following impact of a disaster?

7. Following the Hurricane Harvey's impact on Houston and its surrounding counties, the water supply and the sewage systems were damaged or destroyed. Toxic floodwaters exposed citizens to a multitude of dangers. What planning could have mitigated this?

REFERENCES

Al-Madhari, A. F., & Keller, A. Z. (1997). Review of disaster definitions. *Prehospital and Disaster Medicine, 12*(1), 17–21. doi:10.1017/S1049023X0003716X

American Nurses Association. (2010). *Nursing's social policy statement: The essence of the profession* (3rd ed.). Silver Spring, MD: Author.

American Nurses Association. (2011). What is nursing? Retrieved from https://www.nursingworld.org/practice-policy/workforce/what-is-nursing

Atta-ur-Rahman, Shaw, R., Surjan, A., & Parvin, G. A. (2016). Urban disasters and approaches to resilience. In R. Shaw, A. Surjan, A.-U. Rahman, & G. A. Parvin (Eds.), *Urban disasters and resilience in Asia*. (1st ed.; pp. 1–19). Oxford, UK: Butterworth-Heinemann.

Auf der Heide, E. (1989). *Disaster response: Principles of preparation and coordination.* St. Louis, MO: Mosby.

Auf der Heide, E. (1996). Disaster planning. Part II: Disaster problems, issues, and challenges identified in the research literature. *Emergency Medicine Clinics of North America, 14*(2), 453–475. doi:10.1016/S0733-8627(05)70262-5

Auf der Heide, E. (2002). Principles of hospital disaster planning. In D. E. Hogan & J. L. Burstein (Eds.), *Disaster medicine* (pp. 57–89). Philadelphia, PA: Lippincott Williams & Wilkins.

Auf der Heide, E. (2006). The importance of evidence based disaster planning. *Annals of Emergency Medicine, 47*(1), 34–49. doi:10.1016/j.annemergmed.2005.05.009

Auf der Heide, E. (2007). Principles of hospital disaster planning. In D. E. Hogan & J. L. Burstein (Eds.), *Disaster medicine* (2nd ed., pp. 95–126). Philadelphia, PA: Lippincott Williams & Wilkins.

Basher, R. (2006). Global early warning systems for natural hazards: Systematic and people-centred. *Philosophical Transactions of the Royal Society, 364*(1845), 2167–2182. doi:10.1098/rsta.2006.1819

Berggren, R. (2005). Hurricane Katrina: Unexpected necessities—Inside Charity Hospital. *New England Journal of Medicine, 353*(15), 1550–1553. doi:10.1056/NEJMp058239

Burkle, F. M. (2006). Population-based triage management in response to surge capacity requirements during a large scale bioevent disaster. *Academic Emergency Medicine, 13*(11), 1118–1129. doi:10.1197/j.aem.2006.06.040

Burkle, F. M. (2007). Complex humanitarian emergencies. In D. E. Hogan & J. L. Burstein (Eds.), *Disaster medicine* (pp. 86–94). Philadelphia, PA: Lippincott Williams & Wilkins.

Burkle, F. M. (2009). Public health emergencies, cancer, and the legacy of Katrina. *Prehospital and Disaster Medicine, 22*(4), 291–292. doi:10.1017/S1049023X0000488X

Burkle, F. M. (2010). Future humanitarian crises: Challenges for practice, policy, and public health. *Prehospital and Disaster Medicine, 25*(3), 191–199. doi:10.1017/S1049023X00007998

Burstein, J. L. (2014). Disaster planning and management. In A. B. Wolfson (Ed.), *Harwood-Nuss' clinical practice of emergency medicine* (6th ed., pp. 1575–1578). Philadelphia, PA: Lippincott Williams & Wilkins.

Connor, S. B. (2014). When and why health care personnel respond to a disaster: The state of the science. *Prehospital and Disaster Medicine, 29*(3), 270–274. doi:10.1017/S1049023X14000387

Cuny, F. C. (1998). Principles of disaster management. Lesson 2: Program planning. *Prehospital and Disaster Medicine, 13*(2–4), 63–79. doi:10.1017/S1049023X0003017X

Danna, D., Bernard, M., Schaubhut, R., & Matthews, P. (2009). Experiences of nurse leaders surviving Hurricane Katrina, New Orleans, Louisiana, USA. *Nursing and Health Sciences, 12*(12), 9–13. doi:10.1111/j.1442-2018.2009.00497.x

Executive Office of the President. (2006). Executive Order 13407 of June 26, 2006: Public health warning system. *Federal Register, 71*(124), 36975–36977. Retrieved from https://www.federalregister.gov/documents/2006/06/28/06-5829/public-alert-and-warning-system

Federal Emergency Management Agency. (2010). Comprehensive Preparedness Guide 101: Developing and maintaining emergency operations plans (Version 2.0). Retrieved from https://www.fema.gov/media-library-data/20130726-1828-25045-0014/cpg_101_comprehensive_preparedness_guide_developing_and_maintaining_emergency_operations_plans_2010.pdf

Federal Emergency Management Agency. (2013). *National response framework* (2nd ed.). Retrieved from https://www.fema.gov/media-library-data/20130726-1914-25045-1246/final_national_response_framework_20130501.pdf

Federal Emergency Management Agency. (2015). NIMS and the incident command system. Retrieved from https://www.fema.gov/txt/nims/nims_ics_position_paper.txt

Federal Emergency Management Agency. (2017a). Disaster declarations by year. Retrieved from https://www.fema.gov/disasters/year

Federal Emergency Management Agency. (2017b). Disaster relief fund: Monthly reports. Retrieved from https://www.fema.gov/media-library/assets/documents/31789

Federal Emergency Management Agency. (n.d.). IPAWS course summary. Retrieved from https://emilms.fema.gov/IS247a/lesson1/IPAWS_Print.htm

Fong, F. H. (2007). Nuclear detonations: Evaluation and response. In D. E. Hogan & J. L. Burstein (Eds.), *Disaster medicine* (2nd ed., pp. 378–401). Philadelphia, PA: Lippincott Williams & Wilkins.

Garshnek, V., & Burkle, F. M. (1999). Telecommunication systems in support of disaster medicine: Applications of basic information pathways. *Annals of Emergency Medicine, 34*, 213–218. doi:10.1016/S0196-0644(99)70231-3

Gordis, L. (2013). *Epidemiology* (5th ed.). Philadelphia, PA: W. B. Saunders.

Haddow, G., & Haddow, K. (2014). *Disaster communications in a changing media world* (2nd ed.). Oxford, UK: Butterworth-Heinemann.

Hendrickson, R. G., & Horowitz, B. Z. (2016). Disaster preparedness. In J. E. Tintinalli (Ed.), *Tintinalli's emergency medicine: A comprehensive study guide* (8th ed.; pp. 23–29). New York, NY: McGraw-Hill.

Hu, Q., & Kapucu, N. (2016). Information communication technology utilization for effective emergency management networks. *Public Management Review, 18*(3), 323–348. doi:10.1080/14719037.2014.969762

Institute of Medicine. (2009). *Guidance for establishing crisis standards of care for use in disaster situations: A letter report.* Washington, DC: National Academies Press.

Institute of Medicine. (2012). *Crisis standards of care: A systems framework for catastrophic disaster response.* Washington, DC: The National Academies Press.

Institute of Medicine. (2015a). *Healthy, resilient, and sustainable communities after disasters.* Washington, DC: National Academies Press.

Institute of Medicine. (2015b). *Regional disaster response coordination to support health outcomes. Surge management: Workshop in brief.* Washington, DC: National Academies Press.

International Federation of Red Cross and Red Crescent Societies. (2017). Resilience: Saving lives today, investing for tomorrow. *World Disasters Report 2016.* Retrieved from http://www.ifrc.org/Global/Documents/Secretariat/201610/WDR%202016-FINAL_web.pdf

Jha, M. K. (Ed.). (2010). *Natural and anthropogenic disasters: Vulnerability, preparedness and mitigation.* Dordrecht, the Netherlands: Springer Science & Business Media.

Joint Commission on Accreditation of Healthcare Organizations. (2017). Guidelines for hospital emergency operations planning. Retrieved from www.jointcommission.org

Kano, M., Wood, M. M., Siegel, J. M., & Bourque, L. B. (2017). Disaster research and epidemiology. In K. L. Koenig & C. H. Schultz (Eds.), *Koenig and Schultz's disaster medicine: Comprehensive principles and practices* (2nd ed., pp. 3–22). New York, NY: Cambridge University Press.

Kapadia, K., & Badhuri, S. (2009). *Proactive planning approach for disaster risk management of megacities.* New Delhi, India: School of Planning and Architecture.

Khan, O., & Pappas, G. (2011). *Megacities and global health*. Washington, DC: American Public Health Association. doi:10.2105/9780875530031

Kim, D. H., Proctor, P. W., & Amos, L. K. (2002). Disaster management and the emergency department: A framework for planning. *Nursing Clinics, 37*(1), 171–188. doi:10.1016/S0029-6465(03)00091-4

Lam, E., McCarthy, A., & Brennan, M. (2015). Vaccine-preventable diseases in humanitarian emergencies among refugee and internally-displaced populations. *Human Vaccines & Immunotherapeutics, 11*(11), 2627–2636. doi:10.1080/21645515.2015.1096457

Landesman, L. Y. (2011). *Public health management of disasters: The practice guide* (3rd ed.). Washington, DC: American Public Health Association.

Landesman, L., & Morrow, C. (2013). Roles and responsibilities of public health in disaster preparedness and response. In F. Novick, C. Morrow, & G. Mays (Eds.), *Public health administration: Principles for population-based management* (3rd ed.; pp. 551–598). Sudbury, MA: Jones & Bartlett.

Lasker, R. (2003). *Redefining readiness: Terrorism planning through the eyes of the public*. New York, NY: The New York Academy of Medicine.

Lechat, M. F. (1979). Disasters and public health. *Bulletin of the World Health Organization, 57*(1), 11–17.

Lechat, M. F. (1990). Updates: The epidemiology of health effects of disasters. *Epidemiology Review, 12*, 192–197. doi:10.1093/oxfordjournals.epirev.a036053

Leonard, R. B. (1991). Emergency evacuations in disasters. *Prehospital and Disaster Medicine, 6*, 463–466. doi:10.1017/S1049023X00038978

Levitin, H. W., & Siegelson, H. J. (1996). Hazardous materials: Disaster medical planning and response. *Emergency Medicine Clinics of North America, 14*(2), 327–347.

Levitin, H. W., & Siegelson, H. J. (2007). Hazardous materials disasters. In D. E. Hogan & J. L. Burstein (Eds.), *Disaster medicine* (2nd ed., pp. 311–325). Philadelphia, PA: Lippincott, Williams & Wilkins.

Lillibridge, S. A., Noji, E. K., & Burkle, F. M. (1993). Disaster assessment: The emergency health evaluation of a population affected by a disaster. *Annals of Emergency Medicine, 22*, 1715–1720. doi:10.1016/S0196-0644(05)81311-3

Lindsay, B. R., & McCarthy, F. X. (2011). Considerations for a catastrophic declaration: Issues and analysis (No. 7-5700). *Congressional Research Service*. Retrieved from https://fas.org/sgp/crs/homesec/R41884.pdf

Lindsay, B. R., & McCarthy, F. X. (2015). Stafford act declarations 1953-2014: Trends, analyses, and implications for Congress. *Congressional Research Service*. Retrieved from https://fas.org/sgp/crs/homesec/R42702.pdf

Merriam Webster's Collegiate Dictionary. (2017). Retrieved from www.merriam-webster.com

National Fire Protection Administration. (2017). *NFPA 1600 standard on disaster/emergency management and business continuity programs*. Quincy, MA: Author.

National Oceanic and Atmospheric Administration. (2017). Billion-dollar weather and climate disasters: Table of events. Retrieved from https://www.ncdc.noaa.gov/billions/events/MI/1980-2017

National Science and Technology Council. (2000). Effective disaster warnings. Retrieved from http://tap.gallaudet.edu/emergency/nov05conference/EmergencyReports/EffectiveDisasterWarnings.pdf

Nedelman, M. (2017). Florida nursing home death toll reaches 12. *CNN*. Retrieved from http://www.cnn.com/2017/09/29/health/florida-irma-nursing-home-deaths/index.html

Parillo, S. J. (1995). Medical care at mass gatherings: Consideration for physician involvement. *Prehospital and Disaster Medicine, 10*, 273–275. doi:10.1017/S1049023X00042163

Physicians for Social Responsibility. (2011, April 26). Physicians for social responsibility cites flawed evacuation zones, nuclear's health risks on Chernobyl anniversary. Retrieved from http://www.psr.org/news-events/press-releases/psr-cites-flawed-evacuation-zones-nuclears-health-risks.html

Potash, M. N. (2008). The struggle for mental healthcare in New Orleans—One case at a time. *Psychiatry, 5*(7), 32–41.

Quarantelli, E. (1983). *Delivery of emergency medical care in disasters: Assumptions and realities*. New York, NY: Irvington.

Rabins, P. V., Kass, N., Rutkow, L., Vernick, J., & Hodge, J. G. (2011). Challenges for mental health services raised by disaster preparedness: Mapping the ethical and therapeutic terrain. *Biosecurity and Bioterrorism: Biodefense Strategy, Practice, and Science, 9*(12), 175–182. doi:10.1089/bsp.2010.0068

Robert, T. Stafford Disaster Relief and Emergency Assistance Act, Pub. L. No. 93–288 (1988).

Rodriguez, H., & Aguirre, B. (2006). Hurricane Katrina and the healthcare infrastructure: A focus on disaster preparedness, response, and resiliency. *Frontiers of Health Services Management, 23*(1), 13–24.

Rudowitz, R., Rowland, D., & Shartzer, A. (2006). Health care in New Orleans before and after Hurricane Katrina. *Health Affairs, 25*(5), w393–w406. doi:10.1377/hlthaff.25.w393

Sabatino, F. (1992). Hurricane Andrew: South Florida hospitals shared resources and energy to cope with storm's devastation. *Hospitals, 66*(24), 26–30.

Save the Children. (2017). Protecting children in emergencies: Escalating threats to children must be addressed (Vol. 1). Retrieved from www.savethechildren.org/site/c.8rKLIXMGIpI4E/b.6191697/k.F89E/Protecting_Children.htm

Schultz, C. H., Koenig, K. L., & Noji, E. K. (1996). Current concepts: A medical disaster response to reduce immediate mortality after an earthquake. *New England Journal of Medicine, 334*(7), 438–444. doi:10.1056/NEJM199602153340706

Smith, K., & Petley, D. N. (2009). *Environmental hazards: Assessing risk and reducing disaster* (5th ed.). New York, NY: Routledge.

Subbotina, K., & Agrawal, N. (2018). Natural disasters and health risks of first responders. In A. J. Masys & L. S. F. Lin (Eds.), *Asia-Pacific security challenges* (pp. 85–122). Cham, Switzerland: Springer.

Tierney, K. J. (2012). Disaster governance: Social, political and economic dimensions. *Annual Review of Environment and Resources, 37*, 341–363. doi:10.1146/annurev-environ-020911-095618

Timbie, J. W., Ringel, J. S., Fox, D. S., Waxman, D. A., Pillemer, F., Carey, C., … Kellermann, A. L. (2012). *Allocation of scarce resources during mass casualty events* (Evidence Reports/Technology Assessments, No. 207). Rockville, MD: Agency for Healthcare Research and Quality. Retrieved from https://www.ncbi.nlm.nih.gov/books/NBK98854/

United Nations, Department of Economic and Social Affairs, Population Division. (2016). The world's cities in 2016: Data booklet (ST/ESA/SER.A/392). Retrieved from http://www.un.org/en/development/desa/population/publications/pdf/urbanization/the_worlds_cities_in_2016_data_booklet.pdf

United Nations International Strategy for Disaster Reduction. (2017). Terminology. Retrieved from https://www.unisdr.org/we/inform/terminology

U.S. Department of Health and Human Services. (2017a). Chemical Hazards Emergency Medical Management. Estimation of protective distance/threat zone. Retrieved from https://chemm.nlm.nih.gov/threatzone.htm

U.S. Department of Health and Human Services. (2017b). Radiation Emergency Medical Management. Radiation control zones and perimeters recommended by various agencies for responding to radiological emergencies. Retrieved from https://www.remm.nlm.nih.gov/zones_radincident.htm

U.S. Department of Homeland Security. (2015). *National preparedness goal* (2nd ed.). Washington, DC: Author. Retrieved from https://www.fema.gov/media-library-data/1443799615171-2aae90be55041740f97e8532fc680d40/National_Preparedness_Goal_2nd_Edition.pdf

U.S. Department of Labor, Bureau of Labor Statistics. (2018). Registered murses. Retrieved from https://www.bls.gov/ooh/healthcare/registered-nurses.htm

Veenema, T. G., Walden, B., Feinstein, N., & Williams, J. P. (2008). Factors affecting hospital-based nurses' willingness to respond to a radiation emergency. *Disaster Medicine and Public Health Preparedness, 2*(4), 224–229.

Waeckerle, J. F. (1991). Disaster planning and response. *New England Journal of Medicine, 324*, 815–821. doi:10.1056/NEJM199103213241206

Wolfson, J., & Walker, G. (1993). *Hospital disaster preparedness: Lesson from Hurricane Andrew*. Tampa: Florida Public Health Information Center, College of Public Health, University of South Florida.

World Health Organization. (2016). 2016 WHO humanitarian response plans. Department for Emergency Risk Management and Humanitarian Response (ERM). Retrieved from http://www.who.int/hac/donorinfo/who_humanitarian_response_plan_2016_may.pdf?ua=1

Zschau, J., & Kuppers, A. (2003). *Early warning systems for natural disaster reduction*. New York, NY: Springer.

2

LEADERSHIP AND COORDINATION IN DISASTER HEALTHCARE SYSTEMS: THE U.S. NATIONAL PREPAREDNESS SYSTEM

Lynn A. Slepski, Mary Pat Couig, Roberta Proffitt Lavin, Susan M. Orsega, and Tener Goodwin Veenema

LEARNING OBJECTIVES

When this chapter is completed, readers will be able to:

1. Describe the U.S. National Preparedness System.
2. List the conditions that must be met before federal response coordination occurs.
3. Describe the basic tenets of the Pandemic and All-Hazards Preparedness Act and the National Health Security Strategy.
4. Describe the National Response Framework (NRF) and the National Incident Management System (NIMS).
5. List the 15 Emergency Support Functions (ESFs) included in the plan, particularly ESF8, Public Health and Medical Services.

EDITOR'S NOTE

The information presented in this chapter has been verified up to the date of submission for publication; however, references and resources frequently change. Readers are encouraged to visit the DHS website at www.dhs.gov/index.shtm, the FEMA website at www.fema.gov, and preparedness page of the HHS at www.phe.gov/preparedness/pages/default.aspx for the most current, available information. Information on low-cost or no-cost training is available at training.fema.gov/.

6. Discuss the purpose and scope of ESF8.
7. Describe federal resources for nurse volunteers, including the National Disaster Medical System (NDMS), the Medical Reserve Corps (MRC), and the Emergency System for Advance Registration of Volunteer Health Professionals (ESAR-VHP).

KEY MESSAGES

Nursing leadership during a disaster or public health emergency demands a broad knowledge base, an understanding of all-hazards preparedness, national emergency healthcare system Frameworks, and individual roles and responsibilities during an event. Recent events have taught us that preparedness is a shared responsibility that requires the involvement of everyone or the "whole community." The whole community includes individuals and families; businesses, including healthcare systems; faith-based groups and disability organizations; nonprofit groups; schools and academia; and all levels of government including federal, state, local, tribal, and territorial.

When the whole community works together, the nation is kept from harm and is more resilient when struck by all types of hazards, including natural disasters such as hurricanes or ice storms, diseases such as pandemics, chemical spills and other man-made hazards, terrorist attacks, or cyberattacks.

All federal planning is based on the whole community which focuses on involving people from all walks of life in the development of national preparedness documents as well as ensuring that *everyone* understands his or her roles and responsibilities and knows how to perform when called upon.

Presidential Policy Directive 8 (PPD-8) established a series of integrated national planning Frameworks, covering prevention, protection, mitigation, response, and recovery. These Frameworks are designed around the whole community concept that leverages all available capabilities in a coordinated and efficient way based on community needs. PPD-8 also refocuses preparedness from the national level back to individual and community preparedness; each community contributes by preparing for the risks that are most relevant and urgent for its members individually.

Public–private sector relationships are critical, especially considering the fact that only 10% of the total workforce is from the public sector, while the remaining 90% span private sector, nongovernmental, and faith-based organizations. The nation's critical infrastructure—water, power, communication, healthcare, and transportation networks—rests largely within the private sector. Community and faith-based groups are key assets, with leadership and communication structures and significant resources in support of disaster response (National Research Council, 2012).

The U.S. National Response Framework (NRF) includes emergency management authorities, policies, procedures, and resources of local, state, and federal governments, as well as voluntary disaster relief agencies, the private sector, and international resources to provide assistance following a natural or man-made disaster. The U.S. Department of Homeland Security's (DHS's) Federal Emergency Management Agency (FEMA) coordinates the NRF to provide supplemental assistance when the consequences of a disaster overwhelm local and state capabilities.

The NRF includes 15 Emergency Support Functions (ESFs), each of which has a designated federal coordinator and primary agency and supporting agencies. Nurses need to be aware of ESF8, Public Health and Medical Services, and its core provisions.

The NRF and the National Incident Management System (NIMS) are related documents designed to improve the nation's response capabilities and incident management. The NRF provides the structure for all-hazards, tiered responses, and the NIMS provides the template for the management of incidents.

Nursing leadership during a disaster or public health emergency demands a broad knowledge base and an understanding of all-hazards preparedness and individual roles and responsibilities during an event.

Nurses in every type of workplace and in every type of position from a new graduate to a nurse in senior healthcare leadership position have a role in ensuring they are personally prepared, the nurses in their workplace are prepared, and that every nurse in their workplace knows and can perform their role in a disaster or emergency.

All disasters begin at the local level. There are many opportunities for nurses to get involved to help strengthen the ability of communities, states, and our nation to be prepared.

CHAPTER OVERVIEW

This chapter explores the U.S. National Preparedness System with an emphasis on healthcare systems' Frameworks for disaster response. Included is a brief review of the key components of federal disaster planning; a detailed overview of the NRF and its changes from previous doctrine; the NIMS; two pieces of foundational disaster health legislation, the Pandemic and All-Hazards Preparedness Act and the National Health Security Strategy; and a description of several medical surge mechanisms including the NDMS, the MRC, and the Emergency System for Advance Registration of Volunteer Health Professionals. Topics discussed include the NRF's purpose, scope, and 15 ESFs, highlighting the importance of ESF8 Public Health and Medical Services in providing supplemental assistance to state and local governments in identifying and meeting the public health and medical needs of victims and communities. Federal definitions of disaster conditions, the basic underlying assumptions of the NRF, and links to the most current information are provided. Issues and challenges related to defining the role of nurses in a disaster situation are discussed. Disaster nursing leadership mandates that nurses have a sound knowledge base in critical management areas, as well as in health policy and public health. The chapter presents suggestions for nursing leadership and opportunities for nursing leadership engagement. Nurses are encouraged to use their skills and expertise for leadership during disaster planning and response as well as during other periods of crisis.

"What we at one time could barely imagine, we must now prepare for as likelihoods. We cannot afford to do otherwise," said Rear Admiral Audrey Manley, Acting Surgeon General of United States Public Health Service (USPHS), at a seminar on responding to the consequences of chemical and biological terrorism in 1995 (U.S. Department of Health and Human Services [HHS], 1995). Six years later, on September 11, 2001, high-jacked Boeing 767 airplanes struck the North and South Towers of the World Trade Center in New York City. What was barely imagined was realized. September 11 reshaped the way the nation's leaders understand our country's vulnerabilities and the importance of disaster response preparedness. In 2005, Hurricane Katrina again tested the nation's ability to respond to disasters. Public health emergencies that can turn into disasters are a fact of life in a world as interconnected as ours. In the past 5 years, we have witnessed outbreaks of diseases such as Asian Lineage Avian Influenza A (H7N9) virus, Ebola virus disease, and Zika virus infection, none of which stayed within a geographical border. During the 2017 hurricane season, towns and cities suffered damages from 10 hurricanes, six of which were major (Category 3 or stronger) in the Atlantic (Erdman, 2017). Areas that were better prepared such as Houston, TX, New Orleans, LA, and Gulfport, MS, fared much better. However, as of late October 2017, the world continues to witness the humanitarian disaster unfolding in Puerto Rico which was ravaged twice in 10 days by Hurricanes Irma and Maria. Four weeks after Hurricane Maria, most of Puerto Rico remained without potable water, food, power, telephone, Internet, and transportation (Dickerson & Ferré-Sadurní, 2017).

As is true for many disasters, healthcare systems, especially hospitals, are the first port of entry for patients. The ability to respond depends on the preparedness of the hospital staff, the department, and the hospital (Kaji, Koenig, & Lewis, 2007). Although nurses are the largest number of health professionals in the United States, most are not prepared to respond to a disaster (Baack & Alfred, 2013). Nurses need to be ready to participate in planning efforts, actual disaster events, mock drills, and training opportunities specific to disaster preparedness.

Recent natural and man-made events have caused the federal government to revisit existing disaster planning and funding. The HHS's Hospital Preparedness Program estimated awards for FY17 were $850,000,000 under the Hospital Preparedness Program—Public Health Emergency Preparedness Cooperative Agreement funds (HHS, 2017a). Public health departments and hospitals continue to implement these grants to effectively expand their medical surge capability, develop and exercise preparedness plans, train staff on disaster response, and purchase equipment such as mobile communications and response medical units. As a result, state and local governments are making changes to their planning and workforce, especially in the area of public health.

In order to actively participate in our nation's plan for emergency preparedness for disasters and other public health emergencies, nurses must have an understanding of the overall National Preparedness System and an awareness of the existing Frameworks for disaster prevention, protection, mitigation, response, and recovery. During a disaster response, the role of nurses may include identifying the event; functioning as a first responder at the scene; working with a rapid needs assessment team to identify requirements; providing patient care by working in a local hospital, Federal Medical Station (FMS), public health department, or field medical team; or assuming a leadership position in the coordination of all of these types of activities. Each of these roles might include planning, leadership skills, policy writing, or research; or managing communications and the media. Knowledge of the disaster life cycle and of the organization of local, state, and federal response plans is critical for nurses to function successfully during these types of events. Leadership roles for nurses here require a unique knowledge base and skills set. Finally, because of the continued restructuring of federal systems for public health and medical response and accommodations for additional national security concerns, nurses need to view some of the information in this chapter as "a moving target" subject to change. To understand how these changes will alter the leadership structure and coordination of efforts of the major disaster health systems, nurses are advised to seek updated information on the Internet websites listed at the end of the chapter.

FEDERAL PREPAREDNESS PLANNING AND EMERGENCY RESPONSE

Local and state responders are best able to handle most disasters and emergencies. Occasionally, the actual or potential impact of an event may overwhelm resources available at the local level. When the scope of a disaster exceeds local and state capability to respond, the federal government may provide supplemental assistance.

In the aftermath of the September 11, 2001, terrorist attacks, there was a need to enhance the way the nation responds to disasters. As such, President Bush established DHS and the Homeland Security Council via an executive order to assist with the planning and coordination of federal efforts to combat terrorism and maintain the domestic security of the United States. Shortly thereafter, the president launched a new series of directives—Homeland Security Presidential Directives (HSPDs)—intended to "record and communicate presidential decisions about the homeland security policies of the United States."

Homeland Security Presidential Directive 5 (HSPD-5) was established in 2003, to enhance the ability of the United States to manage domestic incidents by establishing a single, comprehensive NIMS. It designates the Secretary of Homeland Security as the principal federal official responsible for coordinating federal operations within the United States to prepare for, respond to, and recover from terrorist attacks, major disasters, and other emergencies (White House, 2003). Coordination begins if any one of the following four conditions applies:

1. A federal department or agency acting under its own authority has requested the assistance of the Secretary.
2. The resources of state and local authorities are overwhelmed and federal assistance has been requested by the appropriate state and local authorities; examples include:
   - Major disasters or emergencies as defined under the Stafford Act
   - Catastrophic incidents
3. More than one federal department or agency has become substantially involved in responding to an incident. Examples include:
   - Credible threats, indications, or warnings of imminent terrorist attack or acts of terrorism directed domestically against the people, property, environment, or political or legal institutions of the United States or its territories or possessions
   - Threats or incidents related to high-profile, large-scale events that present high-probability targets such as National Special Security Events (NSSEs) and other special events as determined by the Secretary of Homeland Security, in coordination with other federal departments and agencies
4. The Secretary of Homeland Security has been directed to assume responsibility for managing the domestic incident by the President.

HSPD-5 also directs federal department heads to provide their full and prompt cooperation, support, and resources to the Secretary in protecting national security. In addition to coordinating federal operations and resources, the Secretary establishes reporting requirements and conducts ongoing communications with federal, state, local, tribal, private sector, and nongovernmental organizations to maintain situational awareness, analyze threats, assess the national implications of threats, maintain operational response activities, and coordinate threat or incident response activities.

The Pandemic and All-Hazards Preparedness Act, passed in 2006, amended the Public Health Service Act to require the Secretary of HHS to lead all federal public health and medical responses to public health emergencies. In this legislation, there were many requirements to improve the ability of the nation to respond to a public health or medical disaster or emergency, and it included the creation of the Office of the Assistant Secretary for Preparedness and Response (ASPR) and the requirement to establish a near–real-time electronic nationwide public health situational awareness capability to enhance early detection of, rapid response to, and management of potentially catastrophic infectious disease outbreaks and other public health emergencies. This legislation also tasked HHS/ASPR to disseminate novel and best practices of outreach to, and care of, at-risk individuals before, during, and following public health emergencies (HHS, 2010b).

The NRF, enacted in January 2008, supersedes the National Response Plan and serves as a guide to how the nation conducts comprehensive incident response using an all-hazards approach to respond to natural and man-made disasters (DHS, 2008a). Built on its predecessor, it includes guiding principles that detail how federal, state, local, tribal, and private sector partners, including the healthcare sector, prepare for and provide a unified domestic response through improved coordination and integration. Updated in 2016, the NRF now emphasizes the whole community working together to determine current and future requirements (DHS, 2016).

The purpose of the National Health Security Strategy (NHSS), released in 2009, was to refocus the patchwork of disparate public health and medical preparedness, response, and recovery strategies to ensure that the nation is prepared for, protected from, and resilient in the face of health threats or incidents with potentially negative health consequences (HHS, 2011c). It is the first comprehensive strategy focusing specifically on protecting people's health in the case of a large-scale incident that puts health and well-being at risk. It contains two goals: build community resilience and strengthen and sustain health and emergency response systems. These overarching goals are supported by 10 detailed Strategic Objectives such as "develop and maintain the workforce needed for national health security" and "ensure timely and effective communication." Included with the strategy was the requirement to develop a biennial implementation plan to describe the priority implementation activities to occur in each planning cycle. The NHSS, however, was not accompanied by funding. The authors state, "Since such investments are beyond the scope of a single department, policy, or level of government, the NHSS and implementation documents emphasize coordinating and prioritizing resources across all communities and sectors" (HHS, 2011a).

On March 30, 2011, the President published PPD-8 (Figure 2.1): National Preparedness, directing the development of a national preparedness goal that identifies core capabilities as well as a national preparedness system to guide preparedness for the threats that pose the greatest risk to the security of the nation (DHS, 2011a). These threats include both natural and man-made incidents. What is most different about the approach of this directive is that it states that national preparedness and response require a "Whole Community" approach that shifts the focus from a federal government lead to one that "utilizes the capabilities of federal, state, local, tribal, and territorial

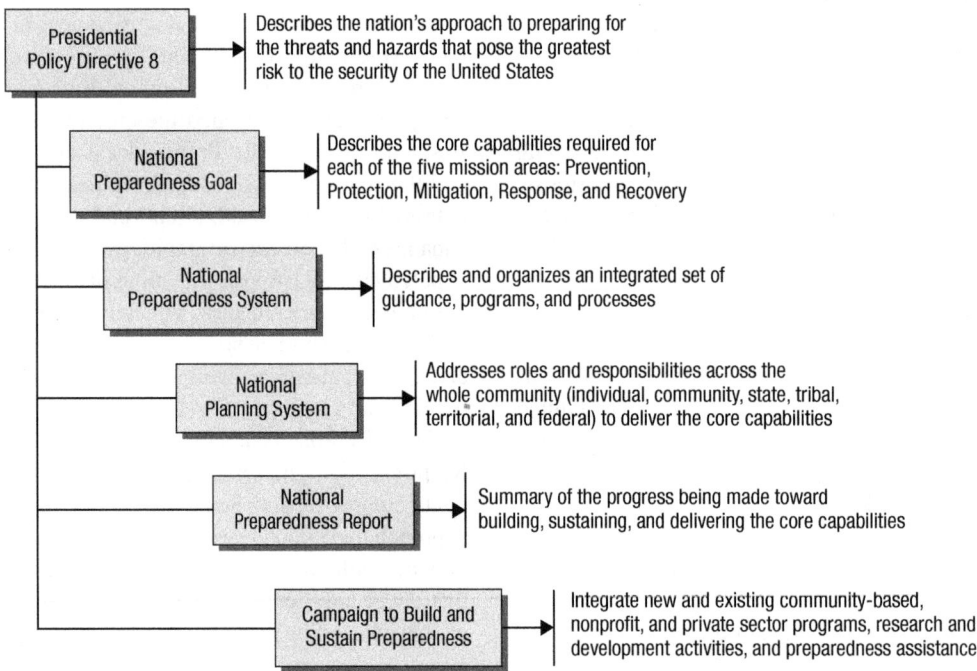

Presidential Policy Directive 8	Describes the nation's approach to preparing for the threats and hazards that pose the greatest risk to the security of the United States
National Preparedness Goal	Describes the core capabilities required for each of the five mission areas: Prevention, Protection, Mitigation, Response, and Recovery
National Preparedness System	Describes and organizes an integrated set of guidance, programs, and processes
National Planning System	Addresses roles and responsibilities across the whole community (individual, community, state, tribal, territorial, and federal) to deliver the core capabilities
National Preparedness Report	Summary of the progress being made toward building, sustaining, and delivering the core capabilities
Campaign to Build and Sustain Preparedness	Integrate new and existing community-based, nonprofit, and private sector programs, research and development activities, and preparedness assistance

FIGURE 2.1 National Preparedness Paradigm.

Source: Slepski, L., Proffit, R., & Veenema, T. G. (2012). Leadership and coordination in disaster health care systems: The U.S. national response Framework. In T. G. Veenema (Ed.), Disaster nursing and emergency preparedness: For chemical, biological, and radiological terrorism and other hazards (3rd ed., pp. 21–44). New York, NY: Springer.

governments, private sector, nongovernment organizations, faith-based and community-based organizations and the American public" (DHS, 2011e, p. 3). The directive charges the Assistant to the President for Homeland Security and Counterterrorism (and not the Secretary of Homeland Security) to coordinate the development of a PPD-8 implementation plan.

The *National Preparedness Goal* (the Goal) was the first deliverable required of PPD-8 and was published on September 29, 2011. It began with the definition of core capabilities required for each of the five mission areas that are necessary to prepare for the specific types of incidents positing the greatest risk of security to the nation. As an example, the response core capability is described as: "Responding quickly to save lives, protect property and the environment, and meet basic human needs in the aftermath of a catastrophic incident" (DHS, 2011c, p. 1). Since 2011, the Goal has been updated once. Today's Goal is very concise: "A secure and resilient Nation with the capabilities required across the whole community to prevent, protect against, mitigate, respond to, and recover from the threats and hazards that pose the greatest risk" (DHS, 2015, p. 1).

The *National Preparedness System* (the System) then is composed of all of the activities needed for strengthening national preparedness and achieving the Goal. The system includes six specific components and provides specific tools and resources to accomplish them. The six components are: (a) identifying and assessing risk; (b) estimating capability requirements; (c) building and sustaining capabilities; (d) planning to deliver capabilities; (e) validating capabilities; and (f) reviewing and updating capabilities. When assessing risk, planners must consider both the likelihood of an incident and the significance of the impact should such an incident occur.

Plans should encompass the most likely and significant risks to a family, organization, or community, and should capitalize on those activities that are "all-hazards" or needed across most scenarios. These components help us understand risk, inform current and future planning and decisions as well as resource allocation, and aid in understanding the progress of the nation (DHS, 2011d).

NATIONAL PLANNING FRAMEWORKS

Much progress has been made from the single NRF to five national planning Frameworks describing how the whole community works together in each of the mission areas: prevention, protection, mitigation, response, and recovery. Each Framework identifies the scope of the mission area and describes the roles and responsibilities, core capabilities, coordinating structures, and relationships to other mission areas. Three core capabilities are shared across all mission areas: Planning; Public Information and Warning; and, Operational Coordination. Each Framework has additional core capabilities as well as unique principles that ground how each mission area is approached. An important inclusion to each Framework was a set of coordinated planning assumptions, an identified common starting point, to assist planners at every level in the development of operational plans that will work across all levels, starting at the individual or organizational level up to the federal interagency (e.g., individual, local, regional state, tribal, territorial, federal), to execute the strategies contained in the Frameworks. The following is a brief description of four Frameworks to be followed by a more in-depth review of response.

The National Prevention Framework. While "prevention" may be a common term, it has a very specific meaning in the context of this Framework and the Goal. This Framework applies only to those capabilities, plans, and operations necessary to avoid, prevent, or stop a threatened or actual act of terrorism. Though the other Frameworks encompass all-hazards, the Prevention Framework focuses only on terrorist activities directed against U.S. soil, and specifically on imminent threats or acts of terrorism for which there is intelligence or information that warns of a specific, credible, and impending threat or ongoing attack on the United States. Because of this specificity, this Framework does not capture the full spectrum of the nation's efforts to counter terrorism. The seven Prevention core capabilities are Planning; Public Information and Warning; Operational Coordination; Forensics and Attribution; Intelligence and Information Sharing; Interdiction and Disruption; and Screening, Search, and Detection. This Framework sets out three principles that guide the development and execution of the core capabilities for Prevention: Engaged Partnerships; Scalability, Flexibility, and Adaptability; and Readiness to Act (DHS, 2013b). One activity that many may be aware of that came specifically from this Framework is the DHS program "If You See Something, Say Something" (DHS, 2010), which encourages the public to be aware and report suspicious activity.

The National Protection Framework. The National Protection Framework provides individual, community private sector, nongovernmental organizations, and governmental leaders with an understanding of the range of activities within the Protection mission area and how the whole community can work together to secure the homeland against acts of terrorism, natural disasters, and other man-made threats or hazards, promoting a secure and resilient nation. The Protection mission area includes actions to deter threats, reduce vulnerabilities, or minimize the consequences associated with an incident, especially involving critical infrastructure protection, cybersecurity, defense against weapons of mass destruction, defense of agriculture and food, health, border, immigration, maritime, and transportation security. The 11 Protection core capabilities are: Planning; Public Information and Warning; Operational Coordination; Access Control and Identity Verification; Cybersecurity; Intelligence and Information Sharing; Interdiction and Disruption; Physical Protective Measures; Risk Management for Protection Programs and Activities; Screening, Search and Detection; and Supply Chain Integrity and Security. Three principles that guide the development and support the execution and deployment of Protection core capabilities are Resilience and Scalability; Risk-Informed Culture; and Shared Responsibility. Protection capabilities are coordinated through existing partnerships at all levels of government and with the private sector, including nongovernmental organizations. These partnerships may cross critical infrastructure sectors and geographical boundaries. They allow for the exchange of expertise and information and provide a source of potential resources through mutual aid and assistance agreements (DHS, 2014).

The National Mitigation Framework. The National Mitigation Framework establishes a common platform and forum for coordinating and addressing how the nation manages risk through mitigation capabilities, saving lives, and reducing property damage. Mitigation reduces the impact of disasters by supporting protection and prevention activities, easing response, and speeding recovery to create better prepared and more resilient communities. Building on a wealth of objective and evidence-based knowledge and community experience, the Framework seeks to increase risk awareness and leverage mitigation products, services, and assets across the whole community. The National Mitigation Framework discusses seven core capabilities required for entities involved in mitigation: Threats and Hazard Identification; Risk and Disaster Resilience Assessment; Planning; Community Resilience; Public Information and Warning; Long-Term Vulnerability Reduction; and Operational Coordination. The four guiding principles for Mitigation include Resilience and Sustainability, Leadership and Locally Focused Implementation, Engaged Partnerships and Inclusiveness, and Risk-Conscious Culture. One example of mitigation is the activities undertaken by the U.S. Corps of Engineers to reduce the flooding potential in New Orleans after Hurricane Katrina. The Corps redesigned levees and installed additional pumping stations decreasing the risk of flooding while at the same time increasing the amount of time local citizens would have to evacuate. Separately, many hurricane-prone areas have adopted building codes that require minimum construction standards for surviving high winds (DHS, 2013a).

The National Disaster Recovery Framework (NDRF). Recovery begins with the response effort and continues until needs have been met. In the days and weeks following a disaster, a range of both short- (e.g., getting people into shelters) and long-term (e.g., rebuilding) activities begin in parallel to get an affected community back on its feet, and to rebuild in a stronger, smarter, and safer manner. It is during the recovery phase that actions to mitigate and reduce future risks are identified. The NDRF provides context for how the whole community works together to restore, redevelop, and revitalize the health, economic, social, natural, and environmental fabric of the community. According to the Goal, eight core capabilities are aligned with the Recovery mission area. These include: Planning; Public Information and Warning; and Operational Coordination. The five capabilities that are unique to the Recovery mission area are: Economic Recovery; Health and Social Services; Housing; Infrastructure Systems; and Natural and Cultural Resources. Because the development of the NDRF began under an earlier initiative, the document is organized a little differently than the other four Frameworks. There are six specific Recovery Support Functions: Community Planning and Capacity Building; Economic; Health and Social Services; Housing; Infrastructure Systems; and Natural and Cultural Resources (DHS, 2011b).

NATIONAL RESPONSE FRAMEWORK

The updated Framework is intended to ensure that everyone—governmental executives, leaders from the private sector and nongovernmental organizations as well as emergency managers and responders—understand response roles, responsibilities, and the relationships required to respond effectively to any type of incident. The Framework includes five principles that form the basis of national response doctrine: engaged partnerships; tiered response; scalable, flexible, and adaptable operational capabilities; unity of effort through unified command; and most importantly, readiness to act (DHS, 2008c). The Framework emphasizes preparedness activities that include planning, organizing, training, equipping, exercising, and applying lessons learned. The Framework is based on three basic premises: (a) resilience begins with prepared individuals and families; (b) communities, tribes, and states are responsible for the safety and security of their residents; and (c) all responses are local and based on layered and mutually supporting capabilities that promote expanded partnerships.

The Framework assigns coordinating and primary federal agencies to each of 15 ESFs used to provide federal support during a response (Table 2.1).

TABLE 2.1 National Response Framework Emergency Response Function Descriptions

ESF	Scope	ESF Coordinator/Primary Agency
ESF-1—Transportation	• Federal and civil transportation support • Transportation safety • Restoration/recovery of transportation infrastructure • Movement restrictions • Damage and impact assessment	Department of Transportation
ESF-2—Communications	• Coordination with telecommunication industry • Restoration/repair of telecommunications infrastructure • Protection, restoration, and sustainment of national cyberspace and information technology resources • Oversight of communications within the federal incident management and response structures	Department of Homeland Security/National Protection and Program Department of Homeland Security/National Protection and Program and Federal Emergency Management Agency
ESF-3—Public Works and Engineering	• Infrastructure protection and emergency repair • Infrastructure restoration • Engineering services and construction management • Emergency contracting support for lifesaving and life-sustaining services	Department of Defense/U.S. Army Corps of Engineers Department of Defense/U.S. Army Corps of Engineers and Department of Homeland Security/Federal Emergency Management Agency
ESF-4—Firefighting	• Coordination of federal firefighting activities • Support to wildland, rural, and urban firefighting operations	Department of Agriculture/Forest Service
ESF-5—Emergency Management	• Coordination of incident management and response efforts • Issuance of mission assignments • Resource and human capital • Incident action planning • Financial management	Department of Homeland Security/Federal Emergency Management Agency
ESF-6—Mass Care, Emergency Assistance, Housing, and Human Services	• Mass care • Emergency assistance • Disaster housing • Human services	Department of Homeland Security/Federal Emergency Management Agency

(continued)

TABLE 2.1 National Response Framework Emergency Response Function Descriptions (*continued*)

ESF	Scope	ESF Coordinator/Primary Agency
ESF-7—Logistics Management and Resource Support	• Comprehensive, national incident logistics planning, management and sustainment capability • Resource support (facility space, office equipment and supplies, contracting services, etc.)	General Services Administration and the Department of Homeland Security/ Federal Emergency Management Administration
ESF-8—Public Health and Medical Services	• Public health • Medical • Mental health services • Mass fatality management	Department of Health and Human Services
ESF-9—Search and Rescue	• Lifesaving assistance • Search and rescue operations	Department of Homeland Security/ Federal Emergency Management Agency Department of Homeland Security/ Federal Emergency Management Agency and U.S. Coast Guard Department of the Interior/National Park Service Department of Defense/U.S. Air Force
ESF-10—Oil and Hazardous Materials Response	• Oil and hazardous materials (chemical, biological, radiological, etc.) response • Environmental short- and long-term cleanup	Environmental Protection Agency Environmental Protection Agency and the Department of Homeland Security/ U.S. Coast Guard
ESF-11—Agriculture and Natural Resources	• Nutrition assistance • Animal and plant disease and pest response • Food safety and security • Natural and cultural resources and historic properties protection and restoration • Safety and well-being of household pets	Department of Agriculture (USDA) Department of the Interior
ESF-12—Energy	• Energy infrastructure assessment, repair, and restoration • Energy industry utilities coordination • Energy forecast	Department of Energy
ESF-13—Public Safety and Security	• Facility and resource security • Security planning and technical resource assistance • Public safety and security support • Support to access, traffic, and crowd control	Department of Justice
ESF-14—Long-Term Community Recovery	• Social and economic community impact assessment • Long-term community recovery assistance to states, local governments, and the private sector • Mitigation analysis and program implementation	Department of Homeland Security/ Federal Emergency Management Agency Department of Agriculture Department of Homeland Security Department of Housing and Urban Development Small Business Administration
ESF-15—External Affairs	• Emergency public information and protective action guidance • Media and community relations • Congressional and international affairs • Tribal and insular affairs	Department of Homeland Security Department of Homeland Security/ Federal Emergency Management Agency

ESF, Emergency Support Function.

Source: U.S. Department of Homeland Security. (2016). *National Response Framework* (3rd ed.). Retrieved from https://www.fema.gov/media-library -data/1466014682982-9bcf8245ba4c60c120aa915abe74e15d/National_Response_Framework3rd.pdf

THE NRF AS IT RELATES TO THE NIMS

The NRF and NIMS (DHS, 2017) work together to improve the nation's incident management capabilities and overall efficiency by ensuring that emergency management and response personnel from different jurisdictions and disciplines can work together to respond to natural disasters and emergencies, including acts of terrorism, by following standardized practices and using common terminology (DHS, 2016). Together, they are designed to ensure that all local jurisdictions retain command, control, and authority over response activities within their areas. As part of the preparedness activities, NIMS encourages the development of mutual aid and assistance agreements, which are mechanisms between agencies, organizations, and governments to help one another by quickly deploying personnel, equipment, materials, and services.

The NIMS provides a template for incident management regardless of size, scope, or cause. The template includes a core set of concepts, doctrines, principles, organizational processes, and terminology. It standardizes emergency management, personnel and resource management procedures, promoting coordination during planning and response. There are five interrelated components: preparedness; communications and information management; resource management; command and control; and ongoing management and maintenance. As an example, preparedness includes assessment, planning, procedures and protocols, training and exercise, personnel qualifications, licensure and certification, equipment certification, and evaluation and revision as the requirements to ensure that the entity is prepared. Use of the NIMS template enables federal, state, local, tribal, and territorial governments, as well as the private sector and nongovernmental organizations, to work seamlessly together effectively and efficiently to prevent, prepare for, respond to, and recover from domestic incidents, regardless of cause, size, or complexity. NIMS standard incident command structures are based on the following three key organizational systems:

1. *Incident Command System (ICS)*: NIMS establishes ICS as a standard incident management organization with five functional areas—command, operations, planning, logistics, and finance/administration—for management of all major incidents. To ensure further coordination, and during incidents involving multiple jurisdictions or agencies, the principle of unified command has been universally incorporated into NIMS. This unified command not only coordinates the efforts of many jurisdictions but provides for and ensures joint decisions on objectives, strategies, plans, priorities, and public communications.
2. *Multiagency Coordination Systems*: These define the operating characteristics, interactive management components, and organizational structure of supporting incident management entities engaged at the federal, state, local, tribal, and regional levels through mutual aid agreements and other assistance arrangements. These systems assist agencies and organizations that are responding by supporting coordination of effort through incident prioritization, critical resource allocation, communications system integration, and information management. The most frequently used systems are Emergency Operations Centers and Multiagency Coordination Groups.
3. *Public Information Systems*: These refer to processes, procedures, and systems for communicating timely and accurate information to the public during crisis or emergency situations.

NIMS is meant to be used at all levels of a response (Figure 2.2). NIMS standard incident command structures are based on the following three key organizational systems:

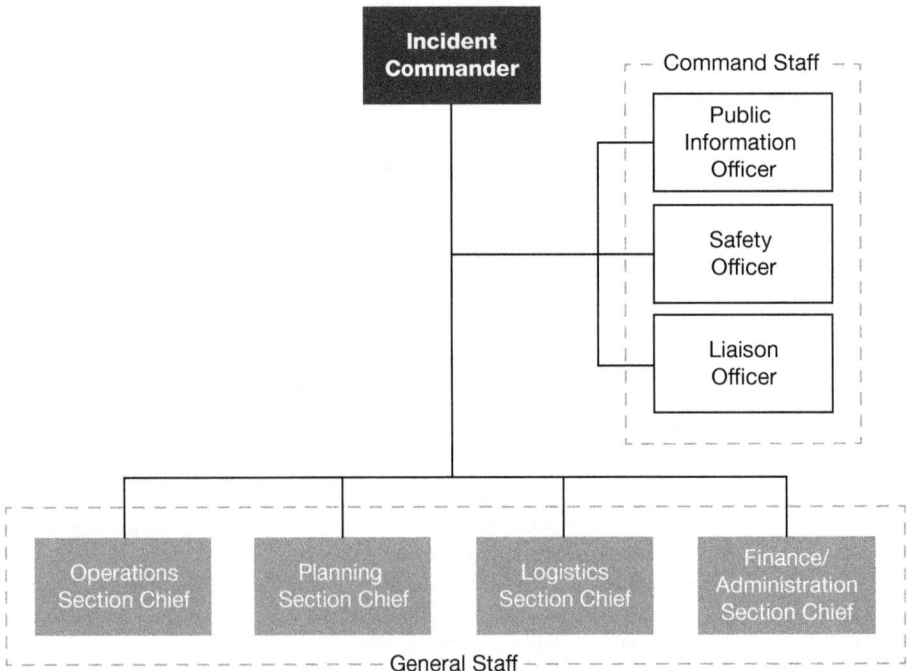

FIGURE 2.2 National Incident Management System (NIMS) incident command organization: Command staff and general staff.

Source: U.S. Department of Homeland Security. (2017, October 10). *National Incident Management System* (3rd ed.). Retrieved from https://www.fema.gov/media-library/assets/documents/148019

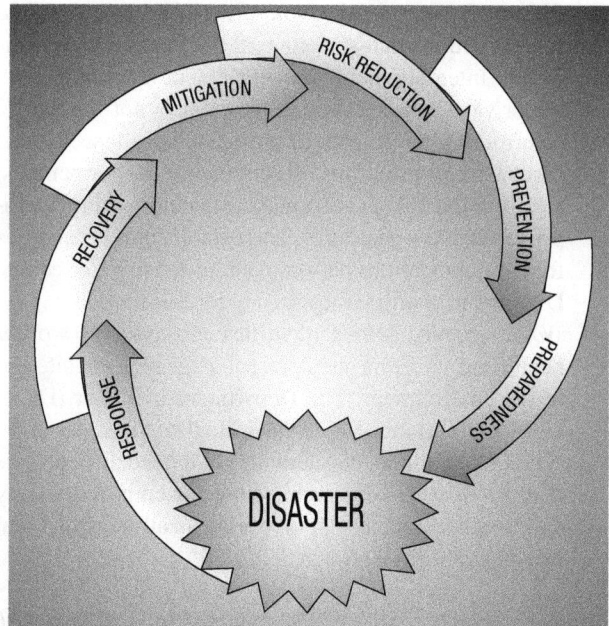

FIGURE 2.3 The disaster life cycle describes the process through which emergency managers prepare for emergencies and disasters, respond to them when they occur, help people and institutions recover from them, mitigate their effects, reduce the risk of loss, and prevent disasters such as fires from occurring.

Source: Federal Emergency Management Agency. (2015). Coastal Hazards Management Course, Slide 31.3.

By setting standard roles, functions, and language, responders know what to expect and how to communicate their needs. Together, the NRF and the NIMS integrate the capabilities and resources of various governmental jurisdictions, incident management and emergency response disciplines, nongovernmental organizations, and the private sector into a cohesive, coordinated, and seamless national Framework for domestic incident management. NIMS benefits include a unified approach to incident management, standard command and management structures, and emphasis on preparedness, mutual aid, and resource management. NIMS activities address each phase of the disaster life cycle (see Figure 2.3).

IMPLEMENTATION OF THE NRF

Consistent with NIMS, the NRF is flexible and scalable depending on the specifics and the magnitude of a threat or an event. The following structures and annexes are the primary, but not exclusive, mechanisms that may be implemented during a catastrophic, multistate earthquake incident.

- *Domestic Readiness Group (DRG)*: The DRG is comprised of senior leaders from all cabinet-level departments and agencies. The White House convenes the DRG on a regular basis to develop and coordinate implementation of preparedness and response policy in anticipation of or during crises such as a catastrophic earthquake to provide strategic

policy direction for the federal response and address issues that cannot be resolved at lower levels.

- *Joint Field Office (JFO)*: A temporary federal facility established near an incident to provide a central point for federal, state, local, and tribal executives with responsibility for incident oversight, direction, and assistance to coordinate protection, prevention, preparedness, response, and recovery actions. Senior federal officials from each of the federal and state stakeholders assemble in the JFO and using ICS work through their home agencies to provide needed resources and support.

- *ESFs*: A functional approach that groups the capabilities of federal departments and agencies into ESFs to provide the planning, resources, and program implementation that are most likely needed during a large-scale invent. Although there are 15 ESFs that can be activated independently or concurrently, key ESFs applicable to the health response during a catastrophic event are as follows:
  - *ESF-5—Emergency Management*: Provides the core management and administrative functions in support of NRF operations. This includes, but is not limited to, activating ESFs; alerting, notifying, and deploying DHS and HHS emergency response teams; information management; and facilitation of requests for federal assistance. FEMA is the ESF5 coordinator.
  - *ESF-6—Mass Care, Emergency Assistance, Housing and Human Services*: Presents the mechanism for coordinating the delivery of federal mass care, emergency assistance, and housing and human services. Mass care includes sheltering, feeding operations, emergency first aid, bulk distribution of emergency items, and collecting and providing information on victims to family members. Emergency assistance includes support to evacuations (which includes registration and tracking of evacuees); reunification of families; provision of aid and services to special needs populations and service animals; support to specialized shelters; support to medical shelters; conventional shelter management; coordination of donated goods and services; and coordination of voluntary agency assistance. Housing addresses postdisaster housing options. Human services use disaster assistance programs to help victims recover their nonhousing losses, disaster unemployment, as well as other types of assistance. This ESF was modified after Hurricane Katrina to also address the requirements for the sheltering and care of pets. Please see the NRF for a full discussion of all of the services addressed in this ESF. FEMA is the ESF6 coordinator.
  - *ESF-8—Public Health and Medical Services*: Provides the mechanism for coordinated federal assistance in response to public health and medical care needs for or during a developing potential health and medical situation. HHS is the ESF8 coordinator.
  - *ESF-15—External Affairs*: Ensures that sufficient federal assets are deployed to provide accurate, coordinated, and timely messages to affected audiences, including governments, the media, the private sector, and the affected populace.

■ *Incident Annexes*: Address contingency or hazard situations requiring specialized application of the NRF. Incident annexes can be implemented concurrently or independently. Examples of incident annexes with applicability to a catastrophic, multistate event are:

■ *Catastrophic Incident Annex*: Establishes the context and overarching strategy for implementing and coordinating an accelerated, proactive, national response to a catastrophic incident with little or no advanced warning, where the need for federal assistance is obvious and immediate. This annex may be activated immediately after the earthquake to push preidentified assets/resources for mass care, public health and medical support, and victim transportation to areas expected to be severely impacted. DHS is the coordinating agency for this annex.

■ *Mass Evacuation Incident Annex*: This annex is intended to be used to augment state, tribal, and local governmental evacuation plans and operations. Impacted state authorities decide on the destinations for evacuees and regulate the flow of transportation assets accordingly. Federal agencies in support of state and local governments ensure that the receiving states agree to accept evacuees in advance of their arrival. Federal contracts include provisions for surface and air evacuation in the form of ambulances, buses, trains, and planes to rapidly move large numbers of persons from the affected area to safe zones. Included in this annex is the requirement that transportation providers must permit passengers with disabilities to be accompanied by their service animals. There are specific considerations to address the needs of children separated from their parents and accommodation for persons with special needs for communication, mobility, medical care, and the maintenance of independence. This annex was modified after Hurricane Katrina to also address the requirements for transportation, sheltering, and care of pets. DHS is the coordinating agency for this annex.

■ *Support Annexes*: Describe the Framework through which common functional processes and administrative requirements necessary to ensure efficient and effective incident management are executed. The actions described in the support annexes are overarching and applicable to nearly every type of incident. Examples of key support annexes that would engage in support of a catastrophic response are:

■ *Critical Infrastructure and Key Resources (CIKR) Annex*: Describes activities taken to protect and restore the 16 critical infrastructure sectors whose assets, systems, networks, whether physical or virtual, are considered so vital to the United States that their incapacitation or destruction would have a debilitating effect on security, national economic security, national public health or safety both within the impacted area and outside the impacted areas. Some examples of critical infrastructure are food and agriculture, energy, water, and transportation. Key resources include governmental facilities, dams, commercial facilities, and nuclear power plants. DHS is responsible for leading, integrating, and coordinating the overall national CIKR effort.

■ *Private Sector Coordination Annex*: Addresses specific federal actions that are required to effectively and efficiently integrate incident management operations with the private sector. This includes, but is not limited to, determining the impact of an incident on a sector and forecasting cascading effects of interdependencies, assisting federal decision makers in determining appropriate recovery measures, and establishing procedures for communications between public and private sectors. DHS is the coordinating agency for this annex.

■ *Worker Safety Annex*: Identifies and assesses worker health and safety hazards present at the incident site and in the environment. The Department of Labor (DOL) and Occupational Safety and Health Administration (OSHA) coordinate the activities of the federal agencies that provide the core architecture for employee safety and health technical support during an all-hazards event or when otherwise directed.

In November 2016, the ASPR released *2017–2022 Health Care Preparedness and Response Capabilities* that details the objectives for the nation's healthcare delivery system, to include healthcare coalitions and healthcare organizations, in regard to preparing, responding, and recovering from emergencies and disasters. The four capabilities are "foundation for health care and medical readiness, health care and medical response coordination, continuity of health care service delivery and medical surge" (HHS, 2016).

ROLES AND RESPONSIBILITIES

Although many agencies and nongovernmental organizations will have responsibilities for assisting in the public health and medical response to a catastrophic multistate earthquake, the following entities described in Table 2.2 have primary roles in disasters.

ESF-8: Public Health and Medical Services

The HHS is the primary agency for ESF-8—public health and medical services, which includes response to a potential or actual public health or medical incident or a developing potential health and medical emergency. In addition to the actual response, these services also include meeting the mental and behavioral health needs and substance abuse considerations of incident victims and response workers. Most important to nurses is ESF-8, or public health and medical services, which provides coordinated federal assistance to communities following a major disaster or emergency or during a developing potential medical situation. HHS is the primary agency for ESF-8. The purpose of ESF-8 is to "supplement state, tribal, and local resources in response to a public health and medical disaster, potential or actual incidents requiring a coordinated federal response, and/or during a developing potential health and medical emergency" (DHS, 2008a). The functional areas addressed by ESF-8 include:

TABLE 2.2 Departmental Roles and Responsibilities

Department	Role/Responsibility
1. Department of Homeland Security	• Overall responsibility for domestic incident management. • Coordinates nonmedical federal response actions. • Coordinates with other federal agencies to develop a public communications plan through ESF-15—external affairs to the NRF. Establishes the Joint Information Center. • Provides logistics support. • Establishes shelters, feeding operations, and distribution centers. • Identifies transportation needs and arranges for use in providing evacuation of victims and urgent airlift and other transportation support of response personnel and resources into the impacted area through ESF-1. • Develops plans and facilitates coordinated incident response planning with the private sector at the strategic, operational, and tactical levels.
2. Department of Health and Human Services (HHS)	• Coordinates medical federal response actions. • Has primary responsibility for public health and medical emergency planning, preparations, and response to an earthquake. • Activates the NDMS, the USPHS responders, and Medical Reserve Corps. • Convenes meeting of ESF8 organizations and provides ESF8 representatives to appropriate multiagency coordinating structures and teams. • Coordinates requests for medical transportation. • Deploys surge medical personnel and teams as needed. • Coordinates assembly and delivery of medical equipment and supplies, including the Strategic National Stockpile.
3. Department of Defense (DOD)	• Provides defense support of civil authorities to all ESFs and support and incident annexes when requested and approved by the Secretary of Defense. Examples of DOD support include, but are not limited to, the following: • Provides support for the evacuation of seriously ill or injured patients to locations where hospital care or outpatient services are available. • Provides available logistical support to health/medical response operations. • Provides available military medical personnel to assist HHS in the protection of public health.
4. Other Agencies and Departments	• Support public health emergencies according to their outlined roles and responsibilities in ESF, support, and incident annexes.

ESF, Emergency Support Function; NDMS, National Disaster Medical System; NRF, National Response Framework; USPHS, United States Public Health Service.

- *Assessment of public health/medical needs*: Includes the needs of at-risk population groups and the healthcare system/facility infrastructure.
- *Enhanced health surveillance*: Monitors the health of the general and medical needs population.
- *Medical care personnel*: Includes medical response capabilities that are internal to HHS (the NDMS, the USPHS, and federal Civil Service Employees) as well as from ESF-8-supporting organizations such as the Department of Defense (DOD), the Department of Veterans Affairs (VA), and civilian volunteers such as the MRC.
- *Health/medical/veterinary equipment and supplies*: Includes equipment and supplies contained within the Strategic National Stockpile (SNS) and may include requested assets from the National Veterinary Stockpile managed by the USDA Animal and Plant Health Inspection Service.
- *Patient evacuation*: Transporting seriously ill or injured patients and medical needs populations from casualty-collecting points in the impacted areas to designated reception facilities.
- *Patient care*: Includes prehospital triage and treatment, inpatient hospital care, outpatient services, pharmacy services, and dental care to victims who are seriously ill, injured, or suffer from chronic illnesses or who need evacuation assistance.
- *Drugs, biologics and medical devices*: Monitoring and ensuring the safety and availability of drugs, biologics and medical devices.
- *Blood, organs, and blood tissues*: Monitoring and ensuring the safety, availability, and logistical requirements of blood, organs, and tissues.
- *Food safety and security*: Information on safety, security and defense of federally regulated foods.
- *Agriculture safety and security*: Maintaining the safety and security of agricultural products (meats, grains, milk, etc.) and ensuring their availability
- *Worker health/safety*: Expert advice and resources to support worker safety and health.
- *Technical support by providing:*
  - All-hazard public health and medical consultation, technical assistance, and support.
  - Behavioral health care through resources and information to support mental and behavioral healthcare.
  - Public health and medical information through resources for federal public health and medical messaging with jurisdictional officials.

- Vector control through resources for assessing, investigating and mitigating vector-borne threats.
- Assistance assessing potable water, wastewater, solid waste disposal and other environmental health issues.
- Mass Fatality Care—Information to assist in the tracking, documenting and respectful management of human remains.
- Veterinary medical support by providing resources to assist with the treatment of sick or injured animals.
- Support to ESF-6 by providing expertise and guidance on the public health issues of the medical needs population.

A basic concept of the NRF is that responding federal resources will operate in coordination with state, local, and tribal entities.

FEDERAL DEFINITION OF A DISASTER CONDITION

For the purposes of the NRF, the federal government defines a disaster condition as follows:

1. A significant natural disaster or man-made event that overwhelms the affected state that would necessitate both federal public health and medical care assistance. Hospitals, nursing homes, ambulatory care centers, pharmacies, and other facilities for medical/healthcare and special needs populations may be severely structurally damaged or destroyed. Facilities that survive with little or no structural damage may be rendered unusable or only partially usable because of a lack of utilities (power, water, sewer) or because staff are unable to report for duty as a result of personal injuries or damage/disruption of communications and transportation systems. Medical and healthcare facilities that remain in operation and have the necessary utilities and staff will probably be overwhelmed by the "walking wounded" and seriously injured victims who are transported there in the immediate aftermath of the occurrence. In the face of massive increases in demand and the damage sustained, medical supplies (including pharmaceuticals) and equipment will probably be in short supply. (Most healthcare facilities usually maintain only a small inventory stock to meet their short-term, normal patient load needs.) Disruptions in local communications and transportation systems could also prevent timely resupply.
2. Uninjured persons who require daily or frequent medications such as insulin, antihypertensive drugs, digitalis, and dialysis may have difficulty in obtaining these medications and treatments because of damage/destruction of normal supply locations and general shortages within the disaster area.
3. In certain other disasters, there could be a noticeable emphasis on relocation; shelters; vector control; and returning water, wastewater, and solid waste facilities to operation.
4. A major medical and environmental emergency resulting from chemical, biological, or nuclear weapons of mass destruction could produce a large concentration of specialized injuries and problems that could overwhelm the state and local public health and medical care system.

NRF CONSIDERATIONS

The authors of the NRF and its predecessors jointly developed a set of considerations or common assumptions to help frame medical response. These include:

1. Resources within the affected disaster area will be inadequate to clear casualties from the scene or treat them in local hospitals. Additional mobilized federal capabilities will be urgently needed to assist state and local governments to triage and treat casualties in the disaster area and then transport them to the closest appropriate hospital or other healthcare facility. Additionally, medical resupply will be needed throughout the disaster area. In a major disaster, operational necessity may require the further transportation by air of patients to the nearest metropolitan areas with sufficient concentrations of available hospital beds, where patient needs can be matched with the necessary definitive medical care.
2. A terrorist release of weapons of mass destruction; damage to chemical and industrial plants, sewer lines, and water distribution systems; and secondary hazards such as fires will result in toxic environmental and public health hazards to the surviving population and response personnel, including exposure to hazardous chemicals, biological substances, radiological substances, and contaminated water supplies, crops, livestock, and food products.
3. The damage and destruction of a major disaster, which may result in multiple deaths and injuries, will overwhelm the state and local mental health system, producing an urgent need for mental health crisis counseling for disaster victims and response personnel.
4. Assistance in maintaining the continuity of health and medical services will be required.
5. Disruption of sanitation services and facilities, loss of power, and massing of people in shelters may increase the potential for disease and injury.
6. Primary medical treatment facilities may be damaged or inoperable; thus, assessment and emergency restoration to necessary operational levels is a basic requirement to stabilize the medical support system.

FEDERAL MEDICAL RESPONSE RESOURCES

A variety of response resources exist across the federal government. Each provides options where nurses can volunteer and make a difference. The following sections briefly discuss some of the major response resources (see Figure 2.4).

National Disaster Medical System. The foundation of ESF-8 is the multiagency (HHS, DOD, VA, and DHS) NDMS, directed by HHS/ASPR. NDMS supports the management and coordination of medical responses to major emergencies and federally declared disasters by working in collaboration with the states and other public and private entities to provide health and human services during public health emergencies for limited periods of time. NDMS provides federal medical response to augment the nation's medical

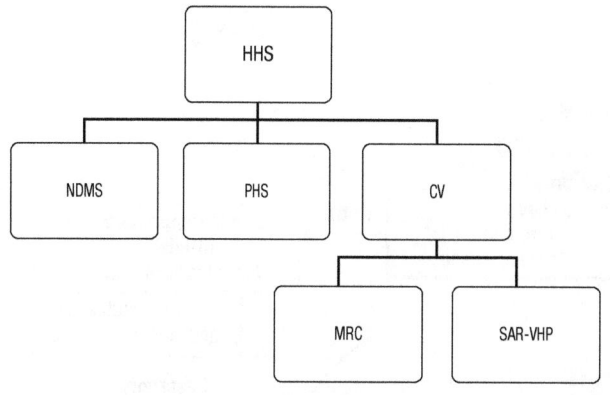

FIGURE 2.4 Federal Medical Response Resources.

CV, Civilian Volunteers; HHS, U.S. Department of Health and Human Services; MRC, Medical Reserve Corps; NDMS, National Disaster Medical System; PHS, Public Health Service; SAR-VHP, System for Advance Registration of Volunteer Health Professionals.

response capability and to support state, local, and tribal authorities through three major missions.

1. *Medical Response:* NDMS provides emergency medical support to a disaster area in the form of personnel, teams and individuals, supplies and equipment.
2. *Patient Movement:* NDMS coordinates arrangements for patients who cannot be cared for locally to be evacuated to predesignated definitive care locations throughout the United States.
3. *Definitive Medical Care:* NDMS has created a network of DOD/VA medical treatment facilities and participating civilian NDMS member hospitals spanning the major metropolitan areas of the country. All hospitals in this network have agreed to accept patients in the event of a national emergency.

The NDMS is designed to care for victims of any incident that exceeds the capability of the state, regional, or federal healthcare system. Some of the events that may require its activation are earthquakes, floods, hurricanes, industrial disasters, a refugee influx, and military casualties from overseas. Team members are intermittent federal employees. Activation of NDMS may be accomplished by a presidential declaration. This authority is granted by the Robert T. Stafford Disaster Relief and Emergency Assistance Act, also referred to as the Stafford Act. When a presidential declaration has not occurred, HHS, under the Public Health Service Act as amended, may request activation of the NDMS (HHS, 2010a). In addition, through the mechanism provided by Emergency Management Assistance Compacts, states may request health and medical teams from another state when either their own resources are overwhelmed or they do not have the particular type of resource available in a nearby jurisdiction (DHS, 2008b; see Figure 2.5).

Disaster Medical Assistance Team (DMAT): A DMAT is a group of professional and paraprofessional medical personnel designed to provide medical care during a disaster or other event. Each team responds rapidly to supplement local resources until other resources can be mobilized or the emergency ends. The team composition includes physicians, nurses, nurse practitioners, physician's assistants,

pharmacists, pharmacy technicians, nurse's aides, mental health specialists, dentists, environmental and laboratory specialists, and emergency medical technicians. In addition, each team has a cadre of logistical and administrative staff as well as technicians such as engineers and radio operators.

Team size and composition will vary according to the mission assignment. Strike teams, as developed during the Atlanta 1996 Summer Olympic Games, are five- to six-member squads, usually made up of medical personnel who can move quickly into an affected area to provide limited medical treatment and assessment. A full team deployment is expected to be 35 to 50 personnel: medical, technical, and support. The full team is usually the configuration that is used for a large event such as a hurricane or an earthquake.

There are highly specialized DMATs that deal with specific medical conditions such as crush injury, burn, and mental health emergencies that can supplement standard DMATs. These other NDMS teams include Disaster Mortuary Operational Response Teams (DMORTs), which provide victim identification and processing and family assistance; National Veterinary Response Teams (NVRT), which provide veterinary services; and an International Medical Surgical Response Team (IMSURT), which can provide surgical and critical care during a disaster or public health emergency overseas.

Teams deploy with enough personnel, supplies, and equipment to be self-sufficient for 72 hours at a fixed or temporary medical care site. In mass casualty incidents (MCIs), their responsibilities may include triaging patients, providing high-quality medical care despite the adverse and austere environment often found at a disaster site, and preparing patients for evacuation. In other types of situations, DMATs may provide primary medical care and may serve to augment overloaded local healthcare staffs. Under the rare circumstance that disaster victims are evacuated to a different locale to receive definitive medical care, DMATs may be activated to support patient reception and disposition of patients to hospitals. DMAT members are required to maintain appropriate certifications and licensure within their disciplines. DMATs are principally a community resource available to support local, regional, and state requirements. When members are activated as federal employees for up to 2 weeks, they are paid and licensure and certification are recognized by all states. In addition, DMAT members have the protection of the Federal Tort Claims Act in which the federal government becomes the defendant in the event of a malpractice claim.

Training plays one of the most important roles in DMAT development. The primary sources of training are federally funded exercises. NDMS, at its annual conferences, offers workshops and training courses for members. More information about the NDMS and its training and education programs can be accessed at www.phe.gov/Preparedness/responders/ndms/teams/Pages/default.aspx. Currently, there are approximately 6,000 professionals registered in the NDMS (HHS, 2017b).

Commissioned Corps of the United States Public Health Service Led by the U.S. Surgeon General, the mission of the U.S. Public Health Service Commissioned Corps is "protecting, promoting, and advancing the health and safety of the Nation." The Commissioned Corps achieves its mission through rapid and effective response to public

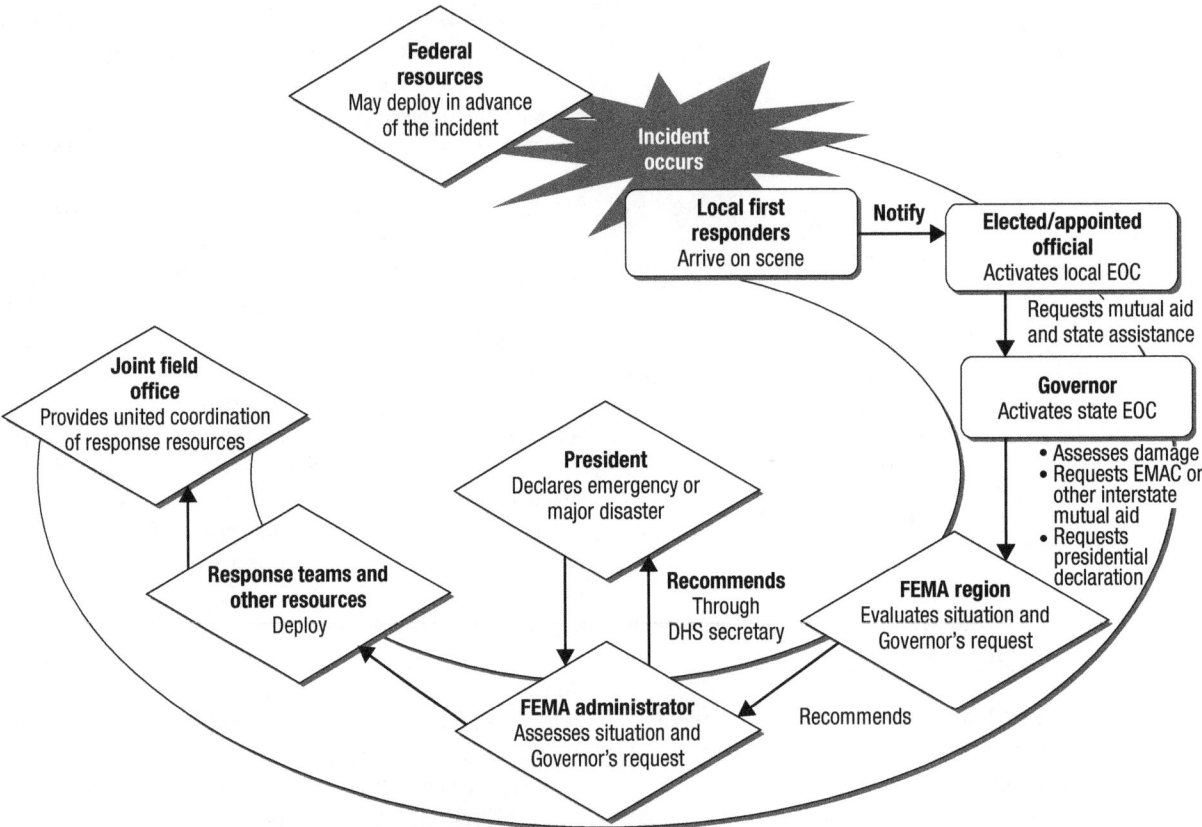

FIGURE 2.5 Federal Support Stafford Act incidents.

DHS, Department of Homeland Security; EOC, Emergency Operations Center; EMAC, Emergency Management Assistance Compact; FEMA, federal emergency management agency.

Source: U.S. Department of Homeland Security. (2008b). *Overview: ESF and support annexes coordinating federal assistance in support of the National Response Framework.* Retrieved from http://www.fema.gov/pdf/emergency/nrf/nrf-overview.pdf

health needs, leadership and excellence in public health practices, and the advancement of public health science. As one of the seven uniformed services of the United States, the corps is a specialized career system designed to attract, develop, and retain health professionals who may be assigned to federal, state, or local agencies or international organizations (HHS, n.d.-c). To accomplish this mission, the agencies and programs are designed to:

- Provide healthcare and related services to medically underserved and disadvantaged populations—such as federally incarcerated prisoners held by the Bureau of Prisons; individuals served by the Indian Health Service such as American Indians or Alaska Natives; and other vulnerable populations with public health needs
- Prevent and control disease, identify health hazards in the environment and help correct them, and promote healthy lifestyles for the nation's citizens
- Improve the nation's mental health
- Ensure that drugs and medical devices are safe and effective, food is safe and wholesome, cosmetics are harmless, and that electronic products do not expose users to dangerous amounts of radiation
- Conduct and support biomedical, behavioral, and health services research and communicate research results to health professionals and the public

- Provide leadership to other nations by leveraging expertise in global health diplomacy to contribute to a safer, healthier world

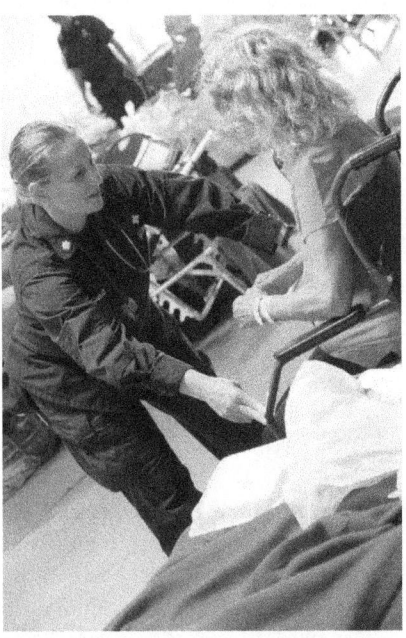

LCDR Sarah Trinidad. Hurricane Irma. Courtesy of Liz Garza.

The Federal Response to Hurricane Katrina: Lessons Learned recommended that, "HHS should organize, train, equip, and roster medical and public health professionals in preconfigured and deployable teams" (HHS, n.d.-a, para 1). This resulted in the implementation of the United States Public Health Service (USPHS) Commissioned Corps tiered response system. The USPHS has seven types of teams (White House, 2006, p. 5):

1. Rapid Deployment Force (RDF): Five RDFs serve on a rotating call basis, with the on-call team capable of deploying within 12 hours of notification. RDF teams have a built-in command structure and can provide mass care at shelters (including FMSs), and staff Points of Distribution and Casualty Collection Points. The RDF can also conduct community outreach and assessments, among other functions.
2. Regional Incident Support Team (RIST): There is one RIST in each HHS region and in the national capital region. They conduct rapid needs assessments, support and direct incoming response assets, serve as a liaison with state, tribal, and local official and on-site incident management.
3. The National Incident Support Teams (NISTs) provide resources and assistance to state, tribal, and local health authorities throughout the United States, usually as the Commissioned Corps component of an Incident Response Coordination Team. The NIST consists of 72 USPHS-trained Commissioned Corps officer responders.
4. Capital Area Provider Teams: These teams provide medical and public health resources and assistance in the National Capital Region during special events and other supported activities.
5. Applied Public Health Team (APHT): The APHT is composed of experts in applied public health and can function as a "public health department in a box." An APHT can deploy within 36 hours of notification and provide assistance in public health assessments, environmental health, infrastructure integrity, food safety, vector control, epidemiology, and surveillance.
6. Mental Health Team (MHT): The MHT consists of mental and behavioral health experts who assess stress and suicide risks within the affected population, manage responder stress, and provide therapy, counseling, and crisis intervention. The MHT can deploy within 36 hours of notification.
7. Service Access Teams (SATs): These teams provide resources and assistance to local health authorities throughout the United States. Each SAT comprises 10 USPHS-trained Commissioned Corps officer responders, enabling scalability and ability to provide only those resources needed.

Department of Defense/Uniformed Services University of the Health Sciences (USUHS). The National Center for Disaster Medicine and Public Health was established in 2008 by HSPD-21 (Public Health and Medical Preparedness) as an "academic center of excellence in disaster medicine and public health" (White House, 2007, p. 38). The National Center functions under a charter from the DOD and the USUHS. It was founded as a collaboration by five Federal Agencies: HHS, DOD, VA, DHS, and the Department of Transportation. Housed within USUHS, the National Center's mission is to lead and coordinate Federal efforts to develop, and coordinate national efforts to develop and propagate core curricula, education, training, and research in all-hazards disaster health. The National Center's vision is to strengthen the national response to natural and man-made disasters or other catastrophic public health events by standardizing core curricula and competencies in disaster medicine and public health education. As a first step, it completed a detailed report on the U.S. Disaster Health Professions Workforce (National Center for Disaster Medicine and Public Health [NCDMPH], 2011).

Modifications were published to the original Framework of core competencies, see Figure 2.6, for disaster medicine and public health to delineate the expectations beginning with core level competencies and moving through professional level, organizational level, and lastly deployment level competencies (Walsh, Altman, King, & Strauss-Riggs, 2014). NCDMPH's 2017–18, strategic plan, not released as of publication, focuses on readiness, education, research, and collaboration and leadership (NCDMPH, n.d.).

Civilian Volunteers. HHS sponsors two programs supporting volunteer efforts in local communities and states: the MRC and the Emergency System for Advance Registration of Volunteer Health Professionals (ESAR-VHP).

The MRC. The MRC is a specialized component of Citizen Corps. It was launched in July 2002 and subsequently authorized by Congress in the 2006 Pandemic and All-Hazards Preparedness Act. As a national network of local groups of volunteers committed to improving the health, safety, and resiliency of their communities, MRC volunteers include medical and public health professionals such as physicians, nurses, pharmacists, dentists, veterinarians, and epidemiologists. Other community members, such as interpreters, chaplains, office workers, and legal advisors, can fill other vital support functions in the units. MRC volunteers supplement existing local emergency and public health resources. MRC units identify, screen, train, and organize the volunteers, and utilize them to support routine public health activities and augment preparedness and response efforts. As of late 2017, there are over 980 MRC units in all 50 states, Washington, DC, Guam, Palau, American Samoa, Puerto Rico, and the U.S. Virgin Islands, with more than 193,000 volunteers. Current units cover 91% of the U.S. population (MRC, 2017). MRC units are organized locally to meet community needs.

The MRC response to the 2005 hurricanes highlights the broad range of services that MRCs can provide. An estimated 6,000 MRC volunteers supported the response and recovery efforts in their local communities in the hardest hit areas. As the storms forced hundreds of thousands of Americans to flee the affected areas, MRC volunteers were ready and able to help when needed and were there to assist as evacuees were welcomed into their communities. These volunteers spent countless

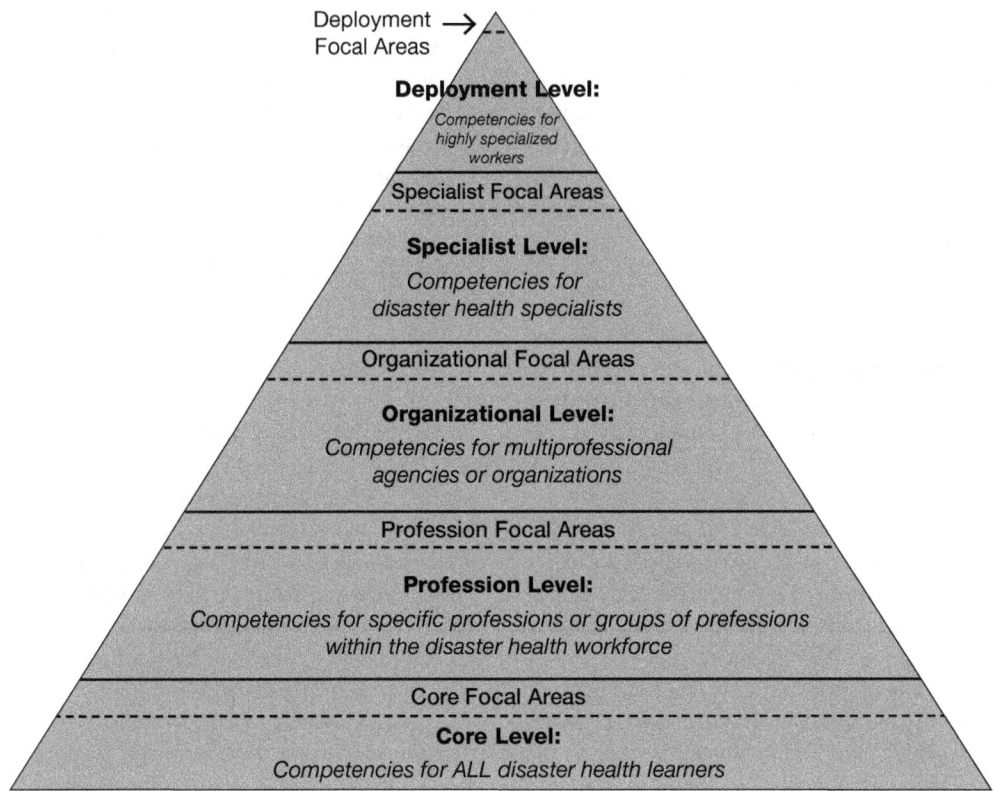

Deployment → Focal Areas

Deployment Level:
Competencies for highly specialized workers

Specialist Focal Areas

Specialist Level:
Competencies for disaster health specialists

Organizational Focal Areas

Organizational Level:
Competencies for multiprofessional agencies or organizations

Profession Focal Areas

Profession Level:
Competencies for specific professions or groups of prefessions within the disaster health workforce

Core Focal Areas

Core Level:
Competencies for ALL disaster health learners

FIGURE 2.6 Disaster Health Competencies.

Source: Walsh, L., Altman, B. A., King, R. V., & Strauss-Riggs, K. (2014). Enhancing the translation of disaster health competencies into practice. *Disaster Medicine & Public Health Preparedness, 8*(1), 70–78. doi:10.1017/dmp.2014.7

hours helping people whose lives had been upended by these disastrous events by:

- Establishing medical needs shelters to serve medically fragile and other displaced people
- Staffing and providing medical support in evacuee shelters and clinics
- Filling in locally at hospitals, clinics, and health departments for others who were deployed to the disaster-affected regions
- Immunizing responders prior to their deployment to the disaster-affected regions
- Staffing a variety of response hotlines created after the hurricanes hit
- Teaching emergency preparedness to community members
- Recruiting more public health and medical professionals who could be credentialed, trained, and prepared for future disasters that may affect their hometowns or other communities

The ESAR-VHP. The ESAR-VHP is a federal program created to support states and territories by establishing standardized volunteer registration programs for disasters and public health and medical emergencies (HHS, n.d.-b). Each state administers its own program, verifying health professionals' identification and credentials so that they can respond more quickly when disaster strikes. By registering through ESAR-VHP, volunteers' identities, licenses, credentials, accreditations, and hospital privileges are all verified in advance, saving valuable time in emergency situations. The system is currently implemented in 47 states and is managed at the state level, where the responsibility for maintaining the database and verifying volunteers' professional credentials lies. Use of ESAR-VHP is variable, which affects the ability to determine the precise numbers of volunteers available for surge and deployments. Because many volunteers are enrolled in more than one volunteer system, it is difficult to determine what assets are available for surge capacity at any given time.

Federal Medical Stations

First used in the aftermath of Hurricanes Katrina and Rita, FMSs are 50- to 250-bed scalable, capacity shelters to care for displaced persons with special health needs that cannot be managed in a general shelter (Walsh, Orsega, & Banks, 2006). Each FMS contains a 3-day supply of medical and pharmaceutical resources to sustain 250 stable primary care–based patients who require bedding services supplied in part from the SNS (https://www.cdc .gov/phpr/stockpile/fedmedstation.htm). FMSs are constructed within structurally intact buildings and can adapt to any 40,000 sq ft area, including an aggregate of multiple buildings. About 48 hours is required from the time of request to the time of delivery within the continental United States. Requests for a FMS are coordinated through the HHS Regional Emergency Coordinators in collaboration with local, state, and tribal agencies.

Fixed facilities, such as the National Institutes of Health, supplement existing FMS capabilities by providing a telemedicine consultation and triage facility to serve as a medical specialty service, allowing providers on the ground to tap into the expertise of National Institutes of Health (NIH) experts in collaboration with 125 medical centers throughout the country (HHS, 2011b). A FMS Strike Team can be deployed to assist with identifying a suitable facility, receiving and staging equipment, and training for the volunteers who will assemble the equipment.

MEDICAL RESPONSE ACTIONS

Federal health and medical assistance is generally categorized into the major functions of prevention, medical services, mental health services, and environmental health. Each of the 15 specific functional areas is contained in one of these categories. When the leader of the national ESF-8 (the ASPR) is notified of the occurrence of a potential major disaster or emergency, the assistant secretary will request HHS and supporting agencies to initiate action immediately to identify and report the potential need for federal health and medical support to the affected disaster area in the following functional areas.

Assessment of Health/Medical Needs

Lead HHS Agency: Office of the ASPR
Action: Mobilize and deploy an assessment team to the disaster area to assist in determining specific health/medical needs and priorities. This function includes the assessment of the health system/facility infrastructure.

Health Surveillance

Lead HHS Agency: Centers for Disease Control and Prevention (CDC)
Action: Assist in establishing surveillance systems to monitor the general population and special high-risk population segments; carry out field studies and investigations; monitor injury and disease patterns and potential disease outbreaks; and provide technical assistance and consultations on disease and injury prevention and precautions.

Medical Care Personnel

Lead HHS Agency: ASPR
Action: Provide federal medical response assets and individual public health and medical personnel to assist in providing care for ill or injured victims at the location of a disaster or emergency. DMATs and FMSs can provide triage, medical, or surgical stabilization, and continued monitoring and care of patients until they can be evacuated to locations where they will receive definitive medical care. Specialty DMATs can also be deployed to address mass burn injuries, pediatric care requirements, chemical injury, or contamination. In addition to DMATs, active duty, reserve, and National Guard units for casualty clearing/staging and other missions will be deployed as needed. Individual clinical health and medical care specialists may be provided to assist state and local personnel. The VA is one of the primary sources of these specialists.

Health/Medical Equipment and Supplies

Lead HHS Agency: ASPR in coordination with DHS/National Response Coordination Center
Action: Provide health and medical equipment and supplies, including pharmaceuticals, biological products, and blood and blood products, in support of DMAT operations and for restocking health and medical care facilities in an area affected by a major disaster or emergency.

Patient Evacuation

Lead HHS Agency: ASPR in coordination with DHS/FEMA
Action: Provide for movement of seriously ill or injured patients from the area affected by a major disaster or emergency to locations where definitive medical care is available. NDMS patient movement will be accomplished primarily by using fixed-wing aeromedical evacuation resources of DOD; however, other transportation modes may be used as circumstances warrant.

In-Hospital Care

Lead HHS Agency: ASPR
Action: Provide definitive medical care to victims who become seriously ill or injured as a result of a major disaster or emergency. For this purpose, NDMS has established and maintains a nationwide network of voluntarily pre-committed, nonfederal, acute care hospital beds in the largest U.S. metropolitan areas.

Food/Drug/Medical Device Safety

Lead HHS Agency: Food and Drug Administration
Action: Ensure the safety and efficacy of regulated foods, drugs, biological products, and medical devices following a major disaster or emergency. Arrange for seizure, removal, and destruction of contaminated or unsafe products.

Worker Safety

Lead Agency: Coordinated by the DOL/OSHA
Action: Assists OSHA in monitoring health and well-being of emergency workers; performs field investigations and studies addressing worker health and safety issues; and provides technical assistance and consultation on worker health and safety measures and precautions.

Radiological/Chemical/Biological Hazards Consultation

Lead HHS Agency: CDC
Action: Assist in assessing health and medical effects of radiological, chemical, and biological exposures on the general population and on high-risk population groups; conduct field investigations, including collection and analysis of relevant samples; advise on protective actions related to direct human and animal exposure, and on indirect exposure through radiologically, chemically, or biologically contaminated food, drugs, water supply, and other media; and provide technical assistance and consultation on medical treatment and decontamination of radiologically, chemically, or biologically injured/contaminated victims.

Mental Healthcare

Lead HHS Agency: Substance Abuse and Mental Health Services Administration

Action: Assist in assessing mental health needs; provide disaster mental health training materials for disaster workers; and provide liaison with assessment, training, and program development activities undertaken by federal, state, and local mental health officials.

Public Health Information

Lead HHS Agency: CDC

Action: Assist by providing public health and disease and injury prevention information that can be transmitted to members of the general public who are located in or near areas affected by a major disaster or emergency.

Vector Control

Lead HHS Agency: CDC

Action: Assist in assessing the threat of vector-borne diseases following a major disaster or emergency; conduct field investigations, including the collection and laboratory analysis of relevant samples; provide vector control equipment and supplies; provide technical assistance and consultation on protective actions regarding vector-borne diseases; and provide technical assistance and consultation on medical treatment of victims of vector-borne diseases.

Potable Water/Waste Water and Solid Waste Disposal

Lead HHS Agency: Indian Health Service

Action: Assist in assessing potable water and waste water/ solid waste disposal issues; conduct field investigations, including collection and laboratory analysis of relevant samples; provide water purification and waste water/solid waste disposal equipment and supplies; and provide technical assistance and consultation on potable water and waste water/solid waste disposal issues.

Victim Identification/Mortuary Services

Lead HHS Agency: ASPR in coordination with DHS/FEMA

Action: Assist in providing victim identification and mortuary services, including DMORTs; temporary morgue facilities; victim identification by fingerprint, forensic dental, and/or forensic pathology/anthropology methods; and processing, preparation, and disposition of remains. Another important function of DMORTs is the provision of family support centers.

Veterinary Services

Lead HHS Agency: ASPR in coordination with DHS/FEMA/ NDMS

Action: Assist in delivering healthcare to injured or abandoned animals and performing veterinary preventive medicine activities following a major disaster or emergency, including conducting field investigations and providing technical assistance and consultation as required.

A BLUEPRINT FOR THE FUTURE FOR DISASTER NURSING

Nursing as a profession has a long history of being creative and visionary in its continuous efforts to meet the needs of patients and their families, regardless of the circumstances. Nursing leadership in tumultuous times, such as throughout the disaster continuum, a public health emergency or an MCI, will also require significant amounts of the same creativity, vision, and advocacy. In 2010, the Institute of Medicine (IOM) (now renamed the National Academy of Medicine) and the Robert Wood Johnson Foundation collaborated to publish a report: *The Future of Nursing: Leading Change, Advancing Health* (IOM, 2011), proposing recommendations designed to advance health in the U.S. population by transforming the role of the nurse in the delivery of care. In January 2016, Veenema et al. (2016) published a call to action for nurses as leaders in disaster preparedness based on the results of planning meetings, semi-structured interviews, and a workshop with nursing experts to "develop a vision for the future of disaster nursing, identify barriers and facilitators to achieving the vision, and develop recommendations for nursing practice, education, policy, and research" (p. 1). The report detailed barriers to implementing the described vision according to personal, organizational, and environmental factors, and detailed recommendations for nursing practice, education, policy, and research. To address the recommendations, advisory, executive, and work committees were formed. Substantial work is underway, including presentations at professional meetings, disaster research projects, social media, and the establishment of the Society for the Advancement of Disaster Nursing (Couig et al., 2017).

LEADERSHIP

The IOM Report (IOM, 2009) called out to prepare and enable nurses to lead change to advance health recommending that *"nurses should be full partners, with physicians and other health professionals, in redesigning healthcare in the United States."* How can we ensure that nurses will ascend to leadership positions in disaster management? Our uniformed service (military and U.S. Public Health Service) nurse colleagues are exemplars for strong leadership in disaster management and public health emergency preparedness. A leader is anyone who uses interpersonal skills to influence others to accomplish a specific goal (Sullivan & Decker, 2001). Leadership (and partnership) is important in forging links and creating connections among organizations and their members to promote high levels of performance, quality outcomes, and the accomplishment of goals. Nurses in leadership positions in *all types of healthcare and public health organizations* can assist with the design of disaster response plans and the development of future change in these organizations. In this capacity, nurses can serve as advocates for communities, and in particular for vulnerable populations such as infants and children, the elderly, the disabled, the mentally ill, and for the safety of other nurses in disaster response. Previous literature describes models for disaster nursing leadership. These models continue to be updated and expanded to meet the challenges of the present and future disasters. Nurses also need to move into leadership positions in politics, public policy, civic administration, educational administration, and emergency management systems. Nurses will have the competencies to be in these positions *if they prepare themselves for them*. Clearly, nursing knowledge of the healthcare process, diagnosis, planning, treatment, and evaluation is an asset. Additional preparation in all phases of disaster planning and management, health promotion, risk reduction, disease prevention and illness and disease management, information and healthcare technologies, and human resource management will prepare nurses for positions of leadership. Effective leadership in disaster management requires personal integrity, strength, flexibility, creativity, and use of collaborative approaches.

Nurse leaders in hospitals, public health, and clinics are in an ideal position to champion disaster preparedness and educational initiatives to improve the readiness of staff. Nurse leaders can work with not only the hospital emergency management team and the state hospital association, but also with a state or local Office of Emergency Preparedness to ensure that the role of nursing is included in the plans. Too often in a major disaster there is a call for more nurses and yet how to recruit, screen, and mobilize nurses is frequently not included in the plans. Nurse executives can manage schedules and implement policies that provide staff with time and continuing education credit for disaster education. Additionally, nurse leaders can work with hospital administration to ensure hands-on exercises that build competence. Finally, they can form academic-practice partnerships to ensure that the skills begin during the educational process and are furthered during practice (Langan, Lavin, Wolgast, & Veenema, 2017).

The American Organization of Nurse Executives (AONE) published guiding principles related to crisis management. The principles included:

- Nurse leaders are trained in media relations and understand the tenets of good communication.
- Leaders are skilled critical thinkers, collaborative, and able to manage ambiguity.
- Nurse leaders project calm, confidence, and authority in all situations. They are also empathetic to how people react to loss, challenges, and uncertainty.
- Nurse leaders are prepared to review and practice the organization's crisis readiness plan with nursing staff.
- The chief nursing officer is a member of the senior leadership team, whose role is clearly defined and sought by colleagues, particularly during a crisis (AONE, 2016).

These principles address the crisis communication; leadership behaviors; leadership skills ("calm, confidence and authority in all situations"), readiness, and the role of the nurse leader (Edmonson, Sumagaysay, Cueman, & Chappell, 2016).

Englebright, a chief nurse executive, stated,

As a large system, all HCA facilities benefit from the after action reports from each disaster response. For instance, in our latest hospital evacuation, we learned that our quarterly drills did not have enough emphasis on command and communication protocols. We plan to use this information to design future drills for all hospitals, to evaluate different communication technology options, and to develop specific training modules. My primary concern is that disaster preparedness is often skimmed over in the business

of the clinical work environment. Training can be concentrated on specific roles such as ED or perinatal staff, leaving much of the nursing workforce unprepared. (Langan et al., 2017, p. 124)

ALL DISASTERS ARE LOCAL

Most disasters begin and end locally and it is for this reason that hospitals, public health departments, businesses, schools, local governments, tribes and communities, need to be prepared to respond. Using FEMA's five national planning Frameworks describing how the whole community should work together in each of the mission areas—prevention, protection, mitigation, response, and recovery (DHS, 2016)—nurses can engage in the entire process of comprehensive emergency management planning or with any of the separate areas. Beginning with personal preparedness, nurses can ensure they are personally prepared with family plans and help support nursing colleagues to become personally prepared. The Ready.Gov website (https://www.ready.gov/) has resources to help people get prepared. Workplace preparedness consists of knowing one's role in a disaster or public health emergency and being educated and trained to respond in that role. Education and training should be based on the results of a hazards vulnerability analysis to determine the highest risks to the workplace and the community. Workplace exercises and drills help determine areas that need to be strengthened. After action reports provide documentation of the exercises, areas for improvement and help ensure program improvement. Community drills are important because they test all the different organizations with roles in the disaster response. The *Boston Marathon Bombing After Action Report* is one example of a comprehensive report of best practices and areas for improvement after a major event (Massachusetts Emergency Management Agency, 2014). In January of each year, prior to the marathon, the appropriate agencies meet to begin planning for the marathon. The comprehensive planning efforts contributed to the coordinated effort and the majority of the injured being transported to hospitals where they received care and survived their injuries.

The priorities of a response are to save lives, stabilize the incident, provide for basic human needs, and protect property and the environment to enable recovery efforts to be fully integrated. The NRF Response mission area includes 15 core capabilities, "planning; public information and warning; operational coordination; critical transportation; environmental response/health and safety; fatality management services; fire management and suppression; infrastructure systems; logistics and supply chain management; mass care services; mass search and rescue operations; on-scene security, protection, and law enforcement; operational communications; public health, healthcare, and emergency medical services; and situational assessment" (DHS, 2016, p. i). Response to incidents should be managed at the lowest level possible. Training, education, and exercises should be based on the core capabilities listed in Table 2.3 and the potential threats as determined by a hazards vulnerability analysis.

To help address the issue of multiple triage methods and lack of integration during a large-scale disaster (Lerner et al., 2008), the Federal Interagency Committee on Emergency Medical Services' (FICEMS) Preparedness Committee developed a concept paper, using available scientific evidence, on the triage

TABLE 2.3 Readiness Competencies

Readiness	Competencies
1. Preparedness and Training-Technical Readiness	Demonstrate personal and family preparedness for disasters and public health emergencies
	Demonstrate knowledge of one's expected role(s) in organizational and community response plans activated during a disaster or public health emergency
	Demonstrate knowledge of personal safety measures that can be implemented in a disaster or public health emergency
	Demonstrate knowledge of surge capacity assets, consistent with one's role in organizational, agency, and/or community response plans
	Demonstrate knowledge of principles and practices for the clinical management of all ages and populations affected by disasters and public health emergencies, in accordance with professional scope of practice
	Demonstrate knowledge of public health principles and practices for the management of all ages and populations affected by disasters and public health emergencies
	Demonstrate knowledge of ethical principles to protect the health and safety of all ages, populations, and communities affected by a disaster or public health emergency
	Demonstrate knowledge of legal principles to protect the health and safety of all ages, populations, and communities affected by a disaster or public health emergency
	Demonstrate knowledge of short- and long-term considerations for recovery of all ages, populations, and communities affected by a disaster or public health emergency
2. Leadership/Partnering and Building Coalitions	Demonstrate situational awareness of actual/potential health hazards before, during, and after a disaster or public health emergency
	Communicate effectively with others in a disaster or public health emergency

Source: Lavin, R., Slepski, L., & Veenema, T. G. (2007). Leadership and coordination in disaster health care systems: The federal disaster response network. In T. G. Veenema (Ed.), *Disaster nursing and emergency preparedness for chemical, biological and radiological terrorism and other hazards* (2nd ed., pp. 25–46). New York, NY: Springer.

Model Uniform Core Criteria (MUCC) (FICEMS, 2014). The MUCC consists of four broad categories (general considerations, global sorting, lifesaving interventions, and individual assessment) and 24 specific criteria which were recommended as model minimum elements for all MCI triage systems. Nurses who may respond to a disaster or public health event should be familiar with the uniform criteria and the local triage system.

CRISIS STANDARDS OF CARE FOR USE IN DISASTER SITUATIONS

In September 2009, the IOM recommended that there was a clear and urgent need for a single national crisis standard of care for states. The Institute of Medicine (IOM, 2009) defined crisis standards of care as

> . . . a substantial change in usual health care operations and the level of care it is possible to deliver, which is made necessary by a pervasive (e.g., pandemic influenza) or catastrophic (e.g., earthquake, hurricane) disaster. This change in the level of care delivered is justified by specific circumstances and is formally declared by a state government, in recognition that crisis operations will be in effect for a sustained period. The formal declaration that crisis standards of care are in operation enables specific legal/regulatory powers and protections for healthcare providers in the necessary tasks of allocating and using scarce medical resources and implementing alternate care facility operations.

Building on the initial work on crisis standards of care, the IOM (2012) published *Crisis Standards of Care: A Systems Framework for Catastrophic Disaster Response*. The report reviews principles for developing the Framework, legal issues, interwoven themes (ethics, palliative care, and mental health), and issues for governments, acute care facilities, emergency medical systems, and other healthcare options that may be established in a crisis and the importance of including the public when a state of crisis is declared. The templates can be used to develop crisis standards of care plans. Additionally, the ASPR Technical Resources Assistance Center Information Exchange (TRACIE) has resources in the following categories—Must Reads; Articles; Guidelines and Strategies; Lessons Learned; Pandemic-Specific Planning; Plans; Tools; and Templates; Studies and Reports; Toolkits; Webinars; and Agencies and Organizations (HHS, 2017c).

RESOURCES FOR DISASTER PLANNING

Disaster response is *not* business as usual—planning for and providing care during an incident requires unique knowledge and skills. Even today, despite this recognition, no state nursing licensing authority in the United States requires continuing education content on disasters (Lippincott Nursing Center, 2017). Only Nevada has a one-time requirement for 4 contact hours related to bioterrorism. Because time constraints and financial barriers are the most significant barriers to emergency preparedness training (Scott, Crumpier, Tolley, Jones, & Wahlquist, 2012), nurses often turn to Internet resources and free or self-paced learning.

The information in Tables 2.4, 2.5, 2.6, 2.7, and 2.8 include applications, courses, online resources, pocket cards, and tools that may be helpful. All hazard plans can be tailored to the

TABLE 2.4 Applications

Topic	Sponsoring Organization	Description	Location
Behavioral Health Disaster Response	Substance Abuse and Mental Health Services Administration	Connects behavioral health responders to evidence-based behavioral health resources for use in the field. Users can access pre-loaded resources when Internet connectivity is limited, locate nearby treatment facilities, search for key materials and share information with colleagues and survivors. Smartphone	http://store.samhsa.gov/apps/disaster/?WT.mc_id=EB_20140311_DISASTERAPP
Blast Injury	CDC	Helps healthcare providers and public health professionals treat injuries, prepare for blast events, and save lives. Smartphone and tablet	https://itunes.apple.com/au/app/cdc-blast-injury/id890434999?mt=8&ign-mpt=uo%3D2
Radiation	FEMA RadResponder	RadResponder provides free software tools for logging, transmitting, storing, analyzing, and presenting environmental radiation monitoring data. Smartphone	https://www.radresponder.net/#resources/apps/index
	HHS REMM	Clinical diagnosis and treatment of radiation injuries. Smartphone	http://disasterinfo.nlm.nih.gov/dimrc/disasterapps.html
Reunification	NLM ReUnite	Ability to upload missing and found person information for family reunification during and after disasters Smartphone	http://disasterinfo.nlm.nih.gov/dimrc/disasterapps.html
	NLM TriagePic	Reporting and tracking tool for use by hospital staff. Allows staff to capture pictures and brief information (name, age, gender, etc.) on victims as they arrive that may be searched by staff for family reunification purposes. Smartphone	https://lpf.nlm.nih.gov/tt.php
OEM Shelter (Previously Shelter View)	American Red Cross	This free application provides quick insight into disaster shelters as they are opened across the United States. Includes location, capacity, current number of shelter residents, last update. Smartphone	https://itunes.apple.com/app/american-red-cross-shelter/id419258261?mt=8
WISER	NLM	WISER provides a wide range of information on hazardous substances, including substance identification support, physical characteristics, human health information, and containment and suppression advice. The system contains information on over 400 chemicals and radiologic agents.	http://disasterinfo.nlm.nih.gov/dimrc/disasterapps.html

CDC, Centers for Disease Control and Prevention; FEMA, Federal Emergency Management Agency; HHS, U.S. Department of Health and Human Services; NLM, National Library of Medicine; OEM, Office of Emergency Management; REMM, Radiation Emergency Medical Management; WISER, Wireless Information Systems for Emergency Responders.

Source: U.S. Department of Health and Human Services. Disaster Apps for Your Digital Go Bag. Retrieved from https://disasterinfo.nlm.nih.gov/dimrc/disasterapps.html (Additional apps can be found in said website.)

TABLE 2.5 Courses/Training

Topic	Sponsoring Organization/ Name	Description	Location
Children and Disasters	NCDMPH	Three online accredited and peer-reviewed training modules: reuniting children in disasters; radiation issues in children; and children's psychosocial needs	https://www.usuhs .edu/ncdmph/ pediatric-preparedness
ICS	FEMA/700a	Introduces the NIMS concept	https://training.fema .gov/is/courseoverview .aspx?code=IS-700.a
	FEMA/100b	ICS introduction	https://training.fema .gov/is/courseoverview .aspx?code=IS-100.b
	FEMA/100.HCb	Similar information on ICS, using healthcare/hospital examples	https://training.fema.gov/ is/courseoverview .aspx?code=IS-100.HCb
	FEMA/200b	Participants learn how to operate efficiently during an incident using ICS. Includes training and resources for supervisors	https://training.fema .gov/is/courseoverview .aspx?code=IS-200.b
	FEMA/200.HCa	Provides training on the ICS to healthcare professionals whose primary responsibility is emergency management, to include middle management within a hospital or healthcare system.	https://training.fema .gov/is/courseoverview .aspx?code=IS-200.HCa
	FEMA/800b	Introduces the concepts and principles of the National Response Framework	https://training.fema .gov/is/courseoverview .aspx?code=IS-800.b
Pandemic Influenza	FEMA/IS-520	Describes the characteristics and effects of a pandemic and steps organizations can take to minimize the effects.	https://training.fema .gov/is/courseoverview .aspx?code=IS-520
Points of Distribution (POD)	FEMA/IS-26	Provides an in-depth look into the planning, operations, and demobilization stages of a POD mission.	https://training.fema .gov/is/courseoverview .aspx?code=IS-26
Preparing for Emergencies and Disasters	National Nurse Emergency Preparedness Initiative	Highly interactive web-based course that provides emergency preparedness training for nurses in practices, incorporating critical thinking involved in performance-level training.	https://nnepi.gwnursing .org/Default.asp?
Public Information Officer	FEMA IS-29	Covers basic information about the role of a state or local public information officer.	https://training.fema .gov/is/courseoverview .aspx?code=IS-29
Radiation Emergency Medical Management	HHS	Includes classroom radiation training courses, online radiation courses, and educational competencies for healthcare professionals.	https://www.remm.nlm .gov/training.htm
Radiologic Emergency Response	FEMA/IS-301	Provides a comprehensive understanding of radiological protection and response principles, guidelines, and regulations.	https://training.fema .gov/is/courseoverview .aspx?code=IS-301
Training and Continuing Education Online	CDC	Free continuing education on a variety of subjects including emergency preparedness. Includes clinician outreach and community activity calls and webinars	https://www2a.cdc.gov/ TCEOnline/

CDC, Centers for Disease Control and Prevention; FEMA, Federal Emergency Management Agency; HHS, U.S. Department of Health and Human Services; ICS, Incident Command System; NCDMPH, National Center for Disaster Medicine and Public Health; NIMS, National Incident Management System.

TABLE 2.6 Online Resources

Topic	Sponsoring Organization	Description	Location
ABC Resource Library	HHS	Includes fact sheets, tools, videos, reports, and partner resources on a variety of topics.	https://www.phe.gov/Preparedness/planning/abc/Pages/resources.aspx
Bioterrorism Agents/ Diseases	CDC	Provides links to over 30 specific agents. Includes diagnosis, treatment, and fact sheets.	https://emergency.cdc.gov/agent/agentlist.asp
Chemical Emergencies	CDC	Provides a list of chemicals by name and category, information for the general public and health professionals.	https://emergency.cdc.gov/chemical/index.asp
Disaster Information Management Research Center	NLM	Includes: • Disaster types and topics • Emergency response tools • Disaster Lit Database—disaster medicine and public health documents available at no cost	http://disasterinfo.nlm.nih.gov/
Disaster Medicine	NCDMPH/ Resilience through Learning	Provides NCDMPH and outside resources on specific all-hazards events including: • Influenza • Wildfires • Winter weather • Hurricanes and typhoons • Earthquakes • Tornadoes • Health emergencies • Explosions and mass gatherings	https://www.usuhs.edu/ncdmph/research-education/resilience-through-learning
Disaster Preparedness and Response	American Nurses Association	Links to documents on: • Mass decontamination • A nurse's duty to respond • Establishing Altered Standards of Care in Disasters	https://www.nursingworld.org/practice-policy/work-environment/health-safety/disaster-preparedness/
	International Coalition for Mass Casualty Education	Includes a set of competencies.	http://www.aacn.nche.edu/leading-initiatives/education-resources/INCMCECompetencies.pdf
	International Council of Nurses	Website includes resources and related publications, disaster response links, emergency care links, and an events list.	http://www.icn.ch/networks/disaster-response-network/
	NLM	Content checked and updated: • Disaster Health Links for 19 topics • Tox Town—an interactive guide to environmental health risks and toxic substances • Medline Plus—information on 700 health topics • Medline Plus en español	https://sis.nlm.nih.gov/dimrc/subjectguides.html
"Do 1 Thing"	Consortium	12-month web-based all-hazards program for individuals and businesses which provides monthly reminders and a progress tracker. Includes fact sheets, brochures, presentations and public service announcements.	http://do1thing.com/
Emergency Management	Joint Commission	Website includes emergency management references, including the link to accreditation standards.	https://www.jointcommission.org/emergency_management_resources_-_general_references/

(continued)

TABLE 2.6 Online Resources (*continued*)

Topic	Sponsoring Organization	Description	Location
Emergency Plans	Department of Homeland Security	Provides guidance on how to develop a family emergency plan which addresses all kinds of emergencies. Includes a 2-page downloadable plan for parents and kids to record important contact information.	https://www.ready.gov/make-a-plan https://www.fema.gov/media-library-data/0e3ef555f66e22ab832e284f826c2e9e/FEMA_plan_parent_508_071513.pdf
Emergency Preparedness	American Red Cross	Information on how to prepare for emergencies. Their disaster research library includes specific information on 25 topics including earthquakes, floods, hurricanes, and winter storms.	http://www.redcross.org/get-help/how-to-prepare-for-emergencies http://www.redcross.org/get-help/how-to-prepare-for-emergencies/types-of-emergencies
	CDC	Information for individuals and families as well as emergency health professionals. As examples, includes information on specific types of emergencies, information for specific groups (older adults, children and their caregivers, people with disabilities or chronic disease), coping with disasters, crisis and emergency risk communications, and recent outbreaks.	https://emergency.cdc.gov/
National Incident Management System (NIMS)	FEMA	NIMS is a systematic, proactive approach to guide departments and agencies at all levels of government, nongovernmental organizations, and the private sector to work together seamlessly and manage incidents involving all threats and hazards—regardless of cause, size, location, or complexity—in order to reduce loss of life, property and harm to the environment.	https://www.fema.gov/national-incident-management-system
National Response Framework, 3rd Edition	FEMA	The *National Response Framework* is a guide to how the nation responds to all types of disasters and emergencies. It is built on scalable, flexible, and adaptable concepts identified in the National Incident Management System to align key roles and responsibilities across the nation.	https://www.fema.gov/media-library/assets/documents/117791
Personal Medical Information Form	CDC	Keep It With You is a temporary record that includes medications, medical conditions, and other related information.	https://www.cdc.gov/disasters/kiwy.html
Public Health Preparedness	National Association of County and City Health Officials	Current initiatives provide detailed information on effective planning and meeting the needs of special populations of five topics: • Medical Countermeasures • Chemical Response • Radiation Preparedness • Pandemic Influenza Planning • Antiviral Distribution and Dispensing	http://www.naccho.org/programs/public-health-preparedness/medical-countermeasures
Radiation Emergencies	CDC	Includes information for the general public and healthcare professionals.	https://emergency.cdc.gov/radiation/index.asp

CDC, Centers for Disease Control and Prevention; FEMA, Federal Emergency Management Agency; HHS, U.S. Department of Health and Human Services; NCDMPH, National Center for Disaster Medicine and Public Health; NLM, National Library of Medicine.

TABLE 2.7 Pocket Cards

Effective Team Formation in a Disaster Setting: The First 15 Minutes	NCDMPH	Practical checklist to help a group that has never worked together before	http://ncdmph.usuhs.edu/Documents/PocketCard_Effective-Team-Formation-in-Disaster-Setting.pdf
Working With Interpreters in a Disaster Setting	NCDMPH	Print ready card includes suggestions on how to prepare for, present information, and evaluate patient interactions using an interpreter	http://ncdmph.usuhs.edu/Documents/PocketCard_Working-with-Interpreter.pdf

NCDMPH, National Center for Disaster Medicine and Public Health.

TABLE 2.8 Tools

Chemical Hazards Emergency Medical Management	National Library of Medicine	Quick identification and treatment of biological and chemical warfare agents. A section on special needs includes information for disabled, hearing and visually impaired persons.	https://chemm.nlm.nih.gov/index.html
emPOWER Map	HHS	Use the map to find the monthly total of Medicare beneficiaries with electricity-dependent equipment claims at the U.S., state, territory, county, and zip code level and turn on "real-time" natural hazard and NOAA severe weather tracking services to identify areas and populations that may be impacted and are at risk of prolonged power outages.	https://empowermap.hhs.gov/
Radiation Emergency Medical Management	HHS	Guidance on diagnosis and treatment of radiation emergencies for healthcare providers.	https://www.remm.nlm.gov/index.html
Wireless Information Systems for Emergency Responders (WISER)	HHS	WISER provides a wide range of information on hazardous substances, including substance identification support, physical characteristics, human health information, and containment and suppression advice. The system contains information on over 400 chemicals and radiologic agents.	https://wiser.nlm.nih.gov/ App available

HHS, U. S. Department of Health and Human Services; NOAA, National Oceanic and Atmospheric Administration.

specific event by incorporating incident-specific information gleaned from trustworthy websites, a concept known as "just-in-time" training or learning.

As recommended by the National Library of Medicine (2014), healthcare professionals should consider the authority, credibility, and affiliation of content developers. Generally, content developed by federal and state governments, major national scientific societies, and professional organizations and international organizations is current and of high quality. Consider when information was created, revised, or last updated when evaluating resources.

When we are better prepared nursing professionals, we can lead, manage, and help our communities recover from disasters better, faster, and stronger. Every small step toward preparedness makes a difference.

SUMMARY

As disasters continue to grow in their magnitude and frequency, disaster response plans will continue to be developed, implemented, evaluated, and modified for use during the next event. Efforts are now refocusing on creating a culture of preparedness where individuals and whole communities understand and plan for the risks that are most relevant and urgent for them individually. The challenge is to convince members of the general public that they play an integral role in preparedness and community resilience.

While the nuances of a disaster response will probably stay consistent, the structure of the federal and state agencies responsible for coordinating the response may continue to change significantly. The economic reality is that the decline in federal programs, grants, and response underwriting may result in fewer resources.

Nurses must remain current about the status of the PPD-8, and its family of Frameworks as well as the organizational responsibilities of collaborating agencies. Every person shares a responsibility in being prepared and in safeguarding the nation from harm.

The U.S. national nursing workforce must address its own issues regarding professional emergency preparedness. Attention to professional issues like crisis leadership, educational preparation for disaster and public health emergency events, advancing nursing science, and establishing or enhancing collaborative relationships with other disaster providers is paramount if we are to be ready when disaster strikes.

In the fall of 2017, portions of the United States were subjected to major hurricanes—Harvey, Irma, and Maria—and raging wildfires. Many lives were needlessly lost because the general population had lost its preparedness focus. In the absence of major storms over the previous 6 years, many had forgotten the potential risks and had neglected to develop or update their individual and family preparedness plans. We, as nurses, need to first take care of ourselves and our families, and then our workplaces, and then our communities. Success in preventing a catastrophe is being prepared and the onus is on each of us.

"Every nurse a prepared nurse." (Society for the Advancement of Disaster Nursing, 2017*)*

STUDY QUESTIONS

1. What is the U.S. National Preparedness System?

2. What conditions must be met before federal coordination occurs during an incident?

3. What tenants are included in the National Health Security Strategy?

4. What do government executives, leaders from the private sector and nongovernmental organizations, emergency managers, and responders need to understand about roles and relationships in the National Response Framework and the National Incident Management System?

5. Which ESF covers sheltering, and who is the lead agency for this function?

6. What is the purpose and scope of ESF-8?

7. What are federal resources for nurse volunteers?

REFERENCES

American Organization of Nurse Executives. (2016). AONE guiding principles: Role of the nurse leader in crisis management. Retrieved from http://www.aone.org/resources/role-of-the-nurse-leader-in-crisis-management.pdf

Baack, S., & Alfred, D. (2013). Nurses' preparedness and perceived competence in managing disasters. *Journal of Nursing Scholarship, 45*(3), 281–287. doi:10.1111/jnu.12029

Couig, M. P., Gable, A., Griffin, A., Langan, J. C., Katzburg, J. R., Wolgast, K. A., … Veenema, T. G. (2017). Progress on a call to action: Nurses as leaders in disaster preparedness and response. *Nursing Administration Quarterly, 41*(2), 112–117. doi:10.1097/NAQ.0000000000000226

Dickerson, C., & Ferré-Sadurní, L. (2017, October 24). Like going back in time: Puerto Ricans put survival skills to use. *The New York Times.* Retrieved from https://www.nytimes.com/2017/10/24/us/hurricane-maria-puerto-rico-coping.html

Edmonson, C., Sumagaysay, D., Cueman, M., & Chappell, S. (2016). The nurse leader role in crisis management. *Journal of Nursing Administration, 46*(9), 417–419. doi:10.1097/NNA.0000000000000367

Erdman, J. (2017, October 14). Atlantic hurricane season 2017 is now seventh most active in history. Retrieved from https://weather.com/en-CA/canada/news/news/2017-10-09-atlantic-hurricane-season-one-of-busiest-october

Federal Interagency Committee on Emergency Medical Services. (2014). National implementation of the model uniform core criteria for mass casualty incident triage. Retrieved from https://asprtracie.hhs.gov/technical-resources/resource/3076/national-implementation-ofthe-model-uniform-core-criteria-for-mass-casualty-incident-triage

Institute of Medicine. (2009). *Guidance for establishing crisis standards of care for use in disaster situations: A letter report.* Retrieved from www.iom.edu/Reports/2009/DisasterCareStandards.aspx

Institute of Medicine. (2011). *The future of nursing: Leading change, advancing health.* Washington, DC: National Academies Press.

Institute of Medicine. (2012). *Crisis standards of care: A systems framework for catastrophic disaster response: Volume 1: Introduction and CSC Framework.* Washington, DC: National Academies Press.

Kaji, A., Koenig, K. L., & Lewis, R. J. (2007). Current hospital disaster preparedness. *Journal of the American Medical Association, 298*(18), 2188–2190. doi:10.1001/jama.298.18.2188

Langan, J., Lavin, R., Wolgast, K., & Veenema, T. (2017). Education for developing and sustaining a health care workforce for disaster readiness. *Nursing Administration Quarterly, 41*(2), 118–127. doi:10.1097/NAQ.0000000000000225

Lavin, R., Slepski, L., & Veenema, T. G. (2007). Leadership and coordination in disaster health care systems: The federal disaster response network. In T. G. Veenema (Ed.), *Disaster nursing and emergency preparedness for chemical, biological and radiological terrorism and other hazards* (2nd ed., pp. 25–46). New York, NY: Springer.

Lerner, E. B., Schwartz, R. B., Coule, P. L., Weinstein, E. S., Cone, D. C., Hunt, R. C., … O'Connor, R. E. (2008). Mass casualty triage: An evaluation of the data and development of a proposed national guideline. *Disaster Medicine and Public Health Preparedness, 2*(Suppl. 1), S25–S34. doi:10.1097/DMP.0b013e318182194e

Lippincott Nursing Center. (2017). Continuing education requirements for nurses by state. Retrieved from http://www.nursingcenter.com/ceconnection/ce-state-requirements

Massachusetts Emergency Management Agency. (2014). After action report for the response to the 2013 Boston Marathon bombings. Retrieved from http://www.mass.gov/eopss/docs/mema/after-action-report-for-the-response-to-the-2013-boston-marathon-bombings.pdf

Medical Reserve Corps. (2017). Find a unit. Retrieved from https://mrc.hhs.gov/HomePage

National Center for Disaster Medicine and Public Health. (n.d.). Vision and mission. Retrieved from https://www.usuhs.edu/ncdmph

National Center for Disaster Medicine and Public Health. (2011). Report on the domestic natural disaster health workforce. Retrieved from https://www.usuhs.edu/sites/default/files/media/ncdmph/pdf/workforceproject2011-b.pdf

National Library of Medicine. (2014). Selection guidelines for non-National Library of Medicine resources. Retrieved from https://disaster.nlm.nih.gov/enviro/envirohealthlinkscriteria.html

National Research Council. (2012). *Disaster resilience: A national imperative.* Washington, DC: National Academies Press.

Scott, L. A., Crumpier, J., Tolley, J., Jones, E. M., & Wahlquist, A. E. (2012). Disaster care provider workforce assessment. *Journal of the South Caroline Medical Association, 108*(3), 80–83.

Slepski, L., Proffit, R., & Veenema, T. G. (2012). Leadership and coordination in disaster health care systems: The U.S. national response framework. In T. G. Veenema (Ed.), *Disaster nursing and emergency preparedness: For chemical, biological, and radiological terrorism and other hazards* (3rd ed., pp. 21–44). New York, NY: Springer.

Society for the Advancement of Disaster Nursing. (2017). Future of nursing: Campaign for action promotes the field of disaster nursing. Retrieved from https://disasternursing.org

Sullivan, E. J., & Decker, P. J. (2001). *Effective leadership and management in nursing* (5th ed.). Upper Saddle River, NJ: Prentice Hall.

U.S. Department of Health and Human Services. (n.d.-a). Readiness and deployment operations group (RedDOG). *Commissioned Corps of the U.S. Public Health Service.* Retrieved from https://dcp.psc.gov/ccmis/ReDDOG/REDDOG_current_teams_m.aspx

U.S. Department of Health and Human Services (n.d.-b). The emergency system for advance registration of volunteer health professionals. *Public Health Emergency.* Retrieved from https://www.phe.gov/esarvhp/pages/about.aspx#

U.S. Department of Health and Human Services. (n.d.-c). U.S. Public Health Service Commissioned Corps. Retrieved from https://www.surgeongeneral.gov/about/corps/index.html

U.S. Department of Health and Human Services, Office of Emergency Preparedness. (1995). *Responding to the consequences of chemical and biological terrorism.* Seminar conducted at the Uniformed Services University of Health Sciences, Bethesda, MD. Retrieved from https://permanent.access.gpo.gov/lps15853/Proceedings.pdf

U.S. Department of Health and Human Services. (2010a). National Disaster Medical System. Retrieved from https://www.phe.gov/preparedness/responders/ndms/Pages/default.aspx

U.S. Department of Health and Human Services. (2010b). Pandemic and All Hazards Preparedness Act. Retrieved from https://www.phe.gov/preparedness/legal/pahpa/pages/default.aspx

U.S. Department of Health and Human Services. (2011a). Frequently asked questions. Retrieved from https://www.phe.gov/Preparedness/planning/authority/nhss/Pages/faqs.aspx

U.S. Department of Health and Human Services. (2011b). Medical assistance. Retrieved from https://www.phe.gov/Preparedness/support/medicalassistance/Pages/default.aspx#fms

U.S. Department of Health and Human Services. (2011c). National Health Security Strategy. Retrieved from https://www.phe.gov/preparedness/planning/authority/nhss/Pages/default.aspx

U.S. Department of Health and Human Services. (2016). 2017–2022 Health care preparedness and response capabilities. Retrieved from https://www.phe.gov/Preparedness/planning/hpp/reports/Documents/2017-2022-healthcare-pr-capablities.pdf

U.S. Department of Health and Human Services, Centers for Disease Control and Prevention. (2016). Federal medical station. Retrieved from https://www.cdc.gov/phpr/stockpile/fedmedstation.htm

U.S. Department of Health and Human Services. (2017a). Hospital Preparedness Program: Public Health Emergency Preparedness Cooperative Agreement, CDC-RFA-TP17-1701. Retrieved from https://www.grants.gov/web/grants/view-opportunity.html?oppId=290860

U.S. Department of Health and Human Services. (2017b). NDMS teams: Working together to provide the best of care in the worst of times. Retrieved from https://www.phe.gov/Preparedness/responders/ndms/ndms-teams/Pages/default.aspx

U.S. Department of Health and Human Services. (2017c). Topic collection: Crisis standards of care. Retrieved from https://asprtracie.hhs.gov/technical-resources/63/crisis-standards-of-care/63

U.S. Department of Homeland Security. (2008a). Emergency Support Function #8—Public Health and Medical Services Annex. Retrieved from https://www.fema.gov/media-library-data/20130726-1825-25045-8027/emergency_support_function_8_public_health___medical_services_annex_2008.pdf

U.S. Department of Homeland Security. (2008b). Overview: ESF and support annexes coordinating federal assistance in support of the National Response Framework. Retrieved from http://www.fema.gov/pdf/emergency/nrf/nrf-overview.pdf

U.S. Department of Homeland Security. (2008c). What's new in the National Response Framework. Retrieved from http://www.fema.gov/pdf/emergency/nrf/whatsnew.pdf

U.S. Department of Homeland Security. (2010, July 1). If you see something, say something. Retrieved from https://www.dhs.gov/see-something-say-something/what-suspicious-activity

U.S. Department of Homeland Security. (2011a, March 30). Presidential Policy Directive 8—National Preparedness. Retrieved from https://www.dhs.gov/presidential-policy-directive-8-national-preparedness

U.S. Department of Homeland Security. (2011b, September 23). National Disaster Recovery Framework. Retrieved from https://www.fema.gov/media-library-data/20130726-1820-25045-5325/508_ndrf.pdf

U.S. Department of Homeland Security. (2011c, October 7). DHS announces first National Preparedness Goal. Retrieved from https://www.dhs.gov/news/2011/10/07/dhs-announces-first-national-preparedness-goal

U.S. Department of Homeland Security. (2011d, November). National Preparedness System. Retrieved from https://www.fema.gov/media-library-data/20130726-1855-25045-8110/national_preparedness_system_final.pdf

U.S. Department of Homeland Security. (2011e, December). A whole community approach to emergency management: Principles, themes, and pathways for action, FDOC 104-008-1. Retrieved from https://www.fema.gov/media-library-data/20130726-1813-25045-0649/whole_community_dec2011__2_.pdf

U.S. Department of Homeland Security. (2013a, May). National Mitigation Framework. Retrieved from https://www.fema.gov/media-library-data/20130726-1914-25045-9956/final_national_mitigation_framework_20130501.pdf

U.S. Department of Homeland Security. (2013b, May). National Prevention Framework. Retrieved from https://www.fema.gov/media-library-data/20130726-1913-25045-6071/final_national_prevention_framework_20130501.pdf

U.S. Department of Homeland Security. (2014, July). National Protection Framework. Retrieved from https://www.fema.gov/media-library-data/1406717583765-996837bf788e20e977eb5079f4174240/FINAL_National_Protection_Framework_20140729.pdf

U.S. Department of Homeland Security. (2015, September). *National Preparedness Goal* (1st ed.). Retrieved from https://www.fema.gov/pdf/prepared/npg.pdf

U.S. Department of Homeland Security. (2016). *National Response Framework* (3rd ed.). Retrieved from https://www.fema.gov/media-library-data/1466014682982-9bcf8245ba4c60c120aa915abe74e15d/National_Response_Framework3rd.pdf

U.S. Department of Homeland Security. (2017, October 10). *National Incident Management System* (3rd ed.). Retrieved from https://www.fema.gov/media-library/assets/documents/148019

Veenema, T. G., Griffin, A., Gable, A. R., MacIntyre, L., Simons, R. N., Couig, M. P., ... Larson, E. (2016). Nurses as leaders in disaster preparedness and response—A call to action. *Journal of Nursing Scholarship, 48*(2), 187–200. doi:10.1111/jnu.12198

Walsh, L., Altman, B. A., King, R. V., & Strauss-Riggs, K. (2014). Enhancing the translation of disaster health competencies into practice. *Disaster Medicine & Public Health Preparedness, 8*(1), 70–78. doi:10.1017/dmp.2014.7

Walsh, T. J., Orsega, S., & Banks, D. (2006). Lessons from hurricane Rita: Organizing to provide medical care during a natural disaster. *Annals of Internal Medicine, 145*(6), 468–470. doi:10.7326/0003-4819-145-6-200609190-00137

White House. (2003, February 28). Homeland Security Presidential Directive/HSPD-5. Retrieved from https://www.dhs.gov/publication/homeland-security-presidential-directive-5

White House. (2006, February 23). The federal response to Katrina: Lessons learned. Retrieved from http://library.stmarytx.edu/acadlib/edocs/katrinawh.pdf

White House. (2007, October 18). Homeland Security Presidential Directive (HSPD) 21. Retrieved from https://www.hsdl.org/?view&did=480002

3

HOSPITAL AND EMERGENCY DEPARTMENT PREPAREDNESS

David Markenson and Sarah Losinski

LEARNING OBJECTIVES

When this chapter is completed, readers will be able to:

1. Describe the importance of hospital and ED preparedness.
2. Understand the threat of internal and external disasters to effective hospital functioning.
3. Describe the essential components of a comprehensive emergency operations plan.
4. Describe the structure and purpose of the Incident Command System (ICS).
5. Differentiate the four phases of emergency planning.
6. List the essential hospital services.
7. Differentiate between daily hospital triage and disaster triage.

KEY MESSAGES

Hospital emergency preparedness is critical to maintaining the integrity of the healthcare system during a disaster.

The capacity of a hospital to continue to function effectively during a disaster will be dependent upon a comprehensive emergency operations plan that covers all phases of the disaster and competent staff who know their roles in executing the plan.

The cornerstone of emergency management is to first protect life, then property, then the environment.

Internal disasters disrupt the effective functioning of the hospital and threaten the safety of patients, visitors, and staff.

The ICS provides a unified structure for leadership during a disaster.

Resource readiness ensures that the hospital and ED will have the appropriate resources (supplies, personnel, equipment, facilities) in the event a disaster occurs.

Disasters create challenges to maintaining standards of care.

The unique needs of children must be accommodated during a disaster.

CHAPTER OVERVIEW

Traditional emergency management focused on the scene of a disaster, field response and resuscitation, followed by recovery. An element of response was the hospital but the emphasis was usually focused on the ED and followed typical emergency management without adaptation to the unique needs of hospitals. With the recent development of healthcare emergency management, the role of not only the ED but also the entire hospital in emergency preparedness has taken on increased emphasis. This chapter provides an overview of hospital preparedness and response through the view of a healthcare emergency manager.

If one looks back more than 30 years, it would be almost impossible to find a hospital role called "hospital emergency management" or even a position for a healthcare emergency manager in a hospital or medical center. Yet, certain aspects of healthcare emergency management responsibilities have always been addressed by hospitals, such as fire safety, backup power, and the ability to handle victims from a mass casualty event. In addition, the public has strong expectations of the roles hospitals should play during times of disaster. Healthcare institutions are expected to provide both emergency care and continuance of the day-to-day healthcare responsibilities regardless of the volume and demand. The public believes that hospitals will have light, heat, air-conditioning, water, food, and communications capabilities, regardless of the fact that the institution may itself be affected by the calamity.

A major change in the way hospitals plan for hazards and vulnerabilities includes a comprehensive emergency management planning process for all hazards rather than planning for specific issues or threats. Additionally, hospitals should look beyond their ED doors and engage community stakeholders, reaching out to local and regional emergency planners to assist in larger community-wide emergency preparedness planning. The interest of nonhospital entities in health system emergency preparedness can be seen through several examples, including emergency management and public health initiatives on mass vaccination, pandemic planning, increasing hospitals' ability to perform decontamination of casualties contaminated with hazardous materials, and so on. For example, there is the Joint Commission on the Accreditation of Healthcare Organizations (JCAHO) change from placing emergency preparedness standards in the Environment of Care section to placing the standards in a separate section with specific goals and requirements, as well as the release of the Occupational Safety and Health Administration (OSHA) document *Best Practices for Hospital-Based First Receivers* (Joint Commission, 2007, 2008; U.S. Department of Labor, 2005).

Emergency management agencies have traditionally been responsible for bringing first responders, government agencies, and community stakeholders together to assist with comprehensive emergency planning or disaster response and recovery. A common cornerstone of emergency management has been to protect life, then property, then the environment. As a result, when conducting emergency planning activities, the health and medical needs of the population are among the most significant and are considered with basic public health and human needs, including sheltering, mass care, sanitation, environmental health, food and water, and other essential services. In addition, as public health professionals, we also believe that population health activities include the mitigation of increased morbidity and mortality during and following a disaster, act of terrorism, or public health emergency.

In healthcare delivery, we attempt to meet community needs by providing a place for preventive medicine, care for chronic medical conditions, emergency medical treatment, and rehabilitation from injury or illness. While a healthcare institution serves the community, this responsibility occurs at the level of the individual. Each individual expects a thorough assessment and treatment if needed, regardless of the needs of others. This approach is different than that practiced by emergency managers, whose goal is to assist the largest number of people with the limited resources that are available. As such, emergency management principles are focused on population, rather than individual, needs. When either planning for a disaster or operating in a disaster response mode, the hospital should be prepared at some point to change its focus from the individual to the community it serves, and to begin weighing the needs of any individual patient versus the most good for the most patients with scarce resources. While the initial planning for emergencies by hospitals is focused on maintaining operations and handling the care needs of actual or potential increased numbers of patients and/or different presentations of illness or injury than is traditionally seen, there is also the need to recognize that at some point during a disaster, act of terrorism, or public health emergency, an imbalance of need versus available resources will occur. At this point, the approach to delivering healthcare will need to switch from a focus on the individual to that of the population. This paradigm shift, one of the core aspects of hospital emergency management, allows the hospital to prepare to maximize resources in disasters and then to know when to switch to a pure disaster mode, utilizing limited and often scant resources to help the most people with the greatest chance of survival.

The healthcare delivery system is vast and comprises multiple entry points at primary care providers, clinics, urgent care centers, hospitals, rehabilitation facilities, and long-term care facilities. The point of entry for many individuals into the acute healthcare system is through the ED. Hospital emergency management activities vary and can be categorized in many ways; however, some common areas of focus within healthcare emergency management include the following:

- Communication
- Surge capacity
- Volunteer management
- Security
- Hazard material (HAZMAT) and chemical, biological, radiological, nuclear, and explosive (CBRNE) preparedness
- Collaboration with public health
- Education and training

- Equipment and supplies
- Worker safety
- Drills and exercises
- ED disaster operations
- Trauma center role

HOSPITAL PREPAREDNESS

Hospitals must have adequate plans to handle both disasters and terrorism within an all-hazards approach to ensure preparedness for any possible event. These plans must also include an effective ICS that incorporates those capable of making decisions. The healthcare facilities responsible for treating victims in a biological, radiological, nuclear, chemical, or explosive event could be strained or overwhelmed. Medical facilities can become inundated with patients if large numbers of victims appear without ambulance transport and pre-entry notification. This situation differs markedly from existing hospital disaster alert systems in which victims are triaged in the field and carefully distributed among available resources to prevent any single facility from being overwhelmed. Along similar lines, victims appearing without full hospital preparation could thwart attempts to isolate contaminated victims from other patients and hospital staff. Large-scale biological, chemical, nuclear, radiological, or explosive incidents may necessitate the use of alternative healthcare sites (e.g., auditoriums and arenas), which requires that healthcare resources be dispersed to areas where victims may not receive optimal care.

The U.S. federal government has recently had a significant influence in reinforcing the importance of disaster preparedness in healthcare facilities. The Centers for Medicare and Medicaid Services (CMS) implemented federal requirements in November 2017, dictating that a number of actions in disaster preparedness must be taken by facilities in order to receive CMS funding and reimbursements (CMS, 2016). The outcome of these requirements has yet to unfold, but with ever-increasing natural disasters and mass casualty incidents (MCIs), these requirements may motivate more facilities to establish quality response plans. This will hopefully decrease negative consequences that result from underpreparedness.

Hazard Vulnerability Analyses

In today's resource-constrained environment, it is not realistic to plan for every conceivable hazard or eventuality that might befall an institution. As such, hospital emergency managers must use the scarce resources available to them to prioritize their efforts to manage hazards and their associated risks.

In its most basic form, a hazard vulnerability analysis (HVA) is a tool that emergency managers employ to screen for risk and plan for the strategic use of limited resources. Healthcare institutions' complex combinations of equipment and hazardous materials, along with an ever-changing population within, including visitors and patients in varied conditions of physical and mental health, make these sites more susceptible to untoward events.

The first step in conducting an HVA is the identification of potential hazard. Doing so offers hospital emergency managers the chance to identify those hazards that are most likely to occur and that will have the greatest impact, in terms of life and economic costs, should they take place. Given current resource limitations (e.g., time, money, and personnel), an HVA helps entities focus their work on those hazards that would be likely to yield the maximum adverse consequences.

Developing the list of potential hazards is best managed through the collaborate surveying of key hospital stakeholders. One method is to distribute, via mail or email, a blank HVA table and ask respondents to list all hazards that could impact the hospital. To assist, the hospital emergency manager can suggest that these be divided between natural (e.g., earthquakes, landslides), technological (e.g., rail accidents and power failures), and intentional hazards (e.g., terrorism).

A common method for organizing potential hazards is to list various types of emergencies and assign scoring values to each one that reflects its likelihood, its impact, and the institution's readiness for the emergency. For instance, a pandemic avian flu outbreak may be scored as very high impact, low likelihood, and intermediate readiness score. A summation or product of the values then assigns a total score to the hazard (pandemic flu). Other hazards on the HVA will also be scored in a similar manner. This allows numeric comparisons between hazards. Certainly, this is a rather arbitrary method that allows much subjectivity in terms of the actual numeric ratings and the validity of the comparisons. However, the strength of this concept is that it does create an organized framework to direct where an institution's emergency management committee's energy and efforts should go. An HVA then lists the mitigation, preparedness, response, and recovery activities necessary for each hazard, with the resultant measures taken to manage each hazard varying for each.

The Hospital Emergency Management Committee

The hospital's emergency management committee should consist of a broad cross section of hospital departments, including clinical, support, operational, and financial units. Qualifications of the committee chairperson should include significant fluency in emergency management principles and practices, familiarity with the ever-changing regulatory and accreditation requirements of this complex aspect of healthcare, and organizational empowerment to enact the hospital emergency management plan and recommendations of the committee. Members should represent all hospital areas, including at a minimum senior leadership, legal, environmental health, security, laboratory, ED, chaplaincy, public affairs, clinical and academic affairs, human resources, occupational health, infection control, engineering, life safety, and housekeeping. Though there is limited literature that outlines the optimal makeup of an emergency management committee, inclusion of clinicians from departments such as nursing, emergency medicine, surgery, medicine, pediatrics, infectious diseases, and employee health should be strongly considered, given the expertise they can offer. Administrative leaders such as the chief executive, chief nurse, chief medical officer, medical staff leadership and department chairs, operating officers, and other senior leaders will also provide leadership to the committee and are important to ensure buy-in and support.

The importance of their presence is immeasurable and sends a significant message to the entire institution that emergency management is a key facet of the hospital's daily operations.

The committee should also interface with representatives from local, state, and federal agencies involved in emergency management, fire protection, law enforcement, and public health and become familiar with the plans made by these agencies. Many hospitals will find it imperative to build alliances with local community groups, nongovernmental organizations, and other grassroots efforts that are the foundation of neighborhood cohesiveness.

Key responsibilities of the hospital emergency management committee include overseeing and guiding the hospital's mitigation, preparedness, response, and recovery efforts. Meetings are held as needed by the institution; however, monthly meetings should be considered feasible and adequate to ensure that changes to the institution's capabilities can be addressed.

Alliance Building and Community-Based Planning

Collaborative emergency management planning between hospitals and their communities is imperative to ensure that all stakeholders, internal and external to the institution, are aware of and familiar with the hospital's emergency management measures. Examples of entities that hospitals should approach for collaborative planning are local and state departments of health, governmental emergency management offices, Centers for Disease Control and Prevention (CDC), Federal Emergency Management Agency (FEMA), and the Department of Health and Human Services.

Most nongovernmental community groups have periodic forums that welcome hospital participation and presentations on emergency management and bolster dialogue in areas such as prioritizing local emergencies and response efforts. Often, these forums offer opportunities for various healthcare institutions (primary, acute, and long-term care facilities), governmental agencies, community organizations, and others to discuss emergency management topics and plans. This may be especially true when planning for large-scale incidents such as tornadoes, earthquakes, and hurricanes, and can prove to be invaluable during training, drills, and exercises. Active participation in these local and regional committees is an essential preparedness function for hospitals.

Hospital Preparedness for Children

The healthcare facilities responsible for treating pediatric victims in a biological, radiological, nuclear, chemical, or explosive event could be strained or overwhelmed. Children are difficult to care for by persons wearing protective equipment, which is essential in the management of biological or chemical events. Protective clothing is bulky and cumbersome; it impedes the ability of persons to perform procedures such as venipuncture on small children. It is imperative that hospitals and the healthcare community develop protocols and equipment that allow for treatment of children, taking into account the restrictions of operating in protective clothing. Examples might include use of intraosseous access to obtain access for medications of

fluids and intramuscular injections when appropriate. This is the case when restrictive clothing or other conditions make intravenous lines not feasible.

It is important that hospitals consider the needs of children in all aspects of emergency preparedness and that these plans are designed to be applicable in any major disaster situation—the so-called all-hazards strategy. This will include, but is not limited to, appropriate types and numbers of pediatric-trained staff, equipment, medications, and decontamination equipment. Plans should account for the screening, triage, or management of patients in ambulatory as well as inpatient situations. In addition, hospitals must be prepared to handle situations in which patients will be cared for as a family unit and not be able to separate, even under dire circumstances such as large-scale quarantine. This will not only require all hospitals to have the capability to handle children, but in turn, pediatric hospitals must be able to potentially care for adult patients who would be staying with their children.

In addition to the pediatric-specific issues of hospital emergency preparedness, one must ensure general hospital emergency preparedness.

PHASES OF EMERGENCY PLANNING

In the classic model of emergency management, there are four phases—mitigation, preparedness, response, and recovery (see Figure 3.1).

Mitigation Measures

As the cornerstone of the healthcare system, the hospital receives the injured, infected, and ill during a major incident. During incidents, healthcare leaders must impart judgment based on the best available data, which are often incomplete, incorrect, or both; remain cognizant of the time-sensitive nature

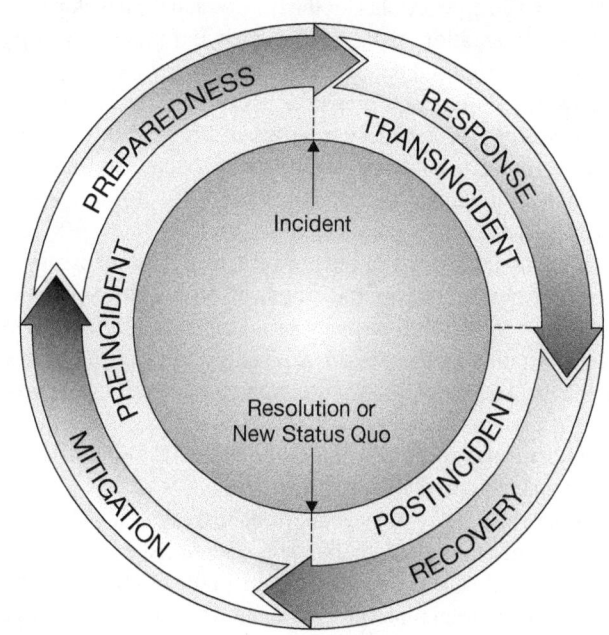

FIGURE 3.1 Phases of emergency management.

Source: Image used with permission from Rains Analytics (2017).

of the issue at hand; and ensure that a well-defined command structure is initiated and remains intact throughout the duration of the incident.

To that end, hospitals must make sustained efforts, either structural or nonstructural, to lessen the likelihood and impact of hazards.

Structural efforts include those that the hospital performs through the construction or alteration of the physical environment through engineered solutions. Examples include employing disaster-resistant construction, structural modifications (e.g., "hardening"), and detection systems (e.g., radiation monitors at the hospital's portals).

Nonstructural mitigation measures are those that the hospital undertakes by modifying human behaviors or processes. These may include regulatory measures, staff awareness, and educational programs.

Typically, mitigation activities are based on a cost–benefit analysis that assesses the costs of both the losses and the necessary action for mitigation against the likelihood of the incident.

The emergency management plan must specify the institution's mitigation efforts and ensure that these elements meld into the other phases of the plan (preparedness, response, and recovery) to ensure a seamless approach.

Preparedness Efforts

To effectively manage the full spectrum of emergency incidents that a hospital may face, hospital emergency managers—in collaboration with the institution's emergency management committee comprising members of every clinical, operational, and financial department—must develop and maintain a comprehensive, effective emergency management plan. In addition to the intellectual and practical importance of maintaining an up-to-date and well-developed emergency management plan, major provisions in the 2017 CMS emergency preparedness requirements include compliance in a risk assessment, maintenance of an emergency plan for the facility, and the development and implementation of facility policies and procedures that support the proposed emergency plan (CMS, 2016).

Hospital emergency preparedness efforts are, by nature, often contrary to the daily realities of hospital operations. Whereas most hospitals operate on stringent budgets and seek to minimize financial losses on unfilled beds, storing unnecessary perishables (e.g., medications, food, and supplies) and reducing unnecessary staffing in excess of providing essential services, emergency management efforts require just the opposite—an increase in many or all of these limited, often taken-for-granted, resources. And given the fact that emergency incidents occur with modest frequency, regardless of scope, intensity, or duration, comprehensive emergency planning is necessary despite the fact that many deem it to draw from, rather than add to, the bottom line.

Some emergency managers erroneously anticipate that in the event of an emergency incident, federal, state, and local resources will be activated to supplement the hospital's ability to respond. As seen time and time again with various incidents, most notably Hurricane Katrina, these outside resources have a time factor for arrival on scene, may be significantly delayed and due to the event may be too unreliable to effectively

be counted upon in emergency planning. While potentially overwhelming to local resources, some incidents may not be large enough to warrant mobilization of resources beyond the immediate response area.

The emergency management plan is the core of the hospital's emergency preparedness activities, which the hospital assumes to bolster its capacity and categorize resources that it may employ before, during, and after an emergency incident. Preparedness efforts range from developing a resource inventory and conducting institution-wide emergency management training, drills, and exercises to leading an institution emergency management committee.

The Response Phase

Often, the most visible and well supported by outside resources of the emergency management plans' activities are those that fall under the response phase. Despite the time and effort that hospitals put into attempting to mitigate and prepare for emergency incidents, reducing to zero the likelihood and consequences of the countless hazards hospitals may face is simply not possible. Consequently, as part of their all-hazards approach, hospitals must spend considerable time *strengthening* their organization's response capacities.

Efforts include those measures taken when an emergency incident occurs and may involve care for patients, staff, and visitors: to limit injuries, loss of life, and damage to the physical environment. Regardless of the scale of the incident, the impact on the institution in terms of physical damage, and the volume of patients it may receive, the public's expectations are that hospitals remain safe havens for all. This significant expectation yields challenges for all involved in the hospital's emergency management work and is the reason that the concept of surge remains an important challenge to stakeholders.

Because the response phase is said to commence as soon as the incident is apparent and conclude when leadership declares it over, it is often the most comprehensive of the emergency management phases.

Hospital emergency managers must remain mindful of the fact that emergency incidents generate patients with physical and behavioral effects whose first impulse is to go to the location in their community that relentlessly dedicates itself to helping those in need: the hospital.

The Recovery Function

The primary goal of recovery efforts is to restore core services and normal operations. From a hospital planning perspective, the institution's recovery actions and implementation activities for its core financial, human resources, and support services should also be addressed.

Given the significant costs associated with incidents that directly impact hospitals, the recovery section of the emergency management plan should also detail its insurance coverage and include copies of the actual insurance certificates, key contact information for agents, and mechanisms to rapidly access funding.

Because emergency incidents often disrupt vital supply chain processes, it is imperative that alternative means for purchasing goods and services to support the hospital's core services be thoroughly outlined, again, with key contact information readily available. Ultimately, the institution's ability to recover from any incident, be it small or large, internal or external, will be based in large part on the recovery planning steps it has in place and activates postincident.

DISASTER STANDARDS OF CARE

An understanding has developed that in order for community healthcare delivery systems to remain viable and effective, community resources changes must occur with respect to the manner in which healthcare is delivered during disasters, terrorism, and public health emergencies. For many years, specific guidelines for healthcare deliverance were assumed or improvised when a disaster response was demanded of healthcare providers. The Institute of Medicine (IOM), which changed its name to the National Academy of Medicine, developed a report in 2009 that defined, for the first time, Standards of Care for healthcare that included the alterations necessary in the face of a disaster. The appropriately named Crisis Standards of Care (CSC) details the services that healthcare providers should deliver, based on their training, the situation, the environment, and the available resources, while keeping in mind the best outcome for the larger population (Hanfling, Altevogt, Viswanathan, & Gostin, 2012).

HOSPITAL DISASTER PLANNING

Every hospital and ED should have a comprehensive emergency plan. In most hospitals, the ED comprehensive emergency plan will be a part of the hospital plan. While the plan is important, the planning process that created the plan is far more important. While the discussion of all considerations in the disaster plan would exceed the scope of this chapter, several key elements for consideration follow.

Surge Capacity

The General Accounting Office (GAO [www.gao.gov]), which changed its name to the Government Accountability Office (GAO) in 2004, finalized reports during 2003 on the public health and hospital preparedness for bioterrorism and emerging infectious diseases. These reports found that most hospitals in the United States do not have the means to care for a surge of patients during a public health emergency. They stated that, based on the national ED diversion rates in urban and suburban areas, shortages in the healthcare workforce, and the general lack of available supplemental medical equipment and supplies in hospitals, the medical community is not prepared to handle a patient surge caused by an infectious disease outbreak or bioterrorism-related event. Though improvements have been made for many EDs across the United States, due to increasing need of response and the Joint Commission requirements, many facilities remain underprepared. Already operating in a state that is stretched to its limits, EDs are chronically understaffed, underresourced, and overused (American Hospital Association,

2010; Kamal et al., 2014). The current state of affairs in the nation's EDs makes it very difficult to prepare for surge capacity when many hospitals cannot effectively handle their daily patient volume.

Referral patterns of patients who present to medical facilities will vary in terms of how they arrive at the facility (emergency medical services [EMS] or self-transport) as well as which facilities they access (hospital ED or physician's office) depending on the type of disaster or public health emergency. In cases of natural disasters, explosions, and acute catastrophic events where there is a clear and defined "scene," many patients will be triaged, treated, and perhaps transported to hospitals or trauma centers by EMS personnel. In cases of bioterrorism or infectious disease outbreaks, patients would normally exhibit minor signs and/or symptoms of an illness (i.e., fever, rash, flu-like symptoms, etc.). These patients may present to their primary care physician or an urgent care center to receive initial diagnosis and treatment. The patients who can be expected to arrive at the ED in these cases would be those who could not access a private physician, those too acutely ill to seek care in an office setting, those referred to the ED by their physicians, and those patients who called EMS for assistance. This latter group would yield the least number of ED arrivals.

Incidents of chemical and biological terrorism as well as pandemic or epidemic incidents of infectious diseases may arguably produce the most significant burden on the healthcare system. A main reason for this is the unpredictable referral patterns of patients who fall victim to a chemical or biological hazard. Although some disaster after-action reports do suggest that even victims of conventional disasters will self-refer to medical facilities, the issues of delayed onset of symptoms, cross-contamination, and person-to-person disease transmission that are associated with a chemical, biological, or radiological incident call for more detailed contingency plans.

At some point during the evolution of a disaster or other public health emergency, patients will converge on acute care hospitals. Studies have consistently shown that despite rigorous planning initiatives, hospitals and EDs are not prepared to handle the mass influx of patients that a bioterrorism event or infectious disease outbreak would produce. During the Sarin attack on the Tokyo subway in 1995, the nearest hospital had 500 patients in the first hour after the incident and more than 20% of its staff was secondarily contaminated. It is important that planners recognize additionally, that in certain catastrophic disasters involving bombings, building collapse, and so forth, mass injuries and a patient surge may not occur as anticipated because of the high rate of mortality. The hospital and all those involved in hospital emergency management must ensure that their hospital has adequate plans for the surge of patients who will arrive during a disaster, terrorism event, or public health emergency.

Staffing

The current state of the U.S. healthcare industry, with its widespread staffing shortages, primarily in the field of nursing, negatively impacts hospital emergency management efforts. Moreover, the supply of healthcare professionals does not meet the demand for even basic healthcare services, so the idea of surge capacity, particularly in light of nursing resources, may be challenging to address. Alternatively, healthcare providers may also act in dual public safety capacities within the community (e.g., hospital-based first responders may also be volunteer firefighters within the community), thus limiting these staffs' abilities to respond in both capacities simultaneously.

Compounding these already weighty challenges, emergency incidents will affect many hospital staff members' willingness to remain at and report for work. During these times, concerns for themselves, their families, and the confidence they have in their own abilities to provide care during times of crisis pervade. Emergency incidents may also hamper staff members' abilities to physically report to their hospital, given impacts on transportation systems and personal obligations such as caring for children, elders, and pets. Institutions must realize that employees prepared on the individual level are better able to help themselves, and, therefore, others. Hospitals, with support of senior leaders, should encourage the utilization of personal preparedness resources that include checklists for food, water, medications, and financial records, and suggestions for pediatric and geriatric preparedness.

It is imperative, therefore, that the hospital emergency management plan addresses the challenges of staffing during crises and that the emergency management committee collaborates with staff to ensure the highest levels of service provision throughout the duration of any incident.

Credentialing

It has been shown that well-meaning volunteers will come to hospitals during crises to offer assistance. Hospital emergency management plans must address the means to screen and place volunteers. Some plans may call for volunteers to register in advance, so that in case of an emergency incident, they will already be conversant with the facility's emergency management plan. To address the accreditation issues in this area, the Joint Commission requires that hospitals have procedures in place to rapidly credential volunteer health personnel. Some states issue healthcare provider identification cards that verify an individual's professional status.

Stockpiling and Logistics

The ability of a healthcare institution to remain self-sufficient to provide and sustain core services without the support of external assistance for at least 96 hours from the inception of an incident, with a goal of 7 days, remains a vexing problem for healthcare leaders.

Unfortunately, the stark realities of lean organizations and just-in-time inventory management are directly counter to effective hospital emergency management planning. While these efforts seek to reduce costs and waste through the delivery of products on an as-needed basis, thin supply chains can lead to shortages of critical material resources such as pharmaceuticals, blood products, oxygen masks, disposables, and ventilators when demand for these goods rises sharply. A simple rule of thumb when developing the stockpiling and logistics section of the hospital emergency management plan is, "If a resource is not accessible by foot, it does not exist."

Resource Inventories

Hospital emergency management plans must include documentation and tracking of equipment, supplies, and resources. These inventories should include medical, nonmedical (e.g., food, linen, water, fuel for generators, and transportation vehicles), personal protective equipment (PPE), and pharmaceutical supplies. The emergency management plan must detail means for replenishing these critical assets and most hospitals will find *Memoranda of Understanding* (MOU) with their supply vendors for use during emergency incidents to be invaluable. Hospitals must be aware of these limitations to the MOUs. In large-scale events, it is likely that regional or state authorities will take over the distribution of supplies and vehicles. Regardless, alternative MOUs with local suppliers who may not be the usual vendor to a hospital would be a wise move.

Another source of resources is neighboring or affiliated hospitals, or hospitals distant from the affected area. Again, MOUs set up in advance give hospitals an advantage in situations where they may be challenged to maintain adequate supplies. These MOUs should also establish methods and timetables for repayment after the emergency incident has been secured.

In the case of pharmaceuticals, some hospitals choose to keep stockpiled caches of commonly used drugs for use in certain emergency incidents. Antibiotics such as ciprofloxacin, doxycycline, bronchodilator drugs, anticholinergic, and cyanide poisoning antidotes may be kept in reserve and used for nonemergency indications before they expire, as long as they are replaced by newer stock when consumed.

Security Issues

Hospitals frequently overlook the need to maintain adequate security of the healthcare facility and overall medical operations as part of both daily operations and emergency planning. The concept of "locking down" or restricting access to a healthcare facility is often contradictory to the typical hospital design and approach of open access to both patients and their families and other visitors. But during a disaster this type of control is essential for many reasons, which include, but are not limited to, control of the flow of patients to the areas where care will be provided, access to the facility only by authorized staff, accounting for staff and patients in times of evacuation, prevention of potentially contaminated patients entering the hospital prior to contaminating staff, other patients and facilities, and prevention of acts of terrorism.

HAZMAT/CBRNE Readiness

There is no question that in the current state of trauma system and public health preparedness that the medical community, while improving, is still ill-prepared to deal with an incident that involves the management and treatment of multiple potentially contaminated victims. Multiple recent reports of hospital preparedness cite decontamination capabilities as a serious weakness of disaster readiness plans. At the request of the CDC, researchers at the University of Alabama Birmingham conducted a study to poll hospital personnel at several facilities on their level of preparedness in the case of a hypothetical "dirty bomb" scenario;

the study found that participants consistently reported that their EDs and larger hospitals were not currently prepared to respond appropriately to such a situation (Becker & Middleton, 2008). Planning for these events has traditionally centered around the fallacy that patients will be decontaminated at the scene by first responders and then be triaged, treated, and transported to the ED. The decontamination process serves a dual purpose. First, it removes the potential agent that is causing harm to the patient, and second, it prevents the spread of secondary contamination to other patients and hospital staff. We have come to realize from recent incidents involving victim contamination that many ambulatory victims will leave the scene and bypass EMS decontamination and triage, seeking medical care on their own.

Throughout the nation, acute care hospitals are unprepared for handling an event involving the release of a nuclear, biological, or chemical (NBC) agent. The most often cited weaknesses are an overall lack of training, lack of PPE, lack of resources and equipment to rapidly and reliably perform preliminary agent detection, and lack of appropriate medical facilities, equipment, and supplies to effectively isolate infectious patients and manage them through the course of their illnesses.

Collaboration and Integration With Public Health

In order for disaster preparedness and response to be successful, it must involve interagency resources and consider the 3Cs of emergency response planning: Collaboration, Cooperation, and Coordination. Public health agencies at the federal, state, and local levels have the responsibility under the National Response Framework (NRF) to coordinate and serve as the lead agency for disasters involving mass care. This may include assisting both hospitals and communities to establish alternate care sites (ACS) where patients can be directed to receive medical treatment during a public health emergency, which will allow a hospital to use its resources to treat higher acuity patients and remain open to handle routine emergencies during a pandemic or other public health emergency.

Equipment and Supplies

In a sentinel GAO report of hospital preparedness (August 2003), the GAO reported several findings on hospital equipment and supply resources. The survey showed that for every 100 beds, 50% of hospitals had fewer than six ventilators, fewer than three PPE suits, fewer than four isolation beds, and could handle only fewer than six patients per hour through a 5-minute decontamination shower, given their current state of preparedness (U.S. GAO, 2003). In addition to PPE issues, hospitals and trauma centers often lack the inventory of equipment and supplies necessary to effectively treat an influx of potentially affected patients. Many hospitals, in a strategy to reduce overall costs, replenish their central supply on a "just-in-time" basis, clearly ineffective in preparing to treat a mass influx of patients. Pharmaceutical access is another concern among healthcare facilities. Maintaining an adequate pharmaceutical stock of essential antibiotics, antidotes, and specialty medications in case of a disaster is often viewed as cost prohibitive due to the shelf life and daily usefulness of certain drugs.

Utilities

Given the expectation that hospitals will provide services to those in need regardless of the impact an incident has on the facility's utility systems, the hospital must outline alternative means of providing for the myriad utilities required to operate the institution.

Ensuring that basic electrical services are provided is often best handled through the use of emergency generators. The specifics of these devices, which vary in size, capability, and cost, will often be outlined by local building codes and regulations, which can be invaluable to hospitals. However, with their functionality come significant support requirements.

Water needed for consumption and essential care activities is a taken-for-granted resource, the consumption volumes of which, when calculated, are staggering. Many hospitals maintain a cache of bottled water for consumption using the baseline metric of three bottles per person per day. Water needed for equipment and sanitary purposes presents additional challenges. The hospital emergency management plan should assist by providing the limits of the facility's water storage tanks and should contain sections on means to provide these services, either with limited water supplies or significant restrictions on the use of water.

Facility Evacuation

Evacuating a hospital is an extremely complex action that requires much advanced planning. For most incidents hospital plans call for shelter in place but one must recognize there are still situations which would require evacuation. Because it is so difficult, it should be reserved for the direst circumstances when the hospital environment cannot support basic care services. Shelter in place or internal evacuation (vertical or horizontal), such as in a fire, will usually involve a relatively limited number of hospital patients and staff, and transfers to specific units. Staff on individual units should be aware of fire escape routes. All staff, clinical and nonclinical alike, must be trained in the principles of evacuation. In an incident where time is limited, ambulatory patients should be moved first with minimal guidance from staff. The greatest efforts should be directed to rapid transport of patients who must remain prone and life-support–dependent patients. Several commercially available evacuation aids, such as Sked stretchers, stair chairs, infant carriers, and Evacusleds™, are available and should be kept for such occasions. However, common hospital resources such as wheelchairs, stretchers, blankets, and Isolettes should also be considered for use during rapid evacuations. The hospital should list the methods used to evacuate people and inventories of the resources and related equipment and supplies needed to also be evacuated.

When time is less pressing, but evacuation is still necessary, hospitals should transport not only the patients, but also the patient's related, relevant medical information and necessary supportive equipment. But there also should be plans for transfer of this information when feasible even for emergent evacuations. If evacuation to a distant alternative care site is warranted, hospital staff may be required to accompany patients to the new site and aid in their care.

Triage systems that are usually used for influx will be reversed for evacuation. The least sick will likely move first, and those who need the most care will likely move later due to the increased complexity of transportation. Staging areas should be developed ahead of time to house the patients awaiting vehicles for transportation to an alternative facility. Ambulatory patients may wait in large spaces, such as those atriums, cafeterias, and auditoriums designated as emergency alternative care sites. Sicker patients would have to be transported to a staging area on the ground floor that has the capability to supply care to the critically ill. In most hospitals this means the ED.

Drills and Exercises

Criticisms regarding drills and exercises are notable throughout the preparedness literature. Comments include statements that exercises are not realistic, drills tend to be conducted with advanced warning on shifts with favorable staffing levels, and with equipment and resource levels at their best, and so forth. Therefore, the drills bias any useful results from the exercise. The purpose of conducting drills and exercises, aside from remaining in compliance with accrediting bodies and CMS requirements, is to assess whether or not a facility is adequately prepared to handle an incident with relatively low probability, but with extremely significant impact on the health system, and to identify areas that need improvement from an operational and planning level (CMS, 2016). Exercises that simply go through the motions or are conducted with limited realism under optimal conditions, or are simply haphazardly conducted to meet regulatory or legal requirements, are futile and worthless assessment tools that will only perpetuate a hospital's state of unpreparedness.

ED Disaster Operations

The importance of the ED's role in disaster and emergency preparedness is discussed in several sources. Among the many strengths of the ED is the ability to integrate two major components of the trauma system: prehospital and definitive care. The ED maintains constant communications with the EMS system and serves as the direct point of entry for prehospital providers into the hospital. ED clinicians represent a critical link in the chain of survival by anticipating the resources that ill and injured patients will need upon arrival at the ED, and initiating appropriate lifesaving medical care until specialty resources become available.

Trauma Centers

The roles of trauma centers during a disaster, terrorism event, or public health emergency are consistent with their daily activities in the treatment of injured patients. Triage and treatment of injured victims after a disaster are frequently discussed as a central role of the trauma center in the aftermath of a disaster. Trauma centers are adept at the care of the injured victim, and are often viewed as the best choice for the triage and treatment of disaster-related injured victims, though they are limited by the resulting

increased overuse of these facilities. Another expectation is that trauma centers and acute care hospitals will be able to treat mass numbers of affected patients as well, including the rapid triage and treatment of all casualties (including those from CBRNE events), decontamination and/or isolation, and quarantine of contaminated or potentially infectious patients. Trauma centers are also expected to have access to essential equipment, supplies, and pharmaceutical agents (Cryer & Hiatt, 2009; Faul, Sasser, Lairet, Mould-Millman & Sugerman, 2015).

ALTERNATE CARE SITES

When planning for surge capacity, hospitals often realize that even creative use of existing space may not meet the needs of the number of ill or injured patients. A common approach to this problem is the planning for ACS. Alternate care facilities function as an extension to the surge planning process, through selection and utilization of locations to serve as a receiving point for patient overflow or those, for instance, who were impacted by exclusion criteria. This type of facility would likely serve patients with a lower level of acuity, chronic ailments, and/or those who require minimal supervised care. The establishment of alternate care facilities incorporates considerations related to the scope of medical care and staffing necessary to support patients using the prescribed standard of care. Alternate care facilities are also supported by disaster standards of care due to decreased numbers of clinicians and the resulting increased caregiver/patient ratio that exceeds recognized standards, for example.

Incident Command System

All emergency preparedness plans must contain an ICS. The ICS tries to avoid historical problems related to MCIs, such as inadequate planning, poor communications, lack of on-scene needs assessment, or triage of patients. In general, besides a command structure, the ICS also implements perimeters and areas to optimize responder safety and patient flow, as well as the preservation of evidence and environment. Additional ICS guidelines and education can be found online at the FEMA ICS Resource Center (training.fema.gov/EMIWeb/IS/ICSResource/index.htm).

The ICS has many potential components and configurations depending on the magnitude, location/terrain, weather, agencies required to be involved, as well as volunteering groups. For didactic purposes, lists and organizational illustrations may be simplistic, so it is important to keep in mind that these frames are very *elastic*, and should be tailored to the specific needs of the MCI.

The ICS has eight principles for adequate operation.

1. *Common terminology* avoids confusion by coordinating terms utilized with different agencies, allowing adequate identification of personnel, areas, equipment, and procedures.
2. *Modular organization* is based upon a "top-down development approach." Starting on the initial phases of the emergency, the Incident Commander will be responsible for the implementation and delegation of duties of the different functional areas, as the situation develops.

3. *Integrated communications* allow the coordination of communications plans, operating procedures, terminology, and common frequencies.
4. *Unified command structure* with one Incident Commander or a Unified Command with more than one agency shares responsibility for the management of the situation. However, the Unity of Command should be followed in which each person reports to one supervisor.
5. *Consolidated action plans*, verbally or written, ideally follow established strategic goals, objectives, and activities.
6. *Manageable span-of-control* in which the number of individuals who report to a supervisor is established, ideally five with a range of three to seven.
7. *Predesignated incident facilities* or zones that clearly indicate areas for command post, search and rescue, staging, decontamination, transport, press, and so forth.
8. *Comprehensive resource management* that coordinates and consolidates independent resources, avoiding cluttering of personnel and communications.

The implementation of the ICS within a hospital facility can be done following similar guidelines, as previously described. One approach to hospital incident command is called the Hospital Incident Command System (HICS). Initially developed in 1993 in California by the County of San Mateo EMS Authority, it has been used more and more nationwide as the basis for the hospital response in these situations. In HICS, besides the designation of hospital personnel as chiefs and leaders in the different positions, there is added to the Command Staff (Information, Liaison, and Safety Officers) a fourth member, as the Medical Officer (Figure 3.2).

Management of a Mass Casualty Situation

One of the most likely events a hospital and ED will have to address is the MCI. The ability to respond to such a situation is based on a good disaster-planning effort with a well-developed all-hazards comprehensive emergency management plan. In addition to the all-hazards plan, it is essential for hospitals and EDs to have a specific annex to the plan to address the MCI. This annex must address some of the unique challenges faced with a MCI.

Initial Evolvement of MCI

There are two distinct phases of care in a mass casualty event (Holcomb, Helling, & Hirshberg, 2001). Initially, during the arrival of casualties, the full magnitude of the event is unknown and the key element is conservation of limited hospital resources and facilities. Stable patients will temporarily receive only minimal acceptable care and will be transferred to other hospital areas awaiting later definitive care. Only critical—but salvageable—patients will have immediate access to key hospital resources such as imaging techniques and operating rooms (ORs).

The element of uncertainty in the first phase becomes even more prominent with the multistaged tactics practiced by Al-Qaeda and associated terror groups. Most recent terror acts were evolving, multistaged events: Such were the attacks on the Twin Towers in both 1993 and 2001, the 2013 Boston Marathon bombings, the 2015 Paris terrorist attacks with coordinated suicide bombings and shootings, 2016 Brussels airport and metro station bombings, and the 2017 London attack on Westminster Bridge and Parliament. Such evolving,

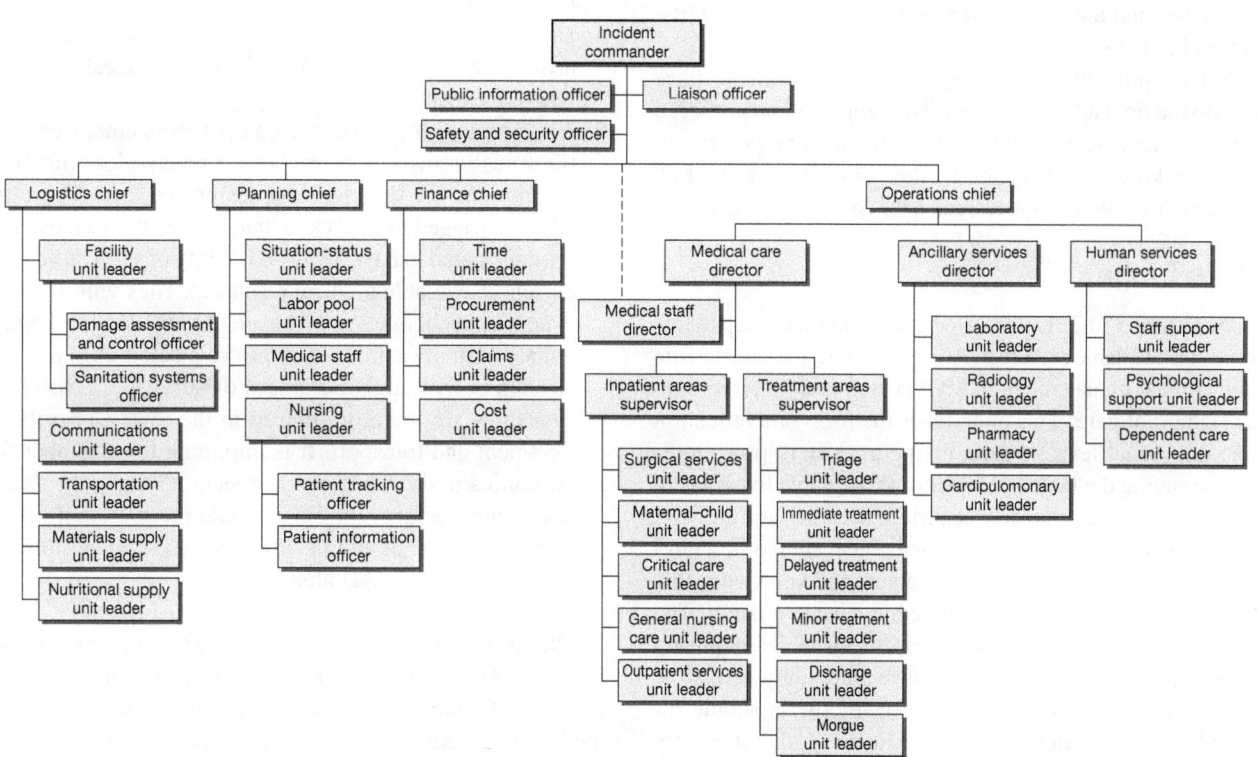

FIGURE 3.2 Hospital emergency Incident Command System organizational chart.

serial assaults in the same geographical area might disrupt any organized approach to manage MCIs, and contingency plans should take this into consideration. To achieve the best results, it is crucial to adhere to the basic principle of prioritization of care to life- or organ-endangering conditions with postponement of care to less severely wounded patients.

The second phase begins after containment of the event and arrival of all casualties. Following secondary triage, a comprehensive, priority-oriented plan for definitive care of all patients can be devised.

Casualties Flow to the Hospital

Casualties flow consists typically of three waves. The first wave, shortly after the event, includes casualties—usually with minor injuries—who evacuate themselves or are brought in by bystanders without previous triage. This wave arrives while the medical facility is still getting organized and most of the casualties arrive in the hospital closest to the scene. This wave can overwhelm any hospital and can practically block its emergency facilities (Bloch et al., 2007). It is therefore vitally important that with first notice, an experienced physician will be positioned in front of the ED to perform primary triage. The second wave consists of casualties with more serious injuries, which were triaged at the scene, may have required extrication and received initial treatment, and were evacuated by EMS transportation. The third wave consists of casualties with more minor injuries and of patients with emotional stress. This wave can persist for several hours to days after the initial event.

Casualties Flow Within the Hospital

Rapid, unobstructed casualties flow within the hospital is crucial. Factors to be considered are the hospital layout, potential bottlenecks, and the number of available trauma teams, ORs, and hospital beds.

The basic principle is a one-way, forward flow from the triage area into the final admitting ward. Therefore, patients proceed in their management track only forward, with no possibility of backtracking. Backtracking or slow flow through the ED, while casualty influx continues, can have chaotic consequences.

Patient Triage

By definition, a MCI is one in which the number of patients exceeds the available resources. As a result, a basic characteristic of the clinical management in MCI is temporary alteration in the standard of care. This often takes the form of a reduction in the individual level of care, giving priority to procedures aimed at saving the largest number of salvageable lives. There is an apparent correlation between triage accuracy and casualty outcome (Frykberg, 2002). The triage officer should be a physician experienced in trauma management and knowledgeable in the hospital's emergency preparedness triage system. The triage officer's role is to rapidly identify casualties requiring immediate interventions and who have potentially reversible injuries. To reduce over triage, the triage criteria should include physiological and anatomical indicators rather than only "mechanism of injury" criteria. In most systems, casualties are triaged into one of four (or five in some systems) categories.

The most commonly recognized categories and the usual colors used to designate them include:

RED	Immediate
YELLOW	Delayed
GREEN	Minimal
GRAY	Expectant (used in some systems)
BLACK	Deceased (or expectant)

A basic explanation of each color-coded category, with examples, is the following:

- *Immediate (Red)*—This includes severely injured patients with a high probability for survival. They need procedures of moderately short duration required to prevent death. Casualties with severe but potentially reversible injuries are the focus of medical efforts. Examples of these circumstances are airway obstructions, accessible hemorrhage, and sometimes emergency amputations.
- *Delayed (Yellow)*—These casualties require operative interventions that may be delayed without compromise of a successful outcome or life endangerment. Temporizing measures include IV fluids, splints, antibiotics, pain management, catheterization, or gastric decompression. Some examples are large muscle wounds, major bone fractures, uncomplicated major burns, head or spinal injuries, and intraabdominal and/or thoracic injuries.
- *Minimal (Green)*—This includes patients without serious injuries to vascular structures or nerves. The walking wounded can usually provide self-care or require only minimally trained personnel. The largest number of casualties belongs to this group.
- *Dead (Black)*—This includes patients found to be dead on arrival (DOA) and casualties with nonsalvageable injuries who are expected to die.
- *Expectant (Gray)*—In five category systems, expectant becomes its own category. These receive low treatment priority and are directed to a designated area. Casualties who are triaged to the "expectant" category are those who are considered to have a low probability of survival with the currently available medical resources. They will likely die even if all available resources are used to care for them. In a mass casualty setting, such effort is better used on other casualties with higher chances of survival. "Expectant" casualties are therefore placed in the lowest priority for treatment and transport. It is important to remember that casualties assigned to the "expectant" category should not simply be ignored. They should receive comfort care or resuscitation should be attempted as soon as sufficient resources become available.

One system for triage that has gained support in the United States is SALT (sort, assess, lifesaving interventions, treatment/transport; Figure 3.3; Lerner et al., 2008). The SALT triage methodology was intended, and designed, to be a national guideline for mass casualty triage in the United States. It was designed to be simple to use and easy to remember. It instructs

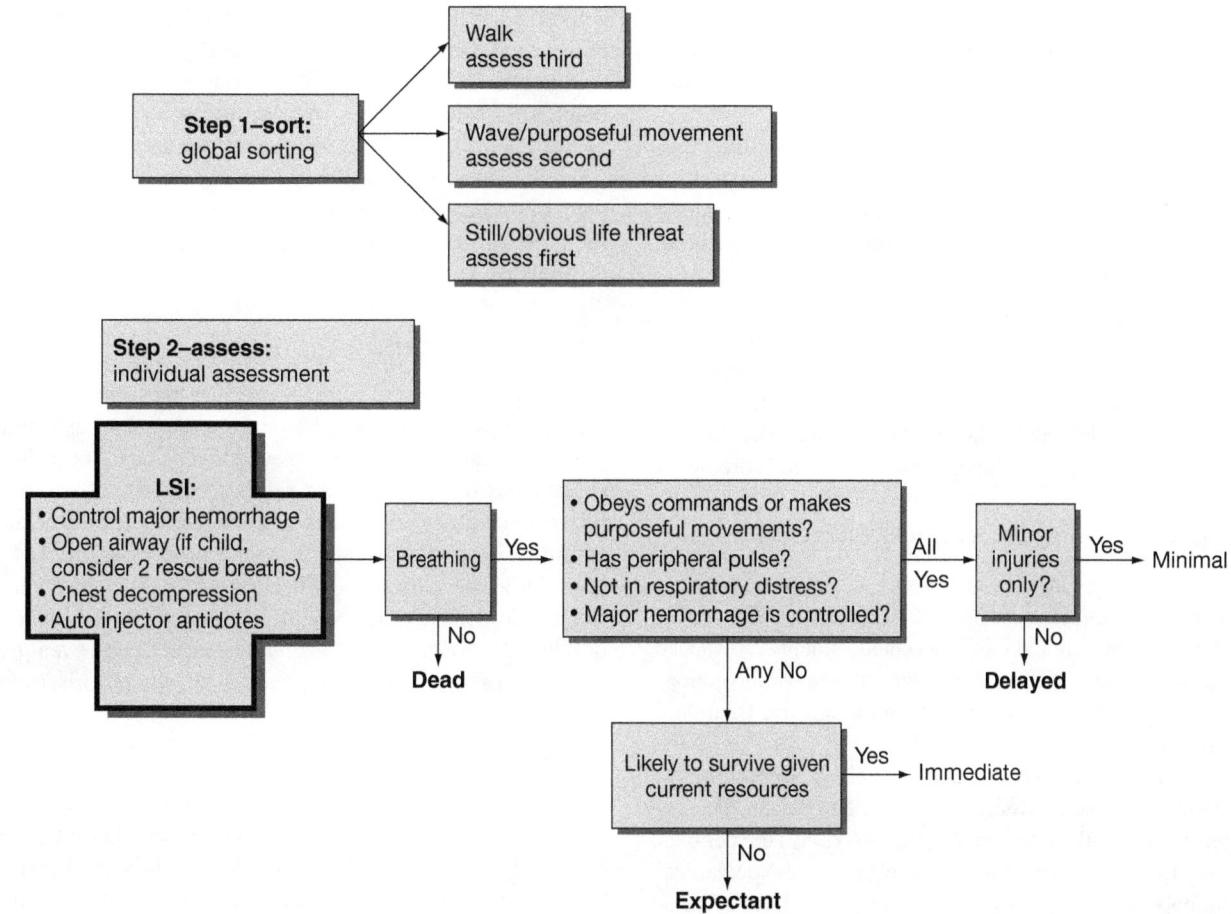

FIGURE 3.3 SALT mass casualty triage.

LSI, lifesaving interventions; SALT, sort, assess, lifesaving interventions, treatment/transport.

Source: Lerner, E. B., Schwartz, R. B., Coule, P. L., Weinstein, E. S., Cone, D. C., & Hunt, R. C. (2008). Mass casualty triage: An evaluation of the data and development of a proposed national guideline. *Disaster Medicine and Public Health Preparedness, 2*(Suppl 1), S25–S34. doi:10.1097/DMP.0b013e318182194e

providers to quickly "Sort" casualties by their ability to follow commands, then to individually "Assess" casualties, to rapidly apply "Lifesaving interventions (LSI)," and assign a priority for "Treatment and/or transport." SALT triage is intended to allow rapid evaluation and sorting of any age patient injured in any type of event. While applicable to different situations, SALT is most suited for scene triage and initial triage of those arriving at the hospital who may not have been triaged.

Step 1: Sort—SALT begins with a global sorting of casualties, prioritizing them into tiers for individual assessment. In this first step, casualties are asked to walk to a designated area. The responder should yell or use a public address system to say: "If you can hear my voice and need help please move to _____." Those who walk to the designated area are the last priority for individual assessment, since they are the least likely to have a life-threatening condition. Specifically, the ability to walk indicates that they are likely to have an intact airway, breathing, and circulation (they are unlikely to have severe breathing difficulties or a low blood pressure because they are able to walk from the scene) and intact mental status (because they are able to follow commands). Those who remain should be asked to wave (or follow a command) or be observed for purposeful movement

(e.g., trying to free oneself or self-treat an injury). The responder should yell or use a public address system to say: "If you can hear my voice and need help, please wave your arm or leg." Those who do not move at all, and those with obvious life threats (e.g., major bleeding) are assessed individually first since they are the most likely to need LSI. Those who wave are the next to be assessed. Those who walked to the designated location are the last to be assessed. It is important to note that the global sorting process will not be perfect. Therefore, every casualty must be individually assessed, even if they are able to walk.

Step 2: Assess—The second step is individual assessment of each casualty, starting with the first priority tier (patients who could not walk to the designated area and did not wave or have an obvious life threat).

Step 3: Lifesaving Interventions—During individual assessment, rapid LSIs are performed but only if they can be provided quickly, can greatly improve a casualty's likelihood of survival, do not require a care provider to stay with the patient, are within the responder's scope of practice, and any equipment that is needed is immediately available. Lifesaving interventions that meet these criteria include the opening of the airway with simple basic airway maneuvers, two rescue breaths in a child, performing needle decompression for casualties with signs of a tension pneumothorax, control of any major hemorrhage using pressure dressing or tourniquet, and providing auto-injector antidotes to casualties with known chemical exposure.

Step 4: Treatment/Transport—After any lifesaving interventions are performed, casualties should be prioritized for treatment and/or transport by assigning them to one of the five triage categories described previously (Immediate, Delayed, Minimal, Expectant, or Dead).

A key point to always remember is that each casualty should be individually assessed as previously described irrespective of the tier, but, starting with those who during global sorting did not move, followed by those who followed the "wave" command, and then those who followed the "walk" command.

Principles of Initial Hospital Management

Treatment priorities in MCI are to save salvageable patients and to prevent complications and future handicaps. Generally, patient management should follow accepted guideline, Advanced Trauma Life Support (ATLS), though only essential interventions are performed in the first phase and comprehensive treatment of all injuries is postponed.

Teamwork is crucial: Teams of a physician and (preferably) two nurses should be preassigned to every ED station. The ED director (or other title based on hospital ICS) plays the conductor's role: He coordinates medical teams, oversees specialists' assignments, sets priorities for transfer to the OR, ICU, or ward, decides about further imaging, and ensures continuous patient flow through the admitting area. An important task is to prevent overcrowding and excessive commotion in the ED. Personnel not directly participating in patient care should be kept away to avoid havoc.

Use of Radiology

The radiology department is a common bottleneck during disasters and should be used judiciously. As a rule, mobile radiography and radiography of the chest, cervical spine, and pelvis are not performed on a routine basis. Point-of-care or bedside sonogram has the advantage of being fast, inexpensive, and noninvasive and, when used effectively by trained professionals, can greatly reduce the pressure on radiology in disaster events. One study, conducted in Guatemala after a mudslide, found 12% of scanned patients with an emergent problem and excluded disease in 42%, greatly saving time and effort on those without pathology (Dean, Ku, & Zeserson, 2007). A bedside abdominal ultrasound, known as a Focused Assessment with Sonography for Trauma (FAST), is also quick and beneficial; but should be used sensibly, that is, in unstable patients, to confirm or rule out intra-abdominal bleeding. Computed tomography (CT) scanning should be reserved for restricted indications and the ED director should make these decisions. Brain CTs are performed only to assist decision making regarding neurosurgery.

Operating Room

The OR is also a major bottleneck. Therefore, its immediate use should be reserved for a few "absolute" indications such as compromised airway or control of active bleeding endangering life or limb. Other surgeries are delayed to later phases.

Once in surgery, the fundamental approach is "damage control." Basically, this situation demands that surgeons, accustomed to expending enormous resources and time on single patients, reset their priorities and rapidly provide only the minimal acceptable care, moving patients quickly through the most needed operative procedures in order to maximize care to as many patients as possible.

Secondary Transport

An important aspect of primary triage at the scene is dividing patient load among available hospitals, taking into consideration "specialty" capabilities such as neurosurgery, burns, or pediatric surgery. Secondary transport refers to transfer of casualties between medical facilities. This is indicated when the primary admitting hospital is unable to provide proper care due to lack of essential specialties, overwhelmed with patient load, unable to provide needed surgery within a reasonable time period, or when the hospital itself is compromised by the event (i.e., nature disaster, hazardous materials event, war/terrorist event).

Reassessment Phase

Following the first phases of the event, all casualties should receive definitive, appropriate treatment. To avoid misdiagnoses and overlooking of injuries, designated teams should perform this reassessment, review every patient's chart, and recommend further investigations or interventions. Once again, decision making and planning should be centralized, taking into consideration individual priorities as well as the entire hospital's capabilities.

Communication and Manpower Control

Rapid staff recruitment is crucial and each hospital should have an effective paging system. Insufficient physician attendance in the ED of a large urban hospital was recorded in the first hours after a major earthquake because physicians were helping their own families and because of lack of communication or transportation. On the other hand, Israeli experience and data from disaster events have repeatedly shown that a large portion of the hospital staff shows up even without being paged. Emergency preparedness plans should allocate a staff waiting area with communication to the event director(s) who will allocate personnel according to needs.

An Emergency Operations Center (EOC) should be manned rapidly in a preestablished location and one which has been pre-equipped for this role. Aside from communication within the hospital, communication (preferably radio) with the EMS forces at the scene is critical. A preestablished communication plan that complies with both state and federal law is now required by the CMS regulations (CMS, 2016).

Information Center and Public Relations

A public information center should be opened as soon as possible. Its telephone lines should be designated in advance and their numbers should be announced by the electronic media after the event. The information center should have software for creating a database of missing persons in a manner that has been prearranged by the hospital and local emergency management and law enforcement agencies. In some cases these agencies may provide staff for this function. As the hospital may be "stormed" by worried relatives, the information center should be located distant from the patient management area.

COMMUNICATION AND INFORMATION TECHNOLOGY ISSUES

Two key elements cited in all evaluations of disaster, terrorism, and public health emergency events are communication and information technology systems. Telecommunications, including telephone, radio, two-way radio, video, facsimile, and digital imaging via satellite transmission, have been used in response to disasters (see Chapter 36). Telemedicine is one technology that can be used not only during the disaster phase but also before and after as a way to educate the community, institute prevention programs, and establish emergency assistance, public health measures, and sanitation services. The use of the Internet and electronic mail can also prove effective. The use of cellular phones is very convenient, but unfortunately, during MCIs (especially in terror acts), cellular networks tend to collapse due to overcrowding and cannot be relied upon. Radio communication is the preferred mode of communication.

By identifying the vulnerabilities in the existing system of healthcare communication systems, we can take steps to address these issues and further increase our health system preparedness. Addressing the vulnerabilities in communication systems and planning how to overcome them is an essential responsibility of a hospital emergency manager. Many of the criticisms of the current health system's communication systems center around the inability to communicate easily with external agencies and share critical information. Disaster after-action reports and exercise-improvement plans almost universally cite poor communication as one of the problems associated with incident management and the event being reviewed.

Infrastructure support is an important consideration when examining whether adequate safeguards are in place to support the systems we will rely upon during a disaster. On September 11, 2001, while one New York City hospital was preparing to treat a large number of (anticipated) casualties from the disaster, they experienced a loss of their computer and information systems (Feeney, Parekh, Blumenthal, & Wallack, 2002). This unplanned event arose because the communication system line that supported their system's infrastructure ran beneath the World Trade Center. Additionally, other reports have cited problems with battery failure and the lack of a prolonged power supply as limiting communication systems' abilities during an event. This example illustrates a major point in emergency communication systems: Hospitals need the ability to connect all significant parties during a disaster or other emergency and the system should be based on a redundant infrastructure. Clearly, from a planning perspective, this would be a desirable option. However, the reality remains that investing in communication

systems is a significant financial burden on already underfunded hospitals and healthcare systems.

Risk communication is often overlooked during the planning phase of an event, and this can lead to frustration and confusion during disaster operations. Risk communication is sometimes the only way for the public to gain an understanding of the scope and severity of an incident. Additionally, risk communication information provided by hospitals may be used to help families of disaster victims find information about their loved ones' condition. Reviews of risk communication have shown that a predesignated public information officer (PIO), who will liaise with the media and the public and who has specific training and experience in giving briefings and fielding questions, should perform all risk communication tasks during disaster operations. Specific elements of risk communication that may be conveyed to the public may include information on evacuations, scope and breadth of the event, where and how to obtain assistance if needed, whom to call for specific information, location of postexposure prophylaxis or vaccination clinics, and what to expect over the next several hours and/or days of the event.

HOSPITAL-BASED DECONTAMINATION AND PEDIATRIC CONSIDERATIONS

For many years, the standard level of preparedness for most hospitals in the case of a patient with a hazardous substance exposure has been the ability to perform a cursory decontamination of the individual in the ED. Many hospitals have a dedicated "decon" or "HAZMAT" (hazardous materials management) room, which has a shower and some equipment to perform this function, but it likely serves as an equipment closet or storage area most of the time. Although most hospitals have considered the need to perform emergency decontamination of victims from a hazardous substances incident, many reports have underscored the lack of hospital preparedness for victims from a HAZMAT-related event.

The process of developing the capability to perform single patient or mass casualty decontamination takes time, effort, and funding. It is easier for hospitals to initiate planning for hazardous substances emergencies when a full-time emergency manager is employed by the healthcare organization; however, this is often the exception rather than the rule in healthcare emergency management. It is also important that pediatricians be involved so the specific needs of children in decontamination are included in the hospital plan. The OSHA *Best Practices for Hospital-Based First Receivers of Victims from Mass Casualty Incidents Involving the Release of Hazardous Substances* document discusses elements of decontamination planning that should be included in the decontamination plan as an annex to the hospital's overall emergency operations plan (OSHA, 2005). Engaging community stakeholders during this process can assist in creating a sound operating plan. Community stakeholders include the local hazardous materials response team, the local office of emergency management, the health department, private companies that use toxic industrial chemicals or materials, and others as appropriate.

Essential elements of the decontamination plan should include the following information:

- Notification procedures for staff to implement if information becomes available that patient decontamination may need to be performed.
- How to contact members of the decontamination team and assemble the staff trained to perform decontamination.
- Site security procedures to lock down the hospital and secure entrances to ensure that all victims who may present to the hospital are routed to a single entrance to minimize the risk of facility contamination.
- Location of decontamination site setup and appropriate criteria for determining when to set up tents and other equipment.
- The appropriate type of PPE and respiratory protection to be used to perform decontamination.
- Triage procedures.
- Functional roles of team members and relevant Job Action Sheets.
- Training requirements of team members and general hospital staff.
- Medical surveillance policies and procedures for team members.
- Communications procedures.
- Staffing configurations and shift rotations for decontamination staff.
- Integration of the team ICS structure into the overall HICS structure.
- Demobilization procedures.
- Cleanup and site restoration plans.

Initial identification of the hazardous material may be impossible until scene responders contact the hospital with the specific nature of the substance. There are, however, ways to determine the general type of substance based on the signs and symptoms reported by victims. Chemical agents are usually associated with an acute or rapid onset of symptoms consisting of irritation or burning of the eyes, mouth, and nose; dizziness or light-headedness; shortness of breath; altered mental status; or loss of consciousness. The rapidity of symptom onset in these victims is the key that will usually point to a chemical exposure. Additionally, the history of present illness will give clues to the nature of the exposure, such as what the victim was doing when the symptoms first began. Victims may report they were at work or in a traffic accident when the symptoms began, suggesting an occupational or accidental exposure.

Current mass casualty decontamination procedures for adults are risky for children. Children have a higher surface area and a more difficult time with temperature regulation; decontamination with room temperature or colder water can lead to dangerous hypothermia. Although hypothermia may be a risk, it is less risky than not decontaminating a child. Young children may be unable to understand the concepts of decontamination and will be unable to comprehend why they must be separated from their family and asked to strip down with strangers. Lastly, response personnel should ensure that

clothing is available for children after decontamination. This includes diapers for infants.

Many shower systems are not suitable for children, who require systems that use warm water and are high-volume but low-pressure. Shower decontamination units designed for young children and infants must be able to accommodate an adult (parent or caretaker) as well as the child. Specific questions to be addressed for pediatric decontamination are:

- Is the water pressure appropriate? Will it injure a child?
- Is the water temperature acceptable? If water is not warm, it may cause hypothermia.
- Can the process handle the nonambulatory child, as well as infants, toddlers, and children with special healthcare needs?
- Does the method and equipment used allow decontamination of a child with a parent or caregiver?
- Will children follow instructions?
- Have mental health concerns been addressed?
- What are the long-term effects of such decisions?

Similar to nonambulatory patients, children will require more time to decontaminate, and require additional staff to assist the child through the decontamination process. Consider the following when decontaminating children:

- Keep children with their families or a caregiver whenever possible.
- Have the child go through the decontamination tent with the parent and allow more time to ensure that both the parent and the child have been washed for a minimum of 5 minutes.
- Be conscious of the increased risk for hypothermia in the pediatric population.
- Take steps to ensure that decontamination water is heated when possible and that blankets and heaters are used in the postdecontamination area.
- Attempt (when possible) to have dry pediatric-specific garments (e.g., gowns, diapers) available in various sizes for use at the decontamination location.

SUMMARY

Hospital and ED emergency management is an essential aspect of modern healthcare. The emergency management activity must be directed by a multidisciplinary group that is central to all activities and reports directly to hospital administrative and medical leadership. This planning effort must focus on all phases of disasters, mitigation, preparedness, response, and recovery. These activities must be based on an all-hazards approach to ensure preparedness for disasters, terrorism events, and public health emergencies. Lastly, these efforts must be inclusive of entire populations and ensure the hospital is able to continue to function during any event to serve its critical resource in the community and serve the entire population.

STUDY QUESTIONS

1. What would be some important personnel positions or departments to include in a hospital emergency management committee? Why would it be important to include these individuals or departments?

2. What would be some specific considerations when planning hospital preparedness for pediatrics?

3. Briefly describe each phase of emergency planning.

4. What is a memorandum of understanding?

5. Please describe how the concept of patient triage in a disaster differs from standard triage practices.

6. What questions may a first responder ask of disaster victims on scene to assist with the sorting phase of SALT triage?

7. What are common communication challenges in a disaster?

REFERENCES

American Hospital Association. (2010). *The State of America's Hospitals: Taking the Pulse.* Retrieved from https://pdfs.semanticscholar.org/presentation/1891/f3f5fc2a19c0d1103143c8357d49379a61b0.pdf

Becker, S., & Middleton, S. (2008). Improving hospital preparedness for radiological terrorism: Perspectives from emergency department physicians and nurses. *Disaster Medicine and Public Health Preparedness, 2*(3), 174–184. doi:10.1097/DMP.0b013e31817dcd9a

Bloch, Y. H., Leiba, A., Veaacnin, N., Paizer, Y., Schwartz, D., Kraskas, A., . . . Bar-Dayan, Y. (2007). Managing mild casualties in mass-casualty incidents: Lessons learned from an aborted terrorist attack. *Prehospital and Disaster Medicine, 22*(3), 181–185. doi:10.1017/S1049023X00004623

Centers for Medicare and Medicaid Services. (2016). *Medicare and Medicaid programs: Emergency preparedness requirements for Medicare and Medicaid participating providers and suppliers.* Federal Register 81 (180). Washington, DC: Centers for Medicare and Medicaid Services, U.S. Department of Health and Human Services.

Cryer, H. G., & Hiatt, J. R. (2009). Trauma system: The backbone of disaster preparedness. *The Journal of Trauma, 67*(2), S111–S113. doi:10.1097/TA.0b013e3181ae9d63

Dean, A. J., Ku, B. S., & Zeserson, E. M. (2007). The utility of handheld ultrasound in an austere medical setting in Guatemala after a natural disaster. *American Journal of Disaster Medicine, 2*(5), 249–256.

Faul, M., Sasser, S. M., Lairet, J., Mould-Millman, N. K., & Sugerman, D. (2015). Trauma center staffing, infrastructure, and patient characteristics that influence trauma center need. *Western Journal of Emergency Medicine, 16*(1), 98–106. doi:10.5811/westjem.2014.10.22837

Feeney, J., Parekh, N., Blumenthal, J., & Wallack, M. K. (2002). September 11, 2001: A test of preparedness and spirit. *Bulletin of the American College of Surgeons, 87*(5), 12–17.

Frykberg, E. R. (2002). Medical management of disasters and mass casualties from terrorist bombings: How can we cope? *Journal of Trauma, 53*, 201–212. doi:10.1097/00005373-200208000-00001

Hanfling, D., Altevogt, B. M., Viswanathan, K., & Gostin, L. O. (Eds.). (2012). *Crisis standards of care: A systems framework for catastrophic disaster response.* Committee on Guidance for Establishing Crisis Standards of Care for Use in Disaster Situations; Board on Health Sciences Policy; Institute of Medicine. Washington, DC: National Academies Press.

Holcomb, J. B., Helling, T. S., & Hirshberg, A. (2001). Military, civilian, and rural application of the damage control philosophy. *Military Medicine, 166*, 490–493. doi:10.1093/milmed/166.6.490

Joint Commission. (2007). Emergency management standards. *Environment of Care News, 10*(12), 2–8.

Joint Commission. (2008). Preparing for catastrophes and escalating emergencies. *Environment of Care News, 11*(1), 1–3, 11.

Kamal, N., Kelly Barnard, D., Christenson, J. M., Innes, G. D., Aikman, P., Grafstein, E., & Marsden, J. (2014). Addressing emergency department overcrowding through a systems approach using big data research. *Journal of Health and Medical Informatics, 5*, 148. doi:10.4172/2157-7420.1000148

Lerner, E. B., Schwartz, R. B., Coule, P. L., Weinstein, E. S., Cone, D. C., & Hunt, R. C. (2008). Mass casualty triage: An evaluation of the data and development of a proposed national guideline. *Disaster Medicine and Public Health Preparedness, 2*(Suppl. 1), S25–S34. doi:10.1097/DMP.0b013e318182194e

U.S. Department of Labor. (2005). *OSHA best practices for hospital-based first receivers of victims from mass casualty incidents involving the release of hazardous substances.* Washington, DC: Occupational Safety and Health Administration, U.S. Department of Labor.

U.S. General Accounting Office. (2003). *Hospital preparedness: Most urban hospitals have emergency plans but lack certain capacities for bioterrorism response.* Report to Congressional Committees, GAO-03-924. Washington, DC: Author.

4

EMERGENCY HEALTH SERVICES IN DISASTERS AND PUBLIC HEALTH EMERGENCIES

Jeremy T. Cushman, Manish N. Shah, and Mahshid Abir

LEARNING OBJECTIVES

When this chapter is completed, readers will be able to:

1. Review common characteristics of the current emergency health services system.
2. Discuss the emergency health services planning necessary for disaster preparedness.
3. Discuss the major emergency health services challenges that must be addressed within a disaster plan.

KEY MESSAGES

The emergency health services system is a complex network of various providers, organizations, and facilities that provide evacuation, stabilization, and redistribution.

The multiple components of the emergency health services system and the complex processes of entry and exit create many potential problems and inefficiencies, particularly when stressed by a disaster.

Paralytic disasters or catastrophic events will severely limit the emergency health services systems' ability to respond.

CHAPTER OVERVIEW

Emergency health services (EHS) constitute a critical element of the medical response to disasters, and their planning is a key component of community disaster preparedness. This chapter reviews the characteristics of the EHS system, the challenges and barriers facing the system, and how these challenges may affect disaster response. Potential solutions are identified, and the EHS planning necessary for disaster preparedness is outlined.

THE EHS SYSTEM

EHS Components

The Emergency Health Services system is a complex combination of various providers and facilities that provide three basic medical functions: evacuation, stabilization, and redistribution. Although organizational structures and resources vary worldwide, the fundamental components of any EHS system are essentially the same. Those components are the prehospital emergency medical services (EMS) system, EDs, and alternate sources of emergency care.

The EMS system traditionally includes all services from the receipt of emergency requests for assistance to the transport of patients to EDs. In most circumstances, EMS dispatchers receive the call for assistance and, in response, send appropriate resources to the patient. Some communities provide maximal EMS response to all patients regardless of their complaint; however, in most areas, dispatchers have special training and follow protocols to triage patients' acuity and provide the appropriate resources given the complaint. The Medical Priority Dispatch System (MPDS) is an example of a commonly used triage system specifically designed to abstract caller information through a question-driven protocol and direct appropriate resources based on that information. Despite the widespread use of MPDS, only limited evaluation has been published on its accuracy and effect on patient outcome (Hettinger, Cushman, Noyes, & Shah, 2013; Shah, Bishop, Lerner, Fairbanks, & Davis, 2005), and there are no studies on the effectiveness of MPDS during disasters.

Through the protocol-driven triage process, dispatchers determine the level and rapidity of response required. EMS providers' scope of practice and positions are dependent on the providers' level of training and certification, and range from emergency medical responder through paramedic, and provide care that can be divided roughly into two levels—basic life support (BLS) and advanced life support (ALS). Generally, BLS providers (e.g., Basic Emergency Medical Technicians [EMT-B], Advanced Emergency Medical Technicians [EMT-A]) can administer oxygen and provide extrication, immobilization, and bleeding control and also assist patients in taking their own medication (e.g., nitroglycerin; Institute of Medicine [IOM], 2015). Some areas allow BLS providers to administer additional medications (e.g., albuterol, naloxone, epinephrine) or perform additional procedures (e.g., continuous positive airway pressure). ALS providers (e.g., EMT-A, Paramedics [EMT-P]) can perform more advanced skills, including intubation, needle thoracostomy, defibrillation, and cardiac pacing, while administering a wide variety of pharmacotherapy, including advanced cardiac life support medications (IOM, 2015). Regional variations in the scope of practice for both BLS and ALS providers exist, requiring planners to be familiar with local community training, standards, and practices. More advanced certifications and scopes of practice also exist for paramedics and reflect additional training such as in hazardous materials (HAZMAT) management, critical care, tactical medicine, aeromedical operations, and community paramedicine.

The second component of the EHS system is the hospital ED. Fundamentally, EDs receive undifferentiated, unscheduled patients, and they evaluate and provide initial diagnosis and management of the patient's presenting condition. EDs have differing diagnostic and treatment capabilities due to a number of factors including staff capacity, community structure, availability of specialized care, and inpatient capability-related resources. Many EDs in the United States are staffed continuously and exclusively by emergency medicine–trained physicians, while other EDs, usually rural, rely on alternative staffing sources such as on an on-call physician or advanced practice providers (e.g., nurse practitioners or physician's assistants; Casey, Wholey, & Moscovice, 2008). Although essential to ED functions, certain types of consult services and support staff may be irregularly or entirely unavailable. For example, a small community hospital may not have specialized care such as neurosurgery, pediatrics, or obstetrics, limiting the level of care provided. Accordingly, the hospital's ED and inpatient capabilities may range from providing basic care to administering specialized, advanced interventions such as trauma, stroke, and cardiac care. Based on the various resources available at the hospital, the EMS system may have protocols in place to direct patients with certain conditions (e.g., trauma or burn) to the most appropriate facility.

Alternate sources of emergency care can come in various forms (e.g., freestanding, urgent care centers, physician offices). Freestanding EDs are becoming increasingly common. Although not attached to hospitals, these facilities have the same capabilities as EDs attached to hospitals, but without immediate access to consultative services (Schuur, Baker, Freshman, Wilson, & Cutler, 2017). Many communities have urgent care centers that provide care for minor illnesses and injuries. Some are equipped to perform laboratory testing and radiographs, provide intramuscular or intravenous medications, or provide more advanced therapies. Physician offices are also an alternate source of emergency care. Some integrated physician practices already evaluate and care for acutely ill patients on site. These practices can provide services such as laboratory, radiographic, or even cardiac stress testing. These sites can and should be considered part of the EHS system because they possess tremendous resources that may be accessed in times of increased patient demand. Finally, telemedicine, defined as the "use of electronic information and communications technologies to provide and support healthcare when distance separates the participants," (IOM, 1996, p. 2) is increasingly being used as an option to deliver emergency care directly to patients in the community, to EDs without subspecialty services (e.g., stroke neurology), and even to EDs to assist with the triage process (Marcin, Shaikh, & Steinhorn, 2015).

Although not part of the traditional EHS system, satellite or surge EDs are preexisting healthcare facilities that can be activated in the event of a disaster to provide emergency care. These sites can include schools, arenas, stadiums, jails, or fairgrounds that have predefined treatment areas for injured or ill patrons or are simply "facilities of opportunity" that lend themselves well to adaption as an emergency care facility (Joint Commission, 2006). Depending on the resources invested, satellite EDs can provide a level of service ranging from simple first aid to advanced care, including radiographic and surgical capabilities or observation units. These facilities have the potential to provide the required level of care for many patients if their capabilities are investigated and integrated into the region's disaster plan (Cheng et al., 2015; Henderson et al., 1994).

Increasingly, EHS systems are employing the use of community paramedicine to bridge the gap between EMS and ED care. These programs utilize existing EMS resources to augment a community's health needs by providing a range of services. These can include screening for vaccination status, depression, and impaired cognition; referring to existing community resources such as home health, nutrition, mobility, and social services; providing safety assessments, clinical assessments, medication reconciliation; and performing limited diagnostic studies (Bennett, Yuen, & Merrell, 2017; McGinnis, 2004). The role and characteristics of community paramedicine programs are rapidly evolving, but the fundamental structure of these programs, as well as the core program characteristics, are in place in many communities. Although a number of barriers to these programs exist, namely regulatory and financial, community paramedicine remains an important resource for population health during a disaster. As an example, during the H1N1 Pandemic the Rochester, New York area used paramedics to vaccinate thousands of emergency responders—a scope of practice not authorized under routine circumstances but expanded given the public health threat.

Standard Operation of EHS

Under ordinary circumstances, entry to EHS in the United States occurs most often when individual patients request assistance through the 911 system or when they present to EDs or urgent care centers. Once in the care of EMS, patients are transported to EDs for further evaluation and treatment. Initial care may be provided on site or en route to the ED. Patients presenting to EDs with limited capabilities, or urgent care centers, may also be transported to other sites for additional or specialized care. Under disaster-related circumstances, patient entry to EHS is sudden and comes in surges, challenging EMS first responders and EDs with the need to adapt resources (e.g., beds, medical supplies, medication) and staffing by surge capacity, or to utilize alternative sources of care within the EHS system with a potentially disaster-compromised infrastructure (U.S. Department of Health and Human Services [HHS], 2014). For instance, a patient suffering a blast injury may initially receive temporizing care in a smaller local or rural ED without trauma services and then be transported to a regional trauma center for admission and more definitive therapy.

Patients exit the EHS system most commonly by being discharged to home or admitted to inpatient units (including observation units). During disaster-related circumstances, patients receiving inpatient hospital services may be assessed, and discharged if identified as safe for discharge to make room for disaster-related patient surge (HHS, 2014). For example, during Hurricane Sandy, hospitals in affected areas reported having patients at a rate nearly 50% higher than normal (HHS, 2014). Hospitals may continue to shelter critically ill or fragile patients without providing care, and patients who need continued care may be evacuated to makeshift hospitals or shelters where continuity of care is possible (HHS, 2014). Patients discharged to home require transportation, which can be a limiting factor during a disaster. For patients admitted to inpatient units, common limitations are the availability of bed space (Asplin et al., 2003; Hoot & Aronsky, 2008) and, if needed, isolation rooms and equipment.

The multiple components of the EHS system and the complex processes of entry and exit create potential points for problems and inefficiencies, particularly when the EHS system is stressed by a disaster. Cooperation and integration among the groups interacting within the EHS system, such as fire and police departments, are critical to preventing or overcoming problems and inefficiencies within the system. Cooperation within organizations, such as between environmental services and nursing, or between different nursing units, is both practical and critical. Community challenges to collaboration for resources (e.g., fuel, transportation, and hospital beds) must be eliminated. Otherwise, the ability to respond to disasters will be limited and communities and patients will suffer (Chavez & Binder, 1996; HHS, 2014).

Current State of EHS

Today, many would consider the EHS system to be operating in disaster mode on a daily basis, with resources being stretched so far it lacks the flexibility to handle a sudden increase in patient volume (American College of Emergency Physicians, 2014; American Hospital Association, 2015). EDs throughout the United States are routinely overwhelmed with "boarders"—patients who cannot leave the ED because of a lack of inpatient beds. Treated and stabilized patients exiting the system lack an appropriate destination and/or the means of getting there (exit block). Thus, the EHS system must divert its resources to caring for stabilized and admitted patients rather than new acutely ill patients. This situation, described by the input–throughput–output conceptual model of ED crowding (Asplin et al., 2003; Hoot & Aronsky, 2008), has exit blocks that cause "entry blocks," which progressively limit the ED's ability to function. Because the input of ED includes EMS output, when the ED's input gets blocked, the EMS output gets blocked, preventing EMS from caring for new patients. This systemic inability to manage throughput and output, and hospitals' inability to recruit capacity due to system pressures, is a dangerous condition at any time and is particularly problematic when responding to a disaster, when input increases dramatically and output is more limited by transportation and resource limitations (Love et al., 2016).

The difficult circumstances under which the EHS system operates is compounded by staff shortages. The national nursing shortage is well described and unlikely to resolve soon (American Association of Colleges of Nursing, 2014). Some areas of the nation, particularly more rural areas, also lack sufficient physician staffing, particularly for specialists. Estimates suggest that by 2025 a shortage of as many as 94,700 physicians will exist in the United States (American Association of Medical Colleges, 2016). Some shortages of EMS staff also exist (National Association of State EMS Officials, 2014). All of these shortages, which are challenges during regular EHS system operations as they impair throughput, can become serious impediments to an EHS system's capability to respond to disasters.

Financial stressors have also adversely affected the EHS system. Providers face increasing labor and supply costs while suffering from a decrease in reimbursement, when reimbursement is even possible. These financial pressures are reflected in the closure of hospitals (particularly safety net hospitals), bankruptcy proceedings for a number of major EMS providers, and decreasing budgets for many EMS agencies. Given these survival challenges, EMS providers have difficulty meeting daily routine operational needs, let alone undertaking other projects such as disaster planning, particularly when these projects are not externally funded (National Association of State EMS Officials, 2015).

The current sickly state of EHS is a challenge. However, the recognized need for improved disaster response provides opportunities for emergency managers to use their preparations to address current challenges as they prepare for potential disasters. By integrating disaster technology, terminology, and actions into routine operations, one can increase their success during a disaster (Auf der Heide, 2006).

MAJOR EHS CONCEPTS ASSOCIATED WITH DISASTERS

EHS typically differentiates between a mass casualty incident (MCI) and a disaster. Any influx of patients from a single incident that exceeds the capacity of the EHS system can be considered a MCI (American Society for Testing Materials [ASTM], 2009; Auf der Heide, 1989; IOM, 2015, p. 132). A bus accident in a small town may quickly become a MCI if the responding EMS agency or local ED resources are overwhelmed. In a metropolitan area, however, an accident of the same magnitude could be considered a routine event, requiring additional transport units and dispersal of patients to multiple hospitals but not to such an extent that it overwhelms the system. This same incident, therefore, affects two EHS systems differently, but in both cases would not constitute a "disaster."

In turn, EHS will typically refer to a "disaster" as a natural or man-made phenomenon that results in the destruction or dysfunction of the available response infrastructure to meet the community's need for healthcare (ASTM, 2009; Auf der Heide, 1989). Thus, in the case of a hurricane or power outage, only a few injured people may require medical care; however, because the health system infrastructure may have been destroyed, the disaster may clearly require outside assistance to meet the healthcare demands of the community. This type of disaster is sometimes referred to as a "paralytic" disaster because it has the potential to eliminate the EHS's ability to respond to any call for services, let alone extra demands for care resulting from the event. This was exemplified by the 2011 Fukushima nuclear accident, earthquake, and tsunami, and by Hurricane Katrina in New Orleans in 2005, which devastated the community healthcare capacity (Berger, 2006; Fukunaga & Kumakawa, 2014).

The EHS system must be prepared for both MCIs and disasters; fortunately, the planning is similar for both. Throughout the rest of the chapter, we refer to MCIs and disasters interchangeably, but the difference is important to appreciate. The variable nature of disasters that occur with widespread differences in cause and impact (e.g., natural or man-made) and the overall characteristics of each disaster result in a complexity that makes disaster planning very difficult; however, there are a number of unifying concepts that can be considered (Brown, Hickling, & Frahm, 2010; Green, Modi, Lunney, & Thomas, 2003).

All disasters have a time component including the length of time in which the disaster occurs, and the amount of time necessary for recovery. For most, the length of time in which a disaster occurs is very short. With an explosion, a shooting, or a tornado, the damage will occur during a brief period and recovery will follow. However, the impact from this type of event can endure, even beyond 3 months (Hougan, Nadig, & Altevogt, 2010; Sheppa, Stevens, Philbrick, & Canada, 1993). In contrast, a biological attack, infectious epidemic, or flood may cause damage over a longer period, with new patients appearing continuously, healthcare resources being limited, and EHS systems being adversely impacted (Morita et al., 2016). For a routinely overwhelmed EHS system, the premise that most disasters cannot be expected is extremely important for preplanning. The EHS system must be capable of rapidly expanding its ability to treat and transfer patients from the field to the ED and from the ED to their appropriate disposition (admission, specialty care, home, or morgue) to effectively respond to the incident at hand.

The types of disasters vary widely. Some result from planned activity, such as the World Trade Center attacks, while others are accidental, such as the Chernobyl meltdown. Still others are natural, such as the Ebola virus disease (EVD) or severe acute respiratory syndrome (SARS) epidemics, the Indian Ocean earthquake and tsunami of 2004, or the Fukushima triple disaster. Damage may be caused by a contagion such as EVD or SARS, a contaminating event such as a chemical release, or kinetic trauma. Disasters may also entail multiple mechanisms of injury. For example, an explosion resulting in kinetic trauma and chemical exposure further complicates both terminology and response. The EHS disaster plan must account for different types of disasters and be flexible depending on the incident. For example, treatment and transport of contagious patients will require significantly different resources compared with that of victims of a building collapse. Some events, such as the Fukushima disaster, may involve large population displacement and destruction of infrastructure, while others are much more localized. The northern California wildfires (2017) were sudden onset, prolonged disaster events that severely challenged the capacity of Fire Fighter and EHS response.

RESOURCES FOR THE EHS SYSTEM

The scope of a disaster, and the resources necessary in the aftermath, can vary greatly and are partially dependent on the characteristics of the disaster's location. A disaster in a rural community may not be considered a major event in an urban area because of the greater resource availability characteristic of urban areas. Conversely, an event that would have an impact in an urban setting may have next to no impact in rural areas because of low population densities. State, regional, and federal support does exist and will likely be made available in the event of a disaster; however, because a required chain of notification must be completed to obtain outside support and because it takes time for state or federal officials to marshal the proper resources, disasters are usually local for the first days (Auf der Heide, 1989, 2006; Kaji & Waeckerle, 2003; U.S. Department of Homeland Security [DHS], 2008). In the first few days, the extent of the support may be limited by the nature of the disaster (e.g., Hurricanes Katrina, Harvey, Irma, and Maria); further, a widespread infectious epidemic may require that resources be dispersed to a number of regions (e.g., SARS), while a purely local disaster could result in state and federal resources being focused only on one location (e.g., Murrah Federal Building Bombing, Oklahoma City; Hirshberg, Holcomb, & Mattox, 2001; E. K. Lee, Chen, Pietz, & Benecke, 2009).

Regional and Federal Assets

A number of regional assets may also be available to the EHS system. The Metropolitan Medical Response System (MMRS) program is one of the better-known local/regional EHS auxiliary programs. This program identifies metropolitan areas that are vulnerable to terrorist events and, through federal grant funding, supports the development of local, organic response capabilities. Member organizations of a comprehensive MMRS program include EMS, fire/HAZMAT, law enforcement, public health, and local hospitals, while other agencies may be involved as is locally appropriate (e.g., emergency management, public works). Funding is used to develop the capability to respond to and mitigate a terrorist event of any type. Basing their organization on the Disaster Medical Assistance Teams (DMATs) that are a part of the National Disaster Medical System (NDMS), some states have developed and funded State Medical Assistance Teams (SMATs). These teams provide statewide medical response capability for disaster mitigation.

The NDMS is also a key organization for the efficacious management of a potentially overwhelming patient load that is associated with a disaster (HHS, 2017). Blockages in patient "outflow" from healthcare facilities will eventually result in barriers to "inflow." By transferring patients out of regions affected by disasters and by providing DMATs (and other important medical assistance services), the NDMS can both decrease inflow and remove blockages to outflow, improving a community's ability to cope with a disaster using its own resources. This is extremely important to facilitate patient movement to capable healthcare facilities outside of the disaster area since NDMS can facilitate movement with resources that the EHS system lacks due to the local demand. Although NDMS resources are constantly prepared

for deployment, the time from notification to patient care is on average 48 to 72 hours. Thus, although the NDMS is an essential resource for large-scale disaster response, it cannot be relied on to provide medical care and operational control during the first days of a large-scale incident. This responsibility falls on local and regional response agencies.

In an attempt to ensure universal availability of medical equipment, pharmaceuticals, and vaccines, the Strategic National Stockpile (SNS) is a federally funded program that maintains a reserve of these items. In the event of disaster, the SNS may be activated to meet critical supply needs, particularly for those items that are rapidly consumed in the early management of patients during a disaster. The request procedure, types of equipment and pharmaceuticals available, extensive distribution requirements of the SNS, and time lag for arrival of the SNS are essential to understand the limitations of this resource and make necessary plans for its effective use (Centers for Disease Control and Prevention, 2017).

PATIENTS' ACCESS TO EHS DURING A DISASTER

The impact of a disaster on EHS will vary based on the characteristics of the incident. For the purposes of this discussion, we will concentrate on a brief and isolated event such as an explosion. When such an incident occurs, the EHS system will immediately experience a large influx of patients accessing the system. It is estimated that the EHS system in a MCI will face a sudden surge of five to ten times the usual number of patients (Adalja et al., 2014; Chen, Cheng, Ng, Hung, & Chuang, 2001; Henderson et al., 1994). The first wave of the influx will present in two ways. One group of first-wave patients will be cared for by EMS when they respond to the scene of the incident and will be transported to health facilities. The second group of first-wave patients will directly present to EDs by foot, personal vehicle, or nonmedical public transport such as bus or taxicab.

After this initial first wave, a second wave of patients will usually follow. These patients are usually more sick or injured than the first wave of "walking wounded" because they needed to be extricated and assisted, actions that take some time to perform. Overall, the majority of patients will arrive via means other than EMS, and the majority of patients will not be critically ill (Auf der Heide, 2006; Henderson et al., 1994; Hirshberg et al., 2001; Hogan, Waeckerle, Dire, & Lillibridge, 1999; Reilly & Markenson, 2010). The number of patients arriving to EDs by non-EMS means should not be underestimated. The Murrah Federal Building Bombing in Oklahoma City had 33% of casualties arrive by EMS, while the Sarin Gas Attacks in Tokyo had only 11% arrive by EMS. Perhaps the most dramatic example is the World Trade Center attacks, where of the 7,364 patients treated at hospitals, only 6.8% (504) arrived via EMS (Auf der Heide, 2006; Reilly & Markenson, 2010).

Upon presentation, each patient must be rapidly triaged. A complete discussion of the various triage algorithms and their advantages and disadvantages is beyond the scope of this chapter; however, some studies have shown that upward of 50% of patients are overtriaged, regardless of whether triage occurs at the ED or on scene (Frykberg & Tepas, 1988; Gutierrez de Ceballos et al., 2005; Israel Defense Forces Medical Corps, 1997; Pesik, Keim, & Iserson, 2001; Ramesh & Kumar, 2010). This overtriage rate is concerning because the triage process exists to distribute resources optimally. If patients are overtriaged, those who need rapid and critical interventions may not receive them and, according to one study, the mortality rate of severely injured patients increases with an increasing overtriage rate (Frykberg & Tepas, 1988; Roccaforte & Cushman, 2007).

Recently, increased attention has been paid to the practice of "reverse triage." Although the precise environment in which this practice should be used has not been defined, nor have there been any studies to validate its use, the concept of reverse triage may become part of the initial management of a large-scale disaster (Satterthwaite & Atkinson, 2010; Tzong-Luen & Chi-Ren, 2005). In brief, there may be certain disasters, such as nerve agent release, in which treatment of the most acutely injured may be futile and require the expenditure of too many limited resources. Instead, those with less severe symptoms should be treated because they have a greater likelihood of survival from exposure to the agent, similar to military triage wherein the least injured are treated first to allow their return to the battlefield (Jenkins et al., 2008; Wiseman, Ellenbogen, & Shaffrey, 2002). Similar triage algorithms have been discussed for victims of infectious agents and blast injuries (Chaloner, 2005; Ramesh & Kumar, 2010). Although a thorough discussion of reverse triage is beyond the scope of this discussion, the disaster planner should be familiar with the concept and the forthcoming literature on this controversial topic.

For EMS, the ED is the typical destination. However, requiring that all patients from a disaster go to an ED is an inefficient use of a community's available resources. To prevent unnecessarily clogging an ED, some disaster plans employ alternate resources for the healthier patients, reserving EDs as primary resources for those who are critically ill. In the attack on the Pentagon on 9/11, an urgent care center across the street from the Pentagon provided significant stabilizing care as well as definitive care for the less injured. Although the center's location was an accident of location rather than planning, it was nonetheless highly effective ("Arlington County after Action Report," 2002; Eastman, Rinnet, Nemeth, Fowler, & Minei 2007).

Even within a destination category, patients are often poorly distributed. One review of 26 disasters found that on average 67% of patients were treated at an ED (Auf der Heide, 1996), even though other EDs were available (HHS, 2014). In the Oklahoma City bombing, seven of 13 hospitals used only the ED to provide services, while the other six triaged appropriate patients to other areas of the hospital (Hogan et al., 1999). Proper distribution of patients is required to ensure that specialized interventions can be delivered to patients requiring those services (Amram, Schuurman, Hedley, & Hameed, 2012; Auf der Heide, 1989; Einav et al., 2004; Hirshberg et al., 2001). In 2000, after a pedestrian bridge collapsed at a NASCAR event in North Carolina resulting in more than 89 injuries, EMS continued to send patients to a local hospital despite that hospital's statement that they could not handle more patients. However, two local trauma centers saw less than 5% of the total patients. This misdistribution occurred because the bridge collapsed across a major road and the responding ambulances arrived

on the north side of the bridge, putting them closer to the local community hospital. Rather than driving back a quarter mile and taking a bypass route, the EMS providers simply drove another half mile to the local hospital, dropped off their patients, and returned to the scene. In this case, significant issues with patient distribution occurred and these challenges have been seen most recently in the Aurora, Colorado (2012); Orlando, Florida (2016); and Las Vegas (2017) mass shootings.

One specific concern relates to the conflict of appropriate patient distribution and the goal of "clearing" all the patients from the scene as quickly as possible. Although critically ill patients certainly require definitive treatment (and thus transport) as quickly as possible, rapidly transporting all patients, including noncritical patients, may have the effect of simply moving the disaster from the scene to the ED. A built-in "pause" to reevaluate the severity of illness and appropriate destination after all critical patients have been transported may alleviate the risk of certain "downstream" elements of EHS being overwhelmed. This is particularly important in potential terrorist events whereby a primary event (e.g., an explosion) may be used as an attractant before a secondary event (larger explosion or biological/chemical agent release) is used to inflict further harm to bystanders and responders. In these cases, EMS may purposely try to evacuate to a casualty collection point before commencing hospital transport. In some cases, however, that casualty collection point becomes the ED and thus it is important that the ED builds in a triage process to ensure its resources are not immediately overwhelmed and access to critical resources for the critical patients is maintained.

Patients accessing the EHS system for reasons different from the disaster itself complicate patient distribution plans. Although many individuals access the system for conditions directly related to the disaster, such as illness or trauma, others have indirect issues, such as loss of electrical power or the inability to obtain needed resources such as oxygen tanks or social services (Adalja et al., 2014; Prezant et al., 2005; Rand, Mener, Lerner, & DeRobertis, 2005). Still others access the system due to psychiatric issues related to the disaster (Jones et al., 2000; North & Pfefferbaum, 2013). Finally, the worried well often access the system for evaluation and reassurance, particularly during chemical or biological exposures. One amusing case was a homeless gentleman well known for regular visits to an ED who presented with concerns regarding the SARS virus during winter 2003 to 2004 (S. M. Schneider, personal communication). Although there was no chance he had been to Canada or the Far East or had been exposed to anyone with SARS, he was still concerned and presented to the ED, thus potentially diverting resources from others.

Even during a disaster, individuals still access the EHS system for routine conditions unrelated to the disaster, although data from the SARS epidemic in Taiwan found a decrease in regular EMS requests during the extended disaster conditions (Ko et al., 2004). Three major challenges exist regarding patients presenting for concerns unrelated to the disaster. The first is ensuring that ill patients continue to access care. A patient having a myocardial infarction should not avoid care due to concerns regarding the disaster. The second is accurately triaging these requests for assistance to allow care in an optimal time at the optimal site. Finally, in the event of a chemical, biological, or infectious exposure, segregating potentially contaminated patients from noncontaminated patients is critical.

In Rochester, New York, and select other cities, the EMS system chose to address these concerns during the 2009 to 2010 flu pandemic by utilizing the 911 dispatch system to prioritize requests for care related to symptoms consistent with the flu by directing noncritical requests for ambulance service to recorded information lines or nursing/physician hotlines. This served to minimize EMS personnel's exposure to potential flu cases, minimize the use of EDs for non-acute complaints, and retain the ability of the EHS system to respond to "routine" requests for service. Other communities addressed these concerns by establishing triage processes to divert patients to makeshift satellite EDs within a hospital or even "drive-thru" EDs that were able to register, triage, assess, and treat low acuity flu cases without having the patient get out of his or her car (Weiss, Ngo, Gilbert, & Quinn, 2010). Obviously, the disaster type will define the ability for systems such as this to be realistic and effective; however, enhancing throughput and minimizing cross-contamination are often required in any disaster response.

MAJOR EHS ISSUES

In the discussion of the current EHS system, a number of major issues for planners have been identified. This section will directly discuss those and related issues while proposing possible solutions.

System Survey

The first major task faced by planners is to assess the current state of the EHS system for the purpose of understanding the potential impact of disasters; to regularly engage EDs and EMS in the disaster planning process; and to determine EHS needs and opportunities for improvement. Significant variability exists in the components of the EHS system. Planners must know the exact capabilities of each component (i.e., ED, EMS, hospital). For the EMS dispatch system, how is dispatch performed and how can it be used to make triage decisions? For EMS, how many ambulances and EMS providers exist? How many can be requested from surrounding regions? How are the destinations of EMS patients determined? For EDs, how many can handle major trauma? Minor trauma? Intensive care patients? How can a massive influx of patients be handled? What alternate sites for care exist? What transportation resources are available for distributing treated patients efficiently to maintain ED inflow and outflow? What alternate shelter sources exist? What preparations for mass decontamination are in place? This survey must be continually repeated to ensure that the latest data are available to planners to inform evidence-based practice.

Resource Availability

Three types of EHS system resources are critical to responding to any sort of MCI or disaster: facilities, personnel, and materials. The modern healthcare system is extremely lean and

in some areas operates over capacity. This results in a system with great difficulty handling sudden changes in volume such as the influenza season, let alone the rapid influx of patients from a disaster. Health facilities serve as the location for patient care and shelter while simultaneously requiring specialized resources for decontamination, isolation, and medical and surgical treatment. However, these facilities may be destroyed, contaminated, or access to them limited, making the health facility both a victim and responder.

Furthermore, the resource availability of EHS systems is further characterized by their "surge capacity," or ability to respond to the sudden increase in patient demands that will result during a disaster. This capacity to respond to increased health demands extends beyond the scope of an individual facility or single ED and is reflective of the wider healthcare system (Agency for Healthcare Research and Quality, 2006; Hick et al., 2004; Watson, Rudge, & Coker, 2013). The availability of facilities and large capital resources are critically important. As mentioned, the current healthcare systems—including the emergency, acute, and chronic care components—are all operating at maximal capacity. However, EMS vehicles, ED and hospital beds, and operating rooms will be needed in differing levels based on the incident (Auf der Heide, 2006; Pesik et al., 2001). For the EMS system, planners must know and address mutual aid issues as many states have plans and processes in place to shift resources between cities in the event of a crisis. Thus, additional ambulances, communications equipment, and maintenance facilities can be deployed throughout the region. In other areas, mutual aid compacts must be in place to allow for the immediate recruitment of as many additional EMS units as are needed (Auf der Heide, 2006). That said, all of these requests take time and the existing "routine" EHS needs must be met. An option to assist disaster planners with transportation needs is to consider alternative vehicles such as buses and wheelchair or stretcher vans to move patients who require minimal medical care within the EHS system as one must assume that all EMS resources (ambulances) will be unavailable.

For the EDs, bed space is a significant issue. Hundreds of hospitals have closed and the remaining EDs are at or exceed capacity and therefore plans to shift the existing patients and open beds must exist. Alternatives such as satellite EDs and nontraditional care sites must be considered and developed (Aghababian, Lews, Gans, & Curley, 1994; Chavez & Binder, 1996; Davis et al., 2005). For hospitals, similar plans are necessary. Specialized resources, such as decontamination rooms and systems, operating rooms, and trauma and burn specialty teams must be sufficiently available (Burgess, Kirk, Borron, & Cisek, 1999; Clarke et al., 2008). It is a matter of concern that most medical directors and hospital personnel feel their sites are not prepared to handle a biological, chemical weapon, or nuclear incident (Becker & Middleton, 2008; Treat et al., 2001).

The chronic care system is of particular concern. Nursing homes and rehabilitation facilities have very high acuity patients. Home health services provide care for ill patients in their homes. Often, these are patients who would have been admitted to the hospital in the past. In the event of a disaster, particularly a prolonged disaster such as an infectious epidemic, these services must be maintained. These patients will otherwise become ED patients, contributing to the burden borne by the EHS system. Data from the Northeast power outage of 2003 found that for one EMS agency in New York, 35% of their requests for assistance were related to chronic care patients who could no longer survive at home without electricity to power equipment such as oxygen concentrators (Rand et al., 2005). Alternate strategies, including the provision of needed supplies to chronic care facilities to circumvent their use of EHS during a disaster, must be planned in advance.

Human resources are a second critical resource and ensuring the availability of personnel—administrative, physician, nursing, and support staff—is a major issue for which many organizations are ill prepared (Hogan et al., 1999; Treat et al., 2001; World Health Organization [WHO], 2011). Large numbers of people are not necessarily needed to respond to the disaster, but individuals with the right expertise are needed. It is imperative to consider not only skilled healthcare staff but also the numerous ancillary staff who ensure proper facility operation such as environmental services, food service, maintenance, and security personnel (Gamboa-Maldonado, Marshak, Sinclair, Montgomery, & Dyjack, 2012). This became clear during the response to Hurricane Katrina when, after the primary healthcare needs were met, many requests through the Interstate Mutual Aid Compact were for "technician" and support staff, not direct patient care providers.

The task of ensuring sufficient human resources is complicated. At baseline, nearly all aspects of the EHS system face staff shortages, particularly nurses (Schneider et al., 2010). The effect of this shortage may be exacerbated during a disaster because of an increased need for both short- and long-term staff and the potential "loss" of staff. Staff may be functionally "lost" if they are impacted by the disaster and cannot work, as they were in the Taiwan earthquake and the SARS epidemic where 236 paramedics were unable to work at the outbreak's peak in Toronto (Chen et al., 2001; Verbeek, McClelland, Silverman, & Burgess, 2004). Staff can also be "lost" if they are required to report for other duties. For instance, many EMTs work at multiple agencies or work in EDs, while others may have National Guard or military reserve duties or may be members of specialty disaster teams. Planners must be careful to take into account each individual's primary reporting site. Staff may also be functionally lost if they become exhausted from a prolonged event. The physical and mental health of staff must be protected and supported to ensure that they can continue to function in potentially difficult circumstances. This requires secure areas for personnel to sleep, relax, bathe, and eat between extended shifts.

Staff may be lost if they are unable to physically get to work. A disaster may destroy or make bridges and roads unusable. Debris, floods, or an energy shortage may prevent use of cars or mass transit. For example, a catastrophic earthquake could destroy all of the bridges and many of the roads, preventing staff from getting to their workplace.

Finally, staff may be lost if they refuse to report to work. Data remain conflicted as to whether staff will report to work during a disaster (Aoyagi, Beck, Dingwall, & Nguyen-Van-Tam, 2015; Narasimhulu et al., 2015). More important to planners are the studies that have identified that certain factors will increase the likelihood that staff will report to work, such as better communication, providing means of transportation, staff and family prophylaxis, and child day care (Aoyagi et al., 2015). These factors must be directly addressed to ensure that sufficient human resources exist throughout the EHS system.

The opposite problem may also develop. The phenomenon of convergent volunteerism is likely to occur and is widely reported for a number of large disasters (Auf der Heide, 2003, 2006; Cone, Weir, & Bogucki, 2003). At the Oklahoma City bombing and the World Trade Center disaster, well-meaning volunteers rushed to help, possibly encouraged by press reports requesting medical assistance. This can prove to be problematic because when convergent volunteerism occurs, not only do professionals need to manage the disaster and maintain scene safety, they also need to maintain scene command, crowd control, security, organization of volunteers, volunteer safety, medical oversight, accountability, liability, patient tracking, and credentialing. As an extreme example, a nurse who responded to the scene with no training for urban search and rescue was killed by falling debris in the hours following the Oklahoma City bombing (Cone et al., 2003).

The final critical resource is material, especially supplies and medications (Hogan et al., 1999; WHO, 2011). If supplies and medications are lost or exhausted because of the nature of the disaster, EHS cannot be provided. Complicating the matter is the need for both sufficient and appropriate supplies based on the type of incident. A traumatic disaster may require large amounts of radiological supplies and bandages, while an infectious disease incident may require laboratory testing supplies and isolation equipment. Most incidents will need medications of various types and all require electricity. Technology- or medication-dependent populations will be particularly affected including dialysis patients, methadone treatment programs, and the lack of pharmacy resources as was seen in such diverse disasters as the Los Angeles earthquakes and Hurricane Sandy (Adalja et al., 2014; Chavez & Binder, 1996). Although the SNS may alleviate some of these pressures depending on the disaster, it will not be available immediately. Furthermore, the SNS is stocked based on expectations and past lessons learned; thus a particular event may have requirements that cannot be met by the SNS alone.

Critical nonmedical supplies, such as fuel to maintain generators, must be maintained in preparation for disaster. Plans must exist for accessing local, regional, and national stores of these items. Equally critical are financial resources, particularly given the poor financial state of EHS and the healthcare system nationally. Even before the disaster occurs, funding must be available for appropriate disaster planning. During the disaster, EHS system components will have to purchase supplies and pay staff. However, disaster insurance reimbursements and federal support will be delayed, leading to a cash-flow problem that could impede the delivery of care, particularly if the disaster is large and prolonged. Finally, after the disaster, funds will be needed to recover. Facilities and equipment may have to be repaired or replaced or decontaminated, while supplies and medications will have to be restocked.

Fortunately, in the United States, the critical resources of facilities, personnel, and material are generally available. However, the situation must be monitored to ensure that changes in the system, such as the closure of hospitals and ED crowding, do not lead to shortages during a disaster. Furthermore, given the tremendous reliance on technology, an incident such as a contaminated water supply, power outage, or disrupted telecommunications system can lead to a dramatic impact on the EHS system and severely strain the available resources (Adalja, et al., 2014; Auf der Heide, 2006; Quarantelli, 1983). As the events in New Orleans after Hurricane Katrina showed, a catastrophic disaster with widespread devastation will create a resource strain and lead to significant shortages in not only the affected area, but the surrounding unaffected communities that respond to assist (Berger, 2006; Nates & Moyer, 2005).

Communication and Coordination

Communication of information and coordination of the response are major challenges due to the current structure of the EHS and healthcare systems. Unlike those found in other countries, the U.S. healthcare system is splintered (W. H. Lee, Chiu, Ng, & Chen, 2002; Stange, 2009). Competing healthcare systems are reluctant to share information and resources because it could place them at a competitive disadvantage. This makes the sharing of medical information from one hospital to the next, or from a private physician's office to the ED, difficult if not impossible (Susman, 2005). As most hospital information systems do not optimally support disaster events, both patient care and documentation of that care become difficult during a MCI or disaster (Landman et al., 2015).

Additionally, the components of the EHS system are not integrated and do not share information and resources well. For instance, the EMS, fire, and other public safety agencies are often splintered without regional integration (Susman, 2005). Furthermore, communication is limited because of technical considerations as agencies often use different radio frequencies that are not compatible with each other. The disaster itself can also complicate the poor preexisting communication and coordination systems (Auf der Heide, 2006; Cone et al., 2003; Garshnek & Burkle, 1999). As a result, it is difficult for any disaster manager to have a good sense of the resources available, the needs of the community, and the evolving MCI. Recognizing this, guidelines and federal grants now exist to support communication interoperability for emergency responders (O'Connor et al., 2004).

Since September 11, the DHS has further developed and required the use of the National Incident Management System (NIMS) for all public safety agencies that request federal grant funds (DHS, 2017). The NIMS structure is used on a daily basis by fire, EMS, and law enforcement agencies for incidents large and small, and its consistent use across prehospital and hospital environments is critical for an effective disaster response. Developed by communications and disaster experts, the system provides an established template to enable and foster communication and coordination and is a foundation for disaster preparedness. All planners must be familiar with NIMS and ensure that those who will be responding to a disaster or MCI—whether hospital or prehospital—are well versed in its use and their role within the NIMS structure. Although a complete discussion of NIMS is beyond the scope of this chapter, there are a few important considerations relevant to its use in EHS.

The Incident Command System (ICS) within NIMS refers to the organization and operation of an emergency response to an incident. ICS has been used for years by fire and EMS agencies to deal with incidents such as a large fire or major motor vehicle crash and has become ingrained in the initial incident management of public safety agencies, making its scalability, flexibility, and familiarity to EHS personnel its greatest strength during an MCI or disaster. ICS is very well developed and excellent for scene-level activity where numerous agencies or teams are working simultaneously. It does not always, however, provide the same level of coordination for scene to EMS to ED communication such as monitoring available resources, tracking, and repatriating patients. These potential problems with ICS were particularly notable during the Singapore Airlines crash in 2000, which resulted in 82 fatalities and where resource and patient misallocation occurred as a result of poor communication and coordination from the scene to healthcare facilities (W. H. Lee et al., 2002). However, by utilizing certain principles of ICS, these hurdles can be overcome as the importance of the unified medical command system was noted as a strength of the response to the collapse of the Versailles Wedding Hall in Jerusalem in 2001 (Avitzour et al., 2004).

Interagency conflicts and interoperability-associated challenges among EHS-involved entities are two aspects of emergency health service response that may impede interagency cooperation and communication. EMS agencies, police and fire departments, hospitals, and others have some overlap in their roles and duties. These overlapping duties can prevent individuals from knowing their roles in a disaster, a key deficiency noted in previous disaster responses. Compounded with overlapping duties are the factors related to interjurisdictional cooperation, differences in entity structure, prior history of conflict or cooperation, the incentives for stakeholders to participate, power and resource imbalances, and leadership (Kaji & Waeckerle, 2003; Kapucu, Arslan, & Demiroz, 2010). These misunderstandings can lead to conflict, impeding the efficiency by which the disaster response can occur. These challenges can be mitigated, however, by taking action to ensure all agencies participate in the evidence-based disaster planning process.

During the planning phase, all agencies must be focused on the overall goal. They must work together, clearly delineating and documenting each agency's roles and responsibilities to help minimize future conflict, and maximize efficient use of resources. This interaction during the planning phase can also allow the staff of the different agencies to achieve a comfort level with each other. This familiarity can help significantly when the agencies must work together during a stressful disaster response. The very structure of NIMS, which incorporates the planning and implementation of the ICS, can also help minimize conflict because within the system lie defined lines of command and responsibility.

Two additional ways to minimize conflict include training and technology. Training will allow those who would respond to a disaster to work together and become more comfortable doing their jobs. The training will also challenge the disaster plan while allowing for the continuing education of those participating (Sweeney, Jasper, & Gates, 2004). If no drills are run, there will be no detection of problems, no achievement of comfort between staffs, and no improvement in the system (Auf der Heide, 2006; Kaji & Waeckerle, 2003). In addition, the drills need to be realistic, without an announced incident, without common knowledge of the start and stop times, and with all agencies participating to ensure an accurate analysis of the system's ability to respond to such a disaster. Training exercises alone are not necessarily sufficient, however (Sweeney et al., 2004). Shortly before the Singapore Airlines crash in Taiwan, the airport had just completed a set of drills; however, a review of the incident found that the responders failed to use the MCI protocols practiced during that training (W. H. Lee et al., 2002).

Modern technology can also help maximize communication and coordination and address issues of staff failing to follow MCI protocols. Human factors have been shown to be influential in the failures of MCI plans and were particularly noted as a failure in the response to the 2000 Singapore Airlines crash (W. H. Lee et al., 2002). To minimize these human factors, computer software or predesigned response plans and protocols can be used to guide both managers and responders in a disaster. These resources can direct the organization and define roles, the activities that must be performed, the notifications that must be made, and various other aspects of the response plan to ensure no components are ignored.

How to Deal With the Influx

During a disaster, the EHS system will face a huge surge in patients. Depending on the type of disaster, the surge will have different patterns. In a single event, such as a plane crash or explosion, there will be a single large surge over the first hours after the incident (Auf der Heide, 2006; Chen et al., 2001; Eastman et al., 2007; Quarantelli, 1983; Wattanawaitunechai, Peacock, & Jitpratoom, 2005). In contrast, a large constant number of patients may be seen in the event of a bioterror attack or emerging infection (Tham, 2004). Most of these patients will be low acuity and need minimal care, but some will be critically ill and require large amounts of resources, particularly specialized resources (Hirshberg et al., 2001). Patients who are indirectly impacted by the disaster, such as the worried well, the chronically ill who can no longer receive their services at home or in a skilled nursing facility, and the mentally ill, will also present. As described previously, the "usual" EHS system patients will also require evaluation and treatment. However, whether the numbers of usual patients will predictably decrease as it did during the SARS epidemic in Toronto is unclear (Verbeek et al., 2004). Actual numbers of usual patients will likely depend on the nature of the disaster itself and the emotional impact the disaster has on the patient population. An effective and important tool to ensure patients' access to healthcare, while minimizing the number of worried well presenting to the EHS system, is to work with media

outlets in advance of the disaster to ensure that an appropriate and accurate message is relayed to the local population.

One source of patient influx will be from individuals calling 911 for assistance, which classically results in EMS responding to all patients. However, in a disaster situation, the proper distribution of EMS resources must be considered as all patients probably do not need an EMS response immediately. Although published data are limited, the evolving literature shows that patients assigned certain MPDS dispatch codes are of lower acuity and thus can receive a delayed response (Shah et al., 2005) and, as mentioned previously, protocols that allow the routing of certain complaints to nontraditional resources (phone hotlines, alternative care sites, etc.) may be developed. All patients also need not be taken to the nearest hospital or to any hospital. Paramedics do undertriage patients when deciding whether a patient needs to get immediate medical care (Neeki et al., 2016; Schmidt et al., 2001). However, the undertriage rate, which ranges up to 10%, while significant during normal operations, may be acceptable during a disaster. This rate could be decreased by involving a physician in the telephone triage decisions. Alternative transport mechanisms should also be considered in disaster scenarios. For example, if a paramedic evaluates the patient and finds that he or she is stable enough to be transported by an alternative mechanism such as a taxi, the paramedic and ambulance would be able to return to service more rapidly. Having paramedics direct patients to alternative destinations such as urgent care centers or physician offices is not currently allowed in most states; however, during a disaster these may be appropriate and effective options in accommodating the increase in EHS demand.

When patients are being transported, proper distribution among all of the hospitals in the system must be considered, particularly hospitals with specialized resources (Amram et al., 2012; Auf der Heide, 1989; Tham, 2004). Systems monitoring the availability of beds and resources and directing the flow of patients should be devised to help the response. Many cities, regions, and/or states employ methods to monitor real-time in-hospital patient bed status data for EMS agencies, public health, and emergency managers to utilize in a disaster. Proper distribution of patients cared for by EMS, regardless of how they are transported to definitive care, is a challenging task that is, in many ways, analogous to the job of air traffic controllers. Ideally, the available resources and incoming demands should be actively monitored to ensure access and distribution of patients to the best possible care.

The second source of influx will be from patients presenting to the ED for care. Instead of providing ED care to all patients in a disaster, other options need to be created to protect the ED for critically ill patients. For some patients, a medical screening exam could be performed, and then they would be either discharged home or transferred to alternate sites for care. These sites could include urgent care centers, physician offices, or other buildings within a medical center. However, when these plans are developed, issues such as potential contamination and available resources must be considered. For trauma, this model has proven highly effective in the Iraq War as death rates for injured soldiers have been almost halved as surgeons perform only those procedures required to prevent death in the first 6 hours and transfer patients to other facilities for definitive care (Gawande, 2004).

To deal with the influx, operations within the ED can be modified to improve the efficiency of care and handle the increased volume. Although a thorough discussion is beyond the scope of this chapter, improving ED efficiency should be undertaken regardless of disaster planning, given their daily crowded condition. Additional treatment space is also needed in the ED to deal with the influx of patients. This space can be generated by improving efflux from the ED. This presents a major challenge as hospitals and nursing homes are full, and during a MCI or disaster, it will likely be difficult to arrange home health services. Regardless of the solutions considered, it is important to note that hospital planning teams seem to overestimate their ability to respond (Hirshberg et al., 2001; McHugh, 2010). Solutions to consider include immediately moving all admitted or stable patients out of the ED and to inpatient floors, allowing the ED to care for inbound critical patients by freeing up space occupied by already stabilized and/or admitted patients. Additionally, canceling elective admission, including surgery, will open a number of beds and free up significant resources; however, health systems may be resistant to do this due to the large financial cost of canceling these procedures. Other solutions include transferring patients to either nursing homes or lower acuity hospitals, or sending specialized resources such as trauma surgeons to other centers to expand their capabilities. Whether these solutions will be possible depends on the nature of the incident, but they and others must be considered and prepared for. Lastly, although the NDMS and its member organizations can move large numbers of patients out of a region to other care facilities, this will take at least 24 hours to begin, requiring at least temporary means for expanding capacity, a requirement that should be an annex to any disaster plan.

Lastly, it is also important to consider the issue of patient decontamination. Many hospitals rely on local fire or HAZMAT resources to decontaminate patients prior to arrival at the ED. This model is almost always effective as the typical HAZMAT or chemical exposure is an isolated event in which a limited access/egress quarantine can be established, and in which patients can be controlled and decontaminated. However, as was demonstrated during the sarin gas attack in Tokyo, in a disaster, there is no control over the scene or scenes. The majority of patients will self-refer to EDs without being decontaminated by EMS (Auf der Heide, 2006; Okumura, Suzuki, & Fukuda, 1998; Okumura, Takasu, & Ishimatsu, 1996).

During a disaster, hospitals must expect to perform decontamination themselves and cannot rely on the fire department or HAZMAT team as those assets will be on scene mitigating the consequences of the disaster. Regional decontamination hospitals are unrealistic as there will still be a large number of self-referred patients who will present to local hospitals (Auf der Heide, 2006). Resources organic to the hospital must be available to perform decontamination and prevent the ED from becoming contaminated. If the patient is allowed into the ED for a screening exam and contaminates the ED, that ED is effectively closed for all patients (not just victims of the disaster) until cleanup is complete. If the ED refuses to allow entry and tells the patient to go to the "decontamination" hospital, then that ED may have committed an Emergency Medical Treatment and Active Labor Act (EMTALA) violation. Therefore, all hospitals must have the capacity to lock down the hospital, restrict access, and perform decontamination of any self-triaged and self-transported victim of a disaster who presents for care.

There are, of course, certain extenuating circumstances. During Hurricane Katrina, there were concerns among treating hospitals that they could unwillingly violate EMTALA obligations simply because of the health and safety considerations existing during the initial days of the disaster. It was only through a formal declaration from the Health and Human Services Secretary at the time that ensured that hospitals could transfer or divert patients away from their facilities due to disaster conditions and would not be penalized for doing so (Leavitt, 2005). Additionally, a process for obtaining EMTALA waivers does exist as promulgated by the Centers for Medicare and Medicaid Services (2009) for disasters and other public health emergencies such as influenza. Exploration of care alternatives should be part of any disaster preparedness initiative but requires significant preplanning and legal counsel.

SUMMARY

Disaster planners have many complicated problems to address, particularly given the current daily stresses on the EHS system. A thorough understanding of the EHS system and its challenges can help ensure that the developed system can work efficiently and safely during a MCI or disaster. This brief overview should provide healthcare personnel an introduction to this large and rapidly evolving topic.

CRITICAL ACTIONS

1. Understand your current system by performing resource evaluations.

2. Understand the impact of different disasters on your EHS system.

3. Regularly engage EDs, EMS, and hospitals in the disaster planning process.

4. Create and test EMS protocols for dealing with a large influx of patients.

5. Create and test community plans for dealing with a large influx of patients.

6. Create and test ED plans for rapid efflux of patients.

7. Create and test communication and coordination plans.

8. Create and test data collection systems, connecting all data from EMS to ED to hospitals.

9. Develop relationships with all participants and agencies that will be involved in a disaster response now, before a disaster occurs.

10. Be aware of the EMS Agenda 2050 and its people-centered mission (emsagenda2050.org).

STUDY QUESTIONS

1. Describe the components of the National Incident Management System (NIMS) that are relevant in emergency health services.

2. How do the types of disasters influence surge capacity?

3. Using the input–throughput–output conceptual model as a guide, describe what often happens when high numbers of patients are in the emergency department (ED).

4. Explain why the terms "mass casualty incident (MCI)" and "disaster" are often used interchangeably.

5. Despite the fact that state and federal assets greatly exceed those of local areas, those assets may not be dispatched at all, or at least until a few days after a major incident. Why?

REFERENCES

Adalja, A. A., Watson, M., Bourhi, N., Minton, K., Morhard, R. C., & Toner, E. S. (2014). Absorbing citywide patient surge during hurricane Sandy: A case study in accommodating multiple hospital evacuations. *Annals of Emergency Medicine, 64,* 66–73. doi:10.1016/j.annemergmed.2013.12.010

Agency for Healthcare Research and Quality. (2006). *Addressing surge capacity in a mass casualty event: Surge capacity and health system preparedness.* Rockville, MD: Author.

Aghababian, R., Lews, C. P., Gans, L., & Curley, F. J. (1994). Disasters within hospitals. *Annals of Emergency Medicine, 23,* 771–777. doi:10.1016/S0196-0644(94)70313-2

American Association of Colleges of Nursing. (2014). Nursing shortage fact sheet. Retrieved from http://www.aacn.nche.edu/media-relations/NrsgShortageFS.pdf

American Association of Medical Colleges. (2016). The complexities of physician supply and demand. Retrieved from https://www.aamc.org/download/458082/data/2016_complexities_of_supply_and_demand_projections.pdf

American College of Emergency Physicians. (2014). The national report card on the state of emergency medicine. Retrieved from http://www.emreportcard.org/

American Hospital Association. (2015). Always there, ready to care: The 24/7 role of America's hospitals. Retrieved http://www.aha.org/content/15/alwaysthere.pdf

American Society for Testing Materials. (2009). *Standard guide for planning for and response to a multiple casualty incident.* West Conshohocken, PA: American Society for Testing Materials International.

Amram, O., Schuurman, N., Hedley, N., & Hameed, S. M. (2012). A web-based model to support patient-to-hospital allocation in mass casualty incidents. *Journal of Trauma and Acute Care Surgery, 72*(5), 1323–1328. Retrieved from https://insights.ovid.com/pubmed?pmid=22673261

Aoyagi, Y., Beck, C. R., Dingwall, R., & Nguyen-Van-Tam, J. S. (2015). Healthcare workers' willingness to work during an influenza pandemic: A systematic review and meta-analysis. *Influenza and Other Respiratory Viruses, 9,* 120–130. doi:10.1111/irv.12310

Arlington County after action report on the response to the September 11 terrorist attack on the Pentagon. (2002). Arlington, VA: Titan System Corporation.

Asplin, B. R., Magid, D. J., Rhodes, K. V., Solberg, L. I., Lurie, N., & Camargo, C. A. (2003). A conceptual model of emergency department crowding. *Annals of Emergency Medicine, 42,* 173–180. doi:10.1067/mem.2003.302

Auf der Heide, E. (1989). *Disaster response: Principles of preparation and coordination.* St. Louis, MO: Mosby.

Auf der Heide, E. (1996). Disaster planning. Part 2: Disaster problems, issues, and challenges identified in the research literature. *Emergency Medical Clinics of North America, 14,* 453–480. doi:10.1016/S0733-8627(05)70262-5

Auf der Heide, E. (2003). Convergence behavior in disasters. *Annals of Emergency Medicine, 41,* 463–466. doi:10.1067/mem.2003.126

Auf der Heide, E. (2006). The importance of evidence-based disaster planning. *Annals of Emergency Medicine, 47,* 34–49. doi:10.1016/j.annemergmed.2005.05.009

Avitzour, M., Libergal, M., Assaf, J., Adler, J., Beyth, S., Mosheiff, R., ... Shapira, S. C. (2004). A multicasualty event: Out-of-hospital and in-hospital organizational aspects. *Academic Emergency Medicine, 11,* 1102–1104. doi:10.1197/j.aem.2004.06.010

Becker, S. M., & Middleton, S. A. (2008). Improving hospital preparedness for radiological terrorism perspectives from emergency department physicians and nurses. *Disaster Medicine and Public Health Preparedness, 2*(3), 174–184. doi:10.1097/DMP.0b013e31817dcd9a

Bennett, K. J., Yuen, M. W., & Merrell, M. A. (2017). Community paramedicine applied in a rural community. *The Journal of Rural Health.* Retrieved from http://onlinelibrary.wiley.com/doi/10.1111/j.1748-0361.2008.00166.x/full

Berger, E. (2006). Charity hospital and disaster preparedness. *Annals of Emergency Medicine, 47,* 53–56. doi:10.1016/j.annemergmed.2005.12.004

Brown, L. M., Hickling, E. J., & Frahm, K. (2010). Emergencies, disasters, and catastrophic events: The role of rehabilitation nurses in preparedness, response, and recovery. *Rehabilitation Nursing, 35*(6), 236–241. Retrieved from http://onlinelibrary.wiley.com/doi/10.1002/j.2048-7940.2010.tb00053.x/full

Burgess, J. L., Kirk, M., Borron, S. W., & Cisek, J. (1999). Emergency department hazardous materials protocol for contaminated patients. *Annals of Emergency Medicine, 34,* 205–212. doi:10.1016/S0196-0644(99)70230-1

Casey, M. M., Wholey, D., & Moscovice, I. S. (2008). Rural emergency department staffing and participation in emergency certification and training programs. *Journal of Rural Health, 24*(3), 253–262. doi:10.1111/j.1748-0361.2008.00166.x

Centers for Disease Control and Prevention. (2017). Strategic national stockpile. Retrieved from https://www.cdc.gov/phpr/stockpile

Centers for Medicare and Medicaid Services. (2009). Emergency Medical Treatment and Labor Act (EMTALA) requirements and options for hospitals in a disaster. Retrieved from https://www.cms.gov/Medicare/Provider-Enrollment-and-Certification/SurveyCertificationGenInfo/downloads/SCLetter09_52.pdf

Chaloner, E. (2005). Blast injury in enclosed spaces [Editorial]. *British Medical Journal, 331,* 119–120. doi:10.1136/bmj.331.7509.119

Chavez, C. W., & Binder, B. (1996). A hospital as victim and responder: The Sepulveda VA Medical Center and the Northridge earthquake. *Journal of Emergency Medicine, 14,* 445–454. doi:10.1016/0736-4679(96)00083-2

Chen, W. K., Cheng, Y. C., Ng, K. C., Hung, J. J., & Chuang, C. M. (2001). Were there enough physicians in an emergency department in the affected area after a major earthquake? An analysis of the Taiwan Chi-Chi earthquake in 1999. *Annals of Emergency Medicine, 38,* 556–561. doi:10.1067/mem.2001.119054

Cheng, B., Shi, R., Du, D., Hu, P., Feng, J., Huang, G., ... Yang, R. (2015). Mobile emergency (surgical) hospital: Development and application in medical relief of "4.20" Lushan earthquake in Sichuan Province, China. *Chinese Journal of Traumatology, 18*(1), 5–9. Retrieved from http://www.sciencedirect.com/science/article/pii/S1008127515000115?via%3Dihub

Clarke, S. F., Chilcott, R. P., Wilson, J. C., Kamanyire, R., Baker, D. J., & Hallett, A. (2008). Decontamination of multiple casualties who are chemically contaminated: A challenge for acute hospitals. *Prehospital and Disaster Medicine, 23*(2), 175–181. Retrieved from https://www.cambridge.org/core/journals/prehospital-and-disaster-medicine/article/decontamination-of-multiple-casualties-who-are-chemically-contaminated-a-challenge-for-acute-hospitals/381D7CDCA60AF40041811FE0E2812EBA

Cone, D. C., Weir, S. D., & Bogucki, S. (2003). Convergent volunteerism. *Annals of Emergency Medicine, 41,* 457–462. doi:10.1067/mem.2003.107

Davis, D. P., Poste, J. C., Hicks, T., Polk, D., Rymer, T. E., & Jacoby, I. (2005). Hospital bed surge capacity in the event of a mass-casualty incident. *Prehospital and Disaster Medicine, 20*(3), 169–176. Retrieved from https://

www.cambridge.org/core/journals/prehospital-and-disaster-medicine/
article/hospital-bed-surge-capacity-in-the-event-of-a-masscasualty-incident/
FB760E42A7D1441838FB34D2EE66ACB1

Department of Homeland Security. (2017). National incident management system. Retrieved from https://www.fema.gov/national-incident-management-system

Eastman, A. L., Rinnert, K. J., Nemeth, I. R., Fowler, R. L., & Minei, J. P. (2007). Alternate site surge capacity in times of public health disaster maintains trauma center and emergency department integrity: Hurricane Katrina. *Journal of Trauma and Acute Care Surgery, 63*(2), 253–257.

Einav, S., Feigenberg, Z., Weissman, C., Zaichik D., Caspi G., Kotler, D., & Freund, H. R. (2004). Evacuation priorities in mass casualty terror-related events: Implications for contingency planning. *Annals of Surgery, 239,* 304–310. doi:10.1097/01.sla.0000114013.19114.57

Frykberg, E. R., & Tepas, J. J. (1988). Terrorist bombings: Lessons learned from Belfast to Beirut. *Annals of Surgery, 208,* 569–576. doi:10.1097/00000658-198811000-00005

Fukunaga, H., & Kumakawa, H. (2014). Disaster management at Soma General Hospital in response to the great east Japan earthquake. *Japan Medical Association Journal, 57,* 331–334.

Gamboa-Maldonado, T., Marshak, H. H., Sinclair, R., Montgomery, S., & Dyjack, D. T. (2012). Building capacity for community disaster preparedness: A call for collaboration between public environmental health and emergency preparedness and response programs. *Journal of Environmental Health, 75*(2), 24–29. Retrieved from https://www.ncbi.nlm.nih.gov/pmc/articles/PMC4651206

Garshnek, V., & Burkle, F. M. (1999). Telecommunications systems in support of disaster medicine: Applications of basic information pathways. *Annals of Emergency Medicine, 34,* 213–218. doi:10.1016/S0196-0644(99)70231-3

Gawande, A. (2004). Casualties of war—Military care for the wounded from Iraq and Afghanistan. *New England Journal of Medicine, 351,* 2471–2475. doi:10.1056/NEJMp048317

Green, G. B., Modi, S., Lunney, K., & Thomas, T. L. (2003). Generic evaluation methods for disaster drills in developing countries. *Annals of Emergency Medicine, 41,* 689–699. doi:10.1067/mem.2003.147

Gutierrez de Ceballos, J. P., Turegano Fuentes, F., Perez Diaz, D., Sanz Sanchez, M., Martin Llorente, C., & Guerrero Sanz, J. E. (2005). Casualties treated at the closest hospital in the Madrid, April 11, terrorist bombings. *Critical Care, 33,* S107–S112. doi:10.1097/01.CCM.0000151072.17826.72

Henderson, A. K., Lillibridge, S. R., Salinas, C., Graves, R. W., Roth, P. B., & Noji, K. (1994). Disaster medical assistance teams: Providing health care to a community struck by Hurricane Iniki. *Annals of Emergency Medicine, 23,* 726–730. doi:10.1016/S0196-0644(94)70306-X

Hettinger, A. Z., Cushman, J. T., Shah, M. N., & Noyes, K. (2013). Emergency medical dispatch codes association with emergency department outcomes. *Prehospital Emergency Care, 17,* 29–37. doi:10.3109/10903127.2012.710716

Hick, J. L., Hanfling, D., Burstein, J. L., DeAtley, C., Barbisch, D., Bogdan, G. M., & Cantrill, S. (2004). Health care facility and community strategies for patient care surge capacity. *Annals of Emergency Medicine, 44*(3), 253–261. Retrieved from http://www.sciencedirect.com/science/article/pii/S0196064404004202

Hirshberg, A., Holcomb, J. B., & Mattox, K. L. (2001). Hospital trauma care in multiple-casualty incidents: A critical view. *Annals of Emergency Medicine, 37,* 647–652. doi:10.1067/mem.2001.115650

Hogan, D. E., Waeckerle, J. F., Dire, D. J., & Lillibridge, S. R. (1999). Emergency department impact of the Oklahoma City terrorist bombing. *Annals of Emergency Medicine, 34,* 160–167. doi:10.1016/S0196-0644(99)70224-6

Hoot, N. R., & Aronsky, D. (2008). Systematic review of emergency department crowding: Causes, effects, and solutions. *Annals of Emergency Medicine, 52,* 126–136. doi:10.1016/j.annemergmed.2008.03.014

Hougan, M., Nadig, L., Stroud, C., & Altevogt, B. M. (Eds). (2010). *Medical surge capacity: Workshop summary.* National Academies Press. Retrieved from https://www.ncbi.nlm.nih.gov/books/NBK32866

Institute of Medicine. (1996). Telemedicine: A Guide To Assessing Telecommunications In Health Care. Washington, D.C.: National Academies Press.

Institute of Medicine of the National Academies, Committee on the Treatment of Cardiac Arrest: Current Status and Future Directions. (2015). In

R. Grahm, M. A. McCoy, & A. M. Schultz (Eds), *Strategies to improve cardiac arrest survival: A time to act.* Retrieved from http://www.nap.edu/catalog.php?record_id=21723

Israel Defense Forces Medical Corps. (1997). *Trauma Division report: Terrorist suicide bombings in Israel 1994–1996: Medical summary* (pp. 10–13). Israel: Tel Aviv.

Jenkins, J. L., McCarthy, M. L., Sauer, L. M., Green, G. B., Stuart, S., Thomas, T. L., & Hsu, E. B. (2008). Mass-casualty triage: Time for an evidence-based approach. *Prehospital and Disaster Medicine, 23*(1), 3–8. Retrieved from https://www.cambridge.org/core/services/aop-cambridge-core/content/view/F6D96F8BCF56693C610DEF8689E8B1D4/S1049023X00005471a.pdf/masscasualty_triage_time_for_an_evidencebased_approach.pdf

Joint Commission on Accreditation of Healthcare Organizations. (2006). Surge hospitals: Providing safe care in emergencies. Retrieved from http://www.jointcommission.org/assets/1/18/surge_hospital.pdf

Jones, T. F., Craig, A. S., Hoy, D., Gunter, E. W., Ashley, D. L., Barr, D. B., ... Schaffner, W. (2000). Mass psychogenic illness attributed to toxic exposure at a high school. *New England Journal of Medicine, 342,* 96–100. doi:10.1056/NEJM200001133420206

Kaji, A. H., & Waeckerle, J. F. (2003). Disaster medicine and the emergency resident. *Annals of Emergency Medicine, 41,* 865–870. doi:10.1067/mem.2003.10

Kapucu, N., Arslan, T., & Demiroz, F. (2010). Collaborative emergency management and national emergency management network. *Disaster Prevention and Management: An International Journal, 19*(4), 452–468. Retrieved from http://www.emeraldinsight.com/doi/full/10.1108/09653561011070376

Ko, P. C., Chen, W., Ma, M. H., Chiang, W., Su, C., Huang, C., ... Lin, F. Y. (2004). Emergency medical services utilization during an outbreak of severe acute respiratory syndrome (SARS) and the incidence of SARS-associated coronavirus infection among emergency medical technicians. *Academic Emergency Medicine, 11,* 903–911. doi:10.1197/j.aem.2004.03.016

Landman, A., Teich, J. M., Pruitt, P., Moore, S. E., Theriault, J., Dorisca, E., ... Goralnick, E., (2015). The Boston Marathon Bombings Mass Casualty Incident: One emergency department's information system challenges and opportunities. *Annals of Emergency Medicine, 66,* 51–59. doi:10.1016/j.annemergmed.2014.06.009

Leavitt, M. (2005, September). *Letter to hospitals.* Washington, DC: U.S. Department of Health and Human Services.

Lee, E. K., Chen, C. H., Pietz, F., & Benecke, B. (2009). Modeling and optimizing the public-health infrastructure for emergency response. *Interfaces, 39*(5), 476–490. Retrieved from https://pubsonline.informs.org/doi/pdf/10.1287/inte.1090.0463

Lee, W. H., Chiu, T. F., Ng, C. J., & Chen, J. C. (2002). Emergency medical preparedness and response to a Singapore airliner crash. *Academic Emergency Medicine, 9,* 194–198. doi:10.1197/aemj.9.3.194

Love, J. S., Karp, D., Delgado, M. K., Margolis, G., Wiebe, D. J., & Carr, B. G. (2016). National differences in regional emergency department boarding times: Are US emergency departments prepared for a public health emergency? *Disaster Medicine and Public Health Preparedness, 10,* 576–582. doi:10.1017/dmp.2015.184

Marcin, J. P., Shaikh, U., & Steinhorn, R. H. (2015). Addressing health disparities in rural communities using telehealth. *Pediatric Research, 79*(1–2), 169–176. Retrieved from https://escholarship.org/uc/item/7rb777w2

McGinnis, K. K. (2004). Rural and frontier emergency medical services: Agenda for the future. National Rural Health Association. Retrieved from https://www.ruralcenter.org/sites/default/files/rfemsagenda.pdf

McHugh, M. D. (2010). Special features: Health policy: Hospital nurse staffing and public health emergency preparedness: Implications for policy. *Public Health Nursing, 27*(5), 442–449. Retrieved from http://onlinelibrary.wiley.com/doi/10.1111/j.1525-1446.2010.00877.x/full

Morita, T., Tsubokura, M., Furutani, T., Nomura, S., Ochi, S., Leppold, C., ... Oikawa, T. (2016). Impacts of the 2011 Fukushima nuclear accident on emergency medical services times in Soma District, Japan: A retrospective observational study. *British Medical Journal Open, 6,* e013205. doi:10.1136/bmjopen-2016-013205

Narasimhulu, D. P., Edwards, V., Chazotte, C., Bhatt, D., Weedon, J., & Minkoff, H. (2015). Healthcare workers' attitudes toward patients with Ebola virus disease in the United States. *Open Forum Infectious Diseases, 3*(1), ofv192. doi:10.1093/ofid/ofv192

Nates, J. L., & Moyer, V. A. (2005). Lessons from Hurricane Katrina, tsunamis, and other disasters. *Lancet, 366,* 1144–1146. doi:10.1016/S0140-6736(05)67460-0

National Association of State EMS Officials. (2014). EMS workforce planning and development: Guidelines for state adoption. Retrieved from https://www.nasemso.org/documents/EMS-Workforce-Guidelines-11Oct2013.pdf

National Association of State EMS Officials. (2015). Emergency medical services domestic preparedness improvement strategy. Retrieved from https://www.nasemso.org/documents/NASEMSO-EMS-Domestic-Preparedness-Improvement-Strategy-29Jan2015.pdf

Neeki, M. M., Dong, F., Avera, L., Than, T., Borger, R., Powell, J. ... Pitts R.(2016). Alternative destination transport? The role of paramedics in optimal use of the emergency department. *The Western Journal of Emergency Medicine, 17*(6), 690–697. doi:10.5811/westjem.2016.9.31384

North, C. S., & Pfefferbaum, B. (2013). Mental health response to community disasters: A systematic review. *Journal of the American Medical Association*, 310(5), 507–518. Retrieved from https://jamanetwork.com/journals/jama/fullarticle/1724280?tab=cme

O'Connor, R. E., Lerner, E. B., Allswede, M., Billittier, A. J., IV, Blackwell, T., Hunt, R. C., ... Wolff, B. (2004). Linkages of acute care and emergency medical services to state and local public health programs: The role of interactive information systems for responding to events resulting in mass injury. *Prehospital Emergency Care, 8,* 237–253. doi:10.1080/312704000255

Okumura, T., Suzuki, K., & Fukuda, A. (1998). The Tokyo subway sarin attack: Disaster management. Part 2: Hospital response. *Academic Emergency Medicine, 5,* 618–624. doi:10.1111/j.1553-2712.1998.tb02471.x

Okumura, T., Takasu, N., & Ishimatsu, S. (1996). Report on 640 victims of the Tokyo subway sarin attack. *Annals of Emergency Medicine, 28,* 129–135. doi:10.1016/S0196-0644(96)70052-5

Pesik, N., Keim, M. E., & Iserson, K. V. (2001). Terrorism and the ethics of emergency medical care. *Annals of Emergency Medicine, 34,* 642–646. doi:10.1067/mem.2001.114316

Prezant, D. J., Clair, J., Belyaev, S., Alleyne, D., Banauch, G. I., Davitt, M., ... Kalkut, G. (2005). Effects of the August 2003 blackout on the New York City healthcare delivery system: A lesson for disaster preparedness. *Critical Care Medicine, 33,* S96–S101. doi:10.1097/01.CCM.0000150956.90030.23

Quarantelli, E. L. (1983). *Delivery of emergency medical care in disasters: Assumptions and realities.* New York, NY: Irvington.

Ramesh, A. C., & Kumar, S. (2010). Triage, monitoring, and treatment of mass casualty events involving chemical, biological, radiological, or nuclear agents. *Journal of Pharmacy and Bioallied Sciences, 2*(3), 239–247. doi:10.4103/0975-7406.68506

Rand, D. A., Mener, D. J., Lerner, E. B., & DeRobertis, N. (2005). The effect of an 18-hour electrical power outage on an urban emergency medical services system. *Prehospital Emergency Care, 9,* 391–397. doi:10.1080/10903120500255909

Reilly, M. J., & Markenson, D. (2010). Hospital referral patterns: How emergency medical care is accessed in a disaster. *Disaster Medicine and Public Health Preparedness, 4*(3), 226–231. Retrieved from https://www.ncbi.nlm.nih.gov/pubmed/21149219

Roccaforte, J. D., & Cushman, J. G. (2007). Disaster preparedness, triage, and surge capacity for hospital definitive care areas: Optimizing outcomes when demands exceed resources. *Anesthesiology Clinics, 25*(1), 161–177. Retrieved from http://www.sciencedirect.com/science/article/pii/S1932227507000031

Satterthwaite, P. S., & Atkinson, C. J. (2010). Using 'reverse triage' to create hospital surge capacity: Royal Darwin Hospital's response to the Ashmore Reef disaster. *Emergency Medicine Journal.* Retrieved from http://emj.bmj.com/content/early/2010/10/28/emj.2010.098087.short

Schmidt, T. A., Atcheson, R., Federiuk, C., Mann, N. C., Pinney, T., Fuller, D., & Colbry, K. (2001). Hospital follow-up of patients categorized as not needing an ambulance using a set of emergency medical technician protocols. *Prehospital Emergency Care, 5,* 366–370. doi:10.1080/10903120190939526

Schneider, S. M., Gardner, A. F., Weiss, L. D., Wood, J. P., Ybarra, M., Beck, D. M., ... Jouriles, N. (2010). The future of emergency medicine. *Academic Emergency Medicine, 17*(9), 998–1003. doi:10.1111/j.1553-2712.2010.00854.x

Schuur, J. D., Baker, O., Freshman, M., & Cutler, D. M. (2017). Where do freestanding emergency departments choose to locate: A national inventory and geographic analysis in three states. *Annals of Emergency Medicine, 69*(4), 383–392.e5. doi:10.1016/j.annemergmed.2016.05.019

Shah, M. N., Bishop, P., Lerner, E. B., Fairbanks, R. J., & Davis, E. A. (2005). Validation of using EMS dispatch codes to identify low-acuity patients. *Prehospital Emergency Care, 9,* 24–31. doi:10.1080/10903120590891651

Sheppa, C. M., Stevens, J., Philbrick, J. T., & Canada, M. (1993). The effect of a class IV hurricane on emergency department operations. *American Journal of Emergency Medicine, 11,* 464–467. doi:10.1016/0735-6757(93)90084-O

Stange, K. C. (2009). The problem of fragmentation and the need for integrative solutions. *Annals of Family Medicine, 7*(2), 100–103. doi:10.1370/afm.971

Susman, E. (2005). Unforeseen after Katrina. *The Lancet Oncology, 6,* 744–746. doi:10.1016/S1470-2045(05)70379-X

Sweeney, B., Jasper, E., & Gates, E. (2004). Large-scale urban disaster drill involving an explosion: Lessons learned by an academic medical center. *Disaster Management and Response, 2,* 87–90. doi:10.1016/j.dmr.2004.06.010

Tham, K. Y. (2004). An emergency department response to severe acute respiratory syndrome: A prototype response to bioterrorism. *Annals of Emergency Medicine, 43,* 6–14. doi:10.1016/j.annemergmed.2003.08.005

Treat, K. N., Williams, J. M., Furbee, P. M., Manley, W G., Russell, F. K., & Stampler, C. D., Jr. (2001). Hospital preparedness for weapons of mass destruction incidents: An initial assessment. *Annals of Emergency Medicine, 38,* 562–565. doi:10.1067/mem.2001.118009

Tzong-Luen, W., & Chi-Ren, H. (2005). Appraisal of field triage in mass casualty incidents in Taipei. *Annals of Disaster Medicine, 3*(2), 69–75.

U.S. Department of Health and Human Services. (2017). Disaster Medical Assistance Teams: Providing the best medical care in the worst of times. Retrieved from https://www.phe.gov/Preparedness/responders/ndms/ndms-teams/Pages/dmat.aspx

U.S. Department of Health and Human Services: Office of the Inspector General. (2014). Hospital emergency preparedness and response during Superstorm Sandy. Retrieved from https://oig.hhs.gov/oei/reports/oei-06-13-00260.pdf

U.S. Department of Homeland Security. (2008). National response framework. Retrieved from https://www.fema.gov/pdf/emergency/nrf/nrf-core.pdf

Verbeek, P. R., McClelland, I. W., Silverman, A. C., & Burgess, R. J. (2004). Loss of paramedic availability in an urban emergency medical services systems during a severe acute respiratory syndrome outbreak. *Academic Emergency Medicine, 11,* 973–978. doi:10.1197/j.aem.2004.03.021

Watson, S. K., Rudge, J. W., & Coker, R. (2013). Health systems' "surge capacity": State of the art and priorities for future research. *The Milbank Quarterly, 91*(1), 78–122. Retrieved from http://onlinelibrary.wiley.com/doi/10.1111/milq.12003/full

Wattanawaitunechai, C., Peacock, S. J., & Jitpratoom, P. (2005). Tsunami in Thailand—Disaster management in a district hospital. *New England Journal of Medicine, 352,* 962–964. doi:10.1056/NEJMp058040

Weiss, E. A., Ngo, J., Gilbert, G. H., & Quinn, J. V. (2010). Drive-through medicine: A novel proposal for rapid evaluation of patients during an influenza pandemic. *Annals of Emergency Medicine, 55,* 268–273. doi:10.1016/j.annemergmed.2009.11.025

Wiseman, D. B., Ellenbogen, E., & Shaffrey, C. I. (2002). Triage for the neurosurgeon. *Neurosurgical Focus, 12*(3), Article 5. doi:10.3171/foc.2002.12.3.6

World Health Organization. (2011). Hospital emergency response checklist. Retrieved from http://www.euro.who.int/__data/assets/pdf_file/0008/268766/Hospital-emergency-response-checklist-Eng.pdf

5

EMERGENCY MEDICAL CONSEQUENCE PLANNING FOR SPECIAL EVENTS, MASS GATHERINGS, AND MASS CASUALTY INCIDENTS

Tener Goodwin Veenema, Paul Arbon, and Alison Hutton

LEARNING OBJECTIVES

When this chapter is completed, readers will be able to:

1. Define emergency management, emergency medical consequence planning, and surge capacity for mass gatherings (MGs) and mass casualty incidents (MCIs).
2. Appreciate the inherent dangers associated with large gatherings of people and the potential for any large crowd to decompensate into an MCI.
3. Describe the importance of preplanning for medical and nursing services for special events involving large numbers of people.
4. Describe a framework for predicting the amount and types of healthcare services (patient presentation rate [PPR]) that will be needed based on type, duration, location of event, and characteristics of the crowd.
5. Understand that characteristics that are recognized to affect the PPR include weather, event type, event duration, crowd mood, crowd density, attendance, age, and alcohol and drug use.
6. Describe the decision making for medical and nursing aid station design and placement.
7. Discuss the importance of communication systems during large events.
8. Know the location of transport vehicles, all escape routes, and how to activate the emergency operations plan.

KEY MESSAGES

Nurses and other healthcare practitioners are frequently called on to provide care to patients at MG events involving large numbers of people.

Increased rates of injuries and illness can be anticipated when large numbers of people gather at concerts, sporting and other MG events.

The characteristics of the event, including event type and duration, crowd characteristics and environmental considerations such as the weather, will determine the amount and nature of anticipated patient encounters.

Extreme heat increases the risk of life-threatening heat-related illnesses at MG events.

Emergency incidents at large MG events may result in MCIs.

MGs are held in difficult settings, which may result in delayed healthcare response.

Pre-event emergency medical consequence planning for any major MG event involving potentially large numbers of people is critical.

The design of nursing services (as a component of the medical care services provided) requires that nurses collaborate with other service providers, such as security, law enforcement, other medical support (fire, hazard material [HAZMAT], and paramedic/emergency medical services [EMS]/ ambulance), and medical practitioner/physician services to ensure integration with other service provision plans.

CHAPTER OVERVIEW

World Cup Soccer, the Super Bowl, Papal Masses, the Hajj, outdoor music festivals—people across the globe gather in large groups to celebrate sports, politics, music, culture, and religion. In recent years, there has been an increased focus on emergency preparedness and medical consequence planning for large-scale MGs. An MG can be defined as "a situation (event) during which crowds gather and where there is the potential for a delayed response to emergencies because of limited access to patients or other features of the environment and location" (Arbon, 2007), presenting a potential hazard to health and safety. Multiple variables interact during an MG event to create the potential for increased illness and injuries to spectators, participants, and staff working at the event. Advanced planning for a comprehensive and appropriate level of health and emergency management response for each type of MG is critical to ensure the health and safety of people attending the event. Emergency medical and public health authorities must anticipate how to provide care to large numbers of injured or ill people throughout the duration of the event. Additionally, any time large numbers of people gather together in one location there is a possibility that a mass casualty incident (MCI) may occur. The role of the nurse during an MCI may require ingenuity, flexibility, adaptability, creativity, and an understanding of the local Incident Command System (ICS).

MASS GATHERINGS AND SPECIAL EVENTS

Nurses and other healthcare professionals worldwide are frequently called on to provide healthcare for large groups of people attending major public events such as political conventions, national special security events (NSSEs),[1] sporting competitions, outdoor music festivals, auto races, and religious gatherings. According to the World Health Organization, an MG is an event "attended by a sufficient number of people to strain the planning and response resources of the host community, state/province, nation, or region where it is being held" (Isla, Endericks, & Barbeschi, 2015). The definition is purposefully not linked to the size of the gathering or the number of people (although this obviously has an impact on the assessment of associated risks) because each community has a different capacity to manage crowds of people, with some systems, for example, airports or marketplaces, managing upward of 100,000 people on a daily basis with minimal difficulties (Isla et al., 2015).

Whether the event draws 1,000 or 1,000,000 people, the risk of illness and injury is ubiquitous and healthcare services will be needed. Although it is not possible to predict with accuracy how much medical and nursing care will be needed at these events, it is essential that adequate patient care services are available and can be provided to casualties in a timely way. Estimates of total numbers of spectator days and projected medical usage rates can be done for these events. Planning should consider all spectators, participants, support staff, and the locations and context of the event. Emergency medical consequence planning and management involves establishing, in advance, a plan to meet the "normal" expected healthcare needs of people at the event and in addition a plan to rapidly

---

[1] In 1998, U.S. President Clinton issued Presidential Decision Directive-62 (PDD-62) *Protection against Unconventional Threats to the Homeland and Americans Overseas,* which designates certain events of national interest as NSSEs. NSSE designation criteria include size of event, anticipated attendance of dignitaries, and any cultural, historical, or political significance that increases its potential as a terrorist target.

expand services to meet a sudden surge in demand for care if an MCI occurs.

MGs can place a strain on the local healthcare system; even the most prepared of events may experience a disaster or MCI, which can overwhelm local healthcare systems and their ability to provide an adequate emergency response (Isla et al., 2015). In the event an MCI occurs, responders must be able to secure the safety of the scene, control crowds, delineate access and evacuation routes, coordinate, collaborate, and communicate across services (police, fire, HAZMAT, and EMS), and rapidly identify the potential for a secondary event (another incident in the same location). Emergency management is defined as:

> [T]he organized analysis, planning, decision making, and assignment of available resources to mitigate (lessen the effect or prevent), prepare for, respond to, and recover from the effects of all hazards. The goal of emergency management is to save lives, prevent injuries, and protect property and the environment if an emergency occurs. (Committee on Evaluation of the Metropolitan Medical Response System Program, 2002, p. 34)

Adoption of emergency management as the conceptual basis for planning healthcare and emergency response for MGs allows for the use of a standardized systems-based approach and unifies all planning and response-related activities. Extending the concepts of emergency management into the healthcare system permits the definition of healthcare emergency management as:

> The science of managing complex systems and multidisciplinary personnel to address emergencies and disasters in health care systems, across all hazards, and through the phases of mitigation, preparedness, response and recovery. (MacIntrye, Barbera, & Brewster, 2009, p. S55)

A framework should be established for comprehensive emergency management that includes: (a) emergency medical consequence planning to enable the delivery of medical and nursing services during the event; (b) a detailed written emergency response plan for rapid action during emergency incidents (including individual patients requiring urgent treatment and evacuation) and surge capacity for MCIs; and (c) associated plans including a communications plan, logistics plan, and transport plan. Planning for healthcare management of injuries and illness outside of the hospital during MGs has many common elements, which are described in this chapter.

HEALTHCARE EMERGENCY MANAGEMENT

Healthcare emergency management is the use of standardized, widely accepted emergency management principles and practices, and application of commonly used concepts and terminology (Figure 5.1). It, importantly, facilitates the integration of healthcare into the larger emergency response system(s) (MacIntrye et al., 2009). It allows responders from a variety of disciplines and backgrounds to communicate, coordinate, collaborate, and cooperate to render a well-organized well-executed response to a mass casualty event.

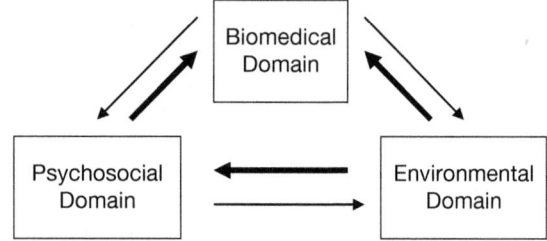

FIGURE 5.1 A relationship model of domains for mass gathering health.

Source: Arbon, P. (2007). Mass-gathering medicine: A review of the evidence and future directions for research. *Prehospital Disaster Medicine,* 22, 131–135. doi:10.1017/S1049023X00004507

EMERGENCY MEDICAL CONSEQUENCE PLANNING

As described in the first two chapters of this book, the most important aspect of special event management is *planning in advance.* Cuny (1998), in a sentinel article, describes three types of advanced planning activities:

1. *Strategic planning*—These are planning activities that focus on preparing the organization for any type of threat or event.
2. *Contingency planning*—These are planning activities related to a site-specific threat that may occur at any time.
3. *Forward planning*—These are planning activities for a known imminent event, for example, an impending snowstorm or rock concert.

Forward planning for a *major event involving potentially large numbers of people* is critical and requires the collaborative and cooperative efforts of the event or venue owner, local health system, ambulance, police department, fire department, selected community agencies, and local governmental officials in the community where the event is to be held. A well-planned event will be able to meet, or at least respond to, the healthcare needs of most who attend. While most of the presenting medical complaints will be minor, provisions must be made to address those health conditions that are potentially life-threatening and require urgent care and evacuation to a tertiary treatment center. Forward planning begins with information collection. When will the event occur? Where will the event be located? What type of audience is expected? What weather conditions are likely? What type of structures will be used to house the event? What types of facilities will be available to healthcare providers working at the event? What types of communication system will be put in place and who will be responsible for it?

Summary information gathering must include identifying: (a) **what** type of event will be held, (b) **where** will it be held (detailed description of the venue[s]), (c) **why** it is being held (e.g., political agenda, religious, cultural experience), (d) **who** is sponsoring the event, and, finally, (e) **who** is expected to attend. It is important to gather as many specific details regarding the event planned as are available.

Risk assessment is a key element in prioritizing and planning and is a continuous process that should occur throughout the period leading up to the MG and during the event. The emergency risk assessment process should be documented and available for later review (Isla et al., 2015). Summary information gathering must include identifying: What hazards exist to create risk to human health? What options exist to mitigate these risks? How can public health be best protected?

The healthcare service commander responsible for organizing and coordinating health services (including nurses as members of the healthcare team) on-site should meet with the individual(s) and agencies in charge of the event well in advance of the date on which the event is scheduled (even years before in some instances, depending upon the anticipated scale of the event). It is important to determine what healthcare providers will be in attendance, and who will be in charge. Some events require physician response teams and other events are aptly handled by nurse, paramedic/EMS, and first aid teams. The contribution of the nurse to the provision of healthcare including scope of practice and clinical practice guidelines should be discussed in advance. The role of the nurse in an MG may range from providing nursing care services along with EMS providers on-site, to the leadership and coordination of all healthcare services for the event, depending on the structure of the on-site care team. The requirements and/or expectations of the sponsoring organization or event owner for levels of medical care must be considered in planning. At times these requirements are very specific and in events such as the Olympic Games, auto-racing events, and extreme sports, these expectations may extend to provision of aerial evacuation and specific aggressive treatments for severe heat exhaustion. Often such requirements form part of the legally binding contract for health services provision.

Police, fire departments, and ambulance services must be involved in all major events planning as they may need to be present during the event to provide a safe environment for participants, spectators, and healthcare providers. Determination should be made as to location and availability of basic life support (BLS) and advanced life support (ALS) services. The intent is to provide a timely response throughout the venue maintaining the "chain of survival" (Ranse, 2006). The design of nursing and other health services requires that nurses and the wider medical team are aware of who will be attending the event in terms of security, crowd control, and other support services. If the use of volunteers (including licensed healthcare professionals) is anticipated, the role and responsibilities of the volunteers should be determined in advance as well as who is responsible for supervising them, providing insurances, and ultimately accountable for their actions.

Paramedics and advanced paramedics will play an integral role in the response and management of MCIs. Preplanning for these events and interdisciplinary education and training can enhance coordination of response efforts and reduce fear and perception of risk of personal harm among responders (Smith, Burkle, & Archer, 2011). Training should review MCI triage principles, the planned location of redundant healthcare sites (frequently external to the venue/site), and safe evacuation skills for healthcare staff during a crowd crush situation.

Healthcare professionals may need to be available before and after the event to provide care for the event staff and for the attendees as they arrive (Leonard & Moreland, 2001) and, at times, planning should include provision of healthcare outside of the event. For example, at music events and during fireworks displays, crowds may form outside of the "official" venue and can be very widespread.

Guidelines

One of the primary challenges for the providers of healthcare at MGs has been the lack of regulations, standards, or formal guidelines to help direct local healthcare clinicians who must supply coverage for the event (Gutman, Lund, & Turris, 2011). The World Health Organization (WHO) has published guidelines (WHO, KC2 2015), the American College of Emergency Physicians and the National Association of Emergency Medical Services Physicians have published position papers regarding their recommendations (Jaslow, Yancey, & Milsten, 2000), and the Event Safety Guide continues to be used in the United Kingdom. However, because of the myriad of variables associated with MGs, the establishment of guidelines remains a daunting challenge (Ranse & Hutton, 2012).

Goals of Emergency Care at Mass Gatherings

Mass gatherings are heterogeneous in terms of size, nature, and duration of the event; venue location and environment; crowd behavior; pervasiveness of recreational substance use; and demographics of the participants and spectators. Nonetheless, the overall goals of medical care at MGs across these parameters are to:

a. Evaluate and stabilize injury and illness in participants, support staff, and spectators involved in the event, consistent with the standard of medical care in the surrounding local community;

b. Preserve the capacity of the local public health and acute medical care systems to serve their local constituents, through pre-event hazard identification, risk assessment, and utilization of these results to mitigate risks, reduce morbidity, and determine appropriate levels of resources and expertise dedicated to the event;

c. Optimally respond to extraordinary or catastrophic events, through utilization of the ICS, as defined in the U.S. National Incident Management System (NIMS) guidelines for the management of MCIs (Schwartz, Nafziger, Milsten, Luk, & Yancey, 2015). (Note: major incident medical management and support and other adaptations of the U.S. ICS model may be used internationally.)

Most patient encounters across all MG event types are generally minor complaints such as headache, fatigue, minor abrasions, lacerations, and sunburn (Hutton, Ranse, Verdonk, Ullah, & Arbon, 2014) and patients requiring transport to the emergency department from MGs generally require minimal medical care beyond supportive management with low rates of hospital admission (DeMott, Hebert, Novak, Mahmood, & Peska, in press). Emergency nurses should maintain readiness in anticipation of patient surge resulting from MGs (Alzahrani & Kyratsis, 2017). Although most MGs are a collection of basically healthy individuals, health problems do appear to occur with increased frequency and the provision of adequate and appropriate care is required. A key decision in the planning process concerns the service that will be provided on the event site and determination of its purpose(s). Will it focus only on urgent response to life-threatening conditions and the evacuation of these casualties, or will it also treat minor conditions on-site, thus alleviating the patient load that would otherwise impact on local hospitals and health services? Does the on-site health service have a role to play in the event of an MCI and if so how will external health services and the local disaster/emergency system coordinate with the in-event health service? In the event of an MCI who will be in charge, and what communications and ICSs will be used? Large-scale catastrophic events require a crucial shift from individual-based care to population-based care through the adoption of an operational process that coordinates decision making at all points of contact (Bostick, Subbarao, & Burkle, 2008). A key benefit of on-site emergency healthcare services is rapid access to the patient, early and effective triage, early stabilization, and preplanned transport to a more definitive level of care. Nurses must, as members of the on-site healthcare team, be prepared to deal with routine minor injuries as well as the urgent response to, for example, sudden cardiac arrest, psychiatric emergency, or precipitous birth.

PREDICTING PATIENT PRESENTATION RATES

Examination of healthcare usage data from previous events provides valuable information in preplanning services for future events and for predicting PPRs. Some of the events that have been historically analyzed include the Olympics, marathons, large stadium events, political conventions, air shows, papal masses, and outdoor music festivals (Gordon, 1988; Kade, Brinsfield, Serino, Savoia, & Koh, 2008; Paul, 1993; Sanders et al., 1986; Thompson, Savoia, Powell, Challis, & Law, 2005). Considerable variation exists in the collection and reporting of data from international MGs, however, making it difficult to determine consensus on key concepts and data definitions (Turris et al., 2016). Nevertheless, review of lessons learned from these events can provide an effective underpinning in planning for future MG events. Collaboration across all jurisdictional and nongovernmental agencies is important, as they may have had previous experience with managing the event and can provide advice as well as assistance. When an event occurs regularly and has been held in the community previously, historical data provide the best indication of patient load and the nature of patient presentations (Zeitz, Zeitz, & Arbon, 2005). Prior event data can be used to calculate an expected PPR and transport to hospital rate (TTHR) for the event. Event health planners should note, however, that changes in timing of the event or in the program of activities can result in altered weather conditions and/or new risks that will alter PPRs and the profile of presenting injuries or illnesses. For events where there has been little prior experience (including new community events), predictive models for PPRs and TTHRs are available that use linear mathematical modeling to consider the crowd, environmental, and venue characteristics (Arbon, 2007).

EVENT TYPE

The nature of patient encounters that can be anticipated is determined largely by the type of crowd, the type of event, and the environmental factors present in the setting where the event

is held (Sampson, 2005). This framework has been described in terms of psychosocial, biomedical, and environmental domains (Arbon, 2004, 2007; see Figure 5.1). Each domain is characterized by key characteristics that will influence the rate of injury and illness. These characteristics are more or less well understood and combine to produce an effect, the PRR. The domains address the following:

- Psychosocial (individual behaviors, collective social dynamic, and culture);
- Biomedical (aggregate spectator age, pre-event health status of attendees, physical activity levels of participants and spectators, physiology of response to extremes of heat or cold, and extent of substance use in the attendees); and
- Environmental (bounded vs. unbounded venue; time-focused vs. extended; seated vs. mobile; local weather; crowd density; type of event; outdoor weather exposure vs. indoor controlled climate).

Crowds attend events based on the specific nature of the gathering, and the type of event is often the best predictor of the characteristics of the people who will be potentially seeking medical care. The type of crowd drawn to attend a rock concert is in all probability quite different from the crowd drawn to attend a political rally or a papal mass (Challenger, Clegg, Robinson, & Leigh, 2010; Hutton et al., 2014). Most people who attend marathons are generally healthy; however, heat exhaustion, muscle injuries, and trauma are common to sporting events, and cardiac arrest can occur (Finn & Coviello, 2011). Characteristics that are recognized to affect the PPR include weather, event type, event duration, crowd mood, crowd density, attendance, age, and alcohol and drug use.

WEATHER

Weather and environmental conditions, such as the terrain and accessibility of the event, are a major factor in determining the types of illnesses and injuries to which the healthcare team will need to respond. The prevailing weather can influence the PPR at events and rapid changes in weather patterns during an MG event are also associated with an increased number of individuals seeking care (Milsten, Seaman, Liu, Bissel, & Maquire, 2003). Long-range weather forecasts and in-event monitoring of weather conditions are a useful adjunct to planning and healthcare response.

Heat

Heat-related illnesses (e.g., heat stroke, blisters, and sunburn) are the most commonly identified environmental health issues for MG events (see Figure 5.2). Use of the heat index (a combined measure of temperature and humidity) is considered to be the most important weather-related determinant and is often used for modeling potential demand for medical services. The demographic characteristics of MG attendees need to be considered. For instance, infants and children, older adults (>65 years), outdoor workers, and athletes are known to be

HEAT-RELATED ILLNESSES

WHAT TO LOOK FOR	WHAT TO DO
HEAT STROKE	
• High body temperature (103°F or higher) • Hot, red, dry, or damp skin • Fast, strong pulse • Headache • Dizziness • Nausea • Confusion • Losing consciousness (passing out)	• Call 911 right away—heat stroke is a medical emergency • Move the person to a cooler place • Help lower the person's temperature with cool cloths or a cool bath • Do not give the person anything to drink
HEAT EXHAUSTION	
• Heavy sweating • Cold, pale, and clammy skin • Fast, weak pulse • Nausea or vomiting • Muscle cramps • Tiredness or weakness • Dizziness • Headache • Fainting (passing out)	• Move to a cool place • Loosen your clothes • Put cool, wet cloths on your body or take a cool bath • Sip water **Get medical help right away if:** • You are throwing up • Your symptoms get worse • Your symptoms last longer than 1 hour
HEAT CRAMPS	
• Heavy sweating during intense exercise • Muscle pain or spasms	• Stop physical activity and move to a cool place • Drink water or a sports drink • Wait for cramps to go away before you do any more physical activity **Get medical help right away if:** • Cramps last longer than 1 hour • You're on a low-sodium diet • You have heart problems
SUNBURN	
• Painful, red, and warm skin • Blisters on the skin	• Stay out of the sun until your sunburn heals • Put cool cloths on sunburned areas or take a cool bath • Put moisturizing lotion on sunburned areas • Do not break blisters
HEAT RASH	
• Red clusters of small blisters that look like pimples on the skin (usually on the neck, chest, groin, or in elbow creases)	• Stay in a cool, dry place • Keep the rash dry • Use powder (like baby powder) to soothe the rash

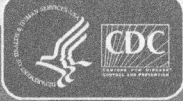

FIGURE 5.2 CDC heat-related illnesses.

CDC, Centers for Disease Control and Prevention.

Source: Centers for Disease Control and Prevention. (2017c). Warning signs and symptoms of heat-related illness. Retrieved from https://www.cdc.gov/disasters/extremeheat/warning.html

more vulnerable to heat-related illnesses than individuals with preexisting illnesses, particularly cardiovascular and pulmonary (Centers for Disease Control and Prevention [CDC], 2017a). Also "visiting" populations can be less prepared and more susceptible to climate conditions (heat, cold, humidity) and altitude. Heat-related illnesses are commonly monitored using syndromic surveillance. In order for this to be effective, medical and emergency personnel need to be appropriately trained to recognize signs of heat-related illnesses, particularly among sensitive populations (Isla et al., 2015).

Heat Rash

Heat rash is commonly referred to as "prickly heat," a maculopapular rash accompanied by acute inflammation and blocked sweat ducts. Heat rash frequently affects areas of the body covered by tight clothing. Initial treatment is the application of chlorhexidine lotion to remove any desquamated skin (talcum powder is not effective).

Heat Cramps

Heat cramps are painful, often severe, involuntary spasms of the large muscle groups used in strenuous exercise. Heat cramps occur after intense physical exertion. They usually develop in people performing heavy exercise in the heat while sweating profusely and drinking nonelectrolyte-containing water. Hyponatremia results and causes cramping in the overstressed muscle. Initial treatment is rehydration with salt-containing fluids. Rehydration will bring rapid relief to patients suffering minor cramps. Patients experiencing severe heat cramps will need intravenous (IV) rehydration therapy. Several sports drinks on the market provide all of the necessary electrolytes to prevent heat cramps. Salt tablets should not be used as they provide inadequate fluid replacement and can be a gastric irritant. Cases of heat cramps are more likely to be seen than cases of heat stroke. However, even well-trained athletes may suffer heat stroke.

Heat Syncope

Heat exposure can cause postural hypotension leading to a syncopal or near-syncopal episode. Heat syncope is believed to result from intense sweating, which leads to dehydration, followed by peripheral vasodilatation. Initial management of the patient with heat syncope involves cooling and rehydration of the patient with oral rehydration solutions (e.g., commercially available sports drinks).

Heat Exhaustion

Heat exhaustion is the precursor to heat stroke. The two conditions appear similar clinically; however, with heat exhaustion, the patient remains neurologically intact. Heat exhaustion presents as headache, nausea and vomiting, dizziness, fatigue, myalgias, and tachycardia. Heat exhaustion is characterized by excessive dehydration and electrolyte depletion. The body temperature may be normal but is generally elevated. Initial therapy involves removing patients from the heat and replenishing their fluids. Mild cases can be treated with oral rehydration; however, moderate to severe (most patients) will require IV fluid replacement therapy. Patients will need several hours of observation prior to being released.

Heat Stroke

Classic heat stroke occurs during periods of sustained high temperatures and humidity. Typical patients are infants, the elderly, and the chronically ill who may not have access to air-conditioning. Sweating is absent in many of those affected. Heat stroke is a medical emergency, and patients need initiation of lifesaving measures and transport to the nearest emergency facility. Exertional heat stroke develops in healthy young persons and is not related to heat waves. Athletes and military personnel are frequently victims due to physical exertion during hot weather conditions. These patients present with marked sweating and are treated in the same manner as patients with classic heat stroke. Immediate intervention is imperative as patients can go on to develop rhabdomyolysis, acute renal failure, hepatic damage, impairment of the central nervous system, and disseminated intravascular coagulation. The initiation of lifesaving measures, including rapid cooling and immediate transport to an emergency facility, is indicated.

Healthcare providers face the same hazards from heat when providing routine care during the summer or a heat wave. During a heat wave, greater stress is placed on both personnel and equipment. Air-conditioning must be provided at the event to provide a safe environment for healthcare providers to give care, to protect medications and equipment, and to provide a cooling mechanism for patients experiencing heat-related illness. The American College of Sports Medicine issued a position statement that strenuous events be postponed or canceled at certain "wet bulb" temperatures, which are derived from a combination of several environmental factors.

Cold

Cold weather decreases the total number of injuries, but it does produce a variety of injuries and illnesses that are unique to colder temperatures. Cold injuries can be divided into local cold injuries and the systemic state of hypothermia. Hypothermia is further classified as mild, moderate, and severe. Local cold injuries include frostnip, frostbite, and chilblains. The CDC website describes the spectrum of cold injuries (CDC, 2017b).

Frostnip

Frostnip is the precursor to frostbite. It is a superficial cold injury without ice crystal formation or tissue damage. Clinically, the involved area is pale from vasoconstriction, and mild burning or stinging is usually felt. Symptoms improve with rewarming, and no long-term tissue damage occurs.

Frostbite

Frostbite can occur anywhere, but it is most commonly observed on the face, nose, ears, hands, and feet. It can be divided into superficial and deep injuries. Erythema, mild edema, and no blisters characterize first-degree frostbite. It is often accompanied by burning and stinging. Second-degree frostbite is characterized by erythema and edema, followed by the formation of clear blisters in 6 to 12 hours.

Hypothermia

Hypothermia is defined as a core temperature of less than 35°C (95°F). While hypothermia can affect any organ system in the body, the most prominent effects are on the neurological and cardiovascular systems. Mild hypothermia is a core body temperature between 32°C and 35°C. In this range of core temperature, patients present with shivering and increased heart rate and blood pressure. Moderate hypothermia is seen with a core temperature between 27°C and 32°C. As the temperature drops below 32°C, progressive slowing of all bodily functions is observed. Shivering ceases between 30°C and 32°C. Decreased mentation develops, and atrial fibrillation or other arrhythmias may occur. Below 28°C, the irritability of the myocardium increases, making the patient more susceptible to the development of ventricular fibrillation.

Hypothermia may occur in settings that do not necessarily involve cold temperatures. It is especially likely in MGs involving water, such as triathlons or citizen swim meets. The presence of rain in a non-water event markedly increases the likelihood of hypothermia.

Other environment-related problems may include sudden thunderstorms, lightning, flooding, and injuries related to low ambient illumination (e.g., tripping and falling).

EVENT DURATION

How long is the event scheduled to last? Will the event occur on a weekend or a weekday? Will it be open after dark? Is the event scheduled to occur in a rural area or in the middle of a large city? Are there people living on the grounds where the event is to occur? How far do participants need to travel to access the event? These factors and many others will influence not only the number of attendees but also the types of medical problems treated (Health and Safety Executive, 2007; Isla et al., 2015). An air show held in rural England presents a very different challenge to healthcare planners than the Molson 500 automobile race held in the streets of Toronto or the Salt Lake speed record challenges held in remote central Australia. Furthermore, the healthcare planning for a 1-day youth soccer tournament differs significantly from planning for a multi-day-long international World Cup Football event. In general, the longer the duration of the event, the greater the number of individuals who will seek care.

Healthcare usage rates may be higher in settings where groups are allowed to move about more freely. Such mobility heightens the risk of minor trauma and exposure- or exertion-related illnesses compared to events where spectators are seated for most of the duration (Arbon, 2007; Michael & Barbera, 1997). Some of the world's largest MGs are spiritual in nature. Among all MGs, the public health issues associated with the Hajj (a 5-day annual pilgrimage to Mecca, Saudi Arabia) is one of the best reported because of its international or even intercontinental implications in terms of the spread of infectious disease. The Hajj routinely attracts 2.5 million Muslims for worship. Planning for and emergency management of the Hajj focuses upon ensuring the health and safety of pilgrims, containment of infectious diseases, and protection of global health security (Memish, Stephens, Steffen, & Ahmed, 2012). Health managers, therefore, need to be aware of the physical or geographical layout as well as the duration of the event. Health planners can assist in this task by ensuring that event staff are aware of the link between injuries and the structures and terrain within the event site and by notifying event staff when they become aware of a hazard or when they receive multiple casualties from the same location. The presence of physical barriers such as ditches, large fields, or fences that would limit movement must be noted. Hazardous areas or access to busy roads should be roped off in advance. If the event is to be held indoors, are there elevators, stairwells, locked doors, or other potential barriers to patient access or evacuation? Where will the healthcare facilities be located? The plan must include provisions for drinking water and sanitation facilities, adequate power supply, and rubbish disposal. Shelter should be a major concern during event planning, especially for outdoor events, lengthy events, or adverse weather conditions. In the event that an MG should decompensate into an MCI, every healthcare provider must be aware of the *entire site layout, location of all escape routes, how to activate the emergency operations plan, and their roles within the plan.*

CHARACTERISTICS OF THE CROWD

What is the actual number and type of people expected to attend? Based on the expected attendance, one can estimate the potential number of patients. If the event involves ticket sales, this number may be easy to obtain. If not, prior similar event attendance may provide a good starting point for estimating the size of the anticipated crowd. What are the characteristics of the people who are expected to attend? Will they be young or elderly? Will they be predominantly male or female? Perhaps the crowd will consist of a combination of both. Will the event attract individuals who may have an underlying medical condition? An example of this would be a walk to raise money for a disease such as asthma or HIV. This will increase the probability of individuals needing care for certain conditions. Will alcohol be sold and consumed at the event? Historical data, as mentioned above, such as previous medical records and event reports can be used to gather information prior to the event (Zeitz et al., 2005).

Crowd density, type, and mood are important and yet predictable variables in MGs and can influence the health needs of attendees (Brown & Hutton, 2013; Hutton, Brown, & Verdonk, 2012). A "crowd" can be defined as a number of people colocated in a specific place for a measurable time period; frequently with common goals and displaying common behaviors. "Thus, a gathering of 20 people standing in close proximity at a specific location to observe a specific event over a one-hour period, who feel united by a common identity and, despite being strangers, are able to act in a socially coherent way, could be considered a crowd" (Challenger et al., 2010, p. 43). Some characteristics of crowds include

- Size—a large group of people;
- Density—people colocated in a particular area, with a particular density distribution;
- Time—individuals who come together in a specific location for a specific purpose over a measurable amount of time;
- Collectivity—crowd members share a social identity, including common goals and interests, and act in a coherent manner;
- Novelty—individuals act in a socially coherent manner, despite coming together in an ambiguous or unfamiliar situation.

Crowd Density

Crowd density is often linked to the purpose of the event and higher crowd densities may lead to increased interactions between individuals (Li, Wu, Matsumoto, & Zhao, 2010). Increased density can foster feelings of claustrophobia, paranoia, or aggression and can incite inappropriate behavior among certain individuals attending large events. Crowd densities combined with crowd mood at the World Cup Football Tournament, and in the chaos that ensued following the Olympic bombing in Atlanta, created dangerous conditions and the potential for additional injuries (Spaaij, 2016).

Crowd Mood

The type of music played at a concert, religious affiliations, political demonstrations, rivalry between competing sports teams, all contribute to creating an emotionally charged event and influence crowd mood.

Social influence on individual audience members exerted by the wider audience can be a very powerful force and can affect different people in different ways with some people more susceptible to this influence than others. Crowd mood and associated behavior has been researched extensively by Reicher (2008); however, only one model exists in the literature that attempts to measure crowd mood in relation to healthcare. Pines and Maslach (1993) developed a matrix to calculate the resources required to support a public event using the audience profile to assess crowd mood. Their model is twofold. First, they use descriptors to clearly identify separate groups (e.g., families, young adults, children, elderly, and rival factions). Second, they attach a rating scale (1–5) to rate these groups (Pines & Maslach, 1993). This rating scale is used to grade the amount of verbal noise, physical movement, and overall audience participation. Even though this scale is over 20 years old, there has not been another developed to assess crowd mood, and the majority of what is written about crowd mood is highly theoretical. Zeitz, Tan, Grief, Couns, and Zeitz (2009) used this model to assess 35 MG events, and found that crowd mood was an important factor in predicting medical workload at MG events, although it did not significantly affect the work of other emergency services, such as police or fire and rescue. Nurses and other health professionals need to be equipped with practical strategies to monitor and measure crowd mood and type, and how these changes may impact on the resultant behavior of a crowd (Hutton, Zeitz, Brown, & Arbon, 2011).

Application of new technologies, such as active monitoring by event command and control centers of social media (emotion analysis) associated with an event in order to preempt incidents, is helping to address this issue (Ngo, Haghighi, & Burstein, 2015).

ALCOHOL AND DRUG USAGE

Patterns of alcohol and drug use have long been associated with certain types of MGs, especially rock concerts and outdoor music festivals and are significant contributors to increased morbidity and mortality (Hutton et al., 2014; Milsten et al., 2003). Studies have shown a 10-fold increase in presentations at events where alcohol is sold when compared to those events which are alcohol-free (Arbon, Bridgewater, & Smith, 2001). The use of drugs and alcohol is therefore one of the most significant biomedical issues of concern at many MGs and is related to other crowd behaviors such as "moshing" and stampedes that result in increased rates of injuries and illness (Raineri & Earl, 2006). Alcohol, drug usage, and dehydration can be expected to be higher among spectators at outdoor sporting events.

MEDICAL AID STATIONS

Careful selection of the location of patient treatment areas is paramount in increasing their effectiveness. The placement of medical and first aid stations should be such that the stations are easily accessible within a reasonable time by all. The size of the event and the site layout will determine the number of aid stations needed. For example, a small indoor event may require only one aid station, whereas an event in a large open field such as an exposition, air show, or automobile race may require multiple stations. All aid stations should be clearly marked with signs. Location and directions to aid stations should be listed in the event program (in all appropriate languages) and announced over the public address system during the event. Aid stations should have tables and sufficient room for equipment, supplies, and personnel. They should have beds or cots for patients to lie down. Ideally, they should be located near sanitation facilities. Ample water and sanitation facilities should be available to all who attend the event. Accommodations must be made for the physically challenged and special accommodations must be made for any high-risk, high-vulnerability groups in attendance.

How will patients access the triage and treatment areas and how will nursing and EMS personnel reach patients unable to ambulate? Depending on the size and scope of the event, provisions should be made for mobile healthcare teams to meet the needs of patients who require urgent assistance or are unable to walk to the aid station. Most patients will present to the station to receive care, but some will be unable to do so. Consideration needs to be given as to what equipment nurses and paramedics may use and in what manner that equipment will be carried. The locations of patient litters or backboards should be logical and easy to access. Specific routes should be marked. Leonard and Moreland (2001) recommend that very large outdoor venues may require the mobile team to have supplies such as IV drugs, a cardiac monitor, intubation equipment, oxygen, and a defibrillator. Patient extrication devices such as golf carts, backboards, or wheelchairs can assist in the removal of patients from the crowd (Leonard & Moreland, 2001). In stadium events, special devices such as stair-climbing stretchers may be required.

TRANSPORTATION CONSIDERATIONS

Ambulance areas should be within easy access of the medical treatment stations. Although transportation considerations may not be the responsibility of the nurse, all healthcare providers should be aware of the plans for transportation and know where transport vehicles will be located. Consideration as to what roads are available for ambulance traffic as well as what physical obstructions ambulances may encounter must be part of the overall planning process. In addition, the plan should consider the number of ambulances that should be kept at the site as opposed to those that are on call. If air medical transportation is necessary, a clear and safe landing zone must be established and maintained. The receiving hospitals for patients should be determined in advance, and mechanisms for notifying these hospitals of incoming patients must be implemented prior to an event. (See Appendix 5.1 for a discussion of guidelines for mass casualty prediction for receiving hospitals.)

Mass casualty triage should be implemented as a systemic multitiered process that incrementally addresses mass casualty care decision making under significant resource constraints (Subbarao et al., 2009) and informs decision making on priorities for transport where patient numbers overwhelm available ambulance resources. Decisions must ensure that appropriate patients are directed to the appropriate site for care; for example, trauma centers, primary care clinics, or pediatric facilities.

COMMUNICATION SYSTEMS

Communication systems must be established so that healthcare providers can communicate with each other, with leadership, and with collaborating partners such as police, fire, security, and local hospitals. Good communication is essential for the successful operation of any large healthcare activity. Communication techniques used in MGs should closely parallel daily communication techniques, used by the healthcare service providers; reflecting a "business as usual approach." As with disasters and MCIs, radios will provide the bulk of the communications. Cellular (mobile) telephones may also be considered, although their use may be limited by the local infrastructure and geographical location of the event. In the event of an MCI, the mobile telephone system may be overwhelmed, although recent MG emergencies such as the London Underground Bombings (2005) and the Manchester Stadium Attack (2017) have demonstrated that these systems can be remarkably robust and both public and emergency responders continued to use mobile telephones during the response (P. Arbon, personal communication, May 10, 2017).

STAFFING

Medical and nurse staffing at MGs requires consideration of expertise levels and types. These should match the nature of demands for medical care that likely will need to be addressed. The specialization of staffing must also match that of medical equipment and pharmaceuticals that are to be dedicated to on-site care. Personnel chosen must be qualified, screened, credentialed, and appropriately trained to resuscitate airway and circulatory life threats that need to be immediately addressed and maintain the quality of care expected in the host community, until delivery to the next most appropriate higher level of care (Schwartz et al., 2015). Nurse and other healthcare practitioner staffing needs will be specifically customized for the event and determined based on a number of factors, including the total number of medical aid stations, the anticipated size of the gathering, the type of event, and the anticipated medical problems that may be encountered. The planned profile of health practitioner coverage will also factor into the nurse staffing needs for the event. Sanders et al. (1986) recommend that healthcare provider staffing for special events accommodate the provision of (a) basic first aid and BLS within 4 minutes, (b) ALS within 8 minutes, and (c) evacuation to a hospital within 30 minutes. Gutman et al. (2011) confirm that despite relatively high PPRs, with adequate staffing, there can be minimal impact on emergency health services.

DOCUMENTATION

A brief written record should be generated for all presentations including the most trivial. A multi-patient record can be used for minor requests—such as bandages and sunscreen—and this ensures that future planning for the event benefits from an accurate picture of demand. A standard and detailed medical record should be kept for all but the most trivial patient encounters. Standard medical record items include demographic data and brief medical history, including medications and allergies, type of illness or injury, treatment rendered, and disposition. Various databases can be used if they are available. Detailed records absolutely must be kept for those patients sick or injured enough to receive medical or nursing assessment and on-site treatment and those who are sent to a hospital. The patient encounter forms should include some description of the location of the incident, mechanism of injury, and any other important variables. The use of handheld digital devices and smartphones for medical record documentation during MG events may expedite and improve record keeping. Patient clinical records should remain confidential, be copied to other healthcare providers if the patient is transferred and kept on file for the legally required period within that jurisdiction. In addition to clinical records, other documentation should include event health plans, emergency response plans, communications and dispatch logs, and event summary or debrief reports.

MASS CASUALTY INCIDENTS

As seen at the Las Vegas Route 91 Harvest Festival, an MG can decompensate into an MCI at any point before, during, or after the scheduled event. Therefore, the fundamentals of healthcare practice during an MG event involving large numbers of people including triage, assessment, diagnosis, and treatment are accompanied by an expectation and heightened vigilance for the unexpected. For example, the 2017 Route 91 Harvest Festival saw 59 people killed, and another 527 injured (Boyle, Henderson, Mendick, Crilly, & Ensor, 2017). The resultant MCI event creates a sudden "surge" of individuals requiring immediate assessment and care. "Surge capacity" implies that after a hazard's impact, the healthcare system will be capable of responding effectively to an unanticipated increase in patient presentations. Nurses must realize that in stressful circumstances such as an MCI, the demand on their skills may be greater and the circumstances unusual; however, the *nursing fundamentals practiced in other settings and during smaller crises will still be applicable.* That said, all nurses providing care during an MG should possess a minimum set of core competencies in disaster nursing. The American Red Cross proposes that disaster nursing is "doing the best for the most, with the least, by the fewest." Advanced preparation of our national nursing workforce for such events is predicated on the belief that mastery of the unique knowledge and skills needed to respond appropriately to such a challenging event as an MCI can improve patient outcomes. Resources may be limited. Time is an important factor. The longer the delay in care for a seriously injured patient, the less chance for recovery. The governing principle is to do the *greatest good for the greatest number of casualties, with the least amount of harm.* MCIs may necessitate consideration of alterations in standards of clinical care (Hanfling, Altevogt, Viswanathan, & Gostin, 2012; Hick, Hanfling, & Cantrill, 2012). The basic principles of disaster nursing during special (events) circumstances and MCIs include the following:

- Rapid assessment of the situation and of victims' immediate nursing care needs (see Appendix 5.1 for further discussion.)
- Security of the scene and assessment of the potential for a secondary disaster
- Mass casualty triage and the initiation of lifesaving measures first
- Knowledge of one's role within the ICS
- The selected use of essential nursing interventions and the elimination of nonessential nursing activities
- Adaptation of necessary nursing skills to a mass casualty situation and the allocation of scarce resources (The nurse must use imagination and resourcefulness in dealing with a lack of supplies, equipment, and personnel.)
- The potential need for decontamination
- Ongoing evaluation of the environment and the mitigation or removal of any health hazards
- Prevention of further injury or illness
- Leadership in coordinating patient triage, care, and transport during times of crisis
- The teaching, supervision, and utilization of auxiliary medical personnel and volunteers
- Provision of understanding, compassion, and emotional support to all victims and their families
- Appreciation of and the knowledge to keep oneself safe during the MCI response

PRACTICE PARAMETERS FOR NURSING CARE

The nursing fundamentals practiced in normal daily situations and during smaller crises will be applicable during an MG event or mass casualty situations. All nurses providing healthcare at MGs must be competent in the basic principles of first aid, including cardiopulmonary resuscitation and the use of the automated external defibrillator. In addition, nurses should possess, within the limits of their license to practice and local regulations, the following competencies:

Nursing Assessments

- Perform a respiratory, airway assessment
- Perform a cardiovascular assessment, including vital signs, monitoring for signs of shock
- Perform an integumentary assessment, including a burn assessment
- Perform a pain assessment
- Perform a trauma assessment from head to toe
- Perform a mental status assessment, including a Glasgow Coma Scale
- Know the indications for intubation
- Know IV insertion and administration of IV medication
- Know emergency medications
- Know the principles of fluid therapy

Nursing Therapeutics and Core Competencies

- Concepts of basic first aid and hemodynamic stabilization
- Disaster triage and transport
- Pain management
- Management of hypovolemia and fluid replacement
- Suturing (if appropriate based on practice parameters) and initial wound care
- Blast injuries/dealing with tissue loss
- Eye lavage techniques
- Decontamination of chemical and radiation exposures
- Fractures/immobilization of fractures
- Management of hemorrhage
- Stabilization of crush injuries
- Movement of patients with spinal cord injury.

In all types of MG event and MCIs, the American Red Cross (*Guidelines for Disaster Nursing* and revised *Disaster Health Services Concepts of Operations,* 2011) states that nurses will be expected to exercise great leadership and discerning judgment in the following:

1. Assessment and triage of patient's condition for priority care
2. Provision of care, treatment, and health protection
3. Appropriate utilization of nursing service personnel
4. Detection of changes in the event environment to organize activities to modify or eliminate health hazards
5. Dealing with mass casualties if necessary

Public Health for Mass Gatherings: Key Considerations by the World Health Organization is an excellent resource for nurses seeking information regarding public health planning, communications, design of emergency services, and psycho-social considerations for MG events and MCIs (www.who.int/ihr/publications/WHO_HSE_GCR_2015.5/en/). Above all, the nurse must ensure his or her own safety throughout the duration of the event.

SUMMARY

Multiple interacting variables combine to create complexity and uncertainty when planning for emergency health consequences during a special event or MG. It is important to recognize that an MG may suddenly become an MCI without any warning, resulting in a "surge" of victims and an immediate need for disaster healthcare services. Understanding the specific details of an event—the type and purpose of the event, the location and duration, the characteristics of the crowd, weather conditions, and the impacts of the presence of alcohol—can be used to predict healthcare usage.

Advanced preparation of the nursing workforce for such events is predicated on the belief that mastery of the unique knowledge and skills needed to respond appropriately to such an event as an MCI can improve patient outcomes. Nurses do need to possess basic core competencies in emergency nursing in order to respond in a timely and appropriate manner and keep themselves safe. Time becomes a major factor in predicting patient recovery—the longer the delay in care for a seriously injured patient, the lesser the chance for a full recovery. Rapid assessment of the situation and nursing care needs, triage, and the initiation of lifesaving measures first, and the selected use of essential nursing interventions, along with the simultaneous elimination of nonessential measures, are the skills needed to successfully manage emergencies outside of the hospital. The governing principle is always to *do the greatest good for the greatest number with the least amount of harm.*

STUDY QUESTIONS

1. You have been asked to participate in the planning for a heavy metal concert to be held in August outside of Paducah, Kentucky. The line-up includes several popular bands and over 10,000 people are anticipated to attend. Outline your top ten priorities for planning and your rationale.

2. You are designing the medical aid stations for this event. Describe how many you will need and what you need for staffing and supplies.

3. Discuss why crowd density and crowd mood are important considerations for mass gathering planning. What steps could be taken in advance to address these factors?

4. Describe the key considerations for public health for mass gatherings according to the World Health Organization.

5. You are working in the emergency department on a Saturday evening when the EMS call comes in that there has been a mass shooting one mile away with an unknown number of victims. Describe what actions you would take and why.

6. Outline the broad communications plan for emergency healthcare services for this event.

REFERENCES

Agency for Healthcare Research and Quality. (2005). Altered standards of care in mass casualty events. Retrieved from https://archive.ahrq.gov/research/altstand

Alzahrani, F., & Kyratsis, Y. (2017). Emergency nurse disaster preparedness during mass gatherings: A cross-sectional survey of emergency nurses' perceptions in hospitals in Mecca, Saudi Arabia. *British Medical Jounral Open, 7*(4), e013563. doi:10.1136/bmjopen-2016-013563

American Red Cross. (2011). Guidelines for disaster nursing. Retrieved from http://www.redcross.org

Arbon, P. (2004). The development of conceptual models for mass gatherings health. *Prehospital and Disaster Medicine, 19*(3), 208–212. doi:10.1017/S1049023X00001795

Arbon, P. (2007). Mass-gathering medicine: A review of the evidence and future directions for research. *Prehospital Disaster Medicine, 22,* 131–135. doi:10.1017/S1049023X00004507

Arbon, P., Bridgewater, F. H., & Smith, C. (2001). Mass gathering medicine: A predictive model for patient presentation and transport rates. *Prehospital and Disaster Medicine, 16*(3), 150–158. doi:10.1017/s1049023x00025905

Bostick, N., Subbarao, I., & Burkle, F. M. (2008). Disaster triage systems for large-scale catastrophic events. *Disaster Medicine and Public Health Preparedness, 2*(Suppl 1), S35–S39. doi:10.1097/DMP.0b013e3181825a2b

Boyle, D., Henderson, B., Mendick, R., Crilly, R, & Ensor, J. (2017, 3 October). Las Vegas shooting kills at least 59 in deadliest ever US gun attack. *Telegraph.* Retrieved from https://www.telegraph.co.uk/news/2017/10/02/las-vegas-strip-shooting-multiple-casualties-reported-near-mandalay

Brown, S., & Hutton, A. (2013). Developments in the real-time evaluation of audience behaviour at planned events. *International Journal of Event and Festival Management, 1*(4), 43–55. doi:10.1108/17582951311307502

Centers for Disease Control and Prevention. (2017a). About extreme heat. Retrieved from https://www.cdc.gov/disasters/extremeheat/index.html

Centers for Disease Control and Prevention. (2017b). Cold related illnesses. Retrieved from https://www.cdc.gov/niosh/topics/coldstress/coldrelatedillnesses.html

Centers for Disease Control and Prevention. (2017c). Warning signs and symptoms of heat-related illness. Retrieved from https://www.cdc.gov/disasters/extremeheat/warning.html

Challenger, R. Clegg, C. Robinson, M., & Leigh, M. (2010). Understanding crowd behaviour, Volume 1.—Practical guide and lessons identified. London, England: The Stationary Office.

Committee on Evaluation of the Metropolitan Medical Response System Program. (2002). F. J. Manning & L. Goldfrank (Eds.), *Preparing for terrorism: Tools for evaluating the metropolitan medical response system program.* Washington, DC: National Academies Press. Retrieved from https://www.ncbi.nlm.nih.gov/books/NBK220771/pdf/Bookshelf_NBK220771.pdf

Cuny, F. (1998). Principles of disaster management. Lesson 1: Introduction. *Prehospital and Disaster Medicine, 13*(1), 88–92. doi:10.1017/S1049023X00033082

DeMott, J., Hebert, C. L., Novak, M., Mahmood, S., & Peksa, G. D. (in press). Characteristics and resource utilization of patients presenting to the emergency department from mass gathering events. *The American Journal of Emergency Medicine.* doi:10.1016/j.ajem.2017.11.006

Finn, S. E., & Coviello, J. (2011). Myocardial infarction and sudden death in recreational masters marathon runners. *Nurse Practitioners, 36*(2), 48–53. doi:10.1097/01.NPR.0000392797.09383.41

Gordon, D. (1988). The pope's visit: Mass gatherings and the EMS System. *Emergency Medical Services, 17*(1), 38–44.

Gutman, S., Lund, A., & Turris, S. (2011). Medical support for the 2009 world police and fire games: A descriptive analysis of a large scale participation event and its impact. *Prehospital and Disaster Medicine, 26*, 33–40. doi:10.1017/S1049023X10000117

Hanfling, D., Altevogt, B. M., Viswanathan, K., & Gostin, L. O. (Eds.). (2012). Crisis standards of care: A systems framework for catastrophic disaster response. Institute of Medicine, Washington, DC: National Academies Press.

Health and Safety Executive. (2007). *The event safety guide: Guide to health, safety and welfare at pop concerts and similar events* (2nd ed.). Edinburgh, Scotland: Author. (Original work published 1999)

Hick, J. L., Hanfling, D., and Cantrill, S. V. (2012). Allocating scarce resources in disasters: Emergency department principles. *Annals of Emergency Medicine, 59*(3), 177–187. doi:10.1016/j.annemergmed.2011.06.012

Hutton, A., Brown, B., & Verdonk, N. (2012). Exploring culture: Audience predispositions and consequent effects on audience behavior in a mass-gathering setting. *Prehospital and Disaster Medicine, 28*(3), 292–297. doi:10.1017/S1049023X13000228

Hutton, A., Ranse, J., Verdonk, N., Ullah, S., & Arbon, P. (2014). Understanding the characteristics of patient presentations of young people at outdoor music festivals. *Prehospital and Disaster Medicine, 29*(2), 160–166. doi:10.1017/S1049023X14000156

Hutton, A., Zeitz, K., Brown, S., & Arbon, P. (2011). Assessing the psychosocial elements of crowds at mass gatherings. *Prehospital and Disaster Medicine, 26*(6), 414–421. doi:10.1017/S1049023X12000155

Isla, N. Endericks, T., & Barbeschi, M. (2015). Chapter 1: Contextual issues and risk assessments public health for mass gatherings: Key considerations. In *Public health for mass gatherings*. Geneva, Switzerland: World Health Organization. Retrieved from http://www.who.int/ihr/publications/WHO_HSE_GCR_2015.5/en

Jaslow, D., Yancey, A., & Milsten, A. (2000). Mass gathering medical care [NAEMSP Position Paper]. *Prehospital Emergency Care, 4*(4), 359–360.

Kade, K. A., Brinsfield, K. H., Serino, R. A., Savoia, E., & Koh, H. (2008). Emergency medical consequence planning and management for national general security events after September 11: Boston 2004. *Disaster Medicine and Public Health Emergency Preparedness, 2*, 166–173. doi:10.1097/DMP.0b013e318184556e

Leonard, R. B., & Moreland, K. M. (2001, January). EMS for the masses. Preplanning your EMS response to a major event. *Emergency Medical Services, 30*(1), 53–60.

Li, W., Wu, X., Matsumoto, K., & Zhao, H.-A. (2010). A new approach of crowd density estimation. TENCON 2010-2010 IEEE Region Conference. IEEE, pp. 200–203.

MacIntrye, A. G., Barbera, J. A., & Brewster, P. (2009). Health care emergency management: Establishing the science of managing mass casualty and mass effect incidents. *Disaster Medicine and Public Health Emergency Preparedness, 3*(Suppl 2), S52–S58. doi:10.1097/DMP.0b013e31819d99b4

Memish, Z. A., Stephens, G. M., Steffen, R., & Ahmed, Q. A. (2012). Emergence of medicine for mass gatherings: Lessons from the Hajj. *The Lancet Infectious Diseases, 12*(1), 56–65. doi:10.1016/S1473-3099(11)70337-1

Michael, J. A., & Barbera, J. A. (1997). Mass gathering medical care: A twenty-five year review. *Prehospital Disaster Medicine, 12*, 305–312.

Milsten, A. M., Seaman, K., Liu, P., Bissel, R., & Maquire, B. (2003). Variables influencing medical usage rate, injury pattern, and levels of care for mass gatherings. *Prehospital Disaster Medicine, 18*, 334–346.

Ngo, M. Q., Haghighi, P. D., & Burstein, F. (2015). *A crowd monitoring framework using emotion analysis of social media for emergency management in mass gatherings*. Australasian Conference on Information Systems, University of South Australia, Adelaide, South Australia.

Paul, H. M. (1993). Pope's Denver visit causes mega MCI. *Journal of Emergency Medical Services, 18*(11), 64–68.

Pines, A., & Maslach, C. (1993). *Experiencing social psychology*. New York, NY: McGraw-Hill.

Raineri, A., & Earl, C. (2006). Crowd management for outdoor music festivals. *Journal of Occupational Health and Safety, 21*(3), 205–215.

Ranse, J. (2006). Cardiac arrest: Can the in-hospital chain of survival be improved? *Australasian Emergency Nursing Journal, 9*(1), 23–27. doi:10.1016/j.aenj.2006.01.002

Ranse, J., & Hutton, A. (2012). Minimum data set for mass-gathering health research and evaluation: A discussion paper. *Prehospital Disaster Medicine, 27*(6), 543–550. doi:10.1017/S1049023X12001288.

Reicher, S. (2008). The psychology of crowd dynamics. In M. A. Hogg & R. S. Tindale (Eds.), *Blackwell handbook of social psychology: Group processes*. Oxford, England: Blackwell.

Sampson, T. R. (2005). Influence of environmental factors on morbidity at mass-gathering sporting events. *Emergency Medicine, 12*(1), 88. doi:10.1197/j.aem.2005.03.246

Sanders, A. B., Criss, E., Steckl, P., Meislin, H. W., Raife, J., & Allen, D. (1986). An analysis of medical care at mass gatherings. *Annals of Emergency Medicine, 15*, 515–519. doi:10.1016/S0196-0644(86)80984-2

Schwartz, B., Nafziger, S., Milsten, A., Luk, J., & Yancey, A. (2015). Mass gathering medical care: Resource document for the National Association of EMS Physicians position statement. *Prehospital Emergency Care, 19*(4), 559–568. doi:10.3109/10903127.2015.1051680

Smith, E. C., Burkle, F. M., & Archer, F. L. (2011). Fear, familiarity and perception of risk: A quantitative analysis of disaster specific concerns of paramedics. *Disaster Medicine and Public Health Preparedness, 5*(1), 46–53. doi:10.1001/dmp.10-v4n2-hre10008

Spaaij, R. (2016). Terrorism and security at the Olympics: Empirical trends and evolving research agendas. *The International Journal of the History of Sport, 33*(4), 451–468. doi:10.1080/09523367.2015.1136290

Subbarao, I., Bostick, N. A., Burkle, F. M., Hsu, E. B., Armstrong, J. H., & James, J. J. (2009). Re-envisioning mass critical care triage as a systematic multi-tiered process. *Chest Journal, 135*(4), 1108–1109. doi:10.1378/chest.08-1891

Thompson, J. M., Savoia, G., Powell, G., Challis, E. B., & Law, P. (2005). Level of medical care required at mass gatherings: The XV winter olympic games in Calgary, Canada. *Annals of Emergency Medicine, 20*, 385–390. Retrieved from www.sciencedirect.com/science/article/pii/S0196064405816609

Turris, S. A., Steenkamp, M., Lund, A., Hutton, A., Ranse, J., Bowles, R., ... Arbon, P. (2016). International consensus on key concepts and data definitions for mass-gathering health: Process and progress. *Prehospital and Disaster Medicine, 31*(2), 220–223. doi:10.1017/S1049023X1600011X

World Health Organization. (2015). *Public health for mass gatherings: Key considerations*. Geneva, Switzerland: Author.

Zeitz, K. M., Tan, H. M., Grief, M., Couns, P. C., & Zeitz, C. J. (2009). Crowd behavior at mass gatherings: A literature review. *Prehospital and Disaster Medicine, 24*(1), 32–38. doi:10.1017/S1049023X00006518

Zeitz, K. M., Zeitz, C. J., & Arbon, P. (2005). Forecasting medical work at mass-gathering events: Predictive model versus retrospective review. *Prehospital and Disaster Medicine, 20*(3), 164–168. doi:10.1017/S1049023X00002399

Appendix 5.1

No-Notice Incidents: Hospital Triage, Intake, and Throughput

April 2018

ASPR TRACIE Tip Sheets: No-Notice Incidents

ASPR TRACIE has developed a series of tip sheets for hospitals and other healthcare facilities planning for no-notice incident response. Our traditional concepts and approaches have not kept pace with real-world incidents in the U.S. and other countries or the challenges the healthcare system faces in managing the resulting extraordinarily large number of casualties. The tip sheets are based on discussions ASPR NHPP and ASPR TRACIE had with healthcare personnel who were involved in the October 2017 mass shooting response in Las Vegas and supplemented with information from other recent no-notice incidents. While there is great variance in the scope and healthcare needs resulting from no-notice incidents, these tip sheets focus on some of the identified challenges.

Triage and Intake

Prepare for Non-Triaged Patients

- During a large-scale incident, emergency medical services (EMS) may not be able to assess, triage, and/or treat all of the casualties at the scene.
- The initial volume of patients may exceed the capacity of available responders and ambulances at the scene, leading to first aid and direct transport by civilians.
- Survivors may flee the incident scene and may not realize their injuries until they reach a safe location or may become injured while escaping. Transports may originate from multiple locations over an extended period of time rather than a single, coordinated incident scene.
- Asymmetric attacks may result in multiple scenes. Hospitals may be targets of a primary or secondary attack.

> Patients arrived to Sunrise via 24 EMS transports and 188 private vehicle transports.

> The Las Vegas incident scene expanded from 17.5 acres to 4 square miles as survivors fled the scene and began to call 911.

Conduct Initial Triage and Intake

- Security personnel should maintain clear vehicle entry points and monitor access to the emergency department (ED). Other entrances to the facility should be controlled. Ideally, law enforcement should be present to support hospital security at the entrance and to provide traffic control.
- Bring essential assets to the ground floor including carts, wheelchairs, personnel, and any designated disaster supplies. Pop the heads up on gurneys so patients are not placed backwards.
- Clear the ED—discharge, cohort existing ED patients requiring additional workup and transport admitted patients to units. Assure each area has a "team leader" appointed.
- Determine in advance which areas of your facility are appropriate for use as expanded ED space and the types of patients that may be accommodated in each of these areas (e.g., post-anesthesia care unit, pre-induction, intensive care unit, procedural areas).
- Appoint an experienced provider to do initial triage. Provide an assistant to tag or mark patients and others to move them to the appropriate area.
- Consider grouping arriving patients by the severity of their injuries.
- Consider bringing deceased patients brought in by loved ones back as expectant rather than black tagging them.
- As part of your planning, develop temporary signs or identify staff who can assist in wayfinding for these expanded spaces. This will reduce confusion among your own staff, your patients and their loved ones, and personnel who are unfamiliar with your facility if you elect to use volunteers or emergency privileging.

> In Las Vegas, many patients attended the festival wearing their entrance wristbands and carrying only cell phones and small amounts of cash. The lack of identification cards in combination with varying levels of alcohol consumption on the final day of the event contributed to challenges in identifying and treating patients.

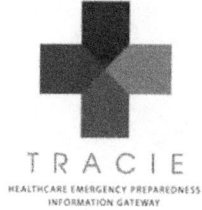

TRACIE
HEALTHCARE EMERGENCY PREPAREDNESS
INFORMATION GATEWAY

Review Your Trauma Alias Process for Patients Who Arrive Without Identification

- Expect that registration and use of electronic systems will not be fast enough to support a rapid influx of large numbers of patients.
- Ensure an adequate supply of paper triage tags and/or paper charts.
- Determine whether patients or accompanying loved ones are able to provide identifying and medical information; be prepared to capture this information for clinical and registration purposes.
- Practice assigning large numbers of trauma aliases to avoid duplication.
- Plan to back up your electronic registration systems in the event wireless networks are overwhelmed.

Stage Personnel and Resources to Manage Initial Treatment Needs

- Consider pairing a nurse with each patient until handoff to the operating room, intensive care unit, or floor. This enables capture of a paper medical record in the event electronic medical records cannot keep pace with the incident and assures that at least one provider knows the patient, and can monitor for changes in condition.

> Sunrise used more than 125 crash carts in the first 3 hours.

- Dedicate providers to each space to continually monitor and reevaluate patients and intervene as needed.
- Dedicate a respiratory therapist for intubation support in the ED. Consider pre-packaged disaster intubation or critical care supply packs for bedside use.
- Dedicate pharmacy personnel and resources in the ED to ensure adequate medication supplies. Automated medication dispensing stations may be unable to keep up with the volume of needed medications.
- Determine a coordinated process for integrating personnel as they arrive in response to requests for additional staffing.

Throughput

Initiate Rapid Discharge of Existing Patients, as Appropriate

- Mobilize hospitalists and intensivists to do rounds and assess inpatient status for potential "surge discharge."
- Identify a single location where discharged patients may wait (e.g., discharge lounge) while other arrangements are made if the incident delays their ability to leave your hospital.

> There were 500 patients in Sunrise prior to the incident. They discharged 184 patients in 15 hours.

Establish a Process for Disaster Patient Flow

- Assure that surgery and ED staff (and potentially anesthesia if available) understand the initial locations of care for critical, moderate, and minor injury.
- Assure a process for triage to CT and to OR. This may involve tags, writing on patient/cart/paper, or simply verbal coordination in smaller departments. Staging areas for CT may be needed (e.g., line up in hallway).
- All critical or moderate patients not requiring immediate CT or OR should be assigned to an inpatient unit or surge area as rapidly as possible (including use of hallway beds). Staff should be available in these areas to re-triage and continue to treat.
- Assure that ED and surgery staff understand priorities for OR (e.g., unstable abdominal injuries first).

Partner With Hospital Incident Command to Expand Capacity

- Move non-incident patients to other areas of the hospital.
- Convert single bed units with two existing headwalls to double capacity.
- Cohort patients where possible.
- Pre-identify units, such as behavioral health, that will have more difficulty rapidly discharging patients.
- Coordinate with other area hospitals to distribute patients and balance loads.

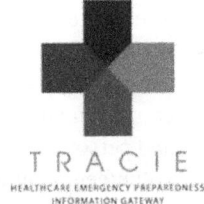

TRACIE

HEALTHCARE EMERGENCY PREPAREDNESS
INFORMATION GATEWAY

Be Prepared for Existing ED Patients to Depart

- Existing (non-incident related) ED patients may leave on their own (or go to an alternate location), recognizing that large numbers of patients with more serious injuries may take precedence.
- While facility planners should not assume this will be the case for all incidents, they should prepare to handle patients who delay care until the following day.

Prepare to Provide Short-Term Assistance to Patients Who Are Treated and Released

- Patients who reside in the area may not have someone immediately available to take them home.
- Patients who are visiting from other areas may not know where or have another place to go.
- Access to and from your facility and throughout the surrounding area may be challenged by perimeter controls and roadblocks.

> Sunrise allowed released patients to wait in the auditorium until other arrangements could be made. UMC arranged transportation to a designated pick-up location.

Related ASPR TRACIE Resources

Tip Sheets in This Series:

Community Response and Media Management
Expanding Traditional Roles to Address Patient Surge
Family Assistance
Fatality Management
Non-Trauma Hospital Considerations
Trauma Surgery Adaptations and Lessons
Trauma System Considerations

Other Resources:

Healthcare Response to a No-Notice Incident: Las Vegas (Webinar)
Hospital Surge Capacity and Immediate Bed Availability Topic Collection
Explosives and Mass Shooting Topic Collection
Incident Management Topic Collection
Pre-Hospital Topic Collection
The Exchange Issue 3: Preparing for and Responding to No-Notice Events

ASPR TRACIE gratefully acknowledges ASPR NHPP staff who provided feedback on these documents and the healthcare personnel from University Medical Center and Sunrise Hospital and Medical Center who responded to the October 1, 2017 no-notice incident in Las Vegas, shared their experiences and insights with staff from ASPR NHPP and TRACIE, and reviewed these tip sheets.

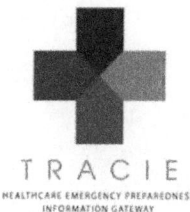

TRACIE
HEALTHCARE EMERGENCY PREPAREDNESS
INFORMATION GATEWAY

6

LEGAL AND ETHICAL ISSUES IN DISASTER RESPONSE

Eileen M. Amari-Vaught, Marilyn M. Pesto, and Kevin D. Hart

LEARNING OBJECTIVES

When this chapter is completed, readers will be able to:

1. Understand the sources of ethical and legal obligations for nurses and nurse administrators.
2. Discover that legal and ethical obligations may be similar, or may change, in the event of a bioterrorist attack or other public health crisis.
3. Explore and identify personal beliefs about disaster response and consider the impact they may have on professional values.
4. Be familiar with major legal and ethical issues related to nurses' responses in a disaster.
5. Become familiar with sources for legal and ethical guidance in the event of a bioterrorist attack and learn when it may be necessary to consult such sources.

KEY MESSAGES

The legal framework for dealing with a bioterrorist attack and the resultant public health crises combine governmental authority at the national, state, and local levels.

States are currently the leading source of legal authority for dealing with a public health crisis, and laws are different in each state.

Staff nurses and nurse administrators need to learn from the legal counsel in their institutions the legal framework for their states.

The American Nurses Association (ANA) *Code of Ethics for Nurses*, ANA Issue Brief, standard ethical theories and principles provide frameworks and guidance for making ethical decisions during disasters.

The broader bioethical framework for dealing with a bioterrorist attack and the resultant public health crises is in flux.

CHAPTER OVERVIEW

This chapter introduces various legal and ethical issues that may arise during a disaster or major public health crisis. It begins with an overview of the legal system and then describes the sources of law and ethical obligations, the importance of the various levels of government in public health regulation, and resources that are available to nurses for legal and ethical advice. The second half of the chapter discusses specific legal and ethical issues that may arise in a public health crisis.

LEGAL AND ETHICAL FRAMEWORK AND BACKGROUND

Introduction to the Legal System

In order to understand how the law will impinge on nursing practice during a public health crisis, it is necessary to recall that in the United States, there are three separate levels of government, all with a role in public health regulation. At the national level, the federal government oversees certain aspects of public health regulation, primarily through executive branch agencies such as the U.S. Department of Health and Human Services (HHS) and the Environmental Protection Agency (EPA). Yet, the U.S. Constitution limits the role the federal government can play in public health, as it grants to the national government only those powers specifically enumerated in the Constitution. Regulating health is not specifically mentioned in these powers and, thus, to operate in this area, the federal government must use one of its other powers, such as the power to raise and spend revenue. The impact of this constitutional restriction, as well as a frequently used method to circumvent it, can be illustrated through an example. Although it would probably not be constitutionally permissible for the federal government to directly impose a mandatory vaccination requirement, it could do the same by requiring all states that receive funds from a federal health program to require the vaccination or face the loss of some funds. The U.S. Supreme Court has recently limited this withholding of federal funding, holding that withdrawal of all federal funding for Medicaid to compel states to participate in expanding Medicaid eligibility under the Affordable Care Act would be unconstitutional (*National Federation of Independent Businesses v. Sebelius*, 2012). Through this use of constitutional power to allocate funds, the federal government could extensively regulate in the public health field, although it generally has not.

As a result of the constitutional division of governmental powers, and in the absence of federal action, it usually falls on the state governments to engage in the primary regulation of public health. State governments are endowed with the complete array of public health powers, including the power to enforce quarantines, require vaccinations, impose disease-reporting requirements, and any other power needed to protect the public's health. This power is generally unlimited, save for the requirement that any public health law, or any other law, must not violate any restrictions imposed by either the state or federal constitutions.

Local governments may also exercise public health regulatory powers, but because local governments are considered "creations of the state," their powers are, in most states, limited to those powers specifically granted by the state government. For example, in most states, a local government (e.g., a city or county) cannot impose a mandatory vaccination law without a law passed by the state legislature granting them this power.

Ideally, the division of responsibility would be based on what makes the most sense in terms of the optimum functioning of the public health system. In practice, there are overlaps and gaps in the division of responsibility. Even more troubling for someone trying to fathom public health policy is that each state is free to adopt its own regulatory scheme, making it difficult to make simple statements about what the law allows or requires nurses—or other health professionals—to do in a public health crisis. In the discussion in the second portion of this chapter, the reader is cautioned to seek professional advice on the law in his or her own state.

EFFECT OF LAW ON NURSING PROFESSIONALS

Law—that is, the rules and regulations under which nurses must carry out their professional duties—can come from many different sources. What most people commonly think of as "law" are what lawyers call "statutes." These are the laws enacted by the legislative body—Congress in the case of the national government and in the case of the states, the state legislatures, often called the "state assembly" and "state senate." These are not the only sources of law governing nurses. Both federal and state agencies (often the departments within the executive branch, e.g., the HHS) typically have the authority to issue regulations, sometimes called "rules," which have the same effect as the statutes the legislative body enacts by governing implementation of such statutes. A third source of law is the decisions of the courts, which interpret the laws enacted by the legislative branch.

All of these sources of law can affect nurses in many different ways. For example, laws may require them to do some affirmative act, such as report new cases of certain diseases to the local or state health department. There may be criminal penalties for those who fail to comply with these requirements. Laws may also give the authority to certain governmental officers to require nurses to either do or refrain from doing something in a particular circumstance. Law can also create certain responsibilities for nurses, such as laws that impose civil liability for the failure to provide professionally adequate care. (Civil liability is when an individual may be required to pay monetary damages to another individual, or in some cases to the government, for failure to comply with a legal obligation.) Negligence is rooted in case law and a nurse can be accused of negligence if a party shows the nurse departed from an accepted standard of care, resulting in injury (Pesto, 1985). Nurses often assume the Good Samaritan law covers them from liability from negligence in times of disaster. It is important for nurses to understand the limitations of the Good Samaritan law, which may cover a nurse's good deed during a sudden emergency, but not always during a disaster. The next section addresses the scope of the Good Samaritan laws.

Unfortunately, because laws are the result of compromises and are meant to cover a broad array of circumstances, some of which the drafters of the laws may not be able to contemplate at the time of writing, legal rules do not always provide a specific course of conduct in a particular situation. Nursing professionals must work with the legal professionals on the hospital's staff when questions arise concerning the proper course of conduct in a particular circumstance.

RELATIONSHIP BETWEEN ETHICAL AND LEGAL OBLIGATIONS

As will be seen in some of the specific situations discussed later in this chapter, there can be different relationships between a nurse's ethical and legal obligations. Ethics refers to the examination of what it means to live a moral life. Morality encompasses the norms people adopt to direct right and wrong conduct (Beauchamp & Childress, 2013). "[T]he connections between moral norms and judgments about policy or law are complicated and ... [the] judgment about the morality of acts does not entail an identical judgment about law or policy" (Beauchamp & Childress, 2013, p. 10). In some cases, the ethical and legal obligations will be coextensive. That is, both what the law and the ethical obligations require will be the same. Breaching patient privacy and confidentiality under normal circumstances is both legally and ethically wrong. In other situations, the legal obligations may be less stringent than what is required ethically of the nurse. The law may require a nurse to report to work during a disaster but a nurse's ethical obligations to her family may supersede her legal obligations depending on the degree of risk to the nurse or the nurse's family (Rutkow, Taylor, & Powell, 2017). In some cases, there may be no legal obligation imposed at all, yet there is an ethical obligation. In this way, ethics operates in tandem with, but often covers more scenarios than, the law. For example, in most states the law does not require a nurse to be a Good Samaritan and stop at an accident scene to provide emergency care, but a nurse may have a strong ethical obligation to stop for a victim with a severe injury that would be merely slightly inconvenient for the nurse to address.

Nurses' ethical obligations come from many different sources, but one formal source is the professional code of ethics. The ANA *Code of Ethics for Nurses* proscribes the ethical obligations of nurses, and expresses the profession's commitment to society (ANA, 2015). In 2017, the ANA issued an updated brief specifically addressing ethical and legal considerations unique to disasters, emphasizing the importance of being personally, ethically, and professionally prepared for a disaster (ANA, 2017). Studying the potential issues in advance is key to this preparation. Nurses can also turn to the broader field of bioethics for additional resources. A discussion of the widely accepted bioethics frameworks will follow in the section of this chapter entitled, "Specific Legal and Ethical Issues."

As the field of bioethics developed, it has reflected issues of import in society, such as abortion, euthanasia, self-determination,

and the ethical conduct of research. Much of contemporary bioethics has roots in the values of individualism and autonomy (Moreno, 2002). Emphasis in bioethics has tended to be on issues of individual rights, personal freedom, and choice; there has been less emphasis on the public good (Gostin, 2002). These values are important to note because they also reflect how resources are allocated, with the vast majority of funds allocated to biotechnology and healthcare and much less to population-based services (Gostin, 2002). Beauchamp and Childress (2013) clarify that respect for autonomy and individual rights do not take priority over other ethical theories as many people have assumed during the past several decades. "We ... do not emphasize individual rights to the neglect or exclusion of social responsibilities and communal goals" (Beauchamp & Childress, 2013, p. ix).

As the focus shifts to public response and public good, leaders in bioethics continue to reevaluate the prominence of autonomy. According to Moreno, "the emphasis on autonomy and individual rights may come to be tempered by greater concern over the collective good" (2002, p. 60). An increased emphasis on the collective good would have profound effects on the delivery of healthcare in the United States (Richards, 2005). Karadag and Hakan (2012) similarly suggest disaster situations "may require a stronger effort to achieve balance between individual and collective rights" (p. 603). Wagner and Dahnke (2015) likewise conclude that the ethical issues unique to disasters are best addressed with greater emphasis on utilitarianism, the goal of producing the greatest good for the greatest number of people in order to achieve the morally right outcome, than principlism. "To say this does not place one outside of or at odds with the ANA Code of Ethics. The pluralistic approach to the construction of the code noted by the ANA makes conceptual and practical room for different approaches that may best fit the specifics of the situation" (p. 301). Wagner and Dahnke (2015) conclude, "Most contemporary ethicists, including bioethicists, perceive utilitarianism as a helpful tool but believe it is incomplete as a general theory on ethics and ethical decision making. However, as a limited theory with potential insight, it can be useful in limited situations such as the crisis of disaster" (p. 304–305).

Thus, scholars of ethical issues in disaster situations emphasize that it is important to be prepared by anticipating in advance potential issues that may arise and by understanding that the routine emphasis on patients' rights over the collective good, common to everyday ethical decision making in healthcare, may need to be reevaluated especially in the unique setting of a disaster.

PROPOSED MODEL STATE ACTS

Even before the events of 9/11, assessments of the country's vulnerability to terrorism and how best to respond to mitigate harms had a nationwide focus (Shalala, 1999). This broadened view has only increased in the wake of Hurricane Katrina (2005), Hurricane Sandy (2012), and several other disasters that occurred in 2016 and 2017, and fears over a pandemic influenza outbreak. The Federal Emergency Management Agency

(FEMA) now has the authority necessary to lean forward and leverage the entire emergency management team in response and recovery efforts including not only government but also the private sector, nonprofits, and citizens.

Following the events of 9/11, the National Governors Association, the National Conference of State Legislatures, the Association of State and Territorial Health Officials, and the National Association of County and City Health Officials recognized the need to revamp state public health laws to increase the ability of states to deal with a public health crisis. Initially, only a few states, either through their statutes or administrative regulations, had adopted legal frameworks to deal with a bioterrorist attack. The Center for Law and the Public's Health at Georgetown and Johns Hopkins Universities drafted a model law, the Model State Emergency Health Powers Act (MSEHPA), to give state governments a clear legal framework for dealing with a public health crisis, particularly one caused by an act of bioterrorism. The model law is one that states are free to adopt or not, and to amend in any way they wish. For example, Maryland has an adaptation of the MSEHPA that was last updated in 2016 (Maryland Code of Public Safety Title 14, 2016).

The MSEHPA grants to the governor of the state the power to declare a public health emergency in the event of a bioterrorist attack (and some other types of events, e.g., a chemical attack or a nuclear accident). The declaration of a public health emergency would give the state health department (or other designated state agency) certain powers during the duration of the public health emergency. The Model Act is structured to reflect five basic public health functions to be facilitated by law: (a) *preparedness,* comprehensive planning for a public health emergency; (b) *surveillance,* measures to detect and track public health emergencies; (c) *management of property,* ensuring adequate availability of vaccines, pharmaceuticals, and hospitals, as well as providing power to abate hazards to the public's health; (d) *protection of persons,* powers to compel vaccination, testing, treatment, isolation, and quarantine when clearly necessary; and (e) *communication,* providing clear and authoritative information to the public. The Model Act also contains a modernized, extensive set of principles and requirements to safeguard personal rights. As such, law can be a tool to improve public health preparedness (Gostin, 2002); the nature and extent of these powers will be discussed in the second part of this chapter.

As of June 2012, 40 states have adopted at least some portion of the Model Act. (For a list of states adopting all or part of the Model Act, see the table at www.networkforphl .org/_asset/80p3y7/MSEHPA-States-TableFINAL.pdf.)

Following Hurricanes Katrina and Rita in 2005, the Uniform Laws Commission proposed a second model uniform act, the Uniform Emergency Volunteer Health Practitioners Act (UEVHPA). Its scope is more limited than MSEHPA. Generally, the UEVHPA would provide some protection from civil liability for volunteer emergency healthcare workers and allow volunteer emergency healthcare workers to work in states other than where they are licensed. As of 2017, 16 states and the District of Columbia adopted versions of the uniform act (see www.facs.org/ahp/uevhpa.html for a list of those states). For example, in 2017, Hurricane Harvey hit the Texas and Louisiana area and Hurricane Irma hit the states of Florida and Georgia. Among the states affected by these two disastrous hurricanes, Texas, Louisiana, and Georgia were listed under the UEVHPA list. Florida was not on the list. The Texas Board of Nursing posted an announcement stating, "any out-of-state nurse with a license in good standing is not required to hold a Texas license in order to practice nursing in a disaster relief effort operation setting" (Texas State Board of Nursing, 2013, "Important Update"). In Florida, the Director of the Division of Emergency Management did take a step during the disaster to enact an emergency order on September 8, 2017 permitting licensed health professionals from other states, as long as they were in good standing, to provide healthcare to disaster victims for 30 days, thus temporarily suspending the statutes during the time of the emergency (Florida State Board of Nursing, 2017). See www.texasdisastervolunteerregistry.org for an example of a disaster volunteer registry.

The Robert Wood Johnson Foundation and the W. K. Kellogg Foundation in a collaborative effort with several state public health officials developed the Model State Public Health Act (MSPHA) in 2003. Unlike the Model Act or the Uniform Act, the purpose of the Turning Point Act is to provide a complete state or local law covering all aspects of public health, including emergency public health measures. To date, 48 states have passed legislative bills or resolutions that are based on or feature provisions that either used actual language from the MSPHA, or are based on some part of its subject matter. (For details on what provisions have been enacted in which states, see www.networkforphl.org/_asset/80p3y7/ MSEHPA-States-Table-022812.pdf).

THE ROLE OF GOVERNMENT IN A PUBLIC HEALTH CRISIS

As stated earlier, the federal government has a somewhat limited role in public health and consequently in managing a public health crisis. The model of federal governmental intervention in public health crises is to assume a subservient role to state and local governments, unless or until the state requests federal intervention. Historically, the health of a population is presumed to be a local/state matter (*Hillsborough County v. Automated Medical Laboratories, Inc.,* 1985). Following the events of 9/11, Congress has focused more federal attention on helping manage a public health crisis. The following sections will outline the present role of local, state, and federal governments in managing a public health crisis.

Although outside the scope of this chapter, international law may also apply. In 2005, the World Health Organization (WHO) passed new international health regulations, which went into effect in the United States on July 18, 2007 (HHS, 2007).

Local Government

In many public health crises arising from a bioterrorist attack or other disasters, local governments—city, town, or county government—will be the first to respond. Most state laws authorize (and some may require) that local governments draft local disaster preparedness plans, to plan the coordination of resources, manpower, and services in the event of an emergency (e.g., see New York Executive Law, § 23 [2011]). There is frequently a provision in state law allowing for the creation in local governments of an agency to deal with emergencies.

In order to deal with emergencies, local governmental executives, such as the mayor of a city, may be authorized by state law to declare an emergency or may request the state governor to declare a state of emergency (e.g., New York Executive Law, § 24[1] [2011] and www.stlouisco.com/lawandpublicsafety/emergencymanagement/basicemergencyoperationsplan). Once the state of emergency is declared, the executive is frequently authorized by state law to suspend certain laws or to put into place special regulations for the duration of the state of emergency. For example, under New York State law, the local governmental executive has the authority, among other powers, to put into place a curfew, prohibit or limit the movement of individuals, and establish emergency medical shelters (New York Executive Law, § 24[1] [2011]).

State Government

Local governments are limited in the resources they can employ in an emergency, and, thus, the state government will frequently become involved when the emergency is large. State law may allow the governor to make this decision on his or her own initiative or at the request of the local executive authority (e.g., New York Executive Law, § 28 [2011] and Missouri Department of Public Safety State Emergency Management Agency [SEMA] sema.dps.mo.gov). The governor may then be authorized to have state agencies provide any assistance needed, including distribution of medical supplies and making use of private facilities to cope with the emergency.

In many states, one of the most important powers that the governor has during a state of emergency is the power to suspend other laws. Each state's law will differ in the exact procedure that must be followed and the extent of the governor's power. When a state government declares, or refuses to declare, a state of emergency, the resources available for response, and how to respond, are controlled by that state's laws. Understanding the relationship between state and federal authorities is an important part of preparing and responding to public health emergencies. As discussed earlier, the MSEHPA would explicitly give governors the power to declare a public health emergency in the event of a bioterrorist attack. These powers would be limited in duration and subject to legislative review.

The states themselves may not have sufficient resources to handle emergencies, and when this occurs, they may request assistance from the federal government. Typically the state governor will request that the president declare all or a portion of the state a federal disaster area, which will allow the use of federal resources to deal with the emergency (42 U.S.C. § 5191[a] [2011]). The president may, under certain circumstances, declare an emergency without a request from the state's governor (42 U.S.C. § 5191 [b] [2011]).

Federal Government

The two primary federal agencies with authority in national emergencies are the Public Health Service (PHS) and the FEMA. When there is a public health and medical services component to the emergency, the PHS, which is within the HHS, is the lead federal agency to coordinate the federal response (Department of Homeland Security [DHS], 2016). The Public Health Service Act of 1944, as amended, is the foundation of the HHS legal authority for responding to public health emergencies. Among other things, it authorizes the HHS secretary to lead all federal public health and medical response to public health emergencies and incidents; to direct the PHS and other components of the department to respond to a public health emergency; to declare a public health emergency; to take such actions as may be appropriate to respond to the emergency consistent with existing authorities; to assist states in meeting health emergencies; and to control communicable diseases (Public Health Service Act, 2016).

The Pandemic and All-Hazards Preparedness Act (PAHPA) amended the Public Health Service Act to give the Secretary of the HHS clearer authority to lead all federal public health and medical responses to public health emergencies. This legislation included many requirements to improve the ability of the nation to respond to a public health or medical disaster or emergency, such as the creation of the office of the Assistant Secretary for Preparedness and Response (ASPR) and the requirement to establish an electronic nationwide public health situational awareness capability to enhance early detection of, rapid response to, and management of potentially catastrophic infectious disease outbreaks and other public health emergencies (PAHPA, 2013).

The PAHPA directed the secretary of the HHS to develop a National Health Security Strategy (NHSS). The NHSS was issued in 2015 to run through 2018. The Strategic Objectives of the NHSS are:

1. Build and sustain healthy, resilient communities.
2. Enhance the national capability to produce and effectively use both medical countermeasures and nonpharmaceutical interventions.
3. Ensure comprehensive health situational awareness to support decision making before incidents and during response and recovery operations.
4. Enhance the integration and effectiveness of the public health, healthcare, and emergency management systems.
5. Strengthen global health security (NHSS 2015–2018, p. 9). Of particular importance to the nursing profession is the NHSS's focus on developing and maintaining the workforce needed for national health security and fostering integrated, scalable healthcare delivery systems.

The second federal agency, FEMA, is designated to coordinate the federal response to a natural or man-made emergency (DHS, 2016). It was created in 1979 by Executive Order. On March 1, 2003, it became part of the DHS following the enactment of the Homeland Security Act (2002). The stated mission of the DHS is to prevent terrorist attacks and reduce our vulnerability to such, as well as to mitigate any effects from attacks (DHS, 2008).

Response to any national emergency requires coordination between various federal agencies (e.g., the DHS and HHS), and among federal agencies, state agencies, local governmental agencies, and nongovernmental entities. Given the overlapping authorities of these various entities, coordination in the event of a national emergency, such as Hurricane Katrina or other disasters, often proves difficult. In an effort to provide better coordination, the DHS issued the National Response Framework (NRF) in January 2008, and a third edition in 2016, to serve as a guide to how the nation conducts comprehensive incident response to natural and man-made disasters (DHS, 2016). It provides guiding principles that detail how federal, state, local, tribal, and private sector partners, including the healthcare sector, prepare for and provide a unified domestic response. The NRF replaced the National Response Plan of 2004 (DHS, 2004).

An important part of the nation's response to disasters is the Emergency Management Assistance Compact (EMAC). EMAC is the first national disaster–relief compact since the Civil Defense and Disaster Compact of 1950 to be ratified by the U.S. Congress. Since ratification and signing into law in 1996 (Public Law 104-321), 50 states, the District of Columbia, Puerto Rico, Guam, and the U.S. Virgin Islands have enacted legislation to become EMAC members.

EMAC offers assistance during governor-declared states of emergency or disaster through a responsive, straightforward system that allows states to send personnel, equipment, and commodities to assist with response and recovery efforts in other states. Through EMAC, states can also transfer services (e.g., shipping newborn blood from a disaster-impacted lab to a lab in another state) and conduct virtual missions (such as geographic information system mapping).

The strength of EMAC and the quality that distinguishes it from other plans and compacts lie in its governance structure; its relationship with federal agencies, national organizations, states, counties, territories, and regions; the willingness of state and response and recovery personnel to deploy; and the ability to move any resource one state wishes to utilize to assist another state.

Law and Ethics

Typical disaster-related issues that challenge traditional legal and ethical thinking include the privacy issues of reporting diseases of epidemic or pandemic proportions, maintaining confidentiality, and issues surrounding a potential quarantine. Mandatory vaccination, treatment refusal, resource allocation, and duty to treat also legally and ethically challenge nurses working in disaster situations. It is important for nurses to think about ethical and legal issues in advance of disasters because sometimes it is the fear of handling these ethical issues that keep healthcare providers from offering their services during disasters. Public health events quickly transform resource-rich environments into settings of austerity and as a consequence produce unique and challenging ethical and legal issues. Healthcare providers are often conflicted between their moral duty to serve disaster victims and their moral duty to safeguard their own health, as well as their family's and even their pet's health (Rutkow et al., 2017). Research studies reveal that healthcare providers are more likely to respond to disasters with appropriate knowledge, sense of role importance, and trust in their organizations (Connor, 2014).

All ethical and many legal issues produce dilemmas. A dilemma is a circumstance in which a person finds himself or herself choosing between two or more actions he or she is morally required to perform, but the actions are actually incompatible with one another (Beuchamp & Childress, 2013). A basic illustration of a moral dilemma is when an impoverished person must choose between stealing food from a grocery store to save his or her starving family or leaving the food only to see his or her family perish (Beauchamp & Childress 2013). One of these obligations must be overridden by the other. The individual draws on his or her knowledge of law, policy, and moral frameworks, weighs them together, and decides the right action. The ANA Issue Brief (2017) acknowledges that "Ethics are certainly not black and white, and in a disaster situation, they become even more blurred" (ANA, 2017 p. 3).

The examples in the next section illustrate common ethical and legal dilemmas faced by nurses working in disaster situations. The ANA (2017) recommends several preparatory steps to aid in the resolution of ethical dilemmas during disasters and notes several policies under development to protect nurses. Individual nurses should be aware of their employer's emergency response plans. Volunteering with a disaster registry would ensure the proper credentialing and training for disaster response. Nurses should know in advance that they may be called to work during a disaster and should make advanced arrangements with family and friends for communication, childcare, or other dependent care. Nurses need to be aware of potential ethical situations that could arise and advocate for systems and protocols that will protect their ethical obligations as nurses. "Future disasters are all but guaranteed to occur. We cannot stop them, but we can be better prepared for them. Creating better systems for nurses to respond, including ensuring ethical and safe environments for response and recovery, will give some assurance that when the call for nurses goes out, there will be a robust answer" (ANA, 2017, p. 5). Two documents the ANA urges nurses to review are UEVHPA at www.facs.org/advocacy/state/uevhpa and Guidance for Establishing Crisis Standards of Care for use in Disaster Situations: A Letter Report (2009) at www.nap.edu/read/12749/chapter/1 for suggestions about ethical policy making.

Nurses working in disasters may find that even after consulting with lawyers or referencing the law, guidelines, policies, and ethical codes, cases remain complex without a clear, definitive moral or legal answer. In such cases, nurses should continue to strive toward an ethical outcome using critical thinking, ethical principles, ethical theories, and trusting their own moral character. Theories such as utilitarianism and principles such as autonomy, beneficence, nonmaleficence, and justice are standard concepts that help providers frame and resolve ethical dilemmas. Autonomy is respect for patient choice, beneficence is the duty to promote good, nonmaleficence is the duty to avoid harm, and justice is the duty to distribute goods fairly or treat others fairly.

Beyond performing the right action or avoiding the wrong action, nurses should think about the role character plays in moral decision making. "What often matters most in the moral life is not adherence to moral rules, but having a reliable character, a good moral sense, and an appropriate emotional responsiveness ... Our feelings and concerns for others lead us to actions that cannot be reduced to merely following rules, and morality would be a cold and uninspiring practice without appropriate sympathy, emotional responsiveness [and] excellence of character" (Beauchamp & Childress, 2013, p. 30).

SPECIFIC LEGAL AND ETHICAL ISSUES

Privacy Issues

Case Example: An outbreak of an infectious disease leads public health officials to believe that a bioterrorist attack has occurred. To avoid panic of the public, however, the officials have made no public announcement of their suspicions. They have requested, however, that nurses be on the alert for new cases of the infectious disease and to report them immediately, along with certain information about the patient. A nurse asks her supervisor if she can legally make such reports.

Reporting of Diseases

Under their police powers, states have the constitutional authority to require healthcare providers to report new cases of diseases. Although such reporting raises an issue concerning patient privacy, the U.S. Supreme Court has upheld the authority of states to require the collection of disease information (*Whalen v. Roe*, 1977).

Each state varies considerably as to which diseases must be reported, to whom the information is reported, who is required to report, and what information they are required to provide concerning the patient. Rapid collection of H1N1 information in hospitalized patients was critical for learning about the nature of this disease but not all states had the ability or resources to collect the data during the H1N1 epidemic. A study showed that of 19 jurisdictions, 37% made postpandemic changes in surveillance after the H1N1 situation by making novel cases reportable, providing access to medical records and expediting the reporting of new diseases (Danila et al., 2015). After experiencing the crisis, many states amended their reporting laws for the benefit of the public. The release of infectious agents as a result of a bioterrorist attack may well be covert, and the release may be discovered only through careful reporting and tracking of disease information. With this in mind, the MSEHPA would, if adopted by a state, allow the state to mandate the reporting and tracking of diseases specified by the state public health agency. In addition, the state could require pharmacies to report unusual or increased prescription rates, unusual types of prescriptions, or unusual trends in pharmacy visits that might accompany a public health crisis.

Nurses should already be aware of the reporting requirements of the state and local governments in the areas where they currently practice. In the event of a public health crisis resulting from a terrorist attack, nurses will need to keep current on any additional reporting requirements that may be imposed by state and local health authorities. If the reporting is anonymous, then there is not concern for confidentiality of the individual. Where the reporting requires the naming of a particular individual, however, this raises both legal and ethical

concerns surrounding the privacy and confidentiality of medical information, which will be discussed in the next section.

Disclosure of Health Information

When health information contains information that would identify the individual, issues are raised concerning both privacy and confidentiality. Frequently, these two terms are used interchangeably (Gostin, 2000, p. 127), but there are technical distinctions between the two. "Privacy" is an individual's claim to limit access by others to some aspect of his or her life (Beuachamp & Childress, 2013; Gostin, 2000, p. 127), whereas "confidentiality" is a type of privacy aimed at preserving a special relationship of trust (Beuchamp & Childress, 2013; Gostin, 2000, p. 128), such as the relationship between medical care provider and patient. A person who gains access to a patient's electronic medical record without authorization violates patient privacy but does not violate confidentiality (Beauchamp & Childress, 2013). A nurse who discloses to a neighbor or colleague that a particular patient told her or him about past drug abuse violates confidentiality. Patient privacy and confidentiality protect patients from harm and give patients control over their personal information. These rules are justified ethically on the basis of autonomy and nonmaleficence (Beauchamp & Childress, 2013). There are also utilitarian reasons for upholding confidentiality and protecting privacy. However, protecting the public good may actually outweigh the legal and ethical obligations nurses have to protect private and confidential information in some circumstances. Additionally, preventing social inequalities of health disparities is another ethically compelling reason to justify breaching privacy and confidentiality in times of disaster (Fairchild & Bayer, 2016).

Medical information can be identifiable not only when it contains the name of the individual, but also when it contains sufficient other information to identify the individual. This would include information such as the person's address, telephone number, Social Security number, date of birth, and other personal characteristics that allow a third person to connect the health information with the individual. When data are collected about individuals within a small geographical area, such as a small town or a zip code, even data such as a person's race or ethnic origin can be sufficient to allow personal identification. Although one U.S. Supreme Court decision appears to recognize a constitutionally protected right to privacy of medical information (*Whalen v. Roe*, 1977), this right is fairly narrow (Gostin, 2000, p. 133) and, thus, any protection of health information must be either the result of federal or state legislative action. Currently there is a complex web of federal and state laws and regulations that govern privacy of medical information.

In the Health Insurance Portability and Accountability Act of 1996 (HIPAA; 42 USC § 1320d-1, 2011), Congress authorized the HHS to issue regulations governing the privacy of health information in the hands of providers. The new regulations provide protection for patient health information that is in the hands of doctors, hospitals, insurance companies, and some other entities. The exact protections and coverage of the regulations are complex and subject to revisions by the HHS (for a summary of the regulations, see www.hhs.gov/ocr/privacy). Generally, the regulations tell providers what protections they must provide for identifiable medical information and when the patient must approve release of medical information. In July 2006, the HHS released a web-based, interactive HIPAA privacy decision tool to assist emergency preparedness planning and HIPAA compliance (accessible at www.hhs.gov/ocr/privacy/hipaa/understanding/special/emergency/decisiontoolintro.html). This valuable tool continues to assist disaster planners to accommodate HIPAA compliance guidelines.

However, though extensive, two provisions of the HIPAA regulations, taken together, remove most public health information from its reach. First, the regulations permit providers to disclose protected information "for public health activities and purposes" to public health authorities (HIPAA; 45 C.F.R. § 164. 512[b], 2011). In addition, another provision of the regulation recognizes that state law will govern the disclosure of medical information for purposes of "public health surveillance, investigation, or intervention" (HIPAA; 45 C.F.R. § 160.203 [c], 2011). Thus, under HIPAA, healthcare providers can still share patient information to prevent or lessen a serious or imminent threat to the public health, consistent with other laws and professional standards. HIPAA also does not affect disclosure by noncovered entities (Centers for Disease Control and Prevention [CDC], 2003, 2015).

The MSEHPA would address the issue of confidentiality in two ways. First, access to health information of a person who has participated in medical testing, treatment, vaccination, isolation, or quarantine programs or "efforts by the public health authority during a public health emergency" is limited. Only persons who will provide treatment, conduct epidemiological research, or investigate the causes of transmission may gain access to this information (MSEHPA, 2001, § 607[a]).

The MSEHPA also addresses limitations on disclosure. Generally, disclosure of health information could not be made without the consent of the individual. Five exceptions are:

1. Disclosure directly to the individual
2. Disclosure to the individual's immediate family members or representative
3. Disclosure to appropriate federal agencies or authorities pursuant to federal law
4. Disclosure pursuant to a court order to avert a clear danger to an individual or the public's health
5. Disclosure to identify a deceased individual or to determine the manner or cause of death (MSEHPA, 2001, § 607 [b])

Nurses have ethical obligations to protect the privacy and confidentiality of the patients with whom they work. The dual obligations of privacy and confidentiality arise out of the fiduciary relationship between a patient and a nurse. Breaches in confidentiality and privacy endanger the patient–nurse relationship and may pose risks to the patient. However, the nurse's ethical obligation to maintain the privacy and confidentiality of the patient is not absolute (ANA, 2015). Under several circumstances, a nurse's obligation to maintain privacy and confidentiality may be superseded by competing obligations in order to protect the patient (e.g., an actively suicidal patient at risk for imminent harm), to protect innocent others (e.g., mandatory reporting of child or elder abuse), and

mandatory disclosure for public health reasons (ANA, 2015). In the context of a disaster response, especially responses to biological or chemical terrorism, disclosures of identifiable patient information may be ethically obligatory.

Quarantine, Isolation, and Civil Commitment

One of the traditional public health tools is government-compelled isolation of persons with infectious diseases. Although often used interchangeably both by public health professionals and in public health laws (Gostin, 2000, pp. 209–210), usually a distinction is made between the terms "quarantine," "isolation," and "civil commitment." Quarantine had its origins in maritime law and practice. It was the forced isolation of a vessel, its crew and passengers, and its cargo for a period—traditionally 40 days—when the vessel was suspected of carrying an infectious disease. Today quarantine is usually considered to be the restriction of the activities of a healthy person who has been exposed to a communicable disease, usually for the period of time necessary for the disease to reveal itself through physical symptoms (Gostin, 2000, p. 210). Isolation, on the other hand, is usually defined to mean the separation of a person known to have a communicable disease for the period of time in which the disease remains communicable. Some make the distinction between "status-based isolation," which is the confinement of infected persons based on their diseased status alone, and "behavior-based isolation," which is the confinement of infected persons who engage in dangerous behavior (Gostin, 2000, p. 210). (For a helpful discussion clarifying quarantine vs. isolation, see CDC, 2005.) Civil commitment is often associated today with proceedings in the mental health system to forcibly confine persons who are mentally ill and a danger either to themselves or to others. More broadly in public health, civil commitment "is the confinement (usually in a hospital or other specially designated institution) for the purposes of care and treatment" (Gostin, 2000, p. 210).

Because of the restriction on a person's liberty, the courts have long had to struggle with exactly when the state can limit an individual's freedom in order to protect the public's health. Today's jurisprudence recognizes the authority of the state to confine a person for public health purposes, but imposes several important limitations. First, there must be a compelling state interest, which means that there must be a significant risk of disease transmission. Second, the intervention must be narrowly targeted to the group that is infectious. Thus, a state-mandated isolation of all in a particular geographical area, which included both those infected and those who were not, would likely be invalid (Gostin, 2000, p. 214). The restriction on free movement must be the least restrictive alternative to achieve the state's health objectives. Finally, there must be procedural fairness in the process used to confine an individual for public health purposes (Gostin, 2000, p. 215), including notice, counsel, a hearing, and a right to appeal.

As can be imagined, in a public health crisis the need to provide procedural protections may conflict with the need to act rapidly to avoid the spread of disease. Thus, the MSEHPA provides for temporary isolation and quarantine without notice, if delay would "significantly jeopardize the public health authority's ability to prevent or eliminate the transmission of a contagious or possibly contagious disease to others" (MSEHPA, 2001,

§ 605[a]). After exercising this emergency power, the public health authority would be required to petition a court within 10 days to continue the isolation or quarantine. The public health authority would also be authorized to seek isolation or quarantine through a judicial proceeding that would provide notice and a hearing for the individuals involved (MSEHPA, 2001, § 605 [b]). The MSPHA has similar provisions concerning the authority of state officials to isolate or quarantine individuals and remains current today (MSPHA, 2003, § 5–108).

A private individual who confines another individual without consent commits a civil wrong (called a "tort"), which could possibly result in the payment of damages. Hospitals that are operated by the government are required to follow constitutionally mandated procedures for isolation and quarantine. Thus, nurses and nurse administrators at both private and public hospitals need to proceed with caution in attempting to restrict the movement of a potentially infectious person. The hospital's legal counsel and the appropriate health official in the state should be contacted to find out how to proceed.

Ethically, the restriction of movement of a potentially infectious person is highly problematic. It violates the core of the ANA *Code of Ethics*, respect for the inherent dignity of individuals, which is the nurse's primary commitment to the patient (ANA, 2015). In the event of a public health emergency, a nurse may have a corresponding obligation to the community. Appeal to the ANA *Code of Ethics* as well as theories and principles of bioethics may help the nurse frame these issues.

The ANA opposed the mandatory quarantining of health professionals returning from West African nations to the United States during the Ebola outbreak in 2014. The state of Maine imposed a 21-day quarantine on Kaci Hickox, an RN who treated patients with Ebola in Sierra Lion. Ms. Hickox arrived at the Newark Airport on October 24, 2014. Ms. Hickox did not meet CDC guidelines for quarantine. In addition to the harms of restricting her liberty, the ANA reported concerns that imposing more restrictive conditions than outlined by the CDC would incite public fear and misinformation, thwarting efforts to recruit healthcare professionals needed to treat Ebola patients in West Africa. Additionally legal and ethical questions arose such as what should law enforcement do when someone under quarantine breaks the order? How much force is permitted to limit the individual's freedom? Is law enforcement trained in infection control enough to safely restrain an exposed or infected individual? Who will provide compensation for a quarantined individual's lost wages while under quarantine? (Rothstein, 2015) Furthermore, other harms associated with quarantine include the harms of social stigma, especially if the individual already belongs to a marginalized group (Desclaux, Badji, Ndione, & Sow, 2017).

Vaccination

Under their police powers, states have the governmental authority to require citizens to be vaccinated against disease. The U.S. Supreme Court, early in the last century, upheld the authority of states to compel vaccination, even when an individual refused to comply with the mandatory vaccination laws (*Jacobson v. Massachusetts*, 1905). All states currently have laws that require

school children to obtain vaccinations against certain diseases, such as measles, rubella, and polio, before attending school. In a public health crisis, however, the question may arise whether the state (or local) government could require an individual to be vaccinated against an infectious agent released into the general population. The state or local government must have the authority to do so. This may arise from a specific grant of authority by the state legislature to mandate vaccinations in the wake of a public health crisis, or the authority may be found in more general grants of authority given specific governmental agencies to protect the public's health. Given that the latter may be too vague to ensure the public health agency's authority to act, both MSEHPA and the MSPHA would specifically grant the state public health authority the power to require vaccination in the event of a declared public health emergency (MSEHPA, 2001, § 603 [a]; MSPHA, 2003, § 5–109).

Mandatory vaccinations impinge on the rights of individuals to freely decide their own healthcare, but, as noted earlier, the courts have generally upheld mandatory vaccinations. Because all laws are subject to the constraints of the federal and state constitutions, which grant protection for religious freedom, mandatory vaccination laws frequently are challenged as violating constitutionally protected religious freedom. The U.S. Supreme Court has upheld laws that require vaccinations before children attend school, even in the face of religious freedom claims. Most states, however, although not constitutionally required to do so, allow exceptions for individuals raising religious objections to mandatory vaccinations. The state courts, however, often strictly construe these rights. Neither the MSEHPA nor the MSPHA contain an exception based on religious objections, although a state adopting the Act would be free to add one if it chose.

A second difficulty raised by mandatory vaccination requirements is that some individuals may react adversely to vaccinations, particularly individuals who have other health conditions or who are taking medications for chronic illnesses. States often recognize this problem and provide exceptions to their mandatory vaccination laws for those who are susceptible to adverse reactions. These provisions vary from state to state. Both the proposed MSEHPA and MSPHA contain such a provision (MSEHPA, 2001, § 603[a]; MSPHA, 2003, § 5–109).

State laws on mandatory vaccination vary considerably in the legal implications for nurses and administrators. Typically, it is the individual who falls within the class required to be vaccinated who bears the legal burden. Thus, laws that condition the attendance in public schools on first having a vaccination for a particular disease typically bar the individual from school if there is no vaccination. Other laws may impose a criminal fine or other criminal penalty on the individual who refuses to be vaccinated. In some cases, state laws may allow for the isolation or quarantine of individuals who refuse to be vaccinated. Some state laws may require that health professionals, including nurses, inform certain patients about vaccination requirements and might possibly require some action, such as notification to a local or state health department, if the vaccination is refused. Nurses will need to check with the legal counsel of their hospital for the specific requirements in their state.

Treatment for Diseases

The U.S. Supreme Court affirmed the right of adults to select the course of treatment for their disease, including the right of adults to refuse treatment. This right is not absolute, however. For example, when children are involved, the courts have consistently upheld the power of the state to step in and require treatment, even in the face of religious objections by the parents to medical treatment (*Prince v. Massachusetts*, 1944). Moreover, most state public health laws contain provisions mandating treatment for certain contagious diseases, such as sexually transmitted infections (STIs) and tuberculosis (Gostin, 2000, p. 218).

As with the authority of the state to mandate vaccination during a public health crisis, there must be some authority granted by the state legislature to the state or local agency to require treatment. In order to clarify the authority of the state public health authority to require treatment in a public health crisis, the MSEHPA would allow mandatory treatment of persons with infectious diseases during a declared public health emergency (MSEHPA, 2001, § 603 [b]). Persons who refuse treatment on grounds of religion, conscience, or health could be isolated or quarantined (MSEHPA, 2001, § 603[b][3]). The MSPHA contains similar provisions (MSPHA, 2003, § 5–107).

Screening and Testing

Case Example: Because public health officials suspect a "stealth" bioterror attack, they request that hospitals secretly test all of their new patients for the suspected contagious disease. The patient is to be notified only if he or she tests positively for the disease, and he or she will be offered standard medical treatment. Reports are to go directly to public health officials. Can a nurse legally or ethically participate in such a program?

Screening and testing are two related, yet distinct, public health tools. "Testing" usually refers to a medical procedure to test whether an individual has a disease. "Screening," on the other hand, might be thought of as testing all the members of a particular population. Although this distinction is important to public health officials, public health laws often use the terms interchangeably or make no sharp distinction between the two.

Laws on testing and screening can take many different forms (Gostin, 2000, pp. 193–194). Some screening or testing laws are compulsory; they apply to anyone who is a member of a particular population. An example is laws that require all pregnant women to be tested for STIs. Other testing or screening laws are conditional on a person receiving some public benefit or service such as laws requiring testing for tuberculosis before a student can attend public schools.

Legal controversy arises in several different situations. First, there is an implied right in the civil law (called a "common-law right") for individuals to consent to all medical procedures, including testing, before it is performed (Gostin, 2000, p. 195). Thus, a medical professional who performs a test without first obtaining consent is open to a lawsuit for monetary damages. Where the medical professional is a governmental employee—for example, nurses working in a local, state, or federal hospital—testing or screening without consent can raise issues based on the constitutional protections against governmental searches and seizures. The court decisions in this area are very complex and often hinge on a host of factors. Generally, if the screening is for public health purposes, rather than for the prosecution of a criminal case, the courts find there is no constitutional problem to screening or testing without consent. For a more complete discussion of the legal nuances in this area, see Gostin (2000, p. 196).

In the event of a public health crisis resulting from a bioterror attack, there may be a public health need to screen the population for a disease. The MSEHPA would allow medical examinations and testing performed by any qualified person authorized by the public health authority (MSEHPA, 2001, § 602 [a]). Persons who refuse the medical examination or treatment could be isolated or quarantined (MSEHPA, 2001, § 602 [c]). The authors of the MSEHPA recognize that testing can cause harm to particular individuals and, thus, require that the tests "must not be such as are reasonably likely to lead to serious harm to the affected individual" (MSEHPA, 2001, § 602 [b]). It is not clear who would make this determination. It may be that this would be left to the discretion of the health professional administering the test. On the other hand, it may be that the public health authority (e.g., the state health department) would issue exceptions for particular classes of individuals. The MSPHA is similar in its provisions for testing and examination (MSPHA, 2003, § 5–106).

Nurses and nurse administrators who are ordered to perform mandatory testing or screening in a public health crisis face both legal and professional ethical issues. Because civil liability for performing a screening test without proper consent can fall on both the nurse and the institution, nurses and administrators must work closely with the legal counsel to ensure they are acting properly in carrying out the testing.

Beyond legal liability, however, is the question of whether nurses may ethically perform mandatory testing, even in the event of a public health crisis, without proper consent. Respect for autonomy is the primary justification for informed consent (Beauchamp & Childress, 2013), effectuated by the ability to give informed consent. Patients have the right to refuse testing and treatments based on the right to self-determination. However, provisions within the ANA *Code of Ethics* leave open the possibility that the right to self-determination may be superseded in the event of a public health emergency. Overriding such a basic right, however, requires compelling justification because of the tremendous risks and harms associated with limiting freedoms.

Professional Licensing

Case Example: In the immediate aftermath of the release of a biological agent in a large city, the city's health professionals are overwhelmed with the number of people they must treat. Nurses from a nearby city, which is in another state, offer to help. In addition, it is proposed that nurses carry out duties normally performed solely by physicians. Can nurses without a current state license "help out" in a public health crisis? Can nurses perform duties and procedures normally outside the scope of their field?

All states require licenses in order for an individual to engage in the practice of nursing. Most states, in addition, recognize different types of nurses such as professional nurses, licensed practical nurses, and nurse practitioners (New York Education Law §§ 6905, 6906, 6910, 2011).

Nurse licensing laws have two effects. The first is to limit the geographical area in which a nurse may practice to the state in which he or she holds a license. The second is to define the scope of practice. State statutes make illegal the practice of nursing within the state by one not licensed to practice in the state (e.g., see New York Education Law § 6512, 2011), including the practice by an individual licensed to practice in another state. During a disaster when a surge of healthcare providers are needed to care for victims in other states, the licensing can slow down the deployment of healthcare workers between states. The MSEHPA would allow the public health authority to appoint healthcare workers from other jurisdictions and to waive the state licensing requirements (MSEHPA, 2001, § 608 [b]). Such appointments would be limited in time to the period of the declared public health emergency (MSEHPA, 2001, § 608[b][1]). The ANA (2010) recommends that nurses read the UEVHPA to review the list of states that have adopted the UEVHPA. The UEVHPA was developed as a response to the immense delays in clearing healthcare providers for practice in other states during the 2005 hurricane season. Victims suffered while awaiting healthcare while volunteer nurses, physicians, and emergency medical technicians waited in long lines, navigating through the bureaucratic channels (UEVHPA, 2007). The UEVHPA clarifies the scope of practice and interstate practice differences. Nurses who wish to volunteer during disasters should register in advance with a public or private registration system to participate (National Conference of Commissioners on Uniform State Laws, 2018).

The MSPHA also allows the use of health professionals who are licensed in another state during the duration of a public health emergency (MSPHA, 2003, § 6–104).

A more difficult legal problem arises if, during a public health crisis, nurses are called on to perform medical services not typically viewed as within the scope of nursing practice. Again, it is difficult to conceive that licensing boards would raise objections in the face of a serious public health crisis. However, practicing outside the scope of their nursing license might subject nurses to civil liability from injured patients. Some states have dealt with this problem through *Good Samaritan* laws, which are covered in the Professional Liability section of this chapter that discusses liability issues. The MSEHPA would relieve out-of-state emergency medical workers of liability for civil damages arising from care provided in a public health emergency, unless the care exhibited a "reckless disregard for the consequences so as to affect the life or health of the patient" (MSEHPA, 2001, § 608[b][3]).

The UEVHPA does not authorize a volunteer health practitioner "to provide services that are outside the practitioner's scope of practice, even if a similarly licensed practitioner in [the state] would be permitted to provide the services." The act contemplates that an appropriate state agency would have the authority to modify the services a practitioner could provide during the emergency, and may do so without prior notice or hearing, as might otherwise be required by state law (UEVHPA, 2007, § 8).

Although this is a dynamic arena, efforts to anticipate and plan for what nurses may be called on to do in the event of an emergency are well under way. Emergency and disaster nurse leaders have identified new core competencies for all nurses regarding emergency preparedness in the event of a disaster or bioterrorism emergency. Nurses who have already completed their basic education have an ethical obligation to update their training to encompass these new core competencies.

A call to act outside of the scope of practice presents a complex dilemma. Not all events can be anticipated and planned for in advance. Nurses may be asked to perform duties not within their normal scope of practice and expertise imposing a risk to the patients. A nurse may be morally justified in taking such action if the nurse takes *due care* to minimize harm. "Due care is taking sufficient and appropriate care to avoid causing harm, as the circumstances demand of a reasonable and prudent person" (Beauchamp & Childress, 2013, p. 154). Ethically and legally, emergency situations often justify risks that would not be justified in a nonemergency situation; for example, high speed emergency vehicles pose a danger to citizens that is outweighed by the potential to save lives (Beauchamp & Childress, 2013). Indeed, a failure to act in such a situation may be ethically unjustified.

Resource Allocation

Despite preparation, a bioterrorist attack or a disaster involving a large number of casualties or casualties in excess of personnel and resources will challenge providers to justly allocate resources. In this case, resources might be medical supplies, antibiotics, antitoxins, pain medications, vaccines, and/or personnel. One aspect of justice in healthcare is the concept of "distributive justice." Distributive justice involves such issues as the fair and equitable allocation of scarce resources (Beauchamp & Childress, 2013). There is currently much debate about the fair distribution of healthcare resources in the United States; disasters provide an even more complex challenge to distributing resources.

Triage is one mechanism for allocating scarce resources in emergency situations. "Triage" is a French word meaning "to sort." Emergency room and military personnel use triage to prioritize treatments of wounded persons. Utilitarian theory, "that we ought always to produce the maximal balance of positive value over disvalue [or] ... the greatest good for the greatest number as determined from an impartial perspective that gives equal weight to the legitimate interests of each affective party" (Beauchamp & Childress, 2013, p. 355) is the ethical basis for triage. The categories by which one sorts, however, can be different. For example, in the military, the practice of triage is to sort the wounded into three groups—the walking wounded, the seriously wounded, and the fatally wounded. The walking and seriously wounded receive immediate attention, the walking wounded so that they may be returned to fight in battle, the seriously wounded to save their lives. Those deemed fatally wounded are given narcotics to be kept comfortable, but their wounds are not treated (Edge & Groves, 1994). In emergency departments and at disaster sites, the wounded are also sorted into categories according to medical need and medical utility (Beauchamp & Childress, 2013). Treated first (triage level 1) are those people who have major injuries and will die without immediate help; second are those whose treatment can be delayed without immediate danger (triage level 2). The third group treated is those with minor injuries (triage level 3), and the last group is those for whom treatment will not be effective. In emergency rooms, treatment for those with minor injuries tends to be delayed because the order of treatment is based only on medical need and medical utility.

Military triage is based on medical need, medical utility, and an additional category, social utility. Social utility is the notion of allocating resources to those who may be the most useful or most valued in a society (Beauchamp & Childress, 2013). In the military, there is a social utility to treating those with minor injuries quickly because to do so serves a larger social purpose of returning soldiers to the battlefield to help win the battle. In contrast, emergency department triage is based on only medical need and medical utility. The use of social utility as a factor in triage decisions in emergency departments is highly problematic.

Treating large numbers of persons after a disaster raises ethical questions for nursing. Clinicians are called to use their expertise to provide maximum benefit to the greatest number of people (Pesik, Keim, & Iserson, 2001). Exactly how to provide the greatest benefit for the greatest number, however, is ethically complex. For example, is it ethically justifiable to treat a nurse with minor injuries (triage level 3) before treating someone with serious but stable injuries (triage level 2)? Typically, level 2 patients would be treated prior to level 3 patients. The argument for treating healthcare persons with priority is that these persons, once treated, will assist in the effort of treating all the casualties. Thus, treating healthcare providers first will serve the larger social goal of saving as many lives as possible. This is based on a judgment of the social utility of a healthcare provider. In an emergency situation, this justification holds "if, and only if, his or her contribution is indispensable to attaining a major social goal" (Beauchamp & Childress, 2013, p. 292).

The use of medical utility to justify triage decisions is well established; however, the use of social utility is more problematic. For example, with the advent of hemodialysis during the early 1960s, the demand for dialysis therapy exceeded the capacity to provide such therapy. Committees were set up to sort through the existing patients and prioritize them for treatment. Criteria for treatment included age, marital status, sex, number of dependents, educational level, future potential, and emotional stability (Edge & Groves, 1994). It is interesting to note that the "committees' choices favored males, Caucasians, and the middle class or above" (Edge & Groves, 1994, p. 175). Choices for dialysis therapy are now based on medical need and medical utility. The use of social utility to justify triage decisions requires extreme circumstances, clear guidelines, and compelling evidence to support that those benefiting will, in turn, fulfill their obligation to enhance the social good.

In addition to raising ethical issues, triage also poses the possibility of legal claims of discrimination by individuals from legally protected populations, including people with disabilities and minorities (Hodge, Garcia, Anderson, & Kaufman, 2009). An executive order issued by President George W. Bush in July 2004 gave priority to people with disabilities in all aspects of emergency preparedness, response, and recovery. In addition, HHS and the Office of Minority Health developed a consensus statement on disaster preparedness for minority communities. The DHS Appropriations Act of 2006 requires the FEMA to address the needs of populations with limited English proficiency during a disaster (Hodge et al., 2009).

Professional Liability

All healthcare professionals, including nurses, are subject to civil liability for providing substandard healthcare. Malpractice liability is generally a matter of state law, although the law of malpractice liability is very similar in all of the states. A nurse may be held liable, that is, have to pay monetary damages, for providing professional care that is below the standard followed by the profession. Absent special legislation, liability for medical professionals continues, even when they are performing medical care in an emergency situation.

Some states have enacted special legislation, often called "Good Samaritan" laws, which may provide immunity from civil liability for persons when they render care in emergency situations (Pesto, 1985). For example, a Florida statute limits the liability of a nurse (or other medical professional) for emergency care or treatment rendered gratuitously (i.e., without compensation) either at the scene of an emergency outside of a hospital or in response to a situation arising out of a declared state of emergency. Some other states have similar laws, although they may be limited to care rendered at the scene of an accident. Other states do not limit the liability for nurses rendering emergency care. It is important for nurses to know the Good Samaritan laws in their own states in order to avoid being held liable for negligence for intending to perform a good deed during an emergency or disaster. A nurse can be held liable for negligence if he or she deviates from the accepted standard of care, resulting in injury.

The MSEHPA only partly addresses this problem. It provides that the liability of out-of-state emergency healthcare providers is limited (MSEHPA, 2001, §§ 608[b][3] and 804). It does not directly address the liability of emergency healthcare providers working in their own state who apparently could be covered by the existing liability rules, including any Good Samaritan laws that might exist. Knowledge of the Good Samaritan laws of the state is important for protection from liability. For a summary of the state Good Samaritan laws, see www.heartsafeusa.com/forum/99/state-laws-legislation. This site presents a summary of each state's Good Samaritan laws but nurses should read the complete state laws before volunteering during an emergency as they may not cover care provided during emergencies.

Good Samaritan laws differ widely between states and no two states have the same Good Samaritan law. In general, the Good Samaritan laws cover nurses who (a) provide care at the scene of the emergency and (b) where no relationship or duty existed prior to the emergency (Pesto, 1985). The Good Samaritan laws generally delineate the type of care the state allows at an emergency scene but are not comprehensive enough in their current form to cover the types of care needed at the scene of a disaster such as the ongoing care that victims of Hurricane Katrina needed in 2005 (Howie, Howie, & McMullen, 2012). "[A] nurse who happens upon a disaster unexpectedly, where there has been no previous planning, and sets about to render aid or nursing care will probably be immune from liability . . . [but] a nurse who has been designated as part of a response team and is called accordingly in response to a disaster, whether it be to render aid in a shelter or a hospital, is probably not protected under the Good Samaritan Statute" (Pesto, 1985, pp. 377–378). Another way to understand the Good Samaritan laws is to think about the following situation: If a nurse hears about a volcanic eruption and arrives on the scene to provide care but harms a victim, she or he would most likely be immune from liability based on the Good Samaritan laws; but if a nurse is part of a response team and arrives at a shelter to provide care for victims of the same volcano eruption and harms a patient, she or he may not be immune from liability based on the Good Samaritan law (Pesto, 1985) but may be immune based on other acts or policies. Nurses who volunteer for disasters may also worry if there will be ramifications for their current position. Electing to volunteer for emergencies may depend on the nurse's confidence in his or her job security, especially if the disaster necessitates a long absence from work. The ANA wrote a position statement, "Registered Nurses' Rights and Responsibilities Related to Work Release During a Disaster" (2002a) and "Work Release During a Disaster Guidelines for Employees" (2002b). These position statements help guide both volunteers and employers.

The UEVHPA provides two options that limit, but do not eliminate, individual liability of volunteer health providers during declared emergencies. One option would hold volunteer workers free of liability for an act or omission in providing services. The second option would also hold volunteer workers free of liability for acts or omissions in providing services, but only if they received less than a specified amount of payment (e.g., $500). Neither option limits liability for (a) willful misconduct or wanton, grossly negligent, reckless, or criminal conduct; (b) an intentional tort; (c) breach of contract; (d) a claim asserted by a host entity or by an entity located in this or another state that employs or uses the services of the practitioner; or (e) an act or omission relating to the operation of a motor vehicle, vessel, aircraft, or other vehicle.

The MSPHA also limits civil liability for death or injury caused by any nongovernmental persons and employees and agents of such persons in the performance of a contract with, and under the direction of, the state or its political subdivisions, or who renders assistance or advice at the request of the state or its political subdivisions, except in the event of gross negligence or willful misconduct (MSPHA, 2003, § 6–105).

Another potential area of civil liability for nurse administrators is failure to adequately plan for an emergency situation (Hodge et al., 2009). While it is more typically the legal entity of the healthcare facility that is held liable, administrators at all levels face at least the potential of civil liability for failure to adequately plan for an emergency (Hodge et al., 2009).

Provision of Adequate Care

Case Example: The local television news carries a story that a rash of human-to-human transmission cases of avian flu has occurred in the region, resulting in five deaths to date. Nurses and other staff begin calling in "sick." When contacted by supervisors, the nurses admit they are afraid to come in to work because of fears of a possible pandemic and the danger of spreading flu to their families (as healthcare workers they received vaccinations, but their families were not similarly protected). What legal recourse does a hospital have if staff refuse to work during a public health crisis? What liability does the institution face if it operates in the absence of adequate staff? What ethical issues does calling in sick raise for the nurse and the institution?

The relationship between nurses and hospitals legally is the same as between any other employer and employee. Aside from the exceptions discussed in the following, the relationship is viewed as an "at-will contract." This means that the hospital can set the terms and conditions of employment and is free to dismiss an employee for any reason (except as this right is modified by state or federal statutes, e.g., laws against racial discrimination). Likewise, the employee, here the nurse, is free to leave the employment to go elsewhere for any reason, and technically without even giving notice, although custom usually prevails here.

This at-will relationship can be modified in two different ways. One is by statute, which will be discussed in detail later, and the other is by private contract between the hospital and the nurse. Although it is probably a rare practice in the field, hospitals and nurses can sign employment contracts that spell out the duties and responsibilities of the two parties, and that modify the typical at-will relationship. No doubt more common are contracts negotiated between unions representing the nurses and the hospital itself. Such contracts often spell out the terms and conditions of the job, including hours of work, limits on required overtime work, and disciplinary procedures to be followed if an employee fails to comply with the conditions in the contract.

Both the traditional at-will relationship and a contractual relationship can be modified by statute. As pointed out earlier, state and federal statutes prohibiting racial discrimination in employment trump the generally unfettered right of the employer to dismiss an employee with or without cause. The same is true of other statutes prohibiting employment discrimination on the basis of gender and disability. State statutes could, in theory, limit the number of hours that a nurse works, as well as require a nurse to come into work in the event of an emergency.

The MSEHPA contains a provision that would give the state the authority to mandate that healthcare providers assist "in the performance of vaccination, treatment, examination, or testing of any individual as a condition of licensure, authorization, or the ability to continue to function as a health care provider" in the state (MSEHPA, 2001, § 608[a]). The model act also contains a general provision that would give the public health authority the power to set rules and regulations necessary to implement the provisions of the act (MSEHPA, 2001, § 802), and it is possible that this would allow the state to enact further rules concerning the duty of healthcare workers to report for work in a crisis through its regulatory power.

The MSPHA allows state or local public health agencies to require in-state healthcare providers to assist in the performance of vaccination, treatment, examination, testing, decontamination, quarantine, or isolation of any individual as a condition of licensure, authorization, or the ability to continue to function as a healthcare provider in the state (MSPHA, 2003, § 6–104).

The ANA (2017) acknowledges that some states have laws requiring licensed healthcare professionals to respond and report to work during a disaster. Refusal to comply with this law could be punishable. Some nurses may take this risk if they believe it will put their safety in jeopardy. If nurses are not confident that they will be safe, then they may not feel confident reporting to work, regardless of the requirement (O'Boyle, Robertson, & Secor-Turner, 2006). The ANA prefers that policy makers and governing bodies write protocols addressing the legal protection, license verification, liability standards, and definition of the scope of practice during a disaster.

In dealing with staffing requirements during a public health crisis, nurses and nurse administrators will need to seek advice about the exact legal nature of the relationship between the nurses and the hospital or other employing agency. Employee policies regarding hours of work and refusals to work should be reviewed, and this is particularly critical if there is a contract (either individual or a collective union contract) governing the conditions of employment. In addition, legal advice will be needed concerning any state requirements about mandatory work and the hours of employment.

A second legal issue surrounding staffing is liability for failing to maintain adequate nursing staff during a public health crisis. Generally, all hospitals may be held civilly liable if they fail to maintain adequate staffing and an individual is injured as a result of the inadequate staffing (Pozgar, 1999, p. 265). There is no hard-and-fast standard as to what constitutes adequate staffing, and the courts are likely to allow hospitals a large degree of discretion in determining whether staffing is adequate, particularly in the event of a public health crisis. Nonetheless, if at some point sufficient numbers of nursing staff fail to report for work, administrators will need to consider whether the staffing is so insufficient that the quality of care will suffer.

Selected Ethical Issues

Historically, nurses have responded quickly during public health emergencies. The events following 9/11 provide a case in point. Hospitals in and around New York City mobilized disaster teams, ready to receive casualties. In New York City, nurses saw the World Trade Center collapse and immediately reported to work (New York State Nurses Association, n.d.). Across the state and in neighboring states, nurses mobilized to receive casualties. This response was, in part, the routine disaster plan of every hospital in the New York City region, but above and beyond disaster plans, nurses went to work. Within hours the New York State Nurses Association was fielding calls from nurses across the country volunteering

to help out in any way they could. Under other conditions, nurses responding to a disaster may face great personal risk. Do nurses have an obligation to care for patients with highly communicable diseases when that care will put nurses at risk for contracting the disease? In conflict are two competing sets of values—professional values that may urge treating the patient and personal values that urge care of the self. The first provision in the code of ethics states that "[t]he nurse practices with compassion and respect for the inherent dignity, worth, and unique attributes" (ANA, 2015, p. 7). However, in the interpretation of the second provision, the ANA has recognized that there may be times when conflicts of interest arise and have urged nurses to try and resolve issues so that patients' safety and patients' interests are not compromised. For example, in 2006, two U.S. nurses were charged with murder following Hurricane Katrina for administering analgesics and sedatives to elderly patients who expired before the hospital could be evacuated. In 2003, nurses in Taiwan and Canada were reluctant to come to work due to real and perceived fears of contracting severe acute respiratory syndrome (SARS). They did not trust that their health organizations had adequate infection control measures or were fully disclosing the risks associated with caring for these patients.

Resolutions to this dilemma have varied, and there is no consensus. At issue is just how much risk a professional is obligated to assume. One solution offered calls for the establishment of an upper limit of risk beyond which healthcare providers would no longer be obligated to provide care for such patients; rather, continued care would be optional (Beauchamp & Childress, 2013). Illustrating the lack of consensus among professional organizations, Beauchamp and Childress point out that some organizations have urged courage, while others have emphasized that caring for patients who may pose a high risk to healthcare providers is optional. In the past, some professionals have volunteered to assume high risks and care for patients, while others have chosen not to volunteer.

Early on in the AIDS epidemic when the risks and mechanisms for transmission were unknown, some physicians and nurses were reluctant or refused to care for patients with AIDS (Bormann & Kelly, 1999; Levine, 1991). One practical solution was to rely on volunteers who would care for patients with AIDS. Now that the mechanism of transmission is known and the risk of contagion from occupational exposure is extremely small, the immediate issue seems to have resolved. Relying on volunteers may provide an immediate solution in a disaster situation, but it does not resolve the greater dilemma of limits to nurses' professional obligations to care for patients.

Nurses have obligations to employers, and employers have obligations to nurses. U.S. workers, especially those in healthcare, face potential hazards in the workplace associated with airborne chemical, biological, or radiological terrorism (National Institute for Occupational Safety and Health [NIOSH], 2004). Healthcare institutions have an ethical obligation to protect the safety and health of those who work in the institution. Following the events of 9/11, NIOSH developed specific recommendations for the assessment and improvement of building safety

(NIOSH, 2002). These included guidelines to address such issues as physical security, ventilation and filtration, maintenance, administration, and training. These recommendations were designed to decrease the likelihood of, or mitigate the harms caused by, a terrorist attack. In 2004, NIOSH issued "Protecting Emergency Responders: Safety Management in Disaster and Terrorism Response" in order to provide more detailed guidelines for the protection of healthcare providers and emergency responders from injury, disability, and death resulting from disasters (NIOSH, 2004).

SUMMARY

The legal and ethical issues related to disaster response are complex, rapidly changing, and occurring at a time of great transition in our society. In this chapter, we reviewed the basic legal and ethical issues related to disaster response.

Nurses have a privileged position of trust in society. In the event of a disaster or terrorist attack, nurses are and will continue to be in the forefront of the effort to mitigate victims' suffering with skill and compassion. It is their obligation to stay informed about the rapidly changing legal and ethical issues associated with emergency and disaster preparedness and response. Keeping current will help nurses to act efficiently and effectively under conditions of duress.

STUDY QUESTIONS

1. Describe the three levels of government and their anticipated roles in a public health crisis. What problems can be anticipated given the different roles of each level of government? What might be the potential benefits?

2. How does the protection of private health information differ depending on whether it is being used for public health purposes or other purposes?

3. In the event of a bioterrorist attack and a resulting public health crisis, how might the legal rules governing nurses change, and what governmental officials would be most likely to make these changes?

4. What is the difference between screening and testing? Is this distinction important in public health laws governing mandatory screening or testing?

5. In the event of a public health emergency, could nurses legally practice in a state where they are not licensed? Explain your answer.

6. If a nurse justifies his or her decision to respond to help victims of an earthquake in his or her own state on the Good Samaritan laws, how would you respond? If a nurse justifies

her or his decision to respond to victims of an earthquake in another state on the Good Samaritan laws, how would you respond? What other acts or policies should a nurse review if volunteering to help in a disaster?

7. What is the connection between a nurse's legal obligations and a nurse's ethical obligations? Give two examples, besides the examples in the chapter, where the legal and ethical obligations might not be identical. How can a nurse resolve such a conflict?

8. How might the notion of social utility become useful in emergency response triage? What are the dangers of introducing social utility into emergency responses?

9. If a nurse feels that responding to a disaster would put herself or himself at personal risk, is that nurse ethically obligated to respond? Explain and justify your answer. How might a nurse administrator legally compel a nurse to respond?

10. Describe two provisions from the ANA *Code of Ethics* that may be in conflict when a nurse is asked to quarantine a patient.

11. When may it be ethically justifiable for a nurse to act outside her or his scope of practice?

12. Describe three ways a nurse can become ethically prepared for a disaster. What type of preparation is most important to you personally?

13. What role does courage play in taking legal or ethical action in a disaster? Explain how a nurse may cultivate the characteristic of courage.

REFERENCES

American Nurses Association. (2002a). Registered nurses' rights and responsibilities related to work release during a disaster [Position statement]. Retrieved from https://www.nursingworld.org/~4af848/globalassets/practiceandpolicy/work-environment/health--safety/disast.pdf

American Nurses Association. (2002b). Work release during a disaster—Guidelines for employers [Position statement]. Retrieved from https://www.nursingworld.org/~4af83e/globalassets/practiceandpolicy/work-environment/health--safety/wrkrel.pdf

American Nurses Association. (2015). *Code of ethics for nurses with interpretive statements.* Washington, DC: Author. Retrieved from http://www.nursingworld.org/Code-of-Ethics

American Nurses Association. (2017). Who will be there? Ethics, the law, and a nurse's duty to respond in a disaster [Issue brief]. Retrieved from http://www.nursingworld.org/MainMenuCategories/WorkplaceSafety/Healthy-Work-Environment/DPR/Disaster-Preparedness.pdf

Beauchamp, T. L., & Childress, J. F. (2013). *Principles of biomedical ethics* (7th ed.). Oxford, UK: Oxford University Press.

Bormann, J., & Kelly, A. (1999). HIV and AIDS: Are you biased? *American Journal of Nursing, 9*(99), 38–39.

Centers for Disease Control and Prevention. (2003). HIPAA privacy rule and public health. *Morbidity and Mortality Weekly Report, 52,* 1–12. Retrieved from https://www.cdc.gov/mmwr/preview/mmwrhtml/m2e411a1.htm

Centers for Disease Control and Prevention. (2005). *Fact sheet on legal authorities for isolation/quarantine.* Retrieved from https://www.cdc.gov/sars/legal/fs-legal.html

Centers for Disease Control and Prevention. (2015). FAQs about HIPPA privacy rule. Retrieved from https://www.cdc.gov/nhsn/hipaa/index.html

Connor, S. B. (2014). When and why health care personnel respond to a disaster: The state of the science. *Prehospital and Disaster Medicine, 29*(3), 270–274. doi:10.1017/S1049023X14000387

Danila, R. N., Laine, E. S., Livingston, F., Como-Sebeti, K., Lamers, L., Johnson, K., & Barry, A. M. (2015). Legal authority for infectious disease reporting in the United States: Case study of the 2009 H1N1 influenza pandemic. *American Journal of Public Health, 105*(1), 13–18. doi:10.2105/AJPH.2014.302192

Department of Homeland Security. (2004). National response plan. Retrieved from https://www.hsdl.org/?abstract&did=450766

Department of Homeland Security. (2016). *National response framework* (3rd ed.). Retrieved from https://www.fema.gov/media-library-data/1466014682982-9bcf8245ba4c60c120aa915abe74e15d/National_Response_Framework3rd.pdf

Desclaux, A., Badji, D., Ndione, A. G., & Sow, K. (2017). Accepted monitoring or endured quarantine? Ebola contacts' perception in Senegal. *Social Science and Medicine, 178*, 38–45. doi:10.1016/j.socscimed.2017.02.009

Edge, R. S., & Groves, J. R. (1994). *The ethics of health care: A guide for clinical practice.* Albany, NY: Delmar.

Fairchild, A. L., & Bayer, R. (2016) In the name of population well-being: The case for public health surveillance. *Journal of Health Politics, Policy and Law, 41*(1), 119–128. doi:10.1215/03616878-3445650

Florida Board of Nursing. (2017). Gov. Scott declares state of emergency to prepare Florida for Hurricane Irma. Retrieved from http://floridasnursing.gov/latest-news/important-notice-due-to-hurricane-irma

Gostin, L. O. (2000). *Public health law: Power, duty, restraint.* Berkeley, CA: University of California Press.

Gostin, L. O. (2002). At Law: Law and ethics in a public health emergency. *Hastings Center Report, 32*(2), 9–11. doi:10.2307/3528516

Health Insurance Portability and Accountability Act of 1996, 42 U.S.C. § 1320d-1 (2011).

Health Insurance Portability and Accountability Act Regulations, 45 C.F.R. pt. 160.203(c) (2011).

Health Insurance Portability and Accountability Act Regulations, 45 C.F.R. pt. 164.512(b) (2011).

Hillsborough County v. Automated Medical Laboratories, Inc., 471 U.S. 707 (1985).

Hodge, J. G., Jr., Garcia, A. M., Anderson, E. D., & Kaufman, T. (2009). Emergency legal preparedness for hospitals and health care personnel. *Disaster Medicine and Public Health Preparedness, 3*(Suppl. 1), S37–S44. doi:10.1097/DMP.0b013e31819d977c

Homeland Security Act of 2002, Pub. L. No. 107–296, 116 Stat. 2135 (Nov. 25, 2002).

Howie, W. O., Howie, B. A., & McMullen, P. C. (2012). To assist or not assist: Good Samaritan considerations for nurse practitioners. *The Journal for Nurse Practitioners, 8*(9), 688–692. doi:10.1016/j.nurpra.2012.07.002

Jacobson v. Massachusetts, 197 U.S. 11 (1905).

Karadag, C. O., & Hakan, A. K. (2012). Ethical dilemmas in disaster medicine. *Iran Red Crescent Medical Journal, 14*(10), 602–612. doi:10.9790/1959-0602079093

Levine, R. J. (1991). AIDS and the physician-patient relationship. In F. G. Reamer (Ed.), *AIDS and ethics* (pp. 188–214). New York, NY: Columbia University Press.

Maryland Code Public Safety Title 14 - Emergency Management. (2016). Retrieved from https://law.justia.com/codes/maryland/2016/public-safety/title-14

Missouri Department of Public Safety. State Emergency Management Agency. Retrieved from http://sema.dps.mo.gov

Model State Emergency Health Powers Act. (2001). The Turning Point Public Health Statute Modernization Collaborative. Retrieved from https://www.law.asu.edu/sites/default/files/multimedia/faculty-research/centers/phlp/turning-point-model-act.pdf

Model State Public Health Act. (2003). The Turning Point Public Health Statute Modernization Collaborative. Retrieved from http://www.turningpointprogram.org/Pages/pdfs/statute_mod/MSPHAfinal.pdf

Moreno, J. D. (2002). Bioethics after the terror. *American Journal of Bioethics, 2*(1), 60–64.

National Conference of Commissioners on Uniform State Laws. (2018). Uniform Law Commission. Emergency Volunteer Health Practitioners Act. Retrieved from http://www.uniformlaws.org/Act.aspx?title=Emergency%20Volunteer%20Health%20Practitioners

National Federation of Independent Business v. Sebelius (2012).

National Institute for Occupational Safety and Health. (2004). *Protecting emergency responders: Safety management in disaster and terrorism response (V3)*. Cincinnati, OH: Author.

National Institute for Occupational Safety and Health, and Centers for Disease Control and Prevention. (2002). *Guidance for protecting building environments from airborne chemical, biological, or radiological attacks.* Cincinnati, OH: NIOSH. Retrieved from https://www.cdc.gov/niosh/docs/2002-139

New York Education Law, § 6512 (2011).

New York Education Law, § 6905 (2011).

New York Education Law, § 6906 (2011).

New York Education Law, § 6910 (2011).

New York Executive Law, § 23 (2011).

New York Executive Law, § 24(1) (2011).

New York Executive Law, § 28 (2011).

New York State Nurses Association. (n.d.). NYSNA honors 9/11 heroes. Retrieved from https://www.nysna.org/nysna-honors-911-heroes#.WrINKCOZNp8

O'Boyle, C., Robertson, C., & Secor-Turner, M. (2006). Nurse's beliefs about public health emergencies: Fear of abandonment. *American Journal of Infection Control, 34*(6), 351–357. doi:10.1016/j.ajic.2006.01.012

Pandemic and All Hazards Preparedness Act. (2013). Retrieved from https://www.congress.gov/bill/113th-congress/house-bill/307

Pesik, N., Keim, M. E., & Iserson, K. V. (2001). Terrorism and the ethics of emergency medical care. *Annals of Emergency Medicine, 37*(6), 624–646. doi:10.1067/mem.2001.114316

Pesto, M. M. (1985). Legal implications of nursing practice in a major disaster. In L. M. Garcia (Ed.), *Disaster Nursing: Planning, Assessment and Intervention.* Rockville, MD: Aspen Systems Corp.

Pozgar, G. D. (1999). *Legal aspects of health care administration.* Gaithersburg, MD: Aspen.

Prince v. Massachusetts, 321 U.S. 158 (1944).

Public Health Service Act. (2016). Retrieved from https://legcounsel.house.gov/Comps/PHSA-merged.pdf

Richards, E. (2005). Bird flu and the law [forum]. *Jurist.* Retrieved from http://www.jurist.org/forum/2005/12/bird-flu-and-law.php

Rothstein, M. A. (2015). Ebola, quarantine and the law. *The Hastings Center Report, 45*(1), 5–6. doi:10.1002/hast.411

Rutkow, L., Taylor, H. A. & Powell, T. (2017). Employer requirements to work during emergency responses: Key ethics considerations. *Journal of Law, Medicine and Ethics, 45*(S1), 73–76. doi:10.1177/1073110517703330

Shalala, D. E. (1999). Bioterrorism: How prepared are we? *Emerging Infectious Diseases, 5*(4), 492–493. doi:10.3201/eid0504.990402

Texas State Board of Nursing. (2013). Retrieved from http://www.bon.state.tx.us/index.asp

Uniform Emergency Volunteer Health Practitioners Act. (2007). Retrieved from https://www.facs.org/advocacy/state/uevhpa

U.S. Department of Health and Human Services. (2007). New international health regulations enter into force in the United States. Retrieved from http://www.hhs.gov/news/press/2007pres/07/pr20070718a.html

Wagner, J. M. & Dahnke, M. D. (2015). Nursing ethics and disaster triage: Applying utilitarian ethical theory. *Journal of Emergency Nursing, 41*(4), 300–306. doi:10.1016/j.jen.2014.11.001

Whalen v. Roe, 429 U.S. 589 (1977).

World Health Organization Health Assembly resolution WHA58.3. (2005). "International Health Regulations," adopted May 23, 2005.

42 U.S. Code § 5191 (a) (2011).

42 U.S. Code § 5191 (b) (2011).

DISASTER MENTAL HEALTH AND HIGH-VULNERABILITY POPULATIONS

7

IDENTIFYING AND ACCOMMODATING HIGH-RISK, HIGH-VULNERABILITY POPULATIONS IN DISASTERS

Elizabeth A. Davis, Rebecca Hansen, Lori Peek, Brenda Phillips, and Sarah Tuneberg[*]

LEARNING OBJECTIVES

When this chapter is completed, readers will be able to:

1. Define and apply the concept of high-risk, high-vulnerability populations to disaster contexts.
2. Identify the social populations most at risk when disaster strikes and offer an intersectional analysis that explains how overlapping population characteristics may increase or decrease the vulnerability of an individual in a disaster.
3. Understand how stakeholder involvement is essential throughout all phases of a disaster to identify and validate gaps, solutions, and unresolved issues regarding vulnerability.
4. Identify varying systemic levels where medical intervention can reduce disaster vulnerability.

KEY MESSAGES

High-risk, high-vulnerability populations refer to groups who have the greatest probability of being exposed to disaster and who have the least capacity to anticipate, cope with, resist, or recover from

---

[*] The authors are listed alphabetically to denote equal contributions.
This fourth edition chapter updates and expands the chapter in the previous editions. The current authors wish to acknowledge the contributions of three authors from the earlier chapter editions: Jane Kushma with Jacksonville State University, Jennifer Mincin with SUNY Empire State College, and Alan Clive, who was formerly with FEMA and has since passed away after a long and noble fight against cancer.

the event, including: the poor, racial and ethnic minorities, immigrants and non-native speakers, women, children, the elderly, and persons with disabilities. Here, such individuals are viewed as possibly having particular medical issues.

By using a systems approach, it is possible to think beyond traditional medical models and influence the social, economic, and policy structures that induce vulnerability.

Anticipatory planning and preparedness actions are key drivers to successful response and recovery outcomes. Such actions do not necessarily require significant effort or expense, and can be integrated with routine activities.

Awareness of possibilities for action is enhanced when individuals understand and personalize the risks they face in their community.

CHAPTER OVERVIEW

Some populations are more vulnerable and at higher risk from disasters than other populations. This chapter will help you identify high-risk, high-vulnerability populations and understand their potentially unique needs in a disaster context. Employing an ecosystems approach across the life cycle of a disaster, you will explore potential strategies to reduce vulnerability, provide necessary assistance or accommodation, and build the capacity of individuals, families, caregivers, agencies, and organizations, and the community. Case studies, tips, and tools are included to help you apply what you learn.

DEFINING AND UNDERSTANDING VULNERABILITY

Disasters in the United States and around the globe have caused widespread loss of life, destruction of built and natural environments, significant economic damage, and prolonged suffering and hardship among survivors. Photographs of flooded communities submerged under murky waters, of historic structures turned to rubble in earthquakes, and of homes and businesses flattened during tornadoes can leave the impression that disasters are "equal opportunity events." Decades of social science research, however, provide substantial evidence to the contrary. Consider the following:

- In 1987, a tornado destroyed nearly half of Saragosa, TX. Home to about 400 people, virtually all of the families in this small west Texas town were of Mexican descent and the majority spoke only Spanish. Yet, the residents received no culturally appropriate official warnings and messages that were disseminated through the Spanish-language media that members of the community typically used were poorly translated (Aguirre, 1988). After failing to take shelter, 30 people ultimately died and 120 sustained injuries (Tierney, Lindell, & Perry, 2001).
- The 1988 Armenian earthquake killed perhaps as many as 25,000 people. About two-thirds of the total deaths were

children and adolescents who were in classrooms in inadequately designed schools at the time of the quake (Miller, Kraus, Tatevosyan, & Kamechenko, 1993).

- In the 3 years following the 1995 Great Hanshin (Kobe) earthquake in Japan, the proportion of low-income elderly men and women living alone in temporary governmental housing increased substantially. The elders who were most socially isolated suffered from the highest rates of sickness and depression and were at elevated risk for suicide and increased rates of alcoholism and suicide (Kako & Ikeda, 2009; Otani, 2010). In response, a nursing college volunteered in the "kasetu" used for elderly survivors. There, they encountered isolated seniors with increased rates of alcohol and suicide. Out of concern for increased deaths (called "kodokushi" or death alone and unnoticed), they moved residents into "kasetu" on the grounds of the nursing college (Kako & Ikeda, 2009).
- Among the approximately 1,300 persons who perished in New Orleans in Hurricane Katrina in 2005, 67% were at least 65 years old. Prior to the storm, this group represented just 12% of the population (Sharkey, 2007). In Orleans parish, the mortality rate among Black adults was 1.7 to 4 times higher than among White adults (Brunkard, Namulanda, & Ratard, 2008).
- Superstorm Sandy, which struck the East Coast in 2012, highlighted that Black and Latino populations disproportionately reside in the census tracts within three miles of the storm surge zone. In addition to seeing a direct and disproportionate impact on people of color, public and subsidized housing residents were also disproportionately affected. In Connecticut and New Jersey, roughly half of the public housing and subsidized housing units within storm-affected census tracts were "highly impacted" by storm surge or other storm damage (Haas Institute, 2016).

In this chapter, we use the term "high-risk, high-vulnerability populations" to refer to the people with a higher probability of being exposed to disaster who also face barriers to anticipate, cope with, resist, or recover from the event (also see Fordham, Lovekamp, Thomas, & Phillips, 2014; Mileti, 1999; Wisner, Blaikie, Cannon, & Davis, 2004). What can the previous examples and the myriad other cases that are now part of the ever-growing disaster research literature teach us about human vulnerability to disasters?

First, some groups in society are more prone than others to damage, loss, and suffering in the context of differing hazards (Wisner et al., 2004). The poor, racial and ethnic minorities, immigrants and non-native speakers, women, children, the elderly, and persons with disabilities are among those most at risk to the adverse impacts of disaster (see Phillips, Thomas, Fothergill, & Blinn-Pike, 2010). Although these groups differ in many ways, they often lack access to vital economic and social resources, have limited autonomy and power, and have low levels of social capital (Barnshaw & Trainor, 2007; Morrow, 1999). They also, for various sociohistorical and economic reasons, tend to live and work in the most hazardous regions and in the lowest-quality buildings, thus further exposing them to risks of morbidity and mortality associated with natural hazards (Cutter, Bryan, & Shirley, 2003; Sutley, van de Lindt, & Peek, 2017a, 2017b).

Second, the aforementioned demographic characteristics—socioeconomic status, race, gender, age, disability—intersect in complex and dynamic ways that may increase or decrease the vulnerability of any given member of a social group (Phillips & Morrow, 2007). For example, although African Americans experienced higher mortality rates than Whites in Hurricane Katrina, not all African Americans were equally at risk. Race interacted with age, gender, and evacuation status, resulting in Black men over 75 years of age who did not leave the city before the hurricane landfall being significantly overrepresented among the dead in Orleans parish (Brunkard et al., 2008; Sharkey, 2007).

Third, over the past decade, there has been some movement away from simple taxonomies or checklists of "vulnerable groups" to a concern with what Wisner et al. (2004, p. 15) refer to as "vulnerable situations." This approach emphasizes vital *temporal* and *geographical dimensions* to examining vulnerability and the social contexts and circumstances in which people live (also see Fothergill & Peek, 2015). The thousands of children who died in the Armenian earthquake may not have lost their lives had the disaster not happened during the school day. Extensive loss of life among women and children from the 2004 Indian Ocean tsunami occurred as they waited on the shore to process fish brought home by their husbands who survived the event at sea. In one Indian school for children with disabilities, nearly all perished. This approach also reminds us that people may become more or less vulnerable depending on their age and stage of development, or due to injuries, pregnancy, or other temporary health conditions (Peek, 2013).

Fourth, when trying to understand why disasters happen and who is affected most, it is crucial to recognize that it is not only "natural" hazards that cause them (Wisner et al., 2004). Disasters are the product of social, political, and economic environments that structure the lives and life chances of different groups of people.

Models for Understanding Vulnerability

When considering high-risk, high-vulnerability populations, two schools of thought, or models, are used to frame the discussion that follows. Note that these models—medical and functional—are derived from a disability-focused approach but can be applied to other high-risk, high-vulnerability groups. To be most effective, however, a balanced use of both methodologies will likely have the most benefit when preventing harm or minimizing the consequences of disasters.

Medical Model

This model is derived from disease, trauma, or health conditions that disrupt what is considered to be "normal" functionality—physically, mentally, or socially. It has implications for public health programming and policy development as it places emphasis on treatments and interventions that manage, reduce, or prevent the debilitation, disease, or condition. But in the realm of high-risk, high-vulnerability planning or response to a disaster, the model is limiting because it does not fully consider the social, cultural, and economic roots of vulnerability nor does it adequately account for capability, ability, and self-direction during disaster. The medical model has been critiqued as ignoring sociopolitical dimensions that marginalize people with medical or disability conditions and overlooking the potential capacity of populations if barriers to full participation and independence are removed (Tierney, Petak, & Hahn, 1988).

Functional Model

The functional model, also called the "social model," moves the focus from categorizing deficits at an individual level, such as found in the medical model, to understanding the vulnerability in the context of the built, social, and political environment. The core principle in the functional model is how it places the onus on society and not on the individual to intervene and make systemic changes that will benefit all people, especially those with support needs in the areas of communication, health, functional independence, support and safety, and transportation. In the realm of disaster, this approach attempts to enable individuals the same opportunities to access services or to take self-determined actions during disaster. So within the disaster life cycle (preparedness, response, recovery, and mitigation), while it is imperative that all individuals take on a responsibility to plan to the best of their abilities, it is equally important that professionals and the overall response system become and remain fully inclusive and sufficiently flexible to actively address barriers, collaborate with stakeholders, and utilize resources effectively.

Currently, the Federal Emergency Management Agency's (FEMA's) "whole community" philosophy is promulgated on the functional model just outlined. As such, FEMA suggests that planning for everyone ensures the exclusion of no one. This means knowing one's community demographics as intimately as possible, beyond a surface level of statistical and census information. Working with direct service providers and others in the community serves as the firm foundation of an effective and stand-alone emergency management program or one within a healthcare organization. For example, this could include activities such as:

- Working with durable medical supply vendors to map higher levels of oxygen delivery to homes
- Partnering with public utilities to identify electrically dependent customers

- Working with immigrant advocacy groups to determine non-native language usages and the best ways to reach people with information
- Supporting domestic violence program organizations to identify security and safety concerns for women and children not easily reached
- Collaborating with local health departments and community clinics to take into account higher area reliance on emergency rooms for standard health needs as an indicator of economic conditions

Using a whole community approach in all phases of emergency management helps to reduce vulnerability and lessen the impact of disasters.

Application

In the medical profession, the medical model represents a common approach as health conditions denote pathology and lead professionals to identify appropriate interventions and treatments. The functional model expands and transforms the medical approach allowing for additional analysis of social systems, providing the opportunity to work more closely with community members, and recognizing that not all health conditions are isolated but instead interwoven with the economic, social, political, racial realities of people's lives. Thus, an appreciation and application of both models are necessary to be most effective.

To demonstrate the need to understand a wider social context, consider that one 87-year-old person may be completely capable of self-sustaining actions in a disaster once provided the appropriate information on which to act, while another person of the same age may have multiple health or medical conditions preventing self-care. The latter may be economically capable of compensating for the physical conditions by utilizing private care support services. So age is not a singular fact; nor is health; nor is economics.

To demonstrate the need for interventions that are more inclusive, consider that another 87-year-old person is deaf or hard of hearing and critical instructions are transmitted in spoken English only via loudspeaker, causing a barrier to understanding, being able to take action and engage in self-protection. If that same person receives printed information, sign language interpretation, or by other alternative ways, then he or she is more likely to take action that results in self-protection. Similarly, imagine the challenges faced by a person with limited English proficiency. Again, providing information in multiple languages and formats will result in a higher likelihood that persons at risk will be empowered to take appropriate action desired because they received the necessary information and messaging.

When acting in the midst of a disaster or within the following short-term recovery period, using a functional rather than a purely medical model can also improve the triage process. Once past the acute medical need, a functional model will enable nurses and others to anticipate resources needed to further facilitate recovery and help prevent adverse outcomes. For instance, after being evacuated from an area, priority should then be put on reuniting a medically healthy individual with his or her service provider (e.g., a home health aide or family member) to facilitate self-reliance, independence, and help more quickly move the person out of the disaster system. Consider also a situation when a culturally competent nurse can quickly identify that a woman will require a female provider due to religious beliefs, expediting her care while meeting her cultural and religious requirements. Such practices acknowledge that once individual abilities and needs are recognized, barriers to medical care and self-protection can be overcome, providing greater access to care by more people. In short, the functional model promotes efficacy in patient assessment and efficiency in provision of care.

Understanding Vulnerability Systematically as a Basis for Intervention

By understanding vulnerability systematically, it is also possible to identify points of intervention. One such approach considers the "ecosystem" that comprises various levels from the individual to the broader society (Brofenbrenner, 1979; Garbarino, 1992). At each ecosystem level, numerous conditions can be identified that increase or decrease the vulnerability of people, households, neighborhoods, communities, and even societies. The value of using the ecosystem framework for understanding vulnerability is clear: it explains why some people suffer disproportionately in disaster while, importantly, suggesting pathways toward action within each systemic level. Moreover, this framework highlights the complex, dynamic, and interactive nature of vulnerability in both pre- and postdisaster contexts. As such, this section provides an overview of each level of the ecosystem coupled with relevant examples. The chapter's concluding section draws upon the ecosystem approach to offer intervention strategies.

The first level of the ecosystem, the *microlevel*, includes individuals, households, and families. Here, vulnerability may result from interaction between an individual's unique personality, disposition, and physical and psychological status, and the practices, resources, and circumstances of the family situation and the household in which the person lives. As a consequence of the interaction between these variables, people experience different types of risk and degrees of exposure based on various conditions. Social isolation represents one such condition; it can cause people to miss disaster warnings or influence the potential for an individual to experience malnutrition and depression (Norris, Friedman, & Watson, 2002; Norris et al., 2002). Central to microlevel vulnerability, then, is the understanding that social networks represent a critical resource to reducing exposure. In short, when individuals have people around them who care about them, they are more likely to hear a warning and be able to take protective action. Social networks, though, may be compromised by income levels, advanced age, disability, and medical conditions. Surviving on entitlement checks, such as social security or supplemental security income, means a wait at the end of the month until funds arrive. Limited income reduces capacity to afford ready kit items including extra medications, gasoline for evacuation, or funds to survive away from home. During response and especially during recovery, people also compete for limited resources (Comfort et al., 1999; Peacock & Ragsdale, 1997; Poulshock & Cohen, 1975). The microlevel also considers exposure levels, which have historically been higher among low-income, minority, and elderly populations, who are more likely to live in or near floodplains in less hazard-resistant and older housing not built to current hazard codes. By focusing on the microlevel, healthcare providers can increase awareness and supply critical information or resources to reduce the impact, assist with the response, and facilitate the recovery of high-risk populations.

In the second, *meso-level* tier, organizations operate to reduce the impact of disasters. Traditionally, such organizations include emergency management agencies and, increasingly, healthcare providers. Pandemics represent one such interorganizational concern with efforts being made recently to establish accessible points of distribution for countermeasures. But a wider array of partners is possible at the meso-level. Consider the places and ways in which healthcare organizations can distribute information at healthcare offices, outreach clinics, and home health agencies (Phillips, 2010). Such efforts can be leveraged by partnering with advocacy and community-based organizations (CBOs). In this regard, consider the potential to influence people's daily lives through their immediate environment, from laundromats, senior centers and schools, to grocery stores, pharmacies, barbershops, beauty salons, churches, and other places of worship. For their part, meso-level organizations can also amass resources to distribute across inequitable access points experienced by households marginalized economically by medical, disability, and aging-associated costs.

The more abstract *exo-level* focuses on policy. Until Hurricane Katrina, many efforts in the United States to enact policies specific to people with disabilities and medical concerns largely failed to garner widespread attention. Post-Katrina, much has happened. The simple existence of a postdisaster housing plan for the FEMA, which includes the needs for disability advocacy and representation in housing planning, serves as one such example. Indeed, legislation in 2011 created FEMA's Office on Disability Integration and Coordination (ODIC). Under that Office, FEMA has developed a cadre of 285 disability integration experts including advisors, American sign language interpreters, and certified deaf interpreters, along with an integration specialist in each FEMA region to coordinate organizational and systemic change in this area. The Federal Highway Administration (2009) represents another example of a step forward with the publication of its guidance document detailing effective evacuation practices for medically fragile populations. In 2016, the U.S. Departments of Justice, Health and Human Services (HHS), Housing and Urban Development, Homeland Security, and Transportation jointly issued guidance to state and local governments engaged in emergency management activities regarding complying with nondiscrimination and civil rights laws. This guidance is further evidence of exo-level activity and the advancement in this area as it pertains to meeting the needs of high-risk, high-vulnerability people and populations in disasters.

The *macro-level* encompasses historical, cultural, and geographical factors that influence social vulnerability. Historic patterns of racism and legally enforced segregation have marginalized some populations into risky areas, including floodplains and areas requiring relocation due to climate change (Bronan & Pollock, 2017; Cutter, 2006). The historic communities of Princeville, North Carolina (first town incorporated in the United States by African Americans) and the Lower Ninth Ward of New Orleans (over 95% African American pre-Katrina) both sustained catastrophic damage from hurricane-related floods. In Princeville, segregation on the floodplain side of the river meant that the predominantly older population, with a majority being African American and female, sustained heavy damage in 1999 and again in 2016 in Hurricane Matthew. In New Orleans, the Lower Ninth Ward also suffered some of the highest water damage with only one-fourth of its predominantly older and African American population back at the 5-year anniversary of the storm in 2010. A legacy of political marginalization in the community created the macro-level context for the higher loss of life and reduced rate of return (Phillips, Stukes, & Jenkins, 2011).

The potential impact of a systematic, successful intervention strategy across all these aforementioned levels can be considerable. The challenge lies in individual and collective willingness to address vulnerabilities and undertake specific interventions. Toward that end, the healthcare sector plays a significant role in each level and can offer considerable human capital that can be leveraged to reduce vulnerability. With a focus exclusively on patients, without concern for organizational intervention, policy attention, and cultural-level change, we will not see change in human vulnerabilities.

USING AN EQUITY AND EMPOWERMENT LENS

When implementing the ecosystem model of vulnerability, using an Equity and Empowerment Lens can assist in understanding how decisions, policies, procedures, and strategies can impact high-risk, high-vulnerability populations and individuals. Adapted by the Multnomah County, Oregon Mass Shelter Access and Functional Needs Task Force, the Equity and Empowerment Lens can be useful to nurses in many applications and settings. As is done through a camera, a lens helps bring ideas into focus or widen perspectives to see things not seen before.

Equity establishes an expectation to *provide the resources everyone needs to be successful* and differs from equality, which is *treating everyone the same*. While both equity and equality are strategies to promote fairness, equality works only if everyone has the same needs and starts from the same place.

Achieving equity in emergencies and disasters requires practitioners to engage more fully in evaluating and understanding the unique needs of high-risk, high-vulnerability community members. The Equity and Empowerment Lens asks users to consider four domains—People, Place, Process, and Power. Within each domain, a series of questions help the user consider who is affected by the decision; what benefits and burdens could yield; and what actions could mitigate and minimize potential burdens. The full version of the Equity and Empowerment Lens tool and guidance can be found at multco.us/diversity-equity/equity-and-empowerment-lens.

Within this framework, the *People* domain refers to individuals, groups, communities, or populations. When evaluating the People domain, consider which communities are impacted by the decision, policy, or plan under consideration. Ask who wins and who loses.

The *Place* domain refers to the physical space and also the social relationships and meaning attached to a physical location that give it context and value. Practitioners should consider the pros and cons and associated impacts of Place and its context within community.

EQUALITY VERSUS EQUITY

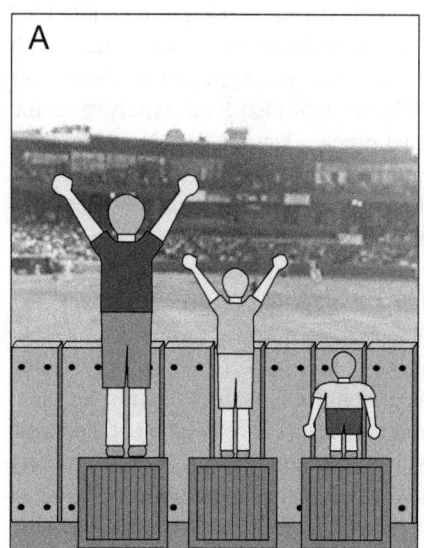

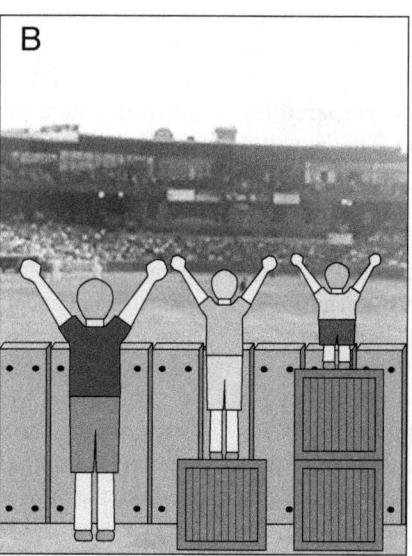

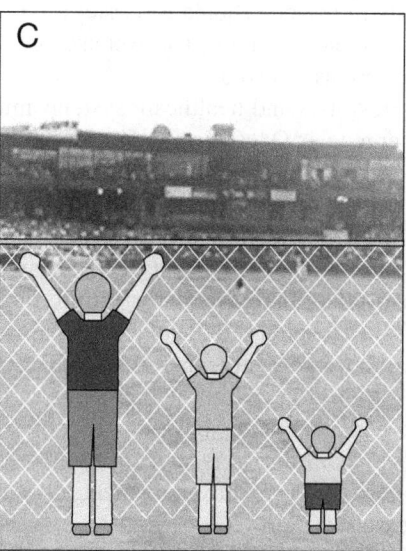

In the first image, it is assumed that everyone will benefit from the same supports. They are being treated equally.

In the second image, individuals are given different supports to make it possible for them to have equal access to the game. They are being treated equitably.

In the third image, all three can see the game without any supports or accommodations because the cause of the inequity was addressed. The systemic barrier has been removed.

FIGURE 7.1 Equality versus equity.

Sources: Panels A and B reproduced with permission from Craig Froehle, PhD. Panel C, Office of Diversity and Equality, Multnomah County, Washington.

The *Process* domain encompasses the policies, plans, and decision-making structures. Process questions consider methods to engage and build relationships to create a more inclusive, respectful, and aware process. In Process, *how* is as important as *what* and *why*.

Lastly, the *Power* domain addresses who is making decisions and who is impacted by those decisions. Similar to process-related questioning, when working through the Power domain, consider methods to engage and build inclusive and respectful relationships. Again, *how* is as important as *what* and *why* questions within this domain. When thinking about Power, consider how the issue under consideration shifts power dynamics to better integrate voices and priorities of underrepresented individuals or communities.

THE LIFE CYCLE OF DISASTERS

Any disaster, whether natural or man-made, can be viewed as having a *life cycle* with certain distinct stages (Mileti, 1999), including: acting to improve readiness to respond (*preparedness*); taking immediate actions after a disaster has occurred to protect life, property, and the environment (*response*); restoring functions and dealing with the aftermath of the disaster to return to a predisaster state or an improved state (*recovery*); and engaging in efforts to lessen the effects of a disaster (*mitigation*).

While the life cycle stages of disaster are distinct, and are described in this section as such, the process is not linear.

Actions within phases can and do overlap and influence outcomes within phases.

This section provides suggestions for addressing and integrating within each stage of a disaster the needs of high-risk, high-vulnerability populations. Examining each stage, consider the following:

- How does this information apply to particular specialties of nursing practice?
- How can professional expertise and experience working with high-risk, high-vulnerability patients link into the disaster planning arena?
- What steps can be taken at a particular healthcare setting to improve integration of emergency-related needs of high-risk, high-vulnerability populations in each phase?
- How can nurses, as trusted members of a community, leverage their professional role to enhance disaster resiliency in the community? How can nurses serve as change agents to inspire and empower patients, coworkers, and partners to take necessary steps to increase their own resiliency?

Preparedness

Preparedness involves planning and getting ready for disasters by individuals, families, organizations, businesses, and communities. The state of preparedness includes the following contexts: recognizing the specific hazards that pose a threat, understanding the associated risks and potential impacts, and identifying suitable strategies and actions to take to be ready to respond should a disaster occur. Planning, personal preparedness, training, and exercises are vital to all strategies and actions involved.

Hospitals and healthcare systems must be prepared for emergencies (McGlown & Robinson, 2011). The Hospital Preparedness Program (HPP), funded by the Assistant Secretary for Preparedness and Response (ASPR) for the U.S. HHS, supports states, territories, and municipalities to improve surge capacity and enhance community and hospital preparedness for public health emergencies. "From Hospitals to Healthcare Coalitions: Transforming Health Preparedness and Response in Our Communities," is the program's first comprehensive report, identifying the advances states have made in preparing hospitals for all types of disasters. According to a May 2011 report, a majority of U.S. hospitals meet all-hazards preparedness measures (HHS, 2011).

Additionally, in 2006, the Centers for Medicare and Medicaid Services (CMS) issued guidance to assist nursing homes and long-term care facilities in complying with Federal requirements regarding emergency preparedness and response. In 2012, the HHS issued a report evaluating progress made by nursing homes and long-term care facilities in achieving emergency preparedness and response requirements since the issuance of the guidance. The report found that though most facilities had written emergency plans and training that complied with Federal requirements, significant gaps persisted (HHS, 2012). For example, nursing homes face challenges with unreliable transportation contracts, lack of collaboration with local emergency management, and concerns about what to do with residents who developed health problems during an emergency.

In November 2016, the CMS issued a final rule "Emergency Preparedness for Medicare and Medicaid Providers and Suppliers." The rule establishes a national emergency preparedness requirement to ensure adequate planning for both natural and man-made disasters and coordination with Federal, state, tribal, regional, and local emergency preparedness systems. Nurses can anticipate engaging in emergency preparedness activities such as developing emergency plans and participating in training and testing as a result of the CMS emergency preparedness rule.

Personal Preparedness

Nurses can encourage individuals and families to take steps toward greater preparedness. In many communities across the United States, organizations have found ways to integrate personal preparedness education and training into their everyday programs. For example, as part of the formal discharge process, nurses can walk patients through emergency-related considerations to help them prepare for emergencies. In some cases, individuals and families will return home with capabilities and limitations that may differ from what they know. These individuals will have to make changes in terms of everyday life and in disaster planning. Some home healthcare agencies have added personal preparedness as part of their assessment

and often educate their patients, consumers, or families during home visits. Posing questions such as: What transportation arrangements have you made if you need to leave your home? and What equipment and supplies do you need to have with you ready to take in an emergency? can help individuals start to formulate a plan. Nurses can also lend expertise to the development of personal preparedness materials and training to ensure that information is provided in multiple modalities, that critical information and resources are included, and that information is delivered in a way that makes it accessible and understandable. Something as simple as including a disaster preparedness checklist in annual reviews or distributing materials in multiple, accessible media can enhance awareness and spur personal change (Phillips, 2009; see Case Study 7.1). Using the Equity and Empowerment Lens as a foundation for these conversations can help nurses ensure consideration of the whole person including the social, economic, racial, and community realities that may influence their personal preparedness. And in some cases, it can be a great service for nurses and others who are supporting this preparedness effort to remind individuals to include their service animals and their well-being in all disaster planning as well.

It is also necessary that agencies inform clients how the agency will operate in an emergency in order to sustain services. Such information will help clients to create more realistic plans for a disaster and to identify alternate ways to receive assistance.

Personal preparedness is also key for nurses and healthcare providers as first-line responders. Ensuring that health professionals and their families are disaster ready stabilizes and sustains services to high-risk, high-vulnerability populations within a community. Personal preparedness should include identifying alternate routes and means of transportation to work, planning emergency caregiving (e.g., for children or elderly family members) with neighbors or friends, and having emergency supplies stocked at home.

Organizational Planning and Preparedness

Individual governmental agencies, not-for-profit organizations, faith-based organizations, schools, and businesses that work directly with high-risk, high-vulnerability populations need business continuity plans as well. Thus, healthcare providers should create plans to sustain services postdisaster. Planning teams should include staff from different programs and levels, facility managers, patients/clients, clinical staff, social workers, partners, vendors, and other critical community-based partners. Encouraging a wide and deep set of groups to work together will lend expertise and validate the process, so that plans they generate capture appropriate strategies, problem areas, or gaps, and result in more informed, creative, and realistic solutions.

- **_Emergency Plans_**: The emergency plans of an agency explain the role and actions of the organization in responding to the specific needs of that agency in a disaster, as well as the role that the agency will play in a community-wide response to a disaster. The following are some examples of emergency-related planning issues that pose challenges to planners and questions that should be answered in the planning process.

Notification: How will patients/clients/students be notified during an emergency? Will the agency be making home visits/phone calls to check in on people? What kinds of alternate communication methods will be utilized to ensure that patients/families/caregivers can receive and understand information and follow instructions?

Evacuation: How will patients/clients/students evacuate who have mobility disabilities and are unable to use the stairs? Will specialized evacuation equipment be purchased? What kind of vehicles will be needed to evacuate people and relocate to another location? What kind of facility will be safe to evacuate patients/clients/students based on their medical and functional needs? Will staff accompany people to an evacuation site? Will a service animal be accompanying the individual as well?

■ ***Continuity of Operations Plans (COOPs)***: A COOP works in tandem with emergency plans and specifically addresses how the entity will continue to carry out critical functions during an emergency or other disruption. For agencies that provide critical medical services to individuals such as dialysis, cancer treatments, physical or occupational therapy, or methadone, the ability to continue services with little or no disruption will directly impact the patient's/client's resiliency to disaster.

Essential Functions: What functions of the agency are critical? What functions provide critical care/assistance to individuals/families? How will these be staffed and carried out during different types of emergencies?

Staffing: How will staff be notified of the situation? What kind of responsibility do they have to the agency versus their own family? Where are they located and how can they communicate with the agency, where should they report, and so forth?

Organizations and individuals serving vulnerable populations have historically been left out of the planning efforts making it very difficult to join or coordinate during response to a disaster. In a report written just a few weeks after Hurricane Katrina hit the Gulf Coast, 87.5% of CBOs interviewed said that they did not know how to link with the emergency management system (National Organization on Disability [NOD], 2005). This can have devastating impacts on the populations that CBOs serve during nondisaster times. When organizational planning is inclusive, CBOs can be brought to the table and have a fuller opportunity to offer many valuable resources and community connections that may be needed during response.

Training and Exercises

Training and exercises are part of every emergency management planning process in that they prepare professionals and the public to test plans and to identify gaps, alternate strategies, and need for improvement. One important initiative, the National Nurse Emergency Preparedness Initiative (NNEPI), has recognized the role that nurses play in emergency preparedness. Their "Nurses on the Front Line" is a highly interactive, web-based course developed to provide emergency preparedness training for nurses working in a wide variety of settings. (To learn more about this initiative and the course, visit https://nnepi.gwnursing.org/). As demonstrated in this course, nurses are often part of training and exercise activities, and can advocate for and integrate issues pertaining to high-risk, high-vulnerability populations. Some ways that this can be done include:

■ ***Training***
  Include awareness curricula in training for staff to deepen understanding of working with diverse and at-risk populations. Include specific information about emergency-related issues.

  Conduct cross-training with emergency management agencies to deepen knowledge of emergency management structure and in particular how that sector integrates high-risk and high-vulnerability populations.

  Conduct cross-training with agencies and organizations that work directly with high-risk, high-vulnerability populations to better understand ways of serving members of those groups, as well as identifying resources and expertise that may be needed.

  Invite people with expertise in high-risk, high-vulnerability populations to help develop training materials and integrate the issues into existing training curricula.

  Train staff on particular roles in an emergency and how to specifically advocate for and address emergency-related needs of high-risk, high-vulnerability populations in their care.

  Be sure that space where training is held, instruction/presentation, and materials are available in accessible formats. Ensure that accommodations allow greater access and participation. Provide childcare and hold meetings at times when large segments of the target population will actually be available.

■ ***Exercises***
  Involve staff from varying levels of practice, settings, and expertise within the agency to participate in planning exercises as they bring valuable perspectives to the process.

  At the exercise development phase, integrate issues that will test the capacity to address the needs of high-risk, high-vulnerability populations; include these as part of the plan objectives and identify evaluation markers in order to assess this aspect of the exercise.

  Utilize individuals who make up diverse populations to actually "play" and test the system as that will allow for more authenticity and reality-based outcomes.

  The Los Angeles County of Emergency Management Drills and Exercises Guidance for Inclusive Emergency Planning provides strategies, resources, and guidance, including training vignettes, regarding establishing and executing a collaborative, inclusive exercise design and execution process that better addresses the needs of high-risk, high-vulnerability populations (available at lacoa.org/PDF/IEP%20Drill_and_Exercise_Guide_08202014.pdf).

Response

The response phase of the disaster life cycle encompasses the period during and immediately after a disaster occurs. FEMA defines response as the immediate actions to save lives, protect property and the environment, and meet basic human needs. Response also includes the execution of emergency plans and actions to support short-term recovery (FEMA, 2008).

Collaboration

Response to a disaster also requires collaboration among governmental and public partners that make up the response network. In terms of addressing high-risk, high-vulnerability populations, those working in the health sector will necessarily coordinate response within their sector, but must also work closely with other key partners, including:

- Governmental agencies encompassing emergency response, transportation, housing, environmental protection, public works, public assistance, and disability and senior services, among others;
- Private and public sector agencies including congregate care facilities, utility companies, CBOs, faith-based organizations, and businesses, among others.

Because of their exposure through the healthcare sector, nurses have a distinct understanding of the diversity of the community and the impact that disasters can have during the response phase. As nurses are dispersed throughout the community in many different kinds of health and caregiving settings, hospitals, public health departments, schools, or other entities, there is a reach and relationship with diverse communities that can come only from working directly with that community. Utilizing these opportunities to help identify resources—possibly not planned for or known to the formal response system—will be invaluable during an actual response. Understanding existing communication protocols and systems also will allow nurses to bring their unique skills and understanding of diverse populations to the response arena.

By working on an interdisciplinary or integrated planning committee, nurses can share their experience and advocate for their patients. The result? A more complete and enriched plan with emergency tactics, strategies, and plans that more effectively and efficiently meets the needs of the whole community. Such integrated planning committees, often organized out of local emergency management agencies or healthcare coalitions, are often looking for diverse membership, including nurses. By reaching out to their local emergency management agency, nurses can provide valuable insights for planning around high-risk, high-vulnerability populations.

Response Activities

This section highlights a few key response activities to demonstrate ways that nurses can better work with, support, and advocate for high-risk, high-vulnerability populations in their care and within their communities during the response phase. Actual activities will vary based on several factors, including area of practice, disaster roles and responsibilities, personal experience, and access to resources, among others.

- *Notification and Communication*: There is no one-size-fits-all solution to communicating with patients and their families

and other potentially vulnerable populations during a disaster. Instead, using a multiple modality approach that overcomes different barriers is more likely to reach more people at a time when it is critical. The particulars will differ depending on the setting (hospital, outpatient, inpatient, at-home, residential) and should be tailored to and appropriate for addressing the needs of those involved. The following are some suggestions to consider:

- Use sign language interpreters on-site or remotely via the web.
- Use language interpreters, included through remote access or through a language bank.
- Create internal communications systems that are customized to patient and staff needs.
- Integrate augmentative and alternate communication systems ranging from options that are low-tech (e.g., pointing board with symbols, pictures, and words) or conversely, high-tech communications devices (e.g., a voice output communication aid [VOCA]).
- Ensure that alarm and notification systems provide notifications in multiple ways such as aural, visual, vibrating, through notification systems (i.e., texts), and so forth.
- Utilize different forms of technology to communicate to a wider variety of age groups—television; landline emergency alerts; cell phones; email; texting; and social media.
- Match staff communication skills (e.g., proficiency in a language) with needs.

- *Temporary Healthcare or Shelter Sites*: During the response phase it is possible that alternate care and shelter sites are opened. Steps can be taken to ensure that sites accommodate different needs through coordination with the agency coordinating the operations, the facility manager(s) and on-site staff, agencies working within the site, and external organizations or businesses that can provide resources. Nurses can help to advocate for and identify accommodation needs. The following are some ways to account for diverse needs.

- Ensure that sites meet physical and programmatic accessibility standards. The U.S. Department of Justice (DOJ) offers a shelter checklist based on accessibility standards (DOJ, 2007).
- Systematically identify needs of individuals with the individual/caregiver/family (e.g., during intake or triage) and put a standard operating procedure in place for meeting accommodation requests.
- Find ways to offer space that is separate from the main congregate space such as quiet rooms; supervised children's areas; supervised areas for persons with dementia, Alzheimer's disease; gender-specific areas; breastfeeding areas; examination or counseling areas that are private; and so forth.
- Develop ways to refrigerate medications and/or specialized food.
- Locate power supplies for those using oxygen machines, power wheelchairs, or other electrically dependent durable medical equipment. This may include alternate locations (e.g., fire stations) where people can regenerate equipment.

- Have durable medical equipment on hand such as canes, wheelchairs, walkers, medical/specialty cots.
- Identify organizations and other suppliers with supply and equipment resources (e.g., medical supply stores, assistive technology organizations, generator supply companies).
- Establish memorandum of understandings (MOUs) with skilled staffing (nurses, social workers, physical and occupational therapists, psychologists, personal care assistants, sexual assault counselors, et al.) that can provide expertise and support operations at the site.
- Utilize multiple modalities to communicate with those at site.

- **Decontamination:** Undergoing decontamination operations can challenge high-risk, high-vulnerability populations. There are specific steps that can be taken to mitigate risk, injury, and/or trauma that can all cause deteriorating conditions and limit independence. The following are examples of ways to mitigate the impact:
  - Identify strategies for decontaminating and/or replacing durable medical equipment, consumable medical supplies, and/or augmentative communication equipment and reconnecting them with owners.
  - Systematically identify needs (with the individual, caregiver, and/or family) and put a standard operating procedure in place for addressing these needs.
  - Practice strategies for decontaminating service animals and/or pets and reconnecting them with owners.
  - Utilize multiple modalities to communicate with those at the site.
  - Establish ways to respect privacy and/or safety concerns of the individual.
  - Offer gender-specific decontamination operations.
  - Craft strategies to address medication needs.
  - Work with caregivers to help support their children through the process.

Although it is critical for nurses to anticipate the needs of patients/clients, it is equally critical for nurses to listen carefully to patients and fully grasp their specific needs. This can be extremely challenging in a high-pressure emergency response environment, where needs are great and may be life-threatening and when there is a shortage or depletion of resources. As such, plan in advance. However, if such planning has not been done or only in a limited way, then ensure that there is flexibility, openness, and communication with those in need to find solutions to help mitigate physical and psychological injury or loss of life.

Recovery

Ideally, recovery in the disaster cycle is characterized by actions that help to restore functioning at predisaster levels, often described as a return to a sense of "normalcy." In practice, however, this rarely occurs, since disasters can forever alter conditions, and another term, "new normal," is often employed (Phillips, 2015a, 2015b). Recovery activities begin once the immediate danger has passed, when lifesaving and life-preserving activities begin to wind down, and when emergency needs have been met. Recovery activities that occur in the short term include restoring utilities,

removing debris, and providing temporary housing. Long-term recovery efforts involve repairing and rebuilding damaged infrastructure, restoring routines and mental health functioning, and redeveloping communities. In some cases, communities may attempt to "build back better" and improve quality of life and sustainability. Greensburg, Kansas, for example, decided to build back as a "green" town with all buildings reconstructed to meet LEED-platinum standards after a devastating tornado leveled 95% of its structures. Such efforts should consider how to enhance life for high-risk, high-vulnerability populations.

One of the most important lessons of disaster recovery is that investing some time thinking about recovery *before the disaster strikes* pays tremendous dividends in a disaster's aftermath. Although it is still relatively rare for communities to engage in predisaster "recovery planning," anticipating demands, organizing resources, and determining a basic recovery strategy can lead to greater efficiency, adaptability, and reduced vulnerability. Such foresight is useful for individuals and families as well as organizations and communities.

High-risk, high-vulnerability populations often experience complex recovery-related issues that can overlap and have compounding effects that influence access to recovery assistance and the actual ability to recover. Postdisaster needs will often extend longer into the recovery period and require additional and specialized assets to resolve. Some of the common needs to facilitate recovery include:

- Access to one or more necessary health-related services such as monitoring, daily or regular interventions/treatments, physical/occupational therapies, psychological treatment and counseling
- Access to appropriate housing (e.g., accessible housing or supervised settings) that allow for maximum independence and safety
- Need for resources that are not often identified in recovery programs such as assistive devices, technologies, or other specialized equipment (lifts, ramps, etc.; see Box 7.1)
- Availability of childcare and/or adult daycare services, which free up time allowing for caregivers to identify recovery assistance, find jobs, secure housing, and so forth
- Access to schools and transportation to schools that allow children to return to a sense of routine and normalcy while parents can return to work
- Access to public transportation and to accessible transportation for transportation-dependent populations and persons with disabilities
- Access to recovery information in different languages but also targeting information to hard-to-reach groups such as socially/culturally isolated populations
- Mental health services to support predisaster and postdisaster psychiatric issues
- Access to necessary prescribed medicine to manage predisaster health conditions so as to avoid diminished health status

Given the vast diversity of populations, there are many different barriers that might prevent someone from accessing these aforementioned needed services or resources, including: lack of information about recovery agencies in general and about providing assistance to high-risk, high-vulnerability populations

BOX 7.1 Assistive Technology

In recovery, access to assistive technologies can be critical for some in resuming independence, self-reliance, and functionality. Often in the chaos of disaster, assistive technology (AT) can be destroyed, damaged, or lost, or the disaster itself causing the need for AT not used before, results in greater vulnerability and trauma for the person experiencing the loss of functionality. For health professionals and emergency management, linking to programs as described below can help facilitate connecting someone with necessary AT.

Under the Assistive Technology Act, the Rehabilitation Services Administration—a component of the U.S. Department of Education's Office of Special Education and Rehabilitative Services (OSERS)—funds a statewide AT program in each of the 50 states and six territories, and the majority of these programs support AT device reuse activities.

For many people with disabilities, AT is an essential support to daily living. A person may depend on a wheelchair, walker, special computer keyboard, speech-generating device, or other AT device at home, at school, or at work. AT is a broad descriptor for anything from low-tech (e.g., a transfer board on which a person can slide from a wheelchair into the backseat of a car) to high-tech equipment (e.g., speech reader software) and constantly emerging new technologies including wireless and wearable technologies (Bennett, Phillips, & Davis, 2017).

Reuse of AT is emerging as one of the ways to make AT more available. To the extent that AT reuse is practiced today, it is generally done through device exchange programs, device recycling programs, or device refurbishment programs. Hundreds of organizations around the country, large and small, are involved in AT reuse. From state agencies to nonprofits, to hospitals, to churches, there are AT reuse programs in all parts of the country that meet all kinds of needs.

Until recently, there was weak coordination or networking of and among these programs to ensure an efficient and effective system for getting used AT into the hands of those who need it. However, with the realization of the important role AT can play, especially during the recovery phase in disaster, this is changing. The reality is that with proper identification of immediate need for access to AT postdisaster and a proper match to available AT, those affected by disaster can more quickly regain independence. It must be noted, however, that even if AT is provided for someone

in particular; providers impacted by the disaster who are no longer available to offer services; lack of professional services and expertise in the area; no list available to identify alternate providers in new temporary or permanent communities; lack of health insurance access; lack of information in different languages or pertaining specifically to the needs of different groups; and no transportation or access to recovery centers, schools, childcare providers, and so forth.

With increased awareness of likely needs and barriers, nurses can help advocate during the recovery planning process and during

in the immediate aftermath of a disaster, this might still only be a "quick fix" requiring proper evaluation, fitting, customization, and so on for a more permanent solution.

There are three levels to viewing AT and disaster recovery. The first is at the individual level. If people who use AT on a regular basis actually incorporated their AT into the predisaster planning, then the recovery process is greatly improved. This can be as simple as keeping a record of equipment make, model, and funding program, for example, along with other important documents in the event that their AT is damaged, destroyed, or lost during a disaster.

The second is at the nexus of care level and here is one place nurses can play a role. It means that those in contact with people who use AT can advise of the importance of taking those necessary preparedness steps but also as professionals learning how to identify ways to utilize AT in unconventional ways during a disaster until appropriate solutions can be put back in place. This might mean learning how to switch a power chair into manual use mode, or realizing that with Velcro attached to utensils, a person can independently feed him or herself, or that a picture communication board or chart using pictorials can assist in communication until power-sourced technology can be restored. Any care professional can become involved at this level including certified rehabilitation counselors, AT professionals, speech language pathologists, occupational therapists, physical therapists, and the like. In fact, many of these professionals actually have added disaster preparedness to their code of ethics and/or responsibilities. Nurses often find themselves engaged across these lines of care providers and are well positioned to tie all the skills together to benefit a disaster survivor.

The third level is a systems network level. This is where nurses and other emergency professionals should reach out to the local AT network to find matches of AT in the existing reuse programs that can be redirected for needed matches during the first phases of recovery postdisaster. It is the AT network that is best suited to help with those matches but also to logistically coordinate the quality review before materials are brought in to be sure they will not cause further harm and are appropriate for immediate reuse. Because AT reuse is already a supported mission of the AT system, it is a perfect example of bringing assets to the recovery table that may not have been thought of as disaster specific under usual circumstances.

an actual recovery to ensure the inclusion of populations that might otherwise go with little or no support postdisaster. Nurses can also start to craft interim solutions such as clustered care or a single intake process for multiple uses to reduce the physical and emotional impact to high-risk, high-vulnerability disaster survivors.

Recovery Programs

In the United States, recovery from disaster is predominantly based on a model dependent on individual insurance. In addition to homeowners' and renters' insurance, assistance for individuals affected by a disaster has historically come from public and private aid. Many community groups and organizations mobilize to provide assistance when disaster strikes. Sometimes communities will receive a Federal disaster declaration making Federal disaster assistance available to help with individual and family recovery.

The Robert T. Stafford Disaster Relief and Emergency Assistance Act authorizes the president to issue major disaster or emergency declarations in response to catastrophes that overwhelm local and state governments. Such declarations result in the distribution of a wide range of Federal aid to individuals and families, certain nonprofit organizations, and public agencies. Congress appropriates money to the Disaster Relief Fund for disaster assistance authorized by the Stafford Act, which is administered by FEMA within the Department of Homeland Security (DHS).

Federal disaster assistance may be offered in the form of cash payments or other direct assistance to individuals, families, and businesses in an area whose property has been damaged or destroyed and whose losses are not covered by insurance. This assistance is meant to help with critical expenses that cannot be covered in other ways. The assistance is not intended to restore damaged property to its condition before the disaster. While some housing assistance funds are available through the FEMA Individuals and Households Program, most disaster assistance from the Federal government is in the form of loans administered by the Small Business Administration (SBA). That said, many high-risk, high-vulnerability individuals will not qualify as they fail to meet loan criteria such as home ownership.

Grants may also unintentionally leave high-risk, high-vulnerability individuals at a disadvantage. The additional costs needed to make a home functional may not fall within the financial range of a grant such as installing a ramp, lower kitchen counters, or accessible bathroom configurations. Such basic necessities are often not calculated into funds guidelines, as was the case post-Katrina Road Home program (Browne, 2015). To meet such needs, voluntary organizations and faith-based groups often form community-based, long-term recovery committees as a way to address unmet needs. Nurses may be in a position to identify gaps in service delivery and call these to the attention of appropriate service providers and/or such newly formed committees.

Usually, unmet needs are addressed through a case management process in the long-term recovery committee, another area where nurses can exert influence. The purpose of case management is to help plan, coordinate, monitor, secure, and advocate on behalf of patients or clients. Case management in a disaster must take into account the unique practice environment in the aftermath of disasters that can involve difficult environmental conditions presenting additional challenges for patients, caregivers, and providers. Such conditions might include infrastructure losses, disruption of operations, communication challenges, and so forth. In addition, an influx of services and resources sent to the disaster area can pose additional access and coordination challenges. People who have experienced a disaster need to think through their daily experience, consider how their needs may have changed, and determine how to move forward, often in collaboration with service providers. The Post Disaster Personal Assessment Tool (Appendix 7.1) can be used with individuals/

families to identify recovery needs including housing, medical services, education, social services, among others.

In a study of the largest disaster case management effort in U.S. history following Hurricane Katrina, Stough, Sharp, Decker, and Wilker (2010) found that the disaster recovery process is typically more complex and lengthy for persons with disabilities. In addition, they noted that recovery requires negotiation of a service system that is often ill-prepared for disability-related needs. In particular, they identified accessible housing and transportation as barriers to recovery (Kelman & Stough, 2015; Phillips, 2015a, 2015b). Factors that supported recovery included case manager individual effort and advocacy skill, agency collaboration, and client motivation and persistence. They concluded that disaster recovery is enhanced by case managers who have disability expertise, including knowledge about the needs of individuals with disabilities and services to help. By application, this lesson can be applied to other high-risk, high-vulnerability populations.

Mitigation

Mitigation is widely regarded as the "single best step that can be taken to safeguard human wellbeing" (National Council on Disabilities (NCD), 2009). FEMA (2008) defines mitigation as:

> Activities providing a critical foundation in the effort to reduce the loss of life and property from natural and/or manmade disasters by avoiding or lessening the impact of a disaster and providing value to the public by creating safer communities. Mitigation seeks to fix the cycle of disaster damage, reconstruction, and repeated damage. These activities or actions, in most cases, will have a long-term sustained effect. p. 50)

Mitigation may entail structural and nonstructural measures that are taken to reduce risk, increase resiliency, and have a long-term impact on community well-being. *Structural mitigation* includes measures taken to alter the built environment in an effort to reduce risk and become more resilient to disasters. *Nonstructural mitigation* includes many different types of activities or measures that are just as critical to reducing risk as structural changes. The following are some examples of mitigation measures that can reduce the impact of disasters on high-risk, high-vulnerability populations.

- *Structural mitigation examples*:
  - Harden existing facilities and build new structures—hospitals, clinics, residential care facilities—to withstand likely hazards such as tornadoes, hurricanes, or flooding. This may prevent damage resulting in injury/death and/or the need for evacuation.
  - Identify facilities that may support response and recovery operations (e.g., a shelter or recovery assistance site) and identify ways to harden and stock these sites.
- *Nonstructural mitigation. examples*:
  - Protect critical supplies and keep them in safe areas. For example, in areas likely to experience earthquakes, tie and secure cabinets, containers, and shelves. Identify suppliers who can quickly restock supplies, identify supplies that will be difficult to replace, and identify strategies for keeping these in an off-site cache if possible.

- Install alarm systems that will immediately alert someone of a potentially hazardous condition—such systems may detect smoke, fire, carbon monoxide, or a radiological occurrence, for example.
- Create redundancies to ensure that medical records and other critical documentation is backed-up at an off-site location. Keep records in safe positions; rather than keeping them in a basement that is likely to flood, move them to a higher floor.
- Create a redundant system for internal communications as well as communicating with external sources.
- Purchase and maintain appropriate insurance that is specific to protecting against hazards. FEMA offers flood insurance for flood damage to properties, residences, and buildings through the National Flood Insurance Program (NFIP).
- Educate staff and patients/clients on mitigation measures that are important for them to take.

According to FEMA, every dollar spent on mitigation saves society an average of four dollars. FEMA offers the Mitigation Best Practices Portfolio on its website with several examples of local and state mitigation efforts (FEMA, 2011).

Although the value of mitigation is widely acknowledged, there are still gaps in terms of implementation, guidance, and information on mitigation best practices, particularly in regard to high-risk, high-vulnerability populations. For example, as of September 30, 2015, only 117 of the 566 Indian tribes recognized by the U.S. government had FEMA-approved disaster mitigation plans. This means that more than three-quarters of all tribes are ineligible to apply for FEMA grants and cannot receive Federal funding for disaster mitigation projects (Carter & Peek, 2016). In 2009, the NCD conducted research to evaluate how well disability issues have been integrated into emergency management research and practice. In terms of mitigation, NCD (2009) reported that:

> It is clear that research has failed to address the question of mitigation for people with disabilities in any meaningful manner. Scant evidence exists in practitioner materials either. (p. 193)

When implementing mitigation measures, it is best to integrate issues pertaining to high-risk, high-vulnerability populations at the hazard vulnerability assessment and initial planning levels. The following are some considerations to take into account when involved in mitigation measures. First, utilize a universal design approach when taking mitigation measures that require alteration or purchase of physical space, equipment, or products. The concept of universal design is the design of products and environments to be usable by all people, to the greatest extent possible, without the need for adaptation or specialized design to ensure greater accessibility and usage (Livable for a Lifetime, n.d.). The universal design approach is important because several factors may act as barriers preventing individuals and families from taking mitigation measures such as:

- Lack of time, education, or understanding to implement measures
- Lack of funds to act on mitigation measures such as purchasing insurance, shuttering windows, making structural changes

to homes, building a safe room, and buying and stockpiling extra supplies of food, medications, and other goods
- Having limited or no physical capacity to carry out the measures without assistance
- Living in substandard rental housing that is in a constant state of disrepair, but the owner refuses to act on behalf of the tenant

Second, to develop sustainable mitigation programs that effectively support high-risk, high-vulnerability populations, as with the other phases already noted above, it is critical to involve key stakeholders in the community who can represent the diversity of interests of this population. This kind of collaboration is absolutely necessary to validate working assumptions, identify barriers, create meaningful and sustainable measures and solutions that meet the needs of diverse communities, and to help educate constituents.

Third, mitigation measures can benefit schools, hospitals, shelters, clinics, and other service sites, and congregate care facilities, reducing impact to facilities as well as patients/clients. These types of facilities, which provide services to some of the most at-risk populations, will help to minimize the physical and emotional toll of disasters and allow for continuity of services that are so necessary to a community after a disaster.

Guiding Principles

Nurses can help to reduce the risk and increase the resiliency of individuals and families who are considered high-risk, high-vulnerability populations. The following principles are meant to guide nurses when working toward a more inclusive approach to emergency programs in all phases of disaster.

- *Professional Continuing Education*: Continually learn about ways to improve the integration of high-risk, high-vulnerability populations in emergency management programs during all phases of disaster. Provide training for staff and clients on emergency preparedness as well as opportunities for cross-training with partner organizations and agencies on emergency plans and procedures.
- *Involvement*: Build sustainable relationships with individuals and organizations that represent high-risk, high-vulnerability populations. Collaborate to identify and validate needs, solutions, and resources to lessen the impact of disasters on individuals, families, and communities.
- *Assessment*: Establish informal and formal assessments to measure the integration of high-risk, high-vulnerability populations in emergency programs.
- *Flexibility*: Programs and plans must be flexible to allow for improvement and change toward a greater outcome in serving high-risk, high-vulnerability populations in all phases of disaster.
- *Building Capacity*: Create plans, build resources, train staff and clients, and exercise plans to build capacity of individuals, families, and communities. For those visiting nurses or others providing in-home service delivery, this can be an extremely beneficial way to ensure directed awareness and planning takes place to mitigate further risks for certain persons.

- *Coordination*: Coordinate resources, information, and plans across organizations, governmental agencies, and health systems to maximize resources and more effectively meet the needs of individuals, staff, organizations, and communities in all phases of disasters.
- *Collaboration*: Apply the nursing perspective and skills knowledge in a related position not necessarily as a practicing nurse. This could be by establishing a rotation into a local emergency management office as a planner.
- *Anticipation*: When functioning on scene during a disaster, articulate anticipated near future impacts for your charge even if not part of the immediate medical response. Nurses can make a difference for disaster survivors by treating them for the immediate medical condition but not ignoring the secondary conditions of lost housing to return to or the missing community support systems, for instance.
- *Agents of Change*: Nurses know their community. They cross over many specialty skills areas to touch people directly. Nurses are in a position to be advocates on scene and during recovery for the holistic approach to those impacted by disaster because they are trusted agents to the individual as well as part of the care services team.

Conditions Fostering Change

It has only been over the past one to two decades that planning work to address unique disaster-related impacts on high-risk, high-vulnerability groups has become a central focus, and thus these groups remain underserved in many aspects of emergency management. During the Obama Administration, FEMA and the U.S. DOJ shifted their paradigm when it comes to whole community planning, as already discussed. And while there is a great deal of emerging data internationally about gender impact in disaster and climate change and aging, for instance, in the United States the shifts have been most notably influenced by the disability rights focus of the functional model.

But certain conditions have encouraged great preparedness for these populations. In the wake of the 9/11 attacks, FEMA gathered information about the response to what was then categorized as the "special needs population" and codified this in a focused after-action report (AAR) ordered by the Federal coordinating officer (Mackert & Davis, 2002). That was the first time a full AAR was dedicated completely to this issue at the Federal level. This was paired with a Congressional Subcommittee on Aging hearing of the same focus held in New York City. While enlightening, the more time that passed since the events of 9/11, the dimmer the attention on these concerns had become. It was not until the tragic loss of life among the elderly at Saint Rita's Nursing Home and real-time images of frail elderly in hospital gowns and socks lying in the streets in the hours, days, and weeks post-Katrina that the attention was focused again on the most vulnerable in our society. Following Katrina, legislation led to the creation of a position of national disability coordinator in DHS; the National Advisory Council (NAC) was established and had representation of several specific stakeholder groups on it; among other actions. This built on some of the post-9/11 changes such as the creation of an Interagency Coordinating Committee (ICC) as articulated in Executive Order 13347 signed by then President George W. Bush but the depth and breadth of the attention and

subsequent actions lasted longer and was much more public. It was during the work done on the ICC that the DOJ took on the task of drafting its Americans with Disabilities Act (ADA) Best Practices Tool Kit for state and local governments outlining their obligations under the ADA. As applied to the practice of emergency management countrywide, of particular focus is Chapter 7, Emergency Management Under Title II.

More recently, evidence of a stronger attention at least in part on certain groups sometimes classified as high-risk, high-vulnerability has emerged in the legal arena. The ADA was signed into law by President Bush in 1990 and was reenacted in 2008. The ADA was a culmination of many years of rights-based movement for people with disabilities and the broader reaching piece of civil rights legislation since the famed Civil Rights Act in 1964. It is under the provisions of Title II and Title III that most of the issues pertaining to emergency management, provision of emergency services, and thus by extension much of the work done by the nursing profession are covered and the DOJ maintains the authority to enforce the ADA. The DOJ is now routinely including language about equitable application of emergency response for people with disabilities into all its Project Civic Access settlements with local jurisdictions and agencies.

In addition to DOJ settlements, there has been an increase in the number of legal challenges to disaster planning efforts in an endeavor to make them more inclusive of and responsive to the needs of people with disabilities. In these class actions in California, New York City, and Washington, DC among others, the plaintiffs represent a group of persons who assert the claim that the government for the city or county in which they reside has not taken their specific needs into account in the planning doctrines and thus they will be unequally impacted when the disaster response system and responders directly cannot address their needs. The outcomes of the current actions are mixed at this time. Whether changes and forward movement in the places involved in litigation are a result of terms of a settlement between parties or a result of actions ordered by a court, there still remains no common approach across the nation. Because these actions are litigated and/or negotiated to address specific concerns in particular places and account for resources, allocations, and conditions in that place alone, it has not always been possible for others to simply replicate the results with success. While the resulting advances are embraced by the community, its advocates, and even the governments involved, it remains to be seen how this may change planning in other areas and for other high-risk, high-vulnerability populations over time and geography in a consistent way.

Under the Obama administration, the role and responsibilities of the NDC were subsumed into the then-newly created ODIC established by former FEMA Administrator Craig Fugate. ODIC is now in a position to spearhead many changes and improvements in the way the disaster services community applies its efforts for people impacted by emergencies, including also the development of new regional integration specialists across the country in all 10 FEMA regions and also the issuance of guidance for response activities such as sheltering operations. It is in the fully integrated shelter provision that nurses and other health professionals will see newly crafted roles.

We see via the abbreviated chronology above the progress toward a "whole community" approach to planning and response.

The nursing profession and its individual practitioners would be well advised to watch this trend to anticipate and get ahead of the ball when it comes to their disaster-related roles and responsibilities as they pertain to all parts of the community they serve. And with every change in administration, watch for ways to identify opportunities to continue the work regardless of direct project funding priorities and/or policy shifts.

EXAMPLES ORGANIZED AROUND THE ECOSYSTEM MODEL

The ultimate goal of an ecosystemic framework is to inculcate change at various systemic levels (see Figure 7.2) and across various time points in the disaster life cycle. In this section, we offer case examples where the micro-, meso-, and exo-levels can be influenced by medical providers, particularly nursing professionals, to reduce vulnerability. Beyond impacting the human condition by reducing injuries and deaths, an ecosystemic approach can reduce patient inflow during a disaster by mitigating harm before it occurs.

Microlevel Example: Personal Preparedness

At the microlevel, the emphasis is on building capacity of those at highest risk. By encouraging personal, household, and familial preparedness, those at risk can stand more ready to take protective actions (shelter in place, evacuation), assist themselves and others, move through response time periods, and recover expeditiously. Though many materials and tools exist for personal-level preparedness, medical providers can participate in personal readiness efforts by educating patients and the broader public on preparedness issues. The summer of 2011 serves as a good example. In the heart of the United States, a heat dome built and stayed in place causing temperatures to soar and remain in place for a record number of days. Those at highest risk included senior citizens, people who were homeless, and those who had to earn their livelihood outside, particularly low-income workers. Programs initiated to reduce risks included educational efforts to raise awareness of the potential for heat-related illnesses. Emergency managers, elder

care providers, first responders, and the media all collaborated to alert the public through traditional and social media and encourage them to check on those at risk. Cooling centers opened for seniors and individuals who were homeless with some communities providing transportation.

Hurricanes Katrina and Rita also generated new attention to those at risk and in need of medical care. Late evacuations meant that people died in assisted living facilities for Katrina. Heavier than expected evacuation for Rita led indirectly to a nursing home bus catching on fire and causing the deaths of nearly 30 residents. More recently, 18 nursing home residents and a caregiver died when an EF5 tornado destroyed over one-third of Joplin, Missouri in the spring of 2011. At the microlevel, these case examples suggest the minimum action steps:

- Educate those at risk in medical care situations about local hazards and appropriate responses. Home healthcare agencies can reach out to those living at home. Medical providers supporting congregate populations can do the same with residents and their families. Experience demonstrates that having one's family around during a disaster event can reduce exposure and mortality. By educating people about area shelters and their ability to meet medical needs, it may be possible to spur evacuation among those with the greatest medical needs (Fernandez, Byard, Lin, Benson, & Barbera, 2002).
- Encourage personal preparedness to the greatest extent possible. Efforts can vary from keeping a Vial for Life on hand (Public Health Agency of Canada, 2008) to a fully developed preparedness kit consistent with federally recommended standards so that individuals can survive on their own for a time (www.ready.gov, also available in languages other than English).
- Identify a means to secure area hazard information and recommendations. In Oklahoma, OK-Warn offers low-cost messaging for people who are hard of hearing or deaf.
- Create a personal plan to evacuate or respond as directed. This means embedding patients in a medical provider and/or social network to assist them. The City of New Orleans, in the aftermath of Katrina, has moved toward such a community-based effort specifically for seniors.

Meso-Level Example: Safe Centers in Alabama

After Hurricane Katrina in 2005, the Alabama Department of Senior Services in partnership with the U.S. Administration on Aging, Alabama Emergency Management Agency, Alabama Department of Economic and Community Affairs, and the City of Guin introduced and began to implement the concept of Safe Centers within the State of Alabama. The Safe Center concept combines a senior center that is used daily and known by the community with a Safe Center that will provide a place of respite for seniors in the event of a disaster.

The first Safe Center was completed in 2008, and as of April 2014, Alabama had created a total of 41 Safe Centers/rooms across the state; some are full freestanding structures while others are smaller scale or even a safe room within a facility. Some of the features of the Safe Center include the following:

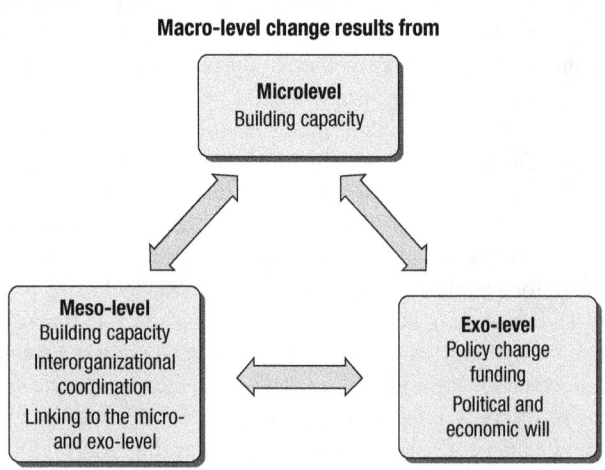

Macro-level change results from

Microlevel
Building capacity

Meso-level
Building capacity
Interorganizational coordination
Linking to the micro- and exo-level

Exo-level
Policy change
funding
Political and economic will

FIGURE 7.2 Change and the ecosystem model.

- Generator power and extra wall outlets can be used to operate light medical equipment such as portable oxygen machines.
- Designated area(s) for seniors in the early stages of Alzheimer's or dementia are available. Each Safe Center has a satellite telephone to ensure communication after storms and other natural disasters.
- Safe Centers are designed according to FEMA standards to withstand hurricane and tornado force winds, floods, and other hazardous conditions in the geographic area.
- All have similar architecture and the same light blue roof color. If a senior from south Alabama is visiting family in north Alabama, he or she can look for the blue roof and know the Safe Center is there to serve after a disaster. This feature also makes it easier for first responders to identify and locate centers.
- Caches of appropriate supplies and shelf-stable meals are rotated on a regular basis.
- Full showering and laundry facilities are available in the event seniors need to stay for an extended period of time.
- Teams of trained volunteers are on call to support staff at the Safe Center in the event of an emergency.

This is a best practice because it:

- Can potentially save lives and lessen the impact of a disaster
- Is a wise use of public resources as it serves the dual purpose of a place for daily senior activities and a hardened facility with disaster protection features
- Allows local municipalities an opportunity to maximize resources under tornado warnings
- Is a replicable practice that goes beyond the state of Alabama and beyond senior centers
- Is a place of comfort and safety for seniors within high-risk communities

The centers have already been tested through real events:

One of our centers used their Safe Room this spring when the tornado sirens went off while attendees were there. Some were exercising, some playing cards, etc., but when the siren went off everyone made it to the Safe Room in 30 seconds. The seniors were glad they were protected at the center. (Collins, Coman, & Black, 2011)

Exo-Level Example: FEMA Trailers and Housing Policy

Policy change in the field of emergency management tends to develop in response to issues and concerns that result after disaster. Lawsuits also change policy. This was the situation following Hurricanes Katrina and Rita in 2005, when a class action discrimination lawsuit (*Brou v. FEMA*) was filed against FEMA and the DHS because of a shortage of accessible FEMA trailers (e.g., trailers with wheelchair ramps, maneuvering room, accessible bathrooms and kitchens). The settlement involved FEMA establishing a call-in process to request accessible trailers and as a result, FEMA provided over 1,000 new accessible trailers and modified over 200 other trailers.

This lawsuit not only set new policy in terms of the Katrina/ Rita recovery, but also influenced part of the development of FEMA's National Disaster Housing Strategy (released in 2009). Through the added pressure from advocates and other Federal partners such as the NCD, the integration of disability issues continues to be addressed in new disaster housing policy and guidance documents. In 2009, the NCD published the report, "Effective Emergency Management: Making Improvements for Communities and People with Disabilities." In this report, the NCD recommends that the outcomes of the lawsuit not be lost. Part of the housing policy development integrates disability organizations, advocates, and people with disability in identifying temporary housing options; empowers these groups to participate in FEMA housing efforts and have a role during disaster activations; establishes a hotline for case management for temporary and permanent housing assistance; encourages expertise within the case management system working with people with disabilities; and allows for postevent evaluations as a result of this policy change.

The NCD report itself offers a good example of how organizations can influence and change policy. In addition to producing this report, the NCD testified to Congress on the findings and recommendations to ensure a broader and ongoing awareness.

Macro-Level Example: Muslim Americans— Targeting and Tolerance after 9/11

Following 9/11, Muslim Americans experienced the most severe wave of backlash violence in their collective history. Civil rights organizations recorded thousands of incidents of anti-Islamic harassment, hate crimes, and vandalism in the months after the terrorist attacks. Federal officials surveilled and raided mosques and froze the assets of several major Islamic charities. Muslim, Arab, and South Asian men were arrested and deported, often without their family members' knowledge of their whereabouts (for a complete discussion of the backlash, see Peek, 2011).

The targeting of vulnerable racial and ethnic minorities during times of national emergency has long been an unfortunate feature of U.S. life. Thus, it is not surprising that many commentators drew parallels between the post-9/11 treatment of Muslim Americans and the experiences of Japanese Americans who were interred during World War II. Both groups, already marginalized, were quickly stereotyped as the "enemy" and subsequently experienced severe violations of their civil rights.

But there are also many differences between the Japanese American and Muslim American experiences. The internment of 120,000 persons of Japanese descent—two-thirds of whom were U.S. citizens—without trial or hearings represents one of the most egregious deprivations of liberty in our national history. The violations that Muslim Americans experienced, while extreme, were on a different scale. The fact that millions of Muslim Americans were not rounded up, stripped of their possessions and property, and imprisoned indefinitely speaks to the *macro-level, systemic changes* that have occurred in the decades since World War II. More currently, a proposed travel ban on Muslim-dominant countries has generated heated debate.

These changes in the social and political climate in the United States—and in particular the strengthening of minority rights—have resulted from, among other things, grassroots advocacy work, the civil rights movement, and many Federal-level policy changes such as the passage of the 1964 Civil Rights Act. These micro-, exo-, and meso-level changes and many others help account for why Muslim Americans, and advocates who worked on their behalf, were able to find a voice after 9/11 and to issue calls for tolerance. At the same time, the ongoing discrimination and prejudice that Muslims continue to face speaks to the often slow and unsteady process of macro-level change (Peek & Meyer, 2016).

SUMMARY

The term "high-risk, high-vulnerability populations" refers to people with a higher probability of being exposed to disaster and who also face challenges in anticipating, coping with, resisting, or recovering from disaster. Vulnerability is a complex phenomenon that is influenced by many social, economic, cultural, and other characteristics. Both the traditional medical model and more recent functional model offer approaches for understanding and addressing vulnerability in a disaster. In addition, understanding vulnerability *systematically* using an ecosystem framework allows for more precise identification of points of intervention at the micro-, meso-, exo-, and macro-levels. The *disaster life cycle* is another useful concept for exploring vulnerability and structuring activities related to the routine disaster phases of mitigation, preparedness, response, and recovery. Contemporary collaborative approaches such as FEMA's *whole community* philosophy emphasize inclusive planning, broad stakeholder engagement, and community resilience as critical factors for success. Healthcare organizations and nursing professionals are key actors in a whole community approach to reducing vulnerability to disaster, particularly for high-risk populations.

REFERENCES

Aguirre, B. E. (1988). The lack of warnings before the Saragosa Tornado. *International Journal of Mass Emergencies and Disasters, 6*(1), 65–74. Retrieved from http://www.ijmed.org/articles/133/download/

Barnshaw, J., & Trainor, J. (2007). Race, class, and capital amidst the Hurricane Katrina diaspora. In D. L. Brunsma, D. Overfelt, & J. S. Picou (Eds.), *The sociology of Katrina: Perspectives on a modern catastrophe* (pp. 91–105). Lanham, MD: Rowman & Littlefield.

Bennett, D., Phillips, B. D., & Davis, E. (2017). The future of accessibility in disaster conditions: How wireless technologies will transform the life cycle of emergency management. *Futures, 87*, 122–132. doi:10.1016/j.futures.2016.05.004

Brofenbrenner, U. (1979). *The ecology of human development: Experiments by nature and design.* Cambridge, MA: Harvard University Press.

Bronan, R., & Pollock, D. (2017). Climate change, displacement and community relocation: Lessons from Alaska. Norwegian Refugee Council. Retrieved from https://www.nrc.no/globalassets/pdf/reports/nrc-alaska_relocation-screen.pdf

Browne, K. E. (2015). *Standing in the need: Culture, comfort, and coming home after Katrina.* Austin: University of Texas Press.

Carter, L., & Peek, L. (2016). Participation please: Barriers to tribal disaster mitigation planning. *Natural Hazards Observer, 40*(4). Retrieved from https://hazards.colorado.edu/article/participation-please-barriers-to-tribal-mitigation-planning

Collins, I. B., Coman, J., & Black, R. (2011, April 18). *Just Build It: The Nuts and Bolts of Safe Centers.* Workshop presented at the National Hurricane Conference in Atlanta, GA.

Comfort, L., Wisner, B., Cutter, S., Pulwarty, R., Hewitt, K., Oliver-Smith, A., . . . Krimgold, F. (1999). Reframing disaster policy: The global evolution of vulnerable communities. *Global Environment Change Part B: Environmental Hazards, 1*(1), 39–44. doi:10.3763/ehaz.1999.0105

Cutter, S. (2006). The geography of social vulnerability: Race, class, and catastrophe. Retrieved from http://understandingkatrina.ssrc.org

Cutter, S., Bryan J. B., & Shirley, W. L. (2003). Social vulnerability to environmental hazards. *Social Science Quarterly, 84*(2), 242–261. doi:10.1111/1540-6237.8402002

Federal Emergency Management Agency. (2008). National response framework: Glossary and acronyms. Retrieved from https://www.fema.gov/pdf/emergency/nrf/nrf-glossary.pdf

Federal Emergency Management Agency. (2011). FEMA's mitigation best practices portfolio. Retrieved from https://www.fema.gov/mitigation-best-practices-portfolio

Federal Highway Administration. (2009). Evacuation of special needs populations. Retrieved from http://ops.fhwa.dot.gov/publications/fhwahop09022

Fernandez, L. S., Byard, D., Lin, C. C., Benson, S., & Barbera, J. A. (2002). Frail elderly as disaster victims: Emergency management strategies. *Prehospital and Disaster Medicine, 17*(2), 67–74. doi:10.1017/s1049023x00000200

Fordham, M., Lovekamp, W., Thomas, D. S. K., & Phillips, B. D. (2014). Understanding social vulnerability. In D. S. K. Thomas, B. D. Phillips, W. E. Lovekamp, & A. Fothergill (Eds.), *Social vulnerability to disasters* (2nd ed., pp. 1–32). Boca Raton, FL: CRC Press.

Fothergill, A., & Peek, L. (2015). *Children of Katrina.* Austin: University of Texas Press.

Garbarino, J. (1992). *Children and families in the social environment* (2nd ed.). New York, NY: Aldine De Gruyter.

Haas Institute. (2016). *Examining the impact of hurricane Sandy on marginalized populations.* The Haas Institute for a Fair and Inclusive Society, University of California-Berkeley. Retrieved from https://haasinstitute.berkeley.edu/sites/default/files/Hurricane-Sandy-and-Marginalized-Populations-2.pdf

Kako, M., & Ikeda, S., (2009). Volunteer experiences in community housing during the Great Hanshin-Awaji Earthquake, Japan. *Nursing and Health Sciences, 11*(4), 357–359. doi:10.1111/j.1442-2018.2009.00484.x

Kelman, I., & Stough, L. (Eds.). (2015). *Disability and disaster: Explorations and exchanges.* London, UK: Palgrave Macmillan. Retrieved from https://www.palgrave.com/us/book/9781137485991

Livable for a Lifetime. (n.d.). Universal design definition and principles. Retrieved from http://livableforalifetime.org/pdf/Universal%20Design%20Principles.pdf

Mackert, R., & Davis, E. (2002). *Report on special needs—Issues, efforts and lessons learned.* New York, NY: Federal Emergency Management Agency.

McGlown, K. J., & Robinson, P. D. (Eds.). (2011). *Anticipate respond recover: Healthcare leadership and catastrophic events.* Chicago, IL: Health Administration Press.

Mileti, D. S. (1999). *Disasters by design: A reassessment of natural hazards in the United States.* Washington, DC: Joseph Henry Press.

Miller, T. W., Kraus, R. F., Tatevosyan, A. S., & Kamechenko, P. (1993). Post-traumatic stress disorder in children and adolescents of the Armenian earthquake. *Child Psychiatry and Human Development, 24*(2), 115–123. doi:10.1007/BF02367264

Morrow, B. H. (1999). Identifying and mapping community vulnerability. *Disasters, 23*(1), 1–18. doi:10.1111/1467-7717.00102

National Council on Disability. (2009). *Effective emergency management: Making improvement for communities and people with disabilities.* Retrieved from http://www.ncd.gov/publications/2009/Aug122009

National Organization on Disability, Emergency Preparedness Initiative. (2005). Report on special needs assessment for Katrina evacuees project report. Retrieved from https://www.preventionweb.net/files/9005_katrinasnakereport.pdf

Norris, F. H., Friedman, M. J., & Watson, P. J. (2002). 60,000 disaster victims speak: Part II. Summary and implications of the disaster mental health research. *Psychiatry, 65*(3), 240–260. doi:10.1521/psyc.65.3.240.20169

Norris, F. H., Friedman, M. J., Watson, P. J., Byrne, C. M., Diaz, E., & Kaniasty, K. (2002). 60,000 disaster victims speak: Part I. An empirical review of the empirical literature, 1981–2001. *Psychiatry, 65*(3), 207–239. doi:10.1521/psyc.65.3.207.20173

Otani, J. (2010). *Older people in natural disasters: The Great Hanshin Earthquake of 1995*. Kyoto, Japan: Kyoto University Press.

Peacock, W. G., & Ragsdale, K. A. (1997). Social systems, ecological networks and disasters: Toward a socio-political ecology of disasters. In W. G. Peacock, B. H. Morrow, & H. Gladwin (Eds.), *Hurricane Andrew: Ethnicity, gender, and the sociology of disasters* (pp. 20–35). New York, NY: Routledge.

Peek, L. (2011). *Behind the backlash: Muslim Americans after 9/11*. Philadelphia, PA: Temple University Press.

Peek, L. (2013). Age. In D. S. K. Thomas, B. D. Phillips, W. E. Lovekamp, & A. Fothergill (Eds.), *Social vulnerability to disasters* (2nd ed., pp. 167–198). Boca Raton, FL: CRC Press.

Peek, L., & Meyer, M. (2016). When hate is a crime: Temporal and geographic patterns of anti-Islamic hate crime after 9/11. In D. W. Harper & K. Frailing (Eds.), *Crime and criminal justice in disaster* (3rd ed., pp. 247–270). Durham, NC: Carolina Academic Press.

Phillips, B. D. (2009). Special needs populations. In K. Koenig & C. Schultz (Eds.), *Disaster medicine* (pp. 113–132). Cambridge, UK: Cambridge University Press.

Phillips, B. D. (2010). *Disaster recovery*. Boca Raton, FL: CRC Press.

Phillips, B. D. (2015 a). *Disaster recovery* (2nd ed.). Boca Raton, FL: CRC Press.

Phillips, B. D. (2015b). Inclusive emergency management for people with disabilities facing disaster. In L. Stough & I. Kelman (Eds.), *Disability and disaster* (pp. 31–49). London, UK: Palgrave Macmillan.

Phillips, B. D., & Morrow, B. H. (2007). Social science research needs: Focus on vulnerable populations, forecasting, and warnings. *Natural Hazards Review, 8*(3), 61–68. doi:10.1061/(ASCE)1527-6988(2007)8:3(61)

Phillips, B. D., Thomas, D. S. K., Fothergill, A., & Blinn-Pike, L. (Eds.). (2010). *Social vulnerability to disasters*. Boca Raton, FL: CRC Press.

Phillips, B. D., Stukes, P. & Jenkins, P. (2011). Freedom hill is not for sale and neither is the Lower Ninth Ward. *Journal of Black Studies, 43*(4), 405–426. doi:10.1177/0021934711425489

Poulshock, S., & Cohen, E. (1975). The elderly in the aftermath of disaster. *The Gerontologist, 15*(4), 357–361. doi:10.1093/geront/15.4.357

Public Health Agency of Canada. (2008). Second international workshop on seniors and emergency preparedness workshop report. Retrieved from http://publications.gc.ca/collections/collection_2009/aspc-phac/HP25-9-2008E.pdf

Sharkey, P. (2007). Survival and death in New Orleans: An empirical look at the human impact of Katrina. *Journal of Black Studies, 37*(4), 482–501. doi:10.1177/0021934706296188

Stough, L. M., Sharp, A. N., Decker, C., & Wilker, N. (2010). Disaster case management and individuals with disabilities. *Rehabilitative Psychology, 55*(3), 211–220. doi:10.1037/a0020079

Sutley, E., van de Lindt, J. W., & Peek, L. (2017a). Community-level framework for seismic resiliency, part I: socioeconomic characteristics and engineering building systems. *Natural Hazards Review, 18*(3), 04016014. doi:10.1061/(ASCE)NH.1527-6996.0000239

Sutley, E., van de Lindt, J. W., & Peek, L. (2017b). Community-level framework for seismic resiliency, part II: Multi-objective optimization and illustrative examples. *Natural Hazards Review, 18*(3), 04016015. doi:10.1061/(ASCE)NH.1527-6996.0000230

Tierney, K., Lindell, M. K., & Perry, R. W. (2001). *Facing the unexpected: Disaster preparedness and response in the United States*. Washington, DC: Joseph Henry Press.

Tierney, K., Petak, W. J., & Hahn, H. (1988). *Disabled persons and earthquake hazards*. Boulder: Institute of Behavioral Science, University of Colorado.

U.S. Department of Health and Human Services. (2011, May 5). Majority of U.S. hospitals meet all hazards preparedness measures [News release]. Retrieved from http://www.phe.gov/Preparedness/planning/hpp/Documents/hpp-healthcare-coalitions.pdf

U.S. Department of Health and Human Services. (2012). *Gaps continue to exist in nursing home emergency preparedness and response during disasters: 2007–2010* (Report OEI-06-09-00270). Retrieved from https://oig.hhs.gov/oei/reports/oei-06-09-00270.asp

U.S. Department of Justice. (2007). ADA best practices toolkit for state and local governments, Chapter 7, Addendum 2. Retrieved from http://www.ada.gov/pcatoolkit/chap7shelterprog.htm

Wisner, B., Blaikie, P., Cannon, T., & Davis, I. (2004). *At risk: Natural hazards, people's vulnerability, and disasters* (2nd ed.). New York, NY: Routledge.

ADDITIONAL RESOURCES

Administration on Aging. Disaster preparedness: Home and community-based services for people with dementia and their caregivers. Retrieved from http://www.aoa.gov/

American Psychological Association. Managing traumatic stress: Tips for recovering from disasters and other traumatic events. Retrieved from http://www.apa.org/helpcenter/recovering-disasters.aspx

American Red Cross. (2006). Disaster preparedness for people with disabilities. Retrieved from http://www.disastersrus.org/mydisasters/disability/disability.pdf

Association of State and Territorial Health Officials. (2008). At-risk populations and pandemic influenza: Planning guidance for state, territorial, tribal, and local health departments. Retrieved from http://www.astho.org/Infectious-Disease/At-Risk-Populations/At-Risk-Populations-and-Pandemic-Influenza-Planning-Guidance/

Federal Emergency Management Agency. Disaster assistance: A guide to federal recovery programs. Retrieved from http://www.fema.gov/pdf/rebuild/ltrc/recoveryprograms229.pdf

Federal Emergency Management Agency's Office of Disability Integration and Coordination. Retrieved from https://www.fema.gov/about/odic. Includes the document, *Guidance on planning for integration of functional needs support services in general population shelters*.

National Commission on Children and Disasters. (2010). *2010 report to the President and Congress*. Retrieved from https://archive.ahrq.gov/prep/nccdreport/nccdreport.pdf

National Council on Disability. Includes resources and reports on disability and emergency management including the *Effective emergency management: Making improvements for communities and people with disabilities and a state of housing in the 21st century: A disability perspective*. Retrieved from http://www.ncd.gov/policy/emergency_management

National Resource Center on Advancing Emergency Preparedness for Culturally Diverse Communities. Retrieved from http://www.diversitypreparedness.org. Includes reports, articles, links, and other resources about diversity and emergency preparedness.

New York City and State Bar Associations. A Guide to the Use of Service Animals in New York State. Retrieved from http://documents.nycbar.org/files/guide-to-the-use-of-service-animals-in-new-york-state.html. Includes information and guidance regarding service animals.

Pass It On Center. Retrieved from http://www.passitoncenter.org. It offers general information about AT; AT reuse locations; emergency management and AT materials; knowledge base collection.

U.S. Department of Homeland Security's National Nurse Emergency Preparedness Initiative. Retrieved from https://nnepi.gwnursing.org/Default.asp?

U.S. Department of Justice. ADA best practices toolkit for state and local governments, Chapter 7: Emergency management. Retrieved from http://www.ada.gov/pcatoolkit/toolkitmain.htm

U.S. Department of Transportation Federal Highway Administration, Office of Operations. (2009). Evacuating populations with special needs: Routes to effective evacuation planning primer series. Retrieved from http://ops.fhwa.dot.gov/publications/fhwahop09022/index.htm

University of Kansas Research and Training Center on independent offers training. Retrieved from https://www.train.org, including *Planning for disaster-related risk and functional needs of people with disabilities: Train-the-trainer* (course #1026720), *Planning for disaster-related risk and functional needs of people with disabilities* (course #1026403), *ready, willing, & able (course #1020884),* and *Animal emergency preparedness: How to keep your service animals and pets safe in natural and manmade disasters (course #1025307).*

Yale School of Public Health, Center for Public Health Preparedness. (2011). Emergency preparedness planning toolkit for diverse populations. Retrieved from https://www.aha.org/system/files/content/11/OMHDiversityPreparednessToolkit.pdf

CASE STUDY 7.1

Parish Nurse as Evacuation Advisor

Joanne C. Langan, Associate Professor, Saint Louis University School of Nursing

HOME EVACUATION: TO GO OR NOT TO GO IN HURRICANE KATRINA

Mr. and Mrs. Harrison survived Hurricane Camille which made landfall on the Gulf Coast of the United States during the 1969 hurricane season as a Category 5 hurricane. It moved through the area quickly and dropped only moderate amounts of precipitation in most areas.

Nearly 35 years later, Mr. and Mrs. Harrison are still living on the Gulf Coast of Mississippi. Mr. Harrison is 82 years old and in relatively good health and still drives. Mrs. Harrison is 80 years old and has dementia and is 6 months post-cerebrovascular accident (CVA). They live in a close-knit subdivision but their two daughters live in northern Mississippi. They have two small dogs. A parish nurse visits them once each month.

It is late August and they have heard of an impending storm, Katrina, that "might be a big one." Mr. Harrison states, "We survived Camille. There is no way we are leaving this time." Mrs. Harrison has slurred speech and difficult mobility. She tells him that she is afraid to stay in the house during the storm.

1. You are the parish nurse. What would you advise this couple?
2. What are some of the community resources that you might share with them?
3. How would you assure them that a shelter is a safe, temporary solution?
4. What should they take with them to the shelter, should they decide to evacuate?
5. If they decide to shelter in place, what are the minimal supplies that they must have readily available?
6. What would you advise them to do with their small dogs if they decide to shelter in place, or if they decide to go to a shelter?

CASE STUDY 7.2

Older Adults in Disaster: 2017 Northern California Wildfires

In disaster after disaster we see that people with disabilities and others with access and functional needs, including older adults, bear a disproportionate burden. Older adults are far more likely than other people to become sick, injured, or die as a result of a disaster, regardless of the type of event (United Nations Department of Economic and Social Affairs, 2011). It is not their age that inherently makes them especially vulnerable, but instead physical conditions such as mobility limitation and hearing loss and social features such as isolation and poverty that cause excess morbidity and mortality (Adams, Kaufman, Van Hattum, & Mood, 2011).

This reality was terribly illustrated in the 2017 Northern California wildfires. Of the 43 people known to have died, the average age was 79 years (Nix, 2017). Reports indicate that most were found inside their homes, unable to escape the fast-moving flames. At least two individuals were wheelchair users and two others were reported by their families to be confined to their beds.

Older adults in nursing home or other care settings also show an elevated vulnerability, even though they are under the care of others including staff with medical training. An estimated 215 people died in hospitals and nursing homes in Louisiana following Hurricane Katrina in 2005, most of them older adults (Brunkard, Namulanda, & Ratard, 2008). Following Hurricane Irma in 2017, 12 people died in a rehabilitation center that had lost power and was unable to keep patients cool (Frisaro, 2017).

In working with older adults, nurses should be cognizant of their elevated disaster risk and, when possible, engage them in conversation regarding personal protection, practical preparedness, and social preparedness. Additionally, nurses should be cognizant of the physical and social vulnerabilities that older adults face in disaster and work to assist their older adult patients in staying healthy and safe before, during, and after any disaster.

REFERENCES

Adams, V., Kaufman, S. R., Van Hattum, T., & Moody, S. (2011). Aging disaster: mortality, vulnerability, and long-term recovery among Katrina survivors. *Medical Anthropology*, *30*(3), 247–270. doi:10.1080/01459740.2011.560777

(continued)

CASE STUDY 7.2 (continued)

Brunkard, J., Namulanda, G., & Ratard, R. (2008). Hurricane Katrina deaths, Louisiana, 2005. *Disaster Medicine and Public Health Preparedness, 2*(4), 215–223. doi:10.1097/DMP.0b013e31818aaf55

Frisaro, F. (2017, September 29). 12th Death from Florida Nursing Home that lost power in Irma. *Time Magazine*. New York, NY. Retrieved from https://www.usnews.com/news/best-states/florida/articles/2017-09-29/12th-death-from-nursing-home-that-lost-power-ac-during-irma

Nix, J. (2017, October 25). California fire damage totals. *Mother Jones Magazine*. Retrieved from http://www.motherjones.com/environment/2017/10/california-fires-damage-total

United Nations Department of Economic and Social Affairs. (2011). Current status of the social situation, well-being, participation in development and rights of older persons worldwide. New York, NY. Retrieved from http://www.un.org/esa/socdev/ageing/documents/publications/current-status-older-persons.pdf

CASE STUDY 7.3

Vulnerable Elderly and Vulnerable Infrastructure: The Case of Hurricane Irma and the Rehabilitation Center at Hollywood Hills 2017

Hurricane Irma, which hit South Florida in September 2017, was an exceptional storm in terms of its size, its duration, the geographic area affected, and the damage it wrought. Florida's governor declared a state of emergency on September 4; over the ensuing days, as the hurricane picked up strength and the forecasts and warnings became dire, mayors across the state began to declare mandatory evacuation orders. In the end, hundreds of thousands of Floridians took to the highways, making it the largest evacuation in the state's history.

Some Floridians, however, did not evacuate because the risk the evacuation posed was perhaps higher than staying in place. Among those who remained to ride out the storm included over 140 patients at the Rehabilitation Center at Hollywood Hills. In the end, 8 elderly patients perished in that nursing home facility, and an additional 3 died after being evacuated to a nearby hospital.

What happened at Hollywood Hills serves as yet another cautionary tale for the high costs that the most vulnerable pay when infrastructure fails. In this case, a transformer box was knocked out that led to the failure of the air conditioning in the facility. When the backup generator failed to power up that air conditioning, the heat in the facility rose to excruciating levels, with some of the patients who perished having recorded body temperatures ranging from 107° to 109°F.

It is true that as people age their bodily systems that are designed to ward off the damaging effects of heat break down. The consequences often include higher susceptibility to dehydration, heat exhaustion, respiratory conditions, and cardiac arrest. But the story of the deaths at Hollywood Hills

are not just about the physical vulnerability of people. The real story is about the physical vulnerability of infrastructure that is meant to serve humanity and the failure to pass strict regulations.

In this case, the nursing home facility had an emergency preparedness plan, and they had a backup generator. But due to lax regulations, the generator was not powerful enough to keep the air conditioning on. The plan was not robust enough to ensure that there were adequate medical personnel on site to care for such a high number of vulnerable elderly. And the local and state response was not rapid enough to save the lives of the most vulnerable among us. Now, criminal charges are pending against the facility, which has a long history of safety violations, and its owner, a medical doctor who has previously been charged with fraud.

This case should serve not just as a cautionary tale, but as a catalyst to prioritize facilities and critical infrastructure that serves the most vulnerable among us. Nurses are at the front line and even under such circumstances should consider inserting themselves into the facility disaster planning efforts; demand periodic review of such plans; help identify areas for improvement; and continue to advocate for their patients by being involved.

Sources: Gabler, E., Fink, S. & Yee, V. (2017). At Florida Nursing Home, many calls for help, but none that made a difference. *The New York Times*, September 23. https://www.nytimes.com/2017/09/23/us/nursing-home-deaths.html; http://www.slate.com/blogs/the_slatest/2017/09/25/governor_rick_scott_s_office_deleted_voicemails_from_the_florida_nursing.html; http://www.npr.org/sections/thetwo-way/2017/09/14/550996932/8-die-at-florida-nursing-home-after-irma-leaving-a-host-of-questions

Appendix 7.1

The Post-Disaster Personal Assessment Tool

The following tool can be used by a nurse, caseworker, and others who are assisting survivors with recovery. Staff would go through the form together. This tool takes into account important health, social, educational, and other critical areas for a person who is in the recovery process, and helps to prioritize areas that need to be addressed to begin recovery.

Consider what's important to you about where you live . . .

After a disaster occurs, this tool will help you consider the things that are the most important to you about where you live. Once you have completed this assessment, you can compare this list to what is available, or what is likely to be available soon in your neighborhood. After completing this form, the results can also inform you and your case manager as you make informed and safe decisions about temporary housing options or long-term relocation decisions that meet your most important needs.

This "snapshot" should give you a better idea of what weight to give certain factors when considering your housing options. You may add to this list anything else you consider important and still use this tool to help you get a better picture.

SELF-ASSESSMENT

Indicate in the spaces below:

1. **Independent**
2. **Needs some assistance**
3. **Needs full assistance**

____ Walking   ____ Cooking
____ Climbing stairs   ____ Bathing
____ Vision   ____ Housekeeping
____ Shopping   ____ Others (specify here):

EVERYDAY ACTIVITIES

Rank each item below by how important the service is to you:

1. **(Not important)**
2. **(Somewhat important)**
3. **(Very important)**

Services

____ Grocery store within walking distance   ____ Accessible public
____ Other goods and retail within walking distance ____ Library
____ Pharmacy within walking distance   ____ House of worship
____ Bank within walking distance   ____ Friends/family

Schools

____ Day Care   ____ Elementary School   ____ College level
____ Pre-K   ____ Middle School   ____ Specialty School (e.g., trade school, school for the blind)
                       ____ High school

Healthcare

____ Hospital with emergency care
____ Access to primary doctor, clinic, etc.
____ Access to medical specialist, support (cardiologist, radiology center, etc.)
____ Dialysis center

(continued)

Appendix 7.1 (*continued*)

Support/Care Services

____ Home-based care agency (nurses, home attendants, physical therapy, etc.)
____ Meals (congregate or delivered programs)
____ Senior center

Housing Options

____ Rental availability
____ Fully accessible unit/location
____ Elevator building
____ Proximity to public transportation system
____ Assistive living community

____ Housing stock for purchase
____ On-site parking
____ Doorman building

After ranking the importance of the items just listed, circle the items that you know are in your community. Then consider:

- How many "very important" items are circled? Will they be available in your neighborhood soon?
- Do you have enough support and are you safe if you do not have some of the "very important" items that you need in your neighborhood?
- Do you need more information about your neighborhood before you can make a decision?
- Do you need to talk to a case manager about this before you make a decision?

Any other notes:

Source: EAD & Associates, LLC. http://www.eadassociates.com © 2011, author.

Appendix 7.2

Think Before You Speak or Write: Polite Communication

The words one chooses to use when referring to people with disabilities in oral and written communication often carry either a positive or a negative connotation. Therefore, adopting the following suggestions will help others know that you respect people with disabilities and may also encourage people to think and act more appropriately toward others.

PUT PEOPLE FIRST

The person should always come first. An individual has abilities as well as disabilities. Focusing on the person emphasizes the status we share, rather than conditions we presently do not. Thus, say "the person who has a disability," rather than "the disabled person." Similarly, it is better to refer to "people with disabilities" than to "the disabled" or "the handicapped."

EMPHASIZE ACTION

People with disabilities, even severe ones, can be quite active. Thus it is better to say "President Franklin Roosevelt used a wheelchair and occasionally walked using braces and crutches" rather than "he was confined to a wheelchair," or "the wheelchair-bound president," or "the president was in a wheelchair."

DO NOT SENSATIONALIZE, PITY, OR CHARACTERIZE

Avoid words like "afflicted," "crippled," "handicapped," and "victim" when referring to a person with a disability. Also, remember that people are more than their disabilities. Instead of saying that "President Roosevelt suffered from asthma," "Helen Keller was handicapped by blindness," "Peter Stuyvesant was an amputee," or "Moses was afflicted with a speech impairment," do say "Einstein had a learning disability," "Napoleon had epilepsy," "Alexander Graham Bell was hard of hearing," or "Marlee Matlin is an actress who is deaf."

AVOID INAPPROPRIATE WORDS

Words have enormous power in shaping how we view the world and how we view one another. As such, it is very important that we work together to use currently acceptable language out of respect and care for those with whom we work, serve, and encounter on a day-to-day basis.

When it comes to the current state of the disability field—like many other areas of research and practice—acceptable terminology is often changing to fit with our times. "Handicapped," for instance, has gone the way of "invalid" and "crippled" and is no longer viewed as an appropriate term to refer to a person with a disability. "Differently abled" and "physically challenged" are fad phrases which have not gained general acceptance among people with disabilities and, in fact, offend many. "Special" when used to refer to people with disabilities, is a rather backhanded compliment—everyone is special in some way—and use of that term as an alternative to "different" is as inappropriate as using the latter term. Words like "wheelchair person" simply should not be used. People without current disabilities, when referred to in contrast to people with disabilities should be referred to as "people without disabilities" rather than as "able bodied" or "normal" since a person with a disability may be more "abled" than others with respect to pertinent activities. Of course, in some contexts, when quoting from an old statute or referring to a particular entity by name, use of some words which otherwise should be avoided may be necessary. For example, the Federal Rehabilitation Act uses the term "handicapped" and schools have "Committees on Special Education" (an improvement over the former "Committees on the Handicapped"). At the time when some organizations were formed and laws were written, few people had yet considered the important role of inclusive language in encouraging inclusion.

POINTS TO KEEP IN MIND

- Physical disability does not imply a mental disability or childishness.
- Different means of communication do not mean low intellectual ability.
- Disabilities can occur to anyone at anytime in life.
- Some disabilities can be temporary or episodic.
- Don't be afraid to encounter someone with a disability.

NOTE ON LANGUAGE REFERRING TO THE "ELDERLY"

There are several terms used to refer to the "elderly" that are used interchangeably, depending on the agency or organization. Common terms include "seniors," "elderly," "the aging," and "older persons." Often the title used in the name of the agency or organization will indicate the appropriate term to use while working with that entity (e.g., the Administration on Aging uses the "aging" primarily in speech and written materials).

By choosing words which convey a positive image of our colleagues, clients, and friends, we begin to break down often unconscious attitudinal barriers to their integration and meaningful participation in society.

Source: Adapted from Leeds, M.H. (1990). *Rights and responsibilities—People with disabilities in employment and public accommodations.* New York, NY: Mark H. Leeds, Esq.

8

HUMAN SERVICES IN DISASTERS AND PUBLIC HEALTH EMERGENCIES: SOCIAL DISRUPTION, INDIVIDUAL EMPOWERMENT, AND COMMUNITY RESILIENCE

Juliana Sadovich and Jonathan D. White

LEARNING OBJECTIVES

When this chapter is completed, readers will be able to:

1. Define the concepts of human services and human security.
2. Identify the role of nurses in human services during disasters.
3. Describe the key actions nurses can take to support human services in disasters.
4. Discuss the relationship of health to the concepts of social well-being and empowerment.
5. Discuss the role of case management in disasters.

KEY MESSAGES

As nursing theory commonly focuses on social well-being (as an aspect of the health of individuals, families, communities, and populations), it is thus consistent with the theory that nurses have a role in human services in disasters.

Although disasters are caused by a variety of man-made or natural events, it is not the magnitude of an event that makes it a disaster but its impact on human populations.

Human services may be defined as the ensemble of systems, both governmental and nongovernmental, whereby assistance is provided to individuals and families in order to address needs they cannot meet solely with their own resources; needs specified in Maslow's hierarchy.

Nurses are a vital link to putting people in touch with the disaster case management system, or whatever other mechanisms exist in the community to link individuals and families impacted by disasters with human service programs, resources, and services that can assist them in meeting their needs.

CHAPTER OVERVIEW

This chapter describes the relationship of nursing and human services in disasters. It also provides an overview of the societal impact of disasters and frames the role of human services in emergency preparedness, response, and recovery. Using nursing theories as a framework, the chapter discusses the role of nursing in the promotion of individual and community well-being in the aftermath of disasters. Finally, the chapter provides an overview of disaster case management, including the role of the federal government, the case management model, and the role of nursing within the model.

It is an axiom of emergency management theory that, although disasters can be caused by a variety of man-made or natural events, it is not the magnitude of that event, but its impact on human populations that makes any event a disaster. A climactic process such as a hurricane or a seismic event such as a tsunami is not a disaster if it has no impact upon people or their communities. The magnitude of the disaster is not measured by hurricane category, seismic intensity, or bioterror agent category, but by the constellation of actual harms sustained by individuals and communities. Disaster preparedness, response, recovery, and mitigation are all dimensions of the effort to lessen the extent and severity of such adverse impacts.

In considering disaster impacts, health is a fundamental domain for assessment and intervention. However, much of the extant literature on disaster health issues focuses on a narrow construction of health—the treatment of injury and illness. Although the recent growth of the disaster behavioral health field has expanded this focus to include the treatment of physiological and psychological injury and illness, there remains a tendency to limit disaster health to a model of healthcare system approaches to disease and trauma. Such a perspective is at odds with a long tradition in nursing that views health as an integral relationship of physiological health, behavioral health, and social well-being. Smith (1981) identified four dimensions of health: the absence of illness, the ability to perform one's role, the capacity to adapt, and the pursuit of eudemonistic well-being.

If we view disaster health impacts not in terms of mortality and morbidity figures alone, but through the lens of the nursing profession's more comprehensive understanding of health, a critical reality comes into sharp focus: the greatest impact of any disaster is the impact on social well-being. Whether a community has been leveled by war or by earthquake, the resulting social disruption is remarkably the same: infrastructure is lost, economy is damaged, people are displaced, and lives are changed. A disaster, by definition, entails social disruption, which in turn adversely impacts the self-sufficiency and functioning of individuals and families and the stability and viability of communities. These negative impacts on individual, household, and community functioning lead to problems of unmet basic human needs. Responding to those needs and empowering individuals, families, and communities to meet them in the long term constitute the field of *human services in disaster*. This chapter introduces concepts of human services in disaster and explores the humanitarian impact of disasters and how nurses can lessen crisis for the individual, family, and community.

HUMAN SERVICES "UNDER CLEAR SKIES"

Approaching questions of human services in disasters requires a clear understanding of the functions of human service systems "under clear skies"—how human services operate in communities in a predisaster environment. "Human services" have been "broadly defined ... [as] approaching the objective of meeting human needs through an interdisciplinary knowledge base, focusing on prevention as well as remediation of problems, and maintaining a commitment to improving the overall quality of life of service populations" (National Organization for Human Services, 2009). Abraham Maslow established a theory of the hierarchy of human *needs* (Maslow, 1954, 1970). Based on this prioritization, Maslow grouped and ordered human needs into categories according to their primacy (Figure 8.1). For the purposes of this chapter, we define human services as the ensemble of systems, both governmental and nongovernmental, whereby assistance is provided to individuals and families in order to address needs at any level in Maslow's hierarchy that those individuals and families cannot meet solely with their own resources.

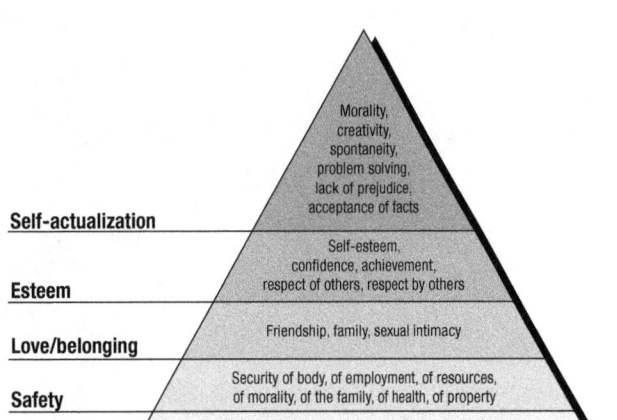

FIGURE 8.1 Maslow's hierarchy of needs.

Although human services (or the synonymous term, "social services") is popularly associated with programs for low-income households, there are both means-tested (low-income-triggered) and non–means-tested (for all income levels) human service systems. Examples of means-tested human services include governmental and nonprofit efforts such as Temporary Assistance for Needy Families (TANF), which provides direct cash assistance; or means-tested programs targeted to a specific need, such as Supplemental Nutrition Assistance Program (SNAP, better known as Food Stamps); the Women, Infants and Children (WIC) program, and community-run food banks, which help meet the need for food; the Low Income Home Energy Assistance Program (LIHEAP), Section-8 subsidized housing, and community homeless shelters, which help meet sheltering (including heating and cooling) needs; and Medicaid, which helps meet the need for healthcare services (Administration for Children and Families [ACF], 2011; Centers for Medicare and Medicaid Services, 2011; Food and Nutrition Service, 2011).

Other human service programs help individuals address unmet needs that occur in the population at all income levels, such as child care systems, child welfare systems, aging services, systems to provide supports for individuals with access and functional needs, and domestic violence prevention and service programs. Populations routinely served by human systems include economically disadvantaged individuals, children and youth, older adults, refugees, and survivors of family or sexual violence.

HUMAN SECURITY

"Human security" is a fundamental concept for the analysis of human services in disasters. Globally, human service needs are the same, but there are great disparities in different nations' human service system's infrastructure to meet those needs. In many developing countries, the primary human service system is not local or national, but is the international humanitarian aid system. The United Nations, in concert with international humanitarian aid agencies, responds to disasters internationally. In 2000, the United Nations, seeking a more effective framework for the humanitarian aid system, developed the concept of human security, which focused on individuals rather than

on the government or on the state. This concept is based on the need for a new paradigm of security that is associated with two sets of dynamics (United Nations, 2003). First, human security is needed as a response to the complexity and interrelatedness of the new security threats of the 21st century, including civil violence; chronic and persistent poverty; environmental and health threats; involuntary population displacements; and illicit trafficking of drugs, arms, and people. These threats have transnational dimensions and exceed traditional notions of security. Second, human security is required as a concerted, comprehensive approach that utilizes the wide range of new opportunities for tackling these threats in an integrated manner. Human security threats require a new consensus that acknowledges the linkages and interdependencies between development, human rights, and national security (United Nations, 2003).

Human security is defined as safety from chronic threats, such as discrimination, unemployment, or environmental degradation, and protection from sudden crises, including economic collapse, environmental disasters, acts of violence, or epidemics. Human insecurity can result from human actions, natural events, or an interaction of human decisions and natural processes (United Nations, 2003). Human security is focused on the vital core of the individual, distinguishing "human security" from "human development," a term that is not linked with disasters (Burd-Sharps, Lewis, & Martins, 2009).

Evidence supports the efficacy of a human security focus in promoting recovery. For example, lessons learned from the December 2004 Asian tsunamis identified that early social, psychological, and community interventions resulted in better individual, family, and community outcomes. The social interventions were identified as services to promote survivor normalization and well-being. These services included the provision of information, temporary housing, family tracing, keeping families together, and early reopening of schools. It was found that psychological support more often was effective when based on local culture, local idioms of distress, and locally acceptable ways of coping and dealing with grief (Chandra, Pandev, Ofrin, Salunke, & Bhugra, 2006).

These findings were consistent with Silove and Steel (2006), who stated the starting point for psychosocial recovery is to ensure that the general emergency management plan is oriented toward an approach that empowers the community to recreate a cohesive and secure society. Understanding the early traumatic stress reaction as a normative survival response encourages an approach to identifying those who need immediate professional intervention, particularly in contexts where resources and skills are scarce (Silove & Steel, 2006).

WHAT IS SOCIAL WELL-BEING?

The idea that disasters create stress within individuals, families, and communities is not new. In 1962, Hill and Hansen, in *Man and Society in Disaster*, stated "disasters create the possibility of changed individuals in changed families within a changed community" (p. 200). The results of these changes are stress and crisis. In this context, coping mechanisms are often ineffective in dealing with changing conditions brought on by the crisis. Four stages of crisis have been identified. Warning, the first stage, is defined as the signs of approaching danger. With impact, the second stage, anxiety heightens. Reorganization, the third stage, occurs at some point during or after impact. In this stage, individuals aspire to work out solutions and to escape the crisis. Change, the fourth stage, occurs when the main threat has passed. It is at this stage that communities are able to focus on rebuilding (Hill & Hansen, 1962).

Using Maslow's hierarchy of needs (Maslow, 1954) as a theoretical foundation, we know that the individual has baseline requirements to sustain life. Once such basic needs are satisfied, the individual can seek a state of self-actualization. The hierarchic theory is often represented as a pyramid, with physiological needs at the base. The pyramid then ascends through safety needs; the need for love, affection, and belonging; the need for esteem; and, at the apex, the need for self-actualization. Maslow believed that, if the environment were right, people would develop straight and beautiful, thus actualizing the potentials they inherited. Maslow also believed that the only reason people would not ascend to self-actualization is because of the socially produced barriers to individual development (Boehm, 2010).

In disaster situations, minority groups—defined by socioeconomic status, race, or ethnicity—usually suffer the most. Lower-income individuals are more likely to live in older and less well-constructed housing, have less insurance protection from loss, and have less access to relief resources (Owen, 2004). Davis, Wilson, Brock-Martin, Glover, and Svendsen (2010) identified that the medically underserved population continues to have a disproportionate impact to disasters. According to the United Nations International Strategy for Disaster Reduction (UNISDR) (www.unisdr.org), in both developing and developed nations, poor people suffer a greater economic impact related to disasters when compared to nonpoor individuals from the same countries. Women and children were found to be 14 times more likely to die than men during disasters (Leoni & Radford, 2011). Most of the 3.3 billion deaths resulting from disasters in the last 40 years have occurred in poor countries. Economically disadvantaged groups also suffer the greatest long-term consequences of disasters, often rendering them more vulnerable to future disasters. The actual scale, in local terms, of economic loss in poor countries is much greater than a mere equivalency in currency of more prosperous nations; thus, for example, the damage from the Indian Ocean tsunami in 2004 cost about $10 billion, compared to $130 billion for Hurricane Katrina, although more people lost livelihood and homes in the tsunami (Leoni & Radford, 2011).

Human development literature gives us an insight into social well-being. In 1959, Erikson conceptualized human development as a process of solving developmental tasks. The goals for attaining and maintaining autonomy and independence relate to socioeconomic status and social integration. As a result, life experiences or disadvantages in socioeconomic status can result in reducing health and social well-being (Davis et al., 2010).

The concept of well-being refers to optimal psychological functioning and experience. Well-being comprises two general approaches: hedonic and eudemonic (Ryan & Deci 2001). The hedonic approach focuses on happiness, and it defines well-being in relationship to attaining pleasure and avoiding pain. The eudemonic approach focuses on meaning and self-realization, and it defines well-being as the degree to which a person is fully functioning (Pinquart & Sorensen, 2000).

EMPOWERMENT

Empowerment is a concept central to the domain of human services, particularly human services in disasters. Fundamentally, all human service systems exist to augment the capabilities individuals already possess without fostering dependence or undermining the self-determination of the client receiving services (Chesler & Hasenfeld, 1989). In the case of disaster human services, the empowerment takes place at the micro-level (individual/family) and the mezzo-level (community). Systems for human services in disasters are designed to promote stabilization and viability at the community level as well as self-sufficiency and human security at the individual and family levels. Access to resources to meet immediate needs and tools to restore the level of independence and autonomy are necessary to participate in long-term recovery. Disaster human services are not something done to take care of clients, but rather they are means made accessible to clients to take care of themselves. The intervention of federal and state agencies and of voluntary organizations active in disaster is necessarily time-limited and partial; the capability of communities to take care of themselves is the horizon of actual disaster recovery.

Norris and Stevens (2007) found that community resilience emerges from four primary sets of adaptive capacities. These capacities are economic development, information and communication, social capital, and community competence. They defined social capital as the aggregate of resources linked to social networks. Community competence was identified as collective action with problem-solving and decision-making skills that arise from collective efficacy and empowerment.

The promotion of empowerment, whether for the individual, family, or community, is a foundational element in emergency management, although it is not a term generally used. The Federal Emergency Management Agency (FEMA) mission is "to support our citizens and first responders to ensure that as a nation we work together to build, sustain, and improve our capability to prepare for, protect against, respond to, recover from, and mitigate all hazards." The focus on empowerment within FEMA lies in two of their largest programs—Individual Assistance and Public Assistance. These programs provide funding to individuals, communities, and states to recover from the impacts of disasters (FEMA, 2011). Volunteer organizations, such as the Red Cross, provide assistance to families focused on meeting basic human needs and social needs. Volunteer organizations and federal, state, and local governmental social service agencies provide a variety of resources to the population impacted by disasters.

HUMAN SERVICES IN DISASTER RESPONSE AND RECOVERY

Human services play a critical role in disaster response and recovery. Two distinct processes define the ways that natural, technological, or intentional disasters transform the landscape of human service needs in impacted populations. First, because disasters can disrupt the infrastructure by which communities meet community members' human needs, those disruptions in systems upon which individuals depend can put human service systems' clients at significant risk until the human service infrastructure can be reconstituted. For example, if a working mother of two preschoolers loses access to child care services when a tornado destroys much of her community's child care capacity, she will likely be unable to work to support her family, even if her job site is intact and has power, until the child care infrastructure is reconstituted. A civil engineer who lived entirely independent using a wheelchair and paratransit services before the disaster may become unable to work, shop, or seek routine medical treatment if the disaster shuts down accessible mass transportation.

Second, disaster impacts create new human service needs that did not exist before the disaster event. For example, the human service needs of an affluent family will be radically changed, likely for a significant period of time, by an earthquake that levels the family home, the children's school, and both parents' jobsites; in a matter of seconds, the family has fundamentally lost its stability and self-sufficiency, and will now require significant human service interventions to meet basic needs related to economic and physical security. Three key drivers of new disaster-caused human service needs are the extent and duration of evacuations and mass movements, critical and social infrastructure damage, and work/wage disruptions. These three manifestations of the social disruption wrought by disaster impacts give rise to many new human service needs by depriving survivors of access to their ordinary means to meet their own needs at all levels of Maslow's hierarchy.

Within Maslow's hierarchy, it is possible to recognize specific disaster human service systems operating to address needs and promote empowerment at every level of the hierarchic pyramid. At the bottom level of physiological needs is the emergency provision of shelter, food, potable water, and clothing—the primary objectives of the Emergency Support Function-6 (ESF-6, Temporary Housing, Mass Care, Emergency Services, and Human Services) and the classical understanding of the term "human services" in the emergency management world. At the next level up, that of security needs, relevant human services include domestic violence prevention/services, child protection, income maintenance/cash assistance benefits, and some employment (including nonlivelihood, improvised employment, e.g., the Vessels of Opportunity employment opportunities in oil cleanup available to Gulf Coast States fishermen when the 2010 Deepwater Horizon Oil Spill shut down the fisheries). Rising still higher, at Maslow's level of love/belonging needs, human services with key equities include community stabilization programs, family reunification systems, and the reconstitution of community-based social networks. At the level of esteem needs, human service systems can be integral to efforts at restoration of independent living for those with access and functional needs, at promoting economic self-sufficiency, and at return to livelihood employment (rather than "whatever work is available," a return to one's own vocation). Last, at the highest level of self-actualization needs, human services play a decisive role in restoration of community pride, economic opportunity, and social justice in the long-term disaster-recovery process. Significantly, while at every level of human need there is a role for human services, the higher the level of need, the more direct community involvement and empowerment is required to meet that need in disaster recovery.

In recent disasters and public health emergencies in the United States, the role of human services programs in response and particularly in recovery efforts has grown significantly (White, 2014). Following Superstorm Sandy in 2012, a critical mission in the states of New York and New Jersey was the reconstitution of the early childhood care and educational systems—child care facilities and Head Start Centers—in order to enable family and community economic recovery. Child care system recovery was also a critical focus after the Joplin, Missouri, tornado disaster of 2011. In these and other recent disasters, Children and Youth Task Forces, partnerships focused on the population needs of children, coordinating efforts by human services, emergency management, and public health and medical systems, convened by state government with support from the Administration for Children and Families (ACF), played decisive roles in the recovery effort (ACF, 2013). In Superstorm Sandy, other critical human services efforts emerged, focused on older adults and power-dependent individuals.

THEORIES SUPPORTING THE ROLE OF NURSES IN HUMAN SERVICES

Theoretical frameworks (or models) of nursing provide a unique perspective; they are similar in the view that nursing is focused on the health and well-being of individuals and populations. Traditionally, the focus of nursing has been on the person or population rather than disease. The writings of Florence Nightingale are relevant in the discussion of nursing in disasters. In her book, *Notes on Nursing: What It Is and What It Is Not*, Nightingale stated, "All the results of good nursing may be spoiled or utterly negative by on defect, petty management, or in other words, by not knowing how to manage that what you do when you are there, shall be done when you are not there" (Nightingale, 1898/2010, p. 35). This statement is consistent with the focus of empowerment in community development. Certainly, her stated position related to harm, "Apprehension, uncertainty, waiting, expectation, fear of surprise, do a patient more harm than any exertion" provides a linkage between lack of understanding and harm (Nightingale, 1898/2010, p. 35). Nightingale's writings demonstrate her view that nursing has a role in social well-being and empowerment.

The multitude of nursing theories provides a variety of perspectives for the promotion of health of individuals, families, communities, and populations along the health continuum. The common focus of nursing theories is the understanding that social well-being is an element of the health of individuals, families, communities, and populations. Thus, it is consistent with nursing theory that nurses have a role in human services in disasters.

The nursing model of transitions can be used as a framework to operationalize the role nurses have in meeting the human services needs in disasters. The concept of "transition" is defined as a passage or movement from one state or condition to another. Three types of transitions have been defined: developmental, situational, and health-illness. The model of transitions suggests that nurses should view the pattern of responses and identify the vulnerabilities and critical needs during transition. Using the concept of transition, nursing interventions are aimed at supporting individuals to create conditions conducive to healthful outcomes (Schumacher & Meleis, 1994).

Evidence-based practice in the field of disaster mental health supports the model that addressing the concrete human services needs of disaster survivors is a critical primary intervention to reduce the prevalence of long-term psychological illness or injury in impacted populations. Operationally the provision of disaster mental health services is integrated with systems to address human service needs caused by the disaster for, as Myers and Wee (2005) explain, "the aim will be to provide human services for problems that are accompanied by emotional strain" (p. 31). The stressors attendant concrete losses and unmet human needs, of the type that human services in disasters are designed to address and mitigate, are critical risk factors in postdisaster psychological injury and illness. Norris et al. (2002) determined that human service needs—"chronic problems in living"—were fundamental to risk of serious psychological impairment following disaster impacts. From a public health standpoint, effective and prompt human service response to a disaster has a primary intervention role in limiting mortality and morbidity due to the behavioral health sequelae of disaster events. Hawkins and Maurer (2010) determined that disaster survivors' efforts to regain what they believed to be security had both psychological and concrete dimensions, and took place both as individuals coped with stressors and as neighborhoods and communities reconstituted themselves. In practice, behavioral health interventions at the population level, and the foundations of economic recovery and psychological recovery for individuals, families, and communities are dependent upon adequately addressing significant gaps in human service needs early in the response and recovery effort. In other words, both psychological and economic recovery of the community are hastened and made more comprehensive by strategic human service response planning and operations. Programmatic systems for human services are integral to disaster recovery, although their effective utilization to promote community recovery is impeded if there is not effective multisectoral integration of human services, public health, and emergency management systems—organized around population-level survivor requirements, rather than institutional, agency, or disciplinary boundaries (White, 2014). Nurses are well positioned to help implement community-level multisectoral efforts across these systems.

THE ROLE OF NURSES IN HUMAN SERVICES

The role of nursing in human services during disasters is to understand that individuals impacted by disasters will experience some level of psychosocial disruption, to screen for human service issues, and to provide appropriate referral. The nurse will likely be the healthcare professional who will interact at some level with the greatest amount of the impacted population. This opportunity for interaction places the nurse at the forefront of healthcare for the impacted population of a disaster.

Nurses providing care to disaster survivors in treatment settings such as hospitals, clinics, or skilled nursing facilities (SNFs) can play a critical role in assessment and referral of patients and families to human service systems that can help

to meet their needs. In hospital settings, problem identification has long been a key aspect of the nursing role through nurses' biopsychosocial assessments, their bedside care relationships with patients and families, and their role in discharge-planning processes. Nurses who become aware of unmet human needs that have been caused or exacerbated by disasters have the opportunity and the responsibility to assist their patients through appropriate referrals for multidisciplinary action to address those needs. In most cases, this will mean a referral to the hospital social worker, or, if that is not an option, to social services in the broader community.

It is important to differentiate between "assessment" and "screening" in the disaster context. In the social service literature, the concept of screening versus assessment is clear. The screening is rapid identification of potential issues across the landscape of human services. Nursing can use these same tools to understand what, if any, human service issues are present for the individuals, families, communities, or populations of interest. Screening for risk factors and comprehensive assessment of needs are processes rooted in the biopsychosocial–spiritual assessment model, in which it is understood that the biomedical, cognitive–emotional, cultural, socioeconomic, and spiritual contexts in which a patient is situated each influence one another and shape the overall experience of health and illness, to which nursing or other health disciplinary interventions respond (Sulmasy, 2002). In the context of the suddenly volatilized social context of disaster survivors—those for whom basic features of the social and physical environment may have been radically altered by disaster impacts—it is particularly important to bring to assessment of needs a systems theory lens that considers the micro- (individual), meso- (community), and macro- (national/global) level phenomena informing the patient's biopsychosocial situation. Nursing assessment of disaster survivors' needs cannot presume the existence of social and environmental "givens," such as a stable place to live, continuous access to necessary or critical infrastructure, or uninterrupted enjoyment of a 21st-century American standard of living. Consideration of patients' physiological and behavioral health needs for nursing treatment will be most effective in a broader context of systems theory-informed biopsychosocial–spiritual assessment.

Admissions or episodes of care do not occur in isolation; the admission, treatment, and discharge of hospital patients take place in a larger social and medical context. Disaster impacts can significantly alter the social environment out of which patients come into an acute care setting, and back into which they are discharged. Nursing discharge planning must factor in the human service needs and gaps that can render a previously viable discharge plan unsafe for patients.

The role of nursing in human services during disasters consists of three elements. Understanding the potential human service issues for people within the disaster impact area is the first element. The second element is screening for human service needs as the individuals transition between pre- and postdisaster realities. Nurses working in disasters irrespective of the location must screen individuals during care contacts for any human service issues. Problem identification should be the goal of screening, with the solutions for identified problems being the responsibility of the referral agency. The third element is referral to the appropriate organization. In disasters, the social service agencies are often overwhelmed, either due to a sharp and rapid increase in the numbers of individuals requiring services and/or due to the impacts of the disaster to the physical infrastructure and to the employees of the agency. It is important for nursing to understand their community's emergency management plan related to human services.

CASE MANAGEMENT IN DISASTERS

The case management model is a useful model within disaster management to meet the human service needs of individuals and families. The case management model is in reality not one but an array of models that use an interdisciplinary approach and can be defined as a collaborative process to assess, plan, implement, coordinate, monitor, and evaluate options and services to meet health needs. Case management seeks to understand complex needs and align services to optimize outcomes. Case management began with the development of social casework in the late 1800s. In the 20th century, case management flourished as public health, nursing, and social work disciplines emerged. Perhaps the most important outcome of the use of case management is the decreasing fragmentation and duplication of care while enhancing quality and cost-effective outcomes (Huber, 2002).

The U.S. Congress authorized federal efforts to provide disaster case management (DCM) as part of the Post-Katrina Emergency Management Reform Act (PKEMRA) in 2006. While DCM was new to the federal government as a mechanism to address the human service impact of disasters, this concept has been employed within the volunteer organization community for a number of years. The Disaster Case Management Program (DCMP) is a federal, FEMA-funded program that provides supplemental funding to states, territories, and tribes in presidentially declared disasters with individual assistance authorized. The DCMP provides implementation alternatives including Immediate Disaster Case Management, a time-limited deployment of federally managed services, including the alternative to use ACF's Immediate DCMP; and a state grant for longer-term service delivery and capacity building (ACF, 2015). In disaster recovery, DCM may be provided by federal, state, or local governmental agencies, as well as by Voluntary Organizations Active in Disasters (VOADs) and other nonprofit organizations. DCM has the capability to promote the best outcomes for individuals and families, recognizing that, even if helpful resources exist, if people do not access the system, the benefits cannot be attained.

As a modality of assistance to disaster survivors, DCM addresses three interconnected challenges to recovery: infrastructural, organizational, and behavioral consequences of disaster. These three sets of consequences combine to create heightened challenges for disaster survivors to identify and access resources for recovery. Because disasters affect the social fabric and institutional infrastructure of affected communities, including the steady-state human services systems, the postdisaster environment is one with significant infrastructural challenges for survivors to access services. For example, social service systems may be operating below predisaster functioning levels,

and survivors may face challenges related to transportation or communication getting assistance. The postdisaster social environment also poses organizational challenges to efficient, coordinated delivery of human services assistance to survivors, as the predisaster, steady-state human services systems and the newly arrived disaster-specific assistance systems (brought by FEMA and VOADs, for example) may not be well aligned or coordinated. Third, disaster survivors' ability to access services and resources postdisaster is behaviorally challenged, as a common consequence of disaster-related stress is reduced capacity to navigate complex bureaucratic systems. DCM is designed to address these heightened challenges to accessing assistance by tailoring trauma-informed, disaster-specific services to survivors, and coordinating between diverse human services systems with a person-centered approach to resources.

Nurses can provide that vital link to putting people in touch with the DCM system, or whatever other mechanisms exist in the community to link individuals and families impacted by disasters with human service programs, resources, and services that can assist them in meeting their needs. Understanding and identifying the human service needs of their patients and their families, wherever that interaction occurs, begins the process. Knowing the disaster services within his or her community or area where one is working will provide the nurse with the ability to provide appropriate referrals. As in so many other aspects of nurses' work, nurses are positioned to make a critical difference in the lives of disaster survivors through accurate problem identification in screening and subsequent in-depth assessment, and referral to a multidisciplinary and multisectoral service system that can address unmet human service needs.

SUMMARY

Disasters are events that adversely impact individuals, families, and communities. Nurses, in any care setting, have a unique opportunity to identify human service needs and provide appropriate referrals to human service organizations. This role in promoting social well-being has been a part of the nurse's role throughout history. The key to success for the nurse to implement this role in disasters is to understand the relationship of social well-being to health, screen patients for human service needs, and know where to appropriately refer patients and families to receive the necessary human services.

STUDY QUESTIONS

1. How might human service needs related to a disaster be identified by nurses during the provision of healthcare?

2. How is the picture of health of disaster survivors altered when health is understood integrally as physiological health, behavioral health, and eudemonistic well-being?

3. In what ways can disaster events cause new human service needs or exacerbate needs that existed before the disaster?

4. How are human services linked to professional nursing theory and values?

5. Considering Maslow's hierarchy of needs model, how may we describe the sets of needs that disaster survivors may engage human service systems to meet?

6. Explain the human security model of international relief operations and describe its relevance to domestic disaster response and recovery efforts in the United States.

7. Distinguish means-tested and non–means-tested human service programs and their relation to disaster-caused needs.

8. What are three drivers of new human service needs in the wake of disasters and public health emergencies?

9. What are some key identifiable supports and resources for nurses who assess disaster survivor patients as having unmet disaster-caused needs?

10. What types of impacts are necessary for an event to become a disaster?

REFERENCES

Administration for Children and Families. (2011). ACF services. Retrieved from https://www.acf.hhs.gov/ohsepr

Administration for Children and Families. (2013). Children and youth task forces in disaster: Guidelines for development. Retrieved from https://www.acf.hhs.gov/sites/default/files/ohsepr/childrens_task_force _development_web_0.pdf

Administration for Children and Families. (2015). Immediate disaster case management concept of operations. Retrieved from https://www.acf.hhs .gov/sites/default/files/ohsepr/immediate_dcm_concept_of_operations _conops_feb2015_cleared.pdf

Boehm, A. (2010). The functions of social service workers at a time of war in a civilian population. *Disasters, 34*(1), 261–286. doi:10.1111/j.1467-7717.2009.01128.x

Burd-Sharps, S., Lewis, K., & Martins, E. (2009). *The measure of America*. New York, NY: Columbia University Press.

Centers for Medicare and Medicaid Services. (2011). Overview medicaid. Retrieved from https://www.cms.gov

Chandra, V., Pandev, R., Ofrin, R., Salunke, S. R., & Bhugra, D. (2006). Mental health and psychosocial aspects of disaster preparedness. *International Review of Psychiatry, 18*(6), 493–494. doi:10.1080/09540260601108952

Chesler, M. A., & Hasenfeld, Y. (1989). Client empowerment in the human services: Personal and professional agenda. *Journal of Applied Behavioral Science, 25*(4), 499–521. doi:10.1177/002188638902500413

Davis, J. R., Wilson, S., Brock-Martin, A., Glover, S., & Svendsen, E. R. (2010). The impact of disasters on populations with health and health

care disparities. *Disaster Medicine and Public Health Preparedness, 4*(1), 30–38. doi:10.1017/S1935789300002391

Federal Emergency Management Agency. (2011). About FEMA. Retrieved from https://www.fema.gov

Food and Nutrition Service, U.S. Department of Agriculture. (2011). FNS Supplemental Nutrition Assistance Program (SNAP). Retrieved from http://www.fns.usda.gov/snap

Hawkins, R. L., & Maurer, K. (2010). "You fix my community, you have fixed my life": The disruption and rebuilding of ontological security in New Orleans. *Disasters, 35*(1), 143–159. doi:10.1111/j.1467-7717.2010.01197.x

Hill, R., & Hansen, D. (1962). Families in disaster. In G. Baker & D. W. Chapman (Eds.), *Man and society in disaster* (pp. 185–221). New York, NY: Basic Books.

Huber, D. (2002). The diversity of case management models. *Lippincott's Case Management, 7*(6), 212–220. doi:10.1097/00129234-200211000-00002

Leoni, B., & Radford, T. (2011). *Disaster through a different lens: Behind every effect, there is a cause*. Geneva, Switzerland: United Nations International Strategy for Disaster Reduction.

Maslow, A. (1954). *Motivation and personality*. New York, NY: Harper & Row.

Maslow, A. (1970). *Motivation and personality* (2nd ed.). New York, NY: Harper & Row.

Myers, D., & Wee, D.F. (2005). *Disaster mental health services: A primer for practitioners*. New York, NY: Brunner-Routledge.

National Organization for Human Services. (2009). What is human services? Retrieved from http://www.nationalhumanservices.org/what-is-human-services

Nightingale, F. (2010). *Notes on nursing: What it is and what it is not*. Cambridge, UK: Cambridge University Press. (Original work published 1898)

Norris, F. H., & Stevens, S. P. (2007). Community resilience and the principles of mass trauma intervention. *Psychiatry, 70*(4), 320–328. doi:10.1521/ psyc.2007.70.4.320

Norris, F. H., Friedman, M. J., Watson, P. J., Byrne, C. M., Diaz, E., & Kaniasty, K. (2002). 60,000 disaster victims speak: Part I: An empirical review of the empirical literature, 1981–2001. *Psychiatry, 65*, 207–239. doi:10.1521/psyc.65.3.207.20173

Owen, T. (2004). Challenges and opportunities for defining and measuring human security. *United Nations Disarmament Forum, 3*, 15–24.

Pinquart, M., & Sorensen, S. (2000). Influences of socioeconomic status, social network, and competence on subjective well-being in later life: A meta-analysis. *Psychology and Aging, 15*(2), 187–224. doi:10.1037/0882-7974.15.2.187

Ryan, R., & Deci, E. (2001). On happiness and human potentials: A review of research on hedonic and eudemonic well-being. *Annual Review of Psychology, 52*, 141–166. doi:10.1146/annurev.psych.52.1.141

Schumacher, K., & Meleis, A. (1994). Transitions: A central concept in nursing. *IMAGE: The Journal of Nursing Scholarship, 26*(2), 119–127. doi:10.1111/j.1547-5069.1994.tb00929.x

Silove, D., & Steel, Z. (2006). Understanding community psychosocial needs after disasters: Implications for mental health services. *Journal of Postgraduate Medicine, 52*, 121–125. doi:10.1001/jama.296.5.576

Smith, J. A. (1981). The idea of health: A philosophical inquiry. *Advances in Nursing Sciences, 3*(3), 43–50. doi:10.1097/00012272-198104000-00005

United Nations Office for the Co-ordination of Humanitarian Affairs, Human Security Unit. (2003). *Human security in theory and practice: An overview of the human security concept and the United Nations Trust Fund for Human Security*. New York, NY: Author.

White, J. (2014). Children, youth, and families task forces in recovery. In T. Wizemann, M. Reeve, & B. Altevogt (Eds.), *Preparedness, response, and recovery conditions for children and families: Workshop summary* (pp. 113–115). Washington, DC: Institute of Medicine/National Academies Press.

Administration for Children and Families Disaster Case Management Program: Building Coalitions and Best Practices

Roberta Proffitt Lavin and Tener Goodwin Veenema

OVERVIEW

The immediate aftermath of Hurricane Katrina quickly revealed a desperate need for both social services and medical support for the poor and marginalized victims, whether or not they remained in the impacted area or were relocated. Senior leaders from the ACF proposed the development of a DCMP that was based on their previous positive and successful experience with Refugee Resettlement. The DCMP was envisioned as incorporating the principles of self-determination, self-sufficiency, federalism, flexibility and speed, and support to states.

INTRODUCTION

Case management is a process that assists people in identifying their service needs, locating and arranging services, and coordinating the services of multiple providers. DCM uses the same process to help people recover from a disaster event. The Council on Accreditation says disaster recovery case management services "plan, secure, coordinate, monitor, and advocate for unified goals and services with organizations and personnel in partnership with individuals and families ... [They] include practices that are unique to delivery of services in the aftermath of emergencies and major incidents." Thus, DCM is the formal process of organizing and providing a timely, coordinated approach to assess disaster-related needs, including healthcare, mental health, and human services needs that were caused or exacerbated by the event and may adversely impact an individual's recovery if not addressed.

The Council on Accreditation states that while DCM services may include emergency relief services, they extend beyond the immediate to address long-term recovery needs, such as healthcare, employment, housing, and other social services. DCM facilitates the delivery of appropriate resources and services, works with a client to implement a recovery plan, and advocates for the client's needs to assist him or her in returning to a predisaster status while respecting human dignity. If necessary, DCM helps transition the client with preexisting needs to existing case management providers after disaster-related needs are addressed. This is facilitated through the provision of a single point of contact for disaster assistance applicants who need a wide variety of services that may be provided by many different organizations. In line with the Council on Accreditation standards, DCMPs may directly provide assistance, make

referrals to organizations that have agreed to meet specific client needs, contract with other organizations, or otherwise arrange for individuals and families to receive needed services and resources. In addition, the process of DCM generally includes assessment, recovery planning, service delivery, monitoring, and advocacy.

The purpose of DCM is to rapidly return individuals and families who have survived a disaster to a state of self-sufficiency. This is accomplished by ensuring that each individual with disaster-related needs has access to a case manager who will capture information about the individual's situation. The case manager will then serve as an advocate and help the individual organize and access disaster-related resources, human services, healthcare, and mental healthcare that will help to achieve predisaster levels of functioning and equilibrium. The service is particularly critical in situations where large-scale mortality, injuries, or personal property damage has occurred.

Disaster case management agencies may also work in conjunction with long-term recovery committees to serve their clients. These committees are typically community-based organizations that bring together a variety of local leaders, such as members of voluntary organizations, civic organizations, social service agencies, local churches, and case management agencies. Long-term recovery committees coordinate recovery efforts and provide resources to address the unmet needs of disaster victims when all other resources have been exhausted or when current resources are inadequate based on the victims' recovery plan. These committees often include unmet needs committees or roundtables, at which case managers from member organizations present cases in order to obtain resources for clients in need.

The goal of federally sponsored DCM is to assist vulnerable populations with disaster-related needs in the aftermath of disaster. DCM is intended to be culturally sensitive and accessible without creating barriers. It is not intended to replace an existing state or local program, but rather to provide support when requested by a state and approved by FEMA.

Disaster case management is based on the principles of self-determination, self-sufficiency, federalism, flexibility and speed, and support to states.

1. *Self-Determination*: Individuals and families impacted by a disaster have the same rights and responsibilities as everybody else. Government aid to persons adversely impacted by a disaster should therefore seek to support the self-determination of persons adversely impacted

(continued)

CASE STUDY 8.1 (*continued*)

by a disaster as they seek access to public benefits and consider relocation opportunities. Individuals and families focusing on their own needs, resources, and interests are more likely to achieve favorable results for themselves and for the broader society than when government restricts or directs their choices.

2. *Self-Sufficiency*: The object of disaster case management assistance, including efforts targeted toward persons adversely impacted by a disaster and persons with predisaster vulnerabilities, should be individual and family self-sufficiency. As we seek to provide every necessary benefit to help persons adversely impacted by a disaster recover from the disaster and restart their lives, the measure of our success should not be the number of new entrants into disaster assistance systems or dollars expended. Success should be measured by how quickly and successfully persons adversely impacted by a disaster and persons with pre-disaster vulnerabilities are able to become economically self-sufficient and socially integrated. These new lives may be either in the homes and communities held before the disaster or in new locations selected based on the individual's or family's best judgment of where their goals and aspirations may best be fulfilled.

3. *Federalism*: Our federal system is designed so that states and local governments are often the primary means for administering and delivering public benefits and services to those eligible for them. For efficiency, speed, and to take maximum advantage of existing expertise in matching persons adversely impacted by a disaster with benefits and services, aid should be delivered—to the maximum extent possible—through existing state, local governments, and community social services programs rather than through the creation of new federal institutions or programs. The role of the federal government is to enhance and support existing mechanisms and ensure ongoing quality assurance, taking action to reduce unnecessary impediments to the delivery of assistance to persons adversely impacted by a disaster.

4. *Flexibility and Speed*: Persons adversely impacted by a disaster need immediate access to resources, even if they have lost their documentation. Previous eligibility should continue without interruption and new eligibility should be established quickly. Hence, the federal government should endeavor to provide states and local governments with as much latitude as possible in delivering benefits.

5. *Support for States*: States and localities endeavoring to deliver needed benefits and services to persons adversely impacted by a disaster should not be financially disadvantaged by their compassion and generosity. The federal government, to the extent possible, should endeavor to reduce disaster impact on existing service delivery to citizens by filling gaps within existing systems, coordinating with local entities, and helping connect persons adversely impacted by a disaster to human and medical services. Quickly linking persons adversely impacted by a disaster

to appropriate assistance will reduce the likelihood that they will require more intensive healthcare and social service benefits, thus reducing the impact on states and existing systems (Lavin & Menifee, 2009, pp. 7–8).

BACKGROUND AND SIGNIFICANCE

Following Hurricanes Katrina and Rita, Congress recognized the need for comprehensive DCM services. As a result, in 2006, Congress passed the Post-Katrina Emergency Management Reform Act of 2006 (PKEMRA), which amends the Robert T. Stafford Disaster Relief and Emergency Assistance Act (Stafford Act) and includes a provision to provide DCM[1] services. The PKEMRA §426 Case Management Services states, "the President may provide case management services, including financial assistance, to State or local government agencies or qualified private organizations to provide such services, to survivors of major disasters to identify and address unmet needs." As a result of the devastating damage caused by the storms, the federal government, for the first time, funded several DCM pilot programs. Through PKEMRA, the federal government provided at least $209 million to assist survivors in coping with the devastation and rebuilding their lives, yet deficiencies existed that resulted in poor outcomes for these early programs and illuminated the need for greater coordination and program evaluation in the provision of DCM services (General Accounting Office [GAO], 2009).

Most plans assume that human services will be delivered to those adversely impacted by disaster by existing agencies and that case management will be either delivered by those same agencies or supported by voluntary agencies and faith-based groups within the impacted area. However, in a major disaster that impacts thousands of individuals or families, the ability of those agencies within the impacted area to provide DCM services could be compromised. Therefore, it is necessary to have a plan and to have coalitions built to support states and local communities in a manner that will fill existing gaps identified by the state, until the state is able to implement its own case management program.

---

[1] Disaster case management is the process of organizing and providing a timely, coordinated approach to assess disaster-related needs as well as existing healthcare, mental health, and human services needs that may adversely impact an individual's recovery if not addressed. The objective of disaster case management is to rapidly return children and families who have survived a disaster to a state of self-sufficiency. This is accomplished by ensuring that each child/family has access to a case manager who will capture information about the child/family's situation and then serve as their advocate and help them organize and access disaster-related resources. *Disaster Case Management Implementation Guide*, (ed.), U.S. Department of Health and Human Services Administration for Children and Families (Washington, DC: HHS, 2008), 62.

(*continued*)

The ACF Example: How Are Coalitions Built?

Coalition building requires identifying fragmented coordination, key stakeholders, subject matter experts, and a community of interest. When the proposal to develop ACF DCM was first discussed, leaders from the major faith-based organizations that are active in disasters were invited to a meeting to discuss the project and brainstorm a way forward. It was clear that the first task was to build a trusting relationship and identify shared goals for collaboration. Successful coalition building cannot take place within an existing environment of distrust. Coordination, collaboration, and communication are critical to the achievement of DCM program client outcomes (GAO, 2009). The steps included the following:

- Building a trusting relationship by listening and learning from past communication errors
- Identifying the key stakeholders, their needs, and their goals
- Defining the problem
- Engaging subject matter experts from the beginning
- Assembling the best available evidence across case management programs, including healthcare, wounded warriors, refugee resettlement, and DCM
- Considering all feasible alternatives and presenting them to the stakeholders and refining the alternatives based on input
- Discussing openly and publically the criteria, trade-offs, and possible decisions
- Communicating the process by holding focus groups, interviewing individuals from all levels of DCM, presenting at conferences, and submitting information to the Federal Register to allow public comment
- Endeavoring to reach consensus between federal, state, voluntary organizations, and the faith-based community
- Trusting those that have credibility within the community to do what they do best and what they do everyday—provide DCM

Coalition building began with many hours of active listening to establish a trusting relationship with key stakeholders. Later meetings employed the use of the Delphi process to facilitate the discussion toward consensus surrounding the design of the DCM program.

What the Delphi Process Has Shown

The Delphi technique is a research process that allows communication among groups of individuals to deal with a complex problem and build consensus. The Delphi process for DCM included over 25 organizations (federal, state, local, advocacy organizations, academia, and voluntary and faith-based organizations) that, prior to their involvement, did not agree on a single approach to DCM and did not have a coordinated approach. The Delphi technique was utilized to reach consensus on best practices in DCM, provide input to program design, and help build a coalition that was committed to supporting the program following a disaster. The outcomes of the process included the following:

- Broad consensus on a three-tiered approach to DCM (national, regional, and local)
- Concurrence on the overarching principles of self-determination, self-sufficiency, federalism, flexibility and speed, and support to states
- Support of using registered nurses, especially from the U.S. Public Health Service, as a resource to the case managers when dealing with persons with medical conditions
- Agreement that a federal team needs to deploy quickly, accomplish the initial setup, and maintain a presence until the faith-based organizations can mobilize and assume control on the ground
- Consensus that a cadre of qualified and trained volunteers is essential for the provision of services until the role can be assumed by local agencies
- Identification of AmeriCorps as an essential pool of volunteers for staffing call centers and providing other support
- Identification of the importance of colocation for communication between the DCM teams, the Joint Field Office, the medical teams, and state and local resources as critical
- Realization that outreach, screening, and intakes should begin as soon as the immediate lifesaving measures end—usually within 3 days. The belief that those impacted by disaster are not prepared for human services assistance is not true. The sooner the help arrives, the less likely it is that those impacted will make decisions that will complicate their long-term recovery and financial self-sufficiency
- Concurrence that the team leaders must be trained in the Incident Command System and be knowledgeable of National Incident Management System (NIMS)
- Broad consensus that the people who are in the community every day (Catholic Charities, Luther Social Services, the Salvation Army, etc.) are trusted by the community and should be the public face of DCM
- Broad consensus that ongoing focus groups and public comment periods are essential to maintain trust

Lessons Learned in Building Coalitions

Awareness for the need for DCM at the federal level (within FEMA and ACF) began after a devastating hurricane that left many individuals and organizations feeling that their government had failed them. Two years later, when the decision was made to create a DCM capability with the

(continued)

CASE STUDY 8.1 (*continued*)

support of the federal government (PKEMRA), it was first necessary to rebuild the trust among participating agencies and all those whose lives were touched by the program. Trust is essential to success. The key lessons learned about building trust can be summed up in four rules.

Rule 1: Let the trusted person or organization lead the meetings.
Rule 2: Secrecy (closed meetings and confidential documents) breads mistrust.
Rule 3: The leader in the field must be trusted and communicate effectively.
Rule 4: The local is always more trusted than the outsider and the church is always more trusted than the government.

REFERENCES

General Accounting Office. (2009, July). *Disaster assistance: Greater coordination and an evaluation of program's outcomes could improve disaster case management, GAO-09–561*. Washington, DC: Author.

Lavin, R. & Menifee, S. (Eds.). (2009). *Disaster case management: Implementation guide*. Washington, DC: Administration for Children and Families.

Sulmasy, D. P. (2002). A biopsychosocial-spiritual model for the care of patients at the end of life. *The Gerontologist, 42*, 24–33. doi:10.1093/geront/42.suppl_3.24

9

UNDERSTANDING THE PSYCHOSOCIAL IMPACT OF DISASTERS

Susan M. S. Carlson, Kathleen Coyne Plum, and Elizabeth C. Meeker

LEARNING OBJECTIVES

When this chapter is completed, readers will be able to:

1. Identify the psychosocial effects likely to occur in various types of disasters.
2. Identify the elements of a community impact and resource assessment.
3. Describe the normal reactions of children and adults to disaster.
4. Formulate strategies that helpers can use to assist children and their families in the immediate aftermath of a disaster.
5. Discuss the impact of disaster trauma on first responders and helpers.
6. Describe community reactions to a large-scale disaster.
7. Describe the manifestations of normal grief and mourning.

KEY MESSAGES

No one who is involved in a disaster is left untouched.

Estimating the psychosocial impact of a disaster can help guide the deployment of resources.

Mental health workers need to be members of the disaster response team from the onset and take mental health services to survivors.

A range of psychological and emotional responses to disaster are normal and should not be "pathologized" or "medicalized."

First responders and disaster workers are also vulnerable to stress reactions.

Communities as well as individuals react to disaster.

Noting milestones and anniversaries can facilitate normal grieving among all affected.

CHAPTER OVERVIEW

Involvement in a disaster is a life-altering event, whether one is a survivor, a bereaved family member, a neighbor, or a helper. Although we know that individuals closest to a disaster will be most affected, information about the type and scope of the disaster can enhance estimates of the intensity and duration of the psychosocial resources that will be needed to assist those who will be affected by it. Resistance to psychosocial intervention, however, is such a common reaction among disaster survivors that mental health services must be made readily available and easily accessible to those at greatest risk. Social support, in addition to support from governmental agencies, is essential for survivors. Moreover, mobilization of these services to survivors and the bereaved at their location is paramount to launching a success intervention. All helpers need to know that many types of emotions, thoughts, behaviors, and sensations are normal reactions to a disaster and should not be "pathologized." Outreach provided by well-trained mental health workers is especially crucial for the most vulnerable populations, such as children, the elderly, the medically frail, military veterans, and those with serious mental illness. First responders and other helpers must take special precautions to mitigate the psychological impact of disaster, as secondary traumatization is an ever-present hazard of disaster response. The rituals of normal grief and mourning can help individuals and communities draw on the strengths of the group to promote healing and eventual resolution.

Disasters, by their very nature, are stressful, life-altering experiences, and living through such an experience can cause serious psychological effects and social disruption. Disasters affect every aspect of the life of an individual, family, and community. Depending on the nature and scope of the disaster, the degree of disruption can range from mild anxiety and family dysfunction (e.g., marital discord or parent–child relational problems) to separation anxiety, posttraumatic stress disorder (PTSD), engagement in high-risk behaviors, addictive behaviors, severe depression, and even suicidality. Goldmann and Galea (2014) cite that following a disaster, PTSD may affect 30% to 40% of those who directly experienced the trauma, with children being especially vulnerable. Depression is also a common postdisaster response and was found to be correlated with personal vulnerability and life stressors such as low socioeconomic status (Goldmann & Galea, 2014). Although less frequently studied, substance use is also common following a disaster. A study by Vlahov et al. (2002) after the terrorist attack on the World Trade Center demonstrated almost 25% of New Yorkers reported increased alcohol use, 10% indicated an increase in cigarette use, and 3% reported increased marijuana use. Generalized anxiety disorder (GAD) is also common, as are panic disorders, phobias, suicidality, and somatic symptoms such as headache, abdominal pain, shortness of breath, and fatigue with prevalence of these symptoms varying from 3% to 75% in a literature review performed by Goldmann and Galea (2014). The World Health Organization estimates that 1 in 6 people (10%–15%) who experience a disaster will suffer a mild to moderate mental disorder, and approximately 1 in 30 (3%–4%) will be emotionally impacted to the degree that it interferes with their ability to function (van Ommeren, Hanna, Weissbecker, & Ventevogel, 2015).

While there are common mental health effects across different types of disasters, each disaster is unique and many factors can determine a given disaster's effect on survivors. Natural disasters, such as floods, hurricanes, forest fires, and tornadoes most often result in property loss and dislocation. When physical injury and loss of life are minimal, the incidence of psychiatric sequelae may be reduced. However, subsequent factors such as continuing aftershocks following an earthquake or poor temporary housing conditions can contribute to short-term and long-term traumatic stress. An environmental disaster can lead to a sense of mistrust toward government and business, leading to a sense of helplessness and hopelessness. An example of this is Puerto Rico after the Hurricane Maria in 2017, a level 5 hurricane with sustained gale force winds of 155 mph and severe flooding after the hurricane surge. Routine neglect of the island's infrastructure and ongoing poverty led to angry outlash at the government for the neglect and perpetuated feeling of vulnerability (Dávila & Rushing, 2017). In the case of the 1989 Exxon Valdez oil spill, according to Price (2010), Alaskans who lost their jobs were three times more likely to experience PTSD, twice as likely to experience depression, and three-and-a-half times more likely to have anxiety disorder than those Alaskans who were not affected. In man-made disasters, such as plane crashes and bombings, the sudden loss of life can be overwhelming, and when the presence of symptoms in the short term is very high, the prevalence of disorders in the aftermath is correspondingly high.

Hurricane Katrina was unique in that it was not only a natural disaster but also a man-made disaster in the sense that much of the suffering occurred as a result of delayed or ineffective rescue. The loss of life due to poor preparation and response was stunning. Massive devastation and dislocation led to separation of families. Many victims lost virtually all personal possessions, livelihood, and their support systems. A study of survivors displaced to Federal Emergency Management Agency (FEMA) housing for 8 to 9 months found that 50% met criteria for major depressive disorder, 20% had suicidal ideation, and 14% had increased substance use since displacement (Larrance, Anastario, & Lawry, 2007). In terms of the mental health response, the logistical and financial challenges made it difficult to plan how and where to reach many of the dislocated children and adults. Experts estimated that Katrina's impact on mental health is likely to last years (Voelker, 2006). A study of over 7,000 children affected by Katrina found that during the school year following the disaster, 50% of children had symptoms of PTSD and depression. In the following year, 41% still met the criteria for a referral to mental health services (Osofsky, Osofsky, Kronenberg, Brennan, & Hansel, 2009).

The impact on first responders in these more complicated disasters is also of particular concern. Neria and Shultz (2012) identify those involved in the rescue and recovery profession to be one of the groups at highest risk of developing negative mental health consequences in response to the event. Sakuma et al. (2015) completed a cross-sectional study of PTSD and depression in local disaster relief and reconstruction workers 14 months after the Great East Japan Earthquake of 2011. They found that PTSD prevalence among first responders ranged from 10% to 20%, in contrast with 30% to 40% for direct victims of the disaster (Sakuma et al., 2015). Lack of rest was linked with increased risk for PTSD and depression in municipality and medical workers, while lack of communication was linked with increased PTSD in medical workers and depression in municipality workers (Sakuma et al., 2015). Unfortunately, suicide is far too common in first responders and disaster relief personnel (Antevy & Sobel, 2016).

The mental health effects of any type of disaster, mass violence, or terror attack are well documented in the literature to be related to the intensity of exposure to the event. Documented potential indicators of mental health problems following the event are: sustaining personal injury, death of a loved one due to the disaster, disaster-related displacement, relocation, and loss of property and personal finances (Neria & Shultz, 2012). Goldmann and Galea (2014) identify *predisaster risk factors*: prior mental health problems, female gender, and younger age; *peridisaster risk factors*: degree or severity of disaster exposure (number and intensity of disaster-related events, the type of disaster, duration of exposure, death toll, and proximity to where the disaster occurred); and *postdisaster risk factors*: postdisaster life stressors (job loss, property damage, marital stress, physical health conditions related to the disaster, and displacement) and low level of social supports (pp. 174–176).

In 2001, Hull, Alexander, and Klein found that only 21% of disaster survivors were still meeting diagnostic criteria for PTSD (Aslam & Tariq, 2010). When the disaster involves intentional violence and human maleficence, however, such as with 9/11, rates of probable PTSD may be even higher. According to the National Center for PTSD (U.S. Department of Veteran Affairs, 2016), studies have shown that deliberate violence creates longer lasting mental health effects than natural disasters or accidents.

BIOTERRORISM AND TOXIC EXPOSURES

Bioterrorism has a different profile from that of natural disasters or even sudden violent events, such as bombings and explosions. According to Ursano, Norwood, and Fullerton (2004), "bioterrorism is an act of human malice intended to injure and kill civilians and is associated with higher rate of psychiatric morbidity than are 'Acts of God'" (p. 1). The effects are more uncertain and occur over a longer period of time. Terrorist attacks result in extensive fear, loss of confidence in institutions, feelings of unpredictability about the future, and pervasive experience of loss of safety (Ursano et al., 2004).

The October 2001 anthrax scare was probably designed to be more of a psychological attack than a physical one. In an editorial, Wessely, Hyams, and Bartholomew (2001) note that biological and chemical weapons are notoriously ineffective methods of mass destruction but are much more effective as weapons of terror—by introducing fear, confusion, and uncertainty into everyday life. Fear of biological warfare can lead to mass sociogenic illnesses in which common, everyday symptoms are believed to be signs of biological exposure. Common psychological reactions to bioterrorism (Holloway, Norwood, Fullerton, Engel, & Ursano, 2002) include:

- Horror, anger, or panic
- Magical thinking about microbes and viruses
- Fear of invisible agents or fear of contagion
- Attribution of arousal symptoms to infection
- Anger at terrorists, the government, or both
- Scapegoating, loss of faith in social institutions
- Paranoia, social isolation, or demoralization

Following the anthrax exposures in the United States, many of these psychological reactions were seen around the world. For example, in the Philippines, local clinics were deluged by more than 1,000 people suffering from flu-like symptoms because of rumors that those symptoms were due to bioterrorism.

In response to these incidents, the American Psychological Association [www.apa.org] is now strongly recommending that people limit their exposure to the news media, as overexposure may heighten one's anxiety. Foa et al. (2005) state that reactions can be made worse by sensationalizing in the media and poor transfer of specific recommendations by public officials. They recommend the following interventions to minimize the potential psychological and social consequences of suspected or actual biological exposures:

1. Provide information on the believed likelihood of such an attack and of possible impact
2. Communicate what the individual risk is
3. Clarify that negative health behaviors, which may increase during time of stress (i.e., smoking, unhealthy eating, excessive drinking), constitute a greater health hazard than the hazards likely to stem from bioterrorism
4. Emphasize that the only necessary action against terrorism on the individual level is increased vigilance of suspicious actions, which should be reported to authorities
5. Clearly communicate the meaning of different levels of warning systems when such warnings are issued
6. When issuing a warning, specify the type of threat, the type of place threatened, and indicate specific actions to be taken
7. Make the public aware of steps being taken to prevent bioterrorism without inundating people with unnecessary information
8. Provide the public with follow-up information after periods of heightened alert

COMMUNITY IMPACT AND RESOURCE ASSESSMENT

By brainstorming potential disaster scenarios and the scope of resources anticipated with each scenario, the intensity and duration of the mental health response can also be anticipated. The U.S. Department of Health and Human Services (2004) has promulgated a population exposure model that planners can use to estimate the psychological impact of mass violence and terrorism and, therefore, the resources that might be needed. The model's underlying principle is that individuals who are most personally, physically, and psychologically exposed to trauma and the disaster scene are likely to be affected the most (Figure 9.1). According to Donner and Rodriguez (2011), population growth, most particularly population density and urbanization, has

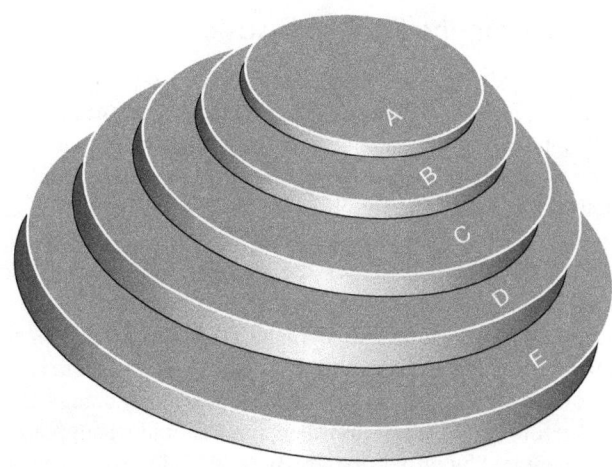

FIGURE 9.1 Population exposure model.

A: Community victims killed and seriously injured; bereaved family members, loved ones, close friends.

B: Community victims exposed to the incident and disaster scene but not injured.

C: Bereaved extended family members and friends; residents in disaster zone whose homes were destroyed; first responders, rescue and recovery workers; medical examiner's office staff; service providers immediately involved with bereaved families; obtaining information for body identification and death notification.

D: Mental health and crime victim assistance providers, clergy, chaplains, emergency healthcare providers, governmental officials, members of the media.

E: Groups that identify with the target-victim group, businesses with financial impacts, community-at-large.

increased vulnerability to disasters. Research comparing the psychological effects of human-caused versus natural disaster has yielded equivocal results. No one type of disaster is "worse" than another, although the number of associated deaths and serious injuries can be expected to have the most significant and longest lasting impact on physical and emotional well-being.

Knowing what the public and private mental health resources are ahead of time is key to effective crisis management. Questions that should be addressed during predisaster planning include:

- *What are the types of disasters that are most likely to occur in my community?* Is this region most vulnerable to natural, technological, toxic, or man-made disasters?
- *Is there a county and state mental health disaster plan?* If so, what does it entail, and how might it support local efforts?
- *What kind of expertise is needed?* Will the anticipated disaster affect a certain age group; racial, ethnic, or religious subpopulation; or individuals having a specific disability, such as hearing impairment, mental illness, dementia, or mental retardation?
- *Who are the qualified mental health professionals in the community who can be called upon in the event of a local disaster?* Do they have a clinical specialty or language proficiency? Who authorizes them and what training do they have/need?
- *What resources can the local American Red Cross chapter provide to responders and/or victims?* Do providers have existing memoranda of understanding with the Red Cross?
- *Is there a team of mental health workers specifically trained in critical incident stress management available to debrief*

rescuers and hospital personnel? How will they be activated? If there is not an identified team, who will be available to provide stress management for rescue/medical personnel?
- *Are there other nonpsychological services that local mental health providers can offer?* For example, are there programs or agencies that could provide space and food for staff or victims?

One reason that medical professionals might be reluctant to include mental health professionals on the team, and a reason that victims do not seek psychiatric consultation, is the concern that emergency mental health intervention implies that emotional distress is equated with mental illness. The World Health Organization (2017) identifies that the stigma of mental illness is still very viable and contributes to limiting access to services following a humanitarian crisis. This is a barrier that needs to be overcome, however, as the immediate mental health response to a disaster should be educationally oriented, not treatment oriented. In the immediate aftermath, before clinically significant psychiatric symptoms emerge, the recommended approach includes: (a) provide a sense of safety, (b) calm anxiety, (c) promote a sense of self- and community-efficacy, (d) encourage connectedness through social supports and bonding with others, and (e) instill hope (Hobfoll et al., 2007).

van Ommeren et al. (2015) point out that it is essential to develop a sustainable community mental health system as part of the recovery process. Several recommendations for the preparedness phase for the mental health and psychosocial support include:

- Embed mental health and psychosocial supports into national health policies, strategies, and emergency preparedness plans
- Identify existing formal and nonformal resources and practices in mental health and psychosocial supports
- Orient staff involved as first responders, healthcare providers, and recovery personnel in "psychological first aid"
- Train and supervise healthcare staff in the management of mental health during emergencies according to the World Health Organization's *Clinical management of mental, neurological and substance use conditions in humanitarian emergencies: mhGAP Humanitarian Intervention Guide (mhGAP-HIG)* (apps.who.int/iris/bitst ream/10665/162960/1/9789241548922_eng.pdf)
- Assemble emergency stocks of essential psychotropic medications, with suggestions of: amitriptyline (or fluoxetine), phenobarbital (or carbamazepine), biperiden, haloperidol, and diazepam
- Develop emergency preparedness plans for people with severe and chronic mental illness who reside in the community

NORMAL REACTIONS TO ABNORMAL EVENTS

Normal reactions to stress and bereavement can and do vary—sometimes even among members of the same family. Factors that affect expressions of stress and bereavement include age, gender, ethnicity, religious background, personality traits, coping skills, and previous experience with loss, especially traumatic loss. Stress symptoms can occur due to secondary exposure, meaning that those experiencing distress need not have been present at the site of the disaster but may have witnessed it secondhand either via media coverage or through retelling of the event by a person who was present. As these reactions can be quite startling and overwhelming to those who have not experienced them before, it is helpful for survivors to hear that their experiences are entirely normal, given the tremendous stress to which they have been exposed (see Box 9.1 for the common reactions of survivors).

BOX 9.1 Common Reactions of Disaster Survivors

EMOTIONAL

Shock, feeling numb
Fear
Grief, sadness
Anger
Guilt, shame
Feelings of helplessness

INTERPERSONAL

Distrust
Conflict
Withdrawal
Work or school problems
Irritability
Loss of intimacy
Feeling rejected or abandoned

COGNITIVE

Confusion
Indecisiveness
Worry
Shortened attention span
Trouble concentrating

PHYSICAL

Tension, edginess
Fatigue, insomnia
Body aches, pain, nausea
Startling easily
Racing heartbeat
Change in appetite
Change in sex drive

Source: U.S. Department of Veteran Affairs: National Center for PTSD. (2010). Mental health reactions after disaster. Retrieved from https://www.ptsd.va.gov/professional/pages/handouts-pdf/Reactions.pdf

---

Resiliency in the Face of Disaster

Because not all survivors of a disaster display symptoms beyond the initial phases of recovery, researchers have become increasingly interested in the factors that might promote resiliency in the aftermath of a devastating disaster. In fact, resilience is often the most commonly observed outcome trajectory after exposure to a potential traumatic event (Bonanno, Rennicke, & Dekel, 2005). Characteristics associated with resilience include family stability, social support, and capacity to tolerate stress and uncertainty. After Hurricane Maria in 2017, feeling abandoned by the federal and local governments, the people of Puerto Rico improvised ways to remain alive without power or running water (Dickerson, 2017). This innovated spirit should be supported and celebrated by professionals. By promoting resilience and coping after disaster, mental health professionals can draw upon the individual's strengths or create the supports needed to ward off lasting symptoms or functional difficulties, and avoid interventions that may actually interfere with one's own inherent resiliency and therefore impede recovery. See Case Study 9.1 for a disaster mental health volunteer's perspective on survivor resilience in the aftermath of Katrina and the 2004 tsunami in Southeast Asia.

SPECIAL NEEDS POPULATIONS

Certain populations affected by disasters may be more vulnerable and therefore require special consideration both in disaster planning and response. In particular, women, older people, children and young people, people with disabilities, and people marginalized by ethnicity are more vulnerable (Sim & Cui, 2015). Formal vulnerability is "the characteristics of a person or group and their situation that influences their capacity to anticipate, cope with, resist and recover from the impact of a natural hazard," in comparison with "differential vulnerability," which takes into account the fact that different populations face different levels of risk and vulnerability (Donner & Rodriguez, 2011, p. 1). Elangovan and Kasi (2014) point out that children along with women, the older population, and disabled persons are the most vulnerable populations (p. 119). Because of this, those suffering in silence may be easily overlooked, and outreach to these vulnerable groups is critical following a disaster or humanitarian emergency.

Children and Youth

While most children are resilient, many children do experience some significant degree of distress. Poverty and parents with mental health challenges put children at higher risk for long-term impairments (McLaughlin et al., 2009). Risk factors for children experiencing stress after an incident include loss of routine and loss/change in caregivers (Elangovan & Kasi, 2014). In instances of terrorism, studies found that children suffer more severe reactions if they are female or know someone who was killed, as well as when children are exposed to higher levels of television coverage, and have parents who suffer a higher level of distress (U.S. Department of Veteran Affairs, National Center for PTSD, 2016). Children who witness or experience war atrocities may experience stress in the form of risk to their physical safety as well as separation from their family members. As refugees, the children can be deprived of food and water, witness violence and harsh living conditions, experience a disruption in their schooling, as well as experience stress in response to relocation in terms of adaptation and acculturation while oftentimes experiencing social exclusion and discrimination (Measham et al., 2014).

A child's response to disaster can be influenced by many factors, including the characteristics of the disaster and exposure to it, individual characteristics, family factors, and the social environment. Of the demographic variables studied, including gender and age, results are inconsistent. Ethnic minority youth may be at greater risk for maladaptive stress reactions; however, the extent to which this may also be due to socioeconomic status, exposure to other traumatic events, and other family factors is unclear. In addition, exposure to other trauma has also been found to contribute to disaster-related posttraumatic stress (Pfefferbaum & North, 2008). For adolescents, perceived social support has been associated with postdisaster adjustment.

The personality and temperament of the child are also associated with risk for psychiatric symptoms. Children often appear to cope well initially, and adverse reactions may not be apparent for weeks to months later. Children who have trauma histories or unstable family lives are particularly vulnerable to reactivation of psychiatric symptomatology. Thus, those having preexisting emotional and family problems will likely need greater support and counseling in the aftermath of a disaster.

It is particularly important for helpers to be aware that there is also a wide range of emotional and physiological reactions that children of differing ages may also display following a disaster. Clearly, children of all ages find comfort and stabilization in the routines of daily life. Family interactions, going to school, playing with friends—these activities provide structure to the child's world. When disasters interrupt this routine, we can expect that children may become scared, anxious, and confused. Interventions that can support consistency and familiarity will help to facilitate adaptive coping and mitigate the impact of trauma. Refer to Table 9.1 for reactions and supportive response by developmental level.

Older Adults

Older adults are particularly vulnerable to loss. Factors such as age and disability affect vulnerability to a disaster. Both of these vulnerability traits are apparent in the elderly population. They are often lacking in social supports, may be financially disadvantaged, and are traditionally reluctant to accept offers of help. Older adults are also more likely to have preexisting medical conditions that may be exacerbated, either directly because of the emotional and psychological stress, or because of disruptions to their care, such as loss of medications or needed medical equipment, changes in primary care providers, lack of continuity of care, or lack of consistency in self-care routines due to relocation. Over 70% of the fatalities from Hurricane Katrina occurred in individuals over age 65 (Donner & Rodriguez, 2011). Older women are at particularly high risk for PTSD in that they live longer than men, are more likely to be widowed, have limited social supports, and are disproportionately more likely to be victims of crimes such

as muggings and robberies (Lantz & Buchalter, 2003). In any event where there is personal loss and disruption in routine, there is an increase in anxiety symptoms. With financial loss and disrupted daily routines, there is an observed increase in PTSD symptoms, while depression is associated with evacuation and relocation in the elderly (Bei et al., 2013).

Loss of irreplaceable possessions—photographs, mementos, and heirlooms—often have even greater meaning and value for older adults and are irreplaceable. Disasters may serve as a reminder of the fragility and ultimate finality of life. Older adults may also be more likely to withhold information or refuse help due to fears of losing their independence. Institutionalization remains a real concern among senior citizens who suffer the trauma of a disaster. The frail elderly are especially vulnerable to relocation stress and may experience exacerbations of chronic health problems. Disorientation can occur when the frail elderly are moved to unfamiliar surroundings, especially without substantial support from caregivers. Visiting psychiatric nurses following a disaster are important as they provide additional screening, support, and follow-up to the relocated elderly without the elderly having to travel to access the resources.

The Seriously Mentally Ill

According to Austin and Godleski (1999), the most psychologically vulnerable people are those with a prior history of psychiatric disturbances. Although previous psychiatric history does not significantly raise the risk of PTSD, exacerbations of preexisting chronic mental disorders, such as bipolar and depressive disorders, are often increased in the aftermath of a disaster. Those with a chronic mental illness are particularly susceptible to the effects of severe stress, as they may be marginally stable and may lack adequate social support to buffer the effects of the terror, bereavement, or dislocation.

Utilizing existing community resources that already have established relationships with this population can be particularly effective. For example, assertive community treatment (ACT) teams played a vital role in maintaining connections with those who were most vulnerable to the effects of stress following Hurricane Hugo. In the 3 months following the hurricane, not one ACT recipient required a psychiatric hospitalization (Lachance, Santos, & Burns, 1994). However, it is vitally important to provide regular visits to those institutions that are providing care to those with severe mental illness following a conflict as neglect and abuse of people in institutions is common in emergencies. Safety, basic physical needs (water, food, shelter, sanitation, and medical care), human rights surveillance, and basic psychiatric and psychosocial care must be provided throughout the crisis (van Ommerer et al., 2015, p. 500).

Cultural and Ethnic Subgroups

Sensitivity to the cultural and ethnic needs of survivors and the bereaved is key not only in understanding reactions to stress and grief but also in implementing effective interventions. Mental health outreach teams need to include bilingual, multicultural staff and translators who are able to interact effectively with survivors and the bereaved. Whenever possible, it is preferable to have bilingual staff or trained translators rather than relying solely on family

TABLE 9.1 Common Reactions in Children and Adolescents in Response to Tragedy and Ways to Help

Common Reactions by Age	Ways for Adults to Help
Infants and toddlers will react to trauma in response to the distress of their caregivers and degree of separation or disruption in relationship and routines. They may demonstrate separation anxiety, become fussy, develop feeding or sleeping problems, and become easily startled.	Provide physical comfort and maintain routines as much as is possible. Maintain safety at all times—safeguard against taking out one's frustration on a colicky or fussy infant by using other familiar caregivers, if necessary.
Preschool children are extremely dependent on routine and will react strongly to any disruption in their daily routine. They may exhibit mild to extreme helplessness, passivity, and a lack of responsiveness to people and things in their environment. A heightened level of arousal, confusion, and generalized fear may be present. Other symptoms of distress include a lack of verbalization, sleep disturbance, nightmares and night terrors, fear of separation and clinging to caregivers, irritability, excessive crying, and neediness. Somatic complaints may include stomachaches, headaches, and nondescript pains. At this developmental stage, children may have a tendency to assume that the disaster is related to something they did or did not do. This age group is also more likely to relive the traumatic experience in play or behavioral reenactments. Resumption of bed-wetting, thumb-sucking, and clinging to parents is not uncommon.	Avoid unnecessary separations from parents. It is okay for parents to allow children of this age to sleep in their parents' room on a temporary basis. Give plenty of verbal reassurance and physical comfort. Monitor media exposure to disaster trauma. Be honest and give developmentally appropriate explanations about the traumatic event. Provide answers to questions using language they can understand. Reassure children that they did nothing that caused the event to happen. Encourage expression through play activities.
School-aged children are more mature, both cognitively and emotionally, but remain highly vulnerable to events involving loss and stress. School-aged children may present with more classical symptoms of PTSD, as well as depressive and anxiety disorders. However, reactions to stress at this age may also include sleep and appetite disturbances, academic problems, and occasionally behavioral difficulties such as oppositional or aggressive conduct. Behaviors more typical of a younger child may also be seen, such as clinginess or whining, while others may react by withdrawing from friends and familiar activities.	Provide extra physical comfort and reassurance; however, gentle, firm limits should be set for acting out behavior if it occurs. Provide reassurance that they are not responsible for the disaster. Tell children that their feelings are normal and that others feel the same way. Use of puppets, dolls, and other "props" facilitates the expression of anxiety-producing emotions among young children. By assisting children to identify sources of stress and loss, and correct distortions in thinking, a more accurate and realistic perception of the event can be developed by the child. Provide structure by encouraging undemanding home chores, physical exercise, and activities.
Adolescents tend to respond to a disaster much as adults do. However, this may also be accompanied by the awareness of a life unlived, a sense of a foreshortened future, and the fragility of life (Shaw, 2000). Adolescents may also exhibit a decline in academic performance, rebellion at home or school, or delinquency, as well as somatic complaints and social withdrawal. Adolescents may feel a strong need to make a contribution to the recovery effort and find meaningful ways to "make a difference."	In addition to the extra attention and consideration afforded to younger children, teens should be encouraged to resume regular social and recreational activities, and to participate in community recovery work should they so desire. Parents should avoid insisting that they discuss their feelings with them but should encourage them to discuss their disaster experiences with peers or significant adults in their lives.

PTSD, posttraumatic stress disorder.

members because of privacy concerns and the importance of maintaining appropriate family roles and boundaries. The availability of written materials in other languages can also increase access to information for those who do not speak English as their primary language, and can serve as a reminder of information only partially understood at a time of great stress. Many online resources have materials written in languages other than English, and predisaster planning should include identifying known ethnic groups in the community in order to have those materials accessible as needed.

Understanding the local norms, history, and politics can be important in providing culturally appropriate services. Five principles for incorporating culturally sensitive emergency care during a disaster include: understanding that culture is the predominant force in people's lives, that dominant culture serves people in various ways, people have both personal identities and group identities, diversity within cultures can be vast and significant, and that each individual and each group has unique cultural values and needs (Bergeron, 2015). It is often the case in large-scale transportation disasters, such as those involving airplanes, that there are individuals of different cultures. Understanding and addressing the cultural needs of survivors and the bereaved can be complicated by a lack of cultural competence on the part of the responders, as well as separation from usual supports and familiar environments on the part of survivors and the bereaved.

Disaster Relief Personnel

The list of those vulnerable to the psychosocial impact of a disaster does not end with the survivors and the bereaved. Often victims can include emergency personnel: police officers, firefighters, military personnel, Red Cross mass care and shelter workers, cleanup and sanitation crews, the press corps, body handlers, funeral directors, staff at receiving hospitals, and crisis counselors. For example, cleanup and recovery workers at the World Trade Center site were found to suffer debilitating consequences of their work, including depression, drug use, and PTSD, which points to the need to include all personnel contributing to the response efforts in similar preparations as given to first responders (Johnson et al., 2005).

Some studies of PTSD among firefighters and other first responders have found the frequency of PTSD to be 10% to 20%, and that those at greatest risk were those whose occupations were least likely to have disaster training (Sakuma et al., 2015). Clearly, stress-induced symptoms are a hazard of disaster work and can lead to absenteeism and burnout, as well as difficulties in family, work, and social life, and physical and psychiatric disorders. Box 9.2 lists the common stress reactions experienced by disaster workers.

Those medical personnel receiving disaster victims and families at local hospitals can also be affected by the intense emotions of those seeking help. Often, nurses and other medical personnel report for emergency duty after having worked their regular shift. These workers not only treat injured survivors but also provide needed services to the families of the injured.

BOX 9.2 Common Stress Reactions by Disaster Workers

PSYCHOLOGICAL

Denial
Anxiety and fear
Worry about the safety of self or others
Anger
Irritability
Restlessness
Sadness, moodiness, grief, depression
Distressing dreams
Guilt or "survivor guilt"
Feeling overwhelmed, hopeless
Feeling isolated, lost, or abandoned
Apathy

BEHAVIORAL

Change in activity level
Decreased efficiency and effectiveness
Difficulty communicating
Outbursts of anger, frequent arguments, irritability
Inability to rest or "let down"
Change in eating habits
Change in sleeping patterns
Change in patterns of intimacy, sexuality
Change in job performance
Periods of crying
Increased use of alcohol, tobacco, and drugs
Social withdrawal/silence
Vigilance about safety of environment
Avoidance of activities/places that trigger memories

COGNITIVE

Memory problems
Disorientation
Confusion
Slowness of thinking and comprehension
Difficulty calculating, prioritizing, making decisions
Poor concentration
Limited attention span
Loss of objectivity
Unable to stop thinking about disaster
Blaming

PHYSICAL

Increased heart/respiratory rate/blood pressure
Upset stomach, nausea, diarrhea
Change in appetite, change in weight
Sweating or chills
Tremor (hands/lips)
Muscle twitching
"Muffled" hearing
Tunnel vision
Feeling uncoordinated
Proneness to accidents
Headaches
Muscle soreness, lower back pain
"Lump" in the throat
Exaggerated startle reaction
Fatigue
Menstrual cycle changes
Change in sexual desire
Decreased resistance to infection
Flare-up of allergies and arthritis
Hair loss

Source: Myers, D. (1994). *Disaster response and recovery: A handbook for mental health professionals* (SMA Publication No. 94–3010). Washington, DC: U.S. Department of Health and Human Services.

This includes identifying cultural needs, obtaining translators if needed, and facilitating connections to relief organizations. Through all of this, staff must manage their own emotional reactions to the disaster. Secondary traumatization is a hazard that comes with exposure to the horrific stories of the bereaved and injured. Hospital personnel are also subject to the stress of increased workload due to increased admissions and discharges related to triage to make room for the trauma victims, and the need to communicate timely information not only to families but also the request for interviews from members of the media. In addition, the number of individuals requiring treatment does not end with impact—many people will sustain serious injuries in the process of disaster cleanup.

Nurses and other medical professionals may be afraid to show their emotions during the disaster and therefore will often experience profound emotional reactions afterward. There may be a sense of emotional "letdown" followed by an "emotional rollercoaster," in which emotions may vacillate between the euphoria of saving a life to the sadness or anger of losing lives. Psychological first aid and debriefings can assist staff by normalizing these reactions and helping to facilitate staff in identifying their natural support system. Such groups ought not only include doctors and nurses but also x-ray personnel, laboratory staff, and housekeeping. The stress on hospital workers may also continue for some time after the disaster, as those with psychological and physiological manifestations of trauma begin to seek assistance for symptoms they can no longer deny or ignore.

In addition, ongoing support for the mental health counselors at the disaster site is crucial. A study by Lesaca (1996) found that at 4 and 8 weeks after a 1994 airline disaster, trauma counselors experienced significantly more symptoms of PTSD and depression than a comparison group. Fortunately, the only significantly increased symptom after 12 weeks was avoidance behaviors, specifically of situations that aroused memories of the crash.

Vicarious traumatization was a significant problem, however, among mental health disaster workers in the Oklahoma City bombing aftermath (Call & Pfefferbaum, 1999). The impact of the traumatic scenes and the intense emotions of the survivors led to increased physical illness, psychological distress, and absenteeism. Experience in Oklahoma indicates that a mental health consultant, separate from those providing direct services, ought to be brought in to provide support to staff, so as not to discourage open sharing of personal feelings and reactions. The use of early career therapists, with little personal or professional experience in dealing with bereavement, was viewed as a mistake by the authors. They recommend that therapists be mature, culturally sensitive, and trained in specific techniques, such as psychological first aid. Similarly, a recent study of counselors responding to the 9/11 terror attack found that higher levels of secondary traumatic stress was associated with a heavier prior trauma caseload, less professional experience, younger age, longer lengths of assignment, and more time spent with child clients, firefighters, or clients who discussed morbid material (Creamer & Liddle, 2005). This indicates that potential recruits need to be informed of the potential risk of secondary traumatic stress; those at risk should have lower risk assignments whenever possible, and ongoing monitoring of counselor exposure to risk should occur at regular intervals during the course of deployment.

COMMUNITY REACTIONS AND RESPONSES

It is important to understand common responses and needs after a disaster, regardless of the type of disaster. It is important to recognize:

1. Everyone who sees or experiences a disaster is affected by it in some way.
2. It is normal to feel anxious about your own safety and that of your family and close friends.
3. Profound sadness, grief, and anger are normal reactions to an abnormal event.
4. Acknowledging your feelings helps you recover.
5. Focusing on your strengths and abilities helps you heal.
6. Accepting help from community programs and resources is healthy.
7. Everyone has different needs and different ways of coping.
8. It is common to want to strike back at people who have caused great pain. (Department of Homeland Security, 2016, "Understand Disaster Events")

For children, schools provide a key opportunity for outreach as teachers and principals are in contact with students throughout the day, and they are in an excellent position to disseminate information, allow expression of feelings, screen children for unusual difficulties, and make referrals when indicated. Both over- and underexposure to the disaster are potential pitfalls that schools can avoid with consultation from professionals. The first step, however, is to have established a preexisting, warm, open consulting relationship between mental health professionals and the schools. Minimally, mental health professionals can work with principals and teachers to see that schools have the latest information about reactions of children to disaster and supplement school counselors on-site when large numbers of children are anticipated to need crisis intervention. In addition, professionals can provide guidance about the age-specific strategies that might be used in discussing a community-wide disaster. The National Child Trauma Stress Network provides a Child Trauma Tool Kit for Educators (2008) that contains many helpful strategies for assisting children after exposure to a traumatic event. Screening of requests for resources and assistance by a committee that includes a disaster mental health professional can assist schools in identifying resources consistent with their needs as well as accepted standard practices.

Large-group preventive techniques for children have been used for some time in California during the aftermath of community-wide trauma (Eth, 1992). This type of school-based intervention occurs as soon after the event as possible, and follows three phases:

1. Preconsultation—identifying the need; preparing the intervention with school authorities
2. Consultation in class—introduction, open discussion (fantasy), focused discussion (fact), free drawing task, drawing or story exploration, reassurance and redirection, recap, sharing of common themes, and return to school activities
3. Postconsultation—follow-up with school personnel and triage/referrals, as needed

(See Case Study 9.2 for an example of a school mental health consultation in the wake of community-wide response to a victim of murder.)

Mourning, Milestones, and Anniversaries

The normal process of mourning is often facilitated by the use of rituals, such as funerals, memorials, and events marking key time intervals, such as anniversaries. It is important to include the community in the services, as well as the immediate family members. Community-wide ceremonies can serve to mobilize the supportive network of friends, neighbors, and caring citizens and provide a sense of belonging, remembrance, and letting go, as was recently demonstrated after the 2017 Las Vegas shootings where 58 victims were killed and over 400 wounded by a shooter (Munks, 2017). Websites and social media groups link the bereaved and can also provide special support during important anniversaries or milestones. Ceremonies or memorials in schools should be developmentally appropriate and involve students in the planning process. Websites and pages to be created in the aftermath of a disaster serve as a place for people, both directly and indirectly impacted, to express their condolences and offer support.

Many different terms have been used to describe grief and grieving. Understanding the various nuances in meaning can be helpful in properly identifying and labeling the experiences and reactions of survivors and relatives of the deceased. Grief is the internal, emotional response to loss, affliction, or regret. It is a normal reaction and is experienced by virtually all disaster survivors. Mourning is the external expression of grief as seen in traditional or creative rituals, especially for the dead. Disaster survivors may also mourn other losses, such as material possessions, homes, and jobs. Bereavement is the state of having lost something, whether it be significant others, significant things, or a sense of self and well-being. It is generally ascribed to family members of disaster victims. Depression refers to a state of feeling sad or, more specifically, is an emotional disorder marked by sadness, inactivity, difficulty in thinking and concentrating, and feelings of dejection. Feeling sad is a common reaction to disaster, but clinical depression is a much less frequent occurrence, depending on the nature of the disaster (see Box 9.3 for a list of the normal manifestations of grief).

Working with the bereaved is a common need following virtually every disaster because loss is such a predominant theme. Grief counselors facilitate the normal process of mourning by assisting individuals to express emotions, begin to detach from the deceased, and eventually, to reinvest in life—including the possibility of another close relationship. The phases of the mourning process have much in common with the emotional phases of disaster recovery, and Worden (1982) has identified specific tasks that need to be accomplished at each phase of mourning for successful resolution:

Period of shock, or "numbness." The task is to accept the reality of the loss (as opposed to denying the reality of the loss).

Reality, or "yearning," and "disorganization and despair." The tasks are to accept the pain of grief (as opposed to not feeling the pain of the loss) and to adjust to an environment in which the deceased is missing (as opposed to not adapting to the loss).

Recovery, or "reorganized behavior." The task is to reinvest in new relationships (as opposed to not loving).

One indicator of mourning coming to an end is when one is able to think of the deceased person or loss without

---

BOX 9.3 Normal Manifestations of Grief

FEELINGS

Sadness
Anger
Guilt and self-reproach
Anxiety
Loneliness
Fatigue
Helplessness
Shock (most often after sudden death)
Yearning (for the deceased person)
Emancipation
Relief
Numbness

THOUGHTS

Disbelief
Confusion
Preoccupation
Sense of presence
Hallucinations

PHYSICAL SENSATIONS

Hollowness in stomach
Tightness in chest
Tightness in throat
Oversensitivity to noise
Sense of depersonalization/derealization
Breathlessness, shortness of breath
Weakness in muscles
Lack of energy
Dry mouth

BEHAVIORS

Sleep disturbance
Appetite disturbance
Absentmindedness
Social withdrawal
Avoiding reminders (of deceased)
Dreams of deceased
Searching, calling out
Restless overactivity
Crying
Treasuring objects
Visiting places/carrying objects of
    remembrance

Source: Worden, J. W. (1982). *Grief counseling and grief therapy: A handbook for the mental health practitioner.* New York, NY: Springer Publishing.

pain or the intense physical sensations. Another is when the survivor can reinvest his or her emotions into life and the living. In some ways, however, mourning never ends; only as time goes on, it manifests itself less frequently and with less intensity. Old losses are mourned again with each new loss and life transition.

SUMMARY

The psychosocial impact of a disaster and the resources that will be needed to respond to the disaster can be estimated based on data from past experiences with a variety of natural and man-made disasters. Normal reactions to abnormal events include a range of distressing thoughts, emotions, sensations, and behaviors, which are different than the characteristics of a mental illness. However, early outreach can set the stage for those at risk of a psychiatric disorder to accept help in the future, should it be needed. Children display a variety of reactions that are normal given the extreme nature of the stressor and their level of emotional and cognitive maturity. Mental health responders must be culturally competent and attuned to the needs of special populations. In addition, they, along with first responders, disaster workers, and healthcare personnel, are particularly vulnerable to stress-induced symptoms and secondary trauma. Work groups, schools, and entire communities not only react to a disaster but also serve as a conduit for support and psychoeducational information. There is no timetable for grief, and expressions of mourning and bereavement reflect the characteristics of the person, the loss, and the disaster.

STUDY QUESTIONS

1. What are the common psychosocial effects following a major disaster?

2. What are the common psychological reactions to bioterrorism?

3. Describe the normal reactions of children to disasters. Describe the normal reactions of adolescents to disasters.

4. What types of strategies should be used to protect the emotional and psychological well-being of children?

5. Identify populations that may have special needs for mental health services following a disaster. How would you attempt to meet these needs?

6. What types of reactions do disaster relief workers experience?

7. How can nurses help other nurses deal with the emotional aftermath of a disaster?

8. Describe the purpose of mourning, milestones, and anniversaries in dealing with the aftermath of a disaster.

INTERNET ACTIVITIES

1. Go to the American Academy of Child and Adolescent Psychiatry website at www.aacap.org. Review the section on "Disaster: Helping children cope," and also find the "Facts for Families Guide"; scroll down, click "view all" then "next" until you come to the topic "Terrorism and war: How to talk to children." What are some factors you might need to consider when answering a child's questions about terrorist attacks? What are some suggested supports you might incorporate?

2. Go to the Center for the Study of Traumatic Stress website at www.centerforthestudyoftraumaticstress.org. Click on "Fact Sheets," then click on "Information for Healthcare Provider" and "Preparedness." Then click on "Addressing the Needs of the Seriously Mentally Ill in Disaster." What are some of the losses that a person with a serious mental health disorder may experience during a disaster that is different than the average disaster victim? What are some of the symptoms that are of particular concern and warrant immediate referral?

3. Go to the American Academy of Experts in Traumatic Stress home page at www.aaets.org. Under the "Publications" button, click on the dropdown, "The Trauma Stress Library" and then click on the article, "The role of counseling in an emergency response recovery plan." What are the four signs that a person requires trauma support? Should supervisors insist that all medical and first responder personnel undergo counseling support? Include a rationale for your response.

USEFUL LINKS

American Academy of Child and Adolescent Psychiatry. *Disaster resource center.* www.aacap.org

American Psychiatric Association. *Disaster psychiatry.* www.psych.org

American Psychological Association. *Natural disasters.* www.apa.org

National Association of School Psychologists. *Natural disasters.* www.nasponline.org

National Center for PTSD. *Resources for providers.* www.ptsd.va.gov

Substance Abuse and Mental Health Services Administration. *Resources to help cope with a traumatic event.* www.samhsa.gov

The National Child Traumatic Stress Network. *Psychological first aid.* http://nctsn.org

The National Child Trauma Stress Network. *Child Trauma Tool Kit for Educators* http://nctsn.org/resources/audiences/school-personnel/trauma-toolkit

World Health Organization. *Clinical management of mental, neurological, and substance use conditions in humanitarian emergencies.* http://apps.who.int/iris/bitstream/10665/162960/1/9789241548922_eng.pdf

REFERENCES

Antevy, P., & Sobel, R. (2016). From devastation to determination: The heavy burden of pediatric care in the field. *EMS World.* Retrieved from http://

www.emsworld.com/article/12187196/from-devastation-to-determination-the-heavy-burden-of-pediatric-care-in-the-field

Aslam, N., & Tariq, N. (2010). Trauma, depression, anxiety and stress among individuals living in earthquake affected areas. *Pakistan Journal of Psychological Research, 25*(2), 131–148.

Austin, L. S., & Godleski, L. S. (1999). Therapeutic approaches for survivors of disaster. *Psychiatric Clinics of North America, 22*(4), 897–910. doi:10.1016/S0193-953X(05)70132-5

Bei, B., Bryant, C., Gilson, K.-M., Hoh, J., Gibson, P, Komiti, A., ... Judd, F. (2013). A prospective study of the impact of floods on the mental and physical health of older adults. *Aging and Mental Health, 17*(8), 992–1002. doi:10.1080/13607863.2013.799119

Bergeron, W. P. (2015). Considering culture in evacuation planning and consequence management. *Journal of Emergency Management, 13*(2), 87–92. doi:10.5055/jem.2015.0222

Bonanno, G. A., Rennicke, C., & Dekel, S. (2005). Self-enhancement among high-exposure survivors of the September 11th terrorist attack: Resilience or social maladjustment? *Journal of Personality and Social Psychology, 88*(6), 984–998. doi:10.1037/0022-3514.88.6.984

Call, J. A., & Pfefferbaum, B. (1999). Lessons learned from the first two years of Project Heartland, Oklahoma's mental health response to the 1995 bombing. *Psychiatric Services, 50*(7), 953–955. doi:10.1176/ps.50.7.953

Creamer, T. L., & Liddle, B. J. (2005). Secondary traumatic stress among disaster mental health workers responding to the September 11th attacks. *Journal of Traumatic Stress, 18*(1), 89–96. doi:10.1002/jts.20008

Dávila, A., & Rushing, K. (2017, October 2). "People are getting desperate" in Puerto Rico as federal response not equal to the crisis [Web log post]. Retrieved from https://earthjustice.org/blog/2017-september/people-are-getting-desperate-in-puerto-rico-as-federal-response-not-equal-to-the-crisis?gclid=EAIaIQobChMI8dD7nrj61gIVXZ7ACh09KA5tEAMYAiAAEgJZa_D_BwE

Department of Homeland Security. (2016). Coping with disaster. Retrieved from https://www.ready.gov/coping-with-disaster

Dickerson, C. (2017, October 16). Stranded by Maria, Puerto Ricans get creative to survive. *The New York Times.* Retrieved from https://www.nytimes.com/2017/10/16/us/hurricane-maria-puerto-rico-stranded.html

Donner, W., & Rodriguez, H. (2011). Disaster risk and vulnerability: The role and impact of population and society. Population Reference Bureau. Retrieved from http://www.prb.org/Publications/Articles/2011/disaster-risk.aspx

Elangovan, A. R., & Kasi, S. (2014). Psychosocial disaster preparedness for school children by teachers. *International Journal of Disaster Risk Reduction, 12,* 119–124. doi:10.1016/j.ijdrr.2014.12.007

Eth, S. (1992). Clinical response to traumatized children. In L. S. Austin (Ed.), *Responding to disaster: A guide for mental health professionals* (pp. 101–124). New York, NY: American Psychiatric Press.

Foa, E. B., Cahill, S. P., Boscarino, J. A., Hobfall, S. E., Lahad, M., McNally, R. J., & Solomon, Z. (2005). Social, psychological, and psychiatric interventions following terrorist attacks: Recommendations for practice and research. *Neuropsychopharmacology, 30,* 1806–1817. doi:10.1038/sj.npp.1300815

Goldmann, E., & Galea, S. (2014). Mental health consequences of disasters. *Annual Review of Public Health, 35,* 169–183. doi:10.1146/annurev-publhealth-032013-182435

Hobfoll, S. E., Watson, P., Bell, C. C., Bryant, R. A., Brymer, M. J., Friedman, M. J., ... Ursano, R. J. (2007). Five essential elements of immediate and mid-term mass trauma intervention: Empirical evidence. *Psychiatry, 70*(4), 283–315. doi:10.1521/psyc.2007.70.4.283

Holloway, H. C., Norwood, A. E., Fullerton, C. S., Engel, C. C., & Ursano, R. J. (2002). The threat of biological weapons: Prophylaxis and mitigation of psychological and social consequences. *Journal of the American Medical Association, 278*(5), 425–427. doi:10.1001/jama.1997.03550050087038

Johnson, S. B., Langlieb, A. M., Teret, S. P., Gross, R., Schwab, M., Massa, J., ... Geyh, A. S. (2005). Rethinking first response: Effects of the clean up and recovery effort on workers at the World Trade Center disaster site. *Journal of Occupational and Environmental Medicine, 47*(4), 386–391. doi:10.1097/01.jom.0000158722.57980.4a

Lachance, K. R., Santos, A. B., & Burns, B. J. (1994). The response of an assertive community treatment team program following a natural disaster.

Community Mental Health Journal, 30(5), 505–515. doi:10.1007/BF02189066

Lantz, M. S., & Buchalter, E. N. (2003). Posttraumatic stress disorder: When older adults are victims of severe trauma. *Clinical Geriatrics, 11*(4), 30–33.

Larrance, R., Anastario, M., & Lawry, L. (2007). Health status among internally displaced persons in Louisiana and Mississippi travel trailer parks. *Annals of Emergency Medicine, 49,* 590–501. doi:10.1016/j.annemergmed.2006.12.004

Lesaca, T. (1996). Symptoms of stress disorder and depression among trauma counselors after an airline disaster. *Psychiatric Services, 47*(4), 424–426. doi:10.1176/ps.47.4.424

McLaughlin, K. A., Fairbank, J. A., Gruber, M. J., Jones, R. T., Lakoma, M. D., Pfefferbaum, B., ... Kessler, R. C. (2009). Serious emotional disturbance among youths exposed to Hurricane Katrina 2 years postdisaster. *Journal of the American Academy of Child and Adolescent Psychiatry, 48*(11), 1069–1078. doi:10.1097/CHI.0b013e3181b76697

Measham, T., Guzder, J. G., Rousseau, C., Pacione, L., Blais-McPherson, M., & Nadeau, L. (2014). Refugee children and their families: Supporting psychological well-being and positive adaption following migration. *Current Problems in Pediatric and Adolescent Health Care, 44,* 208–215. doi:10.1016/j.cppeds.2014.03.005

Munks, J. (2017, October 15). Thousands walk on strip to remember Las Vegas shooting victims. *Las Vegas Review-Journal.* Retrieved from https://www.reviewjournal.com/local/the-strip/thousands-walk-on-strip-to-remember-las-vegas-shooting-victims

National Child Traumatic Stress Network Schools Committee. (2008). Child trauma toolkit for educators. Retrieved from http://nctsn.org/resources/audiences/school-personnel/trauma-toolkit

Neria, Y., & Shultz, J. M. (2012). Mental health effects of Hurricane Sandy: Characteristics, potential aftermath, and response. *Journal of the American Medical Asssociation, 308*(24), 2571–2572. doi:10.1001/jama.2012.110700

Osofsky, H. J., Osofsky, J. D., Kronenberg, M., Brennan, A., & Hansel, T. C. (2009). Posttraumatic stress symptoms in children after Hurricane Katrina: Predicting the need for mental health services. *American Journal of Orthopsychiatry, 79,* 212–220. doi:10.1037/a0016179

Pfefferbaum, B., & North, C. (2008). Children and families in the context of disasters: Implications for preparedness and response. *The Family Psychologist, 24,* 6–10. doi:10.1901/jaba.2008.24-6

Price, M. (2010, September). A mental health crisis unfolds: Psychologists' research points the way to healing after the Gulf oil spill. *Monitor on Psychology, 41*(8), 16.

Sakuma, A., Takahashi, Y., Ueda, I., Sato, H., Katsura, M., Abe, M., ... Matsumoto, K. (2015). Post-traumatic stress disorder and depression prevalence and associated risk factors among local disaster relief and reconstruction workers fourteen months after the Great East Japan earthquake: A cross-sectional study. *BioMed Central Psychiatry, 15,* 58. doi:10.1186/s12888-015-0440-y

Shaw, J. A. (2000). Children, adolescents and trauma. *Psychiatric Quarterly, 71*(3), 227–243.

Sim, T., & Cui, K. (2015). Psychosocial needs assessment and interventions in a Chinese post-disaster community. *Health and Social Work, 40*(4), 329–332. doi:1093/hsw/hiv061

Ursano, R. J. & Norwood, A. E., & Fullerton, C. S. (Eds.). (2004). Bioterrorism: Psychological and public health interventions. Cambridge, United Kingdom: Cambridge University Press. Retrieved from https://books.google.com/books?hl=en&lr=&id=qKPofdNV2C8C&oi=fnd&pg=PA2&dq=Psychological+responses+to+bioterrorism&ots=s4M-_1xosb&sig=5-N1wJKkp8tJZeSR9q4d6BFKJ0A#v=onepage&q=Psychological%20responses%20to%20bioterrorism&f=false

U.S. Department of Health and Human Services. (2004). *Mental health response to mass violence and terrorism: A training manual* (HHS Pub. No. SMA 3959). Rockville, MD: Center for Mental Health Services, Substance Abuse and Mental Health Administration.

U.S. Department of Veteran Affairs: National Center for PTSD. (2016). Mental health reactions after disaster. Retrieved from https://www.ptsd.va.gov/professional/trauma/disaster-terrorism/terrorist_attacks_and_children.asp

van Ommeren, M., Hanna, F., Weissbecker, I, & Ventevogel, P. (2015). Mental health and psychosocial support in humanitarian emergencies.

Eastern Mediterranean Health Journal, 21(7), 498–502. doi:10.26719/2015.21.7.498

Vlahov, D., Galea, S. Resnick, H., Ahern, J., Boscarino, J. A., Bucuvalas, M., ... Kilpatrick, D. (2002). Increased use of cigarettes, alcohol, and marijuana among Manhattan, New York residents after the September 11th terrorist attacks. *American Journal of Epidemiology, 155*(11), 988–996. doi:10.1093/aje/155.11.988

Voelker, R. (2006). Katrina's impact on mental health likely to last years. *Journal of the American Medical Association, 294*(13), 1599–1600. doi:10.1001/jama.294.13.1599

Wessely, S., Hyams, K. C., & Bartholomew, R. (2001). Psychological implications of chemical and biological weapons. *British Medical Journal, 323,* 878–879. doi:10.1136/bmj.323.7318.878

Worden, J. W. (1982). *Grief counseling and grief therapy: A handbook for the mental health practitioner.* New York, NY: Springer Publishing.

World Health Organization. (2017). Addressing the silent impact of war: WHO expands mental health care services across Syria. Retrieved from http://www.emro.who.int/syr/syria-news/who-expands-mental-health-care-services-across-syria.html

---

CASE STUDY 9.1

A Personal Perspective on the Resilience of Katrina and Tsunami Survivors

Lynne MacConnell

In September 2005, I spent 2 weeks as an independent volunteer at Kelly Air Force Base in San Antonio, Texas, where between 2,000 and 4,000 Katrina evacuees were cared for daily. I worked along with local professionals in a satellite mental health clinic at the base. We spent time "roaming" in the huge dormitories to talk with folks informally, provide support, and identify individuals and families who might benefit from more specific services in the clinic itself. In the clinic, we provided assessments of mental health needs; arranged for assistance with practical matters such as securing prescriptions; provided counseling around issues such as insomnia, flashbacks, and anxiety; and provided support as people "told their stories" of horror.

The people we worked with in the clinic included people with severe and persistent mental illness who were being treated prior to Katrina. Many of these folks came seeking refills of their medications, or depot injections for their antipsychotics, knowing that their stress level was leading to potential or current exacerbation of symptoms. Others, without any previous psychiatric history, came seeking help for symptoms they had never experienced before. Many told of sleepless nights, increasing anxiety and agitation, poor appetite, and feelings of depression and uncertainty about the future.

The severity of these symptoms in the aftermath of the flooding and the chaotic and uncertain rescue conditions was compounded by the living conditions in the dorms. Several hundred people slept in each dorm with cots laid head to head and side by side, with no provision for privacy and no screen against the noise of such crowded conditions. Despite what these evacuees had experienced prior to their arrival and during their stay in the shelter situation, their overall response was generally one of gratitude for the help they were receiving. People I had not worked with approached me in the hallways and dorms to say, "Thank you for what you are doing." Individuals in the clinic were uniformly grateful for the assistance they were offered. Most of these folks had lost everything they had owned; some were still awaiting word on what had happened to other family members; and many already knew they had lost loved ones. Most were uncertain about what their future held.

The stories of two individuals with whom I worked stand out for me. One was a 60-year-old gentleman named Donald who was diagnosed with schizophrenia. He appeared outside the clinic door one morning. He appeared exhausted, discouraged, and anxious. He was reluctant to come in but agreed to talk with me in the hallway. He related that he had been seen in the clinic a week earlier and been given prescriptions for his antipsychotic medication. The prescriptions had been sent to the emergency pharmacy, but as he went daily to pick up his medications, he had been told that either the medications were not ready or that he was no longer in the computer. Donald had not slept for several nights, which he attributed in part to not having his medication. I invited him to come into the clinic and register so we could give him new prescriptions. He just shook his head no and said, "It wouldn't do any good this time either." I was able to keep him talking to me in the hallway long enough so that eventually he began to relate to me in a way that allowed me to convince him to come in for new prescriptions and start over.

While he was waiting to be seen by the psychiatrist, he overheard me talking with another staff member about how to distribute a large number of Beanie Babies that a friend had sent with me to San Antonio. When I finished talking, Donald motioned for me to come sit by him again in the waiting area. He said, "I couldn't help overhearing what you were saying. Do you think I could have a couple of those dolls for my wife? She is diabetic and depressed and I think those Beanie Babies would help to cheer her up." Of course I replied that he could have the dolls. The next day, while roaming in the dorms, I came across the cots where Donald and his wife were staying. He called me over to meet his wife and she expressed her gratitude for the dolls propped up on her pillow. The expressions on their faces represented the return of hope for this couple and the love of a man for

(continued)

his wife in the midst of despair. Fortunately, by this time, he had also obtained the medication that he needed.

The second story is that of Robin. Robin was 53 years old and had no previous psychiatric history. As she registered, she began to cry, with silently flowing tears and then with her body convulsing with sobs. She was unable to talk. After sitting with me in this state for several minutes, she started to choke out phrases, "I can't take a shower," "I can't flush the toilet," "I can't be around water." I said, "You were in the floodwaters?" She described walking from her home for 3.5 days looking for food for her children. She was in water up to her neck. The water was murky so she couldn't see her feet. Several times she lost her footing and started to slip under the waters. Since she couldn't swim, she was terrified that she would drown and that her children would be left alone. Now she couldn't be near water, she couldn't sleep, and she was afraid of letting her children see how afraid she was.

As Robin told her story, she began to calm down and respond to support. I was able to assure her that her reactions were normal, that it was alright to cry in front of her children and thereby give them permission to express their emotions. After some time she was able to tell me something about her life prior to Katrina, her work as a cook in a four-star hotel, her accomplishment of buying a house for her family the previous year, and her love of her family. Robin clearly responded to an opportunity to tell her story, to understand that her reactions were normal in an abnormal situation, and to identify her strengths from the past for use in the future.

Three months after my work in San Antonio, I traveled to India with a team of 16 nonprofessional short-term missionaries. Our task was to be family for 52 tsunami orphans at Christmastime and to be with them during the first anniversary of their losses. On the plane over, I wondered to myself what we could possibly do to help these children, most of whom did not speak English. I had no experience working professionally with children, and my role on this trip was not a professional one. Once we arrived at the orphanage, however, the children from our team led the way in connecting immediately with the orphans, without language, on the playground.

Taking our lead from them, the adults broke out toys and games we had brought with us. Soon we were laughing and hugging and playing together. The next day, one of the children told us through an interpreter, "We are so happy you came to be with us all the way from America and we were amazed that you adults took time to play with us." Other "play" opportunities included taking the children to a Pizza Hut, which they had never before experienced, and treating them to a day at a water park, where they began to learn that water could be fun instead of a terrifying and deadly experience. More serious activities included asking the children to draw their experience of the tsunami and then explain their pictures to us. The pictures were graphic and horrifying, but the children clearly found release in the activity and in talking about their experiences in the presence of people they knew cared about them.

We also participated with the children in a memorial service on the first anniversary of the tsunami, the last day of our stay. I had been asked to talk about my personal experience of grief and loss in the death of my husband in the same week as the tsunami. I shared some of my experience while also emphasizing the differences in their losses being so unpredictable, sudden, and premature. Knowing the burden of guilt that many carried in addition to their grief, I emphasized the normalcy of guilt as part of grief and the importance of finding ways to resolve that sense of guilt. As I talked about this piece of guilt, the children's eyes were glued to me with what seemed a sense of connection and relief. I thought of the story one boy of 8 had told of holding the hands of two siblings, aged 1 and 2 and his inability to hold on to them through the swirling waves. And of the boy of 14 who was so traumatized by his inability to save his grandparents who drowned before his eyes, that he was mute for 4 months when he first arrived at the orphanage.

In the week we spent at the orphanage it was clear that although the children were still scarred by their heavy burdens of grief and guilt, they were healing. They were responding to the day-to-day care provided (often in better living conditions than they had ever experienced, since they were untouchables from poor fishing villages along the coast), to the love of people who truly cared for them, to the structure of education that most had not enjoyed before, and to the therapeutic interventions that were being provided.

School-Mental Health Collaboration

Kathleen Coyne Plum

In early 1997, a 6-year-old girl named "Samantha" disappeared, allegedly on her way to school. Missing posters were visible throughout this rural western New York County. The entire community responded by participating in several large-scale search efforts in subzero weather. When the ground thawed that spring, her body was found by a farmer plowing his field late on the Friday before Memorial Day weekend. The girl's mother's boyfriend was the prime suspect in the murder.

The school already had a previous working relationship with the county mental health provider and opened the school on Saturday for counseling. That Saturday also provided an opportunity for mental health professionals, the principal, and teachers to develop a comprehensive and collaborative strategy for assisting children the next school day. A letter was drafted to parents, informing them of the event and the plans the school had made. Bus drivers also received information about the tragedy and what to do if a child had a problem. A mental health intensive case manager for children and youth and the school psychologist, who lived in the neighborhood, rode the school bus Tuesday morning; the principal greeted the children as they exited the buses. Teachers and retired teachers from that school were visible, friendly faces in the hallways. Retired teachers were also available to spell teachers who may have themselves felt drained or in need of a break.

The principal held a crisis meeting with teachers Tuesday morning before class, with mental health counselors present to provide information and answer questions. Access to the building was monitored, and the press was given information only through designated spokespersons (the principal and the mental health coordinator). Memory boxes were created in classrooms, in which students could submit writings or drawings expressing their feelings about Samantha. A sundial was later selected as a permanent memorial for the elementary school courtyard. At the end of the day on Thursday—the day of the memorial service for the family, the school, and the community—a debriefing was held with teachers and counselors that focused on a review of how the situation was handled. Overwhelmingly, teachers felt that the event had gone smoothly and that children and parents seemed to find the experience supportive and emotionally beneficial.

Five mental health counselors were available to meet with individuals or groups referred by teachers on the Saturday after Samantha's body was found, the first day back to school, and the day of the memorial service. Forty-seven children received 58 contacts; 7% of contacts included a parent; 24% occurred on an individual basis; and 69% occurred in a group setting. Almost half of contacts (49%) resulted in a referral to the school psychologist for ongoing monitoring and counseling. By far, most of the children referred were girls (79%). Elementary and middle schoolers, being housed in the same building, were equally affected.

A range of emotions, behaviors, and issues were manifested by the children during contacts with the counselors. Those most commonly encountered were sadness; fear, anxiety, or worry; loss and grief (present as well as past); vulnerability or lack of safety; guilt; powerlessness; anger and frustration; clinginess; teasing or provocative behavior; physical aggression; confusion; withdrawal; listlessness; difficulty concentrating; parental divorce, conflict, violence, or drug use; flight (wanting to go home); and fidgetiness or hyperactivity.

This poem, written by the second-grade class and their teacher, and poignantly read at the memorial service by two little girls, illustrates the effect of a traumatic event on the most vulnerable:

Little Girls
Little girls are full of giant-sized dreams,
happiness, and joy.
Little girls give us reasons to love and laugh.
Little girls play with their friends in a fun way.
Little girls make us believe in yesterday.
Little girls are proud of who they are and what
they can be.
Samantha will always be a little girl.

10

MANAGEMENT OF THE PSYCHOSOCIAL EFFECTS OF DISASTERS

Susan M. S. Carlson, Elizabeth C. Meeker, Kathleen Coyne Plum, and Tener Goodwin Veenema

LEARNING OBJECTIVES

When this chapter is completed, readers will be able to:

1. Discuss the role of the mental health professional on the disaster team.
2. Describe the psychosocial training needs of all disaster responders.
3. Describe helpful interventions for use with survivors of a disaster.
4. Identify the symptoms that warrant an immediate mental health referral.
5. Describe the hallmarks of acute stress disorder (ASD).
6. Discuss the possible benefits and dangers of psychological debriefing.
7. Identify assessment criteria for complications of grief and stress.
8. Discuss the presentation of posttraumatic stress disorder (PTSD) in children and adults.
9. Identify evidence-based practices for the treatment of PTSD.

KEY MESSAGES

Psychiatric nurses play a critical role on disaster response teams.
Many events are primarily mental health disasters.
Psychological triage identifies those at greatest risk for psychiatric complications.
Crisis intervention and social support are key elements of psychological first aid.
ASD experienced in the immediate aftermath of a disaster increases risk for later PTSD.

Early identification and intervention of psychiatric disorders can prevent subsequent disability.
Cognitive behavioral therapy for ASD may speed recovery and prevent PTSD.
Managing psychosocial effects after impact may become a long-term treatment goal for several years postdisaster.

CHAPTER OVERVIEW

The management of psychosocial effects begins with a sound plan to mitigate the adverse impact of the disaster on the emotional, cognitive, and behavioral capacity of the individual. Involvement of mental health professionals, such as psychiatric nurse practitioners and clinical nurse specialists, should begin with the development of the community or agency disaster plan. Utilizing "psychological first aid" through assistance with problem solving, stress management, and "normalization" of the emotional response can prepare the individual for the challenges yet to be faced, and in some instances, prevent frustration from escalating to maladaptive or dangerous behaviors. Also, when symptoms reach the severity of a diagnosable psychiatric disorder, early identification and treatment are essential if the individual's decline in social and occupational functioning is to be contained and quickly reversed. Longer-term psychological recovery can take months to years, depending on the scope and nature of the disaster. Cognitive behavioral therapies have been found to be an effective treatment of acute stress reactions as well as posttraumatic stress. Psychological debriefing, when used as an educational tool, can assist first responders to share feelings and coping strategies, although rigorous research into the effectiveness of debriefing is generally lacking. Evaluation through a postdisaster review process is the key to understanding the effectiveness of mental health services for individuals and groups, as well as the strengths, weaknesses, and gaps in the response of the mental health services as a system.

A mental health disaster plan is an essential part of any community disaster plan. The response of the public mental health system to the Twin Towers disaster on September 11 (9/11) was exceptionally rapid and extensive, primarily because of the planning that had occurred in anticipation of possible Y2K terrorism during the New Year's Eve celebration at Times Square in Manhattan. Within an hour of the first plane crashing into the World Trade Center, the mental health disaster command team was set up in Manhattan at the Port Authority. Mental health workers initially manned Ground Zero, as well as the family assistance centers around the clock. After the initial impact, mental health workers were available during peak times. Once it became evident that there were very few bodies to be recovered, local and regional psychiatric centers that had initially cleared facility space to be used as temporary morgues, instead provided food and beds for rescuers who otherwise might not

have had even minimal nourishment and rest during the first feverish days of search for survivors.

It is essential to ensure that rescuers do not deplete their psychological reserves, and that they get adequate sleep and food. This stress reduction strategy needs to be constantly promoted among the workers who become so absorbed in their mission that they fail to take care of their own basic needs. Within the Red Cross system, certified mental health disaster counselors have the authority and the obligation to recommend that volunteers showing signs of psychological distress take a break, and if warranted, can take them off duty against their wishes. In extreme cases, volunteers may be deemed unfit for work and sent home before their tour is up.

Because of the tremendous scope of the Twin Towers disaster, and the fact that there were so few physically injured to care for, 9/11, in actuality, was primarily a mental health disaster. Experience with such disasters has served only to emphasize the importance of recruiting, screening, and training mental health professionals, paraprofessionals, and volunteers in order to have the personnel necessary to respond to the specific short- and long-term needs of those exposed to the disaster (Box 10.1).

BOX 10.1 A Summary of Disaster Mental Health Response Principles

1. No one who experiences a disaster is untouched by it.
2. Most people pull together and function during and after a disaster, but their effectiveness is diminished.
3. Mental health concerns exist in most aspects of preparedness, response, and recovery.
4. Disaster stress and grief reactions are "normal responses to an abnormal situation."
5. Survivors respond to active, genuine interest and concern.
6. Disaster mental health assistance is often more practical than psychological in nature (offering a phone, distributing coffee, listening, encouraging, reassuring, comforting).
7. Disaster relief assistance may be confusing to disaster survivors. They may experience frustration, anger, and feelings of helplessness related to federal, state, and nonprofit agencies' disaster assistance programs. They may reject disaster assistance of all types.

Source: Center for Disease Control and Prevention. (2005). *Disaster mental health primer: Key principles, issues and questions.* Retrieved from https://stacks.cdc.gov/view/cdc/29151/cdc_29151_DS1.pdf

THE MENTAL HEALTH RESPONSE TEAM

Designation of a mental health coordinator is a crucial first step in the formulation of a team. This is the person who will manage and coordinate the mental health response from the command center, decide what resources are needed, activate appropriate mental health agencies, and assign staff to locations such as neighborhood centers, Red Cross shelters (when requested), family assistance centers, schools, hospitals, and so on. This person also monitors field reports regarding the ongoing needs of victims, workers, and counselors, and adapts the plan as events unfold.

The mental health coordinator may also serve as a consultant to agencies or designate a member of the administrative team to provide this function. Based on experience in Oklahoma City, the consultant should be someone other than direct line staff. The immediate responders deployed by the coordinator may include mobile crisis teams, case managers, professionals, and volunteers who have been preapproved. Most Red Cross chapters or regions have a Disaster Mental Health (DMH) team which is made up of independently licensed master's level (or higher) mental health professionals including psychiatrists, psychologists, licensed clinical social workers, marriage and family therapists, professional clinical counselors, nurses with specialty certification, school psychologists, and school counselors. Members of these teams respond at the local level supporting smaller responses like storm-related events and can also be deployed to larger relief operations outside their local area. Within the mission, the DMH team supports not only those directly affected by disaster, but other relief operation volunteers (American Red Cross, 2013). A field coordinator may supervise the staff providing direct services to victims, and provide reports to the command coordinator.

Psychiatric nurses and psychiatrists are particularly well suited as members of the medical team, as they can also be alert to organic mental disorders caused by conditions such as head injuries, toxic exposures, preexisting illnesses, dehydration, or hyper-/hypothermia. Because nurses have a tradition of practice in homes, in schools, and other natural settings, they tend to be readily accepted by members of the community. Agencies and staff that will be activated for counseling and treatment upon referral from the on-site counselors also need to begin preparations for the influx of individuals and the type of psychiatric symptomatology they are most likely to see, based on the estimates of the command coordinator.

Paraprofessionals and volunteers play an extremely vital role in disaster response and recovery. They may be indigenous workers known to the community affected by the disaster, and may share ethnic or religious backgrounds. Psychiatric intensive case managers are critical in maintaining a bridge with the community. In the ensuing aftermath, it is the case manager who provides that consistent, familiar link for children and families in the neighborhood needing referrals for additional services.

Following demobilization, the mental health coordinator conducts a review of the mental health response both separately and in conjunction with the entire disaster response team—medical, rescue, public safety, communications, and transportation. Reviewing the adequacy of the predisaster plan in light of the actual response not only helps to strengthen future planning but also brings a sense of closure to the participants. This procedural review is in addition to the psychological debriefing that may be provided to workers at demobilization.

RECRUITMENT, SCREENING, AND TRAINING

One major task of the mental health coordinator in the planning phase is to recruit and prescreen potential volunteers and staff for credentials, so that they can be a part of the team from the very beginning of the event.

Not everyone, however, is suited for disaster work. Temperament and personal preference must also be taken into account. Those who cannot tolerate the uncertainty and chaos inherent in disaster work ought to consider being available for counseling referrals in a hospital or clinic setting, rather than being part of the immediate response team in the field. Matching the skills and aptitude of individuals with the phase of disaster response can avoid potential pitfalls. Keep in mind, however, that last-minute changes in immediate responders may be necessary if an individual is personally involved in the disaster or is in acute distress for other personal reasons; in such cases, the individual might need to excuse himself or herself. Easing the sense of guilt that those in the helping professions feel when they are unable to respond is an important stress reduction strategy.

Over 90% of the American Red Cross responders are volunteers (American Red Cross, 2017). The Red Cross Disaster Action Team (DAT) Academy is a *free* program that trains individuals to respond and recover from a disaster. The DAT is charged with the initial response for most, if not all, disaster events. Most governmental agencies deploying mental health counselors rely on state-licensing criteria to assure minimum competency. Well-qualified mental health professionals, who have a variety of skills in assessment and intervention, are suited for most types of disaster work; however, the U.S. Department of Health and Human Services (HHS) recommends additional training for all potential responders (medical, mental health, human services, citizen volunteers, et al.) in several areas:

- An understanding of disaster concepts and disaster recovery
- The needs of special populations (i.e., children, the elderly, people with disabilities, ethnic populations)
- Disaster stress symptomatology: normal reactions and when/where/how to refer
- Helpful skills and styles of relating (listening, problem solving, crisis intervention)
- Self-help and stress management skills for disaster survivors
- Recovery resources (HHS, 2015)

There are many reasons, therefore, to rely on well-qualified, as well as well-prepared, mental health practitioners. In the aftermath of 9/11, many well-intentioned but poorly prepared individuals presented themselves as volunteer counselors. Such individuals may actually hamper the work of qualified professionals and rescue personnel and introduce the risk of further traumatizing victims rather than mitigating the effects of the traumatic event. Mental health professionals responding to a disaster need to be familiar with general assessment and intervention strategies and be prepared psychologically and physically for the arduousness of the work. It is crucial that mental health professionals be aware of their own strong emotional reactions to the disaster and the impact it would have on their work, and that they also have access to support and counseling. Perhaps most importantly, mental health workers need to be culturally competent to work with the population they are serving (i.e., know the language, spiritual beliefs, and rituals surrounding loss and bereavement), and need to be briefed about local referral resources. When needed, the mental health professionals on the team can also provide consultation to volunteers and paraprofessionals in instances where a greater knowledge of psychopathology is indicated in the assessment or management of adverse responses.

DISASTER MENTAL HEALTH INTERVENTIONS

Psychological First Aid

Once exposure to a disaster has already occurred, efforts must then be directed toward the reduction of psychological harm. Psychological first aid (PFA) is an evidence-informed approach to assist and support survivors in the immediate aftermath of a disaster. There has recently been a revived interest in PFA, with the main goal being to relieve immediate distress and prevent or minimize the development of pathological sequelae (Math, Nirmala, Moirangthem, & Kumar, 2015, p. 3).

Because most survivors who express early symptoms of distress are likely to recover normally, the goal of the immediate mental health response is to reduce distress, assist with current needs, and promote adaptive functioning. PFA provides a framework to prepare survivors and the bereaved for the emotional challenges that lie ahead, and to identify those individuals and families needing additional follow-up and referral. Education about the normal reactions to extreme stress and traumatic bereavement is an important strategy at both the community and individual levels.

Other steps that can be taken immediately to reduce potential psychological harm include:

The prevention of re-traumatization—limit the number of persons with whom victims must interact in order to receive services, as well as reduce the amount of red tape required. "Telling the story" can be a source of trauma for some individuals; therefore, forcing someone to tell his or her story is contraindicated.

Prevention of new victims—limit the number of people exposed to the sights, the sounds, and the smells of a disaster site, whenever possible. Those who do not need to be at the disaster site should be discouraged from witnessing any of the horror of the aftermath.

Prevention of "pathologizing" distress—avoid labeling normal reactions as pathological to prevent symptoms from being interpreted as a medical condition or disorder that requires treatment. Provide anticipatory guidance about the emotional, cognitive, behavioral, and physiological responses survivors are likely to experience in the coming weeks and months, normalize these reactions, and help survivors to regain perspective and self-confidence. If prepared for these responses, individuals will be less likely to become frightened or overly worried by them.

Identification of individuals showing signs of acute distress—Those who may need immediate medical intervention include individuals with obvious and active physiological stress reactions (exceedingly frantic, panicky, or extremely anger) or individuals who are profoundly shut down (numb, dissociated, disconnected).

Crisis Intervention

Substance Abuse and Mental Health Services Administration [SAMHSA] (2015a, 2015b) recommends that "crisis intervention services should be considered as a first line of emergency management for those potentially affected by large-scale community disasters ... These interventions are meant to 'lend' survivors the strengths needed to decrease their fear responses (thereby calming themselves) and access immediate care and support, allowing them to move to the next stage of recovery" (p. 1). Crisis intervention is still the mainstay of disaster counselors. Crisis intervention is a technique used to assist persons whose coping abilities have been overwhelmed by a stressful event. Most survivors at some point in the evolution of a disaster experience a level of stress so overwhelming that their usual coping is inadequate to meet the need. Two key tools of the crisis/disaster worker are *active listening* and *problem solving*. Active listening allows the disaster worker to establish a sense of respect and trust and to better understand the survivor's situation and needs.

Because survivors are often so overwhelmed by their situation, it is difficult for many to know where to start. Thus, counselors may advise survivors not to make any new or big decisions while undergoing a crisis. While some are immobilized by the stress, others may feel pressured to take some action. Helping individuals to prioritize their energies can be very beneficial, as some might find themselves spending inordinate amounts of time on things they cannot control, while not taking necessary action in matters where they can make a difference to themselves and their families. Counselors at the site of Family Assistance Center in Manhattan found that both they and the survivors had varying tolerances for not being in control, and so there was no "cookie-cutter" approach to help survivors cope with the trauma.

Social Support

Social support networks can provide important affective and material aid that mitigates the adverse effects of disaster trauma (van Ommeren, Hanna, Weissbecker, & Ventevogel, 2015). Thus, mobilizing the natural social support system of family, friends, the faith-based community, and coworkers can be one of the most helpful interventions in the aftermath of a disaster. However, because disruption of one's natural supports is inherent in most disasters, this can require the development of innovative and creative approaches. Social isolation is one of the psychological threats inherent in most disasters as roads may be blocked, landline and cell phone services interrupted, as well as access to the Internet limited. This was the case with Hurricane Harvey in 2017 when more than 3,500 people were rescued from flood waters over 6 days (Cirillo, 2017), and with the northern California wildfires where people fleeing left cell phones and computers behind in their hurry to evacuate and where cell service was disrupted due to cell towers being destroyed by the fires (Nelson, 2017).

The mutual support provided by the trapped Somerset, Pennsylvania coal miners in 2002 played an important role in their survival. They worked as a team to assist the person most vulnerable at the moment, whether that threat was physical (hypothermia) or psychological (hopelessness and despair). This disaster also illustrates how the community members supported one another and the rescuers throughout the ordeal.

The bonds that develop as a result of a disaster can be particularly strong. The bereaved families from the plane that crashed near Somerset, Pennsylvania on 9/11 responded with reciprocal gestures of support to the coal mining community that had so recently responded to their own profound loss with compassion and assistance. Thus, survivors of a disaster can draw great comfort and emotional strength by sharing their experiences with one another, even if not previously acquainted.

Psychological Triage

One of the most important roles of the mental health professional in the immediate aftermath of a disaster is to identify which individuals are most at risk for psychiatric complications and to make referrals for further mental health evaluation and treatment when indicated. Psychiatric difficulties seem to follow a dose-related trajectory—those closest to the event are at greatest risk.

Factors increasing the risk of ASD and PTSD in someone suffering a sufficient precipitating event include the following:

- Loss of a loved one in the event
- Significant injury from the event
- Witnessing of horrendous images
- Dissociation at the time of the traumatic event
- Development of serious depressive symptoms within 1 week that last for 1 month or longer
- Numbness, depersonalization, a sense of reliving the trauma, and motor restlessness after the event
- Preexisting psychiatric problems
- Previous trauma
- Loss of home or community
- Extended exposure to danger
- Toxic exposure
- Absence of social supports, or social supports who were also traumatized and thus are incapable of adequate emotional availability (Lubit, 2016, "Etiology")

Targeting interventions to those at greatest risk is both more efficient and more effective than attempting to provide mental health interventions to everyone who has been exposed.

Mental Health Referrals

Reactions to stress and bereavement should be assessed in greater detail for the presence of a mental disorder if they are significantly distressing to the individual or impair an important aspect of social or occupational functioning. Referrals to a mental health professional ought to be made when one or more of the following symptoms are present (DeWolfe, 2000):

Disorientation—dazed; memory loss; inability to give date or time, state where he or she is, recall events of the past 24 hours, or understand what is happening

Depression—pervasive feelings of hopelessness and despair, unshakable feelings of worthlessness and inadequacy, withdrawal from others, inability to engage in productive activity

Anxiety—constantly on edge, restless, agitated, unable to sleep, frequent frightening nightmares, flashbacks and intrusive thoughts, obsessive fears of another disaster, excessive ruminations about the disaster

Psychosis—hearing voices, seeing visions, delusional thinking, excessive preoccupation with idea or thought, pronounced pressure of speech (e.g., talking rapidly with little content continuity)

Inability to care for self—not eating, bathing, or changing clothes, inability to manage activities of daily life

Suicidal thoughts or plans—expressing indirect or direct thoughts of harming self

Other behaviors of concern—problematic use of alcohol or drugs, domestic violence, child abuse, or elder abuse

Even if a referral is not accepted at the time it is initially made, the trust that has been established early in the aftermath can be crucial to later follow-up.

Factors that may influence whether trauma exposure progresses to PTSD include one's natural resilience, genetic loading, the type of trauma, whether the trauma is natural or man-made, past traumas, and psychiatric comorbidities (Matthews & Mossefin, 2006).

ACUTE STRESS DISORDER

Although a variety of psychiatric disorders may be seen in the aftermath of a disaster, within the first month of a traumatic event, ASD is the disorder most likely to be encountered by the disaster response team. Again, those in closest proximity to the event are at greatest risk. Although lack of social supports, history of childhood traumas, and poor coping skills may increase likelihood of the disorder, ASD can develop in a child or an adult having no predisposing conditions, particularly if the stressor is extreme. Because the likelihood of developing PTSD is elevated for those having ASD, assessment of individuals for the presence of ASD is key to identifying those at high risk for future complications. The prevalence of ASD following exposure to a traumatic event varies greatly, depending on the severity and persistence of the trauma.

Characteristic of the disorder is the development of anxiety, dissociation, and other symptoms occurring within 1 month after the trauma, lasting a minimum of 2 days. If symptoms persist longer than 4 weeks posttrauma, a diagnosis of PTSD should be considered.

The American Psychiatric Association's *Diagnostic and Statistical Manual of Mental Disorders, Fifth Edition (DSM-5)*, lists five specific diagnostic criteria for ASD.

The first criterion is exposure to actual or threatened death, serious injury, or sexual violation in one (or more) of the following ways:

- Directly experiencing the traumatic event(s)
- Witnessing, in person, the event(s) happening to others
- Learning that the event(s) occurred to a close family member or close friend (in cases of actual or threatened death of a family member or friend, the event[s] must have been violent or accidental)
- Experiencing repeated or extreme exposure to aversive details of the traumatic event(s) (e.g., first responders collecting human remains or police officers repeatedly exposed to details of child abuse)

The second criterion is the presence of at least 9 of 14 symptoms from any of five categories—intrusion, negative mood, dissociation, avoidance, and arousal—beginning or worsening after the traumatic event(s) occurred.

Intrusion symptoms include the following:

- Recurrent, involuntary, and intrusive distressing memories of the traumatic event(s); children may engage in repetitive play during which themes or aspects of the traumatic event(s) are expressed
- Recurrent distressing dreams in which the content or affect of the dream is related to the event(s); children may experience frightening dreams without recognizable content
- Dissociative reactions (e.g., flashbacks) in which the individual feels or acts as if the traumatic event(s) were recurring
- Intense or prolonged psychological distress or marked physiological reactions in response to internal or external cues that symbolize or resemble an aspect of the traumatic event(s)

Negative mood consists of the following:

- Persistent inability to experience positive emotions (e.g., inability to experience happiness, satisfaction, or loving feelings)

Dissociative symptoms include the following:

- Altered sense of the reality of one's surroundings or oneself (e.g., seeing oneself from another's perspective, being in a daze, or feeling that time is slowing)
- Inability to remember an important aspect of the traumatic event(s), typically resulting from dissociative amnesia and not from other factors (e.g., head injury, alcohol, or drugs)

Avoidance symptoms include the following:

- Efforts to avoid distressing memories, thoughts, or feelings about or closely associated with the traumatic event(s)
- Efforts to avoid external reminders (e.g., people, places, conversations, activities, objects, or situations) that arouse distressing memories, thoughts, or feelings about or closely associated with the traumatic event(s)

Arousal symptoms include the following:

- Sleep disturbance (e.g., difficulty falling or staying asleep or restlessness during sleep)
- Irritable behavior and angry outbursts (with little or no provocation), typically expressed as verbal or physical aggression toward people or objects
- Hypervigilance
- Problems with concentration
- Exaggerated startle response

The third *DSM-5* diagnostic criterion for ASD is that the duration of the disturbance is 3 days to 1 month after trauma exposure. Although symptoms may begin immediately after a traumatic event, they must last at least 3 days for a diagnosis of ASD to be made.

The fourth criterion is that the disturbance causes clinically significant distress or impairment in social, occupational, or other important areas of functioning.

The fifth and final criterion is that the disturbance cannot be attributed to the physiological effects of a substance (e.g., a medication or alcohol) or another medical condition (e.g., mild traumatic brain injury) and cannot be better explained by a diagnosis of brief psychotic disorder.

ASD may progress to PTSD after 1 month, but it may also be a transient condition that resolves within 1 month of exposure to traumatic event(s) and does not lead to PTSD. In about 50% of people who eventually develop PTSD, the initial presenting condition was ASD. Symptoms of ASD may worsen over the initial month, often as a consequence of ongoing stressors or additional traumatic events (American Psychiatric Association [APA], 2013).

POSTTRAUMATIC STRESS DISORDER

PTSD is a response to a recognizable, serious stressor that is characterized by specific behaviors. At present, in the general population, prevalence rates range between 5% and 10% (U.S. Department of Veterans Affairs [USDVA], National Center for PTSD, 2016a). A diagnosis of PTSD requires that several criteria be met. To be diagnosed with PTSD, an adult must have all of the following for at least 1 month:

- At least one re-experiencing symptom
- At least one avoidance symptom
- At least two arousal and reactivity symptoms
- At least two cognition and mood symptoms

Re-experiencing symptoms include:
- Flashbacks—reliving the trauma over and over, including physical symptoms like a racing heart or sweating
- Bad dreams
- Frightening thoughts

Re-experiencing symptoms may cause problems in a person's everyday routine. The symptoms can start from the person's own thoughts and feelings. Words, objects, or situations that are reminders of the event can also trigger re-experiencing symptoms.

Avoidance symptoms include:

- Staying away from places, events, or objects that are reminders of the traumatic experience
- Avoiding thoughts or feelings related to the traumatic event

Things that remind a person of the traumatic event can trigger avoidance symptoms. These symptoms may cause a person to change his or her personal routine. For example, after a bad car accident, a person who usually drives may avoid driving or riding in a car.

Arousal and reactivity symptoms include:

- Being easily startled
- Feeling tense or "on edge"
- Having difficulty sleeping
- Having angry outbursts

Arousal symptoms are usually constant, instead of being triggered by things that remind one of the traumatic events. These symptoms can make the person feel stressed and angry. They may make it hard to do daily tasks, such as sleeping, eating, or concentrating.

Cognition and mood symptoms include:

- Trouble remembering key features of the traumatic event
- Negative thoughts about oneself or the world
- Distorted feelings like guilt or blame
- Loss of interest in enjoyable activities

Cognition and mood symptoms can begin or worsen after the traumatic event, but are not due to injury or substance use. These symptoms can make the person feel alienated or detached from friends or family members (National Institute of Mental Health, 2016).

Symptoms usually begin early, within 3 months of the traumatic incident, but sometimes they begin years afterward. Symptoms must last more than a month and be severe enough to interfere with relationships or work to be considered PTSD. The course of the illness varies. Some people recover within 6 months, while others have symptoms that last much longer. In some people, the condition becomes chronic.

PTSD in Children

Children and teens can have extreme reactions to trauma, but their symptoms may not be the same as adults. In very young children (less than 6 years of age), these symptoms can include:

- Wetting the bed after having learned to use the toilet
- Forgetting how to or being unable to talk
- Acting out the scary event during playtime
- Being unusually clingy with a parent or other adult

Older children and teens are more likely to show symptoms similar to those seen in adults. They may also develop disruptive, disrespectful, or destructive behaviors. Older children and teens may feel guilty for not preventing injury or deaths. They may also have thoughts of revenge (National Institute of Mental Health, 2016).

INTERVENTIONS WITH SPECIAL POPULATIONS

Children and Youth

It is important when working with children to modify one's language to match the child's developmental level using direct and simple language. For young children it can be helpful to crouch down to their eye level. It can be helpful to assist children with identifying their feelings by providing labels (i.e., mad, sad, worried, scared). It is important to encourage them to express their concerns and ask questions. Adolescents are likely to be more responsive to adult-like requests to address their feelings, concerns, and questions. It is normal for children and adolescents to regress either behaviorally or in their language or speech. It can be helpful to educate parents and caregivers about normal reactions and reinforce use of these strategies to help provide ongoing support to their child(ren).

Children's Disaster Mental Health Concept of Operations Model

The National Children's Disaster Mental Health Concept of Operations (NCDMH CONOPS; Schrieber, 2011) is a resilience-enhancement strategy used by local communities, regions, and states to build a comprehensive mental health response for children and families. Developed at the Terrorism and Disaster Center at the University of Oklahoma Health Sciences Center, the NCDMH CONOPS is the first national model for building a comprehensive response for children in disasters leveraging evidence-based rapid triage and intervention strategies combined with novel DMH incident command strategies. The NCDMH CONOPS includes a continuum of triage-driven, evidence-informed, and evidence-based response strategies including basic PFA delivered by parents, teachers, and other community members.

The NCDMH CONOPS outlines a strategy for "seamless" preparedness, response, and recovery operations. It contains essential elements necessary for an interoperable, coordinated next-generation Incident Command System (ICS) response for the mental health needs of children that can be immediately adopted by local communities, counties, regions, and states to protect its children affected by disasters and terrorism incidents.

The NCDMH CONOPS was supported in part by the Terrorism and Disaster Center at the University of Oklahoma Health Science Center, a member of the National Child Traumatic Stress Network.

Older Adults

Older adults may have experienced previous challenges and coped successfully. It can be helpful to inquire how they have coped with past adversities and remind them of what has worked in the past. However, some older adults may not have grieved or healed from previous stressors, making them more vulnerable to the stress of the current situation. It is important to be aware of preexisting physical limitations and assess the need to replace lost equipment (canes, wheelchairs, hearing aids, glasses). In addition, older adults may also have preexisting medical conditions and may need access to medication and/or supplies, such as oxygen. While developing a plan to address immediate needs, older adults may be reluctant to take "handouts." It can be helpful to acknowledge their contribution to family and community and frame any assistance as an opportunity for the community to give back. It can be particularly distressful for older adults who may have loss of items of sentimental value that are irreplaceable, and this grief should be recognized and acknowledged.

Individuals With Mental Illness

Shelters usually house many individuals, have minimal privacy, and can be loud and busy. For individuals with preexisting mental illness this could potentially exacerbate symptoms and may require special provisions. A DMH worker can help to identify individuals with preexisting mental illness and advocate on their behalf for accommodations such as a quieter location with less stimulation. In addition, DMH workers can assist with linkage to their ongoing mental health providers, and can also facilitate access to medications, if necessary.

Cultural, Ethnic, and Religious Subgroups

When working with individuals from cultural, ethnic, and religious subgroups, it is important to be sensitive to roles of family members, such as who is considered the head of the family or decision maker. If using an interpreter or translator, make sure to look at the person to whom you are talking instead of the individual translating. Also, be aware of the role of community as there may be suspicion and distrust of outsiders, and help may usually be accepted only from within the community. If possible, attempt to work with community support providers who have established relationships with these subgroups.

Disaster Relief Personnel

Disaster relief personnel can also be susceptible to the stress associated with the traumatic exposure of the disaster itself as well as the disaster response efforts. However, disaster workers will often deny that they are experiencing stress and do not want to appear "weak" or unable to "handle it." DMH workers are in a good position, as members of the larger response team, to observe other workers and monitor disaster-related reactions. It is important to provide support through casual interactions—get to know their role in the disaster response, listen to their concerns, and create opportunities to be approachable. When a worker does reach out for support, it is helpful to identify a space that offers some confidentiality. Providing PFA, including education about typical stress reactions and importance of self-care, can be a helpful intervention (Table 10.1).

FATIGUE MANAGEMENT

The U.S. National Response Team (NRT) developed a document to address worker fatigue during large-scale disaster operations such as the Oklahoma City bombing; the 9/11 World Trade Center attacks; anthrax contamination; the Columbia Space Shuttle Recovery; and Hurricanes Katrina, Rita, and Wilma. The document is intended to serve as a hands-on manual to assist organizations with the development of programs and plans to address fatigue issues among disaster workers (NRT, 2009). NRT recommends use of an incident-specific fatigue management plan that includes a list of personnel, brief description of the event and site conditions, identification of fatigue risk factors present (work hours and rest periods, living conditions, nature of work), management and administrative support, potential emotional stress, controls to be implemented (worker

TABLE 10.1 Psychological First Aid (PFA) Core Actions

1. *Contact and Engagement*	To respond to contacts initiated by affected persons, or initiate contacts in a nonintrusive, compassionate, and helpful manner.
2. *Safety and Comfort*	To enhance immediate and ongoing safety, and provide physical and emotional comfort.
3. *Stabilization* (if needed)	To calm and orient emotionally—overwhelmed/distraught survivors.
4. *Information Gathering: Needs and Current Concerns*	To identify immediate needs and concerns, gather additional information, and tailor PFA interventions.
5. *Practical Assistance*	To offer practical help to survivors in addressing immediate needs and concerns.
6. *Connection with Social Supports*	To help establish brief or ongoing contacts with primary support persons or other sources of support, including family members, friends, and community help resources.
7. *Information on Coping*	To provide information (about stress reactions and coping) to reduce distress and promote adaptive functioning.
8. *Linkage with Collaborative Services*	To link survivors with needed services, and inform them about available services that may be needed in the future.

Source: National Child Traumatic Stress Network and National Center for PTSD. (2006). *Psychological First Aid: Field operations guide* (2nd ed.). Retrieved from https://www.ptsd.va.gov/professional/manuals/manual-pdf/pfa/PFA_2ndEditionwithappendices.pdf

education, advanced planning, work hours and rest periods, transportation, living conditions, recuperation provisions, and healthcare services), and the evaluation schedule.

WHEN GRIEF AND STRESS GO AWRY

Mental health services will remain in place long after the initial impact. After the rescuers and disaster workers have demobilized and returned to their homes and routines, grief and trauma counselors face the task of promoting the healing process and treating those who develop psychiatric symptoms that have not abated with time. In Oklahoma City, counselors were still providing services to survivors more than 5 years after the bombing. More than 30 years after the Attica uprising, family members and survivors were receiving psychological services for persistent or previously undetected PTSD and traumatic grief symptoms.

The hallmark for diagnosing a psychiatric disorder is that the symptoms are significantly distressing, or cause impairment in social, occupational, or other daily-life functioning. This is more difficult to assess in a disaster, as normal daily-life functioning is substantially disrupted because of the event. Practitioners often have to rely on the individual's subjective report or that of the family that the symptoms experienced are not consistent with family/cultural norms, and are causing significant distress or impairment in daily functioning.

Many types of psychiatric disorders can be seen in the aftermath of a disaster. One of the most common is PTSD; others include adjustment disorders, substance use disorders, major depression, complicated bereavement, and generalized anxiety disorders. Marital discord and domestic violence can be exacerbated in an environment of extreme stress, and all clinicians should be alert to the hallmarks of spousal, child, or elder abuse. Among children, other psychiatric difficulties encountered posttrauma include depression and separation anxiety. In addition, adolescents may display disruptive behaviors consistent with a conduct disorder (e.g., fighting, destruction of property, stealing, running away) in the months or years following traumatic stress, and thus, the connection to the traumatic event is often missed. While anniversaries can be a time to share emotions and focus on the future, they can also be a time in which distressing symptoms are easily reactivated.

TRAUMATIC GRIEF (COMPLICATED BEREAVEMENT)

Grief can be determined to be traumatic when it follows a loss that is sudden, violent, or is accompanied by extreme and intense emotional distress. In such cases, the grief can be unrelenting and overwhelming. Those experiencing a loss through sudden or violent death are often left with a feeling of unreality about the loss. Involvement with protracted medical or legal investigations can delay the grieving process. Feelings of guilt tend to occur when the death is sudden, as does the need to blame someone for what happened. The sense of helplessness is often profound, as it represents an assault on

one's sense of power and orderliness. The complications of grief usually present in one of three ways:

Chronic—prolonged, extensive; person not able to get back to life

Delayed—the pain not experienced until sometime later; minor event triggers an intense grief reaction

Masked—a physical symptom (e.g., headache, gastrointestinal distress) or disturbance of conduct or behavior (e.g., delinquency, depression; APA, 2013)

Symptoms of complicated bereavement may include:

- Guilt about things other than actions taken or not taken by the survivor at the time of the death
- Thoughts of death other than the survivor feeling he or she should have died with the deceased person
- Morbid preoccupation with worthlessness
- Marked psychomotor retardation
- Prolonged and marked functional impairment
- Hallucinatory experiences other than thinking he or she hears the voice of, or transiently sees the image of the deceased person

Treatment with medications for depression or anxiety has been found to be beneficial and can prevent subsequent disability. Psychotherapies and medications used for the treatment of major depression and PTSD have also been found to be useful in the treatment of the traumatically bereaved.

Evidence-Based Practices in the Treatment of ASD and PTSD

Cognitive behavioral intervention during the acute aftermath of a disaster for ASD has been found to yield positive results in preventing subsequent posttraumatic psychopathology. Treatment for PTSD typically begins with a detailed evaluation and development of a treatment plan that meets the unique developmental needs of the individual. Generally, PTSD-specific treatment is begun only when the individual is safely removed from the trauma or crisis situation. In persons who are currently experiencing violence (acts of war), abuse (physical, sexual, or emotional), or a disaster, immediate removal from the situation is the first step in managing the crisis. Persons who are severely depressed or suicidal, experiencing extreme panic or disorganized thinking, or in need of drug or alcohol detoxification need to have these crisis problems addressed as part of the initial treatment phase.

Use of PFA is recommended by the National Center for PTSD by focusing on reducing ongoing adversity, promoting safety, attending to practical needs, enhancing coping, stabilizing survivors, and connecting survivors with additional resources to help mitigate the consequences of the traumatic events/disaster (USDVA, National Center for PTSD, 2016a).

Pharmacotherapy (medication) can reduce the anxiety, depression, and insomnia often experienced with PTSD, and in some cases may help relieve the distress and emotional numbness caused by trauma memories. The National Institutes of Health reports that the most studied medications for treating PTSD include antidepressants, which may help control PTSD symptoms such as sadness, worry, anger, and feeling numb inside. Antidepressants and other medications may be prescribed along with psychotherapy. Other medications may be helpful for specific PTSD symptoms. For example, although it is not currently FDA approved, research has shown that Prazosin may be helpful with sleep problems, particularly nightmares, commonly experienced by people with PTSD (National Institute of Mental Health, 2016).

Exposure therapy can help people face and control their fears. It gradually exposes them to the trauma they experienced in a safe way. It uses imagining, writing, or visiting the place where the event happened. The therapist uses these tools to help people with PTSD cope with their feelings (National Institute of Mental Health, 2016).

Cognitive restructuring is a form of therapy that helps people make sense of the bad memories. Sometimes people remember the event differently than how it happened. They may feel guilt or shame about something that is not their fault. The therapist helps people with PTSD look at what happened in a realistic way (National Institute of Mental Health, 2016).

Previous studies (Matthews & Mossefin, 2006; Russell, 2008; Schubert & Lee, 2009) have summarized the evidence supporting psychotherapy models in PTSD using the American Psychiatric Association Practice Guideline for the Treatment of Patients with ASD and PTSD as follows:

Recommended With Substantial Clinical Confidence (Level I)
Cognitive behavioral therapy
Psychoeducation
Supportive techniques

Recommended With Moderate Clinical Confidence (Level II)
Exposure techniques
Eye movement desensitization and reprocessing
Imagery rehearsal
Psychodynamic therapy
Stress inoculation

May Be Recommended in Some Cases (Level III)
Present-centered group therapy
Trauma-focused group therapy

Not Recommended (No Evidence)
Psychological debriefings
Single-session techniques

Utilizing Technology as an Adjunct to Intervention and Treatment

With the growing utilization of technology in daily life, there is opportunity to incorporate these tools/applications (apps) to support interventions and treatment. HelpGuide.org, www .helpguide.org/, offers tips and tools for managing both generalized stress and PTSD symptoms. One app that has been created is called "PTSD Coach." The app contains 17 tools that individuals can use to learn about PTSD and how to manage symptoms. PTSD Coach was created by the USDVA's National Center for PTSD in partnership with the Department

of Defense's National Center for Telehealth and Technology (USDVA, National Center for PTSD, 2017). Another app, "Breathe 2 Relax," created by the National Center for Telehealth and Technology, can be used as a stress management tool to support deep diaphragmatic breathing, helping to reduce the fight or flight response. Federal Emergency Management Agency has an app available that contains safety tips and an interactive emergency kit list. The American Red Cross also has an app available through digital media stores (go to www.redcross.org/ prepare/mobile-apps for the list of providers). While these tools are not designed to replace professional intervention, they are easily accessible and can be used to support adaptive coping for those experiencing traumatic stress symptoms (Disaster Ready.org, 2014).

CRITICAL INCIDENT STRESS MANAGEMENT

According to the National Center for PTSD, Critical Incident Stress Debriefing (CISD) is a formalized, structured method whereby a group of rescue and response workers reviews the stressful experience of a disaster. CISD was developed to assist first responders, such as fire and police personnel; it was not meant for the survivors of a disaster or their relatives. CISD was never intended as a substitute for therapy. It was designed to be delivered in a group format and meant to be incorporated into a larger, multicomponent crisis intervention system labeled Critical Incident Stress Management (CISM). CISM includes the following components:

- Precrisis intervention
- Disaster or large-scale demobilization and informational briefings (town meetings)
- Staff advisement, defusing, CISD
- One-on-one crisis counseling or support
- Family crisis intervention and organizational consultation
- Follow-up and referral mechanisms for assessment and treatment, if necessary (USDVA, National Center for PTSD, 2016b)

The Debriefing Controversy

In general, psychological debriefing has not been found to reduce psychological distress or prevent PTSD (Schwarz & Kowalski, 1992; Wilson, Raphael, Meldrum, Bedosky, & Sigman, 2000). There are several studies that suggest that debriefing may actually produce harm (Math et al., 2015). Specifically, individual, single-session debriefing can no longer be recommended according to a study by Rose, Bisson, Churchill, and Wessely (2002). In their review of 15 randomized control trials, not only did single-session, individual debriefing fail to reduce distress or prevent the onset of PTSD in the longer term (1 year), but some trials reported a significantly increased risk of PTSD among those receiving debriefing. It is hypothesized that this type of debriefing has a negative effect on some people because of *secondary traumatization*. Another hypothesis is that individual debriefing may represent a *medicalization* of normal distress, therefore increasing the expectancy of developing symptoms among those who otherwise would not have done so. Finally, it may be that because shock and denial are normal and protective responses to an overwhelming event, interventions that challenge dissociative and distancing defenses during this time period may be counterproductive.

A study by Rose, Bisson, Churchill, and Wessely (2002) did *not* include group debriefing, crisis intervention, or "postvention" (psychological intervention following a completed suicide). However, the use of resources to identify and treat those with recognizable psychiatric disorders—such as ASD, depression, and PTSD—ought to continue, with an emphasis on *early detection* of those at risk of developing psychological disorders. *Follow-up assessment* should be increasingly viewed as important, and the use of screening and treatment programs need to be developed and brought to the most vulnerable groups where they live or work. Rescuers should be debriefed *as a group*, in which participation is voluntary and occurs only when the group is no longer exposed to traumatic conditions.

SUMMARY

The mental health response to a disaster must be a well-coordinated effort that draws on a variety of professionals, paraprofessionals, and volunteers who have been prescreened and specially trained for this work. In the immediate aftermath, the goal of mental health intervention is to facilitate normal coping, to treat those with immediate needs, and to begin to identify those at risk for psychiatric disorders in the ensuing weeks, months, or years. Although mental health interventions have not been shown to prevent psychiatric disorders once exposure to a traumatic event has occurred, research continues to search for strategies that can mitigate harmful effects. Management of the psychosocial effects of disaster will continue long after the initial impact. PFA is an evidence-informed approach designed to reduce distress in the immediate aftermath of a disaster and foster adaptive functioning and coping. Major depression and PTSD can be disabling consequences of exposure to disaster among those of any age group and, thus, early diagnosis and treatment are critical to the prevention of future disability. There is a growing body of research identifying that effective treatment for PTSD and cognitive behavioral approaches along with exposure therapy are most likely to be beneficial.

STUDY QUESTIONS

1. What factors determine risk for psychiatric complications in the event of a disaster, and why?

2. What is the role of a mental health coordinator in disaster planning, response, and review?

3. What topics should be included in predisaster planning for mental health services?

4. What immediate psychiatric symptoms warrant referral to a mental health professional?

5. What techniques can medical professionals use to provide psychological assistance to adults in the immediate aftermath of a disaster?

6. Under what circumstances might psychological debriefing be appropriate? When is debriefing contraindicated?

7. What is traumatic grief, and how is it treated?

8. What are the manifestations of PTSD in adults and children? What are the common treatment options?

INTERNET ACTIVITIES

1. Go to the American Academy of Child and Adolescent Psychiatry website, www.aacap.org. In the "search box" type in: *Disaster Resource Center.* Click on *Helping Children After a Disaster.* What are the warning signs that a child is having serious problems coping with grief after a disaster?

2. Go to the National Center for Posttraumatic Stress at www.ptsd.va.gov/ and click on "For Professionals." Using the Search PTSD Site button on the right side of the screen, choose the drop down "For Professionals" and below that type in a search for "Disasters and Domestic Violence." Is there any support for the concern about an increase in domestic violence in the aftermath of a disaster? Based on those findings, what steps, if any, should be taken in the aftermath of a disaster?

3. Go to SAMHSA Disaster Technical Assistance Center Supplemental Research Bulletin: Disaster behavioral health interventions inventory at: www.samhsa.gov/sites/default/files/dtac/supplemental-research-bulletin-may-2015-disaster-behavioral-health-interventions.pdf. In the table of contents, find the topic *Eye Movement Desensitization and Reprocessing (EMDR).* What is *dual stimulation?* What is the role of the clinician during EMDR? What are the general goals when employing EMDR with a posttrauma patient?

USEFUL LINKS

American Academy of Child and Adolescent Psychiatry. *Resources for Families, Disaster Resource Center.* www.aacap.org
Disaster Distress Helpline (Substance Abuse and Mental Health Services Administration): www.samhsa.gov/find-help/disaster-distress-helpline
■ Call 1-800-985-5990 toll-free (24 hours a day, 7 days a week)
■ Text TalkWithUs to 66746 to connect with a trained crisis counselor
HelpGuide.org. www.helpguide.org/

The Dougy Center. *Grief Resources.* www.dougy.org
National Association of School Psychologists. *Information for Educators (Crisis and Safety—Providers & Researcher).* www.nasponline.org
National Center for PTSD. *For Professionals.* www.ptsd.va.gov
National Child Traumatic Stress Network. *Terrorism and Disasters.* www.nctsn.org
National Library of Medicine (NLM) Coping with Disasters, Violence and Traumatic Events: disasterinfo.nlm.nih.gov/dimrc/coping.html
Substance Abuse and Mental Health Services Administration of the Health and Human Services Department. *A mental health response to disaster.* www.mentalhealthamerica.net/sites/default/files/MHA%20Disaster%20MH%20All.pdf
SAMHSA Disaster Technical Assistance Center Supplemental Research Bulletin: Disaster behavioral health interventions inventory. www.samhsa.gov/sites/default/files/dtac/supplemental-research-bulletin-may-2015-disaster-behavioral-health-interventions.pdf

REFERENCES

American Psychiatric Association. (2013). *Diagnostic and statistical manual of mental disorders* (5th ed.). Arlington, VA: American Psychiatric Publishing.
American Red Cross. (2013). Red Cross mental health team helps people cope during disaster. Retrieved from http://www.redcross.org/news/article/Red-Cross-Mental-Health-Teams-Help-People-Cope-During-Disaster
American Red Cross. (2017). Become a volunteer. Retrieved from http://www.redcross.org/volunteer/become-a-volunteer?gclid=CMmdgKnwwNQCFUpuMgod1gkETw&gclsrc=ds&dclid=CPWcjqnwwNQCFURLAQodyBsHIg#step1
Centers for Disease Control and Prevention. (2005). Disaster mental health primer: Key principles, issues and questions. Retrieved from https://stacks.cdc.gov/view/cdc/29151/cdc_29151_DS1.pdf
Cirillo, C. (2017, August 29). With death toll at 30, storm makes 2nd landfall. *The New York Times.* Retrieved from https://www.nytimes.com/2017/08/29/us/hurricane-harvey-storm-flooding.html
DeWolfe, D. J. (2000). *Field manual for mental health and human service workers in major disasters* (Publication No. ADM 90–537). Rockville, MD: U.S. Department of Health and Human Services.
Disaster Ready.org. (2014). Top mobile apps for disaster preparedness and response. Retrieved from https://www.disasterready.org/blog/top-mobile-apps-disaster-preparedness-and-response#.WULx3OvysdU
Lubit, R. H. (2016). Acute stress disorder. In D. Bienenfeld (Ed.), *Medscape.* Retrieved from http://emedicine.medscape.com/article/2192581-overview#a5
Math, S. B., Nirmala, M. C., Moirangthem, S., & Kumar, N. C. (2015). Disaster management: Mental health perspective. *Indian Journal of Psychological Medicine, 37*(3), 261–271. Retrieved from http://www.ijpm.info/article.asp?issn=0253-7176;year=2015;volume=37;issue=3;spage=261;epage=271;aulast=;type=0
Matthews, A. M., & Mossefin, C. (2006). The "date" that changed her life. *Current Psychiatry, 5*(2), 75–91.
National Child Traumatic Stress Network and National Center for PTSD. (2006). *Psychological First Aid: Field operations guide* (2nd ed.). Retrieved from https://www.ptsd.va.gov/professional/manuals/manual-pdf/pfa/PFA_2ndEditionwithappendices.pdf

National Institute of Mental Health. (2016). *Post-traumatic stress disorder.* Retrieved from https://www.nimh.nih.gov/health/topics/post-traumatic-stress-disorder-ptsd/index.shtml
National Response Team. (2009). Guidance for managing worker fatigue during disaster operations: A technical assistance document. Retrieved from https://www.cdc.gov/niosh/topics/oilspillresponse/pdfs/NRT-Fatigue-for-Emergency-Workers.pdf
Nelson, L. J. (2017, October 16). For families of dozens missing in California wildfires, "it's emotional limbo." *Los Angeles Times.* Retrieved from http://www.latimes.com/local/lanow/la-me-fire-still-missing-20171018-story.html
Rose, S. C., Bisson, J., Churchill, R., & Wessely, S. (2002). Psychological debriefing for preventing post traumatic stress disorder (PTSD). *Cochrane Database of Systematic Reviews,* (2), CD000560. doi:10.1002/14651858.CD000560
Russell, M. C. (2008). Scientific resistance to research, training and utilization of eye movement desensitization and reprocessing (EMDR) therapy in treating post-war disorders *Social Science and Medicine, 67*(11), 1737–1746. Retrieved from http://linkinghub.elsevier.com/retrieve/pii/S0277953608004796?via=sd&cc=y
Schrieber, M. (2011). *National children's disaster mental health concept of operations.* Oklahoma City: Terrorism and Disaster Center at the University of Oklahoma Health Sciences Center.
Schubert, S., & Lee C. W. (2009). Adult PTSD and its treatment with EMDR: A review of controversies, evidence, and theoretical knowledge. *Journal of EMDR Practice and Research, 3*(3), 117–132. doi:10.1891/1933-3196.3.3.117
Schwarz, E. D., & Kowalski, J. M. (1992). Malignant memories: Reluctance to utilize mental health services after a disaster. *Journal of Nervous and Mental Disorders, 189*(12), 767–772.
Substance Abuse and Mental Health Services Administration. (2015a). A mental health response to disaster. Retrieved from https://www.mentalhealthamerica.net/sites/default/files/MHA%20Disaster%20MH%20All.pdf
Substance Abuse and Mental Health Services Administration. (2015b). Disaster Technical Assistance Center supplemental research bulletin: Disaster behavioral health interventions inventory. Retrieved from https://www.samhsa.gov/sites/default/files/dtac/supplemental-research-bulletin-may-2015-disaster-behavioral-health-interventions.pdf
U.S. Department of Health and Human Services. (2015). Enhancing public health, healthcare and emergency management systems. Retrieved from https://www.phe.gov/Preparedness/planning/authority/nhss/Pages/systems-integration.aspx
U.S. Department of Veterans Affairs, National Center for PTSD. (2016a). Helping Survivors: Long-term treatment interventions following disaster and mass violence. Retrieved from https://www.ptsd.va.gov/professional/trauma/disaster-terrorism/disaster_tx_longterm.asp
U.S. Department of Veterans Affairs, National Center for PTSD. (2016b). Types of debriefing following disasters. Retrieved from https://www.ptsd.va.gov/professional/trauma/disaster-terrorism/debriefing-after-disasters.asp
U.S. Department of Veterans Affairs, National Center for PTSD. (2017). Moblie app: PTSD coach. Retrieved from https://www.ptsd.va.gov/public/materials/apps/ptsdcoach.asp
van Ommeren, M., Hanna, F., Weissbecker, I., & Ventevogel, P. (2015). Mental health and psychosocial support in humanitarian emergencies. *Eastern Mediterranean Health Journal, 21*(7), 498–502. doi:10.26719/2015.21.7.498
Wilson, J. P., Raphael, B., Meldrum, L., Bedosky, C., & Sigman, M. (2000). Preventing PTSD in trauma survivors. *Bulletin of the Menninger Clinic, 64*(2), 181–196.

11

UNIQUE NEEDS OF CHILDREN DURING DISASTERS AND OTHER PUBLIC HEALTH EMERGENCIES

Michael Beach and Patricia Frost

LEARNING OBJECTIVES

When this chapter is completed, readers will be able to:

1. Discuss the epidemiology of disaster-related injuries and illnesses in children.
2. Compare and contrast the physical and psychosocial differences of children and adults exposed to natural disasters; public health emergencies; and explosive, radiological, biological, or chemical agents.
3. Describe the assessment and treatment of children following natural disasters and exposure to nuclear, biological, or chemical agents in the field, emergency department, and hospital setting.
4. Discuss the care of children living in shelters or refugee settings following a disaster.
5. Apply pediatrics-related disaster resources to one's own disaster preparedness plans.

KEY MESSAGES

Pediatric injury and illness patterns following exposure to explosive, radiological, biological, and chemical agents may be different from those in adults.

Children have physiological and anatomical differences from adults that make them more susceptible to injury.

Children are disproportionally affected by disasters and exhibit significantly higher mortality rates than adults.

Treatments for pediatric exposure to radiological, biological, and chemical agents may be different than those for adults.

Children are likely to experience significant adverse emotional and psychological consequences associated with traumatic and disaster events.

Nurses must be prepared to care for children at the disaster scene, in the emergency department, in the hospital, and at shelters or refugee camps.

Pediatric-specific resources are available to assist nurses and other healthcare professionals in disaster preparedness, mitigation, response, recovery, and evaluation.

CHAPTER OVERVIEW

Although it is well understood that infants, children, and adolescents have unique physiological and psychosocial needs during and after disasters and public health emergencies, significant gaps exist in the area of disaster preparedness for children. Children's injury and illness patterns following exposure to radiological, biological, and chemical agents are different from the patterns assessed in adults and require stabilization and transfer to pediatric specialty centers. Treatment options used for adults in these scenarios may be untested, inappropriate, require modification, or simply be unavailable for children. Children with functional and access needs are known to require special attention to assure their chronic healthcare needs are addressed. Nurses and healthcare professionals must be aware of pediatric considerations during disaster response and must be prepared to modify their approaches accordingly. This chapter discusses the epidemiology of disaster-related injuries and illnesses in the pediatric population. The physiological and psychosocial aspects of children applicable to disaster and public health emergencies are described. Injury and illness patterns following natural, explosion, radiological, biological, and chemical disasters are discussed, and current treatment recommendations are offered. Interventions from field through emergency department and hospitalization care are addressed. Pediatrics-related resources for disaster planning are included.

In 2015, the U.S. Census Bureau estimated that there were approximately 73.6 million children younger than 18 years of age residing in the country (U.S. Census Bureau, 2015) with 23.9 million under the age of 5 years. Real-world events have demonstrated that children and families are frequently involved in natural or man-made disasters or public health emergencies at home, school, work, or play. Children have been shown to have higher rates of mortality and morbidity compared with adults affected by a disaster. Children are also likely to be victims of terrorist acts, and these acts may even be targeted specifically at children. Incidents such as the Sandy Hook shootings, where children were the primary targets, affected not only the community involved but also the nation as a whole. Disasters, acts of terrorism, and public health emergencies are a reality. Nurses and healthcare professionals need to be prepared to care for infants, children, and adolescents when these events arise in their communities.

EPIDEMIOLOGY OF PEDIATRIC INJURIES AND ILLNESSES DURING DISASTERS AND PUBLIC HEALTH EMERGENCIES

Natural Disasters

Earthquakes

A report concerning the 2013 Lushan Earthquake (Jiang et al., 2013) showed 34 children under the age of 14 were admitted to the West China Hospital, 67% had variable limb fractures, and 29% had traumatic brain injuries. During the response to the 2010 earthquake in Haiti, there were 471 pediatric patients out of a total of 796 patients treated. During the first 10 days of the response, 91% of the patients were assigned to the trauma group. Eighty-eight percent required specialized orthopedic care (Gamulin, Armenter-Duran, Assal, Hagon, & Daver, 2012).

On March 11, 2011, a magnitude 9.0 earthquake and ensuing tsunami hit the coast of Japan resulting in severe damage to the Fukushima No. 1 nuclear complex resulting in a large release of radioactive contaminates into the environment as a result of reactor meltdown. During the disaster, children accounted for over 6.5% (Yonekura, Ueno, & Iwanaka, 2013) of the 19,000 dead and missing. The resulting nuclear crisis forced over 10,000 children to be evacuated from their homes near the nuclear reactor. Reports from Disaster Medical Assessment Teams (DMATs) deployed to the region noted that 29.5% of disaster victims in the field DMAT clinics were children (Yonekura et al., 2013).

Hurricanes/Tornados

In August 2005, Hurricane Katrina ravaged the Gulf Coast, displacing thousands of American citizens and crippling the infrastructure of cities and states. This Category 5 hurricane disrupted utilities, food distribution systems, healthcare services, and communications in Louisiana and Mississippi (Daley, 2006). Hurricane Rita struck immediately following Katrina, compounding the devastation and taxing relief efforts. According to the Center for Missing Persons, 400,000 people were dispersed to 48 states; of these, 5,000 children were reported missing. The last of the missing children were reunited with their parents 6 months later (Gausche-Hill, 2009; Save the Children, 2015).

Tornados and severe storms affect the Central Plains area of the United States. Following a tornado in Tuscaloosa, Oklahoma in 2011, one adult hospital served 800 patients with 100 of them being children, many unaccompanied by parents and unidentified (Kanter, 2012). From the same tornado, Chern et al. (2011) reported 15 patients were treated at a children's hospital requiring significant neurosurgery including 11 cranial, two spine, and two peripheral surgeries.

In October 2012, Superstorm Sandy affected over 24 states. When Sandy made landfall in New York and southern New Jersey, over 23,000 sought shelter. Post event, it was found that children living in homes that experienced minor damage were at particularly high risk for psychological and emotional issues (National Center for Disaster Preparedness, New York University College of Global Public Health, Rutgers School of Social Work, 2015).

In 2017, Hurricane Harvey devastated Houston, Texas and the surrounding area with unprecedented flooding; Hurricane Irma struck Florida with significant damage to the Florida Keys; and Hurricane Marie impacted over 3 million people in Puerto Rico and the U.S. Virgin Islands. Medical care, housing, utilities, and the basic functions of life were disrupted for children and families in each location.

Floods

Effects of global warming have dramatically increased the frequency of severe weather events including flooding. In September 2013, Boulder, Colorado experienced heavy rainfall of over 14.5 inches in less than 48 hours prompting military helicopter evacuations of stranded children and their families (Rice, 2013). The United Nations International Strategy for Disaster Risk Reduction (UNISDR) estimated that in 2015 there would be 346 climate-related global disasters, affecting 98.9 million people and resulting in 22,773 deaths.

Public Health Emergencies

One of the most notorious public health emergencies is the 1918 influenza pandemic. In the United States alone, during the 17 weeks of its outbreak, the Spanish influenza killed 670,000 people, with some 25 million citizens becoming ill from the disease; worldwide, in the 10 months of the pandemic, Spanish influenza killed between 21 and 40 million people (Iezzoni, 1999). While infants and children were stricken and succumbed to this disease, the age group with the highest mortality was the 15- to 40-year-olds (Iezzoni, 1999). There was no known cure; and it was reported that children at New York City's Roosevelt Hospital were housed on the hospital's screened roof, wrapped in blankets and hot water bottles and left to breathe in the cold, salty air. While the public deemed the treatment to be "barbarous and cruel," mortality rates did drop in patients receiving this treatment (Iezzoni, 1999).

In 2009, H1N1 emerged as a novel virus disproportionally affecting children and pregnant women. During the pandemic, pediatric regional centers surged to capacity. Both vaccines and antiviral therapy were limited for children. Community hospitals experienced up to a 30% surge in emergency department (ED) patients while pediatric centers reported up to a 50% surge. The highest incidence of infections was in school-aged children with the highest hospital rates among those 5 to 24 years of age (Children's Hospital Los Angeles, 2012).

Historically, large-scale exposure to radiation occurred following the detonation of atomic bombs in Japan, fallout from atomic bomb tests, nuclear reactor accidents (e.g., Chernobyl and Japan following the 2011 earthquake and tsunami), and the release of material from radiotherapy devices (Mettler & Voelz, 2002). Such releases resulted in thousands of children and adults being exposed to high levels of radiation and suffering from long-term consequences, such as various types of cancers. Children and adolescents, as well as fetuses, are particularly susceptible to developing malignant thyroid cancer (Waselenko et al., 2004).

In 2001, 11 people in the United States were diagnosed with confirmed or probable cases of cutaneous anthrax (Inglesby et al., 2002). One of these victims was a 7-month-old infant, who probably contracted the spores at his mother's workplace (Freedman et al., 2002). The previously healthy infant experienced severe systemic illness, despite early antibiotic therapy and hospitalization.

Smallpox is a deadly disease that plagued humanity for hundreds of years. In most outbreaks, children were most often infected because adults were protected by immunity from vaccine-induced or previous smallpox infection (Henderson et al., 1999). Large outbreaks in schools were uncommon because the smallpox virus is not transmitted until the rash appears; by this time, infected children were confined to bed because of their symptoms (Henderson, 1999). Smallpox has been eradicated, but it is suspected that the virus remains in laboratories.

Since 2012, vaccine-preventable diseases such as measles and polio-like viruses have reemerged with outbreaks in communities due to and associated with the anti-vaccination movement. This has resulted in numerous community outbreaks and preventable deaths. In August 2014, the World Health Organization (WHO) declared the ongoing epidemic of Ebola virus disease (EBD) in West Africa to be a public health emergency. With a fatality rate of 55% to 60%, the disease could be treated only with supportive care. Population movements both within and across borders and lack of containment measures contributed to the spread of the disease. Infants and children who were suspect Ebola patients or developed symptoms were frequently isolated away from parents and families, interacting with caregivers covered from head to toe in personal protective equipment (PPE) and rarely touched or comforted.

Acts of Terrorism

One of terrorism's defining characteristics is the targeting of noncombatants including children. There have been over 150 terrorist events involving children between 1927 and 2009 (Johnston, 2009). Since 2009, terrorists have increasingly targeted schools. Pediatric injuries and illnesses are found in acts of terrorism. Among 94 children treated for penetrating chest injuries in Turkey over a 6-year period, seven (7.4%) had bomb (shrapnel) injuries; the patients' mean age was 11.51 years (Inci, Ozcelik, Nizam, Eren, & Ozgen, 1996). From 1991 to 2001, 260 patients in Turkey presenting for treatment of terrorism-related open globe injuries were studied (Sobaci,

Akyn, Mutlu, Karagul, & Bayraktar, 2005). The patients' ages ranged from 9 to 47 years (mean age = 22.6 years), with the vast majority being young males. Mine and hand grenades accounted for 62.5% of the injuries, leaving 6.5% of the patients handicapped (Sobaci et al., 2005).

In 1995, during an intentional release of sarin in a Tokyo subway, 16 children (no fatalities) were exposed to the chemical (Committee on Environmental Health [COEH] & Committee on Infectious Diseases [COID], 2000). That same year, 19 children (11.3% of the 168 fatalities) died in the bombing of the Alfred P. Murrah Federal Building in Oklahoma City on April 19, 1995 (Quintana et al., 1997). Sixteen of the children who died were seated by the window of the day care center at the time of the explosion. Among the 19 dead children, 90% sustained skull fractures, with 79% sustaining cerebral evisceration; 37% suffered abdominal or thoracic injuries; 31% had amputations; 47% had arm and 26% had leg fractures; 21% were burned; and 100% had extensive cutaneous contusions, avulsions, and lacerations (Quintana et al., 1997). Forty-seven children sustained nonfatal injuries, with seven requiring hospitalization (Quintana et al., 1997).

Premeditated shootings at schools by students are acts that defy comprehension. School shootings at the Jonesboro School (Jonesboro, Arkansas) on March 24, 1998, resulted in 13 children and two schoolteachers requiring emergency treatment for gunshot wounds; four children and one teacher died from this horrible act (Skaug, 1999). On May 21 of the same year, a 15-year-old student in Springfield, Oregon, opened fire on students in the cafeteria, killing two and injuring 22 (Mitka, 1999). Selected commonalities among the 37 school shootings since 1974 reveal that the 41 shooters involved preplanned the attack; attacked out of revenge or to settle a grievance; and came from a wide range of family backgrounds, academic performances, and social groups (Twemlow, Fonagy, Sacco, O'Toole, & Vernberg, 2002).

In Beslan, Russia, a gang of armed terrorists seized School Number One in Beslan, in North Ossetia, Russia, and held 1,100 students, teachers, and parents as hostages. Over a 53-hour siege, hostages were executed, threatened with being shot, denied food and water, forced to drink urine, and to urinate and defecate where they sat (Parfitt, 2004). During the standoff, a bomb in the sports hall unintentionally detonated. Hostages ran through the debris with the terrorists shooting at them while the security forces fought back (Parfitt, 2004). More than 360 people died, half of them children (Parfitt, 2004).

Acts of War

Many times, the poor of society suffer the most during times of war and turmoil. Slone and Mann (2016) looked at 35 studies that included 4,365 young children and found that posttraumatic stress disorder (PTSD), behavioral and emotional symptoms, sleep problems, disturbed play, and psychosomatic symptoms were prevalent.

Morbidity and mortality plague the pediatric population during mass population movements due to war, famine, drought, or a combination of these factors, predisposing children, adults, and elderly to overcrowding, inadequate sanitation, malnutrition, and diseases against which immunity is lacking. Measles, diarrheal illness, upper respiratory infections, and malaria (Seaman & Maguire, 2005) are the leading causes of morbidity and mortality in displaced pediatric populations. In overcrowded refugee camps, unsanitary conditions, disrupted infrastructures, and the promiscuous defecation of children (Burkle, 1999) contribute to the high rate of communicable diseases. Sadly, in these situations, children under 5 years of age have a disproportionately higher crude mortality rate from infectious diseases compared with older children and adults.

Long-term war-ridden regions such as those found in Syria have reduced life expectancy of resident Syrians by 20 years. More than 75,000 civilians died from injuries incurred in the violence in the first 4 years with twice as many civilians, including many women and children, dying prematurely of infectious and noninfectious chronic diseases for want of adequate healthcare (Sahloul et al., 2016).

PHYSIOLOGICAL CONSIDERATIONS IN PEDIATRIC CARE FOLLOWING A DISASTER OR PUBLIC HEALTH EMERGENCY

Children have physiological differences that, compared with adults, have implications for the signs, symptoms, and severity of illness or injury following disasters or public health emergencies. The body systems likely to be affected in disasters and public health emergencies are reviewed in terms of their anatomy, physiology, and post-exposure considerations.

Pulmonary

Children's faster respiratory rates, higher metabolic rate, as well as greater minute ventilation increase their risk of inhaling a higher dosage or amount of toxic airborne substances including radioactive gases (Chung & Shannon, 2005; Gausche-Hill, 2009; Save the Children, 2015). Sarin, other nerve agents, chlorine, as well as other gases, have high vapor densities, making them heavier than air and more concentrated closer to the ground, leaving infants and small children much more susceptible than their adult counterparts (Bearer, 1995; Gausche-Hill, 2009). Oxygen consumption in infants is 6 to 8 mL/kg/min compared with 3 to 4 mL/kg/min in adults (Chameides & Hazinski, 1998); children exposed to noxious chemicals or vapors would require early oxygen administration.

Tachypnea is a nonspecific sign of respiratory distress (Zaritsky, Nadkarni, Berg, Hickey, & Schexnayder, 2001) and was observed in children and adolescents exposed to mustard gas, probably due to the delicacy of the pediatric epithelial tissues (Momeni & Aminjavaheri, 1994).

Infants and young children have cartilaginous and thus compliant chest walls. This anatomical feature has both medical and trauma implications (Gausche-Hill, 2009; Save the Children, 2015). When a child is in respiratory distress, suprasternal, supraclavicular, infraclavicular, intercostal, or substernal retractions result from the child's increased work of breathing. Respiratory distress could result from exposure to biological or chemical agents, as well as dust and particles from blasts or collapsed buildings. Kinetic energy from blasts, earthquakes, or other forces is easily transmitted to the underlying pulmonary and cardiac tissues, resulting in pulmonary and cardiac contusions leading to pulmonary edema and cardiac arrhythmias. Such contusions may not be readily diagnosed or apparent immediately after injury; therefore, healthcare professionals must have a high index of suspicion for these injuries (Beach, 2010; Gausche-Hill, 2009).

Cardiovascular

A child's estimated blood volume is 80 mL/kg, which is larger than an adult's on a milliliter per kilogram basis and this can result in small amounts of blood loss from trauma decreasing circulating blood volume leading to shock (Gausche-Hill, 2009). Children have greater cardiac reserves and catecholamine responses compared with adults, allowing them to compensate for fluid losses from hemorrhage, diarrhea, or lack of oral intake. However, when this system of compensation fails, shock and cardiopulmonary failure can result quickly in children exposed to severe trauma, biological or chemical agents, or in those sustaining kinetic energy or burn trauma.

Tachycardia is a nonspecific sign for cardiopulmonary distress and along with delayed capillary refill time are important indicators of cardiopulmonary compromise during early stages of shock (Zaritsky et al., 2001). Early in compensated shock, children's vital signs will remain in their age range, or slightly elevated. Hypotension is not observed until the child has lost 20% to 25% of his or her circulating blood volume and is a sign of decompensated shock (Chameides & Hazinski, 1998; Gausche-Hill, 2009; Save the Children, 2015). If fluid stores are not replaced aggressively with intravenous or intraosseous fluids, uncompensated shock ensues and cardiac arrest results. Therefore, children sustaining fluid losses associated with blood loss or dehydration are at risk of dehydration and subsequent cardiopulmonary failure, if untreated.

Integumentary

The skin of infants and children is thinner and more permeable compared with the skin of adults (Gausche-Hill, 2009). They also have less subcutaneous fat than adults. Infants and children have a higher body area-to-weight ratio, predisposing them to greater heat loss through conduction, convection, radiation, and evaporation (Gausche-Hill, 2009). Skin permeability and larger area-to-weight ratio may result in a greater exposure to and absorption of dermal toxicants (COEH & COID, 2000). The rapid onset of dermatological symptoms and dominance of facial involvement in children following exposure to mustard gas may have been accounted for because of these integumentary as well as pulmonary characteristics (Momeni & Aminjavaheri, 1994).

Children are at high risk of hypothermia because of an immature thermoregulatory system and higher surface area-to-mass ratio (Gausche-Hill, 2009). Infants less than 6 months of age do not have fine-motor coordination to shiver and are unable to keep themselves warm; nonshivering thermogenesis occurs where brown fat is broken down to produce warmth (Bernardo & Schenkel, 2003). Shivering is a high-energy-consuming, nonproductive muscular activity initiated for thermogenesis (Bernardo & Henker, 1999). Shivering may not be possible in injured or ill children receiving sedation or neuromuscular blocking agents (Bernardo & Henker, 1999). This has significant impact for decontamination of infants and children (Gausche-Hill, 2009). After children are decontaminated using large amounts of warm water, they will need to be warmed with towels, dry clothes, blankets, radiant heaters, and warm fluids. This is also important for children exposed during inclement weather, and for those infants and children displaced from their homes to shelters or exposed to the environment prior to rescue.

Convection, conductive, and radiant heat loss will occur during entrapment when exposed to floodwaters and when exposed to prolonged rainfall during hurricanes. The convective, conductive, and radiant heat losses will be greater than in adults due to infants' and children's higher body surface area-to-weight ratio. Therefore, access to heating sources, such as heat lamps, blankets, and intravenous fluid warmers will be needed to prevent hypothermia in the pediatric population. These warming measures are also needed to prevent iatrogenic hypothermia and maintain normothermia due to traumatic injuries.

Neonates are at very high risk of morbidity and mortality in disaster events. This is a special population that cannot provide for their own thermoregulation and at extremely small birth weights will not survive without a "neutral thermal environment" either provided as an Isolette or, in extreme conditions, skin to skin contact. Infants lose heat through conduction, convection, radiation, and evaporation. These fragile infants are prone to hypoglycemia, dehydration, and infection due to their immature organ systems.

Musculoskeletal

The long bones of children continue to grow throughout childhood and into adolescence. Physical injury to the growth plate, or physis, can result in growth arrest or deformity. Such injury could occur in children sustaining blast injuries or other traumatic injuries during natural disasters. It has been documented that long bone injuries, particularly of the lower extremities, are prevalent among victims. Among children in Turkey, entrapment following earthquakes resulted in crush injuries, crush syndrome, and subsequent acute renal failure (Donmez, Mral, Yavuz, & Durmaz, 2001; Iskit et al., 2001); children exposed to a bomb detonation sustained long bone fractures and traumatic amputations (Quintana et al., 1997). Among 75 children sustaining peripheral nerve injuries, electromyographic (EMG) findings showed regeneration in brachial plexus damage in 100% of the children at a mean follow-up time of 3.5 months and 62.5% in a mean follow-up time of 7.7 months (Uzun, Savrun, & Kiziltan, 2005). However, compared with adults sustaining peripheral nerve injuries from a disaster, children had higher rates of being buried in debris resulting in compartment syndrome, sustaining peripheral nerve injuries in the lower extremities, and total axonal damage at the first EMG follow-up (Uzun et al., 2005). Brachial plexus regeneration was the most favorable for children and adults, and both groups had similar rates of peripheral nerve regeneration (Uzun et al., 2005).

Young bones are compliant, thereby affording less protection to underlying body organs (e.g., lungs, heart, brain) when external forces are applied. This may lead to significant internal injuries in the absence of bone fractures (Gausche-Hill, 2009; Lynch & Thomas, 2004). Similarly, children's abdominal organs are relatively large and have relatively less protective tissues compared to adults; solid and hollow organ injury from blunt and penetrating trauma forces are likely (Lynch & Thomas, 2004). Along with the large size, the organs in the abdominal compartment are close in proximity, and injuries to several organs can occur from a single penetrating or blunt force (Gausche-Hill, 2009; Lynch & Thomas, 2004).

The head-to-body size ratio is also much larger in children and infants than in adults. The larger head size makes head injuries from explosions, earthquakes, and other potential sources of trauma more likely in children and infants than in adults.

Children's nutritional requirements are greater per kilogram than adults. They drink more milk and eat a more concentrated diet of fruits. These foods are highly susceptible to contamination, particularly radioactive contamination placing children at a much higher risk level than adults. Both general population and medical shelters in real-world events are known not to plan adequately for the nutritional needs of children. Sufficient stores of formula for infants may not be readily available. During the disaster medical response in Haiti, DMATs used wet nurses to provide for infant nutrition as clean water and formula was not readily available and oral electrolyte solution was prepared from limited on-site resources for children presenting with vomiting and diarrhea. In environments where adequate nutrition or quality dietary foods is limited or not available, children are known to suffer from vomiting, diarrhea, constipation, and weight loss.

Cognitive

Protecting oneself from danger is of utmost importance during a natural or man-made disaster. Infants and young children depend completely on adults to provide for their safety and basic needs of life (Gausche-Hill, 2009; Save the Children, 2015). Young children are unlikely to recognize danger or to protect themselves from it (Bernardo, 2001; Gausche-Hill, 2009). Following the release of a chemical or biological agent, children may not have the ability to decide in which direction they should evacuate the area (COEH & COID, 2000). The confusion and disruption present during a disaster may cause extreme levels of fear and anxiety in children and may be magnified when they see their parents experiencing the same levels of fear (Gausche-Hill, 2009; Save the Children, 2015). Such may have been the case in the children exposed to mustard gas during the Iran–Iraq war; these children may not have realized or been informed of the danger of the gas, not protected their faces, and sustained heavy injury to their faces and eyes (Momeni & Aminjavaheri, 1994). Children may not be able to decide how to avoid danger and seek safety in the event of a natural disaster or terrorist attack making them significantly more vulnerable. Also, they may not have the language skills required to provide a clinical history or explain what has happened to them and what injuries they may have sustained.

Cognitive development of the child can be seriously affected by chemical and hazardous materials producing both short- and long-term impacts. During 2014 to 2016, the population of Flint, Michigan experienced one of the worst community contaminations of water supply in the United States. The health effects of lead exposure in children are known to include impaired cognition, behavioral disorders, hearing problems, and delayed growth. This exposure is estimated to affect 6,000 to 12,000 children and resulted in a state of emergency being declared in Michigan.

Nutritional Requirements

Children have a greater growth rate and subsequent higher protein and calorie requirements when compared with adults (Burkle, 2002). In complex emergencies, where displaced populations are without adequate food sources, protein-energy malnutrition can result. Protein-energy malnutrition describes the syndromes characterized by malnutrition and micronutrient deficiency diseases, such as marasmus, kwashiorkor, and marasmic-kwashiorkor (Burkle, 2002). Protein-energy malnutrition is diagnosed when the child's arm muscle circumference is less than the fifth percentile or less than 80% of the reference standard (Burkle, 2002). Children who are malnourished are at risk of secondary infections, which can lead to complications and death (Burkle, 2002). Children at risk of protein-energy malnutrition must receive the rations that meet their requirements for caloric intake, protein, and essential vitamins (Burkle, 2002).

A survey conducted at 7 months after the 2004 tsunami and 3 months after the 2005 earthquake in Indonesia found that among children aged 6 to 59 months, global acute malnutrition (GAM) ranged from 7.8% among nondisplaced children in Banda Aceh to 17.6% among displaced children in Simeulue (Centers for Disease Control and Prevention [CDC], 2006). Severe acute malnutrition (SAM) was highest in Simeulue; 3.4% among displaced children and 1.9% among nondisplaced children (CDC, 2006). These malnutrition levels were below the WHO emergency threshold in Banda Aceh and Aceh Besar but were elevated in Simeulue, a finding that may reflect preexisting malnutrition in this locale (CDC, 2006). Food and drinking water were provided to the majority of the population, although improvements to prevent contamination of drinking water were needed.

Disaster planning at all levels, from personal disaster plans to state and federal levels, must take into consideration the normal nutritional needs of children and the needs of those with particular needs such as special formulas, tube feedings, and other considerations.

Genetic

Exposure to various nuclear, biological, and chemical agents, as well as exposure to natural and man-made disasters, can have genetic implications for children and their future offspring. Following the aftermath of Hurricane Gilbert in Jamaica on September 12, 1988, there was an increase in the incidence of neural tube defects (spina bifida, meningocele, myelomeningocele, and encephalocele) in babies born 10 to 18 months after the hurricane (Duff, Cooper, Danbury, Johnson, & Serjeant, 1991). The incidence increased from a baseline of 1 to 4/10,000 live births in 1980 to 1988 to 3 to 9, peaking at 5 to 7/10,000 live births from July 1989 through March 1990 (Duff et al., 1991). During this same time period, there was a rise in the megaloblastic change in sickle cell patients, probably due to folate deficiency. This increased incidence of neural tube defects was probably due also to folate deficiency, due to its postdisaster nutritional scarcity (Duff et al., 1991).

Mutagenicity and carcinogenicity of mustard gas have been reported, and children exposed to mustard gas should be followed up over time (Momeni & Aminjavaheri, 1994). Following the Gulf War in 1991, unusually high rates of birth defects and rare physical abnormalities in babies fathered by military personnel serving in the Persian Gulf were reported (Doucet, 1994, p. 184). Abnormally high rates of miscarriage and illness in the veterans' partners also were documented (Doucet, 1994). Reported medical conditions in newborns included rare blood disorders, severe respiratory diseases, malformed internal organs, fused fingers, and club feet (Doucet, 1994). Potential multiple causes of these health maladies include the stress of war, infections from sandflies, experimental medication against Iraqi chemical and biological weapons, possible exposure to chemical and biological weapons, fumes from the oil spills and fires, and exposure to depleted uranium shells (Doucet, 1994). In contrast, Araneta et al. (2000) measured the prevalence of selected birth defects among infants born to Gulf War veterans and those born to nondeployed veterans in Hawaii. A data set of 99,545 live births reported to the state of Hawaii Department of Health between 1989 and 1993 was searched for infants born to military personnel. A total of 17,182 infants made up the sample (3,717 born to Gulf War veterans and 13,465 born to nondeployed veterans). A total of 367 infants (2.14/100 live births) were identified as having one or more of 48 major birth defects. The prevalence of these birth defects was similar for Gulf War and nondeployed veterans. Additional longitudinal, epidemiological research is needed among veterans to validate such findings among veterans living throughout the United States.

Immunologic

Newborns and young infants are susceptible to infections due to their underdeveloped immune systems. Therefore, sepsis would be encountered in newborns and infants exposed to biological agents (Nopar, 1967). With young children, there will also be less herd immunity making them more susceptible to infectious disease, as well as a greater potential for reactions to vaccines and more complications of illnesses (Gausche-Hill, 2009).

The thyroid gland is sensitive to the carcinogenic effects of radiation exposure (Rubino, Cailleux, DeVathaire, & Schlumberger, 2002). This is because the thyroid gland concentrates iodine very efficiently, and exposure to radioiodines results in the localization of radioactivity in the thyroid gland (Waselenko et al., 2004, p. w66). The primary route of radioiodine exposure for children close to its release is inhalation, while for children farther from its release, ingestion of contaminated food and

liquids (particularly milk) is the primary route (Waselenko et al., 2004). Radioactive iodine can be absorbed and secreted in human breast milk, placing breast-fed infants at risk of exposure (AAP, 2003). Young age is a risk factor for developing thyroid cancer following radiation exposure; this risk is maximal when radiation exposure occurs in children less than 5 years of age (Rubino et al., 2002). Furthermore, females have a higher incidence of thyroid cancer, both spontaneous and following radiation exposure, compared with males (Rubino et al., 2002). Other risk factors for developing thyroid cancer are a high radiation dose and personal or familial history of radiation-associated tumors (Rubino et al., 2002). Children can be exposed to radioiodines through inhalation or through the ingestion of contaminated food (U.S. Food and Drug Administration [FDA], 2001b). Children have a greater risk for developing cancer when exposed to radiation in utero (Markenson & Reynolds, 2006).

Following the tsunami of 2004, a measles vaccination campaign was enacted, targeting all children aged 6 months to 15 years. Among eligible children aged 12 to 59 months, the percentage receiving measles vaccination ranged from 37.3% of displaced children in Aceh Besar to 58.2% of nondisplaced children in Banda Aceh (CDC, 2006).

Soil-transmitted helminth infections, primarily ascariasis and trichuriasis, were found among children in Aceh Besar and Simeulue, where approximately 75% of school-aged children and half of children aged 6 to 59 months were infected (CDC, 2006). Helminth infection was significantly lower among children in Banda Aceh than among children in the other two districts (CDC, 2006).

CHILDREN WITH FUNCTIONAL AND ACCESS NEEDS

Children with functional and access needs (FAN) will require additional considerations during mass casualty or disaster care. These considerations include decontamination procedures following radiation or chemical exposure for children using wheelchairs, ventilators, or oxygen; and decontamination procedures for children with gastrostomy tubes, tracheostomy tubes, indwelling bladder catheters, and indwelling central venous catheters. Replacement supplies would be needed once the cutaneous decontamination is completed. Such supplies may not be readily available, so provisions must be made to secure these items or to have comparable clean or sterile supplies on hand.

Children who are visually impaired, hearing impaired, and those with cognitive or emotional difficulties will require special care during a disaster response and recovery. Communication will be difficult and require more time. Mass shelters may prove very difficult. Individual care building a trusted relationship and utilizing family or friends when possible are necessary. One of the largest groups of children with FAN are those children on the autistic spectrum. These children experience and interact with the world differently. They can become easily overwhelmed and their families and caregivers should be considered subject matter experts in their care. It is important not to take over the care unless invited by the families. Most families of children with FAN need to be supported in their care. It is not uncommon for FAN children to have multiple chronic and medical conditions that require special diets or replacement medication.

PSYCHOSOCIAL CONSIDERATIONS IN PEDIATRIC CARE

Disasters and public health emergencies are stress-producing events whose impact can last a lifetime. Children are vulnerable to the stresses of evacuation: living in a shelter; losing their homes, schools, parents, pets, and loved ones. The psychosocial changes resulting from a disaster are related to children's developmental stage/age; cognitive level; family's proximity and reactions to the disaster; and direct exposure to, or child's situation during, the disaster (Conway, Bernardo, & Tontala, 1990). Furthermore, children's understanding of natural disasters may be influenced by their magical belief system, religious beliefs, and level of moral development (Belter & Shannon, 1993). The parents and families of children may die or become incapacitated and thus unable to care for their children, or children and families may become separated in shelters or treatment facilities, leading to substantial psychosocial problems (Cieslak & Henretig, 2003).

The effects of children's culture on psychosocial responses to disasters should not be overlooked. Children and families who lose their homes in disasters or acts of war must move to another location, which may mean a different culture, customs, or other life patterns to which they must adjust (Capozzoli, 2002). Such changes occur not only in foreign countries but in the United States as well, where rural families may need to adapt to customs and cultures of urban living, and vice versa.

Children who witness destruction and violence can lose the notion that their home, school, and community are safe places to live and that people are trustworthy. Such notions can create a loss of security, bringing with it fear, anxiety, and horror (Jagodic & Kontac, 2002). Following the 2004 tsunami, many of the children involved feared for their lives, escaped death, and suffered the loss of their families, homes, and communities (Kostelny & Wessells, 2005). Because of the loss of parental and community security, these children were placed at additional risk of sexual exploitation, trafficking, recruitment into armed groups, and dangerous labor (Kostelny & Wessells, 2005).

Young children watching television rebroadcasts of disaster events may believe the event to be happening again and again. Following September 11, 2001, children and adolescents have reported being significantly more worried about coping with stress as compared to before that day (Hagan, 2005). Furthermore, children who witness these intentional acts of violence may experience a greater degree of psychopathology (Hagan, 2005). War, in particular, exposes children to ongoing man-made violence, injury, destruction, and death (Hagan, 2005). In-depth discussions of the psychological and emotional experiences of children following a disaster can be found in Chapters 3 and 6.

There is a growing body of evidence that indicates that children exposed to mass casualty events can experience neurochemical and structural changes within their brains, which may cause PTSD, which may affect them well into their adult lives (Schonfeld & Demaria, 2015). Disaster planning must be prepared to provide mental healthcare and treatment to this population in the aftermath of a disaster.

In a study by Mondal et al. (2013) of children following the Sikkim earthquake in 2011, 84 out of 3,154 children had stress-related symptoms. Static posturing, sleeplessness, anorexia, recurrent vomiting, excessive crying, and night wakenings were common. In a study of children from two schools in Thailand affected by the severe tsunami in 2004, 573 out of 1,615 students showed signs of PTSD. These signs diminished rapidly to 2.7% after a 5-year period (Piyasil et al., 2011). Piyasil et al. (2014) also looked at quality of life after the same event. Fifteen percent of the victims reported a low quality of life and 68.7% reported a moderate quality of life.

PEDIATRIC CARE DURING DISASTERS

One of the earliest attempts at addressing the needs of pediatric patients during disasters occurred during 1967 to 1968 by the AAP Committee on Disaster and Emergency Medical Care. The committee's recommendations were published in 1972, and appear to be the first organized recognition of the special needs of children during disasters and emergency medical care. The publication outlined first aid and rescue; transportation by ground and air; qualification of emergency medical services (EMS) personnel; communication systems; standards for a pediatric ED, including its location, personnel, administration, records, facilities, and functions of the ED area; and equipment, supplies, and medications (American Academy of Pediatrics, 1972). By today's standards, these recommendations are very rudimentary; however, they laid the foundation for the highly specialized pediatric emergency care that is delivered today.

After the September 11 terrorist attacks, the president and Congress established the National Commission on Children and Disasters. This committee was charged with identifying the gaps in the nation's disaster preparedness, response, and recovery for children and make recommendations to close those gaps. The 2009 interim report identified critical deficiencies and, in its 2010 final report to the president and Congress, expanded on those findings. Those findings have served as the basis of legislation and aggressive efforts to assure children are included in disaster preparedness, response, and recovery. Under the Pandemic and Preparedness Reauthorization Act (PAPRA) of 2013, the National Advisory Committee for Children and Disasters (NACCD) was formed and is building on the work of the national commission. However, although excellent guidance, resources, and training opportunities exist, communities, hospitals, and disaster leadership fail to completely integrate children into disaster plans and exercises. It is not unusual for states and communities to do more planning for pets in emergencies than for children.

Pediatric Disaster Triage

In a natural disaster, it is assumed that children would constitute the same proportion of victims as is found in the community;

for example, if one-third of the community consists of children, then one-third of the victims conceivably would be children. A higher proportion of children involved in a disaster would occur if the event included a predominantly pediatric setting, such as a school, school bus, day care or preschool center, children's hospital or rehabilitation center, juvenile detention center, and the like. In either circumstance, children will need to be triaged and treated based on their severity of injury or illness and survivability.

However, it is important for nurses to understand the dynamics of patient surge associated with disasters as hospitals frequently find that walking wounded or those who arrive by personal vehicle are typically the very first to arrive. This requires ED personnel to rapidly perform an initial assessment of the situation, rapidly triage patients, and activate the hospital mass casualty or disaster plan. In 2012, during the Aurora, Colorado mass shooting that occurred at a theater, it was law enforcement who took on the initial role to rapidly transport the most severely injured to nearby hospitals. These hospitals had little or no warning until critical patients began arriving. In active shooter events, EMS ambulances and personnel are restricted from the "hot" zone for scene safety by law enforcement. During a disaster, it is common to have EMS with additional victims as a secondary surge of casualties may need be to be taken to hospitals in immediate proximity to the event.

EMS arriving on scene following a disaster or mass casualty event must have pediatric equipment, supplies, and medications to effectively treat the ill or injured children. Scene safety, field command, and search and rescue attempts are enacted in accordance with predetermined EMS disaster plans. In 2014, a joint policy statement for equipment for ground ambulances was approved by all the major national emergency and pediatric leadership organizations providing national recommendations of equipment for the prehospital care of pediatric patients (AAP, American College of Emergency Physicians, American College of Surgeons Committee on Trauma, Emergency Medical Services for Children, Emergency Nurses Association, National Association of EMS Physicians, and National Association of State EMS Officials, 2014).

In civilian mass casualty triage in the prehospital setting, those patients with the highest severity of illness or injury who can survive are treated first, while the "walking wounded" and the "worried well" are treated last. Triage involves separating the victims into groups of those who need to be treated in the first 12 to 24 hours, those who should be treated in the next 24 to 48 hours, those who can wait longer and those who are either dead or dying and for whom there are not enough resources to save, in light of the other victims and limited resources. Prehospital triage criteria are the primary and secondary trauma surveys—assessing airway, breathing, circulation, and disability. Victims should be reassessed often and a brief head-to-toe assessment performed. This information is documented on a triage tag that remains with the patient.

There are numerous pediatric-specific trauma triage scales, including the Pediatric Trauma Score, Children's Trauma Tool, and Triage-Revised Trauma Score (Lynch & Thomas, 2004). For triage during disasters, the most commonly used is the JumpSTART System. The JumpSTART Pediatric Multiple Casualty Incident Triage is a method that focuses exclusively on the triage of children during mass casualty events and is modeled after the Simple Triage and Rapid Treatment (START) program (Romig, 2002). JumpSTART helps rescuers to categorize pediatric patients into treatment groups quickly and accurately (Romig, 2002). The JumpSTART triage system assesses the victims' airways, vital signs, and level of consciousness categorizing them in the following groups: minor, delayed, immediate, or deceased. The assessment is designed to be completed in less than 60 seconds. Additional information about JumpSTART can be obtained from Lou Romig, MD, at www.jumpstarttriage.com.

Triage of patients during a mass casualty event following an earthquake poses special problems, such as multiple scenes, limited medical resources, an uncertain time to definitive care, delayed evacuation, and lack of outside assistance for at least 49 to 72 hours (Benson, Koenig, & Schultz, 1996). In the field, prehospital triage is focused on quickly identifying and sorting uninjured and walking wounded from those who require expedited transport to the hospital where arriving patients are then re-triaged to determine the need for further intervention. It is essential in such an event that the limited available resources be used to treat and save the largest number of victims. The Secondary Assessment of Victim Endpoint (SAVE) triage was developed to direct limited resources to the subgroup of patients expected to derive the most benefit from their application (Benson et al., 1996). The SAVE triage system assesses survivability in relation to injuries and, on the basis of trauma statistics, applies this information to describe the relationship between expected benefits and consumed resources (Benson et al., 1996). Further details on the SAVE triage are reported in Benson et al. (1996).

Since then, numerous other triage systems have been developed with either a focus on children or are inclusive of children. These include the SMART Triage Tape which incorporates a JumpSTART-like triage approach using a color-coded length-based tape that is designed to provide the responder with a rapid understanding of what physiological signs and symptoms should be considered. Once the child is triaged using this method, he or she is assigned a triage priority from green to black. Green is delayed priority, yellow urgent priority, red immediate priority, and black is dead. Color triage processes are common to the vast majority of triage systems and assist first responders in quickly assessing patient priority to be removed from the scene to definitive care. In 2008, recognizing that there were no evidence-based triage systems yet developed and there was a need to be more consistent in the approach to triage, the CDC worked with stakeholder groups to develop a national standardized triage system. The consensus model recommended was called SALT (Sort Assess Life-Saving Interventions Treatment and Transport). The SALT Mass Casualty Triage system is inclusive of both adults and children; however, the model has not been universally adopted and START and JumpSTART remain the predominant triage methods.

Triage requires an objective assessment of the victim regardless of age, gender, or other complicating factors. This can be difficult. Kouliey (2016) found that objective triage was difficult and complicated by emotional involvement when triaging children and expecting mothers. It was observed that children were consistently over-triaged compared with less injured adults. Koziel et al. (2015) identified other barriers to pediatric triage. These include lacking knowledge concerning pediatric physiology, triaging children with FAN, and emotional reactions such as triaging a child held in the mother's arms.

The purpose of triage in disaster is to manage and allocate resources in response to a disaster or mass casualty event regardless of setting. While triage systems are considered as part of the practice of emergency personnel, there have been a number of evolving triage systems used to help facilities quickly prioritize and respond to an event. One such tool is Triage by Resource Allocation for IN-patient (TRAIN; Lin, Taylor, & Cohen, 2018; Lucile Packard Children's Hospital, n.d.).

TRAIN is evidence based and has been tested in neonatal intensive care units (NICUs), pediatric intensive care units (PICUs), pediatric units, and with OB/GYN and adult patient populations. The hospital-based triage system is designed as a proactive assessment of patients in the hospital either by building the tool into the hospital electronic medical record or a quick paper-based assessment based on the utilization of equipment, medications, and respiratory and medical support. The tool relies on a simple scoring scale that evaluates a patient's transportation needs based on the following criteria: transportation options, life support, mobility, nutrition, and pharmacy. Information from the tool is then used as part of rapid decompression for discharge home or alternative care. The data also help hospitals rapidly determine their medical transportation needs, which is critical to know when making ambulance resource requests in evacuation.

Another important triage system is focused on mental health to assist with the identification of children and adults who are at the greatest risk of adverse outcomes. PsySTART Triage, developed by Dr. Merritt Shreiber, is a mental health triage system that has been tested and commonly used in real-world events. The tool is best used at regular intervals (Schreiber, 2010). PsySTART is very simple screening that relies on the individual's self-report using a checklist scoring system. The checklist can then be used at intervals to assist in helping direct mental health resources to assist individuals in reducing mental and behavioral health sequela such as PTSD, depression, anxiety and, in the case of children, developmental regression.

Prehospital Treatment

During a mass casualty event or disaster, prehospital considerations focus primarily on basic life support and rapid transport to definitive care. Rapid assessment of the prearrest state includes attention to airway, breathing, circulation, and disability (neurologic). More advanced life support including application of oxygen, infusion of intravenous or intraosseous fluids, emergency medications, and maintenance of thermoregulation are initiated at the scene, at a casualty collection point, and during the transport to the hospital ED.

All states have EMS legislation that establishes local regulations that control the extent of services that can be provided by prehospital personnel and the procedures they can perform on children (Sirbaugh & Meckler, 2017). Prehospital personnel vary in their skills and scope of practice. Most EMS providers are trained at the Emergency Medical Technician (EMT) level and provide primarily basic life support treatment. Others are trained at the Paramedic or (EMT-P) level. These personnel have more advanced training including pediatric advanced life support, pediatric trauma life support, and practice advanced medical interventions in the field under state or local operational area EMS Medical Director–approved protocols.

EMS and public safety responders are trained in mass casualty or disaster situations. However, most EMS personnel have limited training and experience in pediatrics. The EMS curriculum varies with EMT-Basic receiving 110 hours of training and 1,000 to 1,200 hours for paramedics. This leaves only a few hours of training dedicated to children. It limits what can be expected of EMS personnel to do when faced with events involving large numbers of injured children to triage and treat. Pediatric intubation, intravenous or intraosseous access, and medication calculation and administration are difficult enough when one critically ill or injured child is involved; multiply that stress and attention to detail by 10 or 20 additional patients, and EMS personnel and resources can become quickly overwhelmed. Therefore, in mass casualty situations, EMS protocols typically focus on basic treatment, such as jaw-thrust and bag-valve-mask ventilation, medication administration via inhalation or intramuscular routes (if indicated), or other basic treatments.

Special considerations may be given for patients found in collapsed structures depending on the resources and personnel available to respond. First responders with special training in extricating victims from collapsed structures are required along with heavy equipment. Patients trapped for prolonged periods of time following earthquakes or building collapses are at an increased risk of contracting an infectious disease. While entrapped, the patient may be contaminated with waterborne and airborne infectious agents, and may be exposed to their own or others' vomit and feces (Goodman & Hogan, 2002). Documenting the approximate duration of entrapment allows ED personnel to anticipate the treatment needs of the patients. For example, in prolonged entrapment, hypothermia, exposure to infectious agents, and crush injuries would be anticipated. The ED would prepare to administer warmed, humidified oxygen and warmed intravenous fluids; administer antibiotics; and prepare for operative management.

Under normal day-to-day conditions EMS personnel function under guidelines and protocols that outline the destination of ill and injured children—that is, designated hospital EDs that have the capabilities to care for critically ill and injured children are utilized. However, during events involving larger numbers of victims, EMS providers are trained to implement mass casualty plans to, when feasible, avoid overloading one hospital with patients (Floyd, 2002). Referral patterns to designated and alternative hospitals during mass casualty situations should be followed to allow for appropriate treatment (Floyd, 2002). During these events, communication between the field, dispatch, and hospitals is key to supporting timely distribution of patients to definitive care. In these emergencies it is not always feasible to take the patient to specialty pediatric hospitals. This reality requires all hospital EDs to be capable of receiving sick and injured children. Most importantly, EMS must plan and exercise mass casualty, disaster triage, and decontamination procedures with hospitals to prepare themselves accordingly, with proper safety equipment and protection. Responders' first instincts are to pick up children and transport them while holding them. In events associated with risks of chemical, radiological, or biological exposure, children must be considered as potentially contaminated *before* EMS and public safety responders hold or touch them, thereby preventing themselves from becoming secondary victims (Hohenhaus, 2005).

Prehospital Medical Transportation and Evacuation

The decision to transport a child by ground or air ambulance from the scene of a mass casualty or disaster event depends on the condition of the child, transportation resources available, the medical capability of transporting personnel, and the desired patient destination. These decisions are determined by the ambulance personnel on scene or, in large events, the incident commander in the field. Typically, ground transport is more readily available than air medical transportation; however, aeromedical personnel are highly trained in the management of critically ill children and may be required to help assure safe transport if there is a long distance between the scene and the receiving facility (Sirbaugh & Meckler, 2017).

In disasters where the hospitals must evacuate, medical transportation resources must be quickly mobilized involving requests for ambulance mutual aid from regional, state, and federal partners due to the number of medical transportation assets required. Most of what is known about patient movement in disaster comes from real-world events such as Hurricanes Katrina and Ike, and Superstorm Sandy where there were numerous controlled evacuations associated with hospital moves. The first known description of a pediatric-specific patient movement plan was associated with the move of Children's Hospital of Colorado relocation of a pediatric hospital's entire population in less than 12 hours. During the planned move, 111 patients were transported 8.5 miles. Sixty-four patients and 32 infants included 24 children on ventilators, three on inhaled nitric oxide, 30 on continuous infusions, and four with external ventricular drains. Thirteen critical care teams were used along with five advanced life support ambulance crews, four SUVs, and one hospital van (Fuzak et al., 2010).

While in the case of a planned hospital evacuation, plans and execution of the hospital move is typically very successfully managed as it benefits from months of careful planning with plenty of resources and personnel to assure safe patient transfer. In no-notice events, the evacuation can be chaotic and hospitals will shelter in place until either they are forced to evacuate or there are sufficient medical transportation resources available to support the evacuation. During Hurricane Katrina, hospitals affected by the storm were faced with moving infants and children many miles away by flatbed trucks, paddleboats, and staff vehicles, requiring the doctors and nurses to accompany the patients under extreme duress. Children's hospitals and their transport teams from across the country were mobilized to support the evacuation of children outside of the federal disaster response system.

However, this is not always the case in events that force immediate evacuation of the hospital such as fire or earthquake.

In these cases, patients are evacuated to predesignated areas on hospital grounds and EMS responders along with hospital leadership coordinate the transport of patients to appropriate facilities. Under these no-notice or short-notice events, there is an increased risk of morbidity and mortality for those children who may require critical interventions. In those conditions, nursing personnel assigned to or caring for the child in the hospital need to be prepared to accompany the child to the receiving facility to assure the patient's safety.

While it is ideal to transport critically ill children using a specialized pediatric transport team, these resources are very limited or may require more time to respond to an acute event. This is why all hospitals need to be prepared to manage sick and injured children for extended periods of time in events where substantial ambulance mutual aid is required. Nurses caring for children in dedicated pediatric specialty centers or community hospitals need to understand that most pediatric specialty care has been increasingly regionalized in the United States and, while this serves to improve the care of children in day-to-day conditions, it creates unintended gaps and challenges when responding to mass casualty and disaster events that are either far away from those specialty resources or the specialty pediatric centers are directly affected. To address this issue the EMS-C program developed a Pediatric Regionalization of Care Primer (Emergency Medical Services for Children Innovation & Improvement Center, n.d.-b) to help communities address the opportunities associated with improving pediatric emergency care. The Pediatric Regionalization of Care Primer is intended to assist state leadership, healthcare professionals, health organizations, and others in understanding the considerations unique to regional pediatric care systems.

Emergency Department Treatment

Over 80% of all hospitals see children in the United States; however, most of these cases are associated with minor injuries or conditions that can be managed without admission or transfer to a pediatric specialty hospital. In emergencies associated with a number of critically injured children, EMS protocols are designed to triage the sickest children to definitive care such as a pediatric trauma center. However, in a disaster or mass casualty situation, all hospitals will be called on to care for ill or injured children of varying degrees of symptom severity. Therefore, all hospital EDs need to be prepared to treat children; likewise, pediatric hospitals must be prepared to treat injured or ill parents and adult family members. As part of their pediatric disaster planning, hospitals should anticipate a lack of prehospital triage; establish protocols for care; create pediatric antidote kits; organize and store pediatric equipment in one setting; and anticipate the need for extra personnel (Hohenhaus, 2005).

When injured children arrive at the ED, they are triaged according to their severity of injury, with those in most critical condition receiving care first. Children with FAN who cannot talk or ambulate should be triaged similar to infants (Hohenhaus, 2005). Triage under disaster circumstances is generally carried out by physicians and nurses to quickly ascertain the numbers of ill or injured children, their severity of injury, and the resources that will be needed to care for them.

TABLE 11.1 Primary Survey of the Pediatric Trauma Patient

Component	Actions
Airway/cervical spine	Assess for patency; look for loose teeth, vomitus, or other obstruction; note position of head. Suspect cervical spine injury with multiple trauma; maintain neutral alignment during assessment; evaluate effectiveness of cervical immobilization and other equipment used to immobilize the spine. The use of rigid C-collars is now considered a potentially dangerous practice. C spine injuries in children are typically rare. Evidence-based practice now encourages spinal stabilization without use of rigid backboards or rigid collars.
Breathing	Auscultate breath sounds in the axillae and throughout the chest area for presence and equality. Assess chest for contusions, penetrating wounds, abrasions, or paradoxic movement.
Circulation	Assess apical pulse for rate, rhythm, and quality; compare apical and peripheral pulses for quality and equality. Evaluate capillary refill; normal is less than 2 seconds. Check skin color and temperature. Note open wounds or uncontrolled bleeding; apply direct pressure or tourniquet as necessary.
Disability (neurologic)	Assess level of consciousness; check for orientation to person, place, and time in the older child. In a younger child, assess alertness, ability to interact with environment, and ability to follow commands. Is the child easily consoled and interested in the environment? Does the child recognize a familiar object and respond when you speak to him or her? Check pupils for size, reactivity, and equality.
Expose	Remove clothing to allow visual inspection of the entire body.

Source: Adapted from Bernardo, L., & Schenkel, K. (2003). Pediatric trauma. In N. Newberry (Ed.), *Sheehy's principles and practice of emergency nursing* (5th ed., pp. 379–400). St. Louis, MO: Mosby-Year Book. Reprinted with permission from Elsevier Science.

After the appropriate level of triage is assigned, emergency health professionals—generally physicians, nurses, and surgeons—complete the primary and secondary surveys of the injured child (Tables 11.1 and 11.2). These surveys allow for the rapid detection of life-threatening injuries and the initiation of lifesaving treatment.

As soon as possible, parents and family members should be permitted to see their children. Emergency personnel should explain to the parents beforehand what they will see and why; such explanations prevent any surprises (Bernardo & Schenkel, 2003). Parents may believe they need permission to touch or talk to their children; they should be encouraged to touch, talk to, and be with their children (Bernardo & Schenkel, 2003). Tell children what will happen before it happens. Children do not like surprises any more than adults do. Prepare them by using feeling terms; for example, "This will feel cold; this will feel heavy; this will smell sweet" (Bernardo & Schenkel, 2003).

The Joint Commission on Accreditation of Healthcare Organizations requires that all patients receive a pain assessment and appropriate pain-relief measures. Various pain scales are available to measure pain in preverbal and verbal children; nurses should administer the scales to determine the child's level of pain and the need for pain-relief measures (Bernardo & Schenkel, 2003). Analgesics may be administered once all injuries are identified and the child is determined to be physiologically and neurologically intact (Bernardo & Schenkel, 2003). Pharmacological management of pain includes narcotic and nonnarcotic analgesics, while nonpharmacological management of pain includes comfort measures such as distraction techniques, progressive relaxation, positive self-talk, and deep-breathing exercises (Bernardo & Schenkel, 2003). Parents and family members can be encouraged to assist their children with pain-relief measures. EDs must also be prepared to meet the psychological needs of pediatric victims. They must provide safe, humane, culturally and developmentally sensitive triage, diagnosis, stabilization, initial management, and treatment for the pediatric population (Schonfeld & Demaria, 2015).

Once life-threatening injuries are stabilized, definitive treatment is initiated. This treatment can include immediate operative management, admission to the intensive care unit, or admission to an inpatient unit. Transfer and transport to a specialized facility, such as a burn center or spinal cord injury center, may be warranted. Transfer is initiated once the patient is stabilized and the receiving hospital agrees to accept the patient. Transport is undertaken by fixed wing aircraft, helicopter, or ambulance, with healthcare professionals experienced in the care of critically injured children accompanying the patient to the receiving facility.

Reunification and Family Assistance Planning

According to Save the Children survey in 2014, 69 million children are separated from parents to attend child care, school, or events as part of normal day-to-day conditions (National Report Card on Protecting Children in Disaster, 2014).

TABLE 11.2 Secondary Survey of the Pediatric Trauma Patient

Component	Action
Head, eye, ear, and nose	Assess scalp for lacerations or open wounds; palpate for step-off defects, depressions, hematomas, and pain. Reassess pupils for size, reactivity, equality, and extraocular movements; ask the child if he or she can see. Assess ears and nose for rhinorrhea or otorrhea. Observe for raccoon eyes (bruising around the eyes) or Battle's sign (bruising over the mastoid process). Palpate forehead, orbits, maxilla, and mandible for crepitus, deformities, step-off defect, pain, and stability; evaluate malocclusion by asking child to open and close mouth; note open wounds. Inspect for loose, broken, or chipped teeth as well as oral lacerations. Check orthodontic appliances for stability. Evaluate facial symmetry by asking child to smile, grimace, and open and close mouth. Do not remove impaled objects or foreign objects.
Neck	Open cervical collar and reassess anterior neck for jugular vein distention and tracheal deviation; note bruising, edema, open wounds, pain, and crepitus. Check for hoarseness or changes in voice by asking child to speak.
Chest	Obtain respiratory rate; reassess breath sounds in anterior lobes for equality. Palpate chest wall and sternum for pain, tenderness, and crepitus. Observe inspiration and expiration for symmetry or paradoxic movement; note use of accessory muscles. Reassess apical heart rate for rate, rhythm, and clarity.
Abdomen/pelvis/genitourinary	Observe abdomen for bruising and distention; auscultate bowel sounds briefly in all four quadrants; palpate abdomen gently for tenderness; assess pelvis for tenderness and stability. Palpate bladder for distention and tenderness; check urinary meatus for signs of injury or bleeding; note priapism and genital trauma such as lacerations or foreign body. Have rectal sphincter tone assessed, usually by physician.
Musculoskeletal	Assess extremities for deformities, swelling, lacerations, or other injuries. Palpate distal pulses for equality, rate, and rhythm; compare with central pulses. Ask child to wiggle toes and fingers; evaluate strength through hand grips and foot flexion/extension.
Back	Logroll as a unit to inspect back; maintain spinal alignment during examination; observe for bruising and open wounds; palpate each vertebral body for tenderness, pain, deformity, and stability; assess flank area for bruising and tenderness.

Source: Bernardo, L., & Schenkel, K. (2003). Pediatric trauma. In N. Newberry (Ed.), *Sheehy's principles and practice of emergency nursing* (5th ed., pp. 379–400). St. Louis, MO: Mosby-Year Book. Reprinted with permission from Elsevier Science.

Given those findings, it should be expected that children and families are likely to be separated immediately after a disaster because of their varying severity of injury or illness, requiring them to go to the facilities most appropriate for their care. As soon as possible, though, children and families should be reunited, and plans for this should be written into hospitals' disaster programs (Conway et al., 1990). Plans should be in place for the activation of support personnel with specialized knowledge in children's mental health needs, such as child life specialists, child psychologists, psychiatrists, and counselors (Conway et al., 1990). Reuniting families can be operationalized on an EMS level or county level through EMS trip reports or other locator systems.

In November 2013, the National Guidance Post-Disaster Reunification of Children: A Nationwide Approach was published providing a comprehensive overview of the coordination processes necessary to reunify children separated from parents and legal guardians in an emergency (FEMA, 2013). While reunifying unaccompanied minors is a priority, it also is complex and requires the coordinated efforts of responders and law enforcement at the local level.

Nurses working in community hospitals should understand what their hospital plan is to support rapid reunification of unaccompanied minors to their appropriate legal guardians. It is recommended that hospitals have a plan to establish a family assistance center to be successful in this process. Hospitals may also need to provide temporary shelter for uninjured unaccompanied children during a disaster until they can be properly reunited with the assistance of law enforcement and child protective services.

Children and families may be discharged to home or to shelters directly from the ED. When they are discharged, families should be given listings of community resources, such as local mental health services, disaster aid services, and hospital/clinic psychiatric services (Conway et al., 1990), thus allowing families the opportunity to follow up with these resources as needed. Families can be given pamphlets or other materials on anticipatory guidance for what their children will experience and how they can promote their children's coping.

Community Hospital Preparedness

Community hospitals are frequently in the role of the first line of defense in disasters and need to be prepared to manage a 20% surge of patients within 4 hours. This can be achieved through implementation of rapid discharge protocols or bed expansion. Routine disaster exercises using the hospital incident command system and participating in operational area disaster and mass casualty exercises will help prepare the facility to manage a rapid influx of injured patients following a real disaster. The hospitals themselves may be damaged and unsafe for patients and personnel and they may have to close their doors. Hospitals that remain open may be faced with caring for large numbers of injured children, and they need to have sufficient resources and trained staff to respond.

Under day-to-day conditions and disaster, the inpatient care of children requires a higher staff-to-patient ratio, especially in the infant population. Infants and children cannot care for themselves, making their care more labor intensive than an adult population. Staff will already be spread thin to care for many patients, including adults and the elderly, who also have special healthcare needs. Parents and family members themselves may be hospitalized and unavailable to provide physical comfort or emotional support. Children may be taken by air transport to specialty hospitals miles away, and uninjured parents may be separated from their children because of impassable roads or the lack of transportation or money. Caring for children under such austere conditions will be challenging for nurses and healthcare professionals.

In each hospital's disaster plan, provisions for the care of large numbers of injured children should be made to assure adequate supplies and staffing. There are numerous resources and guidance in this area and community hospitals should first assess their current capability using the EMS for Children Pediatric Readiness Project Assessment Toolkit (Emergency Medical Services for Children Innovation & Improvement Center, n.d.-a). The toolkit assessment provides an individual hospital with a pediatric centric gap assessment and numerous resources to help address gaps in pediatric care and to enhance disaster capability. A key indicator for success is known to be the assignment of a physician and nurse pediatric champion within each facility to assure improvement occurs over time.

Care in Shelters

In the event of a disaster, families may need to evacuate their homes and go to community-designated shelters or stay with friends or relatives outside of the disaster area. The decision to evacuate to a shelter or alternate safe housing may be based on weather advisories, requests from public safety officials, or self-identified need.

Families that have lived through a natural disaster, such as a hurricane, would likely evacuate to a shelter in the event of a similar situation. Rincon, Linares, and Greenberg (2001) found otherwise in a study conducted 7 years after Hurricane Andrew. In their survey of 325 caregivers whose children were receiving treatment in a pediatric ED, Rincon et al. (2001) reported that only 37% of families living in Dade County during Hurricane Andrew would go to a shelter versus 49% of families who were not living in Dade County at that time. Ninety-six percent of those living in Dade County during Hurricane Andrew who would not go to a shelter in the event of a hurricane evacuation advisory had at least one child under 13 years of age; similarly, 97% of those not living in Dade County during Hurricane Andrew who would not evacuate to a shelter had at least one child under 13 years of age (Rincon et al., 2001). Healthcare and public safety professionals need to be aware that families with children may not evacuate during a disaster and may not be accounted for among families going to shelters or hospitals for care. These families may still require healthcare and would have to be reached through alternative means, such as door-to-door or on-site clinics.

After a disaster, families and children will require mental health services and counseling. Qualified child psychologists, psychiatrists, social workers, and counselors should provide this treatment. To meet children's psychosocial needs following a disaster, healthcare professionals must consider the children's developmental levels, their caregivers, and their families when conducting assessments and providing treatment (Mohr, 2002). Also critical to treatment is an assessment of the nature of the child's exposure to the disaster, the severity of the disaster, and the duration of the trauma or crisis (Mohr, 2002).

Care in Refugee Camps and Camps for Displaced Populations

In war-torn countries, fleeing refugees may be placed in refugee camps until they are free to return to their towns or leave their country. Life in refugee camps provides its own set of circumstances that contribute to the potential for the spread of infectious diseases. Nurses and healthcare professionals must collaborate with public health officials to conduct surveillance for infectious disease outbreaks in these camps. While births and deaths are expected in refugee camps, the mortality rate in displaced populations exceeding 4/10,000/day in children younger than 5 years is a cause for grave concern and investigation (Noji, 2005).

Measles should be suspected in areas where it is endemic and childhood immunization rates are low; signs of measles include fever, cough, mouth sores, and rash. Children under 5 years of age who pass rice water stools with or without vomiting should raise the suspicion of cholera in epidemic areas. *Shigella* is suspected in children with painful bloody stools and fever.

A measles vaccine program, second in priority to the provision of food, can save children at risk of starvation (Burkle, 2002). Vitamin A alone can decrease the mortality rate in starving children up to 50% (Burkle, 2002, p. 50). Current evidence demonstrates that measles vaccination, vitamin A, and insecticide-treated nets can be given to decrease morbidity and mortality (Salama & Roberts, 2005). These interventions should be readily available in complex emergencies (Salama & Roberts, 2005) for infants and children aged 6 months to 5 years (up to ages 12–14 years can be recommended; Noji, 2005). Ideally, 80% of the refugee camp population should receive measles immunization (Noji, 2005). Jablonka et al. (2016) in a study of 678 refugees entering Germany confirmed the need for children to receive the measles, mumps, and rubella (MMR) vaccine. Should meningococcal meningitis be confirmed in an ill person, especially in geographic areas where such epidemics have occurred, a vaccination program is warranted, especially for families and close community contacts. In young children, though, immunity duration is short and does not prevent the spread of the bacteria by carriers.

Coldiron et al. (2017) studied the intermittent treatment of malaria at a refugee camp in Northern Uganda for South Sudanese refugees. Dihydroartemisinin-piperaquine (DP) was distributed at 8-week intervals achieving 90% coverage. The incidence of malaria was reduced in children of all ages while the incidence increased in those not targeted by the intervention.

Mass vaccination is not warranted for typhoid and cholera, as the likelihood of contracting these diseases will occur before the series of immunizations are administered. Treatment of infectious diseases requires a multifaceted approach. Children with bacillary dysenteries should be treated with trimethoprim/sulfamethoxazole. Any outbreak of diarrheal diseases should signal the need to chlorinate the water supplies.

Adequate food must be delivered and distributed to families in refugee camps. In refugee settings, the elderly and unaccompanied minors are at risk of decreased access to food and efforts should be made to get food to these individuals (Burkle, 2002). The most vulnerable to nutritional deficiencies include pregnant women, breastfeeding mothers, young children, people with disabilities, and the elderly (Noji, 2005). Children are placed in feeding programs depending on their nutritional needs and are not discharged until they reach more than 90% of their reference standard (e.g., mid upper arm circumference; Burkle, 2002). The WHO oral rehydration solution is administered when indicated. The results of a double-blinded, randomized, controlled clinical trial indicated that the addition of Benefiber to the WHO oral rehydration solution facilitated recovery from acute watery diarrhea in children (Alam et al., 2000). Benefiber supposedly enhances the colonic absorption of salt and water, thereby improving the course of the diarrheal illness. General food rations should be at 2,100 kcal per person per day and should include sufficient proportions of protein, fat, and micronutrients (Noji, 2005).

Even in refugee settings, children's developmental needs can be met. This includes encouraging children to play; play can help to reduce stress and should be considered a priority along with physical care, treating dehydration, and malnutrition (Raynor, 2002). Play becomes even more important to children in refugee camps (or shelters), where a sense of safety and stability have been restored (Raynor, 2002). Children can use play to express their thoughts and feelings about the disaster. Raynor (2002) describes in detail how to initiate play with children who have been displaced following a disaster. In refugee

settings, interventions to help children must take into account the parents' stresses as well as traditional healing practices of the community (Burkle, 2002).

Long-Term Care Following a Disaster

Large-scale disasters will completely overwhelm the infrastructure of an area; this includes the local healthcare system. This is known as a "catastrophic health emergency." Local hospitals may be affected, being overwhelmed with patients or by significant damage to the physical structure. Providers, including physicians and nurses, may not be able to discharge their normal duties because of injury to themselves or family. This may have a long-term effect on the hospital's ability to serve those in need. Primary care givers will also be affected. Their practice may be completely disrupted. Patients may not be able to financially or physically seek care from those who may have cared for them for years. Free clinics and emergency hospitals provide care free of charge for those in need after a disaster. While this is necessary, in the long term, it may delay the local healthcare system's return to normal (Needle, 2008).

PEDIATRIC CARE DURING PUBLIC HEALTH EMERGENCIES

Exposure to Nuclear and Radiological Agents

Children, like adults, can be exposed to nuclear agents through an attack on a nuclear power plant; they can be exposed to radiological agents through the release of a "dirty bomb" or an unintentional release. The decontamination and treatment of patients exposed to radioactive contaminants are discussed elsewhere in this book (refer to Chapter 30). This section outlines pediatric-specific recommendations for care.

Prehospital Treatment

In the prehospital setting, radioactive contamination can be quickly detected using Geiger counters or dose-rate meters (Mettler & Voelz, 2002). A high index of suspicion for radioactive agents must be maintained. *Pediatric advanced life support protocols always take precedence over radiation issues. It is better to have a dirty patient who is alive than to have a dead clean patient.* The time taken to care for life-threatening injuries will not significantly enhance the impact of the radiation (Beach, 2010). EMS personnel can remove the victims' clothing, resulting in the elimination of 90% of the contamination (Beach, 2010; Jarrett, 1999). EMS personnel must wear protective clothing and gloves, in accordance with their agencies' policies and procedures; when entering highly contaminated areas, respirators must be worn. Surface decontamination can be undertaken in the absence of physical injuries; in the presence of life-threatening injuries, such injuries are stabilized prior to surface decontamination (Mettler & Voelz, 2002). If decontamination occurs out of doors, hot water should be available in the event of near-freezing weather; separate facilities should be established for men and women (Fong, 2002). Infants and young children should remain with their mothers or female caregivers; older children should be decontaminated with the appropriate gender. Contaminated items are placed in labeled plastic bags and properly disposed (Jarrett, 1999; Mettler & Voelz, 2002) or held for law enforcement. Open wounds should be covered until decontamination is completed (Jarrett, 1999).

Emergency Department Treatment

Before patients arrive, the ED must prepare patient care areas to limit the spread of radioactive contamination; security must be in place to prevent unauthorized access. Triage includes a radiological survey to assess dose rate, documentation of prodromal symptoms, and collection of tissue samples for biodosimetry (Waselenko et al., 2004). Children should be given age-appropriate explanations of what is happening to them and what they will feel ("I am going to tickle your nose with this cotton swab").

Parents may not be permitted to see their children until life-threatening conditions are treated and decontamination procedures are completed. Keeping parents apprised of their children's condition is helpful in allaying their anxiety; letting children know that their parents are waiting for them will be comforting to frightened children. Hospitalization is recommended in significant systemic irradiation, disease, or trauma (Fong, 2002).

Definitive Treatment

Should children be exposed to the detonation of a nuclear weapon or the release of radioactive material from a nuclear reactor and iodine is a byproduct of the release, potassium iodide (KI) or iodate would be administered to prevent radioiodine from accumulating in the thyroid gland. KI should be administered immediately or at least within 8 hours postexposure (Chung & Shannon, 2005). KI should be administered with caution in children and adolescents with a known or reported allergy to iodide, as severe allergic reactions have been reported (AAP, 2003; Waselenko et al., 2004). In newborns, KI administration has been linked with transient decreases in thyroxine along with increases in thyroid-stimulating hormone (AAP, 2003). Therefore, newborns who receive KI should have ongoing monitoring of their thyroid function by measuring thyroid-stimulating hormone activity 2 to 4 weeks postadministration of a single KI dose or for longer periods than when one KI dose is administered (AAP, 2003). Because both radioiodine and KI are secreted into human breast milk, lactating women who receive KI should not breastfeed their infants because of the risk of additional exposure to radioiodine from breast milk (AAP, 2003). Public health officials will determine when it is safe to resume breastfeeding and when it is safe to consume produce and milk following a radiological exposure (AAP, 2003).

KI is prepared in tablets, making it easier to store. Infants and children may not be able to swallow tablets. When dissolved in water, the fluid is too salty to drink (U.S. FDA, 2017). To disguise the salty taste of the KI, the tablet can be crushed and mixed with raspberry syrup, low-fat chocolate milk, orange juice, or flat soda (cola; Pelsor, Sadrieh, & Machado, 2002; U.S. FDA, 2017). Nurses or parents can crush one 130-mg KI tablet into small pieces; add four teaspoons of water to the crushed tablet to dissolve it; then add four teaspoons of one of the aforementioned fluids to the mixture making 130 mg per four teaspoons of solution (U.S. FDA, 2002). Each teaspoon contains 30.5 mg of KI. The recommended daily dose for KI in children 4 to 18 years of age is four teaspoonfuls; for children 1 month through 3 years of age, two teaspoonfuls; and for newborns and infants less than 1 month of age, one teaspoonful; 18 years of age weighing 150 or more pounds, eight teaspoons (U.S. FDA, 2017). This daily dosing should continue until the risk of exposure has passed or until other measures, such as evacuation, sheltering, and control of the food and milk supply, have been implemented successfully (U.S. FDA, 2017). Recommendations for continued KI administration should be made by the Environmental Protection Agency, the Nuclear Regulatory Commission, or other governmental agencies involved with assessing the environmental impact of the radioiodine release (AAP, 2003). Overall, the benefits of KI treatment exceed the risks of overdosing, especially in children; however, particular attention to dose and duration of treatment should be afforded to infants and pregnant women (U.S. FDA, 2017).

For children exposed to cesium-137 and thallium, Prussian blue is administered. Prussian blue enhances the excretion of these agents in the stool, thereby decreasing radiation exposure (Chung & Shannon, 2005). The dosage for Prussian blue is 3 to 10 g/d by mouth (0.21–0.32 g/kg/d; Columbia University Mailman School of Public Health National Center for Disaster Preparedness, 2003).

Following exposure to plutonium, curium and americium, chelation with pentetate calcium trisodium (CaDTPA), pentetate zinc trisodium (Zn-DTPA), or dimercapto-propane-1-sulfonic acid (DMPS) can be administered (Chung & Shannon, 2005). Ca-DTPA and Zn-DTPA chelate with metals and are excreted in the urine (Chung & Shannon, 2005). These medications are administered by inhalation or intravenous routes at a dosage of 14 mg/kg IV, up to a maximum of 1 g (Chung & Shannon, 2005).

Children are one of the groups at high risk of psychological effects following terrorist attacks and subsequent exposure to radiation (Mettler & Voelz, 2002; Waselenko et al., 2004). Counseling should be in place to help children cope with the situation and its long-term effects (Fong, 2002; Waselenko et al., 2004).

Exposure to Biological Agents

Children may be exposed to biological agents while at school, at home, or in the community (Rosenfield & Bernardo, 2001). For the most part, signs and symptoms of biological diseases are the same in children and adults: Anthrax and smallpox, though, have different treatment regimens for children and are outlined in Table 11.3. Nurses and healthcare professionals should contact their local health department for current treatment recommendations or refer to the website for the CDC (www.cdc.gov). The CDC classifies biological agents as A, B, or C agents. Category A agents are considered those of the greatest threat due to high morbidity and mortality, as well as the potential ease of dissemination. In category A, there are six agents: anthrax, smallpox, tularemia, plague, viral hemorrhagic fever, and botulism (Beach, 2010). See Table 11.4 for a complete list of biological agents of concern.

In recent years, more pediatric-specific items have been added to the U.S. Strategic National Stockpile (SNS) including a pediatric formulary and materials for compounding tablets and capsules into liquid formulations. Equipment and certain pharmaceuticals are now included. One problem with pediatric-specific pharmaceuticals is that the SNS may stock only items licensed by the U.S. FDA that are used only for their FDA-approved indications. In some instances, FDA indications are lacking for medications used in children exposed to chemical or biological agents; the SNS does not contain therapeutic agents for all indications for children (Markenson & Reynolds, 2006). One approach would be to allow the SNS to include medications for indications that may not be FDA-approved for children provided there is evidence for its use under proper medical supervision (Table 11.5; Markenson & Reynolds, 2006).

Healthcare professionals may experience difficulties in detecting, then treating, children exposed to biological agents. First, physicians may fail to diagnose a disease caused by a biological agent, as such diseases occur rarely or not at all in the United States. Second, if two or more biological agents are dispersed, there may be confusion when diagnoses are attempted. Third, the method of dispersing the biological agent will affect how it enters the body; for example, Q fever, psittacosis, and smallpox can be spread by aerosol attack, while others may occur via natural routes, such as mosquitoes. *A high index of suspicion must be maintained by healthcare professionals when treating children who present with unusual signs and symptoms of infectious or communicable diseases.*

Prehospital Treatment

In the prehospital setting, it is unlikely that EMS personnel will be able to diagnosis a disease caused by exposure to a biological agent. EMS will treat children based on their severity of illness, stabilizing the airways, assisting with breathing and restoring circulatory volume. Pediatric advanced life support

TABLE 11.3 Pediatric Signs and Symptoms Following Exposure to Anthrax

Biological Agent/Disease	Signs and Symptoms	Diagnosis and Treatment	Medication Administration
Cutaneous anthrax	Initial painless papulovesicular lesion surrounded by massive interstitial edema; eschar develops within 2–5 days (Freedman et al., 2002). Systemic symptoms include fever and leukocytosis (in delayed treatment and development of bacteremia; Freedman et al., 2002).	Serum polymerase chain reaction and skin biopsy (Freedman et al., 2002). Hospitalize; monitor electrolyte and hematological status; administer intravenous antibiotics (Freedman et al., 2002).	*Initial Treatment*: Ciprofloxacin or doxycycline; intravenous therapy with multiple antimicrobial agents is recommended (CDC, 2001). In young children under 2 years old, initial therapy should be intravenous and combination therapy with additional antimicrobials considered (CDC, 2001). *Treatment*: Following improvement, begin oral therapy with one or two antimicrobial agents (including either ciprofloxacin or doxycycline) for the first 7–10 days (CDC, 2001). *Remaining time until 60 days*: Amoxicillin is administered for the completion of the remaining 60 days of therapy (CDC, 2001). Amoxicillin dosing in children ≥ 40 kg: 500 mg every 8 hours; children less than 40 kg: 15 mg/kg every 8 hours (total 45 mg/kg/d; U.S. FDA, 2001a).
Systemic (inhalation) anthrax	Fever, myalgia, fatigue, headache, malaise 5–6 days postexposure (Kare, Roham, & Hardin, 2002; Nopar, 1967). Nonproductive cough for 2–3 days, severe respiratory distress, cyanosis, chest pain, diaphoresis, shock, and death over 24–36 hours (Kare et al., 2002; Nopar, 1967).	Chest radiograph (reveals bilateral widened mediastinum; Kare et al., 2002; Nopar, 1967). Hospitalize; support respiratory effort; administer antibiotics.	*Initial Treatment*: Intravenous ciprofloxacin 10 mg/kg/dose every 12 hours (maximum 400 mg/dose) OR 15 mg/kg/dose every 12 hours orally (maximum 500 mg/dose; CDC, 2001), OR intravenous doxycycline 2.2 mg/kg/dose every 12 hours OR orally (maximum 100 mg/dose; CDC, 2001), PLUS one or two additional antimicrobial agents (CDC, 2001).

TABLE 11.4 Biological Agents of Concern by Category

Category A	Anthrax *Bacillus anthracis*
	Smallpox *Variola major*
	Tularemia *Francisella tularenis*
	Plague *Yersinia pestis*
	Viral hemorrhagic fevers *Ebola, Marburg, Lassa*
	Botulinum *Clostridium botulinum toxin*
Category B	Q fever *Coxiella burnetii*
	Brucellosis *Brucella species*
	Glanders *Burkholderia mallei*
	Melioidosis *Burkholderia pseudomallei*
	Viral encephalitis *alphaviruses*
	Typhus *Rickettsia prowazekii*
	Biotoxins *ricin, staphylococcal enterotoxin B*
	Psittacosis *Chlamydia psittaci*
	Food safety threats *Salmonella*
	Water safety threats *Vibrio cholerae*
Category C	Emerging threat agents *Nipah and hantavirus*
	Multidrug-resistant tuberculosis
	Tick-borne encephalitis
	Tick-borne hemorrhagic fever virus
	Yellow fever

Source: Committee on Environmental Health and Committee on Infectious Diseases. (2000). Chemical-biological terrorism and its impact on children: A subject review. *Pediatrics, 105,* 662–670. doi:10.1542/peds.105.3.662

TABLE 11.5 Recommended Dosing for Selected Pediatric Exposures

Disease Exposure	Medication	Dosage
Inhalation anthrax postexposure prophylaxis	Amoxicillin	80 mg/kg/d in 3 divided doses; maximum 500 mg/dose
Inhalation anthrax	Ciprofloxacin	10–15 mg/kg every 12 h; not to exceed 1 g/d
Tularemia treatment	Ciprofloxacin Gentamicin	15 mg/kg every 12 h; not to exceed 1 g/d IV or IM 6–7.5 mg/kg/d in 3 divided doses (every 8 h)
Tularemia prophylaxis	Ciprofloxacin	15–20 mg/kg every 12 h; not to exceed 1 g/d

IM, intramuscular; IV, intravenous.

Source: Centers for Disease Control and Prevention. (2002). *The national pharmaceutical stockpile (NPS) program.* Atlanta, GA: Author.

protocols would be followed, and in mass casualty settings, triage would occur with rapid transport of those with the highest illness severity. EMS personnel would don PPE, such as masks and gloves, as part of their standard procedures for universal precautions. Children and their families may need to be kept together or separated, depending on the location and duration of the exposure to the biological agent.

Emergency Treatment

In the ED, attention is turned toward pediatric life support protocols to maintain the child's airway, breathing, and circulation. Personal protective equipment, such as masks and gloves, are worn. Depending on the symptoms, blood, urine, and other cultures may be obtained, as well as blood specimens for laboratory analysis. Pharmacological therapy may be initiated. ED staff would alert their local public health agency of any symptoms that are suggestive of intentionally released biological agents.

Children may be separated from their parents and family members if they are deemed to be contagious. If children are quarantined, parents may not be able to visit. Young children may experience separation anxiety and they may not respond to staff members. More caregivers may be wearing strange gowns and masks which may add to the child's fear. It is important to know which diseases are contagious person to person requiring special precautions and those not contagious. Anthrax, tularemia, and botulism are not contagious person to person and require only standard personal protection equipment (Beach, 2010). Ebola is very contagious, requiring special precautions. Nurses and healthcare professionals must be able to distinguish separation anxiety and fear of abandonment from a worsening neurological status. Children who are quarantined require extra staff for their care because they cannot care for themselves, and their health condition must be closely monitored. Plans for the care of quarantined children and families must be included in community and hospital disaster planning.

Definitive Treatment

Anthrax

At this time, anthrax vaccine absorbed (AVA) is licensed for use in individuals 18 to 65 years of age (Inglesby et al., 2002). While no data are available for children, it is likely that the AVA would be safe and effective in children, based on experience with other inactivated vaccines (Inglesby et al., 2002). The American Hospital Formulary Services recommends that ciprofloxacin and other fluoroquinolones not be used in children younger than 18 years of age because of a link to transient arthropathy in a small number of children (Inglesby et al., 2002). However, Inglesby et al. (2002) recommend that ciprofloxacin be used as a component of combination therapy for children diagnosed with inhalation anthrax, weighing the risk of arthropathy versus anthrax infection. Postexposure prophylaxis or mass casualty exposure requires the use of monotherapy with fluoroquinolones (Inglesby et al., 2002). These guidelines remain in effect at this writing (Beach, 2010).

The AAP recommends that doxycycline not be used in children less than 9 years of age because of retarded skeletal growth in infants and discolored teeth in infants and toddlers (Inglesby et al., 2002). Because of the serious nature of anthrax infection, however, it is recommended that doxycycline, instead of ciprofloxacin, be used in children if antibiotic susceptibility testing, exhaustion of drug supplies, or adverse reactions preclude the use of ciprofloxacin (Beach, 2010).

In a contained casualty setting, children with inhalation anthrax can receive intravenous antibiotics; in a mass casualty setting and as postexposure prophylaxis, children can receive oral antibiotics (Inglesby et al., 2002). Doxycycline is dispensed in a tablet that children may not be able to swallow; however, it can be ground and mixed with food or drink to make it palatable. Palatable foods and drinks for mixing doxycycline include chocolate pudding, chocolate milk, low-fat chocolate milk, simple syrup with sour apple flavor, apple juice with table sugar, and low-fat milk (Yu et al., 2002). Amoxicillin can be used in the 60-day antimicrobial prophylaxis period in infants and children when the anthrax involved in the exposure is determined to be susceptible to penicillin (CDC, 2001).

Botulism

Botulism is usually tied to a common food source, such as a family picnic or particular restaurant. If no common source can be identified, then an intentional release of possible inhaled botulism toxin must be considered (Beach, 2010). While there is a licensed trivalent equine botulinum antitoxin available through the CDC, its administration is unlikely to reverse the disease in children who are symptomatic (Henretig, Cieslak, & Eitzen, 2003). The antitoxin does prevent the advancement of symptoms and should be administered as soon as possible (Beach, 2010). Botulism Immune Globulin Intravenous (human), a pentavalent investigational vaccine, is available through the California Department of Health Services for administration in infantile botulism.

Avian and Seasonal Influenza

Oseltamivir phosphate (OP) (Tamiflu®) is approved for treatment for treatment of children 1 year of age and older if symptoms are less than 2 days old.

Ricin

Ricin is a category B agent but due to recent activity, it has become an agent of greater concern. Ricin is an extract of the castor bean. As a toxin it enters the cell and disrupts the large ribosomal subunit ribonucleic acid (RNA) affecting rapidly dividing cells such as the gastrointestinal (GI) tract. It is a versatile agent, which can be ingested, inhaled, or injected. Ingestion causes GI upset, gastroenteritis, vomiting, hemorrhage, cardiovascular collapse, and shock. Inhalation presents as respiratory distress and necrotizing pneumonitis and injection produces cardiovascular collapse and rapid shock. Treatment is supportive. A vaccine is under development.

Exposure to Chemical Agents

Exposure to chemical agents is likely to occur in public places, such as a school, mass gathering, or mass transportation location. EMS and public safety agencies may be able to identify quickly the involved chemical agent and initiate appropriate treatment. Children's signs and symptoms may differ from those of adults, and, as in biological agent exposures, a high index of suspicion for chemical exposure is needed. For example, when exposed to a cholinergic agent (nerve agent), children may be less likely to present with miosis and glandular secretions, and they may exhibit only neurological symptoms (Rotenberg & Newmark, 2003). The comparison of signs and symptoms of mustard gas exposure in children and adults is outlined in Table 11.6. Chemical agents are generally dispersed to incapacitate; these agents can be life-threatening to children

TABLE 11.6 Comparison of Mustard Gas Exposure in Children and Adults

Factor	Children	Adults
Onset of clinical manifestations	4 hours	8–24 hours
First symptoms	Cough, vomiting	
Face, neck symptoms (conjunctivitis, photophobia, erythema)	78%	32%
Genitalia involvement	42%	70%
Appearance of bullae	Early	Late
Severity of ophthalmic manifestations	93%	Not reported
Pulmonary and gastrointestinal symptoms	Children (78%) Adolescents (69%)	11%

Source: Momeni, A., Aminjavaheri, M., (1994). Skin Manifestations of Mustard Gas in a Group of 14 Children and Teenagers: A Clinical Study. International Journal of Dermatology Volume 33, Issue 3.

with chronic illnesses, and, if inhaled, chemical agents may cause life-threatening pneumonitis (Markenson & Reynolds, 2006). Chapter 28 addresses chemical exposures; the pediatric considerations are given in this chapter.

Prehospital Treatment

Upon arrival at the scene of a chemical release, EMS, in conjunction with hazardous materials teams, assess the situation and identify potentially exposed individuals. Based on their findings, skin decontamination may be warranted. As in radiological exposures, males and females are decontaminated separately, and young children would stay with their mothers, while older children go through same-gender decontamination. In chemical exposures, EMS personnel will wear special protective equipment that covers their entire bodies, and their faces may not be visible through their masks. The EMS and hospital emergency responders in decontamination events can stay in protective gear for limited periods of time before requiring rest, rehydration, and rehab, increasing the need for manpower.

Young children may become frightened and uncooperative at the sight of such heavily dressed, anonymous emergency care providers—having their clothes cut from their bodies and removed by strangers, then being cleansed with sufficient amounts of warmed water to completely rinse the victims after removal of clothing. Solutions such as 0.5% sodium hypochlorite (dilute bleach) should be avoided as they are known to irritate the skin. In addition, the use of soap increases the risk of injury associated with slips, falls, and not being able to hold on to slippery infants or small children. Additional safety measures may be required such as placing infants and very young children in plastic laundry baskets or store carts to move them safely through a decontamination station. For children with FAN, service animals may need to be accommodated and medical devices may need to be temporarily removed or replaced. A successful decontamination results in rapid removal of contaminants and minimizes harmful effects to the patient, responder, receiver, and medical facility. It is always best to maintain the integrity of the family unit when processing children through decontamination stations. It reduces stress and anxiety facilitating cooperation associated with walking naked through a line of others which can cause considerable anxiety and distress. It should be anticipated that although adults may understand the given situation, children are likely to become inconsolable and this will affect how quickly decontamination can be performed. This anxiety will be especially pronounced in a school or other situation where parents or family members are not readily available. As in any situation where there is a predominance of children, additional healthcare providers will be needed to assist children through the decontamination process. Words of encouragement and praise ("You are doing a great job") will be much appreciated. As with adults, decontamination is completed before the initiation of pediatric advanced life support protocols.

The decision to initiate decontamination is an important one and the process requires specialty-trained personnel and adequate manpower. In December 2014, a general guidance document was published by the Department of Homeland Security (2014). In that guidance, it is recommended that water

is the preferred decontaminant and water-based decontamination should be delivered at low pressure (50–60 PSI), high volume, tepid temperature, and with a duration of no longer than 3 minutes to ensure thorough soaking. Abrasive sponges or washcloths should be avoided to reduce micro-abrasions. Additional decontamination guidance is in development for children and pregnant women.

Management of nerve agent exposure includes supportive care, atropine, and pralidoxime. The use of autoinjectors was complicated since the only injectors available were dosed for adults with 2 mg of atropine and 600 mg of pralidoxime. Of these, atropine may now be administered using a pediatric dosed autoinjector since 2004 when the FDA approved Atropen from Meridian Medical Technologies, Bristol, Tennessee, a pediatric formulation of atropine. There remains an absence of a pediatric autoinjector for pralidoxime. Treatment with pralidoxime is essential to address the central nervous system and muscular toxicity of nerve agents. Recommendations now suggest that children weighing 13 kg or more receive the adult autoinjector dose of 600 mg while children weighing less should receive 20 to 50 mg/kg administered from a multidose vial. If a multidose vial is unavailable, they should receive the 600 mg dose from the autoinjector. The autoinjectors can be found in Mark-1 kits (Meridian Medical Technologies, Bristol, Tennessee). Kits with atropine and pralidoxime are approved for use in adults but can be used in older children (Markenson & Reynolds, 2006). There is no pediatric equivalent to the Mark-1 kit, as the Atropen is atropine only, and no pralidoxime in a pediatric dosage has been approved. Pyridostigmine Bromide has been approved by the FDA for use against the chemical agent soman. It must be given prior to exposure. Safety and effectiveness in children have not been established (U.S. FDA, 2017).

Emergency Treatment

Pediatricians and other healthcare providers must be familiar with the signs and symptoms of these and other agents and have developed protocols for rapid diagnosis and treatment. Upon arrival in the ED, patients' field decontamination should be complete, and the emergency personnel can focus on initial assessment, stabilization, and definitive treatment. Should decontamination be initiated at the ED, patient flow should be controlled. Those nurses and physicians trained in decontamination and fitted for the requisite PPE conduct the decontamination. This can be accomplished inside or outside of the ED. Emergency personnel should expect the same reactions to decontamination in young children. Protective masks as well as gas masks impede communication and make verbal communication difficult. Parents and family members may not be able to see their children prior to decontamination and stabilization; social services and other supportive personnel should be readily available to assist parents while they are waiting.

Definitive Treatment

Each class of chemical agents has its own treatment. Treatment specific to children is presented here. Most of the pediatric pharmacological treatments for nerve agent exposure are off-label uses, with pralidoxime chloride for organophosphate poisoning and diazepam and lorazepam for related seizures (Rotenberg & Newmark, 2003). Exposure to nerve agents (e.g., sarin, tabun, soman) and household organophosphates (sevin) requires supportive measures and the administration of atropine and pralidoxime (2-PAM). Pediatric doses are as follows:

- For malathion/sevin exposure:
  - Starting doses for infants and children under 2 years of age is 0.5 mg.
  - For children 2 to 10 years, the dose is 1.0 mg.
  - The dose of pralidoxime chloride is 15 mg/kg.
  - For malathion,
    - Children younger than 2 years receive 0.5 mg.
    - Children 2 to 8 years old receive 1.0 mg; children older than 8 years receive 2.0 mg.
- Diazepam dose, should convulsions occur, is 0.2 to 0.5 mg/kg.
- Sevin:
  - Is 0.05 mg/kg of atropine initially and again at 5- to 10-minute intervals.
  - Diazepam for seizures is 0.2 to 0.5 mg/kg (Sidell, Patrick, & Dashiell, 2000).

Diazepam was traditionally used because of its injectability. Any benzodiazepine may be used. It is important to note that seizures caused by nerve agents are not affected by antiseizure medications such as dilantin and repeated doses of benzodiazepines may be needed (Beach, 2010).

Vesicants such as mustard or lewisite produce erythema, burning, and vesication followed by desquamation of the skin. Victims will develop tingling which will become a burning sensation followed by the sloughing of the skin in 24 hours. For children exposed to vesicants, the skin is washed with a soap and water solution (Lynch & Thomas, 2004). An adsorbent powder can be sprinkled on the skin, allowed to adsorb the mustard, then removed with a moist cloth (Lynch & Thomas, 2004). Airway maintenance is paramount, and endotracheal intubation and mechanical ventilation may be indicated in children with severe exposure to mustard. Eye exposure requires copious flushing with water or normal saline (Lynch & Thomas, 2004). Thorough eye examinations should be performed, and corneal lesions are treated with antibiotics and mydriatic-cycloplegic medication; petroleum jelly applied to the eyelids will prevent them from adhering together (Lynch & Thomas, 2004).

ETHICAL AND LEGAL CONSIDERATIONS IN PEDIATRIC DISASTER CARE

The Emergency Medical Treatment and Active Labor Act (EMTALA) is an antidiscrimination statute, whereby all individuals who present to a hospital ED must receive the same medical screening examination for their signs and symptoms using the same personnel, protocols, and thoroughness regardless of their ability to pay for such treatment (Mitchiner & Yeh, 2002). The term "all individuals" applies to ill or injured children presenting to an ED, with or without a parent or guardian; under EMTALA, they, too, must receive a medical screening examination and stabilizing treatments.

Parental consent is assumed if the patient is not competent to provide consent and an emergency exists. Although no uniform legal definition of "emergency" exists, preserving life, preventing permanent disability, alleviating pain and suffering, and avoiding eventual harm have been used as guidelines for emergency treatment without consent (Guertler, 1997, p. 311).

To delay or deny care because of the lack of parental consent would be a violation of EMTALA. While attempts to locate a parent or guardian are made, emergency care continues. Once life-threatening conditions are stabilized, children may be transferred, should specialty care be required (Hodge, 1999). To transfer unstable patients, or to transfer patients for economic reasons, is a violation of EMTALA (Hodge, 1999). While implied consent will allow a child to be stabilized, consent issues remain unclear concerning nonacute care.

How EMTALA will function or be enforced in a community during a nuclear, biological, or chemical exposure is not known. Conceivably, EMTALA would apply to children seeking emergency care without parental consent (e.g., chemical exposure during school hours). How EMTALA will be enforced in the event of a biological exposure, where one hospital is designated the "clean" hospital and one is the "quarantined" hospital, is unclear. Under EMTALA, "if an individual arrives at a hospital and is not technically in the ED but is on the premises (including the parking lot, sidewalk, or driveway) of the hospital and requests emergency care, he or she is entitled to a medical screening examination" (Mallon & Bukata, 1999, p. 19). During a public health emergency, though, EMTALA does not allow a community to designate hospitals that are "clean" and "exposed"; all hospitals would have to assess, stabilize, and screen any patient who appears on hospital property (Bentley, 2001). As written, EMTALA includes no exception provision where a mayor, governor, or other official could waive its rules for the best interests of the public's health (Bentley, 2001). As a possible compromise, hospitals may be able to comply with EMTALA by providing medical screening examinations at sites elsewhere on the hospital campus (e.g., clinic; Mallon & Bukata, 1999). This action may prevent patients from being turned away. Hospital triage nurses would not be permitted to turn away or refuse to triage patients based on their exposure to nuclear, biological, or chemical agents. To do so would be in violation of the state's emergency health powers act (see Chapter 4 for further discussion).

Since then, substantial guidance has been developed by the National Academies Institute of Medicine workgroups on crisis standards of care. The Crisis Standards of Care: A Systems Framework for Catastrophic Disaster Response was released in 2012 (Institute of Medicine, 2012). Guidance templates were developed for stakeholder groups, local communities, and policy makers to facilitate decision making in conditions where resources are limited and asset allocation difficult.

PEDIATRIC DEATH FOLLOWING DISASTERS AND PUBLIC HEALTH EMERGENCIES

In the aftermath of natural and man-made disasters, children may die from injury and illness. These deaths may occur at the scene, in the ED, or during hospitalization. While the death of one child is traumatic for parents and healthcare professionals, large numbers of children, including entire families, dying during or after a disaster is overwhelming for everyone, including nurses and healthcare professionals. Nothing in professionals' education prepares them for attending to thousands of dead and dying all at one time, or for living in or returning to communities that no longer exist. Among 3,218 middle and high school students surveyed 7 weeks after the Murrah Building bombing in Oklahoma City, over one-third reported the loss of someone they knew (Pfefferbaum et al., 2000). Following the 2004 tsunami, tens of thousands of children became orphans and displaced citizens in a matter of minutes. Similarly, following Hurricanes Katrina and Rita, children found themselves without families, homes, and communities. Nurses and healthcare professionals found themselves without homes, hospitals, and families, too, and remained on duty to care for patients and others left behind.

There are times when children will die in the prehospital and ED setting, despite the prehospital and emergency teams' best efforts. During a pediatric resuscitation, parental presence can be incorporated into care. Should parents choose to be present for their children's resuscitation, ideally, one nurse should stay with them and explain what is happening; this contact may not be possible during a disaster situation. The Emergency Nurses Association advocates parental presence during pediatric resuscitation. Such presence may be beneficial to the child as well as family members. Offering parents and family members time to grieve after the child has died may be difficult in a disaster situation, where rooms, supplies, and staff are scarce. Under these circumstances, emergency personnel can do only what is in the best interests of all involved.

Existing guidelines (Lipton & Coleman, 2000) outline bereavement practices for healthcare professionals to help them plan for and assist families following the sudden deaths of their children. Having guidelines in place to help healthcare professionals cope with the work of caring for many dead and dying children and families is imperative. It may be difficult to enact these guidelines when multiple victims die, but they are a starting point for further disaster planning and discussion for prehospital and emergency care professionals.

PLANNING FOR DISASTERS— PEDIATRIC-SPECIFIC CONSIDERATIONS

The pediatric population has very specific needs which must be incorporated in disaster planning at all levels and all phases of the disaster cycle. Although it is impossible to completely protect children from the impact of disasters, within the mitigation or planning phase of the disaster cycle, families and communities must plan to reduce the impact of disasters on children. National initiatives have been undertaken to improve the care of children in disasters and public health emergencies. In 1995, the Health Resources and Services Administration, the National Highway Traffic Safety Administration, and the Federal Emergency Management Agency (FEMA) identified

seven goals to meet children's needs in disasters. In 1998, these seven goals were developed by the EMS-C program into the document, *Consensus Recommendations for Responding to Children's Emergencies in Disasters* (Ball & Allen, 2000). The full consensus document, including recommendations and action steps, is available through www.ems-c.org.

In 2002, President Bush signed the Public Health Security and Bioterrorism Preparedness and Response Act to initiate a response to bioterrorism preparedness. Unfortunately, the Act's attention to children was minimal, even with the creation of a National Advisory Committee on Children and Terrorism (NACCT). As defined within the Act, the purpose of the NACCT is to assess and provide recommendations to the secretary of the Department of Health and Human Services on the preparedness of the healthcare system to respond to children's needs; changes needed within healthcare and EMS, including protocols, to meet children's needs; and changes, if needed, to the SNS to meet children's needs (Markenson & Redlener, 2004). This committee was not appointed until March 2003 with its charge of issuing a final report in June 2003 (Markenson & Redlener, 2004). To that end, an interdisciplinary consensus conference of pediatric emergency and terrorism professionals was convened to develop evidence-based recommendations on the care of children in disasters and public health emergencies. (One of this chapter's authors served as an expert consultant at the consensus conference.) The recommendations of this conference were submitted to the secretary of Health and Human Services.

At this time, there are two programs that provide funding support to state health departments for coordinating the healthcare system for terrorism preparedness: the Bioterrorism Hospital Preparedness program of the Health Resources and Services Administration and the Public Health Preparedness and Response for Bioterrorism program of the CDC (Markenson & Reynolds, 2006). While both programs mention pediatric preparedness, overall pediatric preparedness activities have been minimal, and there may be plans without pediatrics included (Markenson & Reynolds, 2006). Another program, the voluntary Medical Reserve Corps, does not include pediatric preparedness, nor does the Metropolitan Medical Response System (MMRS). There are other programs that work to educate healthcare providers toward a greater understanding of pediatric needs. The AAP offers training through the Pediatric Education for Prehospital Professionals and the Neonatal Resuscitation Program, and the Emergency Nurses Association offers the Emergency Nursing Pediatric Course. The federal government offers funding through the EMS-C program. This allows for national recognition as an emergency pediatric facility. Participation is voluntary. Since 2007, the EMS-C designation program has evolved to encourage all hospitals to be prepared at the Emergency Department Approval for Pediatrics (EDAP) level. The designation process is typically carried out by the local or state EMS System Authority and is designed to support a coordinated "system of emergency care for children" within the operational area and region. The highest level designated is typically a pediatric specialty center with a PICU and NICU and other specialized pediatric services.

In 2010, the Children's HHS Interagency Leadership on Disasters (CHILD; U.S. Department of Health and Human Services, 2017) working group was established. Its mission was to support integrating the needs of children (birth through age 17) across the national disaster, public health, emergency preparedness, response, and recovery activities. The working group issued its report in February 2017 summarizing key resources supporting these efforts. This is an important step in establishing planning for pediatric victims of disasters. Much work and coordination, at the local, state, and federal levels, continues to assure the proper treatment of children in a time of disaster or terrorism. This book describes the disaster planning and emergency preparedness for people exposed to natural or man-made disasters, acts of terrorism, and public health emergencies. Additional qualifications that should be in place for the pediatric population are highlighted next.

Pediatric Considerations in Healthcare Preparations

Nurses and other healthcare professionals will be pressed into action once a disaster or public health emergency has occurred. Often these caregivers are unfamiliar with caring for the pediatric population and may have concerns about preparing correct dosages of medications and recognizing other pediatric-specific concerns. They should be knowledgeable about, and familiar with, the disaster-relief agencies and groups within their communities and regions (Coffman, 1994). The assumption is made that healthcare will be delivered through its current means of existing hospitals, clinics, and healthcare professionals. Following the 2004 tsunami, as well as Hurricane Katrina, healthcare facilities, staff, and infrastructure were decimated. In the areas affected by the tsunami, the loss of nurses, midwives, physicians, and other healthcare professionals was particularly devastating because these resources were in short supply and high demand before the event (Carballo, Dalta, & Hernandez, 2005). While the infrastructure can be replaced, the recruitment and retention of nurses, physicians, and other healthcare professionals into this area may take years.

After a disaster has struck, nurses may be called on to assist with preventive mental health services; additional education in this area is of great importance. Early postdisaster interventions that nurses can include in their practice include helping children express their fears and concerns through age-appropriate means such as storytelling, drawing, coloring books, dolls, puppets, and toys (Coffman, 1994; Zubenko, 2002). Such media also allow nurses to help clear misconceptions about what occurred and provide accurate and helpful information (Coffman, 1994). Brohl (1996) details interventions that help children to heal emotionally following a disaster or traumatic event. Kostelny and Wessells (2005) report on the establishment of 240 child-centered spaces in tsunami-affected regions of Sri Lanka, India, and Indonesia that include 38,000 children from birth through 18 years of age. These safe places nurture young children's sense of trust and safety and help older children to develop life skills and leadership abilities (Kostelny & Wessells, 2005). The community serves as an active partner in planning and coordinating these centers.

Equipment

For prehospital and in-hospital pediatric emergency care, there are standards and guidelines in place for essential equipment and supplies; for example, the Emergency Nurses Association, as well as the American Academy of Pediatrics and the American College of Emergency Physicians, has published minimum equipment lists that can be obtained online or in reprinted form from published journal articles. Various pediatric equipment systems such as "color-coded" tapes can be used to estimate rapidly a pediatric patient's equipment size and medication dosage based on the patient's length (Hohenhaus, 2001). With the patient supine, the healthcare professional measures the patient's length with the tape; the patient's height corresponds to a color on the tape, which lists the size of emergency equipment and dosage of medications the patient may need. This system can reduce errors in judgment and save time in situations involving multiple injured or ill children. In one clinical trial of simulated pediatric resuscitations, use of such devices was associated with a significant reduction in medication errors and incorrect equipment sizes (Shah, Frush, Luo, & Wears, 2003). Since then, the use of length-based tapes in pediatrics has been adapted by numerous entities to enhance assessment, improve triage, and support competency in the care of children. Such a system may be beneficial to emergency care professionals who do not routinely care for critically ill or injured children and who may be required to do so during a disaster or public health emergency.

Bioterrorist acts resulting in large numbers of infected children will place a strain on the healthcare system. Physicians, nurses, and others will have to administer medications with which they are unfamiliar and untrained (Cieslak & Henretig, 2003), leading to stress. Such medications may not be readily available in pediatric dosages or preparations, and healthcare professionals will have to extrapolate to achieve the recommended pediatric dosage. In some instances, pediatric dosages will not have been established by the FDA, and the CDC and state health departments will need to provide close guidance and monitoring.

The release of a nerve agent near a school would put a strain on local prehospital and in-hospital resources, with airway equipment, supplies of 2-PAM and atropine, and pediatric intensive care beds being quickly used and depleted (Aghababian, 2002). Therefore, healthcare professionals should know how their community accesses the SNS and other resources to obtain medications and supplies in a timely manner. Additionally, hospitals should keep a 48-hour supply of pediatric equipment and pharmaceuticals on hand for their average daily census of pediatric patients, plus an additional 100 patients (Markenson & Redlener, 2004). Stockpiled pharmaceuticals and equipment should be specifically for pediatric use or appropriately substituted for such use (Markenson & Redlener, 2004). Hospital operations and preparedness policies should include pediatric care and treatment guidelines (Markenson & Redlener, 2004).

Education

Nurses and other healthcare professionals will be involved in caring for children following a disaster or public health emergency. Receiving timely and relevant information about the care of children during these times is essential. Participating in hospital preparedness exercises and trainings improves capability. One course available for healthcare professionals is the 2-day Pediatric Disaster Life Support (PDLS) course. This course focuses on the physiological and psychological needs of children following natural disasters and acts of terrorism (Aghababian, 2002). Pediatric life support and advanced pediatric life support courses are available for prehospital and emergency healthcare professionals. At this time, most of these healthcare professionals in EDs have received this training. In the prehospital setting, the Pediatric Education for Prehospital Professionals (PEPP) course as well as pediatric trauma life support for prehospital care provider courses are available. Recommendations for the education of EMS personnel in pediatric care have been established (Pediatric Education Task Force, 1998). School nurses can enroll in the Managing School Emergencies courses offered through the National Association of School Nurses.

In May 2014 the Department of Homeland Security and FEMA authorized the development of the Pediatric Disaster Response and Emergency Preparedness course (Mgt 439). The course is funded through FEMA and is offered to communities through the Texas A&M Engineering Extension Service (TEEX). The training takes a whole community, interdisciplinary approach to prepare attendees to effectively plan and respond to a disaster incident involving children (teex.org/documentsresources/MGT-439-Pediatric-Disaster-Response.pdf).

Nurses and other healthcare professionals may be called away from their communities to care for children following disasters or public health emergencies. They may find themselves in a new culture, with beliefs and practices different than their own. Healthcare professionals must be sensitive to and respectful of the culture and region in which they are called on to provide relief (Capozzoli, 2002).

Recommendations for nurses caring for children in disaster-relief areas are suggested. It is recommended that an adequate number of pediatric nurses be involved in any type of disaster (Margalit et al., 2003) to provide and direct care for children. Nurses should remain mindful of cultural and language barriers even when translators are provided (Margalit et al., 2003). Nurses should encourage breastfeeding whenever possible, because clean water and alternative food sources may not be available (Margalit et al., 2003). Social support for children and families, as well as hygiene and weather-related concerns, should not be overlooked (Margalit et al., 2003).

In disaster conditions where workforce is limited, background-checked volunteers from the community can be trained to assist in providing basic services to children who are receiving treatment in a hospital or shelter or who are displaced from their families. Such training could be incorporated into the hospital's disaster plan. As part of disaster planning, reunification planning should include the purchase of an instamatic camera (Rosenbaum, 1993). In the event of a mass casualty incident, children will be taken to various hospitals and separation from caregivers can occur. Children do not carry personal identification, making it difficult to reunite them with their families. Emergency staff can take a photo of each child who arrives, and this photo can be posted in the "picture room." These photos may be useful to help determine whether their child is in this ED. Social workers will remain with the families during the time they are scanning the photos to provide emotional support when an identification is made (Rosenbaum, 1993). Another consideration is the use of a secure website by the EMS and hospital personnel to locate children and families; photographs taken with a digital camera could be posted, along with the name of the treatment facility. Children displaced from their families in the event of a disaster may become victims of predators; care needs to be taken by healthcare providers to protect children from these predators preventing the child from becoming a victim twice.

After a disaster strikes, families will experience stressors such as loss of their homes, jobs, social networks, and other support systems. Consequently, these losses are risk factors for child abuse and maltreatment. Curtis, Miller, and Berry (2000) reviewed countywide child abuse reports for 1 year before and after Hurricane Hugo, the Loma Prieta earthquake, and Hurricane Andrew. They found that child abuse reports were disproportionately higher in the quarter and half year following Hurricane Hugo and the Loma Prieta earthquake (Curtis et al., 2000). Therefore, parents need to recognize that they will experience stress and that they need to develop appropriate coping strategies to alleviate that stress. Nurses and healthcare and school professionals need to be vigilant for signs of child maltreatment following disasters and to report and follow up accordingly.

Nurses and healthcare professionals must consider the length of time needed for community recovery following a disaster and prepare to live and practice accordingly. Within 7 weeks following Hurricane Katrina, 20.2% of housing units lacked water, 24.5% had no electricity, 43.2% had no telephone service, and 55.7% of households contained one or more members with a chronic health condition (Norris et al., 2006). Among those older than 18 years of age who were surveyed, almost 49.8% reported emotional distress, indicating a potential need for mental health services (Norris et al., 2006). Consequently, the Louisiana Office of Mental Health has established a crisis-counseling program to provide interventions and support to hurricane survivors (Norris et al., 2006). The degree to which pediatric mental health needs are being met has not been reported in the literature.

In the months following the Beslan, Russia, school siege, children and families continue to receive mental health counseling. Many children are afraid of loud noises. Some children try to hide or can sleep only by holding their parents' hands (Parfitt, 2004). Adults report feelings of guilt for not being able to save children held hostage, even if their own children survived (Parfitt, 2004). Counseling is expected to remain in place on an ongoing basis.

SUMMARY

Children will be victims in natural disasters and public health emergencies. Healthcare professionals must be prepared to care for children in the prehospital, inpatient, and follow-up phases of disaster care. Children may experience long-term physical and psychosocial sequelae following a disaster; appropriate follow-up will be indicated. Nurses and healthcare professionals must place a high priority on the needs of children in disasters or public health emergencies and incorporate these needs into their hospital and community disaster plans.

STUDY QUESTIONS

1. Describe pediatric injuries that result from the following disasters: earthquakes, floods, hurricanes.

2. What are the conditions that predispose children living in refugee camps to infectious and communicable diseases?

3. Why are young children at greater risk for injury from inhalation of chemical agents as compared with adults?

4. List, in order, the steps of the primary and secondary pediatric trauma surveys.

5. What special considerations must nurses take when caring for large numbers of injured children hospitalized following a disaster?

6. Which fluids best hide the salty taste of potassium iodide?

7. How do nurses assess for malnutrition in children living in refugee settings?

8. Select one web-based resource listed in this chapter. Log on to the website and obtain pediatrics-related disaster information. How can this information be applied to one's own hospital or community disaster preparedness plans?

INTERNET ACTIVITIES

1. Go to the American Academy of Pediatrics website at www.aap.org. Click on the link on children, bioterrorism, and disasters. Locate AAP-related resources and materials on disasters, bioterrorism, and psychological support of children. Use the hyper link: CHILDisaster NETWORK. Locate family readiness kits.

2. Go to the EMS-C website at https://emscimprovement. center. Type in the key word "disasters" or "bioterrorism." Locate EMS-C-related resources and materials through the hyperlinks.

3. Go to the Federal Emergency Management Agency website at https://www.fema.gov/disaster/4086/updates/fema-kids. Click the icon for FEMA Kids. Locate information on age-appropriate and disaster-related information.

4. Go to the Johnson & Johnson Pediatric Institute website at www.jjpi.com. Click the icons for "Helping the Children" and "When Terrible Things Happen."

5. Go to the American Academy of Child and Adolescent Psychiatry website at http://aacap.org. Click hyperlinks to "Talking to Children about War and Terrorism" and "Disaster Responses."

6. Go to the Sigma Theta Tau, *Online journal of knowledge synthesis in nursing* website at https://www.ncbi.nlm .nih.gov/labs/journals/online-j-knowl-synth-nurs/. Locate articles related to disasters, mental health, pediatrics, and adolescents.

7. Go to the National Institutes of Mental Health website at https://www.nimh.nih.gov/index.shtml. Search: "Helping Children and Adolescents Cope with Violence and Disasters."

8. Go to the National Center for PTSD website at ptsd.va.gov. Click on "Terrorism and Children."

9. Go to TRACIE (Technical Resources, Assistance Center and Information Exchange) at https://asprtracie.hhs.gov and search the TRACIE Pediatric Topic Collection.

10. Go to SAMSHA at www.samhsa.gov and search for coping with traumatic events: resources for children, parents, educators, and other professionals.

SUPPORT PREPAREDNESS

Pediatric, Perinatal and Neonatal Preparedness Resources

National Advisory Committee on Children and Disasters (NACCD):
www.phe.gov/preparedness/legal/boards/naccd/Pages/default.aspx

Illinois Department of Public Health ESF Plan
http://www.dph.illinois.gov/sites/default/files/publications/peds-neo-surge-annex-final-march2017-public-complete-file-031417.pdf

National Pediatric Readiness Project
https://emscimprovement.center/projects/pediatricreadiness/

Emergency Preparedness ChildCare Aware
https://usa.childcareaware.org/advocacy-public-policy/crisisand-disaster-resources/

Listen Protect and Connect (LPC) Psychological First Aid System
https://www.fema.gov/medialibrary/assets/documents/132712

The National Child Traumatic Stress Network
https://www.nctsn.org

204 II Disaster Mental Health and High-Vulnerability Populations

Psychological First Aid for Children and Parents
https://www.fema.gov/media-library-data/1499091995177-9ff6b07a88db5d
  422062efa4fdca9cfe/pfa_parents_and_children.pdf

American Academy of Pediatrics (AAP) Children & Disasters
www.aap.org/en-us/advocacy-and-policy/aap-health-initiatives/Children
  -and-Disasters/Pages/default.aspx

Children & Disasters: Disaster-Related Coalitions
www.aap.org/en-us/advocacy-and-policy/aap-health-initiatives/Children
  -and-Disasters/Pages/Disaster-Networks-Survey-Project.aspx

*American Academy of Pediatrics Healthy
Children.org: Building Resilience*
www.healthychildren.org/English/healthy-living/emotional-wellness/
  Building-Resilience/Pages/default.aspx

Pediatric Mass Casualty Triage JumpSTART
www.jumpstarttriage.com

Radiation Emergency Medical Management (REMM)
www.remm.nlm.gov

Infants and Children Web Page
www.remm.nlm.gov/radiation_children.htm

Pregnant Woman and Fetus Web Page
www.remm.nlm.gov/specialpops.htm#children

Save the Children: Get Ready. Get Safe
www.savethechildren.org/site/c.8rKLIXMGIpI4E/b.8777053/k.F31D/
  Get_Ready_Get_Safe_Disaster_Report_Card.htm

*Technical Resources, Assistance Center, and
Information Exchange (TRACIE)*
https://asprtracie.hhs.gov

*Disaster Information Management Research Center: Health
Resources on Children in Disasters and Emergencies*
www.sis.nlm.nih.gov/dimrc/children.html

*Health Resources on Pregnant Women
in Disasters and Emergencies*
www.sis.nlm.nih.gov/dimrc/pregnantwomen.html

Stanford: Disaster Planning for Obstetrics & Gynecology
http://obgyn.stanford.edu/community/disaster-planning.html

Loma Linda Pediatric Neonatal Disaster Reference Guide
http://cchealth.org/ems/pdf/Pediatric-Neonatal-Disaster-Reference-Guide.pdf

*American Red Cross Pillow Case Project
and Masters of Disasters*
www.redcross.org/get-help/prepare-for-emergencies/resources-for-schools

My Pillowcase Project: American Red Cross
http://ymiclassroom.com/wp-content/uploads/2013/08/pp_workbook.pdf

*Institute of Medicine Preparedness, Response,
and Recovery Considerations for Children and
Families Workshop Summary (Dec 2013).*
www.nationalacademies.org/hmd/Reports/2013/Preparedness-Response
  -and-Recovery-Considerations-for-Children-and-Families.aspx

Mental Health
National Center for School Crisis and Bereavement. www.schoolcrisiscenter.org
Coalition to Support Grieving Students. www.grievingstudents.org
AAP Children and Disasters. www.aap.org/disasters
Coping and adjustment. www.aap.org/disasters/adjustment
National Center for Disaster Medicine and Public Health (Psychosocial Impacts
  of Disasters on Children – online training module). http://ncdmph.usuhs
  .edu/KnowledgeLearning/2013-Learning2.htm

REFERENCES

REFERENCES

Aghababian, R. (2002). Preparing EMS for acts of violence/terrorism involving children. *EMSC* (Emergency Medical Services for Children) *News, 15*(2), 2–3.
Alam, N., Meier, R., Schneider, H., Sarker, S., Bardhan, P., Mahalanabis, D.,... Gyr, N. (2000). Partially hydrolyzed guar gum-supplemented oral rehydration solution in the treatment of acute diarrhea in children. *Journal of Pediatric Gastroenterology and Nutrition, 31*(5), 503–507. doi:10.1097/00005176-200011000-00010
American Academy of Pediatrics, American College of Emergency Physicians, American College of Surgeons Committee on Trauma, Emergency Medical Services for Children, Emergency Nurses Association, National Association of EMS Physicians, & National Association of State EMS Officials. (2014). Equipment for ground ambulances. *Prehospital Emergency Care, 18*(1), 92–97. doi:10.31 09/10903127.2013.851312
American Academy of Pediatrics, Committee on Disaster and Emergency Medical Care. (1972). *Disaster and emergency medical services for infants and children.* Evanston, IL: Author.
Araneta, M., Destiche, D., Schlangen, K., Merz, R., Forrester, M., & Gray, G. (2000). Birth defects prevalence among infants of Persian Gulf War veterans born in Hawaii, 1989–1993. *Teratology, 62*(4), 195–204. doi:10.1002/1096-9926(200010)62:4<195::AID-TERA5>3.0.CO;2-5
Ball, J., & Allen, K. (2000). Consensus recommendations for responding to children's emergencies in disasters. *National Academies of Practice Forum, 2*(4), 253–257.
Beach, M. (2010). *Disaster preparedness and management.* Philadelphia, PA: F.A. Davis
Bearer, C. (1995). How are children different from adults? *Environment and Health Perspective, 103*(Suppl. 6), 7–12. doi:10.1289/ehp.95103s67
Belter, R., & Shannon, M. (1993). Impact of natural disasters on children and families. In C. Saylor (Ed.), *Children and disasters* (pp. 85–103). New York, NY: Plenum Press.
Benson, M., Koenig, K., & Schultz, C. (1996). Disaster triage: START, then SAVE—A new method of dynamic triage for victims of a catastrophic earthquake. *Prehospital and Disaster Medicine, 11*(2), 117–124. doi:10.1017/S1049023X0004276X
Bentley, J. (2001). Hospital preparedness for bioterrorism. *Public Health Reports, 116*(Suppl. 2), 36–39. doi:10.1016/S0033-3549(04)50139-5
Bernardo, L. (2001). Pediatric implications in bioterrorism. Part 1: Physiologic and psychosocial differences. *International Journal of Trauma Nursing, 7*(1), 14–16. doi:10.1067/mtn.2001.112152
Bernardo, L., & Henker, R. (1999). Thermoregulation in pediatric trauma: An overview. *International Journal of Trauma Nursing, 5,* 101–105. doi:10.1016/S1075-4210(99)90057-3
Bernardo, L., & Schenkel, K. (2003). Pediatric trauma. In L. Newberry (Ed.), *Sheehy's principles and practice of emergency nursing* (5th ed., pp. 379–400). St. Louis, MO: Mosby-Year Book.
Brohl, K. (1996). *Working with traumatized children: A handbook for healing.* Washington, DC: CWLA Press.
Burkle, F. (1999). Fortnightly review: Lessons learnt and future expectations of complex emergencies. *British Medical Journal, 319*(7202), 422–426. doi:10.1136/bmj.319.7207.422
Burkle, F. (2002). Complex humanitarian emergencies. In D. Hogan & J. Burstein (Eds.), *Disaster medicine* (pp. 47–54). Philadelphia, PA: Lippincott Williams & Wilkins.
Capozzoli, J. (2002). Psychological relief: An overview—The Balkan experience. In W. Zubenko & J. Capozzoli (Eds.), *Children and disasters: A practical guide to healing and recovery* (pp. 6–33). New York, NY: Oxford University Press.
Carballo, M., Dalta, S., & Hernandez, M. (2005). Impact of the tsunami on healthcare systems. *Journal of the Royal Society of Medicine, 98*(9), 390–395. doi:10.1258/jrsm.98.9.390
Centers for Disease Control and Prevention. (2001). Recommendations for antimicrobial prophylaxis for children and breast-feeding mothers and

treatment of children with anthrax. *Journal of the American Medical Association, 286*(21), 2663–2664. doi:10.1001/jama.286.21.2663-JWR1205-2-1

Centers for Disease Control and Prevention. (2006). Assessment of health-related needs after tsunami and earthquake—Three districts, Aceh Province, Indonesia, July–August, 2005. *Morbidity and Mortality Weekly Report, 55*(4), 93–97.

Chameides, L., & Hazinski, M. (1998). *Textbook of pediatric advanced life support.* Dallas, TX: American Heart Association, American Academy of Pediatrics.

Chern, J. J., Miller, J. H., Tubbs, R. S., Whisenhunt, T. R., Johnston, J. M., Wellons, J. C. 3rd, … Oakes, W. J. (2011, December). Massive pediatric neurosurgical injuries and lessons learned following a tornado disaster in Alabama. *Journal of Neurosurgical Pediatrics, 8*(6), 588–592. doi:10.3171/2011.9.peds11207

Children's Hospital Los Angeles. (2012). *H1N1 pandemic influenza planning considerations for pediatric patients.* HPP Partnership Grant HFPEP070014-01-00. Los Angeles, CA: Author.

Chung, S., & Shannon, M. (2005). Hospital planning for acts of terrorism and other public health emergencies involving children. *Archives of Diseases in Children, 90,* 1300–1307. doi:10.1136/adc.2004.069617

Cieslak, T., & Henretig, F. (2003). Ring-a-ring-a-roses: Bioterrorism and its peculiar relevance to pediatrics. *Current Opinion in Pediatrics, 15,* 107–111. doi:10.1097/00008480-200302000-00018

Coffman, S. (1994). Children describe life after Hurricane Andrew. *Pediatric Nursing, 20*(4), 363–375. Retrieved from https://www.researchgate.net/publication/15312976Children_describe_life_after_Hurricane_Andrew

Coldiron, M. E., Lasry, E., Bouhenia, M., Das, D., Okui, P., Nyehangane, D., … Grais, R. F. (2017, May). Intermittent preventative treatment for malaria among children in a refugee camp in Northern Uganda: Lessons learned. *Malaria Journal, 16*(1), 218. doi:10.1186/s12936-017-1869-x

Columbia University Mailman School of Public Health National Center for Disaster Preparedness. (2003). *Pediatric preparedness for disasters and terrorism: A national consensus conference.* Executive summary for conference held February 2003 in Washington, DC: Agency for Healthcare Research and Quality.

Committee on Environmental Health and Committee on Infectious Diseases. (2000). Chemical-biological terrorism and its impact on children: A subject review. *Pediatrics, 105,* 662–670. doi:10.1542/peds.105.3.662

Conway, A., Bernardo, L., & Tontala, K. (1990). The effects of disasters on children: Implications for emergency nurses. *Journal of Emergency Nursing, 16*(6), 393–395.

Curtis, T., Miller, B., & Berry, E. (2000). Changes in reports and incidence of child abuse following natural disasters. *Child Abuse and Neglect, 24*(9), 1151–1162. doi:10.1016/S0145-2134(00)00176-9

Daley, W. (2006). Public health response to Hurricanes Katrina and Rita—Louisiana, 2005. *Morbidity and Mortality Weekly Report, 55*(2), 29–30.

Department of Homeland Security. (2014). Patient decontamination in a mass chemical exposure incident: National planning guidance for communities. Retrieved from https://www.dhs.gov/sites/default/files/publications/Patient%20Decon%20National%20Planning%20Guidance_Final_December%202014.pdf

Donmez, O., Mral, A., Yavuz, M., & Durmaz, O. (2001). Crush syndrome of children in the Marmara Earthquake, Turkey. *Pediatrics International, 43,* 678–682. doi:10.1046/j.1442-200x.2001.01469.x

Doucet, I. (1994). Desert storm syndrome: Sick soldiers and dead children? *Medicine and War, 10,* 183–194. doi:10.1080/07488009408409164

Duff, E., Cooper, E., Danbury, C., Johnson, B., & Serjeant, G. (1991). Neural tube defects in hurricane aftermath. *Lancet, 337,* 120–121. doi:10.1016/0140-6736(91)90785-n

Emergency Medical Services for Children Innovation & Improvement Center. (n.d.-a). Pediatric readiness: Readiness toolkit. Retrieved from https://emscimprovement.center/projects/pediatricreadiness/readiness-toolkit/

Emergency Medical Services for Children Innovation & Improvement Center. (n.d.-b). Pediatric Regionalization of Care Primer. Retrieved from https://emscimprovement.center/resources/publications/pediatric-regionalization-of-care-primer

Federal Emergency Management Agency. (2013). Post disaster reunification of children—A nationwide approach. Retrieved from https://www.fema.gov/media-library/assets/documents/85559

Floyd, K. (2002). Pediatric considerations in disasters. In D. Hogan & J. Burstein (Eds.), *Disaster medicine* (pp. 16–22). Philadelphia, PA: Lippincott Williams & Wilkins.

Fong, F. (2002). Medical management of radiation accidents. In D. Hogan & J. Burstein (Eds.), *Disaster medicine* (pp. 237–257). Philadelphia, PA: Lippincott Williams & Wilkins.

Freedman, A., Afonja, O., Chang, M., Mostashari, F., Blaser, M., Perez-Perez, G., … Borkowsky, W. (2002). Cutaneous anthrax associated with microangiopathic hemolytic anemia and coagulopathy in a 7-month-old infant. *Journal of the American Medical Association, 287*(7), 869–874. doi:10.1001/jama.287.7.869

Fuzak, J. K., Elkon, B. D., Hampers, L. C., Polage, K. J., Milton, J. D., Powers, L. K., … Wathen, J. E. (2010). Mass transfer of pediatric tertiary care hospital inpatients to a new location in under 12 hours: Lessons learned and implications for disaster preparedness.. *Journal of Pediatrics, 157*(1), 138–143.e2. doi:10.1016/j.jpeds.2010.01.047

Gamulin, A., Armenter-Duran, J., Assal, M., Hagon, O., & Daver, R. (2012, June). Conditions found among pediatric survivors during the early response to natural disaster: A prospective case study. *Journal of Pediatrics Orthopedics, 32*(4), 327–333. doi:10.1097/BPO.0b013e31825197ec

Gausche-Hill, M. (2009) Pediatric disaster preparedness: Are we really prepared? *Journal of Trauma and Acute Care Surgery, 67*(2), S73–S76. doi:10.1097/TA.0b013e3181af2fff

Goodman, C., & Hogan, D. (2002). Urban search and rescue. In D. Hogan & J. Burstein (Eds.), *Disaster medicine* (pp. 112–122). Philadelphia, PA: Lippincott Williams & Wilkins.

Guertler, A. (1997). The clinical practice of emergency medicine. *Emergency Medicine Clinics of North America, 15*(2), 303–313. doi:10.1016/S0733-8627(05)70300-X

Hagan, J. F., Jr., Committee on Psychosocial Aspects of Child and Family Health, & Task Force on Terrorism. (2005). Psychosocial implications of disaster or terrorism on children: A guide for the pediatrician. *Pediatrics, 116,* 787–795. doi:10.1542/peds.2005-1498

Henderson, D. (1999). The looming threat of bioterrorism. *Science, 283,* 1279–1282. doi:10.1126/science.283.5406.1279

Henderson, D., Inglesby, T., Bartlett, J., Ascher, M., Eitzen, E., Jahrling, P., … Tonat, K. (1999). Smallpox as a biological weapon: Medical and public health management. *Journal of the American Medical Association, 281*(22), 2127–2137.doi:10.1001/jama.281.22.2127

Henretig, F., Cieslak, T., & Eitzen, E. (2003). Biological and chemical terrorism. *Journal of Pediatrics, 141*(3), 311–326. doi:10.1067/mpd.2002.127408

Hodge, D. (1999). Managed care and the pediatric emergency department. *Pediatric Clinics of North America, 46*(6), 1329–1340. doi:10.1016/S0031-3955(05)70188-7

Hohenhaus, S. (2001). Is this a drill? Improving pediatric emergency preparedness in North Carolina's emergency departments. *Journal of Emergency Nursing, 27*(6), 568–570. doi:10.1067/men.2001.119686

Hohenhaus, S. (2005). Practical considerations for providing pediatric care in a mass casualty incident. *Nursing Clinics of North America, 40,* 523–533. doi:10.1016/j.cnur.2005.04.014

Iezzoni, L. (1999). *Influenza 1918: The worst epidemic in American history.* New York, NY: TV Books.

Inci, I., Ozcelik, C., Nizam, O., Eren, N., & Ozgen, G. (1996). Penetrating chest injuries in children: A review of 94 cases. *Journal of Pediatric Surgery, 31*(5), 673–676. doi:10.1016/S0022-3468(96)90672-7

Inglesby, T., O'Toole, T., Henderson, D., Bartlett, J., Ascher, M., Eitzen, E., … Tonat, K.; For Working Group on Civilian Biodefense. (2002). Anthrax as a biological weapon, 2002: Updated recommendations for management. *Journal of the American Medical Association, 287*(17), 2236–2252. doi:10.1001/jama.287.17.2236

Institute of Medicine. (2012). Crisis standards of care: A systems framework for catastrophic disaster response. Washington, DC: National Academy of Sciences. Retrieved from http://www.nationalacademies.org/

hmd/reports/2012/crisis-standards-of-care-a-systems-framework-for-catastrophic-disaster-response.aspx

Iskit, S., Alpay, H., Tugtepe, H., Ozdemir, C., Ayyildiz, S., Ozel, K., & Dagli, T.E. (2001). Analysis of 33 pediatric trauma victims in the 1999 Marmara, Turkey Earthquake. *Journal of Pediatric Surgery, 36*(2), 368–372. doi:10.1053/jpsu.2001.20719

Jablonka, A., Happle, C., Grote, U., Schleenvoigt, B. T., Hampel, A., Dopfer, C.,... Behrens, G. M. (2016, December) Measles, mumps, rubella, and varicella seroprevalence in refugees in Germany in 2015. *Infection, 44*(6), 781–787. doi:10.1007/s15010-016-0926-7

Jagodic, G., & Kontac, K. (2002). Normalization: A key to children's recovery. In W. Zubenko, & J. Cappozzoli (Eds.), *Children and disasters: A practical guide to healing and recovery* (pp. 159–171). New York, NY: Oxford University Press.

Jarrett, D. (1999). *Medical management of radiological casualties* (1st ed.). Bethesda, MD: Military Medical Operations Office, Armed Forces Radiobiology Research Institute.

Jiang, X., Xiang, B., Liu, L.-J., Liu, M., Tang, X.-Y., Huang, L.-G., ... Xin, W.-Q., (2013). Clinical characteristics of pediatric victims in the Lushan and Wenchuan earthquakes and experience of medical rescue (abstract only). *Zhongguo Dang Dai Er Zhi, 15*(6), 419–422.

Johnston, W. R. (2009). Terrorist and criminal attacks targeting children. Retrieved from http://www.johnstonsarchive.net/terrorism/wrjp39ch.html

Kanter, R. K. (2012). The 2011 Tuscaloosa tornado: Integration of pediatric disaster services into regional systems of care. *Journal of Pediatrics, 161*(3), 526–530. doi:10.1016/j.jpeds.2012.02.016

Kare, J., Roham, T., & Hardin, E. (2002). Plague and anthrax: Ancient diseases, modern warfare. *Topics in Emergency Medicine, 24*(3), 77–87.

Kouliey, T. (2016). Objective triage in the disaster setting: Will children and expecting mothers be treated like others? *Open Access Emergency Medicine, 8*, 77–86. doi:10.2147/OAEM.S96913

Koziel J. R., Meckler G., Brown L., Acker D., Torino M., Walsh B., & Cicero M. X. (2015, April–June). Barriers to pediatric disaster triage: A qualitative investigation. *Prehospital Emergency Care, 19*(2), 279–286. doi:10.31 09/10903127.2014.967428

Lin, A., Taylor, K., & Cohen, R. (2018). Triage by resource allocation for INpatients: A novel disaster triage tool for hospitalized pediatric patients. *Disaster Medicine and Public Health Preparedness*, 1–5. doi:10.1017/dmp.2017.139

Lipton, H., & Coleman, M. (2000). Bereavement practice guidelines for health care professionals in the emergency department. *International Journal of Emergency Mental Health, 2*(1), 19–31.

Lucile Packard Children's Hospital. (n.d.). Preplanning disaster triage for pediatric hospitals: TRAIN toolkit. Retrieved from http://www.acphd.org/media/270195/hospital%20disaster%20triage%20pediatric%20planning%20train%20toolkit%20x.pdf

Lynch, E., & Thomas, T. (2004). Pediatric considerations in chemical exposures: Are we prepared? *Pediatric Emergency Care, 20*(3), 198–205. doi:10.1097/01.pec.0000117931.65522.48

Mallon, W., & Bukata, R. (1999). COBRA/OBRA and EMTALA. *Topics in Emergency Medicine, 21*(2), 17–27.

Margalit, G., Goldberg, A., Rosen, Y., Tekes-Manova, D., Golan, M., Benedek, P.,...Bar-Dayan, Y. (2003). Recommendations for pediatric nursing requirements at a field hospital based on the Israel Defense Forces' experiences following the 1999 Turkish earthquake disaster. *Australian Emergency Nursing Journal, 6*(1), 15–18. doi:10.1016/S1328-2743(03)80005-6

Markenson, D., & Redlener, I. (2004). Pediatric terrorism preparedness national guidelines and recommendations: Findings of an evidence-based consensus process. *Biosecurity and Bioterrorism: Biodefense Strategy, Practice, and Science, 2*(4), 301–319. doi:10.1089/bsp.2004.2.301

Markenson, D., & Reynolds, S. (2006). The pediatrician and disaster preparedness. *Pediatrics, 117*(2), e340–e362. doi:10.1542/peds.2005-2752

Mettler, F., & Voelz, G. (2002). Current concepts: Major radiation exposure— What to expect and how to respond. *New England Journal of Medicine, 346*(20), 1554–1561. doi:10.1056/NEJMra000365

Mitchiner, J., & Yeh, C. (2002). The emergency medical treatment and active labor act: What emergency nurses need to know. *Nursing Clinics of North America, 37*(1), 19–34. doi:10.1016/S0029-6465(03)00080-X

Mitka, M. (1999). Learning lessons from true-life school trauma. *Journal of the American Medical Association, 281*(3), 220–221. doi:10.1001/jama.281.3.220-JMN0120-3-1

Mohr, W. (2002). Understanding children in crisis. In W. Zubenko & J. Cappozzoli (Eds.), *Children and disasters: A practical guide to healing and recovery* (pp. 72–84). New York, NY: Oxford University Press.

Momeni, A., & Aminjavaheri, M. (1994). Skin manifestations of mustard gas in a group of 14 children and teenagers: A clinical study. *International Journal of Dermatology, 33*(3), 184–187. doi:10.1111/j.1365-4362.1994.tb04977.x

Mondal, R., Sarkar, S., Banerjee, I., Hazra, A., Maiumder, D., & Sabui, T. (2013, August). Acute stress-related psychological impact in children following devastating natural disaster, the Sikkim earthquake (2011) India. *Journal of Neuroscience Rural Practice, 4*(Suppl 1): 519–532. doi:10.4103/0976-3147.116434

National Center for Disaster Preparedness, New York University College of Global Public Health, Rutgers School of Social Work. (2015, April). *Person report: The Sandy child and family health study*. Briefing Report No. 2. Center for Disaster Preparedness Person report: The Sandy Child & Family Health Study. Retrieved from http://ncdp.columbia.edu/microsite-page/sandy-child-and-family-health-study/scafh-publications-reports

National Report Card on Protecting Children in Disaster. (2014). Retrieved from https://secure.savethechildren.org/atf/cf/%7B9def2ebe-10ae-432c-9bd0-df91d2eba74a%7D/SC-2014_DISASTERREPORT.PDF

Needle, S. (2008). Pediatric private practice after Hurricane Katrina: Proposal for recovery. *Pediatrics, 122*(4), 836–842. doi:10.1542/peds.2007-2307

Noji, E. (2005). ABC of conflict and disaster: Public health in the aftermath of disasters. *British Medical Journal, 330*, 1379–1381. doi:10.1136/bmj.330.7504.1379

Nopar, R. (1967). Plagues on our children: The threat of biological warfare. *Pediatrics, 6*, 63–73. doi:10.1177/000992286700600201

Norris, F., Speier, A., Henderson, A., Davis, S., Purcell, D. W., Stratford, B. D.,... Daley, W. R. (2006). Assessment of health-related needs after Hurricanes Katrina and Rita—Orleans and Jefferson Parishes, New Orleans Area, Louisiana, October 17–22, 2005. *Morbidity and Mortality Weekly Report, 55*(02), 38–41.

Parfitt, T. (2004). How Beslan's children are learning to cope. *The Lancet, 364*(9450), 2009–2010. doi:10.1016/S0140-6736(04)17532-6

Pediatric Education Task Force. (1998). Education of out-of-hospital emergency medical personnel in pediatrics: Report of a national task force. *Annals of Emergency Medicine, 31*(1), 58–64. doi:10.1016/S0196-0644(98)70282-3

Pelsor, F., Sadrieh, N., & Machado, S. (2002). *Palatability evaluations of potassium iodide solid dosage tablets ground and mixed in drinks*. Rockville, MD: U.S. Food and Drug Administration.

Pfefferbaum, B., Gurwitch, R., McDonald, N., Leftwich, M., Sconzo, G., Messenbaugh, A., & Schultz, R. A. (2000). Posttraumatic stress among young children after the death of a friend or acquaintance in a terrorist bombing. *Psychiatric Services, 52*, 386–388. doi:10.1176/appi.ps.51.3.386

Piyasil, V., Ketumarn, P., Prubrukarn, R., Ularntinon, S., Sitdhiraksa, N., Pithayaratsathien, N.,...Sanguanpanich, N. (2011, August). Post-traumatic stress disorder in children after tsunami disaster in Thailand: A 5-year follow-up. *Journal of the Medical Association of Thailand, 94*(Suppl 3), S138–S144.

Piyasil, V., Thammawsi, T., Tasri, L., Chaiyakun, P., Ketumarn, P., Pityaratsatian, N.,...Ularntinon, S. (2014). Quality of life and happiness of students in the disaster area: 6 years after the Tsunami at Taky Pa Distric, Phang Nga, Thailand. *Journal of the Medical Association of Thailand, 97*(Suppl 6), S547–S551.

Quintana, D., Parker, J., Jordan, F., Tuggle, D., Mantor, P., & Tunell, W. (1997). The spectrum of pediatric injuries after a bomb blast. *Journal of Pediatric Surgery, 32*, 307–311. doi:10.1016/S0022-3468(97)90199-8

Raynor, C. (2002). The role of play in the recovery process. In W. Zubenko & J. Cappozoli (Eds.), *Children and disasters: A practical guide to healing and recovery* (pp. 124–134). New York, NY: Oxford University Press.

Rice, D. (2013). Lethal blend of weather, geography caused Colorado Floods. *USA Today*. Retrieved from https://www.usatoday.com/story/weather/2013/09/15/colorado-floods-weather/2816051

Rincon, E., Linares, M., & Greenberg, B. (2001). Effect of previous experience of a hurricane on preparedness for future hurricanes. *American Journal of Emergency Medicine, 19*(4), 276–279. doi:10.1053/ajem.2001.22668

Romig, L. E. (2002). Pediatric triage, a system to JumpSTART(Pediatric version of Simple Triage And Rapid Treatment) your triage of young patients at MCIs. *Journal of Emergency Medical Services, 27*(7), 52–58, 60–63.

Rosenbaum, C. (1993). Chemical warfare: Disaster preparation in an Israeli hospital. *Social Work in Health Care, 18*(3/4), 137–145. doi:10.1300/J010v18n03_13

Rosenfield, R., & Bernardo, L. (2001). Pediatric implications in bioterrorism. Part II: Postexposure diagnosis and treatment. *International Journal of Trauma Nursing, 7*, 133–136. doi:10.1067/mtn.2001.118900

Rotenberg, J., & Newmark, J. (2003). Nerve agent attacks on children: Diagnosis and management. *Pediatrics, 112*(3), 648–658. doi:10.1542/peds.112.3.648

Rubino, C., Cailleux, A., DeVathaire, F., & Schlumberger, M. (2002). Thyroid cancer after radiation exposure. *European Journal of Cancer, 38*(5), 645–647. doi:10.1016/S0959-8049(02)00009-6

Sahloul, M. Z., Monla-Hassan, J., Sankari, A., Kherallah, M., Atassi, B., Badr, S., . . . Sparrow, A. (2016). War is the enemy of health. Pulmonary, critical care, and sleep medicine in War-Torn Syria. Annals of the American Thoracic Society, 13(2), 147–155. doi:10.1513/annalsats.201510-661ps

Salama, P., & Roberts, L. (2005, May 28). Evidence-based interventions in complex emergencies. *The Lancet, 365*(9474), 1848. doi:10.1016/S0140-6736(05)66613-5

Save the Children. (2015). Still at Risk: US Children 10 years after Hurricane Katrina. 2015 National Report Card on Protecting Children in Disasters, pp. 1–24. Retrieved from https://secure.savethechildren.org/atf/cf/%7B9def2ebe-10ae-432c-9bd0-df91d2eba74a%7D/DISASTERREPORT_2015.PDF?v=5PscySTART-cdms02142012

Schonfeld, D. J., & Demaria, P. T.; The Disaster Preparedness Advisory Council and Committee on Psychosocial Aspects of Child and Family Health. (2015). Providing psychosocial support to children and families in the aftermath of disasters and crises. *Pediatrics, 136*(4), e1120–e1130. doi:10.1542/peds.2015-2861

Schreiber, M. (2010). The PsySTART disaster mental health triage and incident management system. Retrieved from http://www.smrrc.org/PDF%20files/psystart-cdms02142012.pdf

Seaman, J., & Maguire, S. (2005). The special needs of children and women. *BMJ, 331*(7507), 34–36. doi:10.1136/bmj.331.7507.34

Shah, A., Frush, K., Luo, X., & Wears, R. (2003). Effect of an intervention standardization system on pediatric dosing and equipment size determination. *Archives of Pediatric and Adolescent Medicine, 157*, 229–236. doi:10.1001/archpedi.157.3.229

Sidell, F. R., Patrick, W. C., & Dashiell, T. R. (2000). *Jane's chembio handbook.* Alexandria, VA: Jane's Information Group.

Sirbaugh, P. E. & Meckler, G. (2017). Prehospital pediatrics and emergency services. UpToDate. Retrieved from https://www.uptodate.com/contents/prehospital-pediatrics-and-emergency-medical-services-ems

Skaug, W. (1999). The Jonesboro school shootings: Lessons for us all. *Pediatrics, 103*(1), 156. doi:10.1542/peds.103.1.156

Slone, M., & Mann, S. (2016). Effects of war, terrorism and armed conflict on young children: A systematic review. *Child Psychiatry and Human Development, 47*(6), 950–965. doi:10.1007/s10578-016-0626-7

Sobaci, G., Akyn, T., Mutlu, F., Karagul, S., & Bayraktar, M. (2005). Terror-related open-globe injuries: A 10-year review. *American Journal of Ophthalmology, 139*(5), 937–939. doi:10.1016/j.ajo.2004.11.009

Twemlow, S., Fonagy, P., Sacco, F., O'Toole, M., & Vernberg, E. (2002). Premeditated mass shootings in schools: Threat assessment. *Journal of the American Academy of Child and Adolescent Psychiatry, 41*(4), 475–477. doi:10.1097/00004583-200204000-00021

U.S. Census Bureau. (2015). United States census. Retrieved from http://www.census.gov

U.S. Department of Health and Human Services. (2017). 2014–2015 report of the Children's HHS Interagency Leadership on Disasters (CHILD) Working Group: Update on departmental activities. Retrieved from https://www.phe.gov/Preparedness/planning/abc/Documents/child-2014-2015.pdf

U.S. Food and Drug Administration. (2001a, December 17). Commentary on non-labeled dosing of oral amoxicillin in adults and pediatrics for post-exposure inhalational anthrax. Retrieved from http://www.fda.gov/Drugs/EmergencyPreparedness/BioterrorismandDrugPreparedness/ucm072106

U.S. Food and Drug Administration. (2001b). FDA's guidance on protection of children and adults against thyroid cancer in case of nuclear accident.

U.S. Food and Drug Administration. (2002). Home preparation procedure for emergency administration of potassium iodide tablets to infants and small children. Retrieved from https://www.fda.gov/Drugs/EmergencyPreparedness/BioterrorismandDrugPreparedness/ucm072261.htm

U.S. Food and Drug Administration. (2017). Pyridostigmine bromide information page. Retrieved from https://www.fda.gov/drugs/emergencypreparedness/bioterrorismanddrugpreparedness/ucm130341.htm

Uzun, N., Savrun, F., & Kiziltan, M. (2005). Electrophysiologic evaluation of peripheral nerve injuries in children following the Marmara earthquake. *Journal of Child Neurology, 20*(3), 207–212. doi:10.1177/08830738050200030701

Waselenko, J., MacVittie, T., Blakely, W., Pesik, N., Wiley, A., Dickerson, . . . Dainiak, N. for Strategic National Stockpile Radiation Working Group. (2004). Medical management of the acute radiation syndrome: Recommendations of the Strategic National Stockpile radiation working group. *Annals of Internal Medicine, 140*, 1037–1051. doi:10.7326/0003-4819-140-12-200406150-00015

Yonekura, T., Ueno, S., & Iwanaka, T. (2013). Care of children in a natural disaster: Lessons learned from the Great East Japan earthquake and tsunami. *Pediatric Surgery International, 29*, 1047–1051. doi:10.1007/s00383-013-3405-6

Yu, L. X., Nguyenpho, A., Roberts, R., Machado, S., Schuirmann, D., Anello, C., & Hussain, A. (2002). Palatability evaluations of doxycycline solid dosage tablets ground and mixed in food or drinks. Food and Drug Administration Center for Drug Evaluation and Research. Retrieved from http://www.fda.gov/cder/drug/infopage/penG_doxy/doxy_food.htm

Zaritsky, A., Nadkarni, V., Berg, R., Hickey, R., & Schexnayder, S. (Eds.). (2001). *Pediatric advanced life support: Instructor's manual.* Dallas, TX: American Heart Association.

Zubenko, W. (2002). Developmental issues in stress and crisis. In W. Zubenko & J. Cappozzoli (Eds.), *Children and disasters: A practical guide to healing and recovery* (pp. 85–100). New York, NY: Oxford University Press.

12

DISASTER NURSING IN SCHOOLS AND OTHER COMMUNITY CONGREGATE CHILD CARE SETTINGS

Cheryl K. Schmidt, Devin Terry, Dona M. Friend, Shannon Finley, Joy Jennings, Susan Roettinger Ritchie, Kelly J. Betts, and Jody Bryant

LEARNING OBJECTIVES

When this chapter is completed, readers will be able to:

1. Identify gaps in local, state, and federal emergency response plans related to caring for children in schools and other community congregate child care settings.
2. Discuss the recommendations of the *National Commission on Children and Disasters: 2010 Report to the President and Congress*, including the 2015 *Save the Children* update.
3. Describe strategies to protect children during disasters in the following settings: elementary and secondary schools, child welfare agencies, juvenile justice settings, child care settings, colleges and universities, and churches.
4. Discuss roles nurses may play in collaborating with community agencies to develop plans to help them prepare for, respond to, and recover from disasters.

KEY MESSAGES

Children comprise nearly 22.9% of the U.S. population, over 73.6 million (ChildStat.gov, 2017); on weekdays, over 90%, or over 66 million of those children are in schools or child care settings.

Prior to the 2010 *National Commission on Children and Disasters Report*, state and local emergency managers were not required by federal law to meet the unique needs of children in their disaster plans. Children were considered "at risk," "vulnerable," or "special needs" populations, so their needs were addressed in annexes, if at all. Several of the Report's recommendations have been met, but the majority have been only partially met or not met at all.

Many organizations have developed detailed guidelines for schools and other community congregate child care settings to follow in developing plans to protect children during and after disasters.

The challenge remains to motivate facilities to adopt the published guidelines, especially in the absence of state or federal regulations requiring emergency plans.

The United States House of Representatives passed the Homeland Security for Children Act (HR 1372) on April 25, 2017, which puts into place many safeguards to further protect children during times of domestic crisis and emergency.

CHAPTER OVERVIEW

This chapter guides nurses in a variety of community settings to develop plans that intentionally integrate children in preparedness, response, and recovery activities during disasters. These guidelines are based on the recommendations published in the Agency for Healthcare Research and Quality's National Commission on Children and Disasters: Interim Report (2009) and Final Report (2010) to the president and Congress (see Appendix 12.1: Index to Recommendations and Responsible Entities). The National Commission was an independent, bipartisan body which identified gaps and in 2010 made recommendations to the president of the United States and Congress. In this chapter, several of these recommendations will be applied to schools and other community congregate child care settings, with specific strategies suggested for implementing the recommendations.

The National Commission was established under the Kids in Disasters Well-being, Safety and Health Act of 2007 to conduct a comprehensive study of the needs of children (0–18 years of age) related to preparation for, response to, and recovery from all hazards (National Commission, 2010). The Interim Report, published in 2009, indicated that children comprised nearly 25% of the U.S. population, over 75 million (America's Children, 2009); on weekdays, over 90%, or 67 million of those children were in schools or child care settings (National Commission, 2010, pp. iv–v), and 88% of low-income children live in counties designated as high risk (Save the Children, 2008). In 2017, the percentage of children in the U.S. population dropped to 22.9% or 73.6 million, with over 66 million in schools or child care settings (ChildStats.gov, 2017), but there are still significant numbers of children separated from their families several hours each day. Despite these figures, state and local emergency managers have not been required by federal law to meet the unique needs of children in their disaster plans. Children are considered "at risk," "vulnerable," or "special needs" populations, so their needs are addressed in annexes, if at all. As an example, the Commission noted examples of "benign neglect" of children during the 2009 H1N1 influenza outbreak. Because children were affected at higher rates (Centers for Disease Control and Prevention [CDC], 2009), many schools and day care facilities were closed, creating major disruptions for families, small businesses, and communities. If these schools and day care settings had well-developed plans in collaboration with other community entities responsible for emergency preparedness, different decisions might have been made during the pandemic.

The National Commission's 2010 Report listed 25 major recommendations and 81 sub-recommendations. As of July 2015, only 17 of those 81 recommendations had been met, 44 were partially met, and 20 had not been met. The ones which had not been met included the need for government funding (Save the Children, July 2015). The Commission described circumstances that make children at higher risk for complications during and after disasters (see Box 12.1). All organizations must consider these needs when planning to care for children before, during, and after disasters. The remainder of this chapter will provide specific suggestions to prepare various settings to provide optimum care for children.

GROWTH AND DEVELOPMENTAL/ COGNITIVE CONSIDERATIONS

When organizations are preparing for children during disasters, it is important to consider the various growth and developmental needs of children. According to Schonfeld and Demaria (2015), approximately 14% of U.S. children between the ages of 2 and 17 years have been exposed to a disaster in their lifetimes. The difference between children and adults in times of disaster is that children are vulnerable to traumatic events due to their lack of experience, skills, and resources to act independently and be able to meet their emotional, social, and developmental needs (Schonfeld & Demaria, 2015). Therefore, what children need during a time of disaster is not therapy, but community-based, developmentally appropriate activities to help restore their sense of safety and hope, and address the developmental needs to ensure a healthy recovery (Kostelny & Wessells, 2005).

Children who experience traumatic events related to disasters have some degree of behavioral symptoms, and adjust to the event depending on their age and developmental status (Hagan et al., 2005) (Tables 12.1 and 12.2). The psychological adjustment of the child can range from a transient reaction to a

BOX 12.1 Children's Unique Needs in Disasters

Children are not simply small adults. Throughout this report, the Commission notes children's unique vulnerabilities in disasters that must be addressed in disaster management activities and policies. For example:

- Children may experience long-lasting effects such as academic failure, PTSD, depression, anxiety, bereavement, and other behavioral problems such as delinquency and substance abuse.
- Children are more susceptible to chemical, biological, radiological, and nuclear threats and require different medications, dosages, and delivery systems than adults.
- During disasters, young children may not be able to escape danger, identify themselves, and make critical decisions.
- Children are dependent on adults for care, shelter, transportation, and protection from predators.
- Children are often away from parents, in the care of schools, child care providers, Head Start, or other child congregate care environments, which must be prepared to ensure children's safety.
- Children must be expeditiously reunited with their legal guardians if separated from them during a disaster.
- Children in disaster shelters require age-appropriate supplies such as diapers, cribs, baby formula, and food.

Source: Reprinted with permission from National Commission on Children and Disasters. (2010, October). *2010 Report to the President and Congress* (p. 20). AHRQ Publication No. 10-MO37. Rockville, MD: Agency for Healthcare Research and Quality.

more severe, prolonged psychological reaction. This prolonged reaction can lead to prolonged consequences of posttraumatic stress disorder (PTSD). Approximately 16% of children who have been exposed to a traumatic event have developed PTSD worldwide, according to a meta-analysis documented by Alisic et al. (2014). Children respond to a traumatic event in many different ways. These cognitive and emotional responses to a traumatic event have been associated with the risk of developing PTSD. The cognitive and emotional responses that may present are (a) high levels of anger about the traumatic event, (b) increased levels of rumination and catastrophizing, (c) high levels of avoidance and suppression of trauma-related thoughts, and (d) dissociation during and after the event (McLaughlin, 2016). Most children who are provided with adequate support and have the internal resources will develop new skills that they can use to cope with future adversity (Schonfeld & Gurwitch, 2012). Activities that are encouraged during sheltering or in disaster-safe houses help children to gather a sense of safety when surrounded by caring adults they trust. Age-appropriate activities also promote a sense of normalcy during usual play routines, such as singing, games, and dancing. Children are especially ritualistic in their daily activities and need to have a sense of routine to feel comfortable in their environment (Bowden & Greenberg, 2010). Teens can take part in the activities of younger children and can lead activities, read, and play with the children. This will give teens a sense of engagement and responsibility to promote their sense of identity.

Chapter 32 in this textbook discusses in detail how to provide for the unique needs of children during disasters and other public health emergencies. As a quick resource for organizations planning for disasters, we include a table listing key elements regarding growth and developmental considerations for children and young adults (Table 12.3).

TABLE 12.1 Stages of Response to Trauma or Disaster in Children

Stage and Time Period	Description of Behaviors
Stage 1 occurs immediately after the disaster or traumatic event.	Reactions of fright, disbelief, denial, grief, and feelings of relief if loved ones have not been harmed. Altruism may be displayed and this will sometimes help the child develop resilience or be a marker of resilience in the child.
Stage 2 can occur from a few days after the disaster to several weeks posttraumatic event or disaster.	Initial reactions lead to regression in many young children and manifest in behaviors that represent anxiety, depression, sadness, fear, hostility, and aggressive behaviors; apathy, withdrawal, and sleep disturbances. The child may act out behaviors during play or socialization.
Stage 3 occurs when the child continues to have abnormal coping behaviors longer than 1 month postevent. Children who experience long-term distress are at risk of posttraumatic stress disorder or delinquent behaviors later in life.	Long-term behaviors escalate from Stage 2. These children will need psychosocial counseling from a mental health specialist.

Source: Adapted from Hagan, J. F.; the Committee on Psychosocial Aspects of Child and Family, and the Task Force on Terrorism. (2005). American Academy of Pediatrics Clinical Report: Psychosocial implications of disaster or terrorism on children: A guide for the pediatrician. *Pediatrics, 116*(4), 787–795. doi:10.1542/peds.2005–1498

TABLE 12.2 Common Symptoms of Adjustment Reactions in Children and Adolescents After a Disaster

Sleep problems	• Difficulty falling or staying asleep • Awakes frequently • Hard to wake up in the morning • Other sleep disruptions such as bedwetting or nightmares
Eating problems	• Loss or increased appetite
Mood changes	• Sadness or depression • Anger • Worries or fears
Changes in school performance	• Difficulty concentrating on tasks • Difficulty retaining new information • Decrease in overall academic performance
Substance abuse	• New onset or exacerbation of alcohol, tobacco, or drug use
Risk-taking behaviors	• Increased sexual behavior or promiscuity • Other reactive risk-taking behaviors
Somatization	• Increased physical symptoms such as stomachaches, headaches, or other physical symptoms or pain
Developmental or social regression	• May become isolated and not as social as before; may be less patient or tolerant of change, revert to bedwetting, or become behaviorally disruptive

Source: Adapted from Schonfeld, D. J., & Demaria, T.; Disaster Preparedness Advisory Council and Committee on Psychosocial Aspects of Child and Family Health. (2015). Providing psychosocial support to children and families in the aftermath of disasters and crisis. *Pediatrics, 136*(94), e1120–e1130. doi:10.1542/peds.2015-2861

Elementary and Secondary Schools

Children, both those living with a disability and those who are not, may lack the capability to make formalized critical decisions to escape danger during an actual emergency. Considering the special healthcare needs of children and a child's inherent dependency on adults for protection, emergency disaster plans that offer specific recommendations for children are crucial. As of May 2016, between 2014 and 2026, total public school enrollment in pre-K through grade 12 is projected to increase by 3% (from 50.0 million to 51.4 million students), with changes across states ranging from an increase of 39% in the District of Columbia to a decrease of 15% in New Hampshire (National Center for Education Statistics, 2017). When a child is dropped off at school or another child care facility, many parents and guardians assume that there are emergency plans in place to safeguard children. Unfortunately, literature disproves this assumption and highlights serious gaps in local, state, and federal preparedness standards (Save the Children, 2013b). Most (86.3%) school superintendents reported having a response plan, but fewer (57.2%) have a plan for prevention. Most (95.6%) have an evacuation plan, but almost one-third (30%) had never conducted a drill. Almost one quarter (22.1%) have no disaster plan provisions for children with special healthcare needs, and one quarter reported having no plans for postdisaster counseling. Almost half (42.8%) had never met with local ambulance officials to discuss emergency planning (Graham, Shirm, Liggin, Aitken, & Dick, 2006). Urban school districts were better prepared than rural districts on almost all measures in the survey. The results of a September 2012 study revealed that children with disabilities are especially vulnerable in disaster situations, and advocated

that written national disaster preparedness standards be mandated for all facilities caring for children (Save the Children, 2013a). Considering that young children and children with disabilities may not be able to understand directives given during the chaos of an actual emergency, formalized disaster plans should be practiced routinely and intra-agency response should occur when practiced. The national outcry for local, state, and federal agencies to address problems identified in school disaster preparedness plans has been a key focus area of the National Commission. In the recommendations for working with families of diverse backgrounds, outreach workers must be sensitive to language differences and cultural needs. Children are often thrust into the role of interpreter if their parents and relatives are not fluent in English. This responsibility may require skills beyond the child's current stage of development and be too stressful for the child. The outreach worker can relieve the child of this responsibility by seeking out adult interpreters for the family (Substance Abuse and Mental Health Services Administration, 2013). Stages of Response to Trauma or Disaster in Children are listed in Table 12.1.

Preparedness

"Each year, approximately 49.8 million students attend public elementary and secondary schools, and 5 million students attend private schools" (Rebmann, Elliott, Artman, VanNatta & Wakefield, 2016, p. 794). Since the likelihood of a child being in a school-based setting during a disaster event or an active shooter situation is real, the National Commission on Children and Disasters (2010) stressed that federal and state support is necessary to help schools ensure that children are protected

TABLE 12.3 Review of Psychosocial and Cognitive Development by Age Group

Age	Psychosocial Developmental Stage	Cognitive Developmental Stage	Disaster Preparedness
Infant (0–1 year)	*Trust Versus Mistrust* • Caregiver responds to infant by meeting the needs and creating a trusting environment.	*Responds With Reflexes and Basic Circular Movements* • Responds with reflexes to external stimuli with random body movements • Becomes aware of the environment and follows sounds • Beginning hand–eye coordination • Beginning development of object permanence	• Keep an emergency stock of the following items: diapers, formula, bottles, water for mixing formulas, wipes, blankets, age-appropriate clothing, and toys. • Create a way to transfer infants to a safe place in the event of a weather-related disaster or earthquake. • Identify each infant by using a wrist or ankle band, or in an equally effective manner.
Toddlers (1–3 years)	*Autonomy Versus Shame and Doubt* • Develops autonomy. If forced to do something not able to master, may develop a sense of shame and self-doubt.	*Invention of New Meanings* • Trial and error activities • Basic concept of causality • View of self as separate from others • Develop object permanence	• Keep an emergency stock of the following items: diapers, formula, bottles, water for mixing formulas, wipes, baby food, blankets, age-appropriate clothing, and toys. • Ensure that each child has on closed-toe shoes. • Identify each child with a wrist or ankle band, or in an equally effective manner. • Assess for risk factors of PTSD and provide mental health counseling for those at risk.
Preschool (3–6 years)	*Initiative Versus Guilt* • Initiative is completed when the child is able to carry out a plan of action. Believes that wants and actions are sound. If child punished for expressing his/her desires, may feel guilt.	*Preconceptual–Conceptual Stage* • Egocentric in thoughts and feelings • Understand literal instructions • Play becomes social • Imitation important • Use of words to express thought	• Keep an emergency stock of coloring books, reading books, crayons, markers, flash cards, and board games. • Be consistent with behavior modification, as some children will act out during stressful events. • Allow children to socialize and play in groups and create songs, dances, and other games that can be played without props. • Assess for risk factors of PTSD and provide mental health counseling for those at risk.
School-aged (6–12 years)	*Identity Versus Inferiority* • Acquires reading, writing, math, and social skills. Develops industry. If compared with others or made to believe he/she is inadequate, then feelings of inferiority will occur.	*Intuitive Stage* • Logical reasoning develops • Able to reverse thinking • Able to understand joking or teasing • Likes to collect and classify objects	• Give older school children tasks and small jobs that they can be responsible for during the sheltering process. • Allow children to socialize and play in groups and create songs, dances, and other games that can be played without props. • Be consistent with behavior modification, as some children will act out during stressful events. • Assess for risk factors of PTSD and provide mental health counseling for those at risk.

(continued)

TABLE 12.3 Review of Psychosocial and Cognitive Development by Age Group (*continued*)

Age	Psychosocial Developmental Stage	Cognitive Developmental Stage	Disaster Preparedness
Teens (12–19 years)	*Identity Versus Role Confusion* • May make impulsive choices, starts to think about future roles of vocation; inability to make decisions may lead to role confusion.	*Formal Operations* • Acquires conceptual thinking skills • Uses scientific approach • Ability to solve complex verbal problems • Can set short- and long-term goals	• Assess for risk factors of PTSD and provide mental health counseling for those at risk. • Allow teens to help care for the younger children if emotionally able. • Assign duties to the teens to promote identity and role assurance.
College age (19–25 years)	*Intimacy Versus Isolation* • Intimate relationships are developed. Fear and anxiety about relationships may lead to isolation.	*Formal Operations* • Acquires conceptual thinking skills • Uses scientific approach • Able to solve complex verbal problems • Can set short- and long-term goals	• Same interventions as teens and adults.

PTSD, posttraumatic stress disorder.

Source: Adapted from Bowden, V. R., & Greenberg, C. S. (2010). *Children and their families: The continuum of care* (2nd ed.). Philadelphia, PA: Lippincott, Williams & Wilkins.

during disaster events and throughout the reunification process with their families according to federally recommended practices. At least 62% of school districts reported facing challenges to the implementation of their emergency plans, citing lack of properly trained staff, lack of equipment, and lack of practice with community-based first responders during drills (National Commission on Children and Disasters, 2010, p. 91). The United States Department of Education Office of Safe and Healthy Students (OSHS) is responsible for managing the Readiness and Emergency Management for Schools (REMS) program, which offers schools direct assistance in developing individualized comprehensive emergency management and disaster planning programs (REMS, 2017). The REMS program offers a variety of free resources, such as virtual and live training sessions, to help schools identify needs and develop comprehensive written disaster plans that incorporate all of the federal preparedness recommendations from predisaster planning through reunification plans with families (National Commission on Children and Disasters, 2010). The U.S. Department of Education (2008) recommends that schools include a vulnerability assessment during their preplanning phase to factor in functional access limitations and the needs of students living with a disability. During the preplanning process, schools should also apply for federal and state funding to obtain resources and create disaster-safe rooms on their campuses. In rural Arkansas, several school districts have included "safe rooms" in their emergency plans, and often call on volunteer fire departments in the area to open those rooms to the community during tornado warnings. Schools and other academic settings should continuously monitor the unique needs of children attending their facilities and plan ahead to offer equitable access to all students following a disaster. Schools should integrate the

resources offered through the REMS program to build individualized disaster plans that are site specific and offer equal accessibility to all students, staff, and visitors. School systems should be encouraged to partner with the REMS education collaborative virtual community. This group of educational practitioners, from all over the nation, meet online to engage with each other while sharing best practices for emergency and disaster preparedness (REMS, 2017).

Another consideration for children attending school is the protection of personally identifiable information. The U.S. Department of Health and Human Services (HHS, 2017) stresses that healthcare professionals understand that the Health Insurance Portability and Accountability Act of 1996 (HIPAA) protects the privacy of individually identifiable health information even in disaster situations, but many may not know that, at schools, health information is also protected under the Family Educational Rights and Privacy Act (FERPA). Since private schools are not federally funded, they are not subject to the federal laws that protect the privacy of student educational records (U.S. Department of Education, 2011). During disaster situations in schools that obtain federal funding, the disclosure of student information to outside parties is still protected and is critically important to consider when formulating emergency disaster plans. However, according to the U.S. Department of Education (2010), there may be several exceptions to FERPA that apply during emergency and disaster situations. School directory information, such as basic contact information, may be disclosed to emergency management agencies trying to locate legal guardians, without the consent of the parent or student (U.S. Department of Education, 2011). Under the health and safety emergency provisions of FERPA, school administrators may determine that it is necessary to disclose nondirectory information to appropriate parties in direct connection with an emergency to protect the safety of students, staff, and visitors in the school (U.S. Department of Education, 2011). But disclosure is strictly limited to the time of the emergency and must be documented in the educational records to whom, what threat, and when the information was disclosed (U.S. Department of Education, 2010). It is important to remember that students with special medical needs may be separated from their families during disasters, and school administrators may need to immediately disclose medical information to public health officials, law enforcement, or healthcare providers to expedite care of that child. FERPA, under the health and safety provision, confirms that those parties would typically be considered appropriate (U.S. Department of Education, 2010). The legalities associated with HIPAA and FERPA, along with the possible exceptions during disasters, offer clear evidence that consideration for health information should be written into all school emergency disaster plans. National and state standards should be practiced during local emergency drills to ensure privacy was maintained and allow open discussion, during the drill debriefing, when potential breaches in confidentiality are identified.

The National Education Association Healthy Futures (NEAHF) organization developed a school crisis guide, created by educators, offering practical suggestions for use before, during, and after an emergency or disaster (n.d.). The National Education Association (NEA) stresses key elements of a district-level emergency preparedness plan that include: crisis prevention activities; identification of a crisis response team with specific roles identified; research-based violence prevention programs and safety policies in place; clear internal and external communication avenues; school safety assessments updated regularly; crisis response policies and procedures; and written plans for recovery (NEAHF, n.d.). Each of the key elements identified, along with trained school personnel and an incident command system aligned with local emergency response personnel, is designed to make school safety an intentional part of every day. The NEAHF (n.d.) recommends memoranda of understanding (MOU) be developed and implemented with community emergency response partners to allow continuity of operations during and after a crisis or disaster situation at school (p. 4).

In many schools, the role of administration and government recommendations are evident in the overall preparedness plan, but nurses must advocate for children to become active participants in their school's emergency disaster plans. An easy way schools can integrate disaster preparedness and safety information into their classroom curriculum, for all students, is to encourage teachers to incorporate programs offered through the American Red Cross and the FEMA. For example, the American Red Cross *Masters of Disaster* curriculum is a series of learning modules for grades K–8 tailored to specific grade ranges and intended to provide safety information to children about disasters (American Red Cross, 2017a). Each ready-to-use lesson plan offers hands-on learning activities, disaster preparedness vocabulary terms, and summary activities to increase disaster safety education in school classrooms. Allowing children of all ages and abilities the opportunity to

actively process what their responses would be in the event of a fire, tornado, hurricane, or shooter on campus will facilitate adherence to established school procedures by eliminating some of the inherent fear. These learning modules are available online or through any local American Red Cross chapter in the United States. Another program developed by the American Red Cross is called the Pillowcase Project. In this program, children learn how to prepare for and respond to disasters, then decorate special pillowcases provided through the Walt Disney Corporation with pictures of what items they would put in the pillowcase to quickly evacuate from a disaster area (American Red Cross, 2017c). For students who choose a more independent learning or online learning environment, FEMA's Ready Kids may be a good solution. Ready Kids is an interactive disaster preparedness program available online that offers games, learning activities, and allows children to progress at their own pace (FEMA, 2017).

Another American Red Cross program designed to help schools, businesses, and other community-based agencies examine their level of disaster preparedness and enhance community resiliency is called The American Red Cross Ready Rating Program (2017b). This free program is designed to allow organizations a systematic method to assess their entire disaster preparedness plans and generates a scorecard after the assessment has been completed. It offers best practice tips to organizations based on their identified weaknesses and then suggests implementation strategies to correct the weaknesses. According to the American Red Cross Ready Rating Program (2017b) businesses, organizations, and schools will continue with automatic free membership renewal if the organization assessment scores show yearly improvement from baseline. This program helps agencies document their preplanning for disasters, which should minimize the adverse effects of a disaster or emergency. Many companies who offer insurance coverage to school-based agencies require documentation of the written emergency disaster plan, but many agencies lack the documentation of the recommendations posed by the 2010 Report to the President and Congress (National Commission on Children and Disasters, 2010).

Nurses have the specialized training necessary to assess the needs of all children under their care while attending school. Nurses should remain educated about current disaster preparedness recommendations and how they affect the vulnerable populations attending school. They should be asked, by administration, to serve on disaster-planning committees to help ensure constant preparedness on campus. Specific examples of how nurses can help school-based settings prepare for disasters include:

1. Nursing students may be invited to collaborate with school nurses to assess the disaster preparedness levels of local schools. If schools are not prepared, the nursing students could offer to assist the schools to develop or expand their plans as a community health nursing project.
2. Nurses and nursing students can volunteer to participate in a school's vulnerability assessments, with one of their key responsibilities being to examine functional access requirements and how the schools are meeting the needs of students living with various disabilities.

3. Nurses and nursing students can volunteer their services to any disaster organization, such as the American Red Cross, any state's Office of Emergency Management, or through their state's Department of Health. Nurses who obtain the appropriate national, state, or local volunteer training stand ready to deploy in cases of disasters or public health emergencies and help manage the surge capacity of the response teams (Veenema et al., 2016, p. 194).

Response

The psychological impact of disasters can have catastrophic consequences on children and adults. Following a disaster, children may be suffering from disruption in basic services at home, homelessness, and/or transportation issues; added to the fact that children often pick up feelings of anxiety from adults, a child's grief response is often magnified. Emotional trauma is an expected sequela following any disaster, and healthcare professionals are trained to assess for the subtle changes in behavior that may indicate poor coping in children; however, teachers and school administrators are not. "Psychological first aid is the practice of recognizing and responding to the emotional needs of people presenting in the wake of a disaster" (Grindlay & Breeze, 2016, p. 207). The National Commission noted that school personnel receive little training in how to recognize, support, and promote adjustment in children following a disaster or emergency event (National Commission on Children and Disasters, 2010). School-based settings must ensure qualified professionals are available to offer the emotional first aid that children require during the response phase.

School personnel should be aware of community mental health resources and have contact information written into the school emergency disaster plans. Since children suffer long-lasting mental and physical effects following a disaster, school personnel should partner with community-based nurses and mental health professionals to monitor for PTSD, behavioral problems, along with signs or symptoms of anxiety and depression. The National Commission recommended mental health training tools be developed for teachers, mandatory statewide training requirements be implemented, and requirements for supporting children following crisis situations become a part of the certification/recertification process (National Commission on Children and Disasters, 2010). Although teachers and school personnel should be educated to recognize basic pediatric mental health issues, it does not suggest these individuals should offer mental health treatment (NEAHF, n.d.). Schools should ensure that trained mental health professionals are available to treat students on campus following crisis situations, emergencies, or disasters.

Recovery

The impact of large-scale disasters on children and schools is tremendous. Following Hurricane Katrina in 2005, it is estimated that more than 1 million people left their homes and more than 300,000 children were enrolled into new schools all around the country (Save the Children, 2015). During the 2017 hurricane season, Hurricane Harvey threatened nearly 3 million children in Texas and Louisiana (Save the Children, 2017b). Hurricane Maria displaced nearly 700,000 children in Puerto Rico alone (Save the Children, 2017a). As many as 62% of all school districts in the United States confirm that they lack needed training, resources, and the expertise to prepare for and manage during disasters (Save the Children, 2015, p. 16). Disaster planning for the recovery phase is essential because schools often sustain damage to facilities, lose necessary equipment, and lose revenue and fiscal resources for normal operation during disaster situations. Regardless of the difficulties posed by a disaster, schools must open quickly to facilitate a positive learning environment and some return of normalcy back into the community. According to Save the Children (2015), "Schools (K–12) are the first line of defense for more than 57 million children every day. In addition, schools can serve as a central hub for children who need services following a disaster" (p. 16). School disaster plans should aim for their campuses to be a one-stop resource zone to facilitate getting children necessary mental and physical health services during the recovery phase.

A major problem hindering schools serving as that one-stop resource hub is that there are no dedicated federal or state funds to support rapid recovery of schools back to full operation. Schools apply for recovery money in a variety of ways. The Stafford Act allows funding for the repair of public and nonprofit private school buildings, as well as replacement of the contents (National Commission on Children and Disasters, 2010). Congress can also pass Acts which authorize one-time grant assistance for areas impacted by large-scale disasters, as with the Hurricane Education Recovery Act (HERA) offered after Hurricane Katrina. This grant-funded assistance can be used to maintain school operations, obtain school supplies, replace equipment, and hire additional staff to meet the mental health needs of the students during the recovery phase of the disaster (National Commission on Children and Disasters, 2010). An additional mechanism by which schools are funded by the federal government following a disaster is through the Education for Homeless Children and Youth (EHCY) program. Since students who are displaced by disasters may be considered tenuously housed or homeless, EHCY funds may be available to school districts to assist with transportation, outreach programs, immunizations, tutoring, counseling, school supplies, and case management activities (National Commission on Children and Disasters, 2010).

Schools are charged with providing care, shelter, and protection for children during their time at the facility; but how many have plans to expeditiously get children back to their legal guardians after a disaster strikes? Six months after Hurricane Katrina, the last of over 5,000 displaced children were reunited with their families (Save the Children, 2013b). The National Commission found 56% of school districts had no plans for providing education to students in the event schools were closed for an extended period of time, and many plans had no mention of accommodating students with special needs (National Commission on Children and Disasters, 2010, p. 91). Baker and Baker (2010) stressed that children with special needs are no better prepared for disasters than the general population and few families had made plans for continuity of medical care following a disaster (p. 244). Based on these identified problems, it is imperative that schools have tracking and reunification procedures written into their emergency preparedness plans. School directory information, on students and all employees, should be saved to an encrypted external hard drive so school personnel can hook up a laptop and have key information readily available in cases of evacuation. This would increase child safety and diminish liability concerns about allowing children to leave with unauthorized individuals following the disaster event or crisis situation.

Even though cell phone towers often do not function properly in disasters and land-based phone lines may be out, communication during disasters is essential and many local emergency plans include the use of HAM radios or satellite phones. Schools should have this equipment on hand and practice using them regularly with other local emergency response agencies. Other communication modalities, such as emergency text messaging alerts, text critical school alerts, handheld radios and updated websites, should be implemented through the disaster plan with school personnel, community emergency responders, and family members of the children participating in training exercises regularly. Grindlay and Breeze (2016) stress that consideration should also be given to communication equipment's battery life, storage, maintenance, and, when all other communication methods fail, to designated people who can be used as runners to move critical information. These elements should be addressed specifically in the school disaster plans. Parents and/or guardians should have their role in the reunification process clearly delineated and should have electronic accessibility to updated disaster plans at all times via the school's website. Faculty, staff, students, and families should practice every step of the emergency disaster plan, including the reunification process, with local first responders on a routine schedule (Lee et al., 2008). Practice is the only way that children, with or without special needs, understand their roles during emergency situations and quickly respond to the safety strategies in place for their protection.

Child Welfare Agencies

Professionals working in a child welfare setting should be knowledgeable about disaster preparedness and have plans developed for all employees to follow when disaster strikes. This section will discuss the recommendations for evidence-based disaster plans based on the recommendations published by the Agency for Healthcare Research and Quality's *National Commission on Children and Disasters: 2009 Interim Report to the President and Congress* (October 2010).

Preparedness

Continuity of Operations Plan (COOP) disaster management and recovery integrates the needs of all supervised children. This plan should address minimally the components focused upon in the Child and Family Services Improvement Act of 2006 (Child Welfare Information Gateway, 2016, pp. 2–3) as well as incorporating recommendations from the Justice Working Group on Children and Disasters implemented by the Department of Justice (Save the Children, 2015, p. 17).

1. Coordinate management with federal, state, and local agencies.
2. Educate staff members about their roles during a disaster and how to carry out the plan.

3. Identify, locate, and continue availability of services for children under state care or supervision who are displaced or adversely affected by disaster.
4. Respond to new welfare cases in areas adversely affected by a disaster and provide services.
5. Remain in communication with caseworkers and other essential child welfare personnel who are displaced because of disaster.
6. Preserve essential program records.
7. Continue funds for children and families during the recovery of a disaster.
8. Coordinate services and share information with other states.

Ancillary goals may need to be developed depending on the facility's location and special requirements. For example, continuous communication should be developed with courts and the judicial system that make decisions related to the care of juveniles in state care (Gatowski & Sophia, 2008). When developing a facility's COOP, the goal should be to return to operation within 12 hours after a disaster strikes, with COOP operations sustaining themselves for up to 30 days. When developing a recovery COOP, agencies need to keep in mind that there may be severe damage to the structural safety in the area directly affected by the disaster.

Child welfare agencies must take a leadership role in the development of disaster planning and the COOP. This is done jointly with the juvenile and family courts, child advocates, volunteers, and other community resources (Gatowski & Sophia, 2008). Finally, child welfare agencies should make allowances that set a standard higher than the minimal guidelines by: (a) providing annual staff training, including implementation of the plan; (b) coordinating with emergency management services to integrate the child welfare disaster plan and COOP with other local and state COOPs; (c) coordinating with high stakeholders to implement the child welfare COOP training and drills; (d) developing a plan to address the high emotional needs of children that are found after the impact of a disaster; (e) requiring best practice emergency planning for all entities in child welfare (foster families, kinship care providers, residential and group care facilities); and (f) implementing the state plan at local levels and collaborating to get the local plan(s) integrated into the state plan (National Commission on Children and Disasters, 2010). COOPs developed with best practices and coordination of local and state agencies and governments will reduce the chances of children being displaced or stranded in locations after a disaster without provisions or medical attention.

When developing the agency's COOP, close attention should be paid to the children's needs related to education, health, mental health, substance abuse, probation, and case processing (National Commission on Children and Disasters, 2010). The National Council of Juvenile and Family Court Judges, in collaboration with the American Bar Association, have developed template tools to help with this process (Portune & Gatowski, 2008, p. 67). This COOP should be overseen and reviewed by the state's juvenile justice agencies for statewide coordination and disaster planning that flows well across the system. This can be accomplished by developing a State Coalition for the planning of the COOP, using representatives from the high stakeholders involved.

The National Commission on Children and Disasters recommends that coalitions or child welfare agencies take at a minimum these basic steps (2010):

1. Perform a gap analysis for the agencies involved. Assess for shortcomings and best practices in all juvenile agencies.
2. Develop a training program that will assist agencies in implementing the plan as well as ensuring all staff have adequate knowledge of their roles in the plan.
3. Coordinate and support management and review of the COOP with state emergency management teams and key stakeholders.

The Annie E. Casey Foundation produced a free toolkit as a resource guide for child welfare agencies' disaster preparedness. This toolkit is for the assessment of existing plans, direction in performing the agency's gap analysis, budget, development of new plans, response, and recovery (www.aecf.org/m/resourcedoc/AECF-DisasterPreparednessResourceGuide-2009.pdf). Facilities need to perform an assessment of the potential disasters in their area. Creating a COOP for the most potential disasters will limit the hard work and enhance the benefits to actual threats to the system. Using the list of recommendations from the Annie E. Casey Foundation will provide step-by-step topics: assess agency preparedness and evaluate current disaster management plans; determine the most likely threats to the facility; assign duties to staff/professional employees; articulate the disaster plan so that it is available to all employees; develop financial security for the employment of the disaster plan annually; ensure that the agency plan is coordinated with agencies at the local, state, and federal levels (sheriff's office, state troopers, FBI); address within the COOP where the agency can relocate if the main office is affected; carry out education with the family and friends of clients to ensure they have disaster plans; include plans to protect families of employees who may become essential during the act of a disaster; ensure all employees have personal disaster plans; incorporate adequate communication systems that will function in the case of a disaster; address how the agency will maintain vital records in the stages of disaster; consider admission into the agency from out-of-state residents due to the effects of the disaster; proactively consider how to budget for disaster management; and hold annual or semiannual drills in which the agency enforces the COOP from beginning to end with an evaluation/participant debriefing at the end of the drill (The Annie E. Casey Foundation, 2009, pp. 4–6).

Response

Child welfare agencies must ensure they have practiced disaster management activities and operations that provide for those under their supervision prior to a disaster. Disasters may not be predictable; there may be warnings of a potential tornado, but no notification of a potential bioterrorist targeting the area. Agencies need to hold drills so all employees are familiar with the COOP. Note that all disaster drills that will involve young children need to take into consideration the age of the participants. If theatrical makeup or dramatic injuries will be used, participants may need to be older children or teenagers to prevent emotional distress of younger participants.

Carrying out drills even in the absence of essential participants is vital, as well as when everyone is on campus. The agency needs to have experience with adapting the COOP in the midst of disaster, because there is no guarantee that all vital participants will be onsite when disaster strikes. Assistant Secretary Marketa Gautreau of Louisiana speaks about "rigid flexibility" the Office of Community Services had to uphold during Hurricanes Katrina and Rita in 2005 in response to the magnitude of the disaster and the involvement of several state agencies (The Annie E. Casey Foundation, 2009).

Clients and families may report to an agency after the occurrence of a disaster with vital needs related to the disaster. They may have had to evacuate without clothing, financial assistance, or members of their family. The agency's COOP needs to address how they are going to manage clients' and families' needs during disasters. The Annie E. Casey Foundation suggests using direct deposit for all financial deposits for all clients and families to help prevent the occurrence of financial distress during a disaster. This will provide continuity in payment and clients' and families' ability to access their money away from their home. Having personnel on hand to perform a thorough intake related to client and family needs as they report to an agency after a disaster will allow for adequate assessment and interventions in the beginning of the response. This will promote normal functioning and influence the ability of clients and families to begin the recovery phase after a disaster (O'Brien, Webster, & Herrick, 2007).

When responding to a disaster, agencies need to be aware of the possibility of new referrals into the child welfare system. These children may or may not present to the agency with guardians. Agencies should prepare for those situations where a child advocate needs to be assigned for the protection of a minor. These children may or may not know if their current guardian is alive due to becoming separated from him or her during the disaster. Plans on how to locate children who are in need of services, but do not report directly to the agency, need to be included in each agency's COOP. Facilities may need financial assistance when trying to implement a new disaster preparedness system as encompassing as the one described in this section. Financial means can be obtained via the Human Resources and Services Administration (HRSA).

Recovery

When developing the recovery plan in an agency COOP, agencies should consider the workload that will likely be placed on existing employees during and in the months following a disaster. Agencies need to think about employees who may not be able to report to work due to the disaster, and how that will affect the implementation of the COOP. After disaster strikes, there is a lot of confusion; taking steps to minimize confusion within collaborating agencies will decrease the time spent on discussing issues such as welfare jurisdiction.

When developing an agency COOP, it is very easy to focus solely on clients and families, but agencies should be reminded to consider their staff and professional employees' assessment of needs. Assessments for mental health needs and support systems should be provided during the recovery phase. Remember that staff and professional employees will most likely have been affected by the same disaster. They may be worried about loved ones who are missing or victims of the disaster. Workers will also begin to develop side effects from compassion fatigue if intervention is not taken (The Annie E. Casey Foundation, 2009).

Workers during a disaster tend to put others first and take poor care of themselves, at times developing compassion fatigue. Workers may become apathetic to the cause, neglect caring for themselves, and in long-term studies even turn to substance abuse trying to deal with the tragedies they witnessed (Compassion Fatigue Awareness Project, 2010). Agencies can provide assistance for their staff and professional employees by using leadership within the agency; ensuring proper daily operations; debriefing opportunities on an ongoing basis; and by providing mental health treatment. Providing moral support and counseling opportunities may prevent further harm from compassion fatigue (The Annie E. Casey Foundation, 2009). Developing an agreement with specific health professionals is one recommendation during the writing and development phase of the COOP. This will help fill any of the healthcare gaps that may be brought on by the health professional shortage in the area directly related to the disaster. Holding educational opportunities for healthcare providers related to compassion fatigue, PTSD, depression, and childhood mental disorders will help after a disaster when mental health professionals may be overwhelmed by their caseloads and clients have to seek care from their primary care provider (PCP). Educating about mental health stigmas will ensure that more individuals affected by disaster are comfortable seeking help when they notice signs and symptoms related to mental healthcare needs (The Annie E. Casey Foundation, 2009).

Coordination of not only mental health, but clients' and families' needs for physical healthcare is also essential. Ensuring adequate treatment options are provided either when sheltered in place or evacuated is a goal that may require coordination with outside providers. Physical care needs to incorporate all aspects of health: nutritional, injury prevention, wellness, illness, and sleep/rest. If clients and families have had to evacuate to a new location, they may not have adequate supplies for special diets (i.e., diabetic, gluten-free, and low fat). Residents in the area not directly affected by the disaster may prepare meals for clients and families that may not meet nutritional restrictions of certain individuals. In a new setting, agencies need to be able to provide a safe, quality environment for clients and families. Making sure that the location is safe for all ages can be done during the development of the agencies' COOP. Will there be medical personnel on site to assess any complaints of injury or illness, or will everyone be referred to the local emergency department? What if the local healthcare facility was destroyed or damaged during the disaster? Will there be staff on site to educate clients and families how to maintain wellness during disaster? Rearranging clients' and families' schedules so all members can obtain needed sleep and rest will have a significant effect on both physical and mental health needs and adaptations.

While still operating under the recovery phase of the agencies' COOP, action to find adequate housing for clients' and families' needs should be initiated. Many disasters may leave clients and families permanently without housing. Having a safe place for shelter is the long-term goal of all child welfare agencies. If the direct area has sustained major damage, church, school, or Red Cross shelters may have to remain open until housing (apartments, hotel rooms, etc.) can be located nearby or rebuilt in the area. When clients and families are displaced during a disaster, getting to and from school can become a major issue for these individuals. After a disaster, if a school is in session, communication with the proper authorities for transportation to and from school will help ensure continuity of education for children affected by disasters. Communicating with the local schools with the addresses of shelters, relocation addresses for agencies, and so forth, prior to disaster striking, will promote a smooth transition in the COOP. Maintaining attendance in school will help children keep a regular schedule in the days following the disaster.

Local foster parents may be unable to foster children after a disaster. One recommendation is having a backup plan with surrounding counties and states communicating potential needs for foster parents. Meanwhile, supporting local foster parents is needed to enable them to continue their services to the children they may have in their care at the time of a disaster. Funding may be available for these families at the federal level, but families should not plan on that.

At the end of the disaster response and recovery phases, agencies should hold debriefing sessions to assess what in the COOP went well and what needs to be changed or updated. These sessions should always be held after drills to provide feedback, and needed changes made prior to the occurrence of an actual disaster. All information should be communicated in an open and direct fashion so that all old copies of the COOP are deleted and the whole agency is trained on the new development that may occur after these debriefing sessions. COOPs should be reviewed on a routine basis, at least annually with drills.

Juvenile Justice and Residential Settings

Nationally, in 2015, more than 48,043 juvenile offenders were placed in facilities outside their homes (The Annie E. Casey Foundation, 2017). Considering the high number of children residing in non-home-based facilities, it would be prudent to have a national, comprehensive disaster plan in place to provide for the care, welfare, and recovery of these children before, during, and after a disaster. Although a baseline level of disaster planning is required for state child welfare agencies, federal law does not require juvenile justice systems to develop and implement disaster plans (National Commission Report, 2010; Save the Children, Still at Risk: U.S. Children 10 years After Hurricane Katrina, 2015 National Report Card on Protecting Children in Disasters).

With that statement in mind, there is a vast need to ensure that these children receive the same care and benefits that a child-sensitive disaster plan would provide for any child in this nation. In the best of circumstances, all children have unique characteristics requiring the care of their varied and special needs. In a disaster situation, children's needs change and adults must be aware of and be able to provide for these needs. Children in the juvenile justice system have special needs both emotionally and judicially. They often enter the system as victims of past traumas. In many cases, these traumas have played into the delinquent acts that have caused them to enter into this system (Ko et al., 2008, p. 400). Many of these children may have started out in the child welfare system, moving from foster home to foster home, resulting in frustration, anger, and hopelessness, possibly leading to delinquent behavior. The recommendations for children in the child welfare system can apply equally to the children who end up in the juvenile justice system. However, once they become offenders and are adjudicated in the system, or are awaiting a formal hearing, additional precautions need to be taken to protect these children and the communities in which they live. In disaster situations when court records are destroyed or misplaced, these children may be temporarily or inadvertently placed in adult detention facilities, placing them at further risk. For example, during the 2005 hurricanes, New Orleans safely transferred some of the 16,000 children in the juvenile justice system to Baton Rouge, but others were trapped for days in an adult-populated Orleans Parish Prison without food, water, or medical care (National Commission Report, p. 106), illustrating the need for a well-coordinated system, such as the COOP described in the previous section.

Preparedness

When these children are faced with a disastrous situation, they need the juvenile justice system to create a clear and precise plan that provides for their care, safety, and recovery while maintaining their rights as minors. This responsibility rests with many agencies that are interconnected with the juvenile justice system. The juvenile justice system works with prisons, law enforcement agencies, detention centers, probation officers, residential centers, group homes, training schools, and rehabilitation centers, as well as the state welfare system. The task of creating a workable plan that communicates with these varied agencies is monumental.

In an effort to guide each state in creating a plan for the juvenile justice system, the *National Commission on Children and Disaster Report* (2010) has put forth the following recommendations, with explanations:

Recommendation 8.2 states that state and local juvenile justice agencies and all residential treatment, correctional, and detention facilities that house children should adequately prepare for disasters. To accomplish this recommendation,

> Congress should require state and local juvenile justice agencies and all residential treatment, correctional, and detention facilities that house children to have comprehensive disaster plans in place. [Furthermore,] the Department of [Homeland Security/Federal Emergency Management Agency] (DHS/FEMA) and [Department of justice] (DOJ) should support disaster planning for state and local juvenile justice agencies and residential treatment, correctional, and detention facilities that house children, by providing funding, technical assistance, and training. (p. 106)

Many of the stakeholders who collaborated with the National Commission (p. 177) in developing the Report should be engaged in developing specific plans in their local communities to respond to the physical safety and emotional well-being requirements of children in the state's care. Community-based organizations which provide education, health, mental health, and substance abuse services should be involved in developing the plans in collaboration with courts, probation services, and emergency management officials. State-level agencies should provide oversight and consultation to local jurisdictions as needed.

> Recommendation 8.3 states that the Department of Health and Human Services (HHS) and the Department of Justice (DOJ) should ensure that juvenile, dependency, and other courts hearing matters involving children adequately prepare for disasters. (p. 109)

Recommendation 8.3 deals with the court system itself, as opposed to the agencies caring for children. Hurricanes Katrina and Rita demonstrated that many courts for children and youth in the juvenile justice system lacked comprehensive disaster plans. In the 2005 hurricanes, judges could not be contacted, and critical court records were lost during that disaster, as well as the 2008 tornados and floods in Iowa (p. 109). Communication was disrupted, resulting in unnecessary delays for children in the system. The entire court system needs to review these problems and develop strategies to prevent future disruptions, using funds available through the proposed National Juvenile Delinquency Court Improvement Program. After developing plans, the courts should participate in annual disaster exercises with local or state community agencies and stakeholders (pp. 108–109).

In response to the *National Commission on Children and Disaster Report of 2010*, the U.S. Department of Justice, Office of Justice Programs (2011), has published a document to guide juvenile justice residential facilities in preparing for, responding to, and recovering from emergencies and disasters. This document, *Emergency Planning for Juvenile Justice Residential Facilities*, is the first comprehensive planning guide to offer guidance to individual residential facilities as they prepare their own disaster plans for the care of children, youth, and families during an emergency (U.S. Department of Justice, 2011).

Response

These recommendations in the *National Commission on Children and Disaster Report* must be fully integrated into federal, state, and local disaster plans operationalized within the juvenile justice system throughout the nation. In 2015, a report, "Still at Risk: U.S. Children 10 Years After Hurricane Katrina," was published by Save the Children. It is a national Report Card on Protecting Children in disasters. The results of their research indicate that the three recommendations specific for Juvenile Justice System fall short and remain only partially met or completely unmet in most instances (Save the Children, 2015).

Professional nurses who practice in a variety of settings would be able to contribute a vast amount of information, expertise, and creativity in the preparation of disaster plans on all levels. Daughtery and Blome (2009) explored strategies to guide child welfare agencies in disaster planning, many of which can be adapted for children in the juvenile justice system. For example, nurses may participate in the broader community by:

- Working with local and state juvenile justice systems as advocates for this population of children, insuring that they are not forgotten and their rights are upheld
- Working within professional nursing organizations, educating other nurses, enlisting support, and networking with other professionals
- Becoming members of local, state, and county boards, and committees entrusted with the creation of the disaster plan
- Becoming disaster preparedness educators within local agencies and organizations such as the Red Cross
- Becoming members of community partners/agencies/organizations to ensure that a larger pool of advocates has been created and is willing to help with the issues evolving in an emergency/disaster situation

Nurses working in any one of the agencies housing or caring for the juvenile justice population would have specific responsibilities to the residents that would include:

- Providing disaster preparedness education for staff and residents
- Providing sufficient practice of the disaster plan
- Ensuring there are plans for both sheltering-in-place and during evacuations
- Ensuring each offender's record is protected and filed in a system not only in hard copy, but also electronic and stored securely in more than one off-site location
- Ensuring the general population is protected from any dangerous or illegal acts the juvenile justice population might commit if it escaped from the system (This could be accomplished by a unique tracking system being used, that is, Global Positioning System [GPS] ankle bracelets.)
- Ensuring postdisaster care is provided

An example of a plan well executed just before the landfall of Hurricane Harvey (2017) in a juvenile justice detention center is described by Cargo (2017). The author writes that as Hurricane Harvey bore down on the city of Victoria, Texas, the hurricane disaster plan at the Victoria Regional Juvenile Justice Center was put into effect. Inmates were evaluated to determine those able to return to their homes from those who would need to be transported to another facility. Those able to return home were allowed to do so only if they lived in a non–disaster-declared county and they had not been accused of a violent crime. Those not able to return to their families were transported to a facility safe from the disaster-declared area. A supervisor at Victoria Regional Juvenile Justice Center describes how the staff members were affected by leaving their own families and how the juveniles became even more anxious as the storm neared and transportation to a new facility became a reality. The supervisor shared a quote from a staff member, "They were anxious; they didn't know where they were going. Being separated from their family when locked up here causes anxiety, and you do something like that and it messes up their whole routine" (Cargo, 2017). Twenty-six juvenile inmates were evacuated along with 12 staff. The evacuation took 7.5 hours. This demonstrates the effectiveness of a hurricane disaster plan when used by a knowledgeable and practiced administration and staff.

Recovery

Physical and psychological care is essential for all children after a disaster. Children in the juvenile justice system will require special considerations when planning this care due to their detention status. All traditional methods should be employed, similar to other children in this country. In the future, technology such as wireless sensors may be useful for tracking the movements and whereabouts of juvenile justice detainees and probationers, and also could be used for tracking meaningful life information. This technology has been piloted in a small group of elderly persons. The types of information recorded included factors that reflect physical and mental health (Berke, Choudhury, Ali, & Rabbi, 2011). This technology, combined with the technology being used for the offenders' probations, could be used for the provision of after-disaster care. However, the cost of the devices, personnel to monitor and evaluate the information gathered, and the need to update electronic systems with emerging technology will financially burden the juvenile justice system. Other cost-effective methods must be put in place to ensure care for this population.

Child Care Settings

Records indicate that over 12 million children aged 6 years and younger spent time in some type of child care setting in 2015 (National Association of Child Care Resource and Referral Agencies, 2009). According to the National Child Care Information and Technical Assistance Center and National Association for Regulatory Administration (2009)

> there are more than 400,000 licensed child care facilities in the United States including 110,000 child care centers, 147,000 small family child care homes, 50,000 large family child care homes and 18,000 other types of child care facilities. In addition, there are thousands of child care programs which are not licensed by the states because they are administered by religious organizations, the military services, or government organizations or are not required to be licensed because of the limited number of children in care or hours they operate, including informal arrangements where a friend, relative or neighbor of the parent or parents provide child care. When an emergency occurs or a disaster strikes during the hours when children are in care, the children are totally dependent on the program to protect them from harm. (p. 4)

During disasters, FEMA has the ability to reimburse local and state organizations that provide emergency services. After Hurricane Katrina, FEMA denied reimbursement to Mississippi for the $1.65 million the state spent serving over 2,700 evacuee children, stating "emergency child care services did not qualify as an eligible Category B Emergency Protective Measure" (National Commission, Final Report, p. 38). However, if child care is not provided, families cannot easily clean up their damaged property, apply for disaster benefits, search for housing and employment, and begin to rebuild their lives. Also, those who volunteer or work during disaster relief efforts need a safe child care setting for their children.

Preparedness

In the wake of Hurricane Harvey in August 2017, an estimated 40% of child care and early education centers were damaged or destroyed in Houston alone. Save the Children staff worked with local educational partners across Texas to help restore these centers quickly (Save the Children, 2017a). According to a recent report (Save the Children, 2017b), only 30 states require licensed child care settings to develop written plans addressing evacuation, reunification efforts, and accommodation of children with special needs during disasters. All states should adopt regulations requiring disaster planning to address the needs of children.

One of the largest early education settings in the country is Head Start, which enrolled over 1.2 million children in FY 2015 (Office of Head Start, 2016). In 2014, the Office of Head Start updated the *Head Start Emergency Preparedness Manual*, which guides staff in developing emergency preparedness plans (Administration for Children and Families, 2009). The Manual was based on an earlier manual published by the American Academy of Pediatrics, the American Public Health Association, and the National Resource Center for Health and Safety in Child Care, called *Emergency/Disaster Preparedness for Child Care Programs: Caring for Our Children National Health and Safety Performance Standards: Guidelines for Out-of-Home Child Care Applicable Standards* (Emergency, n.d.). The Office of Head Start recommends that during the preparedness stage of disasters, Head Starts or child care centers should identify the specific types of disasters that may affect them.

The National Commission Report (2010) includes several recommendations regarding protecting children in child care and early education settings. The minimum recommendation requires state child care regulatory agencies to: "1. include planning, training and exercising requirements within the scope of the state's minimum health and safety standards for child care licensure or registration, and 2. develop statewide child care plans in coordination with state and local emergency managers, public health, child care regulatory agencies and child care resource and referral agencies" (p. 81).

Child care centers should have the freedom to write their own disaster plans that work for their setting, environment, and clients, as long as the minimum standards are met. Child care centers should be encouraged to have parental input as to how the parents would like their children handled during and following a disaster until reunification is possible. Regulatory agencies should also have examples of disaster plans to provide child care centers for those who ask for them. This would increase compliance. The American Red Cross *Masters of Disaster* plan for grades K–8 could serve as a template and be rewritten to incorporate children of the preschool age. Developmentally appropriate interventions would be necessary. Once a disaster plan is developed, practice drills should become as common as the age-old fire and tornado drills practiced at schools.

Response

During a disaster, the normally competent child caregiver who could previously comfort a single child may be overwhelmed by the special needs of up to 10 overwhelmed, traumatized children. The *Head Start Emergency Preparedness Manual* (2015) recommends that a decision tree be written for staff to follow during a disaster. The decision tree is detailed and tells the staff how and where to evacuate, how to help protect and provide for basic needs of the preschooler during the disaster, and how to notify parents to plan reunification with their child. A written well-known plan for contacting parents or guardians could possibly give relief to the child care workers. A collaborative agreement with other agencies and community groups, such as churches, the Red Cross, or other schools could be prearranged to assist affected child care centers. Lessons learned from Hurricane Katrina brought to the forefront the need to help identify younger children who may be displaced from their families during disasters. A method for identifying children in child care settings is very important. Use of armbands or picture ID badges with a scan card that holds contact information for the child and parent could possibly be incorporated into disaster plans.

During and following a disaster, it is highly likely that there could be a need for a temporary (make-shift) child care center. The centers will serve not only to care for their regular clients, but also for workers and volunteers with children who need care to continue in volunteer efforts. One of the problems with temporary disaster child care accommodations is that they do not always meet minimum regulatory standards. The regulatory agencies must understand that meeting the basic standards may not be possible during the immediate aftermath of a disaster and exempt the temporary shelter from those requirements if the highest possible standards are met by the shelter. For example, the requirement of having a ratio of 1:10 faculty to preschoolers may not be possible because of the limited number of volunteers available.

Recovery

Another National Commission Report (2010) recommendation is for Congress and federal agencies to improve the capacity to provide child care services in the immediate aftermath of, and recovery from, a disaster. During many disasters, permanent structures and buildings are destroyed. This is not unique to family homes, but also applicable to businesses, schools, and child care centers. Recovery for communities depends on the rebuilding of these vital structures. Parents need to return to work, and others may need to rebuild their homes or businesses. Child care during the recovery stage of a disaster is vital for the recovery of the community. Federal and state agencies should be preemptive in policies for providing emergency funding and reimbursement of child care during this stage of recovery.

Hurricane Katrina sheds light on the need to rewrite some of the existing policies to include this essential need under reimbursement for families. Recovery has been slow in Louisiana since Katrina. Part of this can be linked to a slow rebuilding of child care centers as evidenced by the National Commission, Final Report. The Report states "in St. Bernard Parish in Louisiana, the number of child care centers dropped from 26 before Katrina to only 2 by 2007" (p. 38). The population of this area is still far behind the pre-Katrina time. Communities may also be preemptive by encouraging churches and community groups to have written plans on how to help provide support and assistance for community recovery following disasters.

The mental health of individuals is a very important aspect of disaster preparedness and recovery. Children, especially younger ones, depend on their parents or guardians for survival, even in routine daily life. The American Red Cross has always had the practice of keeping children and their families together while in shelters following disasters. This practice of keeping families together or children with at least one parent aids the families' recovery time and eases the burden on the shelter staff when a parent or parents can care for their children. The overall mental health of the child and parent is improved when this is possible.

Universities/Colleges

Universities and colleges enroll students of all ages, including those less than 18 years of age. Adolescence is commonly used to describe the transition stage between childhood and adulthood; there is actually no one scientific definition of adolescence or set age boundary found in the literature. In fact, students who attend postsecondary schools are often somewhere along the continuum between middle (14–18) and late (19–24) adolescent physical, cognitive, and socio-emotional development. Adjusting to the academic, social, and organizational demands of college is difficult for most students; however, older adolescents have an increased independent function, the ability to think ideas through, increased concern for others, and increased emotional stability (American Academy of Child and Adolescent Psychiatry, 2015).

The College/University Environment

There are more than 4,700 2- and 4-year public and private institutions of higher education (IHEs) in the United States, totaling over 20 million students and over 1 million faculty members, staff, and visitors. The record college enrollments have been driven by both increases in the traditional college age population and rising enrollment rates. In 2016, this constituted an increase of about 5.2 million since fall 2000, about 11.7 million females compared with 8.8 million males (National Center for Education Statistics, 2017).

Every IHE has a commitment to ensure the safety and general welfare of those on their campuses, and to provide appropriate policies, procedures, and strategies to maintain a safe campus. College and university campuses often cover large geographical areas, and sometimes even resemble small towns or cities with the full extent of services in their vicinity (medical centers, sports complexes, residential centers, businesses, etc.). These structural and environmental characteristics pose challenges for access control, monitoring movements, defining boundaries for facilities and grounds, standardizing procedures and decision-making processes, and prioritizing resource allocations. IHE governance is also highly complex and decentralized; decision making can be slow and hinder campus response to a crisis. Also, most IHEs have open access and are geographically integrated into the surrounding community. At any one time, students and others are dispersed around the campus in classrooms, common areas, cafeterias, offices, dormitories, and other facilities. Unlike secondary education, most college campuses include residential facilities in which students live throughout the year; they are often home to many out-of-state, international, and married students (FEMA, 2013). IHEs serve primarily adult students who are capable of making decisions on their own, but the campus population is perpetually in flux, changing from day to day, semester to semester, and year to year. Some students commute to and from campus, others attend class virtually, resulting in a dispersed population (FEMA, 2013). All of these factors impact how an IHE plans, responds to, and recovers from a campus or community-wide emergency.

Student Health Concerns

College students' health needs are different from their younger counterparts; those over 18 years of age are considered adults capable of making decisions on their own, which are often complicated by issues surrounding HIPAA and FERPA regulations. Ninety-five percent of college counseling center directors surveyed said that the number of students with significant psychological problems is a growing concern in their center or on campus. Anxiety is the top presenting concern among college students (41.6%), followed by depression (36.4%) and relationship problems. On average, 24.5% of clients were taking psychotropic medications and 21% of counseling center students present with severe mental health concerns (American Psychological Association, 2013). These facts must be taken into consideration when planning the recovery phase of postemergency/hazard situations. On the other hand, young adults are ideal volunteers during a disaster because of their ability to participate in the preparedness, response, and recovery phases of disasters. Colleges and universities should capitalize on the strengths of their students by educating them about disaster preparedness, then inviting them to assist in developing emergency plans.

Emergency Planning Guidelines

In 2011, the American College Health Association (ACHA) outlined guidelines for campus health services in the event of an emergency or disaster that use national preparedness and response systems and an "all-hazards" approach. The guidelines are in the process of revision to include specific training resources, clarification of which situations can be considered emergencies under the Clery Act, and a revision and expansion of the Psychological Impact of Crisis. Recognizing that few campuses have the ability to manage mass critical incidents alone, these guidelines recommend colleges work together with campus and community partners to effectively manage emergencies. Nurses in the community can work with college health professionals to provide medical, psychological, and public health expertise, training exercises, and membership in institutional emergency management teams (ACHA Guidelines, 2017).

Other emergency planning guidelines available to IHEs include:

- FEMA—*Building a disaster resistant university* (DRU; FEMA, 2003), a "how-to" guide compiled with the real-life experiences of six universities and colleges across the country. This guide is still used today by many IHEs.
- FEMA—*Guide for developing high-quality emergency operations plans for IHEs* (FEMA, 2013), which incorporates international students into IHE emergency management and planning. This guide replaces the Action Guide for Emergency Management at IHEs from 2009.
- U.S. Department of Education—*A guide to school vulnerability assessments: Key principles for safe schools* (2008). This guide is still in use today and is intended to assist schools with the implementation of an effective vulnerability assessment process.

- U.S. Department of Homeland Security—*Academic Resource Catalog* (U.S. Department of Homeland Security [DHS], 2017b). This catalog is updated yearly and serves as a guide to the DHS programs and resources available to the academic community promoting campus preparedness, including cyber security and public awareness campaigns.

IHEs can also find multiple resources at fellow institutions from workshops that share disaster-DRU approaches to real-life disasters (http://scholarworks.uno.edu/dru2013). All of these guidelines recommend an "all-hazards" approach to emergency management, which allows for a more efficient and effective way to prepare for emergencies. All outline the four-phase framework of emergency management: Prevention-Mitigation, Preparedness, Response, and Recovery. An emergency management plan must be comprehensive in design, while also providing for students, faculty, staff, and visitors with special needs (vulnerable populations). IHEs should conduct "tabletop" exercises prior to fully adopting and implementing the emergency management plan. These exercises should cover a wide range of scenarios that may occur on campus, and should be conducted with a variety of partners and stakeholders from the campus and the community.

The CDC's "Preparedness 101: Zombie Pandemic" (CDC, Office of Public Health Preparedness and Response, 2015) could be used as a novel method to get people interested and involved in disaster preparedness (Figure 12.1). The CDC cited reader responses such as the following as proof: "For high school graduation, we are now giving a medical kit and tool bag as gifts." However, Kruvand and Bryant (2015) conducted research which found that while participants enjoyed the humorous zombie material, their positive effect did not lead to greater retention of preparedness information or greater expressed intent to prepare compared to exposure to factual information about emergency preparedness.

IHEs must conduct routine training based on the institution's prevention and preparedness efforts, prioritized threats, and issues highlighted from institutional assessments. Finally, after adoption of an emergency management plan, the information should be disseminated to students, staff, faculty, community partners, and families. The overall goal of this process is to minimize the impact caused by an emergency at the institution and/or within the community.

Until recently, preparation for most colleges has meant identifying ways they could secure themselves in response to disaster. While necessary, that is not enough. Colleges need to play a more significant role in the process of community-wide disaster preparedness and recovery. IHEs have a particular set of strengths and assets that are well suited to assist, and sometimes lead, the disaster preparedness and relief processes. This engagement is also an opportunity for students to participate and learn. While individual situations determine the specific response to be taken, campus leaders and community nurses can be better prepared for disaster recovery by taking these actions:

- Engage in or create a local or regional long-term recovery organization.
- Develop centers for community engagement and/or centers for teaching and learning that lift up service and civically engaged pedagogies (e.g., service learning).

- Partner with the American Red Cross to provide emergency shelter.
- Contact (if religiously affiliated) a denominational disaster response organization to explore partnerships.
- Create and train a student-led Rapid Response Team that can function until official responders arrive.
- Organize students into teams to assess campus buildings for disaster preparedness and share their results with campus staff.
- Develop a campus response plan (focusing on assistance, not just recovery).
- Develop emergency communication strategies, such as cell phone or text message alerts.
- Integrate the campus plan with local and regional response plans.
- Put in place risk-management policies to enable an informed, safe, and quick response.

The American Association of Community Colleges (AACC, 2017) is the primary advocacy organization for the nation's community colleges, representing almost 1,200 2-year institutions and 13 million students. Community colleges have taken the lead in Homeland Security Education, with over 80% of police, fire, and emergency medical technicians (EMTs) receiving their credentials from these institutions. AACC works in partnership with FEMA to raise awareness among community college faculty, staff, and students about

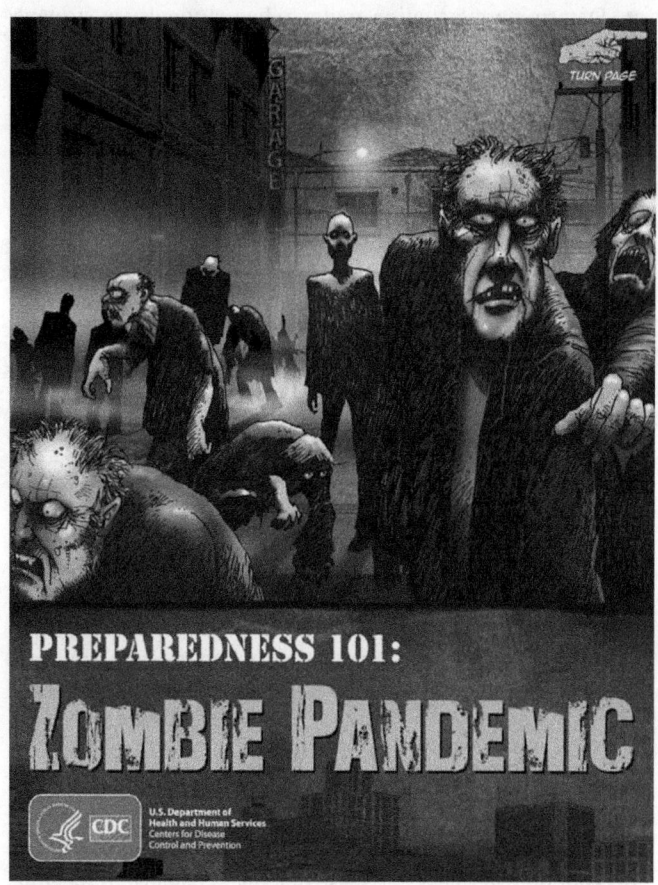

FIGURE 12.1 Preparedness 101.

Source: Centers for Disease Control and Prevention, Office of Public Health Preparedness and Response. (2015). Preparedness 101: Zombie Pandemic. Retrieved from https://www.cdc.gov/phpr/documents/zombie _gn_final.pdf [22–0894]

appropriate actions to take regarding disaster preparedness and response, public health issues, life-supporting first aid, and volunteer service. AACC promotes participation of community college students and administrators on local Citizen Corps Councils to support community-based multisector preparedness planning for all hazards; assists in promoting education, training, and exercises; provides volunteer service opportunities that support first responders, disaster relief, and community safety, to include support for Community Emergency Response Team (CERT) training and other safety courses; and, coordinates national activities, including participation in the National Preparedness Month (FEMA, 2006).

Prevention

Of course, campuses cannot prevent the occurrence of all critical incidents; however, they can take steps within the planning process to identify risk reduction strategies that prevent potential incidents and identify actions that will mitigate the impact of an actual emergency, such as:

- Form behavioral intervention teams to decrease the risk of acts of violence.
- Develop exposure policies and procedures during public health outbreaks.
- Determine evacuation routes when students must leave buildings or other areas of campus.
- Develop plans and collect supplies to allow students and staff to shelter-in-place.

In 2000, FEMA funded a grant program to foster IHE efforts to reduce and manage vulnerability to hazards. When they cut the funding a few years later, several IHEs kept the core concept of a DRU alive. They saw the need for a practical, common sense approach to disaster planning on their campuses. In 2005, the University of Oregon started the DRU listserv (with more than 1,400 members) with the goal to facilitate interdisciplinary communication, discussion, and resource sharing among IHE practitioners charged with making America's campuses more disaster resilient (National Center for Campus Public Safety, 2016). Another interesting approach to prevention of hazards is the partnering of some college/university campuses with the DHS's campaign "If You See Something, Say Something," which is meant to raise public awareness of the indicators of terrorism and terrorism-related crime, as well as the importance of reporting suspicious activity to state and local law enforcement (DHS, 2017c).

Preparedness

Much of the current literature about prevention/preparedness for disasters refers to individual and community efficacy about disaster preparedness, the sense that one is capable of meeting the challenge. Hazards should ideally be viewed as a challenge or problem to be solved, rather than a threat to be faced with few resources. Some IHEs are approaching preparedness in just such a way. The DHS provides an Active Shooter Preparedness ("Run. Hide. Fight.") program for IHIs and others by helping to

enhance preparedness through a "whole community" approach (DHS, 2016). The DHS is also committed to engaging colleges and universities in an effort to foster resilience best practices and to bolster campus emergency preparedness efforts. They are currently in the developmental stages of a Campus Resilience Program that will build upon best practices, lessons learned, and resources already developed to make U.S. colleges and universities more resilient in preparing for campus violence, cyber threats, infectious disease, and other disaster emergency scenarios (DHS, 2017b).

The California Community Colleges (CCC) organization is the largest system of higher education in the nation. It is composed of 72 districts and 113 colleges serving 2.1 million students each year. In March 2017, the CCC Chancellor's Office composed and sent out an Emergency Preparedness Guidelines Memorandum to standardize guidelines for emergency response throughout the state as dictated by a 2015 state law (CCC Chancellor's Office, 2017). An example of how well the state system responds to disaster can be illustrated by the San Bruno fire of 2010 which affected Skyline College, located less than a mile from the epicenter of an explosion. The school immediately called its Campus Crisis Action team together, checked with the police and fire officials to get updates, and made the decision to keep classes in session since the fire was heading away from campus. This prevented additional cars on the streets from students leaving campus, and reduced possible blockages for the city's public safety vehicles trying to respond to the fire. The team also prepared the gym as an emergency evacuation site in the event that they were called upon by the American Red Cross to serve as a shelter.

Many colleges have some type of disaster preparedness information for students available on their websites. For example, the Texas Extension Disaster Education Network (EDEN) has tips for students listing suggestions for developing their own "disaster plans":

- Be aware of the types of emergencies/hazards that can potentially affect your area of residence.
- Plan a meeting with your family, roommates, and coworkers to discuss disaster preparedness.
- Determine how you will exit your apartment, dorm, or house in case of an evacuation. Know at least two ways to get out.
- Plan for several different meeting places. One should be directly outside your living space. The other should be a site away from your neighborhood in the event you cannot return home. Give your family members and roommates a copy of this information.
- Choose an out-of-state contact person. It is often easier to call long distance than locally during an emergency situation. As soon as possible, let the designated person know you are safe. Share this contact person's information with your family and roommates.
- Discuss how to "shelter in place." The type of incident will determine how you should shelter.
- Discuss and practice how to turn off electricity, water, heating/cooling systems, and gas.
- Assemble a disaster supply kit for at home, at work, and in your vehicle (recommended by the Red Cross).
- Take a course in first aid and cardiopulmonary resuscitation (CPR).

- Become familiar with the 2-1-1 Texas Information and Referral Hotline to receive information regarding the closest evacuation routes and access to water, food, and shelter as well as information on other HHS available across the state (Texas A&M AgriLife Disaster Education Network, 2017).

The website also recommends an emergency supplies kit of essential items for the college student (Table 12.4).

College Health Services staff should be prepared to actively participate in emergency management and lead, if appropriate, emergency management efforts. This can be accomplished through several educational and preparedness activities:

TABLE 12.4 Recommended Essential Supplies Kit for a College Student

Essential Personal Supplies

Water: 3-day supply of 1 gallon/person/day	Extra clothes and socks
Food: 3-day supply of nonperishable, ready-to-eat, high nutritive value	Emergency radio: battery, hand-crank or solar powered
Water purification drops or tablets	Weather radio with tone alert: battery, handcrank or solar powered
Prescription medications	Extra pair of eyeglasses or contact lenses
Non-prescription medications: pain relievers, antacids, laxatives, anti-diarrhea, antibiotic cream	First-aid kit/ handbook
Flashlight: batteries, hand-crank or solar powered	Out-of-state contact person's phone number
Extra batteries (in assorted sizes)	Cash for gas purchases, etc.
Extra set of house and car keys	Some form of personal identification
Waterproof matches and candles	Copies of important documents: insurance policies, bank account records, etc.
Sturdy shoes: closed toe/waterproof	

Safety and Comfort

Heavy duty gloves	Extra blankets or pillow
N95 Face Mask	Tent/tarp
Fire extinguisher	Local and state maps
Communication kit: paper, pens/pencils/markers	Addresses/phone numbers for family/friends
Cell phone/phone charger/backup battery	Books/playing cards/games/puzzles

Sanitation Supplies

Toilet tissue	Paper towels
Moist towelettes/baby wipes	Feminine hygiene supplies
Antibacterial hand sanitizer	Shaving cream and razor
Bar soap/liquid detergent	Bath towels/wash cloths
Personal hygiene supplies	Trash can/large trash bags/plastic ties
Shampoo	Household chlorine bleach (disinfect water if necessary)
Toothbrush/toothpaste	

Cooking Supplies

Plates, cups, bowls	Aluminum foil
Camp stove/ fuel tablets (outdoor use only)	Eating utensils

Tools and Supplies

Manual can opener	Duct tape
Adjustable wrench (for shutting off gas)	Chalk (to mark search areas)
Shovel, broom, saw, axe	Rope
Tool kit: screwdrivers, pliers, hammer, crowbar	Knife, razor blades, scissors

Helpful Tips

1. Encrypted flash drives may be used to save copies of personal documents and identification. Back up computer data and take a copy with you on the encrypted flash drive.
2. Organize items into large storage containers for easy access.
3. Waterproof containters are ideal for storing items needing to remain dry.
4. Store water in a separate area to avoid damaging dry items in case of leakage.
5. Check emergency supplies kit every 6 months to ensure that no items have expired.
6. Cover your computer and other electronic equipment with plastic sheeting or large plastic garbage bags (Tulane University Emergency Preparedness and Response, 2017).

Sources: Adapted from Texas A&M AgriLife Disaster Education Network (2017) & U.S. Department of Homeland Security, *Ready* (2017).

- Participating in emergency-planning exercises and drills; coordinating with departments across campus.
- Encouraging staff to seek specialized training in psychological first aid, mass casualty training, and public health threats.
- Providing staff updates regarding emerging infectious diseases or other health threats, recommendations for treatment protocols, and appropriate infection control procedures.
- Encouraging staff to make personal preparedness plans with family so they will be better able to fulfill their roles as responders in the event of an emergency.
- Engaging staff in discussions regarding their anticipated psychological and emotional support needs during and after an event.
- Fitting staff with direct patient care responsibilities with N95 respiratory protection annually and providing in-service training on proper use of personal protection equipment.
- Identifying resources for food and on-campus lodging for health service staff in the event staff cannot or do not wish to commute home.
- Compiling a list of supplies that might be needed for various medical emergencies, such as respiratory protection equipment, gloves, gowns, protective eyewear, medications (antibiotics), disinfectants, potable water, intravenous (IV) fluids, and other trauma supplies.
- Identifying sources of vaccines, antitoxins, immunoglobulin by engaging in discussions with the local and state health departments.
- Maintaining a stock supply of necessary medications and equipment.
- Establishing a plan for continuation of cleaning and waste removal services including triggers to increase the frequency of the scheduling of these services.
- Investigating the feasibility of establishing negative pressure rooms in the campus health service; consulting with the Department of Environmental Health and Safety for assistance.
- Identifying staff roles and responsibilities for all types of critical incidents (ACHA, 2017).

Many believe that to create an emergency preparedness culture in any setting, it must begin with our youth. Trusting them with accurate information and real responsibility helps prepare them for citizenship in the larger community and world, and strengthens the larger community now and in the future.

Response

Response involves taking action to effectively contain and resolve an emergency. Campus officials must activate the emergency management plan; specific actions vary greatly depending on the type, severity, magnitude, duration, and intensity of the event. Effective response requires informed decision making and identification of clear lines of decision authority. Accounting for students, faculty, and staff is one of the most important activities needed. Examples such as Hurricane Katrina and the April 2013 Boston Marathon bombing illustrate the need to incorporate international students into higher education emergency operation plans (REMS, 2017).

The American Academy of Pediatrics Disaster Preparedness Advisory Council (DPAC; 2017) suggests that there are

specific responses seen in adolescents/young adults resulting from loss, exposure to trauma, and disruption of routine: decreased interest in social activities, peers, hobbies, and school; a decreased ability to experience pleasure; decline in responsible behaviors; rebellion and increased risk-taking behaviors; physical complaints; sleep and eating disorders; lack of concentration; and PTSD. DPAC developed a Strategic Plan for Disaster Preparedness (2016–2020) that hopes to promote the resiliency of children through federal, state, and legislative advocacy (DPAC, 2017). Young adults can also respond to hazards/disasters with resilience and a willingness to help meet the needs of their peers and community. Often, they can be a motivational reservoir within the IHE and larger community through active involvement, volunteering, and delegating duties. The 2012 Citizen Corps National Survey on Personal Preparedness in America (FEMA Citizen Corps Research, 2012) indicates that people who volunteered during disasters were more likely to have disaster supplies and a personal/family disaster plan and to be active in training programs for disaster preparedness in the future. Nurses involved in disaster mobilization must be familiar with these anticipated responses and capitalize on the workforce available in an IHE to face the disaster. Preparedness programs can increase awareness and knowledge and increase the emotional resilience of all involved.

Most well-prepared IHEs attempt to communicate thoroughly and often with students before, during, and after a disaster. On August 29, 2005, Hurricane Katrina caused massive destruction in New Orleans, and Tulane University suffered major property damage and losses—estimated at more than $600 million. The university had to close its doors for the fall semester and spend weeks attempting to locate faculty, staff, and students who had evacuated around the country. Tulane University now has an emergency response website, call center, and remote offices to provide regular and accurate updates to the entire campus community (Tulane University, 2017). They also use several methods for students to update their information online (emergency notices website) and via text messaging (Tulane's alert line). Their Hurricane Procedure for students is a detailed plan for responding to a possible flooding/evacuation situation.

The University of California at Berkeley has a visually arresting website (http://oem.berkeley.edu) that outlines "How to Become an Urban Survivalist," giving advice on basic emergency preparedness and response for students. The university also created an emergency preparedness mobile app for students that provides quick access to notifications, shelter-in-place suggestions, and even recommendations for nighttime safety.

On April 16, 2007, Virginia Tech (VT) was the site of one of the deadliest mass shootings in U.S. history. In 2011, the U.S. Department of Education fined VT for failing to issue a prompt campus-wide warning after the first two shootings. In 2014, the Virginia Tech Office of Emergency Management is the first in higher education to obtain national accreditation through the Emergency Management Accreditation Program (valid for 5 years). To qualify, the office adheres to 64 professional standards in areas including emergency planning and procedures; prevention; risk management; training exercises; and communications and warning. The school now offers a

"Be Hokie Ready" website for students, encouraging them to subscribe to VT Phone Alerts, digital VT Desktop or Twitter Alerts, and the LiveSafe mobile app. The app allows users to submit reports of suspicious activity and invite other students to "virtually escort" and monitor their location while walking on campus (VT Office of Emergency Management, 2017).

Recovery

The recovery phase establishes procedures, resources, and policies to assist an IHE and its members to return to functioning after an emergency. It is an ongoing process and will vary based on the nature and scope of the emergency. The ultimate goal is to meet the needs of the people affected and restore the learning environment. Decisions should be made with community and state officials and partners. Restoring the learning environment may involve housing students, conducting classes in off-site locations, and implementing online learning. It is important to communicate these decisions to media, faculty, staff, students, and families in an expedient manner. Also, it is critical to identify the mental health resources to promote psychological and emotional recovery, making sure all those who need these can receive short- and long-term mental health services on and off campus.

Leadership support within the IHE and the community is critical to the success of an emergency planning effort. A collaborative approach building partnerships both inside and outside the IHE system is a key success factor. Community nurses can offer their expertise and knowledge of disaster planning, response, and recovery to the young adults who might be exposed to and survive an emergency on campus or within the larger community.

Churches/Parishes

Churches are valuable resources in the community because of their members' willingness to reach out to others during times of crisis. Most churches and parishes consist of families, so the children in those families must be considered when preparing for disasters. The guidelines discussed earlier in this chapter should apply to children in churches, especially those that operate schools, day care facilities, and other congregate care settings such as Sunday School or Bible Study sessions.

Preparedness

The first step churches should take is to prepare their families for disasters, following guidelines from www.redcross.org or www.ready.gov to create a plan and collect supplies for sheltering in place or evacuating during disasters. Some denominations are well known for their disaster preparedness philosophy. The Church of Jesus Christ of Latter Day Saints (Mormons) has a strong preparedness platform, and provides numerous online resources to help church members become better prepared ("LDS Preparedness," www.ldsemergencyresources.com).

The Southern Baptist Convention has a long history of collaborating with the American Red Cross, the Salvation Army, and other organizations to provide mass feeding and sheltering prior to, during, and after disasters. They have been approved by the public health department in many states to provide food for emergency shelters, and some churches have purchased large trailers filled with convection ovens that can cook thousands of meals each day. There are many online resources available to help churches prepare for disasters, such as Emergency Preparedness for Churches (www.xpastor.org/operations/facility-policy/emergency-preparedness-for-churches).

All churches can take steps to prepare their parishioners for disasters. Our Lady of Fatima Catholic Church in Benton, Arkansas, hosted a disaster preparedness speaker to educate families about how to prepare themselves and their school for disasters. Each class in the parochial school developed a poster and skit related to a specific disaster. One class taught about floods using a Noah's Ark theme. Another class taught about preparing for tornados with a "Wizard of Oz" theme. Other disasters included fires, winter storms, earthquakes, and chemical disasters. The children searched for online resources in preparing their posters and skits, and were excited to help teach each other and their teachers and families how to prepare for different disasters.

Response

Churches are ideal for providing disaster shelters in their communities. The most suitable churches are those with large fellowship halls for setting up sleeping cots and meal areas, handicap accessibility features, showers and large bathrooms, and commercial kitchens. Those that have schools or religious education programs often have child-oriented classrooms which can be used for child care services while the shelter is open. Church members frequently volunteer to serve when the shelter is open, and willingly supplement the American Red Cross and other volunteers staffing the shelter. Church leaders are encouraged to sign a Memorandum of Agreement/Understanding (MOA/MOU) to become a shelter, allowing the Red Cross to assess the suitability of the church prior to a disaster.

Smaller churches may develop coalitions in their communities to share resources. For instance, a church that does not have space for sheltering people affected by disaster could provide child care for volunteers who need that service to fulfill their volunteer roles. Some denominations have recently begun requiring background checks and special training for parishioners who have any contact with children, so it would be ideal for providing volunteers to serve in child care settings.

Recovery

After a disaster, many families seek solace in their community churches. If the church structure itself is damaged during the disaster, church members need to identify alternate locations for services. News reports often show religious services being held in the church parking lot, with the skeleton of the damaged church, possibly a cross or statue, in the background. The stress of the disaster may unite church members more closely, and other churches may reach out to offer comfort, donations, shelter, and even the use of their own church for services during the rebuilding phase. Churches of all sizes and denominations throughout the country typically gather donations of money or supplies to send to damaged churches. After rebuilding, church members may be more motivated to develop disaster plans, gather supplies for sheltering in place, and educate members on how to prepare for future disasters. Children in these churches should be actively involved in the rebuilding and recovery stage, and may take leadership roles in these efforts.

Legislation

The U.S. House of Representatives passed the Homeland Security for Children Act (HR 1372) on April 25, 2017, which puts into place many safeguards to further protect children during times of domestic crisis and emergency. The Homeland Security for Children Act will help strengthen FEMA and the DHS and also increase accountability across government agencies in times of emergency. The legislation seeks to appoint a permanent Children's Needs Advisor to integrate the needs of children into its activities to protect against natural disasters, acts of terrorism, and other man-made disasters. Further, it requires the Undersecretary of Policy at the DHS to review and incorporate any feedback from youth-serving organizations to prioritize and represent the needs of children into department-wide policies. And finally, it forces accountability through regular reports and updates to Congress (Save the Children, 2017a, 2017b).

SUMMARY

This chapter described the recommendations of the *National Commission on Children and Disasters 2010 Report to the President and Congress*, including an update on the status of these recommendations. The Commission identified several gaps in emergency plans for children in schools and other congregate child care settings. Many organizations have developed detailed guidelines for schools and other community congregate child care settings to follow in developing plans to protect children during and after disasters. However, the challenge is to motivate facilities to adopt the published guidelines, especially in the absence of state or federal regulations and funding requiring emergency plans specific to children. This chapter provides specific resources nurses may use to guide agencies in preparing for disasters and developing plans to protect children during the response and recovery phases of disasters.

STUDY QUESTIONS

1. List the 11 recommendations from the *National Commission on Children and Disasters: 2010 Report to the President and Congress*.

2. Describe the results of inadequate planning for schools and day care facilities during the 2009 Pandemic Influenza.

3. Describe a Red Cross program designed to prepare children for disasters.

4. Discuss circumstances in which schools may disclose information about children during disasters under FERPA regulations.

5. List the recommended components of a disaster supply kit for college students.

6. Describe the components of a COOP for organizations.

7. Discuss roles churches may play in disaster response in the community.

INTERNET ACTIVITIES

1. Go to the U.S. Department of Health and Human Services Administration for Children and Families website at https://www.acf.hhs.gov/ohsepr.

2. Go to the FEMA website at www.fema.gov. Enter "Building a Disaster Resistant University" in the search box. Review strategies to prepare universities for disasters.

3. Go to the FEMA website at www.ready.gov/kids. Retrieve the "Ready" resources and review strategies to prepare children for disasters.

4. Go to the U.S. Department of Education website at www2.ed.gov/policy/gen/guid/fpco/pdf/ferpa-disaster-guidance.pdf. Retrieve the document titled FERPA and the Disclosure of Student Information Related to Emergencies and Disasters. Review the type of information that is allowed to be revealed under FERPA regulations during disasters.

5. Go to the Save the Children website at www.savethechildren.org/atf/cf/%7B9def2ebe-10ae-432c-9bd0-df91d2eba74a%7D/Disaster-Preps-Issue-Brief-Final-1.pdf. Review strategies to protect children during disasters.

6. Go to the Readiness and Emergency Management for Schools (REMS) website at http://rems.ed.gov/default.aspx. Review the At-A-Glance Federal Guides to help schools and other academic institutions develop emergency operations plans.

REFERENCES

Administration for Children and Families. (2009). *Head start emergency preparedness manual: 2015 edition*. Washington, DC: U.S. Department of Health and Human Services.

Alisic, E., Zalta, A. K., van Wessel, F., Larsen, S. E., Hafstad, G. S., Hassanpour, K., & Smid, G. E. (2014). Rates of post-traumatic stress disorder in trauma-exposed children and adolescents: Meta-analysis. *British Journal of Psychiatry, 204*, 335–340. doi:10.1192/bjp.bp.113.131227

American Academy of Child and Adolescent Psychiatry. (2015). Adolescent development part II. Retrieved from https://www.aacap.org/AACAP/Families_and_Youth/Facts_for_Families/FFF-Guide/Normal-Adolescent-Development-Part-II-058.aspx

American Academy of Pediatrics Disaster Preparedness Advisory Council. (2017). About us. Retrieved from https://www.aap.org/en-us/advocacy-and-policy/aap-health-initiatives/Children-and-Disasters/Pages/Disaster-Preparedness-Advisory-Council.aspx

American Association of Community Colleges. (2017). Retrieved from https://www.aacc.nche.edu/research-trends/fast-facts

America's Children. (2009). Key national indicators of well-being, 2017. Retrieved from www.childstats.gov/americaschildren

American College Health Association. (2017). Retrieved from http://www.acha.org/ACHA/Resources/Guidelines/ACHA/Resources/Guidelines.aspx?hkey=450d50ec-a623-47a2-aab0-5f011ca437fb

American Psychological Association. (2013). College students' mental health is a growing concern, survey finds. Retrieved from http://www.apa.org/monitor/2013/06/college-students.aspx

American Red Cross. (2017a). Red Cross masters of disaster program. Retrieved from http://www.redcross.org/local/utah/programs-services/masters-of-disaster-program

American Red Cross. (2017b). The American Red Cross Ready Rating Program. Retrieved from http://www.redcross.org

American Red Cross. (2017c). The Pillowcase Project. Retrieved from http://www.redcross.org

The Annie E. Casey Foundation. (2009). Disaster preparedness resource guide for child welfare agencies. Retrieved from http://www.aecf.org/resources/disaster-preparedness-resource-guide-for-child-welfare-agencies

The Annie E. Casey Foundation. (2017). Kids Count Data Center. Retrieved from https://datacenter.kidscount.org/data/tables/42-youth-residing-in-juvenile-detention-and-correctional-facilities#detailed/1/any/false/573,36,867,133,18/any/319,17599

Baker, L. R., & Baker, M. D. (2010). Disaster preparedness among families of children with special health care needs. *Disaster Medicine and Public Health Preparedness, 4*(3), 240–245. doi:10.1001/dmp.2010.28

Berke, E. M., Choudhury, T., Ali, S., & Rabbi, M. Q. (2011). Objective measurement of sociability and activity: Mobile sensing in the community. *Annals of Family Medicine, 9*(4), 344–350. doi:10.1370/afm.1266

Bowden, V. R., & Greenberg, C. S. (2010). *Children and their families: The continuum of care* (2nd ed.). Philadelphia, PA: Lippincott, Williams & Wilkins.

California Community Colleges Chancellor's Office. (2017). Memorandum. Retrieved from http://extranet.cccco.edu/Divisions/FinanceFacilities/EmergencyPreparedness.aspx

Cargo, K. (2017). Victoria Juvenile Center evacuated to Hays County for Harvey. Retrieved from https://www.victoriaadvocate.com/news/2017/oct/05/victoria-juvenile-center-evacuated-to-hays-county-

Centers for Disease Control and Prevention. (2009). 2009 Pandemic Influenza A (H1N1) virus infections. *Morbidity and Mortality Weekly Report*. Retrieved from https://www.cdc.gov/mmwr/preview/mmwrhtml/mm5833a1.html

Centers for Disease Control and Prevention, Office of Public Health Preparedness and Response. (2015). Preparedness 101: Zombie Pandemic. Retrieved from https://www.cdc.gov/phpr/documents/zombie_gn_final.pdf

ChildStats.gov. (2017). America's children: Key national indicators of well-being, 2017. Retrieved from https://www.childstats.gov/americaschildren/demo.asp

Child Welfare Information Gateway. (2016). Disaster planning for child welfare agencies. Retrieved from https://www.childwelfare.gov/pubs/factsheets/disasterplanning

Compassion Fatigue Awareness Project. (2010). What is compassion fatigue? Retrieved from http://www.compassionfatigue.org/pages/compassionfatigue.html

Daughtery, L. G., & Blome, W. W. (2009). Planning to plan: A process to involve child welfare agencies in disaster preparedness planning. *Journal of Community Practice, 17,* 483–501. doi:10.1080/10705420903300504

Federal Emergency Management Agency. (2003). Building a disaster resistant university. Retrieved from https://www.fema.gov/media-library-data/20130726-1457-20490-1338/dru_report.pdf

Federal Emergency Management Agency. (2006). First responders: Community colleges on the front line of security. Retrieved from https://training.fema.gov/hiedu/06conf/06papers/teich,%20carolyn%20-%20aacv-first%20reponders%20-%20frontline%20of%20securit.pdf

Federal Emergency Management Agency. (2013). Guide for Developing High-quality Emergency Operations Plans for Institutions of Higher Education. Retrieved from https://www.fema.gov/media-library-data/20130726-1922-25045-3638/rems_ihe_guide.pdf

Federal Emergency Management Agency. (2017). Ready kids. Retrieved from https://www.ready.gov/kids

Federal Emergency Management Agency Citizen Corps Research. (2012). Personal preparedness survey: 2012 findings. Retrieved from https://www.ready.gov/research

Gatowski, L. P., & Sophia, I. (2008). *Ensuring the unique needs of dependency courts are met in disaster planning efforts: Dependency court planning templates for Continuity of Operations Plans.* National Council of Juvenile and Family Court Judges and the American Bar Association, Center on Children and the Law. Retrieved from https://www.researchgate.net/publication/318100565_Ensuring_the_Unique_Needs_of_Dependency_Courts_are_Met_in_Disaster_Planning_Efforts_Dependency_Court_Templates_for_Continuity_of_Operations_Plans

Graham, J., Shirm, S., Liggin, R., Aitken, M., & Dick, R. (2006). Mass-casualty events at schools: A national preparedness survey. *Pediatrics, 117*(1), e8–e15. doi:10.1542/peds.2005-0927

Grindlay, J., & Breeze, K. (2016). Planning for disasters involving children in Australia: A practical guide. *Journal of Paediatrics and Child Health, 52,* 204–212. doi:10.1111/jpc.13073

Hagan, J. F., Jr., American Academy of Pediatrics Committee on Psychosocial Aspects of Child and Family Health, & Task Force on Terrorism. (2005). American Academy of Pediatrics Clinical Report: Psychosocial implications of disaster or terrorism on children: A guide for the pediatrician. *Pediatrics, 116*(4), 787–795. doi:10.1542/peds.2005-1498

Ko, S. J., Ford, J. D., Kassam-Adams, N., Berkowitz, S. J., Wilson, C., Wong, M., . . . Layne, C. M. (2008). Creating trauma-informed systems: Child welfare, education, first responders, health care, juvenile justice. *Professional Psychology: Research and Practice, 39*(4), 396–404. doi:10.1037/0735-7028.39.4.396

Kostelny, K., & Wessells, M. (2005). Psychosocial aid to children after the Dec 26 tsunami. *Lancet, 366,* 2066–2067. doi:10.1037/0735-7028.39.4.396

Kruvand, M., & Bryant, F. B. (2015). Zombie apocalypse: Can the undead teach the living how to survive an emergency? *Public Health Reports, 130*(6), 655–663. doi:10.1177/003335491513000615

Lee, D. E., Parker, G., Ward, M. E., Styron, R. A., & Shelley, K. (2008). Katrina and the schools in Mississippi: An examination of emergency and disaster preparedness. *Journal of Education for Students Placed at Risk, 13*(2/3), 318–334. doi:10.1080/10824660802350458

McLaughlin, K. (2016). Posttraumatic stress disorder in children: Epidemiology, pathogenesis, clinical manifestations, course, assessment and diagnosis. Up to Date. Retrieved from https://www.uptodate.com/contents/posttraumatic-stress-disorder-in-children-epidemiology-pathogenesis-clinical-manifestations-course-assessment-and-diagnosis?source=search_result&search=posttraumatic%20stress%20disorder&selectedTitle=4~150

National Center for Campus Public Safety. (2016). National higher education emergency management needs assessment. Retrieved from https://blogs.uoregon.edu/cscenter/tag/national-center-for-campus-public-safety-nccps

National Center for Education Statistics. (2017). Fast facts. Retrieved from http://www.nces.ed.gov/fastfacts/display.asp?id=372

National Child Care and Technical Assistance Center and National Association for Regulatory Administration. (2009). The 2007 child care licensing study. Retrieved from https://www.researchconnections.org/childcare/resources/15564/pdf

National Commission on Children and Disasters. (2010, October). *2010 Report to the President and Congress.* AHRQ Publication No. 10-MO37. Rockville, MD: Agency for Healthcare Research and Quality.

National Education Association Healthy Futures. (n.d.). School crisis guide: Helping and healing in a time of crisis. Retrieved from http://healthyfutures.nea.org/wp-content/uploads/2015/05/schoolcrisisguide.pdf

O'Brien, M., Webster, S., & Herrick, A. (2007, February). U.S. Department of Health and Human Services Administration for Children and Families. Disaster preparedness and response. Retrieved from http://muskie.usm.maine.edu/helpkids/rcpdfs/copingwithdisasters.pdf

Office of Head Start. (2016). Head Start program fact sheet. Administration for Children and Families, U.S. Department of Human Services. Retrieved from https://www.acf.hhs.gov/ohs

Portune, L., & Gatowski, S. I. (2008). *Ensuring the unique needs of dependency courts are met in disaster planning efforts: Dependency court planning templates for continuity of operations plans.* Reno, NV: National Council of Juvenile and Family Court Judges and American Bar Association. Retrieved from http://www.ncjfcj.org/sites/default/files/dependency%20 courts%20and%20natural%20disasters%20tab.pdf

Readiness and Emergency Management for Schools. (2017). Incorporating international students into IHE emergency management and planning. Retrieved from http://rems.ed.gov/IHEIncorpIntlStudents.aspx

Rebmann, T., Elliott, M., Artman, D., VanNatta, M., & Wakefield, M. (2016). Impact of an education intervention on Missouri K-12 school disaster and biological event preparedness. *Journal of School Health, 86*(11), 794–802. doi:10.1111/josh.12435

Save the Children. (2008, August). Protecting children during U.S. Emergencies: How safe are our schools and day-care centers when disaster strikes? Retrieved from https://www.savethechildren.org/content/dam/global/ reports/emergency-preparation-disaster-risk-reduction/disaster-preps -issue.pdf

Save the Children. (2013a). Results for children. Retrieved from https://www. savethechildren.org/content/dam/usa/reports/advocacy/annual-report/ sc-2012-annualreport.pdf

Save the Children. (2013b). Unaccounted for: A national report card on protecting children in disasters. Retrieved from https://resourcecentre .savethechildren.net/node/13243/pdf/disaster-report-2013-.pdf

Save the Children. (2015). Still at risk: U.S. children 10 years after Hurricane Katrina. Save the children. Retrieved from http://www.savethechildren .org/atf/cf/%7B9def2ebe-10ae-432c-9bd0-df91d2eba74a%7D/ DISASTERREPORT_2015.PDF

Save the Children. (2017a). Puerto Rico's lack of power and clean water puts hundreds of thousands of children at risk. Retrieved from http://www .savethechildren.org/site/apps/nlnet/content2.aspx?c=8rKLIXM GIpI4E&b=9506653&ct=15004937

Save the Children. (2017b). Save the Children prioritizes recovery of child care centers, schools in Texas in wake of Hurricane Harvey. Retrieved from http://www.savethechildren.org/site/apps/nlnet/content2 .aspx?c=8rKLIXMGIpI4E&b=9506653&ct=15004131

Schonfeld, D. J., & Demaria, T.; Disaster Preparedness Advisory Council and Committee on Psychosocial Aspects of Child and Family Health. (2015). Providing psychosocial support to children and families in the aftermath of disasters and crisis. *Pediatrics, 136*(94), e1120–e1130. doi:10.1542/peds.2015-2861

Schonfeld, D. J., & Gurwitch, R. H. (2012). Children in disasters. In A. Y. Elzouki, F. B. Stapleton, R. J. Whitley, W. Oh, H. A. Harfi, & H. Nazer (Eds.). *Textbook of clinical pediatrics* (2nd ed.). New York, NY: Springer-Verlag.

Substance Abuse and Mental Health Services Administration. (2013). *Tips for talking with and helping children and youth cope after a disaster or traumatic event: A guide for parents, caregivers and teachers.* (HHS Publication No. SMA-12-4732). Washington, DC: U.S. Government Printing Office.

Texas A&M AgriLife Disaster Education Network. (2017). Disaster preparedness for college students. Retrieved from https://texashelp.tamu.edu/browse/ disaster-preparedness-information/college-students

Tulane University. (2017) Emergency preparedness and response. Retrieved from http://www2.tulane.edu/emergency/preparedness/hurricane -procedure.cfm

U.S. Department of Education. (2008). *A guide to school vulnerability assessments: Key principles for safe schools.* Washington, DC: Author.

U.S. Department of Education. (2010, June). *Family Educational Rights and Privacy Act (FERPA) and the disclosure of student information related to emergencies and disasters.* Washington, DC: Author. Retrieved from http://www2.ed.gov/policy/gen/guid/fpco/pdf/ferpa-disaster-guidance.pdf

U.S. Department of Education. (2011, June). *Addressing emergencies on campus.* Washington, DC: ED. Retrieved from https://rems.ed.gov/ docs/ED_AddressingEmergenciesOnCampus.pdf

U.S. Department of Health and Human Services.(2017). Health information privacy. Retrieved from https://www.hhs.gov/hipaa/for-professionals/faq/1068/ is-hipaa-suspended-during-a-national-or-public-health-emergency/index.htm

U.S. Department of Homeland Security (2016). Active shooter preparedness. Retrieved from https://www.dhs.gov/active-shooter-preparedness

U.S. Department of Homeland Security. (2017a). Academic resource catalog. Retrieved from https://www.dhs.gov/publication/academic -resource-catalog

U.S. Department of Homeland Security. (2017b). Campus resilience. Retrieved from https://www.dhs.gov/campus-resilience

U.S. Department of Homeland Security. (2017c). "If you see something, say something" campaign. Retrieved from https://www.dhs.gov/see-something -say-something Virginia Tech Office of Emergency Management. (2017). Retrieved from http://emergency.vt.edu/about.html

U.S. Department of Justice, Office of Justice Programs, Office of Juvenile Justice and Delinquency Prevention. (2011). Emergency planning for juvenile justice residential facilities. Retrieved from https://www.rems .ed.gov/docs/DOJ_EP_JuvenileJusticeFacilities.pdf

Veenema, T., Griffin, A., Gable, A., MacIntyre, L., Simons, N., Couig, M., … Larson, E. (2016). Nurses as leaders in disaster preparedness and response—A call to action. *Journal of Nursing Scholarship, 48*(2), 187–200. doi:10.1111/jnu.12198

Appendix 12.1

Index to Recommendations and Responsible Entities

	President	Congress	Relevant Federal Agencies	States, Tribes, Territories, and Localities	Nongovernmental Entities	Status (2015)*
1. Disaster Management and Recovery						
1.1: Distinguish and comprehensively integrate the needs of children across all inter- and intragovernmental disaster management activities and operations.	X	X	ALL	X	X	PM
• The president should develop a national strategy for children and disasters.	X		ALL			PM
• The executive branch, Congress, and nonfederal partners should prioritize children separately from "at-risk" population categories.	X	X	ALL	X	X	NM
• The executive branch at all levels of government should establish and maintain permanent focal points of coordination for children and disasters, supported by sufficient authority, funding, and policy expertise. FEMA should establish children's integration specialists at the regional level.	X		ALL	X		NM
• The executive branch and nonfederal partners should incorporate children as a distinct priority in base disaster planning documents and relevant grant programs.	X		ALL	X		M
• The executive branch and nonfederal partners should incorporate education, child care, juvenile justice, and child welfare systems into disaster planning, training, and exercises.	X		DHS/FEMA, HHS, ED, DOJ	X		PM
• The executive branch and nonfederal partners should incorporate children as a distinct priority in relevant target capabilities, preparedness training, and exercises, with specific target outcomes and performance measures.	X		ALL	X		PM
• The executive branch and Congress should institute accountability and progress monitoring measures to track implementation of commission recommendations and capability improvements.	X	X	ALL	X		NM
1.2: The president should accelerate the development and implementation of the National Disaster Recovery Framework with an explicit emphasis on addressing the immediate and long-term physical and mental health, educational, housing, and human services recovery needs of children.	X					PM

(continued)

Appendix 12.1 (*continued*)

Index to Recommendations and Responsible Entities

	President	Congress	Relevant Federal Agencies	States, Tribes, Territories, and Localities	Nongovernmental Entities	Status (2015)*
1.3: DHS/FEMA should ensure that information required for timely and effective delivery of recovery services to children and families is collected and shared with appropriate entities.			ALL	X	X	PM
• Governmental agencies and nongovernmental organizations should collect information on children and families necessary to identify and support their immediate and long-term recovery needs.			ALL	X	X	PM
• DHS/FEMA should expand information sharing with appropriate governmental agencies and nongovernmental organizations to enable the delivery of recovery services.			DHS/FEMA			PM
• DHS/FEMA should preidentify and credential additional local and out-of-state voluntary and nongovernmental organizations and networks that provide disaster assistance to children and families.			DHS/FEMA			PM
1.4: DHS/FEMA should establish interagency agreements to provide disaster preparedness funding, technical assistance, training, and other resources to state and local child-serving systems and child congregate care facilities.			DHS/FEMA, HHS, ED, DOJ			PM
2. Mental Health						
2.1: HHS should lead efforts to integrate mental and behavioral health for children into public health, medical, and other relevant disaster management activities.		X	ALL	X		M
• Congress should direct HHS to lead the development of a disaster mental health and behavioral health CONOPS to formalize disaster mental and behavioral health as a core component of disaster preparedness, response, and recovery efforts.		X	HHS			M
2.2: HHS should enhance the research agenda for children's disaster mental and behavioral health, including psychological first aid, cognitive behavioral interventions, bereavement counseling and support, and programs intended to enhance children's resilience in the aftermath of a disaster.			HHS			PM

(*continued*)

Appendix 12.1 (continued)

Index to Recommendations and Responsible Entities

	President	Congress	Relevant Federal Agencies	States, Tribes, Territories, and Localities	Nongovernmental Entities	Status (2015)*
• HHS should convene a working group of children's disaster mental health and pediatric experts to review the research portfolios of relevant agencies, identify gaps in knowledge, and recommend a national research agenda across the full spectrum of disaster mental health for children and families.			HHS			PM
2.3: Federal agencies and nonfederal partners should enhance predisaster preparedness and just-in-time training in pediatric disaster mental and behavioral health, including psychological first aid, bereavement support, and brief supportive interventions, for mental health professionals and individuals, such as teachers, who work with children.			DHS/FEMA, HHS, ED, DOJ	X	X	PM
2.4: DHS/FEMA and SAMHSA should strengthen the CCP to better meet the mental health needs of children and families.			DHS/FEMA, HHS			PM
• Simplify the ISP grant application to minimize the burden on communities affected by a disaster and facilitate the rapid allocation of funding and initiation of services.			DHS/FEMA, HHS			M
• Establish the position of Children's Disaster Mental Health Coordinator within state-level CCPs.			DHS/FEMA, HHS	X		PM
• Formally modify the CCP model to indicate and promote "enhanced services" where the mental health impact is unlikely to be adequately addressed by "typical" CCP services.			DHS/FEMA, HHS			PM
• Include bereavement support and education within services typically provided under CCP.			DHS/FEMA, HHS			NM
2.5: Congress should establish a single, flexible grant-funding mechanism to specifically support the delivery of mental health treatment services that address the full spectrum of behavioral health needs of children including treatment of disaster-related adjustment difficulties, psychiatric disorders, and substance abuse.		X				NM
3. Child Physical Health						
3.1: Congress, HHS, and DHS/FEMA should ensure availability and access to pediatric MCM at the federal, state, and local levels for chemical, biological, radiological, nuclear, and explosive threats.		X	DHS/FEMA, HHS			PM

(continued)

Appendix 12.1 (continued)

Index to Recommendations and Responsible Entities

	President	Congress	Relevant Federal Agencies	States, Tribes, Territories, and Localities	Nongovernmental Entities	Status (2015)*
• Provide funding and grant guidance for the development, acquisition, and stockpiling of MCM specifically for children for inclusion in the SNS and all other federally funded caches, including those funded by DHS/FEMA.		X	HHS			PM
• Amend the Emergency Use Authorization to allow the FDA, at the direction of the HHS secretary, to authorize pediatric indications of MCM for emergency use before an emergency is known or imminent.		X				PM
• Form a standing advisory body of federal partners and external experts to advise the HHS secretary and provide expert consensus on issues pertaining specifically to pediatric emergency MCM.			HHS			PM
• Within the HHS Biomedical Advanced Research and Development Authority, designate a pediatric leader and establish a pediatric and obstetric working group to conduct gap analysis and make research recommendations.			HHS			M
• Include pediatric expertise on the HHS Enterprise Governance Board or its successor and all relevant committees and working groups addressing issues pertaining to MCM.			HHS			M
• Establish a partnership between the proposed MCM development leader and key pediatric stakeholders both within and outside government.			HHS			PM
3.2: HHS and DOD should enhance the pediatric capabilities of their disaster medical response teams through the integration of pediatric-specific training, guidance, exercises, supplies, and personnel.		X	HHS, DOD			PM
• HHS should develop pediatric capabilities within each NDMS region.			HHS			PM
• HHS should establish a "reserve pool" of pediatric healthcare workers to assist in NDMS disaster response.			HHS			PM
• HHS and DOD should establish a pediatric healthcare coordinator on each disaster medical response team and develop strategies to recruit and retain team members with pediatric medical expertise.			HHS, DOD			NM

(continued)

Appendix 12.1 (continued)

Index to Recommendations and Responsible Entities

	President	Congress	Relevant Federal Agencies	States, Tribes, Territories, and Localities	Nongovernmental Entities	Status (2015)*
3.3: HHS should ensure that health professionals who may treat children during a disaster have adequate pediatric disaster clinical training.			HHS, DOD	X	X	PM
• The president should direct the FETIG to prioritize the development of pediatric core competencies, core curricula, training, and research.	X					PM
• The FETIG should support the formation of a Pediatric Disaster Clinical Education and Training Working Group to establish core clinical competencies and a standard, modular pediatric disaster healthcare education and training curriculum.			HHS, DOD			M
3.4: The executive branch and Congress should provide resources for a formal regionalized pediatric system of care to support pediatric surge capacity during and after disasters.	X	X	HHS			PM
• HHS should include pediatric surge capacity as a "required funding capability" in the Hospital Preparedness Program.			HHS			PM
• States and hospital accrediting bodies should ensure all hospital EDs stand ready to care for ill or injured children through the adoption of emergency preparedness guidelines jointly developed by the American Academy of Pediatrics, the American College of Emergency Physicians, and the Emergency Nurses Association.				X	X	PM
3.5: Prioritize the recovery of pediatric health and mental healthcare delivery systems in disaster-affected areas.	X	X	DHS/FEMA, HHS, SBA	X		PM
• Congress should establish sufficient funding mechanisms to support restoration and continuity of for-profit and nonprofit health and mental health services to children.		X				NM
• The executive branch should recognize and support pediatric health and mental healthcare delivery systems as a planning imperative in the development and implementation of the National Health Security Strategy and National Disaster Recovery Framework.	X			DHS/FEMA, HHS, SBA		PM
• HHS should create Medicaid and Children's Health Insurance Program incentive payments for providers in disaster areas.			HHS			NM

(continued)

Appendix 12.1 (continued)

Index to Recommendations and Responsible Entities

	President	Congress	Relevant Federal Agencies	States, Tribes, Territories, and Localities	Nongovernmental Entities	Status (2015)*
• The American Medical Association should adopt a new code or code modifier to the Current Procedural Terminology to reflect disaster medical care to facilitate tracking of these services and as a means for enhanced reimbursement from public and private payers.					X	NM
3.6: EPA should engage state and local health officials and nongovernmental experts to develop and promote national guidance and best practices on re-occupancy of homes, schools, child care, and other child congregate care facilities in disaster-impacted areas.			EPA			PM
• EPA and HHS should expand research on pediatric environmental health risks associated with disasters.			EPA, HHS			PM
4. Emergency Medical Services and Pediatric Transport						
4.1: The president and Congress should clearly designate and appropriately resource a lead federal agency for EMS with primary responsibility for the coordination of grant programs, research, policy, and standards development and implementation.	X	X				NM
• Establish a dedicated federal grant program under a designated lead federal agency for prehospital EMS disaster preparedness, including pediatric equipment and training.		X				NM
4.2: Improve the capability of EMS to transport pediatric patients and provide comprehensive prehospital pediatric care during daily operations and disasters.			DHS, HHS, DOT	X	X	PM
• Congress should provide full funding to the EMSC program to ensure all states and territories meet targets and achieve progress in the EMSC performance measures for grantees, and to support development of a research portfolio.		X				PM
• As an eligibility guideline for Centers for Medicare & Medicaid Services reimbursement, require first response and emergency medical response vehicles to acquire and maintain pediatric equipment and supplies in accordance with the national guidelines for equipment for Basic Life Support and Advanced Life Support vehicles.			HHS			PM
• HHS and DHS should establish stronger pediatric EMS performance measures within relevant federal emergency preparedness grant programs.			HHS, DHS			PM

(continued)

Appendix 12.1 (continued)

Index to Recommendations and Responsible Entities

	President	Congress	Relevant Federal Agencies	States, Tribes, Territories, and Localities	Nongovernmental Entities	Status (2015)*
• HHS should address the findings of the EMSC 2009 Gap Analysis of EMS Related Research.			HHS			PM
4.3: HHS should develop a national strategy to improve federal pediatric emergency transport and patient care capabilities for disasters.			HHS			PM
• Conduct a national review of existing capabilities among relevant governmental agencies and the private sector for emergency medical transport of children.			HHS			PM
5. Disaster Case Management						
5.1: Disaster case management programs should be appropriately resourced and should provide consistent holistic services that achieve tangible, positive outcomes for children and families affected by the disaster.	X	X	HHS, DHS/FEMA	X	X	PM
• The executive branch and Congress should provide sufficient funds to build, support, and deploy a disaster case management system with nationwide capacity.	X	X	HHS, DHS/FEMA			PM
• DHS/FEMA should clarify the transition from federal to state-led disaster case management programs.			DHS/FEMA			M
• Governmental agencies and nongovernmental organizations should develop voluntary consensus standards on the essential elements and methods of disaster case management, including precredentialing of case managers and training that includes focused attention to the needs of children and families.			HHS, DHS/FEMA	X	X	PM
6. Child Care and Early Education						
6.1: Congress and HHS should improve disaster preparedness capabilities for child care.		X	HHS	X		M
• Congress and HHS should require states to include disaster planning, training, and exercise requirements within the scope of their minimum health and safety standards for child care licensure or registration.		X	HHS			M

(continued)

Appendix 12.1 (continued)

Index to Recommendations and Responsible Entities

	President	Congress	Relevant Federal Agencies	States, Tribes, Territories, and Localities	Nongovernmental Entities	Status (2015)*
• Congress should provide HHS the authority to require states to develop statewide child care disaster plans in coordination with state and local emergency managers, public health, state child care administrators and regulatory agencies, and child care resource and referral agencies.		X	HHS			M
6.2: Congress and federal agencies should improve capacity to provide child care services in the immediate aftermath of and recovery from a disaster.		X	DHS/FEMA, HHS, SBA			PM
• DHS/FEMA should revise its Public Assistance regulations to codify child care as an essential service.			DHS/FEMA			M
• Congress should codify child care as an "essential service of a governmental nature" in the Stafford Act.		X				M
• Federal agencies should incorporate child care as an essential service in the National Response Framework, the National Disaster Recovery Framework, the National Disaster Housing Concept of Operations, and Disaster Housing Practitioners' Guide.			DHS/FEMA, HHS, SBA			PM
• Congress should authorize a grant-funding mechanism, such as an emergency contingency fund, to repair or rebuild private, for-profit child care facilities, support the establishment of temporary child care, and reimburse states for subsidizing child care services to disaster-affected families.		X				NM
6.3: HHS should require disaster preparedness capabilities for Head Start Centers and basic disaster mental health training for staff.			HHS			PM
7. Elementary and Secondary Education						
7.1: Congress and federal agencies should improve the preparedness of schools and school districts by providing additional support to states.		X	DHS/FEMA, ED			PM
• Congress and ED should award disaster preparedness grants to state educational agencies to oversee, coordinate, and improve disaster planning, training, and exercises statewide and ensure that all districts within the state meet certain baseline criteria.		X	ED			PM

(continued)

Appendix 12.1 (continued)

Index to Recommendations and Responsible Entities

	President	Congress	Relevant Federal Agencies	States, Tribes, Territories, and Localities	Nongovernmental Entities	Status (2015)*
• DHS/FEMA should partner with ED to provide funding and other resources to support disaster preparedness efforts of state and local educational agencies, including collaborative planning, training, and exercises with emergency management officials.			DHS/FEMA, ED			PM
7.2: Congress and ED should enhance the ability of school personnel to support children who are traumatized, grieving, or otherwise recovering from a disaster.		X	ED			NM
• Congress and ED should award funds to states to implement and evaluate training and professional developmental programs in basic skills in providing support to grieving students and students in crisis and establish statewide requirements related to teacher certification and recertification.		X	ED			NM
7.3 Ensure that school systems recovering from disasters are provided immediate resources to reopen and restore the learning environment in a timely manner and provide support for displaced students and their host schools.		X	DHS/FEMA, ED			PM
• Congress should create a permanent funding mechanism to support recovery for schools and students.		X				NM
• Congress should establish an emergency contingency fund within the Education for Homeless Children and Youth program and expeditiously provide grants to school districts serving an influx of displaced children.		X				NM
• Congress and ED should support the immediate provision of expert technical assistance and consultation regarding services and interventions to address disaster mental health needs of students and school personnel.		X	ED			PM
• DHS/FEMA, ED, and other federal agencies should clarify, consolidate, and publicize information related to the recovery programs, assistance, and services (e.g., transportation to schools) currently available to school systems through the Stafford Act and other federal resources.			DHS/FEMA, ED			PM
8. Child Welfare and Juvenile Justice						
8.1: Ensure that state and local child welfare agencies adequately prepare for disasters.		X	HHS, DHS/FEMA	X		PM

(continued)

Appendix 12.1 (*continued*)

Index to Recommendations and Responsible Entities

(*continued*)

	President	Congress	Relevant Federal Agencies	States, Tribes, Territories, and Localities	Nongovernmental Entities	Status (2015)*
• Congress should request a national assessment of child welfare disaster planning to determine if significant advances have been made since passage of the Child and Family Services Improvement Act of 2006 (CFSIA).		X	HHS			M
• HHS should develop detailed disaster planning criteria by regulation or other formal policy guidance to supplement the basic procedures mandated in CFSIA.			HHS			NM
• Within each ACF regional office, child welfare staff and the region's emergency management specialist should collaboratively review and evaluate the state child welfare disaster plans required by CFSIA and assist states in developing comprehensive plans and meeting their statutory obligations.			HHS			PM
• DHS/FEMA and HHS should provide funding, guidance, and technical assistance to child welfare agencies and encourage collaboration with emergency management, courts, and other key stakeholders.			DHS/FEMA, HHS			PM
8.2: Ensure that state and local juvenile justice agencies and all residential treatment, correctional, and detention facilities that house children adequately prepare for disasters.		X	DHS/FEMA, DOJ	X	X	PM
• Congress should require state and local juvenile justice agencies and all residential treatment, correctional, and detention facilities to have comprehensive disaster plans in place.		X				PM
• DHS/FEMA and DOJ should support disaster planning for state and local juvenile justice agencies and residential treatment, correctional, and detention facilities that house children by providing funding, technical assistance, and training.			DHS/FEMA, DOJ			M
8.3: HHS and DOJ should ensure that juvenile, dependency, and other courts hearing matters involving children adequately prepare for disasters.			HHS, DOJ	X	X	NM
• HHS should include disaster preparedness as a component of the Court Improvement Program for dependency courts.			HHS			NM
• DOJ should include disaster preparedness as a component of the proposed National Juvenile Delinquency Court Improvement Program.			DOJ			NM

Appendix 12.1 (continued)

Index to Recommendations and Responsible Entities

	President	Congress	Relevant Federal Agencies	States, Tribes, Territories, and Localities	Nongovernmental Entities	Status (2015)*
• DOJ and the National Council of Juvenile and Family Court Judges should incorporate disaster preparedness into the Model Courts program.			DOJ		X	NM
9. Sheltering Standards, Services, and Supplies						
9.1: Governmental agencies and nongovernmental organizations should provide a safe and secure mass care shelter environment for children, including access to services and supplies.			DHS/FEMA, HHS	X	X	M
• Implement national standards and indicators for mass care shelters that are specific and responsive to children.			DHS/FEMA, HHS	X	X	M
• Integrate essential age-appropriate shelter supplies for infants and children into shelter planning and fund the addition of child-specific supplies to caches for immediate deployment to support shelter operations.			DHS/FEMA	X	X	M
• Implement common standards and training, including standards for criminal background checks, to mitigate risks unique to children in shelters, such as child abduction and sex offenders.			DHS/FEMA	X	X	M
10. Housing						
10.1: Prioritize the needs of families with children, especially families with children who have disabilities or chronic health, mental health, or educational needs, within disaster housing assistance programs.			DHS/FEMA, HUD, HHS	X	X	PM
• Governmental agencies and nongovernmental organizations should ensure that families with children in disaster housing, especially community sites, have access to needed services and are provided safe and healthy living environments.			DHS/FEMA, HUD, HHS	X	X	PM
• Congress should authorize DHS/FEMA to reimburse state and local governments for providing wraparound services to children and families in community sites.		X				NM
• DHS/FEMA should develop clear written guidance around emergency transportation planning and reimbursement for state and local governments that addresses the recovery needs of children and families.			DHS/FEMA			PM

(continued)

Appendix 12.1 (continued)

Index to Recommendations and Responsible Entities

	President	Congress	Relevant Federal Agencies	States, Tribes, Territories, and Localities	Nongovernmental Entities	Status (2015)*
• Governmental agencies and nongovernmental organizations should identify and promote innovative programs to expedite the transition into permanent housing for families with children.			DHS/FEMA, HUD	X	X	PM
11. Evacuation						
11.1: Congress and federal agencies should provide sufficient funding to develop and deploy a national information sharing capability to quickly and effectively reunite displaced children with their families, guardians, and caregivers when separated by a disaster.		X	DHS, HHS, DOD			PM
• DHS should lead the development of a nationwide information technology capability to collect, share, and search data from any patient and evacuee tracking or family reunification system.			DHS			PM
• DHS should support the development of voluntary consensus-driven standards for data collection and data sharing through a joint federal, nonfederal, and private sector process.			DHS			NM
• Governmental agencies should ensure the collection of appropriate data on evacuated children, particularly unaccompanied minors.			DHS/FEMA, HHS, DOD			M
11.2: Disaster plans at all levels of government must specifically address the evacuation and transportation needs of children with disabilities and chronic health needs, in coordination with child congregate care facilities such as schools, child care, and healthcare facilities.			DHS/FEMA	X		PM

ACF, Administration for Children and Families; CCP, Crisis Counseling Assistance and Training Program; CONOPS, Concept of Operations; DHS, Department of Homeland Security; DOD, Department of Defense; DOJ, Department of Justice; DOT, Department of Transportation; ED, Department of Education; EMS, emergency medical services; EMSC, Emergency Medical Services for Children; EPA, Environmental Protection Agency; FEMA, Federal Emergency Management Agency; FETIG, Federal Education and Training Interagency Group for Public Health and Medical Disaster Preparedness and Response; HHS, Department of Health and Human Services; HUD, Department of Housing and Urban Development; ISP, Immediate Services Program; M, Met; MCM, medical countermeasures; NDMS, National Disaster Medical System; NM, Not Met; PM, Partially Met; SAMHSA, Substance Abuse and Mental Health Services Administration; SBA, Small Business Administration; SNS, Strategic National Stockpile.

Source: Reprinted with permission from the National Commission on Children and Disasters. (2010, October). *2010 Report to the President and Congress.* AHRQ Publication No. 10-MO37. Rockville, MD: Agency for Healthcare Research and Quality.

*Updated status on Recommendations from *Save the Children, July, 2015.*

13

CARE OF THE PREGNANT WOMAN AND NEWBORN FOLLOWING A DISASTER

Kathleen Leask Capitulo and Robbie Prepas

LEARNING OBJECTIVES

When this chapter is completed, readers will be able to:

1. Understand the special needs of the pregnant woman in a disaster situation.
2. Describe the normal physiology and potential complications of pregnancy, childbirth, and postpartum.
3. Identify strategies for managing complications of pregnancy during disaster events.
4. Describe the normal physiology of the newborn and adaptation to extrauterine life.
5. Describe standard obstetrical care during delivery for uncomplicated and complicated childbirth, and strategies for managing childbirth in disasters.
6. Describe prevention strategies for common infectious diseases affecting the woman and newborn.
7. Identify three healing interventions for women and families who experience the death of a mother and/or baby (e.g., maternal death, fetal demise, miscarriage, stillbirth, or neonatal death, during a disaster).

KEY MESSAGES

When a disaster occurs, the special needs of pregnant women and infants need to be addressed in order to prevent excess neonatal and maternal morbidity.

Breastfeeding is important to the survival of newborns and children under age 5, particularly in time of disaster and must be supported without commercial substitutes.

The provision of obstetrical services to the pregnant woman in a clean, safe environment with access to clean water should be a priority throughout the disaster event.

Planning at the local, state, and federal levels of government should accommodate the delivery of services to women and infants during emergencies and disasters.

Nurses play a key role in the care of women and children during disasters.

CHAPTER OVERVIEW

Pregnant women and infants have unique health concerns in the aftermath of a natural disaster, epidemic, or terrorist event. Disruptions in the availability of clean water supply, inadequate access to safe food, exposure to environmental toxins, interruption of access to regular healthcare, shortages of life-sustaining medicines, and crowded conditions in shelters are just a few of the commonly encountered postdisaster challenges. Disasters may alter the environment and limit the availability of clean, secure areas for women to give birth safely. There are numerous potential complications for pregnant women in a disaster including preterm labor, pregnancy-induced hypertension (PIH), infections, and diabetes (Callaghan et al., 2007; Sulaiman, Mohamad, Ismail, Johari, & Hussain, 2016). Additionally, posttraumatic stress disorder (PTSD) has been associated with premature deliveries, increased cesarean rates, and small for gestational age babies in several studies (Lipkind, Curry, Huynh, Thorpe, & Matte, 2010).

Disasters are disruptive events that create challenges for all populations. Among the most vulnerable are pregnant women and newborns. When a disaster happens, the physical environment is altered and resources are constrained creating significant obstacles for nurses who must render obstetric care and provide a safe environment for a newborn (Orlando, Danna, Giarratano, Prepas, & Johnson, 2010).

Globally, natural disasters impact more than 200 million people each year. Additionally, war and armed conflicts impact over 300 million people, (Leaning & Guha-Sapir, 2013).

This chapter prepares nurses with the knowledge and skills they need to care for the pregnant woman and newborn in the field during or following a major disaster event. It includes a review of the course of normal and complicated pregnancy, childbirth, and postpartum/newborn care and implications for care management during disaster.

PHYSIOLOGY OF NORMAL PREGNANCY

Pregnancy is a natural but complex state of health. During pregnancy, a woman's body experiences many changes to support the growth and development of a baby. Some of the major changes include the following.

Hormone levels increase significantly causing nausea and vomiting, which can be particularly problematic in early pregnancy. Suggested treatments include eating small, frequent meals (especially carbohydrates) and avoiding odorous and spicy foods.

Many changes in hormones impact pregnancy. Estrogen is essential for maturation of the fetus's lungs, liver, and major organs. Estrogen regulates progesterone production and maintains pregnancy. Later in pregnancy, it stimulates fetal cortisol production. Without estrogen, a pregnancy would miscarry.

Progesterone creates a nutrient-rich environment in the uterus, necessary for fetal development. It also prevents contractions and causes the mucus plug to form.

Human choriogonadotropin (HCG) rises early in pregnancy. Levels are measured to confirm pregnancy and monitored after a pregnancy loss or hydatidiform mole (an abnormal pregnancy without a fetus), some of which are cancerous, to ensure the absence of fetal tissue.

Relaxin rises and "relaxes" ligaments, increasing pelvic mobility that may lead to aches in the back and hips (What to Expect, 2011).

Circulatory changes occur because the expectant mother's blood volume increases by 3.0 L with an additional 3.5 L of water in the amniotic fluid, the fetus, and the placenta (Cunningham et al., 2010). Increased blood volume requires that a pregnant woman be able to maintain her fluid volume, preventing dehydration, and increase her iron intake, preventing anemia. Prescription or over-the-counter prenatal vitamins provide the essential iron as well as folic acid required for the neurologic health of the unborn baby.

Increased body weight is required to support fetal growth and development. An expectant mother may gain 20 to 40 lbs during pregnancy. Underweight women may need to gain more to support the baby. Weight gain and avoidance of ketosis are important to fetal growth. Ketones are formed during weight loss and can negatively impact fetal growth and brain development. Women should eat a balanced diet, avoiding processed, high salt, and high sugar foods. Emphasize calcium intake to promote fetal bone growth and avoid maternal calcium depletion. Food patterns are cultural. Advise against fasting, even if for religious reasons. Most religions exempt pregnant women from fasting, but they may feel socially compelled to do so if all others in their family are fasting. Emphasize to family and religious elders that fasting can harm both mother and baby (Kridli, 2011). Many cultures have beliefs that are not founded in science, such as the notion that if you have a craving and do not eat the food, your baby will be born with a birth mark looking like the food. Use the opportunity to discuss myths as a teachable moment. Weight gain will change the woman's center of gravity. Advise the mother to wear flat shoes and focus on maintaining good posture when standing.

Rest is essential for pregnant women. As the fetus grows, the weight of the baby puts pressure on the legs and aorta. The growing uterus also limits lung expansion, making it difficult to breathe, particularly when lying down. Advise frequent periods of rest. When sitting, recommend keeping the legs elevated when possible. Some women with sitting jobs place a pillow over a trash can in order to elevate their legs. Advise resting and sleeping in a side-lying position when reclining, as supine position will decrease circulation to the mother because of the baby's weight. Some women experience easier breathing when supine by raising their arms over their heads to expand their lungs upward (Merck Manual, 2011a, 2011b).

PREGNANCY DURING DISASTER CONDITIONS

When a disaster occurs, challenges arise in meeting the physical, emotional, and mental health needs of the pregnant woman. During a disaster, all the normal physical needs of pregnant women are present but healthcare and birthing environments are altered, creating increased challenges for delivery of safe, obstetrical healthcare. When a community is affected by disaster, people have to find alternative ways to accomplish tasks in their altered physical and social environments. Ideally every pregnant woman and healthcare provider should have emergency childbirth kits, emergency shelters should have birth kits, and alternative sites should be stocked with equipment if birth must occur outside the hospital setting. As part of community planning and preparedness efforts for disasters and emergencies,

all communities should consider the special needs of women giving birth. If possible, pregnant women should keep a copy of their medical records with them at all times.

Nurses must be able to create a clean, safe environment for the pregnant woman as well as provide for a safe delivery. Strategies for responding to the potential complications of pregnancy during disaster conditions are also critically important and should consider the emotional and psychological needs of the mother (Box 13.1).

BOX 13.1 Critical Needs in Caring for Pregnant Women During Times of Disaster for Nonobstetric Healthcare Providers

WHAT ARE THE CRITICAL REPRODUCTIVE HEALTHCARE MESSAGES FOR WOMEN AND THEIR HEALTHCARE PROVIDERS?

Pregnancy Awareness

Half of all pregnancies are unplanned; women may not be aware they are pregnant and that they have special healthcare needs. Pregnancy testing must be available to confirm suspicions of pregnancy when there is doubt; the first 8 weeks of pregnancy are critical for organogenesis so it is important for women to have access to healthcare information. Pregnancy prevention requires access to contraception and this can be a problem when access to care has been interrupted.

All pregnant women should receive prenatal care. They need to find an alternate source of routine care if their healthcare facility is closed. Prenatal vitamins should be taken daily. There is no known safe amount of alcohol during pregnancy. Mass vaccination or prophylaxis must consider the special circumstance of pregnancy; live attenuated vaccines such as varicella and measles, mumps, and rubella (MMR) are contraindicated in pregnant women. Influenza vaccine is recommended for all women who are pregnant during the influenza season. A summary of recommendations for adult immunization can be found at: www.immunize.org/catg.d/p2011b.htm and www.immunize.org/catg.d/p2011b.htm

Pregnant women should avoid children with rashes and adults with shingles in order to minimize the potential exposure to varicella.

WHAT ARE THE CRITICAL ISSUES FOR PRENATAL CARE?

General Considerations

Records from prior prenatal care may not be available; providers may have to "start from scratch." Consider giving a copy of prenatal records to patients if care is likely to be episodic or the woman is likely to be transient.

During the First Trimester (before 13 weeks)

First trimester laboratory testing: blood type, Rh type, antibody screen, Hct, Hgb, platelets, rubella, RPR, urine screen/culture, Hgb electrophoresis, PPD, chlamydia/GC, pap smear, and HIV.

During the Second Trimester (from 13 to 26 weeks)

Prenatal visits every 4 weeks. Assess blood pressure, fundal height, weight gain, and address concerns. Consider ultrasound, if available, for confirming due date. Screening for diabetes with glucose challenge test (26–28 weeks).

During the Third Trimester (from 24 weeks to term [greater than 37 weeks])

Prenatal visits every 2 weeks from 28 until 36 weeks. Assess blood pressure, fundal height, weight gain, and address concerns. Prenatal visits every week after 36 weeks.

WHAT SIGNS AND SYMPTOMS REQUIRE EMERGENCY OBSTETRIC SERVICES?

Seek emergency obstetric care for the following:

Preterm (less than 37 weeks) contractions
Contractions every 10 minutes or more (cramping)
Pelvic pressure
Low, dull backache
Abdominal cramps with or without diarrhea
Regular painful uterine contractions at term (increasing in frequency and duration)
Vaginal bleeding and/or severe abdominal pain
Leakage of fluid (obvious or suspected ruptured membranes)
Decreased fetal movement

Source: Centers for Disease Control and Prevention. (2007). Critical needs in caring for pregnant women during times of disaster for non-obstetric health care providers. Retrieved from http://www2.wpro.who.int/internet/files/eha/toolkit/web/Technical%20References/Special%20Populations/CDC%20Caring%20for%20Pregnant%20Women%20During%20Disaster.pdf

COMPLICATIONS OF PREGNANCY

Hypertension, Pregnancy-Induced Hypertension, and Eclampsia

About 10% of pregnant women across the world experience hypertension. Hypertension in pregnancy has been classified into four types: preeclampsia/eclampsia, chronic hypertension, chronic hypertension with superimposed preeclampsia, and gestational hypertension. Symptoms include elevated blood pressure, proteinuria (not always seen), liver dysfunction, clotting dysfunction, renal insufficiency, and in severe cases, pulmonary edema (American College of Obstetricians and Gynecologists [ACOG], 2013). Hypertension that preexists pregnancy must continue to be treated. The obstetric professional should consult an internal medicine provider to select a medication safe for the fetus.

PIH used to be called "preeclampsia." PIH can lead to toxemia or seizures. Today, PIH is known to be more common in first pregnancies and a complex response involving hypertension. Clinical standards for practice include checking the expectant mother's blood pressure on each visit. Nurses should be aware of subtle clinical signs such as increases in blood pressure and other symptoms, including headaches and swelling of extremities. The goal is to normalize blood pressure using sodium restrictions (no processed/canned food) and antihypertensives when necessary. Rest is important. Suggest to the patient lying on left side to optimize placental blood flow. Frequent periods of rest in a quiet environment are helpful. Stress exacerbates PIH, making it a particular challenge to appropriately manage PIH in a disaster. If PIH does not respond to treatment and the mother is near term, consider delivering the baby. Delivery usually resolves PIH.

Eclampsia is a seizure in a pregnant woman, often precipitated by uncontrolled hypertension. It can occur any time in the perinatal period, both before and after delivery. A perinatal seizure is an emergency and requires constant supervision of the patient and intervention from a healthcare professional. During the seizure, the patient must be kept safe and efforts should be made to prevent injury. Consider administering intravenous (IV) medications (e.g., magnesium sulfate) to decrease central nervous system stimulation. Insure that the mother has adequate oxygenation. If the seizure is prenatal, assess the fetus through fetal heart rate monitoring and pH testing of fetal scalp blood if possible. Continuous monitoring of maternal blood pressure, pulse, fetal heart rate, and oxygenation is standard of care. In a disaster, this may be limited to heart rate monitoring of both mother and baby and blood pressure of mother. Delivery is indicated for women at 37 weeks 0 days and for those under 37 weeks with ruptured membranes (ACOG, 2013). Consider delivery once the woman and fetus are stabilized. Toxemia can be manifested in the perinatal period, including postpartum, requiring immediate treatment (Cunningham et al., 2010).

HELLP (*H*emolysis, *E*levated *L*iver enzymes, and *L*ow *P*latelet count) syndrome is a life-threatening syndrome affecting about 25% of women with PIH. The syndrome includes hemolysis, the breakdown of red blood cells; elevated liver enzymes; and low platelets. The syndrome can come on suddenly and without warning. It can lead to liver failure, hepatic coma, and disseminated intravascular coagulation (DIC). HELLP syndrome is an obstetrical emergency requiring transfer to a tertiary care obstetric hospital. If DIC ensues, transfusion of blood plasma and numerous blood products will be required to save the mother's life (ACOG, 2013; Cunningham et al., 2010).

Diabetes Mellitus

Diabetes of pregnancy (gestational diabetes) impacts 3% to 5% of pregnant women. Essentially, it is a "carbohydrate intolerance during pregnancy" further challenged by the need of the pregnant woman to consume more calories, which puts increased demands on the pancreas. The goal in managing gestational diabetes or preexisting diabetes mellitus in pregnancy is to normalize blood glucose (BG). Fasting BG in pregnancy should be 60 to 80 mg/dL and approximately 110 mg/dL 90 minutes after a meal. Treatment includes diet and medications. Good nutrition is essential during pregnancy. For a mother who has diabetes in pregnancy, the diet should include enough calories to enable her to support the baby but must avoid simple sugars and foods with a high glycemic index, such as cookies, anything with simple sugars, juices, sugared soda pop, and baked potatoes. Complex carbohydrates, protein, and water are preferable. BG monitoring is essential for glycemic control. BG should be monitored during fasting, before and after each meal, and at the hour of sleep. If glycemic control is not achieved with diet alone, insulin may be added. Oral medications to lower BG are not used in pregnancy as their goal is to further stimulate the pancreas to produce insulin. In pregnancy, the pancreas is already overworking, thus, it cannot produce more. Synthetic insulin is administered if diet alone cannot normalize the expectant mother's BG. Many women have difficulty giving themselves insulin and testing their own BG. Patient education should be supportive, teaching insulin self-administration, BG testing using a meter, and documenting these data in a log. The expectant mother should also be able to manage a diet low in simple carbohydrates with sufficient protein and calories to prevent ketosis (Cunningham et al., 2010).

Babies of mothers with diabetes mellitus during pregnancy are at risk of macrosomia, large birth weight. These babies may be born with high levels of BG that crossed the placenta during pregnancy causing increased fetal body weight. Babies born to mothers with hyperglycemia may have difficulty maintaining normal BG at birth due to their insulin production to metabolize the maternal BG. These babies require BG monitoring at birth to assess the need for early feedings to provide a sugar source. They are also at higher risk of respiratory distress (Cunningham et al., 2010).

Premature labor affects about one out of eight pregnancies, ending prematurely (before 37 weeks of gestation).

First trimester bleeding/cramping can lead to miscarriage. A miscarriage can be nature's way of addressing a pregnancy with a genetic problem. In the past, bed rest was advised for women with early pregnancy bleeding; however, bed rest has not been found to decrease pregnancy loss (Maloni, 2010). Should a mother miscarry in the first trimester, check that all products of conception are expelled from the uterus. Continued bleeding may require a surgical dilatation and curettage (D&C) to remove conceptus and stop bleeding.

Second trimester complications include painless dilation of the cervix from 18 to 21 weeks of pregnancy and can be indicative of an "incompetent cervix." Treatment includes surgical suturing to make the cervix closed. Traditional treatments, including bed rest and putting the patient in Trendelenburg position (head lower than the feet), have not been found to be effective. Third trimester preterm labor signs and symptoms may include contractions or cramping. Limited activity, bed rest, and hydration should be used to stop the contractions. The woman should be advised to avoid sexual intercourse as seminal fluids contain prostaglandin hormones that can cause uterine contractions. If a premature birth is inevitable, evacuate the mother to a high-risk center prepared to care for a preterm infant. Administration of steroids to the mother 48 hours before preterm birth and administration of surfactant into the neonate's lungs at birth improve lung function (Bookman, Troy, McCaffrey, & Randolph, 2010; Smart & Princivalle, 2011). Oxygen and intubations or mechanical ventilation may be required to support a very low birthweight premature baby.

Bleeding Disorders in Pregnancy

Placenta previa is a condition where the placenta grows over the cervix. The classic symptom is painless bleeding. Under no circumstances should a vaginal exam be done should a previa be suspected as it can cause severe hemorrhage. In 7% of cases of placenta previa, placenta accrete occurs, in which the placenta has abnormal attachment to the uterine blood vessels causing massive blood loss when separated from the uterine wall at delivery. Although a previa may be suspected with the symptom of painless bleeding, diagnosis requires an ultrasound. Cesarean birth is required for a complete previa. Should hemorrhage occur with an accrete, fluid and blood replacement are required, and uterine artery ligation and hysterectomy may be required to stop the bleeding (Cunningham et al., 2010).

Placenta abruptio (placental abruption, abruptio placentae) is the painful separation of the placenta from the wall of the uterus. It can be precipitated by abdominal trauma (e.g., car accident) or building collapse (earthquake). The diagnosis of abruptions is made by ultrasound, if possible. The provider should monitor girth of the abdomen to assess for increased intrauterine bleeding. Bleeding disorders result from massive blood loss and require fluid volume and blood replacement. Delivery by cesarean is indicated if near term or if the bleeding continues (Cunningham et al., 2010).

Uterine rupture or a tear in the uterus are both considered serious emergencies requiring surgical or cesarean delivery. Symptoms may include acute, severe abdominal pain. A rupture during the second stage of labor may be manifested by the presenting head retreating, that is, going back up into the vagina.

Postpartum hemorrhage is the loss of more than 500 mL of blood after the placenta is delivered and occurs in 5% of deliveries. Most women can tolerate perinatal blood loss due to increases in blood and fluid volume associated with pregnancy. Hemoglobin and hematocrit must be monitored in all cases of hemorrhage, and blood/fluid volume replacement should be considered if bleeding persists. The cause of the hemorrhage should also be treated (Cunningham et al., 2010).

Blood Disorders

Idiopathic thrombocytopenia purpura (ITP) is a decrease in platelets. It can be treated with steroids in pregnancy.

DIC is a bleeding emergency that can occur after delivery. Treatment requires multiple units of blood products including fresh frozen plasma, packed red blood cells, and platelets. Management should be in a hospital's ICU. The patient should immediately be evacuated and transferred to a medical center.

Other Medical Conditions in Pregnancy Occurring During a Disaster

Pregnant women may experience other disaster-related medical conditions unrelated to their pregnancy. These conditions should be treated as soon as possible and may include trauma/fractured bones. An obstetric provider should be consulted to insure the safety and well-being of the fetus during any procedure. Surgical conditions and operative procedures may be required to treat conditions such as acute abdomen. Any surgery during pregnancy has the potential to trigger premature labor.

Asthma, lung spasms, and constrictions must be treated to prevent loss of oxygen to the fetus. Steroids and bronchial dilators are preferred (Cunningham et al., 2010). Avoid epinephrine due to increased heart workload. If the mother has allergies that are the source of the compromised lung function, antihistamines can be prescribed.

Fever (hyperthermia) in pregnancy can be a sign of infection. The source of infection should be identified and treated, and the maternal temperature normalized (Cunningham et al., 2010).

ASSESSMENT OF THE PREGNANT WOMAN AND BABY

Assessment of the mother and baby during labor includes:

- *Mother*: vital signs: heart rate, blood pressure, respirations
- *Baby*: fetal heart rate and patterns, baby's position (head down or vertex presentation preferred)

Cardiovascular System

It is very important to identify any early signs of hypertensive states and to intervene immediately. Nursing assessment includes monitoring the pregnant woman's blood pressure, checking a radial pulse, and listening to heart sounds. During a disaster, the nurse may need to improvise equipment and remain vigilant for complaints of headache, visual changes, and epigastric pain.

CHILDBIRTH DURING DISASTERS

During a disaster, supplies and equipment that are normally used during labor and birth may not be available. In these situations, healthcare workers will need to use whatever is available to accomplish the necessary tasks. Required equipment and treatments along with their potential substitutes include:

- *Fetal monitor substitutes*: Fetoscope, stethoscope, and hand on the abdomen should be used (Pfeiffer et al., 2008).
- *Fluids*: Oral fluids and light fluids should be given.
- *Pain control and emotional support*: Human presence, backrubs and massage, bath or shower if available. Movement is extremely important to comfort and to effectively manage labor and birth.

Triage is essential to childbirth in disasters and should include early assessment, urgency determination, and immediate transfer to an appropriate facility. Priority of care should be based on triage acuity viewed in light of current conditions and capacity for safe transport. Documentation and disposition should be made as quickly as possible.

Stages of Childbirth

There are three stages of childbirth, which are as follows.

First Stage (Can Last up to 20 Hours)

- *Phase 1* (*early labor*)—with cervical dilatation from 0 to 4 cm. Walking and hydration are important. The expectant mother should be advised to keep hydrated with small amounts of fluids, as tolerated. Rest in early labor is advised in order to conserve energy for later labor.
- *Phase 2, 4 to 8 cm* (*active phase*)—contractions are 3 minutes apart and last at least 45 seconds. Women are uncomfortable and may benefit from comfort measures (backrubs, cool cloths on head), rhythmic focused breathing, and pain medication, if available.
- *Transition, 8 to 10 cm* (*full dilatation*)—this is the most difficult time in labor, requiring additional support and comfort.

Second Stage: Birth

This stage involves the passage of the baby through the birth canal. Once the mother is fully dilated (10 cm), she can begin pushing.

Key points
The woman should be sitting at a 45° angle or higher or squatting (use gravity). Pushing should be done with the mouth open. Do not instruct her to hold her breath which decreases oxygen for the baby. Pushing should be done only during a contraction.

Third Stage: Delivery of the Placenta

The placenta should be delivered "naturally" during a contraction in which the mother should give one final "big push." The cord should not be pulled. Upon delivery, inspect the placenta to see if it appears to be complete as any pieces left inside the patient can cause bleeding.

Immediately after birth, the provider should put the baby to breast in order that the baby sucks on the mother's nipples, causing the release of oxytocin to contract the uterus, decreasing bleeding. Massage the uterus to promote contraction.

Key points
When managing or assisting at birth, keep the mother calm and comfortable, maintain clean hands and wear gloves,

prepare a bed for delivery (cover it with plastic or a shower curtain), coach the mother through pushing, assess the newborn to ensure breathing on delivery, and cut the cord when it stops pulsating (Williams, 2004).

COMPLICATIONS OF LABOR AND DELIVERY: MALPRESENTATION

During childbirth, it is best if the head emerges first. This is a vertex presentation. The head is usually the largest part of the baby's body. The pressure of the head against the cervix aids in dilatation. Should the baby's buttocks come first, a breech presentation, the cervix may not dilate fully. During a breech delivery it is essential to get the baby's body and head out right after the buttocks are delivered to prevent the cervix from clamping down on the neck and preventing the head from delivery.

Other malpresentations include shoulders and feet. In a "footling breech," the feet come out first. This is more common in a very preterm birth. In a "transverse lie," the baby is lying sideways in the uterus with no presenting part. In malpresentation, an experienced midwife or obstetrician may be able to "rotate" the baby from outside the abdomen, to get it into a vertex position for delivery.

"Back labor" occurs when the fetus's back is lying against the mother's back. During each contraction, the mother may experience significant back pain. A posterior delivery is more challenging to get the face-up baby around the pelvic bones and out of the mother. An experienced midwife or obstetrician may be able to rotate the baby's head during delivery.

CARE OF THE UMBILICAL CORD

The umbilical cord is the fetus's lifeline during pregnancy and delivery. During delivery, as the baby's head is emerging, the neck should be checked to insure that the cord is not around it. Should the cord be around the neck, the provider can lift it off. If it is tight around the neck, the provider may clamp it in two places and cut the cord (between the clamps) in order to deliver the baby.

After delivery, once the cord has stopped "pulsating," the cord should be clamped with a sterile clamp or umbilical tape. Leave about 6 inches of cord next to the baby. A second clamp should be placed near to clamp off the placental blood. The cord should be cut between the two clamps using sterile scissors. A clamp can be placed nearer the umbilicus after childbirth.

Key points
Do not clamp the cord until all pulsating has stopped.
Keep the cord clean and dry to prevent infection.

Physiology of Postpartum Mother and Newborn

Major Considerations Postdelivery

- *Thermoregulation*: Following delivery, it is best to keep mother and newborn together. The baby can be placed directly on the mother's skin and covered. This helps the newborn regulate temperature.

- *Nutrition*: Breastfeeding helps uterine contraction and, if the mother is healthy, is the best and safest nutrition for the newborn.

Assessment of the Newborn

The initial assessment of the newborn includes the APGAR score: infant's heart rate, color, respirations, muscle movement, as well as the weight and length. The APGAR score is helpful to identify infants with low scores who require immediate intervention and resuscitation but are not indicative of long-term neonatal outcomes nor asphyxia. The transition to extrauterine life involves major changes in respiration and circulation for the newborn. The provider should insure that the baby has a patent airway and is breathing. Within the first few minutes of life, the baby is expected to "pink up," losing the blueish tint in the extremities and breathing occurs. Healthy newborns have a heart rate and respiratory rate about two times that of an adult (Cunningham et al., 2010).

Heat loss is another immediate concern. The infant should be dried and remain with the mother, when possible. As the baby drinks breast milk or formula, the gastrointestinal (GI) and urinary systems will produce stool and urine. For the first 2 to 3 days of life, stool is a blackish-green paste called meconium, a product of the fetus ingesting amniotic fluid. Once milk is metabolized, the stool will appear yellowish-brown. Stools of breastfed babies are looser.

SPECIAL ASSESSMENT/CONDITIONS OF THE NEWBORN

The most important aspect of newborn assessment is insuring that the baby is breathing. Normally, newborn respirations are rapid: 30 to 40 breaths/minute. Once the baby takes breaths on its own, its color should go from blue (hands and feet) to pink. If a baby is not breathing on its own, it is important to assess the respiratory status and begin emergency neonatal management and neonatal resuscitation.

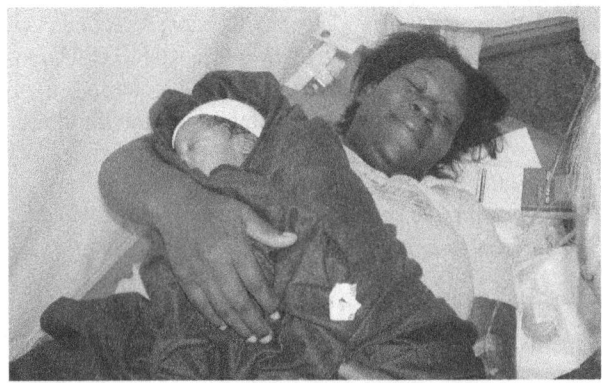

FIGURE 13.1 First baby born at Louis Armstrong Airport during Hurricane Katrina, delivered by Robbie Prepas, CNM.

POSTPARTUM MANAGEMENT IN DISASTERS

Unless the mother or baby is critically ill, it is best to keep the mother and baby together. The mother/baby dyad is the standard for care. In disasters, if evacuation is required, keep the mother and baby together. The mother can hold the infant on her body and be covered for transport. The mother and baby require clean facilities with access to clean water, food, and fluids for the mother. The baby should have a separate, clean sleeping area next to the mother and should be designed in such a way as to prevent falls.

SPECIAL CONSIDERATIONS FOR MOTHER AND BABY IN DISASTERS

Women who give birth and the infants to whom they give birth during disasters will have higher rates of complications than those during nondisaster periods. Crisis situations and emergencies place postpartum women at greater risk of adverse outcomes because of the sudden and prolonged loss of medical support; disruption of normal rest and maternal and infant bonding; and increased risk of trauma, disease, and exposure to civil unrest and violence. There are physiological and anatomical changes in pregnancy; risk of trauma to mother and fetus increases with gestational age (ACOG, 2017; Goodman, 2016).

INFECTIONS AND COMMUNICABLE DISEASES

Prevention of infection is key to perinatal care. The most important intervention to prevent infection is handwashing, a fact that cannot be overemphasized. Perinatal care must be conducted in as clean an environment as possible and all providers who have contact with the mother and infant must wash their hands before each procedure or encounter.

Special Infectious Disease Considerations

Respiratory Isolation

This is required for patients with the following.

- *Varicella (chickenpox)*: Because a pregnant woman's immune system is suboptimal, varicella can pose life-threatening complications including pneumonia. *Note*: Providers should be immune to varicella. Treatment of the virus includes supportive care and respiratory isolation from nonimmune people until the disease has resolved (Harms, 2010).
- *Meningococcal meningitis*: Should a pregnant woman be suspected of having bacterial meningitis, immediate treatment with antibiotics is indicated. Symptoms are a stiff neck and high fever. The diagnosis is confirmed by a spinal tap. Place the patient on respiratory isolation.
- *H1N1 (influenza)*: Requires supportive care including respiratory support and hydration in severe cases. Tamiflu can be given to mitigate the course of the infection. Isolate the patient, using contact precautions.

- *Influenza*: Respiratory support and hydration in severe cases. Tamiflu can be given to mitigate the course of the infection.
- *Pandemic flu*: Cohort the affected patients. Use contact precautions and respiratory isolation (Beigi, 2007).
- *Tuberculosis*: Requires respiratory isolation and supportive care. The mother and affected family should be treated with appropriate antibiotics prior to exposing the baby.
- *Thrombophlebitis*: Blood clots, particularly of the legs, can cause swelling and tenderness. Anticoagulation may be required (Cunningham et al., 2010).
- *Pyleonephritis*: Infections of the kidney cause hyperthermia, bacteriuria, pain, nausea, and vomiting. Kidney infections postpartum are uncommon (Cunningham et al., 2010).

ENVIRONMENTAL CLEANLINESS AND SANITATION

The degree of devastation caused by a disaster will depend on the type, scope, and duration of the specific disaster event. Most commonly, disasters are noted for destroying the existing environment which may include critical components of the healthcare system. When hospitals are impacted, alternative sites must be considered for the provision of obstetrical care. Alternatives may range from satellite/mobile field hospitals to any facility or building that can be located where a safe, clean place for birth can be established. A clean source of water must be available. If not, arrangements should be made to bring water to the site.

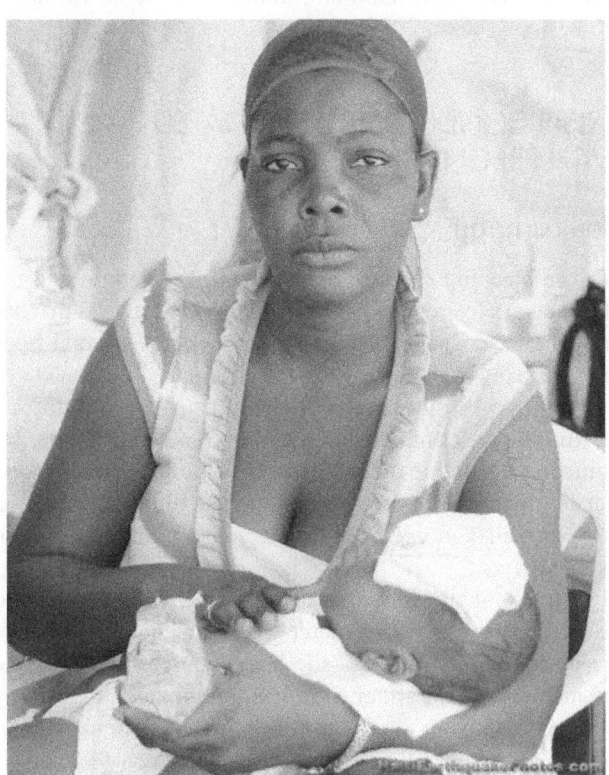

FIGURE 13.2 Haitian mother and daughter after the earthquake.

BIOTERRORISM

A bioterrorist event or a naturally emerging infectious disease outbreak creates additional challenges for the protection of the pregnant woman and fetus. Assessments for exposure to the pathogen as well as the need for vaccinations and/or treatment should be conducted as soon as possible.

TRAUMA IN PREGNANCY

There is a huge challenge in caring for women following a terrorist event: assessment and treatment of the trauma patient and treatment of the pregnant woman. Some injuries may be obvious and others can be severe and it is important to do a full assessment and history of the pregnant woman to ensure the prompt treatment of the trauma patient (James, 2005).

Performing Cardiopulmonary Resuscitation

When planning a trauma response, it is important for all providers to be familiar with the modifications in performing cardiopulmonary resuscitation (CPR) on pregnant women. Ventilating during CPR can be complicated by the increased oxygen equipment and reduced chest compliance in pregnancy. The reduced compliance is due to rib flaring and splinting of the diaphragm by the displaced abdominal contents. In the supine position, the weight of the gravid uterus compresses the large vessels in the abdomen resulting in vena caval and aortocaval syndromes.

BREASTFEEDING AND INFANT NUTRITION

Promoting breastfeeding is always best for mothers and babies, and never more important than during a disaster. The new mother must be kept well hydrated, with large volumes of clean fluids. Both the infant and new mother must *never* receive contaminated fluid. It is essential that all sources of nutrition and supplies *not* be contaminated. If a mother is too sick to feed her baby, ready-to-feed formulas can be used, if available.

Breastfeeding should be initiated immediately upon birth, as long as mother and baby are healthy. Colostrum, a thick yellowish fluid, is first produced by the mother. This helps clean out the baby's GI system and provides antibodies. On the third day postpartum, the mother's breast milk usually "comes in." Breast milk appears thin, and sometimes bluish.

Key to the production of breast milk is adequate nutrition and hydration of the mother. The mother needs increased clean fluids and calories to support breastfeeding. Breastfeeding should be "on demand" at all times and not on a fixed schedule. Common breastfeeding issues include:

- *Latching on*: The baby's mouth should grasp on to the entire nipple, with the jaws on the areola.
- *Inverted nipples*: Should be pulled out to allow the infant to grasp them.

- Babies are initially awake immediately after birth. Thereafter they are sleepy and may need to be stimulated, by rubbing their backs, feet, or blowing gently into their faces.

Breastfeeding Challenges

There are numerous challenges for successful breastfeeding after disaster. In areas within significant environmental damage, people may be living in tents or housed together in large areas, providing little to no privacy. Efforts should be made to identify areas for lactating women and their babies to nurse privately and comfortably. Reducing the stress of breastfeeding is important to support the mother's milk supply. Shawls and scarves should be provided to facilitate breastfeeding (Sulaiman et al., 2016).

Infant Formula

While well-intended companies may donate infant formulas postdisaster, breastfeeding is best. Local conditions, including the lack of refrigeration and a contaminated water supply, may not support the storage and preparation of infant formula. In fact, infant morbidity and mortality is increased when infant formula is distributed in disasters without control or regulation (Sulaiman et al., 2016).

Relactation

For mothers who had stopped breastfeeding or had bottle-fed from birth, relactation is a good option during disaster. Relactation is the resumption of breastfeeding for mothers who have stopped or the initiation of mothers who have not breastfed or even delivered a baby. Since breastfeeding is better and safer than bottle-feeding, women in disasters should consider relactation even if they never breastfed before. Steps to relactation include adequate fluid and calorie intake for the woman, and putting the baby to the breast to suckle every 2 to 3 hours. The nipple stimulation will stimulate milk production. Even if there is not yet milk, the baby should be put to the breast to suck after bottle-feeding. Most women will be able to successfully relactate, including grandmothers and nulliparous women (Bonyata, 2016).

See Appendix 13.1 to this chapter for additional information concerning breastfeeding during a natural disaster.

LACK OF FOOD, MALNUTRITION, AND STARVATION

The availability of safe water and food is essential to survival after a disaster. Natural disasters and long-term wars pose the biggest challenges. A food crisis occurs when the daily supply of food drops severely, below the average food level for the past 3 years and when the food supply declines negatively (Adedeji, Gieck-Bricco, & Kehayova, 2016). For example, the hurricane in Haiti caused food crises; the September 11 terrorist attack in New York did not. Vulnerability to food crises in natural disasters is higher for countries whose financial institutions

are weak, per the World Bank, and where there is low growth in the food supply.

What does one do for food in a disaster? Preplanning is essential. Areas prone to natural disasters should stockpile water and food, including staples and protein. Immediately when a disaster occurs, healthcare professionals should identify sources of food and plan for food for all those in their care and staff. Plans should include storing food for a period of time, allowing for difficult access (Lancet, 2017).

For newborns, the best intervention is breastfeeding. Prudhon, Benelli, Maclaine, Harrigan, and Frize (2017) report that optimizing breastfeeding could prevent 20% of deaths for children under age 5 in natural disasters and conflicts. All mothers should be urged to breastfeed, including those who had stopped or not breastfed. (See the section on Breastfeeding and Relactation.) Formula and breast milk substitutes undermine breastfeeding. Mothers need an adequate supply of clean water, fluids, and food to feed their infants.

Following the Great East Japan Earthquake in 2011, numerous lessons were learned about feeding following a devastating disaster. Building adequate stockpiles of food and water was a challenge. Staff did not know how much food to store and where to store it. Many had inadequate stockpiles as it was difficult to check expiration dates. Researchers recommended that food with longer shelf lives be stored. Key was selection of food items that were tasty. Attempting to serve food that was salted and unappealing was unsuccessful. When planning for the care of women and children, stockpiling good-tasting food and using rolling stock was essential (Amitani, Sudo, Tsuboyama-Kasaoka, Ishikawa, & Sako, 2017).

CRISIS CONDITIONS ASSOCIATED WITH PREGNANCY

Hemorrhage

Profuse bleeding can occur after the infant is born and the placenta is delivered most often from a relaxed uterus that has not contracted. If this type of bleeding occurs, several steps must be taken immediately to save a woman's life.

Massage the uterus through the mother's abdomen to stimulate a contraction. If the uterus fails to contract immediately, do bimanual compression of the uterus using sterile gloves. With a fist in the vagina and other hand on the woman's abdomen, the uterus is compressed between the hands.

At the same time, if medications are available they should be used, such as oxytocin, methergine, or cytotec to stimulate the uterus to contract. Put the baby to breast and/or have the mother or her partner stimulate the mother's nipples by rubbing or sucking to release endogenous oxytocin. Inspect the placenta to see if any fragments have been retained. If so, it will be necessary to manually remove them. *Note*: The women should be transferred to a tertiary center as soon as possible.

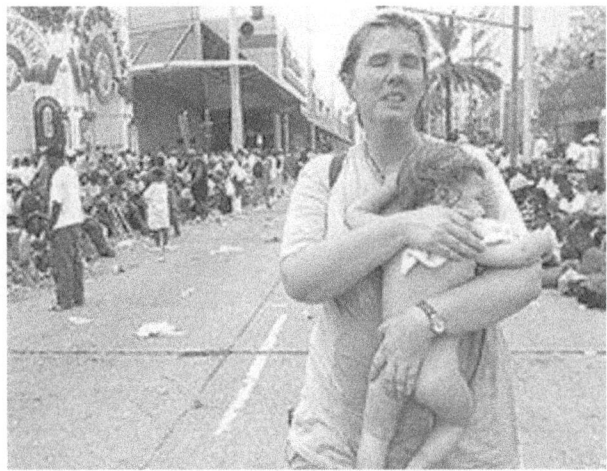

FIGURE 13.3 Mother with toddler during Hurricane Katrina in New Orleans, LA.

INFECTIONS IN POSTPARTUM AND LACTATING WOMEN DURING DISASTERS

Infections can be caused by many organisms, can affect any body system, and can present with a multitude of symptoms. Infections can cause complications such as preterm labor, premature rupture of amniotic membranes, anemia, and congenital malformations. Presenting signs and symptoms of infection include fever, pain, increased pulse, cold or flu-like symptoms, dysuria, abdominal pain, foulsmelling vaginal discharge, and malaise.

Hyperthermia (a temperature greater than 38°C or 100.4°F) soon after childbirth is indicative of a postpartum pelvic infection or genital tract infection. Temperatures greater than 39°C in the first 24 hours after delivery may be signs of an extremely virulent pelvic infection, for example, *Streptococcus A* or *B*. These require immediate treatment with IV antibiotics (Cunningham et al., 2010).

- Some infections can seriously impact on mother and or baby. Many infections can be avoided with basic practices, such as
- Washing hands
- Maintaining a clean environment
- Minimizing the number of vaginal exams of the woman in labor
- Encouraging the woman to urinate hourly while in labor
- Using only sterilized instruments and clean clothes in caring for mother and baby (Women or newborns with infections should be transferred as soon as possible [Keeney, 2004].)

HIV—AIDS

See the WHO bulletin, *Breast is always best, even for HIV-positive mothers* (http://www.who.int/bulletin/volumes/88/1/10-030110/en/).

Zika Virus

The Zika virus is a mosquito-borne virus transmitted by the mosquito *Aedes aegypti*, which also transmits dengue and chikungunya viruses. It is now found around the world in areas with mosquito infections, including Texas, Florida, all of Central America, South America, Central Africa, and South Asia from Pakistan and India on the west to the Philippines, Indonesia, and the Solomon Islands on the east. When the virus infects pregnant women, the fetus is at risk of microcephaly and defects of the eye and brain. Supportive care is the only available treatment available now. However, there is hope that a vaccine will be developed to prevent Zika. Pregnant women and women who may become pregnant are advised not to visit these areas of the world. This includes relief workers; there is no medication or vaccine. Since it is also sexually transmitted, men who have visited a Zika outbreak area should use condoms when having sexual relations to prevent transmission (Centers for Disease Control and Prevention [CDC], 2017; Oduyebo et al., 2016).

Ebola Virus Disease

Known in Africa for decades, Ebola is a devastating virus that is highly communicable though direct contact. The virus causes fever, severe headache, weakness, severe vomiting and diarrhea, abdominal and generalized pain, and massive hemorrhage. Symptoms may appear anywhere from 2 to 21 days after exposure to Ebola, but the average is 8 to 10 days. Recovery from Ebola depends on good supportive clinical care and the patient's immune response. People who recover from Ebola infection develop antibodies that last for at least 10 years. Aid workers and medical personnel have succumbed to the illness while caring for affected cases. Pregnant women should avoid areas with Ebola virus disease (CDC, 2014). Treatment is supportive care (hydration, fluids) with all workers using personal protective equipment (PPE) sealing them from the virus shed by the victims.

In healthcare settings, Ebola is spread through direct contact with blood or body fluids of a person who is sick with Ebola or with objects (e.g., bathroom surfaces, medical equipment) that have been contaminated with infectious blood or body fluids. The virus in blood and body fluids can enter a person's body through broken skin or unprotected mucous membranes

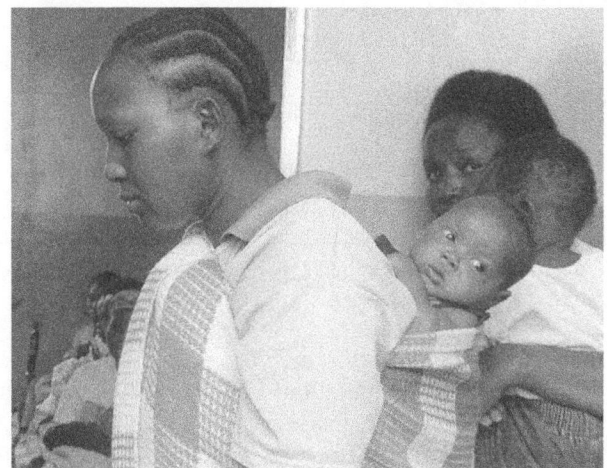

FIGURE 13.4 Mother and baby in Haiti after the earthquake.

in, for example, the eyes, nose, or mouth. For all healthcare workers caring for patients with Ebola, PPE that fully covers skin and clothing and prevents any exposure of the eyes, nose, and mouth is recommended to reduce the risk of accidental self-contamination of mucous membranes or broken skin (CDC, 2015). All PPE must be used in the context of a comprehensive infection control program that follows CDC recommendations and applicable Occupational Safety and Health Act of 1970 (OSHA) requirements, including the Bloodborne Pathogens (29 CFR 1910.1030), PPE (29 CFR 1910.132), and Respiratory Protection (20 CFR 1910.134) standards, and other requirements under OSHA (e.g., the General Duty Clause, section 5[a][1]; and prohibitions against discrimination or retaliation against workers, section 11[c]).

SHELTERS AND PRACTICAL CONSIDERATIONS FOR AUSTERE ENVIRONMENTS

All shelters must be prepared to meet the needs of pregnant women and families with infants. These requirements include:

- A plan to provide prenatal care and well-baby services at the shelter
- A plan to ensure access to a safe environment for safe delivery
- Plans to keep families and infants together and reconnect with families and infants
- An identification system for women and children using ID bracelets
- Health and hygiene needs for mothers and infants and pregnant women that include:
  - *For babies*: ready-to-feed formula, diapers, premature diapers, pacifiers, infant clothes, and breast pumps
  - *For mothers*: sanitary napkins and clean underwear
- Necessary furniture and equipment such as cribs, strollers, and car seats
- Emergency birth kits (ACOG, 2010; CDC, 2011)

DEATH OF THE MOTHER OR INFANT—BEREAVEMENT CONCERNS AND INTERVENTIONS

Despite emergency interventions in a disaster, the death of a mother or infant, whether born or unborn, requires care and special interventions.

Maternal Death

The death of a pregnant woman or new mother is not acceptable in our society. Sudden death of a woman in the perinatal period may be due to:

- *Pulmonary or amniotic embolism.* Treatment of these life-threatening complications is supportive; supporting cardiac and respiratory function.
- *Infection.* Prevention is key, using handwashing, and a clean environment and technique.

- *Bleeding.* Should the mother experience a life-threatening bleeding emergency (e.g., placenta abruption), it may lead to DIC.
- *Accident.* Unexpected death in a disaster.

When the mother dies, it is critical to provide immediate support to the grieving family and provide care for the infant, if healthy.

Perinatal Death

The death of a fetus or newborn, through miscarriage, fetal demise, stillbirth, or neonatal death, is a devastating, life-changing experience. Pregnancy loss is much more common than maternal death. Even if the pregnancy was early, the mother and her significant others may experience grief.

Healing Professional Interventions in Maternal/Perinatal Bereavement

Should a mother and/or her baby die during a disaster, the caregivers should acknowledge the losses, giving value to the life, even if yet to be born (Capitulo, 2005). Additionally, professionals should recognize that their actions should focus on healing, caring, comfort, and support. For surviving family members, what professionals say and do at this vulnerable time will be remembered for a lifetime. The bereaved want to make meaning of the experience. Spiritual rituals, such as baptism for Christians, naming, blessing, and funerals, help them make meaning. If possible, funeral rites and burial rituals should be followed, which may be a challenge in a disaster. Some find support from clergy and have both a dependence on and anger at God (Nuzum, Meaney, & O'Donoghue, 2017).

See Table 13.1, Professional Dos and Don'ts in Bereavement Care (Capitulo, 2005). Which bereavement interventions are healing and which are not?

RETURNING HOME SAFELY

The postpartum woman and newborn must take precautions to stay safe during and after a disaster or emergency event. According to the March of Dimes (2016), potential dangers exist in returning to home after disaster.

Flood Water in Streets and Buildings

Flood water may contain harmful substances such as chemicals, gasoline, or bacteria that could cause serious disease. It is best if children and pregnant women avoid touching or walking in flood water. If individuals do touch the water, they should use soap and clean water to wash the parts of the body that came in contact with it. Whenever possible, people who must come in contact with the water should wear protective clothing, such as gloves and boots. If a woman is pregnant, she should be especially careful not to swallow any floodwater. If she feels sick in any way, she should be encouraged to talk to a doctor, provider, or nurse right away.

TABLE 13.1 Professional Dos and Don'ts in Bereavement Care

Dos	Don'ts

• Inform the family of the death. Use the word "died."
 • Say "I'm sorry."
 • Use the name of the deceased, or in the case of a yet unnamed baby, use the gender, e.g., "baby girl."
 • Provide time for the bereaved to spend with the deceased, unless there is a life-threatening infectious epidemic that requires the deceased being isolated.
 • Provide ways to say "good-bye."
 • Provide memories: a lock of hair, photo, article of clothing, and all associated paperwork are important.
 • Provide appropriate rituals.
   • Spiritual rituals, depending on the family's beliefs, may include religious blessings or rituals, such as baptism. These can be done by a religious person, such as a chaplain, if available. If not, spiritual rituals can be performed by any caring person, including the nurse. Ask the family what they would like to do. Facilitate and organize the rituals. In cases where the body must be isolated, the family can still have rituals and prayers.
   • Wakes and funerals can be done even during a disaster. Even if the bereaved are not spiritual or religious, words of farewell are important in the bereavement process.
   • If showing a deceased body to loved ones, clean the body and present it clothed. If parts of the body are not present, make it as presentable as possible.
   • In mass casualties where individual bodies cannot be viewed, group funerals may be organized.
 • Find other sources of support for the bereaved, including family and friends. After the disaster, the bereaved can be connected to support groups.
 • Know that grief lasts a lifetime, but over time, the bereaved may find peace and keep the death in their hearts.
 • In cases of complicated grief, in which the bereaved cannot function, they should be referred to bereavement counselors or psychologists.
	• Use the word "lost," which implies the deceased will be found.
	 • Make excuses.
	 • Call the baby a "fetus," a "product of conception," or a "specimen."
	 • Rush through the process or limit time with the deceased, whenever possible.
	 • Act as if the death did not happen.
	 • Prohibit collection of mementos and memories, including photographs.
	 • Ban rituals, funerals, and wakes.
	 • Deny spiritual rituals because there is no chaplain; a nurse can pray and perform spiritual rituals.
	 • Deny rituals because you don't know what to do or don't have time. Find another to help.
	 • Deny rituals in the case of mass casualties or infectious diseases.
	 • Show the body full of blood or in pieces.
	 • Show a fetus in a specimen bucket. Place it on a clean cloth or baby blanket.
	 • Ignore the needs of the bereaved. Don't use euphemisms, such as "it's better they died, they were so sick," "you're young; you can have another one." Or "pretend it was a bad dream and didn't really happen."
	 • Pretend that grief doesn't exist or will be short term.

Source: Capitulo, K. (2005). Evidence for healing interventions with perinatal bereavement. *MCN, The American Journal of Maternal–Child Nursing, 30*(6), 389–396.

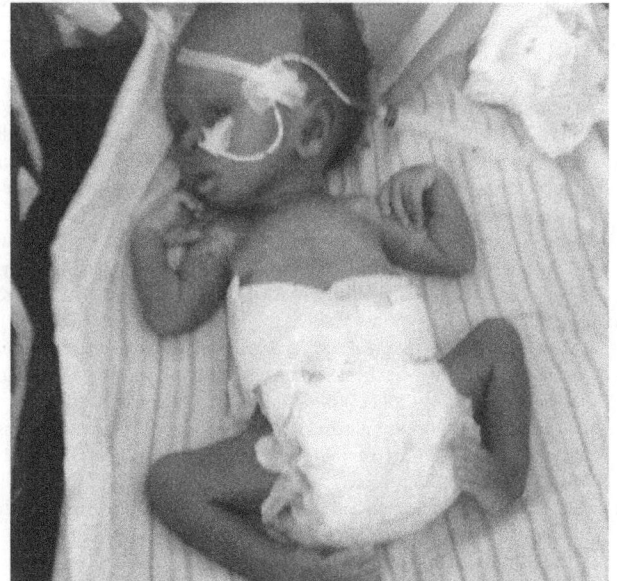

FIGURE 13.5 Abandoned baby in Haiti after the earthquake.

Toxic Exposures During Pregnancy

If a pregnant woman is worried that she may have been exposed to dangerous chemicals or substances during or following the disaster, she should be encouraged to talk to a healthcare provider.

The Organization of Teratology Information Specialists (OTIS, 2018) offers free telephone counseling and a fact sheet on pregnancy and natural disasters to pregnant women worried about toxic exposures (https://mothertobaby.org).

Returning Home

Pregnant women may face several possible dangers when returning home, depending on their individual circumstances and the damage to their homes. If a woman is pregnant and her home has been damaged, it may be best to ask disaster workers, family members, and friends to assist with cleanup. Possible hazards that could threaten her health and pregnancy include:

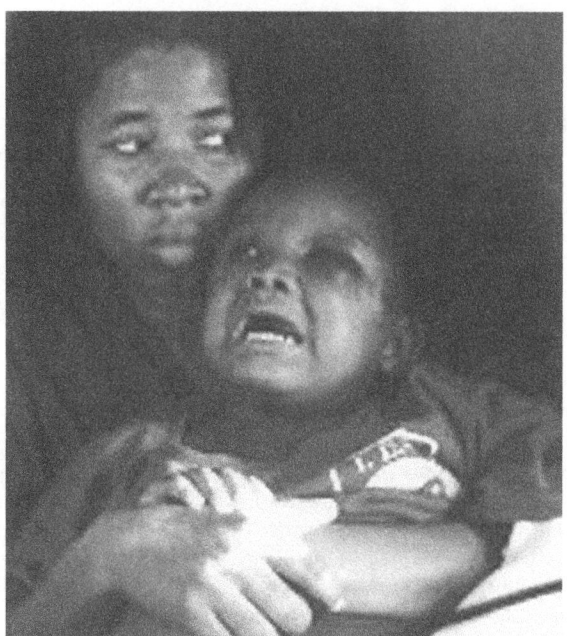

FIGURE 13.6 Young Haitian earthquake victim.

- Pollutants such as bacteria and mold that have contaminated household items
- Hard physical work (e.g., carrying and lifting heavy items)
- Falling while stepping over debris
- Electrical shocks

RISK OF VIOLENCE, ABUSE, SLAVERY, AND HUMAN TRAFFICKING

In disasters, large populations of people may be displaced. Vulnerable populations, including women, teens, and children are at higher risk of abuse following disasters. Postearthquake studies in Haiti found displaced adolescent girls and women at risk of abuse and violence (Sloand et al., 2017). Child and human trafficking and slavery increase after disasters, particularly in impoverished areas. Orphaned children may be taken in as domestic help and are at high risk of physical and sexual abuse. Women and children are particularly at risk of sexual abuse. Slavery and trafficking include forced marriages, work, military services, and sexual abuse and violence (Childs, 2016; Gupta & Agrawal, 2010).

POSTTRAUMATIC STRESS DISORDER

Experiencing a traumatic event such as disaster is a precipitating factor for developing PTSD (North, Oliver, & Pandya, 2012). These researchers studied survivors of 10 major American disasters from 1987 to 1995, including intentionally caused disasters, such as mass shootings and terrorist bombings; natural disasters, such as hurricanes, tornados, floods, and earthquakes; and technological accidents, including plane crashes, hotel disasters, and fires. Participants in the study were 811 survivors of the 10 disasters, with more than 33.3% witnessing injuries or deaths; 33.3% sustaining injuries needing

medical treatment; some having a family or friend killed; and more than 50% knowing someone injured or killed. Of the survivors, 20% had PTSD, 16% had major depressions (with more than half of these having a preexisting depression), and 9% developed an alcohol disorder. PTSD symptoms included numbing and avoidance, and hyperarousal. The type of disaster did not predict the development of PTSD. However, survivors of a disaster, including those sent in to help, are at higher risk of PTSD and professional psychological/psychiatric assessment and intervention.

SUMMARY

Disasters provide substantial challenges to providing care to the pregnant woman and newborn. Rapid assessment and effective appropriate care of the pregnant woman are essential. Establishing a safe and clean environment with access to clean water must be considered a priority whenever possible. Nursing assessments of the physical and psychological needs of the intra- and postpartum woman and newborn should be ongoing throughout the birth process and the duration of the disaster event. Despite the devastation of the event, nurses should strive to provide consistent, optimal levels of care to ensure the best possible outcomes.

REFERENCES

Adedeji, O., Gieck-Bricco, J., & Kehayova, V. (2016). *Natural disasters and food crises in low-income countries: Macroeconomic dimensions* (International Monetary Fund, Working Paper 16/65). Retrieved from https://www.imf.org/external/pubs/ft/wp/2016/wp1665.pdf

American College of Obstetricians and Gynecologists. (2010). Preparing for disasters: Perspectives on women. Committee Opinion No. 457. *Obstetrics and Gynecology, 115*, 1339–1342. doi:10.1097/AOG.0b013e3181e45a6f. Retrieved from http://www.acog.org/Resources_And_Publications/Committee_Opinions/Committee_on_Health_Care_for_Underserved_Women/Preparing_for_Disasters_Perspectives_on_Women

American College of Obstetricians and Gynecologists. (2013). Hypertension in pregnancy. Retrieved from https://www.acog.org/~/media/Task%20Force%20and%20Work%20Group%20Reports/public/HypertensioninPregnancy.pdf

American College of Obstetricians and Gynecologists. (2017). Hospital disaster preparedness for obstetricians and facilities providing maternity care. Committee opinion NO. 726. Obstetrics and Gynecology, 130 e 291-7. Retrieved from https://www.acog.org/Clinical-Guidance-and-Publications/Committee-Opinions/Committee-on-Obstetric-Practice/Hospital-Disaster-Preparedness-for-Obstetricians-and-Facilities-Providing-Maternity-Care

Amitani, Y., Sudo, N., Tsuboyama-Kasaoka, N., Ishikawa, F., & Sako, K. (2017). Meal services after the great east Japan earthquake at nursery schools in a tsunami-affected town: Focus group observations. *Asia Pacific Journal of Clinical Nursing, 26*(2), 308–312. doi:10.6133/apjcn.012016.05

Beigi, R. H. (2007). Pandemic influenza and pregnancy: A call for preparedness planning. *Obstetrics & Gynecology, 109*(5), 1193–1196. doi:10.1097/01.AOG.0000262051.71925.ac

Bonyata, K. (2016). Relactation and adoptive breastfeeding: The basics. *Kelly Mom, Parenting and Breastfeeding.* Retrieved from http://kellymom.com/bf/got-milk/relactation/

Bookman, L., Troy, R., McCaffrey, M., & Randolph, G. (2010). Using quality-improvement methods to reduce variation in surfactant administration. *Quality and Safety in Health Care, 19*(5), e23. doi:10.1136/qshc.2009.034967

Callaghan, W. M., Rasmussen, S. A., Jamieson, D. J., Ventura, S., Farr, S. L., Sutton, P., . . . Posner, S. (2007). Health concerns of women and infants in times of natural disasters: Lessons learned from Hurricane Katrina. *Maternal Child Health Journal, 11*(4), 307–311. doi:10.1007/s10995-007-0177-4

Capitulo, K. (2005). Evidence for healing interventions with perinatal bereavement. *MCN, The American Journal of Maternal–Child Nursing, 30*(6), 389–396. doi:10.1097/00005721-200511000-00007

Centers for Disease Control and Prevention. (2007). Critical needs in caring for pregnant women during times of disaster for non-obstetric health care providers. Retrieved from http://www2.wpro.who.int/internet/files/eha/toolkit/web/Technical%20References/Special%20Populations/CDC%20Caring%20for%20Pregnant%20Women%20During%20Disaster.pdf

Centers for Disease Control and Prevention. (2011). Disaster preparedness: After an event. Retrieved from http://www.cdc.gov/healthywater/emergency/preparedness/after.html

Centers for Disease Control and Prevention. (2014). Ebola virus disease. Retrieved from https://www.cdc.gov/vhf/ebola/symptoms/index.html

Centers for Disease Control and Prevention. (2015). Ebola virus disease, guidance on personal protective equipment (PPE). Retrieved from https://www.cdc.gov/vhf/ebola/healthcare-us/ppe/guidance.html

Centers for Disease Control and Prevention. (2017). World map of areas with risk of Zika. Retrieved from https://wwwnc.cdc.gov/travel/page/world-map-areas-with-zika

Childs, A. (2016). Why child trafficking surges after natural disaster. *The Conversation, CNN.* Retrieved from http://www.cnn.com/2016/03/23/opinions/child-trafficking-natural-disasters

Cunningham, F., Leveno, K., Bloom, S., Hauth, J., Rouse, D., & Spong, C. (2010). *Williams obstetrics* (23rd ed.). New York, NY: McGraw Hill.

Goodman, A. (2016). In the aftermath of disasters: The impact on women's health. *Obstetrics & Gynecology, 2*(6), 29. doi:10.4172/2471-9803.1000137

Gupta, J., & Agrawal, A. (2010). Chronic aftershocks of an earthquake on the well-being of children in Haiti: Violence, psychosocial health and slavery. *Canadian Medical Association Journal, 182*(18), 1997–1999. doi:10.1503/cmaj.100526

Harms, R. (2010). What are the risks associated with chickenpox in pregnancy? Retrieved from http://www.mayoclinic.com/health/chickenpox-and-pregnancy/HO00036

James, D. (2005). Terrorism and the pregnant woman. *Journal of Perinatal and Neonatal Nursing, 19,* 226–237.

Keeney, G. B. (2004). Disaster preparedness: What do we do now? *Journal of Midwifery & Women's Health, 49*(4 Suppl 1), 2–6. doi:10.1016/j.jmwh.2004.05.003

Kridli, S. A. (2011). Health beliefs and practices of Muslim women during Ramadan. *MCN, The American Journal of Maternal–Child Nursing, 36*(4), 216–221. doi:10.1097/NMC.0b013e3182177177

Lipkind, H. S., Curry, A. E., Huynh, M., Thorpe, L. E., & Matte, T. (2010). Birth outcomes among offspring of women exposed to the September 11, 2001, terrorist attacks. *Obstetrics & Gynecology, 116,* 917–925. doi:10.1097/AOG.0b013e3181f2f6a2

Maloni, J. (2010). Antepartum bed rest for pregnancy complications: Efficacy and safety for preventing preterm birth. *Biological Research for Nursing, 12*(2), 106–124. doi:10.1177/1099800410375978

March of Dimes. (2016). Stay safe and prepare for a disaster. Retrieved from https://www.marchofdimes.org/baby/caring-for-your-family-in-a-disaster.aspx

Merck Manual. (2011a). HELLP Syndrome. Retrieved from http://www.medicinenet.com/script/main/art.asp?articlekey=8430

Merck Manual. (2011b). Physical changes during pregnancy. Retrieved from http://www.merckmanuals.com/home/womens_health_issues/normal_pregnancy/physical_changes_during_pregnancy.html

North, C., Oliver, J., & Pandya, A. (2012). Examining a comprehensive model of disaster-related posttraumatic stress disorder in systematically studied survivors of 10 disasters. *American Journal of Public Health, 102*(10), e40–e48. doi:10.2105/AJPH.2012.300689

Nuzum, D., Meaney, S., & O'Donoghue, K. (2017). The spiritual and theological challenges of stillbirth for bereaved parents. *Journal of Religious Health, 56,* 1081–1109. doi:10.1007/s10943-017-0365-5

Oduyebo, T., Petersen, E., Rasmussen, S., Mead, P., Meaney-Delman, D., Renquist, C., . . . Jamieson, D. (2016). Update: Interim guidelines for health care providers caring for pregnant women and women of reproductive age with possible Zika virus exposure—United States, 2016. Atlanta, GA: Centers for Disease Control and Prevention. Retrieved from http://www.cdc.gov/mmwr/volumes/65/wr/mm6505e2.htm

Organization of Teratology Information Specialists. (2018). Fact sheet, pregnancy and natural disasters. Retrieved from https://mothertobaby.org/fact-sheets/natural-disasters/pdf

Orlando, S., Danna, D., Giarratano, G., Prepas, R., & Johnson, C. B. (2010). Perinatal considerations in the hospital disaster management process. *Journal of Obstetrics, Gynecologic & Neonatal Nursing, 39*(4), 466–478. doi:10.1111/j.1552-6909.2010.01158.x

Pfeiffer, J., Avery, M. D., Prepas, R., Summers, L., Wachdorf, C. M., & O'Boyle, C. (2008). Maternal and newborn care during disasters: Thinking outside the hospital paradigm. *Nursing Clinics of North America, 43*(3), 449–467. doi:10.1016/j.cnur.2008.04.008

Prudhon, C., Benelli, P., Maclaine, A., Harrigan, P., & Frize, J. (2017). Informing infant and young child feeding programming in humanitarian emergencies: An evidence map of reviews including low and middle income families. *Maternal and Child Nutrition, 14*(1), e12457. doi:10.1111/mcn.12457

Sloand, E., Killion, C., Yarandi, H., Sharps, P., Lewis-O'Connor, A., Hassan, M., . . . Campbell, D. (2017). Experiences of violence and abuse among internally displaced adolescent girls following a natural disaster. *Journal of Advanced Nursing, 73*(12), 3200–3208. doi:10.1111/jan.13316

Smart, D., & Princivalle, M. (2011). Improving RDS treatment with current drugs. *Journal of Maternal Fetal and Neonatal Medicine, 25,* 1209–1211. doi:10.3109/14767058.2011.634456

Sulaiman, Z., Mohamad, N., Ismail, T., Johari, N., & Hussain, N. (2016). Infant feeding concerns in times of natural disaster: Lessons learned from the 2014 flood in Kelantan, Malaysia. *Asia Pacific Journal of Clinical Nutrition, 25*(3), 625–630. doi:10.6133/apjcn.092015.08

What to Expect. (2011). Your guide to pregnancy hormones. Retrieved from http://www.whattoexpect.com/pregnancy/pregnancy-health/pregnancy-hormones.aspx

Williams, D. (2004). Giving birth "in place": A guide to emergency preparedness for childbirth. *Journal of Midwifery & Women's Health, 49*(4), 48–52. doi:10.1016/j.jmwh.2004.04.030

Appendix 13.1

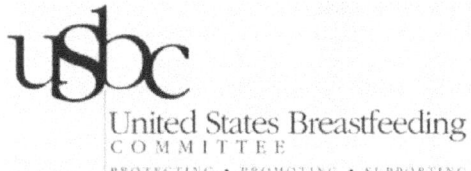

Breastfeeding:
A Vital Emergency Response.
Are You Ready?

BREASTFEEDING SAVES LIVES IN EMERGENCIES

> "While an emergency may be an unplanned event, what we CAN predict is that one will happen. What is unknown is when, where, what type, and how big the emergency will be."
> *Audrey Naylor, MD, DrPH Wellstart International*

Emergencies often occur when least expected, and sometimes when we are least prepared. They can include a wide range of unsettling events, including personal or family crises, public health emergencies (e.g., a flu pandemic), acts of terror and violence, and natural disasters or weather-related events (e.g., floods and blizzards).

Research shows that infants and children are the most vulnerable during emergencies!
- Nearly 95% of infant and child deaths in emergencies result from diarrhea due to contaminated water and an unsanitary environment.
- Infant formula has been linked to an increase in infant disease and death; it can also be contaminated and requires clean water and fuel to sterilize formula, bottles, and nipples. Lack of electricity can also make it difficult to preserve formula.
- Breastfeeding saves lives! Human milk is always clean, requires no fuel, water, or electricity, and is available, even in the direst circumstances.
- Human milk contains antibodies that fight infection, including diarrhea and respiratory infections common among infants in emergency situations.
- Human milk provides infants with perfect nutrition, including the proper amount of vitamins and minerals required for normal growth.
- Breastfeeding releases hormones that lower stress and anxiety in both babies and mothers.
- Mothers who breastfeed are able to keep their babies warm to prevent hypothermia.

MOTHERS *CAN* BREASTFEED IN AN EMERGENCY

- **The safest food in an emergency is the mother's own milk. Donor human milk is the next best option. Mothers who cannot directly feed their babies can also be supported to express their milk.**
- Women who are stressed can continue to make milk. A quiet area that helps mothers relax can help their milk flow to the baby.
- Malnourished mothers can make plenty of milk.
- Even mothers who have already discontinued breastfeeding may be able to restart breastfeeding (known as "re-lactation").
- If a baby (or mother) becomes ill, the *best* thing the mother can do is to continue breastfeeding to provide her baby with human antibodies that fight the illness.
- Support makes the difference!

2025 M Street, NW, Suite 800 ■ Washington DC 20036 ■ Phone: (202) 367-1132 ■ FAX: (202) 367-2132
E-mail: office@usbreastfeeding.org ■ Web site: www.usbreastfeeding.org

(continued)

PROTECTING AND SUPPORTING BREASTFEEDING IN AN EMERGENCY: STRATEGIES FOR RELIEF ORGANIZATIONS, HEALTHCARE PROVIDERS, AND COMMUNITIES

Before an Emergency:
- Provide breastfeeding training for all volunteers who will be assisting in emergency relief efforts.
- Incorporate policies that protect and support breastfeeding in emergencies as part of community emergency preparedness plans.
- Implement the guidelines of the *Operational Guidance on Infant and Young Child Feeding in Emergencies*, developed by the Infant Feeding in Emergencies Core Group (available at www.ennonline.net).
- Identify community resources to assist with breastfeeding, including lactation consultants, medical professionals, lay support groups, and state and local breastfeeding coalitions.

During an Emergency:
- **Feed mothers** so they can properly meet their babies' needs.
- Keep families together.
- Encourage mothers to continue breastfeeding! If a mother is pregnant, encourage her to breastfeed when her baby is born!
- Provide a safe place for mothers to breastfeed or express milk for their babies.
- Help mothers who have questions about breastfeeding to access support (see the following "Who Can Help").
- Do not solicit or accept donations of infant formula. Formula should be used only when the mother has already weaned and relactation is not possible or desired. If formula is used, use only ready-to-feed formula served in a cup (cups are easier to clean than bottles).

WHO CAN HELP

- United States Breastfeeding Coalitions: www.usbreastfeeding.org
- Knowledgeable breastfeeding support personnel:
  - International Lactation Consultant Association members: www.ilca.org/home
  - Local Women, Infants, and Children (WIC) program staff: https://www.fns.usda.gov/wic/women-infants-and-children-wic
  - La Leche League leaders: www.llli.org

ABOUT WORLD BREASTFEEDING WEEK

World Breastfeeding Week, celebrated August 1 to 7 each year in the United States, is an annual global initiative that raises awareness of the vital importance of breastfeeding. The theme is established each year by the World Alliance for Breastfeeding Advocacy. The 2009 theme, "Breastfeeding: A Vital Emergency Response. Are You Ready?" calls upon organizations and individuals in communities everywhere to include breastfeeding support as part of emergency preparedness planning. To learn more about World Breastfeeding Week and to access additional resources, visit the U.S. Breastfeeding Committee's (USBC's) website or the World Breastfeeding Week website at www.worldbreastfeedingweek.org.

ABOUT THE UNITED STATES BREASTFEEDING COMMITTEE

The USBC is an independent nonprofit coalition of 41 nationally influential professional, educational, and governmental organizations. Representing over half a million concerned professionals and the families they serve, the USBC and its member organizations share a common mission to improve the nation's health by working collaboratively to protect, promote, and support breastfeeding. For more information on the USBC, visit www.usbreastfeeding.org.

Adapted from the International Lactation Consultant Association's World Breastfeeding Week materials.

(*continued*)

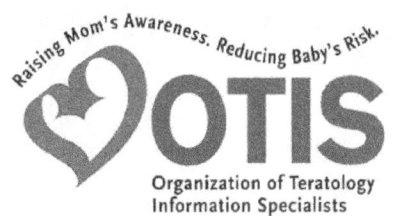

*For more information about the Organization of Teratology Information Specialists or to find a service in your area, call **(866) 626-6847** or visit us online at: **www.mothertobaby.org.***

BREASTFEEDING FOLLOWING A NATURAL DISASTER

The information that follows will help you determine whether certain exposures with which a mother might come in contact following a natural disaster are safe for her breastfed infant. This information should not take the place of medical care and advice from your healthcare provider.

Why is breastfeeding good for my baby?

There are many benefits to breastfeeding. Breast milk is the best source of nutrients for your growing baby. It can also help protect babies from infection. Breastfeeding costs much less than bottle-feeding. It is more convenient because there are no bottles to wash or formula to buy, mix, and refrigerate. If you are breastfeeding during a natural disaster, there is no need to worry about finding safe, clean water to mix formula or to wash bottles. Breastfeeding also can be soothing and reduce stress for both a mother and her baby.

How can I keep my breast milk as safe as possible?

Because many substances enter breast milk in very small amounts, they are not likely to harm a breastfed baby. In many instances, the benefits of breastfeeding far outweigh any risk from an exposure. However, it is important to know to what you are exposed and consider whether it might affect your breastfed baby.

If you notice anything unusual, tell your healthcare provider right away. This is especially important after a natural disaster, when you or your baby could be exposed to things to which you wouldn't usually be exposed.

To what could I be exposed in a natural disaster that might pass to my baby in breast milk?

Vaccinations

Vaccinations are given to protect people from serious diseases. Vaccinations are important for both a mother and a baby for their individual health. All inactivated vaccines and most live vaccines are safe to receive while breastfeeding.

Typical vaccinations you might receive following a natural disaster include hepatitis A, hepatitis B, and tetanus. In most cases, these vaccinations are okay to have while breastfeeding. Other vaccinations might be needed after some disasters. In some areas of the world, particularly in developing countries including Southeast Asia, Bacillus Calmette–Guérin (BCG) is administered. BCG is a vaccine for tuberculosis (TB) disease. Like other supplies and medications in disasters, vaccines may be in short supply (Sulaiman et al., 2016). Check with your healthcare provider and local health officials about which vaccines are recommended if a natural disaster has occurred in your area.

Infections

Some infections are common after a natural disaster. A local infection on a mother's skin usually is not dangerous to a breastfeeding baby. More serious infections such as those caused by West Nile virus, hepatitis A virus, hepatitis B virus, and others can be more complicated. If you think you have an infection, talk to your healthcare provider right away.

In general, mothers who have an infection can continue to breastfeed. If medicines are used to treat infections, it is possible for some medicines to enter breast milk and affect a breastfeeding baby (see the next section). Be sure to drink plenty of liquids when you have an infection or other illness so you don't become dehydrated. If you become severely dehydrated, it might reduce the amount of breast milk you make.

Medicines

It may be necessary to take medicine after a natural disaster if you have an infection or other illness. Many medicines are safe to take while breastfeeding. Other medicines that enter breast milk may affect a breastfeeding baby; for example, some babies are allergic to certain antibiotics that are used to treat infections. Other antibiotics may cause an upset stomach or mild diarrhea in a breastfed infant.

If you need to take medicine for any reason, be sure to tell your healthcare provider that you are breastfeeding so you get the medicine that is right for you and your baby. Watch the baby for side effects while you are taking any medicine. If your baby develops a rash, hives, or if you notice anything else unusual, tell your healthcare provider right away.

You can decrease the amount of medicine in breast milk by timing when you take your medicine and when you breastfeed. Typically it is best to nurse the baby, then take your medicine, and then wait a few hours before you nurse again. Call OTIS to get details about your medication.

Insect Repellant

Using insect repellant is an important way to help protect you from infections spread by mosquitoes. A bite from an infected mosquito could give you a serious illness such as West Nile virus.

(continued)

The most common active ingredient in insect repellant is DEET (*N,N*-diethyl-meta-toluamide). It is not known whether the DEET you put on your skin passes into breast milk. However, only about 6% to 8% of the DEET put on your skin gets into your body. This probably means that very little DEET would get into your breast milk. It is still best to limit the amount of DEET to which you are exposed while breastfeeding. Breastfeeding women should follow the same recommendations that are given for the use of DEET in children. These include applying the insect repellant with DEET to your clothing and only then putting it on exposed skin such as your hands and face. Never apply insect repellant to the breast area. Wash your hands after applying insect repellant and before handling your baby or breastfeeding so that the baby is not exposed to DEET.

Other ways to lower your chance of being bitten by a mosquito include staying indoors during peak times of mosquito activity (overnight from dusk through dawn) and wearing long pants, long-sleeved shirts, a hat, and shoes with socks while outdoors.

Cleaning Agents

Typical household use of cleaning agents is not expected to produce levels in breast milk that could hurt a baby. To help protect yourself, you can wear gloves when using cleaning agents and air out your work area so you do not breathe in the fumes.

Pollutants

Exposure to low levels of environmental chemicals usually is not a reason to stop breastfeeding. If you think that you may have been exposed to high amounts of a harmful chemical, contact your healthcare provider as soon as possible.

If you have been exposed to lead, a blood test can tell whether the level is high. The level of lead in breast milk is similar to that in the mother's blood. However, a mother should not stop breastfeeding unless the level of lead in her blood is very high.

What if I need to give my baby formula?

In most instances, it is fine to continue breastfeeding when a natural disaster occurs. If, however, you must give your baby formula, it is best to use single-serving containers of ready-to-feed formula whenever possible. This is especially important if the water supply is not clean or safe to drink or if the electricity is off. Ready-to-feed formula does not need added water and it does not need to be kept in a refrigerator. Local authorities will tell you if your water supply is safe to drink or to use for cooking or bathing.

If ready-to-feed formula is not available, use bottled water to mix powdered or concentrated formula. If bottled water is not available, use boiled water. Bringing water to a rolling boil for 1 minute will kill most disease-causing organisms, but it will not remove chemicals. If you make formula with boiled water, be sure to let it cool before giving it to your baby.

Do not use water that has been treated with iodine or chlorine tablets to prepare formula unless you do not have bottled water and cannot boil your water. Be sure to clean bottles and nipples thoroughly with bottled, boiled, or treated water before every use. Always wash your hands before preparing formula and before feeding your baby. If you do not have clean water for washing hands, use alcohol-based hand sanitizers.

Where can I find more information on specific exposures to infants through breast milk?

OTIS has fact sheets about many exposures which include information about breastfeeding. La Leche League International provides information about breastfeeding to women affected by natural disasters (www.llli.org; phone: 800-525-3243). The International Lactation Consultant Association maintains a directory of individual lactation consultants who can help with breastfeeding concerns such as reduced milk supply (www.ilca.org).

February 2011.
Copyright by OTIS.
Reproduced by permission.

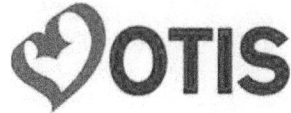

SELECTED REFERENCES

American Academy of Pediatrics. (2015). Infant Feeding in Disasters and Emergencies. Retrieved from https://www.aap.org/en-us/advocacy-and-policy/aap-health-initiatives/Breastfeeding/Documents/InfantNutritionDisaster.pdf

Centers for Disease Control and Prevention. Breastfeeding: Recommendations: Vaccinations. Retrieved from http://www.cdc.gov/breastfeeding/recommendations/vaccinations.htm

Centers for Disease Control and Prevention. Breastfeeding: Infectious diseases and specific conditions affecting human milk. Retrieved from http://www.cdc.gov/breastfeeding/disease/index.htm

Gartner, L. M., Morton, J., Lawrence, R. A., Naylor, A. J., O'Hare, D., Schanler, R. J., & Eidelman, A. I.; American Academy of Pediatrics Section on Breastfeeding. (2005). Breastfeeding and the use of human milk. *Pediatrics, 115*(2), 496–506. doi:10.1542/peds.2004-2491

General Recommendations on Immunization. (2002, February 8). Recommendations of the Advisory Committee on Immunization Practices (ACIP) and the American Academy of Family Physicians (AAFP). *Morbidity and Mortality Weekly Report, 51*(RR-2), 1–36.

World Health Organization. (2002). Breastfeeding and maternal medication. Recommendations for drugs in the eleventh WHO model list of essential drugs. Retrieved from http://whqlibdoc.who.int/hq/2002/55732.pdf

*If you have questions about the information on this fact sheet or other exposures during pregnancy, call **OTIS** at **1-866-626-6847**.*

Section III

GLOBAL DISASTERS AND COMPLEX HUMAN EMERGENCIES

14

DISASTER NURSING AND THE UNITED NATIONS 2015 LANDMARK AGREEMENTS—A VITAL FORCE FOR CHANGE IN THE FIELD OF DISASTER NURSING

Rishma Maini, Joanne Bosanquet, and Virginia Murray

LEARNING OBJECTIVES

When this chapter is completed, readers will be able to:

1. Describe the Sendai Framework for Disaster Risk Reduction (SFDRR) 2015 to 2030, Sustainable Development Goals (SDGs), and the Paris Climate Agreement.
2. Identify important synergies between these agreements and the need for coherence between them.
3. Understand the relevance of these global agreements, particularly the Sendai agreement, for disaster nursing.
4. Understand how nurses can actively engage with these frameworks and provide vital roles, including leadership, in the field of disaster nursing.
5. Describe the roles of organizations such as the International Council of Nurses (ICN), International Confederation of Midwives (ICM), National Nursing Associations (NNAs), and World Health Organization (WHO) structures in coordinating disaster risk reduction efforts.

2015 marked an important year for the adoption of several United Nations (UN) Agreements including the SFDRR 2015 to 2030, SDGs, and the Paris Climate Agreement.

The Sendai Framework is a 15-year nonbinding agreement which recognizes that the State has the primary role to reduce disaster risk but that responsibility should be shared with other stakeholders including local government.

Nurses and midwives have vital roles and responsibilities under the UN landmark agreements of 2015. These include leadership in the development of disaster nursing to reflect the Sendai Framework priorities for action.

Nurses should be encouraged to be part of the agreed local, national, regional, and global mechanisms to address all the needs for disaster nursing from disaster preparedness for understanding risk to effective response and to "Build Back Better" in recovery, rehabilitation, and reconstruction.

Leadership by nurses to support the health and well-being agenda, as part of the implementation of the UN landmark agreements, will be fundamental to achieving success.

CHAPTER OVERVIEW

The Sendai Framework was the first major agreement of the post-2015 development agenda and recognizes that the State has the primary role to reduce disaster risk but that responsibility should be shared with other stakeholders including local governments. Specific emphasis is made on the need to support health and care professionals and particularly disaster nurses to implement resilience-building measures and shift away from managing crises to proactively reducing risks of their occurrence. This chapter will demonstrate how disaster nurses can engage actively and provide leadership that will assist the successful implementation of the recently adopted UN frameworks, particularly the SFDRR.

DISASTERS AND THEIR IMPACTS

A "disaster" is defined as: "a serious disruption of the functioning of a community or a society at any scale due to hazardous events interacting with conditions of exposure, vulnerability and capacity, leading to one or more of the following: human, material, economic and environmental losses and impacts" (United Nations International Strategy for Disaster Reduction [UNISDR], 2017).

Disasters may be human-induced (e.g., armed conflict, environmental degradation, industrial pollution) or natural (e.g., flood, earthquake, drought, and volcano). Any type of disaster, however, can interrupt essential services, such as the provision of health and care services, electricity, water, sewage/waste removal, transportation, and communications, seriously affecting the health, social, and economic networks of local communities and countries long after the disaster has struck (UNISDR, 2017).

Disasters also often result in significant impacts on people's health and well-being, including the loss of many lives. However, deaths, injuries, diseases, disabilities, psychosocial problems, and other health-related impacts can be avoided or reduced by effective risk-management measures involving health and other sectors (World Conference on Disaster Risk Reduction [WCDRR], 2014).

Risk is differentially distributed between and within countries. Vulnerable groups of individuals and communities require special attention during and after a disaster (WCDRR, 2014). Those who experience disaster may suffer from ill health and harm against their person and property (e.g., loss of household possessions, livestock).

It is estimated that women and children account for more than three quarters of all people affected by disaster, and approximately one in five women of childbearing age could be pregnant. (ICM, 2017a, p. 1)

Women as well as underserved groups are particularly ill prepared and have difficulty surviving and recovering from disasters due to discrimination (e.g., age, disability, and culture; Baker & Cormier, 2014; Bolin, 2007; Fothergill, Maestas, & Darlington, 1999). For example, gender inequality may lead to differences in legal status (e.g., land rights), lack of access to education, less mobility (due to family obligations), and economic insecurity, all of which render women particularly vulnerable to the repercussions of disasters.

Figure 14.1 illustrates the impacts disasters have had between 2000 and 2012 in terms of numbers affected, damages, and mortality. In 2015 alone, from 346 reported disasters linked to natural hazards, an estimated 22,500 deaths, 100 million affected, and over $66 billion economic damages were caused (UNISDR, 2015a). Furthermore, while these data refer to large-scale disasters, there are many more smaller scale hazardous events, emergencies, and disasters that affect communities, their health, and livelihoods.

THE 2015 UN LANDMARK AGREEMENTS

In 2015, several landmark UN agreements were adopted by the international community, and included: the SFDRR (2015–2030),

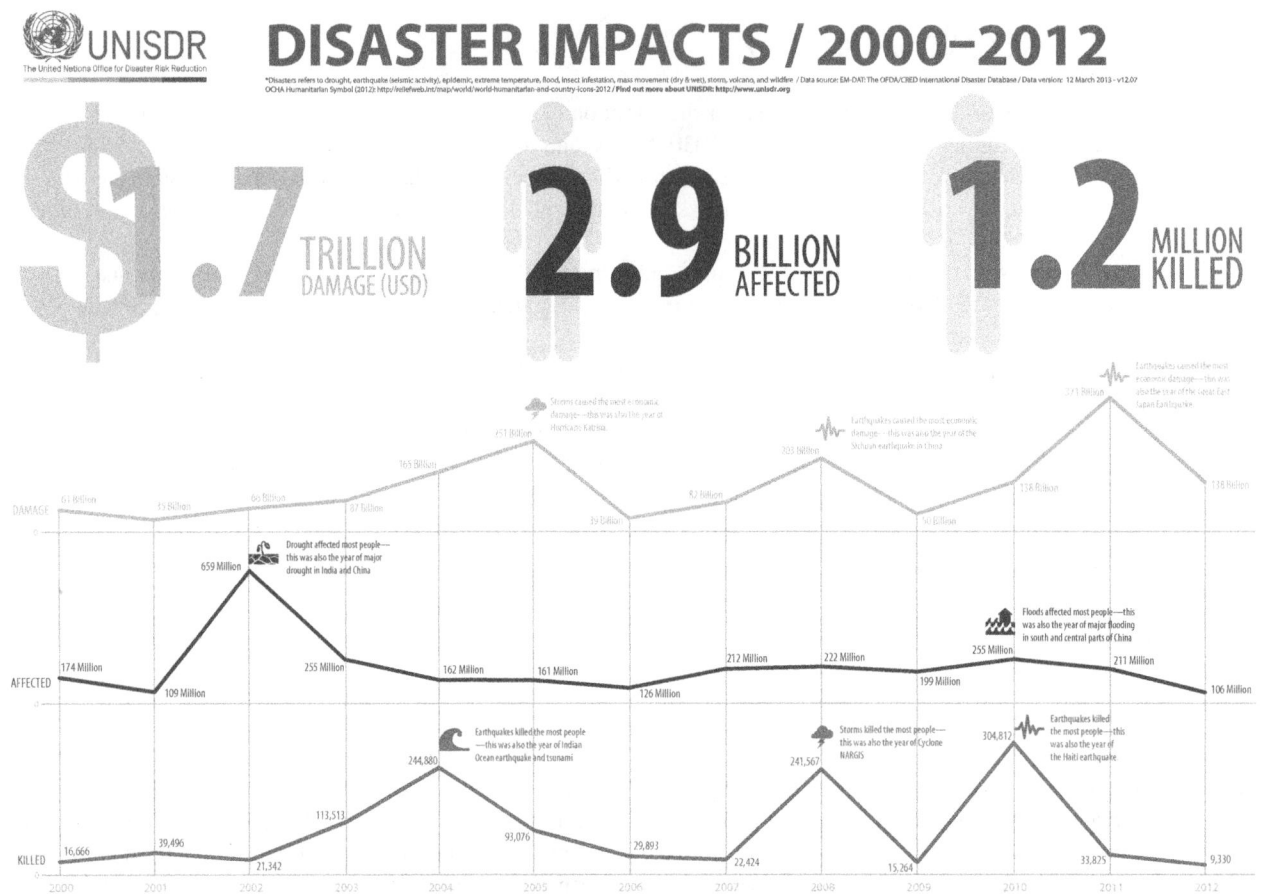

FIGURE 14.1 Summary of disaster impacts 2000 to 2012.

Source: United Nations International Strategy for Disaster Reduction. (2015a). Disasters in numbers. Retrieved from http://www.unisdr.org/files/47804_2015disastertrendsinfographic.pdf

the SDGs, and the Paris Climate Agreement. A brief description of each of these frameworks is offered in Table 14.1.

As illustrated in Figure 14.2, many of these agreements have evolved out of previous incarnations.

Yet, the synchronous adoption of multiple international agreements in 2015 is somewhat unprecedented, and has helped to both create momentum as well as the unique opportunity to coordinate and build coherence across overlapping policy areas (Murray, Maini, Clarke, & Eltinay, 2017). For example, the global increase of natural disasters such as earthquakes, tsunamis, riverine flooding, cyclonic winds, storms, droughts, and heat waves is related to climate change as depicted in Figure 14.3 (Thomas & López, 2015). In this regard, climate change acts as a "force multiplier," exacerbating many of the world's global health challenges (Patz, Frumkin, Holloway, Vimont, & Haines, 2014; Thomas & López, 2015).

Taken together, the UN agreements make for a more complete resilience agenda; building resilience requires action spanning development, humanitarian, climate and disaster risk-reduction areas (Murray et al., 2017). Ensuring coherence between them will serve to strengthen existing risk fragility and resilience frameworks for multihazard assessments, and help develop a dynamic, local, preventive, and adaptive urban governance system at the global, national, and local levels (Murray et al., 2017). Specific emphasis is made on the need to support health and care professionals to implement resilience-building measures and

proactively reduce the risks of disasters, rather than exclusively focusing on the management of crises (UNISDR, 2015b).

THE SENDAI FRAMEWORK FOR DISASTER RISK REDUCTION

The rest of this chapter will focus mainly on the SFDRR and how it applies to the delivery of disaster nursing. The Sendai Framework aims to reinforce the shift in policy and practice of governments and stakeholders from managing disasters and other events to managing disaster risk (UNISDR, 2015b). Rather than focusing exclusively on the response to emergencies, it recognizes that by reducing and managing conditions of hazard, exposure, and vulnerability—while building the capacity of communities and countries for prevention, preparedness, response, and recovery—losses and impacts from disasters can be effectively alleviated (UNISDR, 2015b). Biological hazards such as epidemics and pandemics are also addressed in addition to natural hazards as a key area of focus for disaster risk management.

By 2030, the framework calls for:

The substantial reduction of disaster risk and losses in lives, livelihoods and health and in the economic, physical, social, cultural and environmental assets of persons, businesses, communities and countries. (UNSIDR, 2015b, p. 12)

TABLE 14.1 Description of 2015 UN Agreements

- **The Sendai Framework for Disaster Risk Reduction** 2015 to 2030 was endorsed by the UN General Assembly and adopted by 187 countries at the third World Conference for Disaster Risk Reduction in Sendai, Japan. It puts health at the center of global disaster risk reduction policy and advocates for action to reduce disaster risks for the next 15 years. It is a voluntary, nonbinding agreement with seven global targets, aimed at the reduction of disaster risk and losses in lives, livelihoods, and health (UNISDR, 2015b).
- **The Sustainable Development Goals** represent 17 aspirational "Global Goals" with 169 targets between them, including: the universal call to action to end poverty, protect the planet from climate change, and ensure that all people enjoy peace and prosperity. Target 3.d of the Health Goal is to "strengthen the capacity of all countries, in particular developing countries, for early warning, risk reduction and management of national and global health risks" (United Nations, 2015b).
- The international political response to climate change that began at the Rio Earth Summit in 1992 was complemented with the adoption of the Paris Climate Conference in November 2015. **The Paris Climate Change Agreement** aims to achieve a legally binding and universal agreement on climate and keeping global warming below 2°C (United Nations, 2015a).

UN, united nations; UNISDR, united nations international strategy for disaster reduction.

It specifically advocates for an all-of-society disaster risk-management approach that increases leadership, participation, and risk awareness among marginalized groups including: women, children and youth, persons with disabilities, older persons, indigenous peoples, and migrants (UNISDR, 2015b).

The Sendai Framework also states the need to strengthen disaster risk governance in the management of disaster risk by:

build[ing] awareness and knowledge of disaster risk through sharing and dissemination of non-sensitive disaster risk information and data, contribute to and coordinate reports on local and national disaster risk, coordinate public awareness campaigns on disaster risk, facilitate and support local multisectoral cooperation (e.g., among local governments) and contribute to the determination of and reporting on national and local disaster risk management plans and all policies relevant for disaster risk management. These

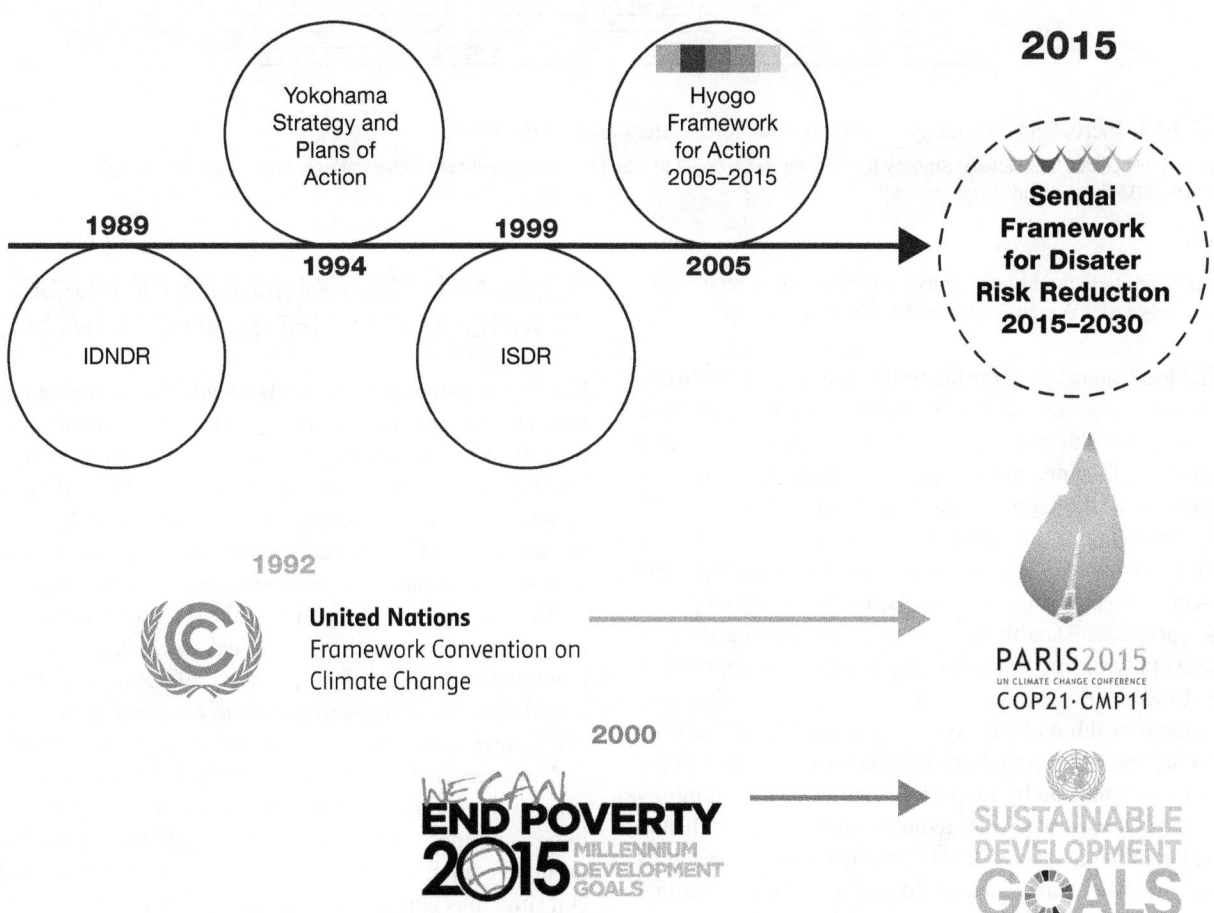

FIGURE 14.2 Twenty-five years of international commitments to disaster risk reduction.

IDNDR, international decade for natural disaster reduction; ISDR, international strategy for disaster reduction.

Source: Reproduced with permission from Maskrey, A. (2015). *Launch of the 2015 Global Assessment Report on disaster risk reduction.* Geneva, Switzerland: United Nations International Strategy for Disaster Reduction.

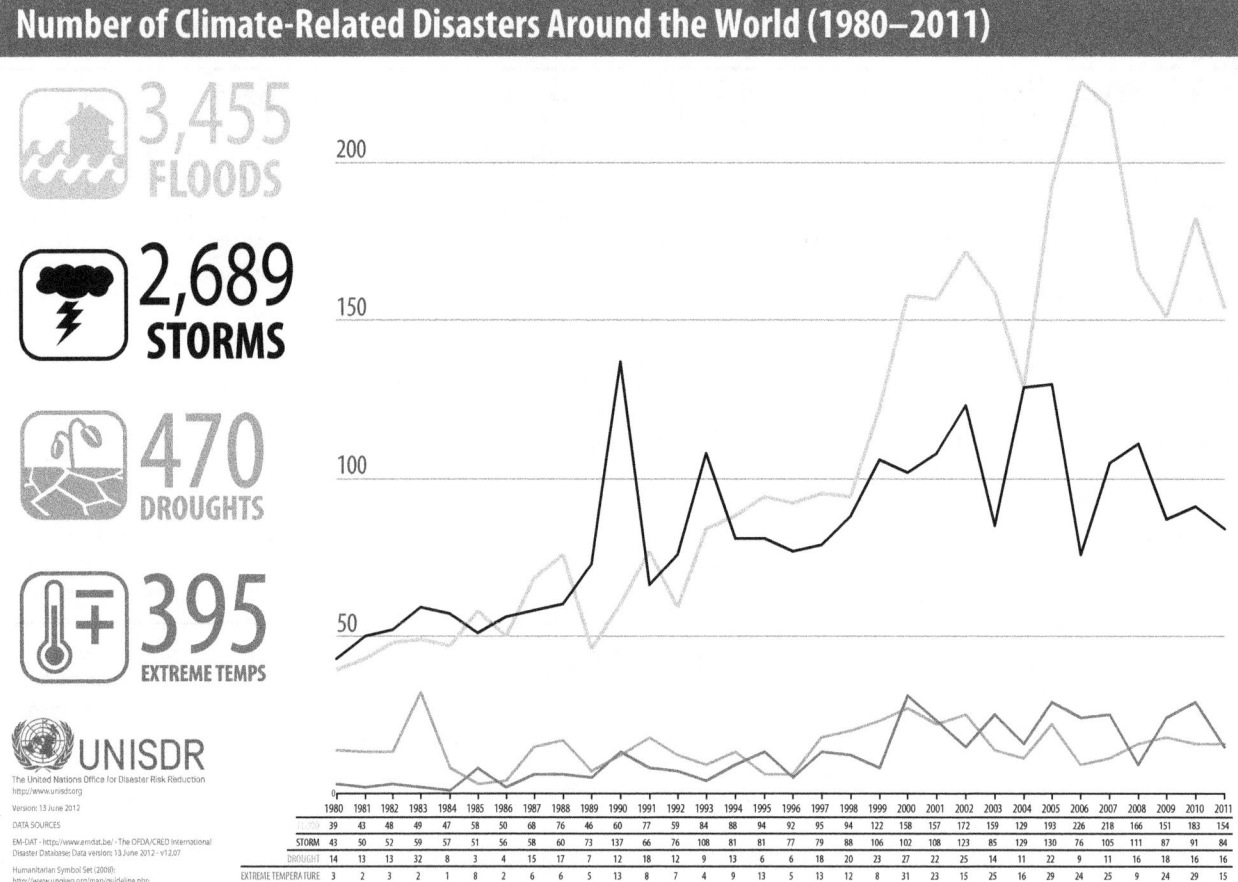

FIGURE 14.3 Increasing frequency of climate-related disasters around the world.

Source: United Nations International Strategy for Disaster Reduction. (2015a). Disasters in numbers. Retrieved from http://www.unisdr.org/files/47804_2015disastertrendsinfographic.pdf

responsibilities should be established through laws, regulations, standards and procedures. (UNISDR, 2015b, para. 27g)

Health is featured as a core theme throughout the framework. Four out of the seven Sendai Framework global targets have direct links to health focusing on: reducing mortality, enhancing population well-being, improving early warning, and promoting the safety of health facilities and hospitals (see Box 14.1).

The Sendai Framework also places strong emphasis on resilient health systems by the integration of disaster risk management into healthcare provision at all levels, and by the development of the capacity of health workers in understanding disaster risk and applying and implementing disaster risk approaches in health work (Bosanquet, 2016).

National health and care systems can be strengthened by promoting and enhancing the training capacities in the field of disaster medicine and by supporting and training community health groups in disaster risk-reduction approaches in health programs. Various competencies exist, including the ICN Framework. There are also a number of recent papers calling for the inclusion of disaster nursing competencies into the undergraduate curricula (Loke & Fung, 2014) but also calls for further rigorous research into this area (Jose & Dufrene, 2014; Veenema et al., 2016).

ROLES AND RESPONSIBILITIES OF NURSES IN IMPLEMENTING THE SENDAI FRAMEWORK

Nursing encompasses autonomous and collaborative care of individuals of all ages, families, groups and communities, sick or well and in all settings. Nursing includes the promotion of health, prevention of illness, and the care of ill, disabled and dying people. Advocacy, promotion of a safe environment, research, participation in shaping health policy and in patient and health systems management, and education are also key nursing roles.

Nurses form the largest healthcare professional group and are the main health professional group in touch with the community. They work in a variety of settings, within and outside health facilities, including in community care such as care homes, rehabilitation units, and supported care facilities.

Nurses are at the front line of service delivery. In many countries, they are either leaders or key actors in multiprofessional, interdisciplinary health teams (WHO, 2013). As the largest group of committed health personnel, they often work in difficult situations with limited resources, playing vital roles when disasters strike, serving as first responders, triage officers and care providers, coordinators of care and services, providers of information or education, and counsellors (Association of

BOX 14.1 Global Targets of the Sendai Framework for Disaster Risk Reduction 2015 to 2030

The Sendai Framework states in paragraph 18 that to support the assessment of global progress in achieving the outcome and goal of the present Framework, seven global targets have been agreed upon.

a. Substantially reduce global **disaster mortality** by 2030, aiming to lower the average per 100,000 global mortality rate in the decade 2020–2030 compared to the period 2005–2015
b. Substantially reduce the number of **affected** people globally by 2030, aiming to lower the average global figure per 100,000 in the decade 2020–2030 compared to the period 2005–2015
c. Reduce direct disaster economic loss in relation to global GDP by 2030
d. Substantially reduce disaster damage to critical infrastructure and disruption of basic services, among them **health** and educational facilities, including through developing their resilience by 2030
e. Substantially increase the number of countries with national and local disaster risk reduction strategies by 2020
f. Substantially enhance international cooperation to developing countries through adequate and sustainable support to complement their national actions for implementation of the present Framework by 2030
g. Substantially increase the availability of and access to **multihazard early warning systems** and disaster risk information and assessments to people by 2030

GDP, gross domestic product.

Source: United Nations International Strategy for Disaster Reduction. (2015b). Sendai Framework for Disaster Risk Reduction 2015–2030. Retrieved from http://www.preventionweb.net/files/43291_sendaiframeworkfordrren.pdf

Women's Health, Obstetric & Neonatal Nursing [AWHONN], 2012; ICN & WHO, 2009).

With their technical skills and knowledge of epidemiology, physiology, pharmacology, cultural-familial structures, and psychosocial issues, nurses can actively contribute in disaster preparedness programs, as well as during disasters. Nurses, as global citizens and team members, can advocate for a significant strategic and leadership role in coordinating and leading health and social disciplines, governmental bodies, community groups, and nongovernmental agencies, including humanitarian organizations.

However, many nurses across the world do not possess the knowledge, skills, and abilities that they will need to be able to participate in a timely and appropriate manner during a disaster response. This issue has significant implications for healthcare systems to mount effective response and recovery initiatives (Veenema, 2016).

The SFDRR 2015 to 2030 recognizes that in order to reduce disaster risk and improve resilience, it is important:

To enhance the resilience of national health systems, including by integrating disaster risk management into primary, secondary and tertiary health care, especially at the local level; developing the capacity of **health workers** in understanding disaster risk and applying and implementing disaster risk reduction approaches in health work; promoting and enhancing the training capacities in the field of disaster medicine; and supporting and training community health groups in disaster risk reduction approaches in health programmes, in collaboration with other sectors, as well as in the implementation of the International Health Regulations (2005) of the World Health Organization (UNISDR, 2015b, para. 30 I)

This call to action offers a major opportunity for health workers, particularly nursing and midwifery professionals, to engage at all levels of disaster preparedness, including risk assessment and multidisciplinary management strategies at all system levels that are critical to the delivery of effective responses to the short, medium, and long-term health and care needs of a disaster-stricken population.

HOW CAN NURSES ACTIVELY ENGAGE IN AND LEAD ON DISASTER RISK REDUCTION AND DISASTER RISK-MANAGEMENT POLICY NATIONALLY AND GLOBALLY?

In order to respond efficiently to disasters, effective use of best available knowledge, innovative thinking, leadership, coordination mechanisms, and partnerships are vital. This requires the engagement of stakeholders at all levels, as well as the breaking down of traditional silos to be replaced by more integrated partnerships that reflect a more holistic approach to risk management.

Disaster nursing and related scientific methods, networks, and communication offer critical assistance to the development of well-informed policies and decisions across all countries. In particular, there is a great need for global leadership in nursing. Nurses are global citizens constituting a professional population of circa 19.7 million nurses and midwives, the majority of whom are women, and are indeed a force for change (All Party Parliamentary Group on Health, 2016).

Nurses Engaging and Leading Nationally

NNAs have a vital role to play at the national level in disaster prevention, mitigation, preparedness, response, and rebuilding/returning to normal. Key activities may include:

Advocacy with government (national and local)
- Actively engaging with governments so that they develop a binding strategy that aims to fulfill the four priorities set out in the SFDRR
- Encouraging governments to plan for responding to the basic needs of nurses in the event of a disaster, ensuring a system is in place that aims to provide food, water, and shelter, as well as continuing with compensation and incentives normally provided for time worked

Evidence-based policy making

- Facilitating the development and implementation of relevant policies, procedures (e.g., disaster simulation exercises, mobilization teams), and legislation (Bosanquet, 2016)
- Promoting nursing and health research on disaster reduction, preparedness, mitigation, response, and recovery. For example, by working with the WHO Collaborating Centre for Nursing in Disasters and Health Emergency Management (WHO, 2017g) and the recently established WHO Thematic Platform for Health Emergency and Disaster Management (Lo et al., 2017)
- Conducting research that addresses key evidence gaps, including disaster health risk profiling of vulnerable groups (e.g., those with chronic illness or disability) and action on strengthening health systems in the context of disasters (Chan & Murray, 2017)

Collaborating and partnering

- Actively participating in supporting institutions and governments to prepare in advance for disaster by assessing potential hazards and vulnerabilities, and by increasing their ability to predict, warn, and respond to disaster (e.g., a national disaster plan, emergency funds)
- Actively participating in strategic planning and implementation of disaster plans ensuring nursing input
- Networking with other professional disciplines, governmental and nongovernmental agencies at local, regional, national, and international levels
- Partnering with independent, objective media, local and national branches of government, international agencies, and nongovernmental organizations

Training/competency development in disasters

- Systematically training nursing personnel to be effective in a crisis/emergency situation (AWHONN, 2012; Veenema et al., 2016)
- Ensuring a register is maintained of trained nurses to ensure rapid deployment of personnel with the appropriate expertise to assist in disasters
- Incorporating disaster preparedness awareness in educational programs at the preregistration and postbasic levels and providing continuing education to ensure a sound knowledge base, skill development, and ethical framework for practice (WHO, 2008); for example, the American Nurses Association considers disaster preparedness and response a part of nursing practice, and strongly recommends registered nurses to take a formal class or certification course in this field (ANA, 2017)
- Raising public awareness of those disasters that their region and country are most likely to experience

Disaster response

- In the short term, assisting in efforts to mobilize the necessary resources (e.g., access to food, water, sanitation, shelter), including helping with emergency medical assistance, giving special attention to vulnerable groups (e.g., the ill, disabled/less abled, homeless, socially or culturally isolated, children, women, and the elderly)
- In the long term, assisting with resettlement programs, psychosocial, economic, and legal needs (e.g., counselling, documentation, mobility)
- For those nurses working in disaster settings, providing as well as being provided with support that meets resilience, daily physical and emotional needs (Knebel, Toomey, & Libby, 2012); health workers who are experiencing human tragedy firsthand may be stressed, fatigued, and trying to provide services with too few resources in physically unsafe circumstances

Nurses Engaging and Leading Globally

The ICN is a federation of more than 130 NNAs representing the millions of nurses worldwide (ICN, 2017). Operated by nurses, ICN works to ensure quality nursing care for all and sound health policies globally (ICN, 2017). ICN has acted in a leadership role to support quality nursing care and education throughout the world. In that role, ICN has identified disaster preparedness and response as essential to providing adequate healthcare and addressing the humanitarian challenges of disasters.

Some of the core values of ICN in responding to disasters are given in Box 14.2:

The ICM is another nongovernmental organization that supports, represents, and works to strengthen professional associations of midwives throughout the world (ICM, 2017b). There are currently 131 Midwives Associations, representing 113 countries across every continent.

At the global level, the ICN and ICM have a key role to play in the implementation of the Sendai Framework, and this work may include:

Advocacy

- Lobbying developmental banks and international financial institutions to integrate disaster prevention and mitigation in their aid programs

---

BOX 14.2 Values of ICN in Responding to Disasters

ICN strongly recognizes that there must be a link between the impact of disasters at all levels and in development of health in all policies.

ICN condemns violations of human rights that often occur during and after a disaster thus further threatening recovery.

ICN promotes strategies that support social justice and equity of access to needed health and social services and calls on governments and disaster risk management organizations to establish the support systems required to address the health needs of health and care workers as well as the disaster casualties.

ICN, international council of nurses.

Source: International Council of Nurses. (2006). Nurses and Disaster Preparedness. ICN Position (under review as of August 2017). Retrieved from http://www.icn.ch/images/stories/documents/publications/position_statements/A11_Nurses_Disaster_Preparedness.pdf

Evidence-based policy making

- Promoting the dissemination and facilitating access to knowledge, information, training, and technology
- Progressing the WHO's *Health in All Policies* framework (WHO, 2014) and other associated international policy drivers such as the SDGs (United Nations, 2015b)
- Encouraging NNAs to develop and/or support a regulatory framework that helps nurses meet regulatory requirements in a timely manner when providing nursing care in an affected jurisdiction

Collaborating and partnering

- Developing, encouraging, and supporting international networks, as disasters do not respect borders
- Supporting international and national coordination of response efforts to reduce duplication of services (e.g., joining Emergency Medical Teams, groups of health professionals providing surge capacity to local health systems during disasters, with agreed standards and quality assurance mechanisms)
- Encouraging NNAs to increase the profession's ability to provide adequate health services before and after a disaster occurs by their participation in prevention, mitigation, preparedness, disaster risk-management, and response operations.
- Assisting countries in their planning by working with strategic partners and regional networks, such as the WHO Collaborating Centres for Nursing and Midwifery, to integrate disaster prevention and impact reduction within the existing machinery and strategies

Training/competency development in disasters

- Ensuring implementation of the ICN Framework of Disaster Nursing Competencies to help strengthen the essential capacities of nurses to deliver disaster and emergency services (ICN & WHO, 2009)
- Ensuring that realistic scenarios are used as the basis for enhancing disaster preparedness for effective response and to "Build Back Better"[1] in recovery, rehabilitation, and reconstruction plans.

Monitoring and evaluating

- Documenting progress made by the ICN toward achieving the 2006 goals (ICN, 2006) and how any unmet goals will be met

ROLE OF THE WORLD HEALTH ORGANIZATION

WHO works with a wide range of partners to improve health outcomes for people at risk of emergencies and disasters,

and these include resources globally for disaster nursing. For example, the WHO provides support for implementing country and community capacities in health and other sectors to manage the health risks associated with emergencies and disasters. This is done in several ways, which include the WHO's commitment to supporting emergency and disaster risk management for health (WHO, 2017a). The WHO provides support globally to countries for a wide range of threats to public health, including: infectious disease outbreaks, unsafe food and water, chemical and radiation contamination, natural and technological hazards, wars and other societal conflicts, and the health consequences of climate change. To help meet these and other challenges, countries are encouraged to strengthen their capacities for emergency risk management incorporating measures for prevention, mitigation, preparedness, response, and recovery. To enable this, in 2011, the WHO developed a partnership to build a WHO Thematic Platform for Health Emergency and Disaster Risk Management (Health-EDRM). There are several outputs from this platform and they include:

- **The WHO Disaster Risk Management for Health Fact Sheets** (WHO, 2017b)

  Disasters and other emergencies often result in significant impacts on people's health, including the loss of many lives. Every new threat reveals the challenges for managing health risks and the effects of emergencies and disasters. Deaths, injuries, diseases, disabilities, psychosocial problems, and other health impacts can be avoided or reduced by disaster risk-management measures involving health and other sectors. These advocacy materials are an introduction for health workers engaged in disaster risk management and for multisectoral partners to consider how to integrate health into their disaster risk-management strategies. The overview places disaster risk management in the context of multisectoral action and focuses on the generic elements of disaster risk management, including potential hazards, vulnerabilities of a population, and capacities that apply across the various health domains. The accompanying fact sheets identify key points for consideration within a number of essential health domains. However, importantly, all health domains are interlinked; each fact sheet should therefore be considered as part of the entire set and in conjunction with the overview.

- **The WHO Thematic Platform for Health-EDRM Research Group** (WHO, 2017f)

  The health disaster research community should engage in the Health-EDRM to provide relevant evidence to support and maximize the global disaster risk-reduction effort. These efforts will be taken forward through the WHO Thematic Platform in Health-EDRM Research Group, which was established in September 2016, and aims to coordinate activity, promote information sharing, develop partnerships, provide technical advice, and facilitate the generation of robust and scientific health research to support the implementation of the Sendai Framework and related global agendas. Disaster nursing colleagues may be interested in engaging with this research platform

---

[1] "The use of the recovery, rehabilitation, and reconstruction phases after a disaster is to increase the resilience of nations and communities through integrating disaster risk reduction measures into the restoration of physical infrastructure and societal systems, and into the revitalization of livelihoods, economies, and the environment."

WHO COLLABORATING CENTERS

In addition, the WHO has developed collaborating centers which are institutions such as research institutes, parts of universities or academies, designated by the director-general to carry out activities in support of the Organization's programs. Currently, there are over 700 WHO collaborating centers in over 80 member states working with WHO on areas such as nursing, health emergency and disaster management, occupational health, communicable diseases, nutrition, mental health, chronic diseases, and health technologies (WHO, 2017c). Two relevant examples of WHO Collaborating Centres for Disaster Nursing are:

- **WHO Collaborating Centre for Disaster Risk Management for Health (Japan;** WHO, 2017d)

    The WHO Collaborating Centre for Disaster Risk Management was first established in 2007. Its Terms of Reference state its mandate is to: promote the nursing and health research on disaster reduction, preparedness, mitigation, response, and recovery from the disaster and similar life-threatening afflictions in the mid to long term; delineate the roles and competencies of nursing professionals involved in various phases of disasters: preparedness, mitigation, response, recovery, and health emergency management; carry out a leading role in the development of an effective national, regional, and global network system for nursing and other health professionals involved in the health emergency management; implement training needs assessments, develop and implement training programs for the public and professionals involved in disasters and emergency management situations and their prevention; and influence the governmental agencies and nongovernmental organizations to promote nursing leadership in the development of nursing on disasters and health emergency management.
- **WHO Collaborating Centre for Public Health Nursing and Midwifery (England;** WHO, 2017e)

    This center was more recently designated in 2016. Its remit is to: support WHO by generating evidence and defining frameworks of practice for nurses and midwives that prevent avoidable illness, protect health, and promote well-being and resilience; support WHO by providing information about the nurses' and midwives' role and impact on maternal and child health; and on request of WHO provide policy advice and technical assistance about public health nursing and midwifery to the regional office and member states.

SUMMARY

2015 was the year during which several notable UN agreements were adopted, and included: the SFDRR, SDGs, and COP21's Paris Climate Conference. The policy areas pertaining to the frameworks are closely interrelated. For example, climate mitigation and adaptation strategies may contribute to reducing the frequency of disasters, which in turn supports sustainable development.

Disasters can result in significant impacts on people's health and well-being, including the loss of many lives. However, deaths, injuries, diseases, disabilities, psychosocial problems, and other health-related impacts can be avoided or reduced by effective risk-management measures.

As the largest group of committed health personnel, nurses have a vital role to play when disasters strike.

This chapter has demonstrated how disaster nurses can both engage actively and provide leadership that will assist the successful implementation of the recently adopted UN frameworks, particularly the SFDRR.

STUDY QUESTIONS

1. Summarize the outcomes of the 2015 UN Agreements, particularly the SFDRR 2015 to 2030, that are particularly relevant for you in your role in disaster nursing practice and leadership.

2. Nurses and midwives should be encouraged to be part of the agreed local, national, regional, and global mechanisms to address all the needs for disaster nursing from disaster preparedness for understanding risk to effective response and to "Build Back Better" in recovery, rehabilitation, and reconstruction—how can you help to implement this?

3. Consider reflecting on a recent disaster and how you would plan to implement the priorities for action within the Sendai Framework to reduce the impact of a future similar disaster.

ACKNOWLEDGMENTS

We thank Howard Catton, Nursing and Health Policy Consultant from the ICN, for his invaluable contributions to this chapter.

USEFUL LINKS

Global Facility for Disaster Reduction and Recovery. (2016). Understanding Disaster Risk. Retrieved from https://youtu.be/O-SWl3J1aQc

International Day for Disaster Reduction—October 13 (Annual). https://www.unisdr.org/we/campaign/iddr

United Nations Office for Disaster Risk Reduction. (2016). The Sendai Framework and the Sustainable Development Goals. Retrieved from https://youtu.be/N6soXnTsgZg

Twitter:

@CDCemergency; @fema; @didrrn; @InclusiveDRR; @ariseinitiative; @UNISDR; @rhea_elena; @ResilienceAF; @UCLIRDR; @PEDRRnetwork; @PreventionWeb; @unescoEARTH; @grp_resilience; @dngl_BBS

#DRR; #SendaiFramework; #Switch2Sendai; #SDGs; #ParisAgreement; #DRRSymposium17

REFERENCES

All Party Parliamentary Group on Health. (2016). Triple Impact—How developing nursing will improve health, promote gender equality and support economic growth. Retrieved from http://www.appg-globalhealth.org.uk/download/i/mark_dl/u/4009611296/4630127784/DIGITAL%20APPG%20Triple%20Impact.pdf

American Nurses Association. (2017). Who will be there? Ethics, the law, and a nurse's duty to respond in a disaster. Retrieved from https://www.nursingworld.org/practice-policy/work-environment/health-safety/disaster-preparedness/be-competent-education

Association of Women's Health, Obstetric & Neonatal Nursing Position Statement. (2012). The role of the nurse in emergency preparedness. *Journal of Obstetric, Gynecologic, & Neonatal Nursing, 41*(2), 322–324. doi:10.1111/j.1552-6909.2011.01338.x

Baker, L. R., & Cormier, L. A. (2014). *Disasters and vulnerable populations: Evidence-based practice for the helping professions.* New York, NY: Springer.

Bolin, B. (2007). Race, class, ethnicity, and disaster vulnerability. In H. Rodríguez, E. L. Quarantelli, & R. R. Dynes (Eds.), *Handbook of disaster research* (pp. 113–129). New York, NY: Springer.

Bosanquet, J. (2016). How disaster response could benefit from nursing expertise. *Nursing Times.* Retrieved from https://www.nursingtimes.net/break-time/how-disaster-response-could-benefit-from-nursing-expertise/7013269.article

Chan, E. Y. Y., & Murray, V. (2017). What are the health research needs of Sendai Framework? *The Lancet, 390*(10106), e35–e36. doi:10.1016/S0140-6736(17)31670-7

Fothergill, A., Maestas, E. G., & Darlington, J. D. (1999). Race, ethnicity and disasters in the United States: A review of the literature. *Disasters, 23*(2), 156–173. doi:10.1111/1467-7717.00111

International Confederation of Midwives. (2017a). Position statement: Health of women and children in disasters. Retrieved from http://internationalmidwives.org/assets/uploads/documents/Position%20Statements%20-%20English/New%20Position%20Statements%20in%202014%20and%202017%20/REVISED%20V2017%20ENG%20Health%20Women%20and%20children%20in%20disasters.pdf

International Confederation of Midwives. (2017b). Who we are. Retrieved from http://internationalmidwives.org/who-we-are

International Council of Nurses. (2006). Nurses and disaster preparedness. ICN position (under review as of August 2017). Retrieved from http://www.icn.ch/images/stories/documents/publications/position_statements/A11_Nurses_Disaster_Preparedness.pdf

International Council of Nurses. (2017). Who we are. Retrieved from http://www.icn.ch

International Council of Nurses, & World Health Organization. (2009). ICN framework of disaster nursing competencies. Retrieved from http://www.wpro.who.int/hrh/documents/icn_framework.pdf (to be reviewed in 2018. Personal correspondence).

Jose, M. M., & Dufrene, C. (2014). Educational competencies and technologies for disaster preparedness in undergraduate nursing education: An integrative review. *Nurse Education Today, 34,* 543–551. doi:10.1016/j.nedt.2013.07.021

Knebel, A. R., Toomey, L., & Libby, M. (2012). Nursing leadership in disaster preparedness and response. *Annual Review of Nursing Research, 30*(1), 21–45. Retrieved from http://lghttp.48653.nexcesscdn.net/80223CF/springer-static/media/springer-downloads/ARNR%20Article-Nursing%20Leadership%20in%20Disaster%20Preparedness.pdf

Lo, S. T. T., Chan, E. Y. Y., Chan, G. K. W., Murray, V., Abrahams, J., Ardalan, A., ... Wai Yau, J. C. (2017). Health emergency and disaster risk management (Health-EDRM): Developing the research field within the Sendai Framework paradigm. *International Journal of Disaster Risk Science, 8*(2), 145–149. doi:10.1007/s13753-017-0122-0

Loke, A. Y., & Fung, O. W. M. (2014). Nurses' competencies in disaster nursing: Implications for curriculum development and public health. *International Journal of Environmental Research and Public Health, 11,* 3289–3303. doi:10.3390/ijerph110303289. Retrieved from https://www.ncbi.nlm.nih.gov/pmc/articles/PMC3987035/pdf/ijerph-11-03289.pdf

Maskrey, A. (2015). *Launch of the 2015 Global Assessment Report on disaster risk reduction.* Geneva, Switzerland: United Nations Office for Disaster Risk Reduction.

Murray, V., Maini, R., Clarke, L., & Eltinay, N. (2017). Coherence between the Sendai Framework, the SDGs, the Climate Agreement, New Urban Agenda and World Humanitarian Summit and the role of science in their implementation, ICSU and IRDR. Retrieved from http://www.irdrinternational.org/2017/05/12/irdr-published-5-policy-briefs-for-2017-global-platform-for-drr

Patz, J. A., Frumkin, H., Holloway, T., Vimont, D. J., & Haines, A. (2014). Climate change: Challenges and opportunities for global health. *The Journal of the American Medical Association, 312*(15), 1565–1580. doi:10.1001/jama.2014.13186

Thomas, V., & López, R. (2015). Global increase in climate related disasters: Asian Development Bank. Retrieved from https://www.adb.org/sites/default/files/publication/176899/ewp-466.pdf

United Nations. (2015a). Paris Agreement (COP21). Retrieved from https://www.preventionweb.net/publications/view/49265

United Nations. (2015b). Transforming our world: The 2030 agenda for sustainable development. Retrieved from http://www.preventionweb.net/publications/view/45418

United Nations International Strategy for Disaster Reduction. (2015a). Disasters in numbers. Retrieved from: http://www.unisdr.org/files/47804_2015disastertrendsinfographic.pdf

United Nations International Strategy for Disaster Reduction. (2015b). Sendai Framework for disaster risk reduction 2015–2030. Retrieved from http://www.preventionweb.net/files/43291_sendaiframeworkfordrren.pdf

United Nations International Strategy for Disaster Reduction. (2017). Terminology. Retrieved from: https://www.unisdr.org/we/inform/terminology

Veenema, T. G. (2016). Strengthening a global nursing workforce: Disaster preparedness and response [Web log post]. *GANM Blogs.* Retrieved from http://ganm.nursing.jhu.edu/strengthening-a-global-nursing-workforce-disaster-preparedness-response

Veenema, T. G., Griffin, A., Gable, A. R., MacIntyre, L., Simons, R. A. D. M., Couig, M. P., ... Larson, E. (2016). Nurses as leaders in disaster preparedness and response—A call to action. *Journal of Nursing Scholarship, 48*(2), 187–200. doi:10.1111/jnu.12198

World Conference on Disaster Risk Reduction. (2014). Health and disasters. Retrieved from http://www.wcdrr.org/uploads/HEALTH.pdf

World Health Organization. (2008). Integrating emergency preparedness and response into undergraduate nursing curricula. Geneva, Switzerland: Author. Retrieved from http://www.who.int/hac/publications/Nursing_curricula_followup_Feb08.pdf

World Health Organization. (2013). WHO nursing and midwifery progress report 2008–2012. Retrieved from http://www.who.int/hrh/nursing_midwifery/NursingMidwiferyProgressReport.pdf

World Health Organization. (2014). Health in all policies. Helsinki statement. Framework for country action. Retrieved from http://apps.who.int/iris/bitstream/10665/112636/1/9789241506908_eng.pdf?ua=1

World Health Organization. (2017a). Emergency and disaster risk management for health. Retrieved from http://www.who.int/hac/techguidance/preparedness/en

World Health Organization. (2017b). Health emergency and disaster risk management fact sheets. Retrieved from http://www.who.int/hac/techguidance/preparedness/factsheets/en

World Health Organization. (2017c). WHO collaborating centres. Retrieved from http://www.who.int/collaboratingcentres/en

World Health Organization. (2017d). WHO collaborating centre for Disaster Risk Management for Health (Japan). Retrieved from http://apps.who.int/whocc/Detail.aspx?cc_ref=JPN-77&cc_region=wpro

World Health Organization. (2017e). WHO Collaborating Centre for Public Health Nursing and Midwifery (England). Retrieved from http://apps.who.int/whocc/Detail.aspx?cc_ref=UNK-277&cc_contact=bennett&

World Health Organization. (2017f). WHO statement to the 2017 Global Platform for Disaster Risk Reduction. Retrieved from http://www.unisdr.org/files/globalplatform/whostatementfinal24may.pdf

World Health Organization. (2017g). WHO collaborating center for nursing in disasters and health emergency management. Retrieved from http://www.coe-cnas.jp/who/eng/about_center/index.html

15

COMPLEX HUMANITARIAN EMERGENCIES

Frederick M. Burkle, Jr.

LEARNING OBJECTIVES

When this chapter is completed, readers will be able to:

1. Define complex humanitarian emergencies (CHEs) as they exist in the modern-day world.
2. Recognize the common thread of public health emergencies in CHEs and the requirements to mitigate preventable mortality and morbidity.
3. Recognize the epidemiological and health profile differences found in CHEs.
4. Recognize the rapidly changing challenges to practice, policy, and public health from future humanitarian crises.
5. Recognize the challenges to nursing, to nursing leadership, and within the current movement to professionalizing the humanitarian profession.

KEY MESSAGES

CHEs, also known as "unconventional warfare," are the most common current form of large-scale violence in the world, resulting in public health emergencies that lead to excess mortality and morbidity.

Indirect, or preventable, mortality and morbidity rates may exceed those arising from the direct violence of warfare itself.

CHEs have severely challenged the capacity and capability of international laws and treaties to protect the most vulnerable of civilian populations.

Health profiles, which are the basis of epidemiological models of CHEs in developing, developed, and chronic/smoldering countries, differ greatly depending on the status of public health infrastructure and social protections.

Future humanitarian crises such as climate change, biodiversity crises, rapid urbanization, and emergencies of scarcity may lead to new CHEs that will further challenge the capacity and capability of the humanitarian community to respond.

Nursing assets remain a dominant force when managing CHEs in the field and at the headquarter level.

Professionalization of the humanitarian professions, especially health providers, will improve accountability and accreditation.

CHAPTER OVERVIEW

Complex humanitarian emergencies (CHEs), the most common human-generated disasters of the past three decades, are defined by the severe breakdown of governance resulting from internal or external conflict. They require an international response to mitigate the immediate and long-term mortality and morbidity and the recovery and rehabilitation of the destroyed essential public health infrastructure and social protections. To best understand the immediate needs of the population at risk, it is important to recognize its epidemiological characteristics. Migration of populations from rural insecurity contributes to the development of rapid and unsustainable urbanization and to the abrupt shift of potential future conflicts to urban environments. These CHEs greatly challenge humanitarian professionals in disaster medicine and nursing in terms of international crises.

DEFINING CHEs

Conventional Warfare

Conventional cross-border wars, such as World Wars I and II, or the 1991 Persian Gulf War, are examples of declared confrontations that occur between nations and arise from chronic hostilities and threats over borders, territory, or resources. Responsibilities and protections of the countries in conflict and those who provide aid and assistance to recover the destroyed health and public health infrastructures and systems are clearly defined by the Fourth Geneva Convention (GC), especially Articles 55 and 56 (International Committee of the Red Cross, 1949).

Unconventional Warfare

During the latter half of the 20th century and currently, more people have been killed by elements within their own country than by outside forces (Brennan & Nandy, 2001). Sovereignty issues limit protections under existing international laws including the United Nations (UN) Charter and the GC. These prolonged political conflicts provoke a variety of unconventional warfare responses that are collectively referred to as CHEs. Of 120 armed conflicts since World War II, 80% were waged by, or against, entities that were not nation-states (Van

Creveld, 2010). The large majority of all nonstate conflicts, ranging from unconventional warfare, terrorism, guerilla warfare, and insurgencies to wars of national liberation, took place in the developing world. Since the September 11 attacks, they have spread to developed countries as well. The term "asymmetrical" war is often used, especially by the military, to recognize that formal military elements are in violent conflict with presumed weaker and less organized belligerents—a situation that differs greatly from conventional warfare where tactics and resources are similar (Tomes, 2004). CHEs typically result in more civilian victims than military, a level that may be as high as 10 civilians for every militant killed (Byman, 2011). Burkle (2008) describes three equal elements of unconventional warfare: the asymmetrical warfare itself, pervasive insecurity that impacts every sector of society, and which characteristically leads to prolonged and often catastrophic public health emergencies (Figure 15.1).

CHEs are defined by the UN as "major humanitarian crises of a multicausal nature that requires a systematic response" (Albala-Bertrand, 2000); adding that they "commonly involve

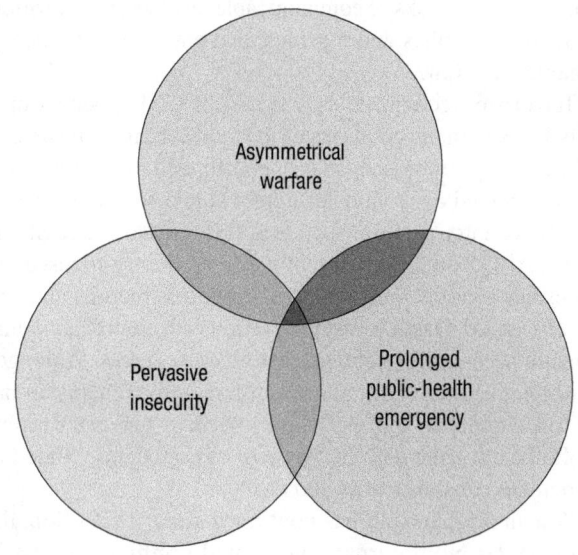

FIGURE 15.1 Current asymmetrical conflicts have three major interdependent and inseparable components that need equal monitoring and measurement.

Source: Reproduced with permission from Burkle, F. M. (2008). Measuring humanitarian assistance in conflicts. *Lancet, 371*(9608), 189. doi:10.1016/ S0140-6736(08)60118-X

a long-term combination of political, conflict and peacekeeping factors." Albala-Bertrand (2000) argues that all CHEs have a *"singular ability* to erode or destroy the cultural, civil, political and economic integrity of established societies" and are internal to existing political and economic structures of the country in conflict. Some organizations include large-scale natural disasters in their definition of CHEs; however, whereas the disaster event may accelerate or catalyze the onset of a CHE, especially in fragile and unstable countries, "they differ from natural disasters and deserve to be understood and responded to as such" (Duffield, 1994).

MAJOR CHARACTERISTICS

CHEs represent the most common human-generated disasters of the past three decades and account for more morbidity and mortality than all natural and technological disasters combined (Brennan & Nandy, 2001). These crises are complicated by a lethal and unpredictable mix of ethnic and religious inequities, poverty, social injustices, cultural incompatibility, pervasive ignorance, racism, oppression, and religious fundamentalism, all of which adversely affect the public health and may result in denied access to the most vulnerable of populations: women, children, the elderly, the disabled, and those with severe mental disorders (Jones et al., 2009). CHEs present risk factors that lead to diminished physical and psychological health (Box 15.1).

No two CHEs are alike, and each will vary in characteristics, intensity, and duration. What is similar is that public health infrastructure and health delivery systems are likely to be the first destroyed and the last to recover. The loss of public health protections, both physical and social, results in a collapse of health services, disease control capacity, poor access to healthcare, outbreaks of communicable diseases, malnutrition, interrupted supplies and logistics, and environmental decay, to name but a few.

Terrorism, recognized as a subset of CHEs, occurs on a daily basis in many countries of the world. In most instances, splinter groups from social movements formed to draw attention to unaddressed economic development and social needs of a specific country perform such acts (Marks, Gorka, & Sharp, 2010). Al-Qaeda differs in that it is not country-focused but represents a global radical Islamic force that recruits and acts worldwide. Al-Qaeda's first motivation is to control a population, not necessarily to obtain territory or resources. Prolonged and organized terrorism as seen in Iraq and Afghanistan has led to a chronic state of pervasive insecurity and catastrophic public health emergencies. The rise of the Islamic State has perpetuated this insecurity and chaos.

War in Afghanistan has continued since 1979, Somalia since 1991. Noninternational armed conflicts persist in Yemen, Libya, South Sudan, Syria, Southwest Turkey, Mali, Myanmar, and Ukraine. There are no clear solutions to both acute and chronic problems facing these fragile countries. However, the state of humanitarian need described in this chapter remains the same regardless of what the catalyst may be for the CHEs.

BOX 15.1 Risk Factors From Complex Humanitarian Emergencies

CHEs produce risk factors that increase both individual and population risk for developing psychosocial and mental health problems and compound the problems for persons with existing psychological conditions. Behavior of neglected and abused mentally ill in a refugee camp setting can lead to an erosive impact on the fragile social fabric of displaced communities. Additional factors include, but are not limited to:

- Poor health and nutrition
- Separation from family and caregivers
- Suboptimum perinatal care, neglect, and under-stimulation of children
- Exposure to chronic communicable diseases that affect the brain
- Risk of traumatic epilepsy
- Exposure to extreme and repeated stress and sleep deprivation

War, conflict, and camp conditions often place those with existing problems at greater risk for:

- Abuse, including gross dereliction, stigma, ostracism, sexual violence
- Child abduction, youth violence/death
- Family separation and displacement
- Neglect or abandonment by family and caretakers
- Exploitation
- Destruction of supportive institutions and services, including psychiatric facilities and medications
- Life-threatening physical illnesses and suicide
- Conditions that foment hatred and revenge
- Unremitting conditions that lead to worsening disability and premature death, especially among the elderly interventions

Common guiding principles and strategies for the humanitarian community in developing interventions for populations exposed to extreme stressors include:

- Contingency planning before the acute emergency
- Assessment before intervention
- Inclusion of long-term development perspectives
- Collaboration between agencies
- Provision of treatment in primary care and community settings
- Access to services for all in need
- Training and supervision
- Monitoring indicators, including project impact

CHEs, complex humanitarian emergencies.

INTERNATIONAL RESPONSE

Only the UN has the legal authority to respond militarily with peacekeeping and peace-enforcement actions (United Nations, 1945). UN Charter language does not adequately address internal conflicts and genocidal actions. The UN-led humanitarian response community—made up of nongovernmental organizations (NGOs), the Red Cross Movement (resources from both the International Committee of the Red Cross and the Federation of Red Cross and Red Crescent National Societies), and UN Agencies such as United Nations International Children's Emergency Fund (UNICEF), World Health Organization (WHO), United Nations High Commission for Refugees (UNHCR), and others—works to protect civilian populations within conflicted countries and on their borders. Civilian protections are included in various legal documents. Such documents include international customary law and treaties that embody obligations for nation-states in International Humanitarian Law and International Human Rights Law, drawn from the GCs of 1949, the GC Additional Protocols of 1977 (where ratified), the Universal Declaration of Human Rights, the International Covenant on Civil and Political Rights, the European Convention and Court on Human Rights, and many others. Unfortunately, CHEs have severely challenged the capacity and capability of these laws to be effective deterrents and provide the necessary protections.

In this regard, the Western-led Coalition military campaign in Afghanistan was not specifically mandated by the UN, but is widely perceived to be a legitimate form of self-defense under the UN Charter. The International Security Assistance Force (ISAF) is a North Atlantic Treaty Organization (NATO)-led security mission established by the UN Security Council (UN News Centre, 2011). The U.S. and Coalition military under the rubric of "stability and reconstruction operations" includes elements of traditional combat, counterterrorism, peacemaking/peacekeeping, counterinsurgency/nation building, monetary development assistance, disaster relief, and direct health interventions (Kem, 2007).

In prior wars and conflicts, health has managed to remain a "soft power" element perceived to be "above politics" (Kickbusch, 2011). This is essential to the expected neutrality and universality of care provided by the humanitarian community and protected under international law and GC mandates. The international humanitarian community, however, has found that the "militarization" of aid and assistance in CHEs provided by the militaries in conflict is both controversial and worrisome (Atwood, 2010). The utilization of health interventions, which has become a major goal of the military in unconventional warfare, both in direct medical care and health infrastructure recovery, is now perceived as a major "hard power" element that some argue has compromised the independence and autonomy that health interventions have previously enjoyed and that is required for the recognition of neutrality (Kickbusch, 2011). Military-led health interventions derived from Provincial Reconstruction Teams have had mixed reviews in Afghanistan, being described as "ad hoc, unevaluated, and ineffective" in "winning the hearts and minds" of the civilian population (Hoekstra & Tucker, 2010). Whereas outcome indicators are routinely required by donors supporting the humanitarian community health interventions, they are not collected or provided by the military—a fault that ultimately interferes with health interventions being properly assessed and transferred to nonmilitary aid organizations.

Data analysis suggests that CHEs have changed substantially over the last three decades, especially in the overall levels of insecurity. Syria and Afghanistan are examples where security assessments and relief strategies have not effectively dealt with worsening security, especially as it impacts civilians and the relief community. In 2016, 158 major attacks against humanitarian operations occurred; 101 aid workers were killed, 98 wounded, and 89 kidnapped (Stoddard, Harmer, & Czwarno, 2017). This mortality number increases for those who have worked for or with NATO powers, although currently all expatriate aid workers are at equal risk even as they routinely pass their duties onto the indigenous aid workers they employ.

MEASURING THE HUMAN COST

Characteristically, CHEs are initially confined within nation-state borders and result in massive numbers of internally displaced populations (IDPs). Political violence and its direct effects on individuals occur first, resulting in death and injury. In time, IDPs experience the additional consequences of being separated from essential public health services, causing an indirect or secondary phase escalation of mortality and morbidity. All indirect consequences are seen as preventable (Burkle & Greenough, 2008).

Without epidemiological studies, we would not know the short- and long-term impact of various forms of political violence (Roberts & Hofmann, 2004). Only when studies were performed in the early 1990s was the dominance of public health consequences and preponderance of civilian victims recognized (Spiegel, Burkle, Dey, & Salama, 2001). The humanitarian community relies on use of *specific* direct and indirect indices to (a) assess consequences including severity of the conflict, (b) measure the impact or outcome of interventions in declining mortality and morbidity, and (c) identify the most vulnerable populations requiring care. Civilians are all too often the forgotten casualties of war and "accepted by all parties involved as unavoidable 'collateral damage' in military operation" (Breau & Joyce, 2011). As such, the Oxford Research Group's recording of casualties of armed conflict program has focused on the legal obligations to record civilian casualties in all theaters of armed conflict. It is evident that governments do not routinely record civilian casualties on any type of systematic basis and those that do so do not publish the records. From both a military and moral point of view, such data are essential to both the analysis of the effects of military practices and to the development of "advanced military policy which aims to avoid and minimize civilian casualties" (Breau & Joyce, 2011). The impact of CHEs will never be known, nor will they receive proper protection, until the binding international legal obligation to record every civilian casualty is followed.

Epidemiological studies detect and verify continued health problems, confirm whether victims are benefiting from aid operations, and catalyze major alterations in the direction of care and health recovery strategies of the international relief community and governmental donors. The lack of local and nation-state capacity in governance, economics, public safety, communications, and transportation works against an efficient and effective recovery and normalization to predisaster health indices.

ASSESSMENTS, DATA COLLECTION, AND ANALYSIS

Assessments define the baseline health status of the population and are critical to identifying the threats faced by the emergency-affected population, including those with epidemic potential. The assessment process engages teams that observe, walk the territory, and talk to the survivors. Population-based cluster sampling follows, including mortality rates for children under age 5 (U5MR), nutritional indices, and crude mortality rates (CMRs) that are then disaggregated for age and gender to determine the most vulnerable of populations in need. In some circumstances, with rapidly shifting populations, less stringent methodologies are implemented, such as "excess mortality." Over time, with improved human and logistical resources available, more exact nutritional indices (weight for height, micronutrient deficiencies, and z-scores [expressed as a deviation from the mean value, such as weight, for a population of children being treated for malnutrition]), infant mortality rates (IMRs), and maternal mortality rates (MMRs), among others, are assessed and monitored.

Direct Indices

Direct effects of political violence result in death, injury, and disabilities, including psychological ones, and there are direct consequences of a lack of protection provided by, and respect for, international humanitarian law. Direct effects are quantitative in nature and are subject to organized attempts to measure (i.e., population-based cluster sampling), and it is easier to find and hold people accountable.

Intervention from outside agencies and organizations is initially driven by reports of battlefield and civilian deaths. Assessment teams use both direct observation and rapid assessment tools to determine the consequences of the conflict on essential public health parameters such as access to and availability of food, water, sanitation, shelter, health, and fuel. Initial assessments focus on measurements for CMRs and U5MRs. As the humanitarian community becomes more established, follow-up surveys include population-based cluster samplings and studies that further disaggregate the CMRs to determine age and gender vulnerability (i.e., infant and maternal mortality and morbidity rates). Ongoing surveys and surveillance ensure that management responses meet Sphere, the Humanitarian Charter and Minimum Standards in Disaster Response (The Sphere Project, 2011) and other essential public health standards.

The operational assumption is that low-cost humanitarian aid, if properly performed and managed, will reduce the direct indicator rates to prewar conflict levels or better within 4 to 6 months. Unfortunately, as the direct effect mortality rates decline, so does outside interest and relief aid from donor agencies and governments, often giving a false assurance of success.

Indirect Indices

Indirect deaths are deaths that would not have occurred without the conflict. They are seen as collateral damage resulting from population displacement, disruption of food supplies, destroyed health facilities and public health infrastructure, and consequences, such as poverty and destroyed livelihoods, that will ultimately account for 90% or more of *overall mortality and morbidity*. Women and children are the most common victims, as are the elderly and those with disabilities. However, no existing data sets measure indirect death tolls, and, except for a few countries, the humanitarian community has no idea of the worldwide extent of indirect deaths from prolonged political violence. In contrast to direct indices, indirect deaths are rarely measured, are more functional and abstract in nature, frequently require qualitative or semiquantitative measures, and are difficult to determine accountability.

EPIDEMIOLOGICAL MODELS

There have been significant improvements in the design and management of humanitarian responses, in part due to the development of quality epidemiological studies and useful measuring tools (Roberts & Hofmann, 2004). Health consequences of CHEs are a predictable combination of:

- Direct effects (e.g., deaths, injuries, human rights abuses, psychological stress, and disabilities) and,
- Indirect effects (e.g., population displacement as refugees or IDPs, interrupted food distribution, destroyed health and public health facilities and infrastructure, and destroyed livelihoods).

Most common *baseline* health indices followed by the humanitarian community are:

- Mortality or death rates
- Morbidity rates
- Nutritional status
- Aid program indicators to ensure predicted impact and outcome
- Age- and gender-specific mortality and morbidity rates critical to determining population vulnerability
- Attack rates and case fatality rates crucial during outbreaks and epidemics

The epidemiological characteristics of CHEs have been studied by Burkle (2006) and are replicated here. For planning and training purposes, the major characteristics can be placed in one of three epidemiological models:

- *Developing Country Model*: for example, Angola, Somalia, Liberia, Afghanistan, and Congo
- *Developed Country Model*: for example, the former Yugoslavia and Iraq
- *Chronic/Smoldering Country Model*: for example, Haiti, Sudan, and Palestine

Epidemiological model data may overlap. The example of Iraq illustrates how a country at war is prone to slip rapidly from a former developed country model to exhibiting health indices similar to those of a less developing country. Over time, deaths from inadequate public health protections exceeded those caused by violence alone.

Overall, communicable diseases, alone or in combination with malnutrition, account for most deaths. Populations without adequate food for health have risen to 1 billion worldwide. Acts of genocide, ethnic cleansing, and torture have been reported in all models. Psychosocial and mental health problems are widespread in CHEs. Services need to be provided through both primary healthcare and community settings. Presentations tend to fall into three categories (Burkle, Chatterjee, Bass, & Bolton, 2008):

- Disabling psychiatric illnesses (new or preexisting illness)
- Severe psychological reactions to witnessed or experienced trauma
- Significant but temporary problems in individuals who are able to cope and adapt once peace and order are restored (This subgroup generally represents the majority of those presenting with symptoms.)

Developing Country Health Profiles

Health profiles (Box 15.2) reflect acute and often severe malnutrition combined with clinical or subclinical micronutrient deficiencies (e.g., vitamins A, C, and B_6 are common, but endemic regional nutritional deficiencies, such as B_1-thiamine and clinical beriberi, will also increase). Seventy-five percent of all communicable disease epidemics in the world occur in CHEs. Direct and indirect effects result in high CMRs and case fatality rates (e.g., measles and malaria in malnourished children), and outbreaks of endemic diseases such as malaria, diarrheal disease and dehydration, acute upper and lower respiratory diseases, meningitis, tuberculosis, vaccine-preventable diseases such as diphtheria and tetanus, and outbreaks of other tropical diseases such as leishmaniasis and leprosy have been reported (Connolly et al., 2004; Gayer, Legros, Formenty, & Connolly, 2007).

Mortality rates can range from 7 to 70 times the baseline levels (region and country-specific baseline rates may be found on websites from WHO [www.who.int], UNICEF [www.unicef .org], ReliefWeb [reliefweb.int], and the Center for Research on the Epidemiology of Disasters [www.cred.be]). Because they do not have parental or adult supervision and protection, orphans and unaccompanied minors may have mortality rates 100 to 200 times

the baseline. Programs must be in place to identify these children among the most vulnerable of populations, but they may not be identified until food distribution and immunization programs requiring cooperation of a parent or responsible adult are instituted in camps for refugees or internally displaced. These children will not receive vital health and nonhealth commodities unless assessment and data collection programs specifically target them.

Assessments may be challenged by absent, incomplete, or markedly outdated baseline demographics; hostile and insecure territory; and rapidly moving and easily lost populations. The methodologies used to determine "excess mortality" rates are appropriate in these CHEs, especially where policy decisions on relief aid must be rapidly determined (Roberts & Despines, 1999). Ninety percent of the deaths result not from violence but from preventable diarrheal disease, malnutrition, and malaria (Roberts & Hofmann, 2004). Though excess mortality studies are useful in defining the extent of the tragedy, they must be followed by more detailed population-based studies as soon as the ground conditions, especially security, allow.

Usually, acute phase priorities of relief programs focus on:

- Supplementary/therapeutic feeding
- Nutritional and health assessments
- Vaccine control measures
- Essential medications
- Surveillance programs

Developed Country Health Profiles

These countries have preconflict health profiles (Box 15.3) similar to those in Western developed countries with relatively healthy populations. Baseline demographics are usually available and are more readily available for population-based assessments. Because an established public health infrastructure, including education and practice of basic hygiene, has been in place for years, epidemics are few. As violence destroys vital infrastructures and health sector workers flee or are killed, the public health consequences rapidly surface alerting the international community to bring in outside resources through WHO teams, health-related NGOs, and the Red Cross Movement.

BOX 15.2 Developing Country Health Profile

- Large majority of mortality and morbidity preventable
- Outbreaks of communicable diseases
- Malnutrition and micronutrient diseases
- Absence of protective public health infrastructure
- Major deficiencies in WHO childhood vaccine protection
- Mental health consequences most often unmeasured and untreated
- Internally displaced and refugee populations
- Weaponry: Usually small arms and machetes; advanced weaponry increasing
- High crude mortality rates
- Higher mortality rates in orphaned and unaccompanied children
- High case fatality rates

WHO, World Health Organization.

BOX 15.3 Developed Country Health Profile

- Occurrence in baseline populations that are relatively healthy
- Demographic and disease profiles similar to those in Western industrialized countries
- Excess trauma deaths from war-related advance weaponry and small arms
- Excess age- and gender-related deaths increase during times of ethnic cleansing
- Few epidemics
- Excess mortality from untreated chronic diseases
- Significant rates of elderly with undernutrition
- Rape, abductions, and psychological traumatic exposures common

Health profiles show high mortality from advanced weaponry that target groups for the purpose of ethnic cleansing and genocide. Studies from Kosovo showed that age- and gender-related mortality increased during times of targeted ethnic cleansing (Spiegel & Salama, 2000). Excess mortality also increases in the elderly who, until the war and conflict, enjoyed an economic status that made medications available for chronic diseases such as hypertension, diabetes, and cancers, a luxury that developing country populations rarely have. The elderly, often unable to or refusing to flee their ancestral homes, may be the most vulnerable for undernutrition. Rape and psychological exposures are common and, when promoted by a warring faction, represent yet another form of ethnic cleansing.

Chronic/Smoldering Country Health Profiles

Health profiles (Box 15.4) result from prolonged degradation (e.g., 55 years in Sudan) of access and availability to many basic services. Cultures are often one of sustained violence. There is a daily struggle to sustain basic health and public health services. Children grow up chronically malnourished and have little access to healthcare and education. Children suffer both chronic stunting and acute malnutrition, which makes them more vulnerable to diseases and their complications. Healthcare workers are most likely expatriates as schools of medicine and nursing no longer exist. Reproductive services such as birth control, safe birthing, and C-section equipment are a luxury.

Studies from Sudan confirmed that peaks of mortality from rebel violence in villages resulted in survivors fleeing to Eastern Chad where little, if any, protective public health infrastructure

---

BOX 15.4 Smoldering or Chronic Country Model Health Profile

- Many years of chronic violence
- Social and political unrest
- Poor maintenance of basic public health infrastructure
- Environmental degradation high
- Little or no access to and availability of health and education
- Below-sustenance-level economy
- Chronic malnutrition and stunted growth
- Children growing up knowing only a culture of violence
- Few indigenous healthcare providers
- Lack of basic reproductive health services
- Organized mental health services generally nonexistent
- Incidents of violent surges resulting in peaks in death rates from direct violence and sudden-onset consequences of chronic conditions (i.e., acute malnutrition and dehydration in children with chronic malnutrition)
- Primarily small arms deaths and wounds, advanced weaponry increasing
- Violent surges increasing internally displaced and refugee populations

---

existed to stem preventable diseases. Gaza–West Bank studies in 1998 and 2003 confirmed widespread chronic malnutrition with macro- and micronutrient deficiencies (Abdeen, Greenough, Chandran, & Qasrawi, 2007). Haiti's environmental degradation is high with forested areas an all-time low of 2% (Library of Congress, 2006). Regional hurricanes directly kill residents but flooding and mudslides in the aftermath kill thousands more because of the lack of protective forest root structures. The 2010 earthquake confirmed that Haiti requires unprecedented root cause developmental and ongoing emergency assistance. Many years and a devastating cholera outbreak later, Haiti still requires assessments of morbidity and mortality and significant humanitarian aid. Assessments must determine the sustainability of restored health services and whether there is enough absorbing and buffering capacity to prevent a slippage back into chaos. The Ministry of Public Health in Afghanistan requires that health assistance conform to a *Basic Package of Health Services* with which all NGOs and others must comply. This has led to an improvement in health indices since 2001 in 85% of provinces where security is maintained (Ministry of Public Health, 2005).

POSTCONFLICT PHASE CONSEQUENCES

Consequences of prolonged CHEs have had a marked effect on Africa and other postconflict regions that are often unappreciated by the outside world. A peace agreement and cessation of shooting marks the beginning of the postconflict transition phase. The transition phase is the most dangerous for indirect mortality and morbidity and will continue until significant development occurs and the prewar resource base of protective infrastructure, good governance, and improving health indices occur (Ghobarth, Huth, & Russett, 2003, 2004). Most postconflict countries have a resource base less than 10% of what existed before the war. With the war declared over, donors lose interest in long-term commitments and in funding NGOs. The risk of continuing death and disability from environmental, communicable, and noncommunicable diseases related to the lack of recovery may continue to exist for a decade more. Mortality in the postconflict phase may far exceed the immediate losses from the war itself. Although declared wars have declined in number, an alarming number of people still experience low levels of conflict intensity where human security is tenuous and weapons, held over from the war, still proliferate and intimidate any meaningful peace process. Unfortunately, when these conditions prevail, 47% of postconflict countries risk returning to war within a decade, a rate that is 60% in Africa (United Nations Development Group, 2004). This occurs because little progress is made in reestablishing governance, reversing economic and health stagnation, and in bolstering an otherwise inadequate public health system. If not corrected, these effects will severely limit the capacity of postconflict countries to rehabilitate themselves (Burkle, 2010).

Despite the cessation of hostilities, subtle and rarely counted mortality and morbidity result from out of work and despondent heads of households, demobilized soldiers, and IDPs who are more likely to suffer suicide, depression, alcohol, and drug abuse. A sensitive marker of the continued community decay and economic and physical insecurity is an increase in *gender-based violence* among intimate partners. Widows from the Iran–Iraq War, the Persian Gulf War, and the 2003 War with Iraq collectively number over 740,000, representing 1 in every 11 Iraqi women. The Iraq Ministry of Women's Affairs reports at least 300,000 widows in Baghdad alone with another 8 million throughout the country. A WHO household survey suggested that 17% of these women are suffering from serious war-related mental illness and 75% are not receiving pensions owed to them. Such burdens inextricably lead to excess mortality and morbidity (Williams, 2009).

Fifty-seven countries, mostly postconflict, currently face a healthcare worker crisis. Sub-Saharan Africa has 11% of the world's population and 24% of the world's burden of disease, yet has only 3% of health workers. Evidence suggests that the burden of intentional and unintentional injuries often arises after a conflict particularly in sub-Saharan Africa and the Middle East. The surgical burden of disease is increasing due to the severe shortage of surgical and anesthetic services and trained professionals (McQueen et al., 2009). This has resulted in an increased use of nondoctors with specific WHO-initiated technical skill education who perform surgery under the supervision of a primary care physician or nurse. In many conflict and postconflict settings, the nursing profession provides the bulk of primary healthcare and basic mental health services (outpatient and inpatient). During the 14 years of ruinous wars in Liberia when less than 20 physicians remained in practice, nurses continued, as they do today, to be the mainstay of primary healthcare.

SHIFTING AID FROM RURAL TO URBAN ENVIRONMENTS

The migration of populations to cities both within the country in conflict and regionally have contributed to rapid urbanization in both Africa and Asia (Figure 15.2).

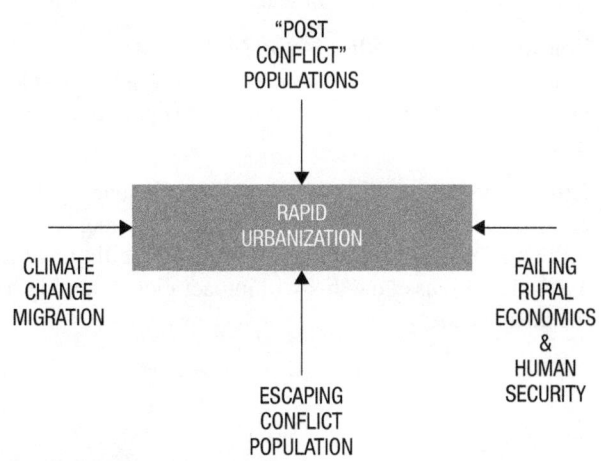

FIGURE 15.2 Rapid urbanization is fueled by populations fleeing conflict, continued postconflict insecurity, climate change migration, and failing economic and human security in rural areas. As such, urban settings in 2008 contained the majority of the world's population, an event that was not anticipated to occur until 2017 to 2020.

Megacities (urban centers with populations over 10 million) in developing countries have shown increasing health inequities and a widening gap between the "have and have not" populations. Rapid urbanization is unsustainable and occurs when the population growth exceeds that of the public health infrastructure, especially water supply, sanitation, shelter, and access and availability of basic health services. Health for many has become a major security issue, especially among the massive numbers of urban squatters who have little or no representation and protections from central governments or the humanitarian community. With sanitation basically ignored, infectious diseases have become more prevalent. The estimated population of Kabul, Afghanistan, in 2001 was 500,000. In 2009, it was over 5 million where most, fleeing the rural insecurity, have become victims of "rapid, unregulated and unequal" urbanization, overstretched health services, and shelters that are "illegal, unplanned and sub-standard" (IRIN, 2009). Conditions are extremely poor in Nairobi, Kenya, where urban settlements contain fleeing populations from eight different regional countries. In Africa, weapons transported to the urban slums have resulted in the rise of predatory gangs and the proliferation of trade centers for the marketing of weaponry for the region. Currently, the highest infant, maternal, and U5 mortality rates are found in these unsustainable urban conclaves where international humanitarian representation is scant and few public health and social protections exist. Rape epidemics and scarcity of shelters, clean water, and sanitation prevail. All the conventional Sphere standards utilized in refugee camps and other conventional wars have long been exceeded. Megacity slums currently report the highest worldwide U5MRs (Burkle, 2010).

FUTURE COMPLEX HUMANITARIAN EMERGENCIES

Mass fatalities from war have occupied our attention during the last three decades and probably prevented serious consideration of looming humanitarian crises. The Global Humanitarian Forum report suggests that "more than 300 million people are already seriously affected by the gradual warming of the earth," a number they claim will double by 2030. The report further warns that 300,000 people per year are already dying due to "gradual environmental degradation and climate-related malnutrition, diarrhea and malaria." Furthermore, the report suggests that climate change threatens "all eight of the Millennium Development Goals that aim to reduce extreme poverty by 2015." About 45 million of the now 1 billion people are estimated to be suffering from chronic hunger due to the direct impact of climate change (Global Humanitarian Forum, 2009).

Paul Collier's "Bottom Billion" based on 1990's population data placed 93% of those in extreme poverty in both low income stable (e.g., Tanzania, Zambia) and fragile conflict-affected (e.g., Congo, Burundi) nation-states (Collier, 2007). Sumner (2011), in tapping into 2007 to 2008 population data, found a significant change: Today, 72% of the bottom billion are now in middle income stable (e.g.,

India, China, Indonesia) and fragile conflict-affected (e.g., Pakistan, Nigeria) nation-states. The implications of the data on aid planning, budgets, and millennium development goals (MDGs) are tremendous, as are the risks for CHEs. Also, these analyses revealed that lower middle income countries, not low income ones, have the highest rate of 1-year-old children without basic three-dose diphtheria, tetanus, and pertussis (DTP3) vaccination coverage (Glassman, 2011). Countries such as India, China, and Indonesia uniquely have both extreme poverty, high infectious disease rates in their "have not" populations, and chronic diseases of old age in their high income "have" populations, a phenomenon rarely seen before in the developing world.

"Emergencies of scarcity" relate to declining access to, and availability of, water, energy, and food. Import-dependent countries like South Korea, Japan, China, and many in the Middle East are actively purchasing land in foreign countries to meet national food security needs (Evans, 2009). Many of these biologically fragile areas in Africa are crucial habitats for plants and animals. Eighty percent of major conflicts have occurred in 23 of the known 34 most biologically diverse and threatened places on earth (Burkle, 2010). War monies commonly come from massive timber harvesting (e.g., Congo and Cambodia). Poor governments pressure farmers, who have no political voice or social protections, to give up their land to foreign investors. Oil energy resources under the Arctic, South China, and Caspian Seas are also being aggressively purchased and tapped. Referred to as "land grabbing," the aggressive competition for resources are considered at risk to provoke "distributional conflicts" that may lead to more demonstrable unconventional crises in the future (Evans, 2009).

PROFESSIONALIZATION OF THE HUMANITARIAN WORKFORCE

Recent CHEs have underscored the need to endorse a process for the accreditation and accountability of providers. A blueprint for professionalizing humanitarian assistance has gained significant worldwide acceptance throughout Europe and North America (Walker, Hein, Russ, Bertleff, & Caspersz, 2010). The international Enhancing Learning and Research for Humanitarian Assistance (ELRHA) project "aims to see a global humanitarian community where humanitarian actors actively collaborate with higher education institutes to develop highly professional responders, share expertise and carry out research that noticeably reduces risk and ensures that those suffering from the impact of crises receive more timely, relevant and sustainable assistance" (n.d., "Our Vision") Currently, 92% of NGOs favor professionalization (Walker & Russ, 2010). Recognizing this trend, professional nursing schools are increasingly offering global health and public health curricula with certificate-, bachelor's-, master's-, nurse practitioner-, and doctoral-level programs. Not surprisingly, for decades, nurses have historically managed, staffed, and sustained the large majority of health projects and missions worldwide.

SUMMARY

CHEs is a composite term that comprises current unconventional warfare and conflicts arising from terrorism, guerilla warfare, insurgencies, and wars of national liberation.

CHEs have emerged as an entity, in part, because the nature of war and conflict has changed considerably in the last three decades. Disaster medicine and nursing are increasingly challenged by political and cultural nuances and the complexities of providing basic healthcare and public health protections in CHEs. The demand on both the expatriate and indigenous health workforce is unprecedented. The nursing profession will have to generate a dialogue with its counterparts in other parts of the world to ensure multidisciplinary global health solutions and research for future humanitarian crises, all of which, as CHEs, will inevitably result in major public health emergencies. Nursing must actively engage in current academically led movements to advance and maintain quality performance, accountability, and accreditation of all humanitarian professionals. Only then will innovative solutions in health, education, human rights, policy, and public health be developed to mitigate the sufferings brought about by CHEs.

STUDY QUESTIONS

1. Provide examples of both direct and indirect mortality and morbidity in complex emergencies and how nursing requirements may differ for each.

2. War and armed conflict in the Middle East are current examples of complex humanitarian emergencies. Explain how climate change and extremes contribute to the onset of conflict.

3. Current refugee and migrant numbers escaping from complex humanitarian emergencies now number over 67 million. They are projected to grow to 140 million within a decade. Discuss how this will impact global nursing for the next decade.

REFERENCES

Abdeen, Z., Greenough, P. G., Chandran, A., & Qasrawi, R. (2007, September 28). Assessment of the nutritional status of preschool-age children during the second Intifada in Palestine. *Food and Nutrition Bulletin, 28*(3), 274–282. doi:10.1177/156482650702800303

Albala-Bertrand, J. M. (2000, October 1–29). *What is a "complex humanitarian emergency"? An analytical essay* (Working Paper No.

420). London, UK: Department of Economics, Queen Mary College, University of London.

Atwood, J. B. (2010). Elevating development assistance. *Prism, 1*(3), 3–12.

Breau, S., & Joyce, R. (2011, June). *Discussion Paper: The legal obligation to record civilian casualties or armed conflict.* London, UK: Oxford Research Group. Retrieved from http://www.oxfordresearchgroup.org.uk/sites/default/files/1st%20legal%20report%20formatted%20FINAL.pdf

Brennan, R. J., & Nandy, R. (2001, June 13). Complex humanitarian emergencies: A major global health challenge. *Emergency Medicine (Fremantle), 13*(2), 147–156. doi:10.1046/j.1442-2026.2001.00203.x

Burkle, F. M. (2006, April–June). Complex humanitarian emergencies: A review of epidemiological and response models. *Journal of Postgraduate Medicine, 52*(2), 110–115.

Burkle, F. M. (2008, January 19). Measuring humanitarian assistance in conflicts. *Lancet, 371*(9608), 189–190. doi:10.1016/S0140-6736(08)60118-X

Burkle, F. M. (2010, May–June). Future humanitarian crises: Challenges for practice, policy, and public health. *Prehospital and Disaster Medicine, 25*(3), 191–199. doi:10.1017/s1049023x00007998

Burkle, F. M., Chatterjee, P., Bass, J., & Bolton, P. (2008). *Guidelines for the psycho-social and mental health assessment and management of displaced populations in humanitarian crises. Public Health Guide for Emergencies.* Geneva, Switzerland/Baltimore, MD: International Federation of Red Cross and Red Crescent Societies/Johns Hopkins University Medical Institutions.

Burkle, F. M., & Greenough, P. G. (2008, October). Impact of public health emergencies on modern disaster taxonomy, planning, and response. *Disaster Medicine and Public Health Preparedness, 2*(3), 192–199. doi:10.1097/DMP.0b013e3181809455

Byman, D. L. (2011). *Do targeted killings work?* Washington, DC: Brookings. Retrieved from https://www.brookings.edu/articles/do-targeted-killings-work

Collier, P. (2007). *The bottom billion: Why the poorest countries are failing and what can be done about it.* New York, NY: Oxford University Press.

Connolly, M. A., Gayer, M., Ryan, M. J., Salama, P., Spiegel, P., & Heymann, D. L. (2004, November 27–December 3). Communicable diseases in complex emergencies: Impact and challenges. *Lancet, 364*(9449), 1974–1983. doi:10.1016/S0140-6736(04)17481-3

Duffield, M. (1994). Complex emergencies and the crises of developmentalism. *Institute of Development Studies Bulletin, 25*(4), 1–15. doi:10.1111/j.1759-5436.1994.mp25004006.x

Enhancing Learning and Research for Humanitarian Assistance. (n.d.). About. Retrieved from http://www.elrha.org/hif/about/background/elrha

Evans, A. (2009). Managing scarcity: The institutional dimensions. Retrieved from http://www.globalpolicy.org/security-council/dark-side-of-natural-resources/other-articles-analysis-and-general-debate/48191.html

Gayer, M., Legros, D., Formenty, P., & Connolly, M. A. (2007). Conflict and emerging infectious diseases. *Emerging Infectious Diseases, 13*(11), 1625–1631. doi: 10.3201/eid1311.061093.

Ghobarth, H., Huth, P., & Russett, B. (2003). Civil wars kill and maim people long after the shooting stops. *American Political Science Review, 97*(2), 189–202. doi:10.1017/s0003055403000613

Ghobarth, H., Huth, P., & Russett, B. (2004). The post-war public health effects of civil conflict. *Social Science and Medicine, 59*, 869–884. doi:10.1016/j.socscimed.2003.11.043

Glassman, A. (2011, April 28). The new bottom billion: Implications for GAVI? *Global Health Policy Blog.* Washington, DC: Center for Global Development. Retrieved from http://blogs.cgdev.org/globalhealth/2011/04/the-new-bottom-billion-implications-for-gavi.php

Global Humanitarian Forum. (2009). *Human impact report: Climate change—The anatomy of a silent crisis.* Geneva, Switzerland: Author. Retrieved from http://www.ghf-ge.org/human-impact-report.pdf

Hoekstra, R., & Tucker, C. E. (2010). Adjusting to stabilization and reconstruction operations. *PRISM, 1*(2), 1326. Retrieved from https://www.humanitarianoutcomes.org/publications/aid-worker-security-report-2017-behind-attacks-look-perpetrators-violence-against-aid

International Committee of the Red Cross. (1949, August 12). *Convention (IV) relative to the protection of civilian persons in time of war.* Geneva, Switzerland: Author.

IRIN. (2009, July 15). Unsafe housing puts Kabul residents at risk. Retrieved from http://www.irinnews.org/report.aspx?ReportId=85286

Jones, L., Asare, J. B., El Masri, M., Mohanraj, A., Sherief, H., & Van Ommeren, M. (2009, August 22). Severe mental disorders in complex emergencies. *The Lancet, 374*(9690), 654–661. doi:10.1016/S0140-6736(09)61253-8

Kem, J. D. (2007, February 7). Stability and reconstruction operations: Connecting the dots between military and civilian efforts. *Small Wars Journal.* Retrieved from http://smallwarsjournal.com/documents/swjmag/v7/kem-swjvol7.pdf

Kickbusch, I. (2011, June 10). Global health diplomacy: How foreign policy can influence health. *British Medical Journal, 342*, d3154. doi:10.1136/bmj.d3154

Library of Congress, Federal Research Division. (2006, May). Country profile: Haiti. Retrieved from https://www.loc.gov/rr/frd/cs/profiles/Haiti.pdf

Marks, T. A., Gorka, S. L., & Sharp, R. (2010). Getting the next war right: Beyond population-centric warfare. *PRISM, 1*(3), 79–96.

McQueen, K. A., Parmar, P., Kene, M., Broaddus, S., Casey, K., Chu, K., . . . Burkle, F. M. (2009, July–August). Burden of surgical disease: Strategies to manage an existing public health emergency. *Prehospital and Disaster Medicine, 24*(Suppl 2), s228–s231. doi:10.1017/s1049023x00021634

Ministry of Public Health. (2005). A basic package of health services for Afghanistan, 2005/1384. Islamic Republic of Afghanistan. Retrieved from http://moph.gov.af/Content/Media/Documents/Monitoring-Evaluation-Policy-Strategy2912201016288921.pdf

Roberts, L., & Despines, M. (1999, June 26). Mortality in the Democratic Republic of the Congo. *Lancet, 353*(9171), 2249–2250. doi:10.1016/s0140-6736(05)76308-x

Roberts, L., & Hofmann, C. A. (2004, October 7). Assessing the impact of humanitarian assistance in the health sector. *Emerging Themes in Epidemiology, 1*(1), 3. doi:10.1186/1742-7622-1-3

Spiegel, P. B., Burkle, F. M., Dey, C. C., & Salama, P. (2001). Developing public health indicators in complex emergency response. *Prehospital and Disaster Medicine, 16*(4), 281–285. doi:10.1017/s1049023x00043430

Spiegel, P. B., & Salama, P. (2000, June 24). War and mortality in Kosovo, 1998–99: An epidemiological testimony. *Lancet, 355*(9222), 2204–2209. doi:10.1016/S0140-6736(00)02404-1

Stoddard, A., Harmer, A., & Czwarno, M. (2017). Aid worker security report 2017: Behind the attacks: A look at the perpetrators of violence against aid workers. Humanitarian Outcomes. Aid Worker Security database. Retrieved from https://www.humanitarianoutcomes.org/publications/aid-worker-security-report-2017-behind-attacks-look-perpetrators-violence-against-aid

Sumner, A. (2011, March 18). *The new bottom billion: What if most of the world's poor live in middle-income countries? Policy Brief.* Washington, DC: Centre for Global Development. Retrieved from http://www.ids.ac.uk/publication/the-new-bottom-billion-what-if-most-of-the-world-s-poor-live-in-middle-income-countries

The Sphere Project. (2011). *The Sphere handbook: Humanitarian charter and minimum standards in humanitarian response.* Geneva, Switzerland: International Federation of Red Cross and Red Crescent Societies. Retrieved from http://www.sphereproject.org

Tomes, R. (2004, Spring). Relearning counterinsurgency warfare. *Parameters, 34*(1), 16–28. Retrieved from http://ssi.armywarcollege.edu/pubs/parameters/articles/04spring/tomes.pdf

UN News Centre. (2011). Afghanistan & the United Nations. Retrieved from http://www.un.org/News/dh/latest/afghan/un-afghan-history.shtml

United Nations. (1945). Charter of the United Nations: Chapter I: Purposes and principles, article 2. Retrieved from https://treaties.un.org/doc/publication/ctc/uncharter.pdf

United Nations Development Group. (2004, February). Report of the UNDG/ECHA Working Group on Transition Issues. Retrieved from http://hdr.undp.org/en/content/human-development-report-2004

Van Creveld, M. (2010). War in complex environments: The technological dimension. *PRISM, 1*(3), 115–128.

Walker, P., Hein, K., Russ, C., Bertleff, G., & Caspersz, D. (2010). A blueprint for professionalizing humanitarian assistance. *Health Affairs (Millwood), 29*(12), 2223–2230. doi:10.1377/hlthaff.2010.1023

Walker, P., & Russ, C. (2010, April). *Professionalizing the humanitarian sector: A scoping study* [Internet]. London, UK: Enhancing Learning and Research for Humanitarian Assistance. Retrieved from http://euhap.eu/upload/2014/06/professionalising-the-humanitarian-sector.pdf

Williams, T. (2009, February 22). Iraq's war widows face dire need with little aid. *The New York Times*. Retrieved from http://www.nytimes.com/2009/02/23/world/middleeast/23widows.html?scp=1& sq=iraq%20widows&st=cse

ADDITIONAL RESOURCES

Burkle, F. M. (2010). Complex public health emergencies. In K. L. Koenig & C. H. Schultz (Eds.), *Disaster medicine: Comprehensive principles and practices* (pp. 361–376). New York, NY: Cambridge University Press.

Burkle, F. M., & Greenough, P. G. (2006). Complex emergencies. In G. R. Ciottone (Ed.), *Disaster medicine* (pp. 43–50). Philadelphia, PA: Elsevier-Mosby.

The Failed States Index. (2017). Annual Report. The Fund for Peace. Retrieved from http://fundforpeace.org/fsi/2017/05/14/fragile-states-index-2017-annual-report

Toole, M. J., Waldman, R. J., & Zwi, A. B. (2001). Complex humanitarian emergencies. In M. H. Merson, R. E. Black, & A. J. Mills (Eds.), *International public health: Diseases, programs, systems, and policies* (pp. 439–514). Gaithersburg, MD: Aspen Publications.

16

NURSING IN DISASTERS, CATASTROPHES, AND COMPLEX HUMANITARIAN EMERGENCIES WORLDWIDE

Pat Deeny and Kevin Davies

LEARNING OBJECTIVES

When this chapter is completed, readers will be able to:

1. Appreciate the scale of disasters and how sociopolitical, economic, and cultural factors contribute to the development of catastrophes and complex humanitarian emergencies worldwide.
2. Determine the contribution of nurses to global aid relief and the range of extended roles that exist for nurses at all levels and stages of the disaster situation.
3. Gain an initial understanding of the necessity for leadership and clinical decision making by nurses in the potentially risk-laden environments that often exist in disaster situations and complex humanitarian emergencies worldwide.
4. Affirm the importance of human rights, cultural awareness, and sensitivity for nurses working in multinational teams or in the care of individuals and communities who fall victim to disaster.
5. Identify the key ethical issues associated with nursing in disaster situations and show increased awareness of the difficulties associated with neutrality and independence.
6. Discuss the key elements of quality assurance in international disaster response and preparedness and how rigorous evaluation contributes to improvements in nursing practice for disaster situations worldwide.
7. Identify transportation and communication as potential major obstacles to relief efforts during disasters.

8. Appreciate that complex emergencies present increased risk to the personal safety of nurses working in disaster relief.
9. Describe the unique challenges for international disaster nursing that are posed by refugee or internally displaced populations requiring care in the acute or recovery phases of disasters.

KEY MESSAGES

In the context of a growing world population, urbanization of nations, and an increasing threat from climate change, disasters worldwide are on the increase. Despite some recent terrible disasters in developed countries, most disasters still occur in the developing world where economic and political factors strongly influence the level of preparedness and capacity for response. As poverty and uneven distribution of wealth is directly linked to disaster vulnerability, sustainable development and building community resilience in poorer countries is the only answer to future risk reduction.

Nurses play a key role in building community resilience, disaster mitigation, response, and recovery. They must continue to alleviate suffering and mitigate loss of life in the acute phase, support communities through mourning and remembrance, and provide education for community resilience building and community recovery. The initial focus on education for rapid and effective disaster response has been laudable, but a fresh impetus for community risk reduction and long-term recovery is now needed worldwide.

Good clinical leadership by nurses in disaster situations is always critical. Knowledge of basic triage techniques, advanced first aid, public health awareness and psychological first aid means that nurses can deal effectively with large numbers of casualties, families and/or groups of displaced people. However, as nurses are not operating in what could be defined as "normal" circumstances and do not have access to resources and professional support structures, clinical decision making can be much more challenging. On the spot decisions have to be made. While Nursing Codes of Conduct support such decision making, nurses need to be clear in advance that professional values and clinical leadership will be tested in disaster situations, especially in other countries and other cultures across the globe.

As is the case with all aid humanitarian relief workers, nurses are accountable for preservation of human dignity. Nurses must be able to operate within the context of the International Red Cross/Red Crescent Code of Conduct and display sensitivity to the political and cultural complexity of disaster situations.

Nurses might have to take an advocacy stance in relation to protection of human rights ensuring that victims are treated according to international humanitarian principles in the Code of Conduct, United Nations Declaration of Human Rights, and the Geneva Conventions. This includes people who may be defined as insurgents, rebels, or terrorists.

Nurses providing aid relief to communities across the world must be aware of the international standards for delivery of aid. These are referred to as the Sphere Standards and are used by aid relief agencies worldwide.

CHAPTER OVERVIEW

Nurses care for nations, communities, families, groups, and individuals worldwide. The changing context of disasters on a global scale provides a backdrop to the discussion on the growth of aid response and the associated contribution of disaster nursing at an international level. Disasters are more often than not caused by natural events but increasingly they have become "complex humanitarian emergencies" due to economic, political, and cultural factors. If the disaster is on a large scale, the term "catastrophe" is sometimes used. With an increased focus on community resilience, care is provided at all levels and across all phases of a disaster. There is a new emphasis worldwide on disaster risk reduction through building community resilience (United Nations [UN], 2015). This invites nurses to work with local communities to reduce vulnerability to disasters. Effective disaster response at an international level requires nurses to have knowledge and skills for work in other cultures. There must be an awareness that clinical leadership and decision making in disaster situations can be outside the normal frame of reference of most nurses. This can present new and challenging clinical situations, which will test nurses to the limit. Specific areas such as communication, transport, personal security, prioritizing the care of victims of disaster, refugee health, and an increased personal, ethical, legal, and cultural awareness are discussed.

Disasters such as floods, famine, earthquakes, armed conflicts, and mass refugee movements are on the increase (Relief Web International, 2017; World Health Organization [WHO], 2017a). This means that many disasters are now defined as catastrophes or complex humanitarian emergencies (Leaning & Guha-Sapir, 2013). Since the time of Florence Nightingale, nurses have contributed at an international level to the care of nations, communities, families, and individuals who have fallen victim to disasters. While local nurses are among the first responders and normally provide most of the care, it is common practice for some nurses to travel abroad to provide assistance to other countries in disaster situations. Disaster, by its definition, normally requires outside help. As the major profession involved in healthcare worldwide, it is recognized that nurses are well placed to make an international contribution to disaster response. Working in all phases of the disaster, nurses contribute to disaster preparedness, response, management, recovery, and overall resilience building to reduce the future impact of future disasters (WHO, 2006).

Although it is a common sight on the international news reports to see nurses working in the world's disaster zones, records of the nursing contribution are scant. A search of the literature reveals that the written nursing contribution to knowledge on disasters and the associated care of victims is small and most of the time it does not go beyond anecdotal accounts from those nurses who experience disasters. Some literature reviews and prepositional papers outline the key issues for nurses in disaster relief worldwide. This chapter in itself is one such contribution. Although these accounts are valuable and point to important needs of victims, communities, and nurses, it seems reasonable to propose that nursing science in relation to disaster relief nursing is still embryonic. This picture seems consistent across the world and is one of the main issues for disaster relief nursing in the 21st century.

This chapter explores the key issues associated with nursing in disasters, catastrophes, and complex humanitarian emergencies worldwide and how the context of aid relief is changing. Slow disasters are also discussed. Outlining the contribution of nurses to global aid relief and the range of nursing roles therein points out the importance of cultural awareness and sensitivity in disaster situations. A case is made for the education of nurses in international groups to foster such awareness and improve competence in working with other cultures and in international teams.

As disasters are normally associated with population displacement and social upheaval, there is always the potential for victims of disasters to feel that dignity is compromised and health as whole human beings is under threat. As key health professionals who value providing a holistic approach, nurses must become advocates for the maintenance of dignity and human rights for those affected by disasters. Ethical challenges are commonplace in disaster situations mainly because of the complexity and mix of political and cultural dimensions that exist in the affected population. This complexity may even exist within international aid relief teams.

As providers of aid relief to communities across the world, nurses must be aware of the need for accountability and quality of care. This is not easy as there is no universally accepted international minimum standards. In the absence of a single universal standard, some international governmental organizations (IGOs) and nongovernmental organizations (NGOs) have developed their own standards. The Sphere Project (2011; presently being rewritten for 2018) has developed universal international minimum standards.

Transportation and communication needs are explored as potential obstacles to successful humanitarian relief efforts and are presented as core knowledge for anyone considering entering the field of disaster nursing. The unique health requirements of displaced persons and refugee populations are described as an example of the types of humanitarian challenges nurses face. Fundamentally, nurses should be aware that most international disasters are now "complex humanitarian emergencies" and are best perceived as volatile situations. As is the case with all humanitarian workers, nurses are in almost constant threat of being robbed, kidnapped, raped, or taken hostage. While road traffic collisions and vehicle accidents predominate, awareness of personal security is critical. The chapter closes with the challenges associated with increased cultural awareness for nursing in disasters worldwide.

SCALE OF DISASTERS WORLDWIDE

Eshghi and Larson's analysis in 2008 of disasters over the previous 105 years (1903–2008) suggests that disasters are on the increase but cautioned against believing that the world has become a more dangerous place. While improved global monitoring systems do contribute to a picture of increasing threat, it would be foolhardy to ignore other major contributing factors. An increasing world population (now at 7.5 billion as we write this chapter; World Population Clock, 2017), increased poverty and hunger coupled with increased urbanization, and a growing threat from climate change all point to the need to see disasters as a major threat to humankind (International Federation of Red Cross and Red Crescent Societies [IFRC], 2017). The Overseas Development Institute highlights that 325 million extremely poor people will be living in the 49 most hazard-prone countries by 2030 (Shepherd et al., 2013). Since the 2004 Indian Ocean Tsunami or Boxing Day Tsunami where an estimated 225,000 were killed in 11 countries and across two continents (WHO, 2017b), fundamental lessons about disaster response were laid down. Wahlstrom identified three main conclusions that may be drawn from the aid relief effort associated with the Indian Ocean Tsunami (Wahlstrom, 2005). These were the affirmation of a truly interdependent world, the need to design an accountability system that can report back quickly to the range of donors involved in a disaster response, and the need for better coordination of the international disaster relief response system. All this should result in affected communities and host governments not being put under as much pressure in the acute phase. In a review of the lessons for public health management in disasters, Nabarro (2005) also suggested new ways to develop public health capacity within disaster management systems in the wake of the tsunami. He proposed that from the WHO perspective it was no longer acceptable to merely observe and analyze. The need to monitor actions that emerged from the analysis of the response to the tsunami indicates that WHO must continue to press world governments on disaster preparedness (Nabarro, 2005). Some of these ideas have been realized in international agreements such as the Sendai Framework (UN, 2015).

It is reasonable to suggest that disasters are probably one of the greatest global threats and challenges to the existence of the human race. This proposition exists even before consideration is given to the increased threat of pandemics. To date, most disasters have been caused by natural phenomena such as drought, windstorms, earthquakes, and floods. For this reason, it is necessary to consider the impact of natural disasters on the world, as it is from this source that the greatest demand is placed on nursing internationally.

The most vulnerable areas are those that very often make up the developing world (perhaps more importantly what one may term the "majority world") and as such have little in the way of resources to cope with any disaster. This is further complicated by the effects of globalization, whereby the wealthier countries are able to exploit further developing technology to become wealthier, and the poorer countries struggle in the wake.

It is important to note, however, that in poorer countries it is more common to experience "slow" or "progressive" disaster events. This is where a disaster occurs over a period of months or years but can have the same devastating consequences as a sudden disaster. In addition, slow disasters often occur in countries that have endemic problems such as malnutrition and disease. Sub-Saharan African countries are a good example of this. Furthermore, the public health impact can be exacerbated by the overcrowding in refugee centers, thereby contributing to increased mortality and morbidity as a consequence of gastrointestinal disease and measles. Chronic malnutrition, chronic dehydration, chronic anemia, chronic malaria, meningitis in the African meningitis belt, HIV/AIDS killing people (or making them orphans who are immunocompromised) results in an ever-increasing vulnerability to pandemic influenza. While HIV/AIDS, malaria, and tuberculosis still remain major foci, the emergence of noncommunicable diseases in poorer countries is becoming equally devastating (Chan, 2017). Furthermore, the fact that 800,000 people across the developed and developing world die each year due to suicide (WHO, 2014) means that poor mental health must be recognized as a slow disaster.

Disaster response is always influenced by global politics and this often sets the context in which agencies have to operate. The passing of the Cold War era has resulted in a new world order or disorder that directly affects the provision of disaster relief nursing. In 2000, Janz and Slead pointed out that aid relief agencies must demonstrate a more reflective learning style and develop new skills to operate in an increasingly hostile and complex world. Described as the "disaster cauldron" by Katoch in 2006, it is clear that disasters are highly volatile and complex situations that require highly trained and specialized people who operate effectively, have a personal resilience and professional competence that enables them to operate within highly challenging and complex care delivery environments.

The delivery of humanitarian aid is an attractive and challenging experience for many of the world's healthcare professionals. Nurses are drawn to relief aid for a number of reasons. The driving force may be religious, humanitarian, altruistic (Asgary & Lawrence, 2014; Carbonnier, 2015),

searching for new experiences, need to attain personal growth or to test personal limits (Bjerneld, Lindmark, McSpadden, & Garrett, 2006; Hunt, 2009). Deployments are usually undertaken under the auspices of an IGO such as the United Nations (UN) or NGOs such as Save the Children International (www.savethechildren.net), World Vision (www.worldvision.org), Concern (www.concern.net), Médicines Sans Frontièrs (www.msf.org), or the International Federation of Red Cross and Red Crescent Societies (IFRC; www.ifrc.org/). The latter works on a system where the National Red Cross Society proposes "delegates" to IFRC.

Additionally, there may be a national or cultural focus to the aid-delivering organization. Most western countries are associated with disaster relief. This, however, is expanding to the Arab countries. Japan as a nation has been striving for some years with a considerable degree of success to become a key player in terms of aid relief delivery and academic pursuit in the field. Aid relief delivery is becoming increasingly culturally diverse. Readers might be interested in the Japanese-led Disaster Nursing Global Leader Program (DNGLP).

GROWTH OF AID AGENCIES AND CONTRIBUTION OF NURSING

The roots of the aid "industry" can be traced back to the Swiss national Henri Dunant who, following the battle of Solferino in 1859, set in motion the processes that resulted in the formation of the International Committee of the Red Cross (ICRC) in 1880 with its distinctive Red Cross insignia. In 1909, 37 IGOs and 176 NGOs were operating worldwide. However, by 1998, there were 260 IGOs and 5,472 NGOs operating. Ryan and Lumley (2000) make two observations regarding this increase: there is an ever-increasing demand; until recently, there was freedom to work in a climate of relative safety. In the 21st century, the numbers continue to exponentially rise with questionable rise in effectiveness. The UN Cluster System (Office for the Coordination of Humanitarian Affairs [OCHA], 2017) has helped to reduce duplication across agencies but overlap is still prevalent. Nurses deploying to the world's disaster zones must be conscious as to how and where the employing agency fits into the UN Cluster (e.g., Oxfam will deal with water, WHO with health).

Nursing has a long association with the care of individuals, groups, and communities that experience disasters. Involved at local, national, and international levels, nurses have, with other healthcare professionals, played a key role in disaster prevention and in the delivery and management of care in disaster situations (WHO & International Council of Nurses [ICN], 2009). The types of roles nurses may hold range from senior managerial and leadership posts to providers of direct care. Such roles exist to assist with not only the preservation of life and maintenance of health during the acute phase, but also during the sequel or recovery phase of the disaster. A critical role is the involvement of nurses in "development work" in countries that are at risk of disasters. This type of work contributes to resilience and capacity building to have mature plans in place in the case of a disaster or indeed prevent disasters from occurring.

The contribution of nursing to disaster response and preparedness is viewed as being immense because nurses are one of the largest groups of frontline workers within the humanitarian community. The ICN holds the view that:

> Nurses with their technical skills and knowledge of epidemiology, physiology, pharmacology, cultural-familial structures, and psychosocial issues can assist in disaster preparedness programs as well as during disasters. Nurses, as team members, can play a strategic role cooperating with health and social disciplines, government bodies, community groups, and non-governmental agencies, including humanitarian organizations. (ICN, 2001; WHO & ICN, 2009)

Despite this perception, critical evaluation of nursing's contribution is scant, with little evidence to confirm that nursing input in disasters at an international level improves health outcomes. Disaster relief is a team affair where nurses contribute to the provision of healthcare in a multinational and multiprofessional environment. On the one hand, it may seem futile to delineate nurses from other professional groups, but on the other, it is valuable to focus on the unique contribution of nursing to this field. Nurses normally have a broad skill base that allows flexibility, adaptability, and creativity to adjust roles and accommodate rapidly changing circumstances. Such attributes are at the hub of working in disasters. As they have the largest numbers worldwide, they also have the largest number of students and thereby provide the greatest future resource for future work in disasters.

There is an immediate need for nurses to carry out valid and reliable evaluative studies that explore and document the value of nursing in this field. While there is widespread recognition of the contribution of nursing at an international level to disaster response and preparedness, more needs to be done in relation to development of a foundation for nursing science in the field. Nursing knowledge in this field is wholly dependent on personal accounts and literature reviews, which are of interest and value, but do not contribute to providing a quantitative empirical base value (see, e.g., Davies & Bricknell, 1997; Davies & Higginson, 2005; Deeny & McFetridge, 2005).

Conducting nursing research during disasters is not easy. There are ethical issues associated with research involving vulnerable groups. Lavin (2006) refers to the difficulties with the Health Insurance Portability and Accountability Act (HIPAA) Privacy Rule in the United States and points out some important legal and ethical issues associated with research in disasters. Our experience of facilitating research programs for master's degree students means that small qualitative studies are the easiest to manage. Interviews, focus groups, and ethnographic methods are the most common tools used and are the easiest to employ when seeking access to another culture and wishing to speak to people who are vulnerable. Personal diaries that constitute contemporaneous accounts could also offer valuable data if a retrospective reflective analysis is applied.

Sorting out the ethical issues in relation to conducting research in disasters is a worthwhile starting point. Ownership of data can be an issue. If data are collected in a community that has just experienced a disaster, the data belong to that community. They should have first call on the dissemination and implementation of findings. Just as in mainstream healthcare

research where participants in the form of patient groups are heavily involved in research, so too should be the case in disaster research. Nurses are in a prime position to develop this process whether they wish to use an action research approach or carry out projects that are immediately applicable to the communities in which they work. Many nurses are closely involved with communities in disasters and could develop the science at the point of practice where it is most required. Although empirical work is scarce at present, it is only a matter of time before nurses carry out empirical studies that contribute to knowledge about nursing in disasters.

DEVELOPMENT OF AN INTERNATIONAL WORKFORCE

Growing global instability has resulted in changes in the nature of international disaster relief efforts. The work effort in disaster relief has increased in its intensity and demand along with a serious increase in risks to the personal safety of international workers. These changes mandate that the preparation of healthcare workers (in this case, nurses) needs to be as comprehensive as possible. It is essential that the individual be as prepared as possible for eventualities that may arise in what may be a potentially volatile and unpredictable environment. Equally, it is essential that the deploying nurse does not become a burden on his or her fellow workers in times of hardship and stress.

Until recently, the preparation for nurses undertaking international relief work was facilitated solely by the employing agency and often in isolation from other agencies deploying to the same area. These courses of preparation are of short duration and concentrate on team building and special role activities. Many of those participating in the past were doing so "to do their part" and considered it a short-term assignment. With the plethora of aid agencies now in place, there has been identified a clear need to ensure that there is comprehensive preparation of nurses undertaking this kind of work as a long-term career option and to ensure professional development in the area. Career development in disaster relief nursing requires a solid academic preparation as well as practical preparation, and many agencies now require master's level qualifications.

When responding to a given disaster of any kind, the need for predeployment intelligence is absolutely crucial if the response is to be in any way meaningful. Of particular importance is the need to have a strong understanding of the culture and cultural norms of the population the disaster response aspires to aid. Due cognizance must be given to the hierarchical structures within communities and the role of gender. To ignore these issues is to court failure. It may be that a traditional needs assessment as undertaken from the Western perspective with Western disaster responses is not what the population either wants or is willing to accept. This is undoubtedly challenging to the Western practitioner, but to respond in a culturally sensitive and community-focused way is to respect the culture within which the work is to be undertaken. Any interventions are far more likely to be successful if designed within the cultural norms of the community that is affected.

Nightingale clearly applied a process of compliance (to her wishes) and not concordance whereas in the 21st century a philosophy of concordance as opposed to compliance is required. Involvement of significant personalities and leaders within a community will ensure a positive attitude in the recipients of the given response. The aim must always be to empower giving maximum ownership of the response to the local community rather than adopting a paternalistic stance. At the completion of the disaster response, relief workers and other healthcare providers will leave, and the community will need to become self-sufficient and sustain the gains that have been made. It is not acceptable to create dependent communities as has happened in the past only to abandon them to the fate of further disasters.

A further critical appointment that needs to be made in any area where there is a language difference is that of the interpreter. An "interpreter" is very different from a "translator," and a clear distinction must be made. A translator is a person who merely states words from one language to another; the interpreter not only conveys words but also adds context and meaning to the words that can be crucial in a culturally sensitive environment. Consider the meaning of the word "terrorist," for instance. This is a culturally defined term dependent on the country in which one is located; one person's terrorist may be another's "freedom fighter." Individuals may consider humanitarian aid to one population or community as preferential treatment. A skilled interpreter can make a very powerful difference when conveying meaning, context, and appropriateness of the discourse with enhanced communication as an outcome.

The importance of predeployment education and training cannot be overemphasized. Most NGOs run in-house preparatory training, which is agency and often mission specific. However, in a world where nurses are pursuing a full career in the provision of aid, there is a need for career development that meets both employment and academic developmental needs. Such programs should be multicultural and multinational in order for those students to experience cultural diversity and its complexities. This experience can then be transferable to the field to positive effect. There is a need for a physical component to the preparation, as often-deployed personnel have to live and work in some very harsh and hazardous conditions where teamwork and mutual support strategies are essential to group harmony and well-being. Survival and coping strategies for living in hostile environments are also valuable and should be included in all training programs.

ETHICAL ISSUES IN DISASTER NURSING

Awareness of the ethical underpinnings of aid relief is critical if nurses wish to participate in such work and be effective in the long term either as practitioners in disaster relief healthcare or as advocates for individuals and communities who experience disaster. Nurses in all parts of the world normally have a focus on the care for individuals, families, groups, and communities and should be accustomed to the ethics underpinning such work. Normal working ethics associated with respect for persons, confidentiality, veracity, fairness, and justice that have now to be applied in a culturally complex world are also applicable in disasters. However, healthcare in disasters requires practitioners not only to continue with their normal ethical practice

but, most importantly, also to be able to modify it to suit the challenge of the environment. Providing healthcare in a disaster situation, especially in another country, is unlike the normal day-to-day environment at home. Disasters are complex and demanding situations that nurses may not have experienced before. There are issues over fair distribution of aid, triage, and prioritizing need. Most importantly, the whole presence of an international aid relief team in a country outside their own is an ethical issue and can have profound impacts on personal ethical stances.

As discussed earlier, recent evidence suggests that altruism and humanitarian values remain as strong motivators for humanitarian workers (Asgary & Lawrence, 2014; Carbonnier, 2015). Despite this, to ensure effectiveness and even survival, it is critical that nurses dispense with naivety that aid relief is only about being altruistic and caring toward those who have experienced loss because of disaster. Aid relief is principally a political action undertaken by those who have resources to help those who do not. Arriving in another country or community with resources in the form of food, water, sanitation facilities, medicine, knowledge, and skills has both cultural and economic impacts. It is critical therefore to ask, Why are we here? What do we want to achieve? It is important to answer the questions fully and honestly, otherwise the ethical tensions experienced in the disaster situation will be more difficult to deal with and may result in difficulties with relationships at all levels. This process of reflection should not be limited to individuals but extend to teams, organizations, and even governments. There is little point in participating in aid relief if the communities and nations who receive the aid do not benefit in the long term. Preserving dignity is about respect and tolerance for all elements of life and culture. As with all helping behaviors, aid has the potential to patronize and mitigate dignity. It is this type of ethical awareness that is needed prior to embarking on any mission to provide aid relief to other nations, communities, families, and individuals. This awareness is almost an ethical principle in that it should be considered when making ethical decisions in disaster relief nursing.

At its core, however, disaster relief nursing is based on the ethic of being humanitarian. The IFRC defines this humanitarian ethic as

> … an ancient and resilient conviction that it is right to help anyone in grave danger. This deeply held value is found in every culture and faith, as well as in the political ideology of human rights. The ideas of the "right to life" and an essential "Human dignity" common to all people are framed in international humanitarian law (IHL), human rights conventions and the principles espoused by humanitarian organizations. (IFRC, 2014)

These values are similar to the values and ethics of nursing worldwide. The International Council of Nurses *Code of Ethics* (ICN, 2000) emphasizes the centrality of respect for human rights including the right to life and to dignity. Appreciating that those who fall victim to disaster are at risk of losing life and having their dignity compromised or removed, it is critical that a full appreciation of the ethics of disaster is accommodated.

Since 2004, the IFRC has recommended that to apply the humanitarian ethic it is necessary to be neutral and independent. Although nurses, irrespective of culture or country, should find it easy to accommodate the ethics of humanitarianism, the reality may be very different. Most disasters worldwide are now complex humanitarian emergencies and are fraught with political, ethical, and tribal conflict. To display respect for the dignity of all groups, it is often difficult to be neutral and independent. Even if an individual nurse or group of nurses claims to be neutral, their nationality, flag under which they operate, passport they hold, color of their skin, or perceived religious beliefs may place them in a particular box that may not be perceived as neutral.

Walker (2006) discusses the need to reflect upon the *Code of Conduct* for the International Red Cross and Red Crescent Movement (see IFRC & ICRC, 1994). He outlines that the *Code* was principally devised for natural disasters and is not as applicable in complex emergencies. In 2004, however, Hugo Slim, the resident scholar and ethicist at the IFRC/Red Crescent, proposed five "moral hazards" aid relief workers should be aware of. These still apply today and are as follows (IFRC, 2014):

- Complicity in abuses (feeding refugees may help armed factions regroup)
- Legitimizing violations (prioritizing aid over investigating rights violations may encourage a climate of impunity)
- Aid's negative effect (too much aid may undermine local markets or depopulate areas)
- Targeting and triage (the neediest may be left to die if others can be more effectively helped)
- Advocacy or access (condemning abuses can mean agencies are expelled)

As is the case in all ethical situations, the most important thing is that the individual practitioner is aware of the consequences of action and inaction. A clear understanding that aid is a political action and aid relief has potential to destroy as well as build for the future is important. Awareness, especially in complex emergencies of the difficulties with neutrality and independence, is very helpful. Most importantly, however, promoting the ethic of humanitarianism not in a naive way but in the context of full political and cultural awareness is critical.

Increased political awareness may come at a price. The case example (Box 16.1) presents a situation where a nurse who is politically aware prior to getting involved in disaster relief experiences an issue when he arrives at the disaster. In this case, the political awareness results in an ethical situation that has the potential to compromise the mission.

> Average rates of mortality tells us only that so many percent will die. Observations must tell us which in the hundred they will be, who will die. (Nightingale, 1860, p. 124)

The need for financial and business governance has been acknowledged by NGOs for several years. Tandon (2013) stated:

> The governance of NGOs focuses on policy and identity rather than the day-to-day issues of the implementation of programs ... governance requires the creation of structure and processes which enables the NGO to monitor performance and remain accountable to its stakeholders. (p. 42)

BOX 16.1 Case Example of a Nurse Experiencing Ethical Conflict in a Disaster Situation

BACKGROUND

John Black has been a charge nurse in Accident and Emergency for over 30 years. Throughout his career, he has always placed a high value on the idea of culturally sensitive care. Recently, the unit in which he works was awarded a quality mark for "Transcultural Care." This was for an accident prevention project with adolescent ethnic groups in inner city housing. He has also been known to advocate for improved public health services for minority groups in his city. He is a member of Greenpeace and Amnesty International.

ISSUE

Recently, he took a leave of absence from work and joined an nongovernmental organization (NGO) that provides healthcare to victims of disasters worldwide. Until he arrives in the country, he is unaware that some of the internally displaced people (IDP) he will be caring for are ex-prisoners of war who were accused of mass rape and torture during the previous political regime in the country. The present

government has given a reprieve for all prisoners in an effort to build peace. John experiences an ethical and professional issue. Can he work in this situation or should he consciously object? Should he ask to be placed in a different part of the country where there is less of a possibility of meeting such people? Should he ask to be sent home?

SOLUTION

Before considering this issue at a personal level, it is necessary to consider the different stakeholder relationships involved. NGOs are normally in a country at the request of the host government, World Health Organization, or the United Nations Office for the Co-Ordination of Humanitarian Affairs (OCHA). Prior to signing up for the mission, John would have been told of these contractual arrangements and should have been briefed on the culture and background of the groups with which he may be involved. It is more likely, however, that the mission had to be organized quickly and there may not have been time to provide this level of information. Disasters are not selective when it comes to victims. A disaster will normally involve a cross section of the society in which it

(continued)

BOX 16.1 Case Example of a Nurse Experiencing Ethical Conflict in a Disaster Situation (*continued*)

occurs. As a nurse, John would be expected to care for all groups irrespective of their backgrounds.

John's departure from the mission may put strain on the relationship with the host government. The media may get hold of John's story, and this may undermine the egalitarian image of the NGO and result in the NGO having to withdraw

from the country. Then again, if the NGO was not aware of this issue in advance, it may be perceived negatively by the donors at home and may have an impact on long-term funding. John's personal feelings should be respected at all times, but he must always be aware of the consequences of his actions and work within the team at all times.

Over the years, an increasing amount of project evaluation has been conducted. The founding of the Active Learning Network for Accountability and Performance (ALNAP) in 1997 provided a central repository for project evaluations and reports. ALNAP produces an annual report based on evaluations, and this information should be used to learn lessons from and improve the quality of care and disaster response. Furthermore, this network provides a valuable resource for existing as well as prospective humanitarian workers. Most of the webinars are open to the public (see www.alnap.org).

In 2002, Rosen argued that a review of working practices is required within humanitarian agencies. It is therefore unsurprising that donors are now demanding an assurance that the myriad of aid agencies delivering humanitarian relief on their behalf are doing so to a recognized and predetermined standard.

A high quality, effective, efficient, and coordinated response to a disaster is required to ensure that the needs of those affected by calamity or armed conflicts are met. It is widely recognized that those affected by disasters have an increased risk of becoming ill or dying from, among other things, diseases associated with inadequate or poor sanitation or water supplies, which are avoidable but often inevitable following a disaster. Therefore, affected individuals may become reliant on the skills of those involved in humanitarian assistance for their survival (see Chapter 19, "Restoring Public Health Under Disaster Conditions," for further discussion). An initial assessment of the disaster area is therefore essential to gain an understanding of the situation or emerging situation, health risks, and population needs.

The *Sphere Handbook*, 3rd edition, published in 2011 and a new edition being published in 2018 (originally launched in 1997) hold the view that the basic human rights of those affected by calamity and conflicts were not being upheld. In 1994, a multidonor evaluation concluded that there were unnecessary deaths in Goma in the Democratic Republic of Congo. Goma was the city that dealt with the massive influx of refugees from the 1994 Rwandan Genocide. This catalyst brought about the Sphere Project. Initially, those involved developed the Humanitarian Charter and followed this with the Sphere Project Minimum Standards in Disaster Response (The Sphere Project, 2011), both of which were derived using input from hundreds of experts from 228 aid agencies from 30 countries (www.sphereproject.org). The Sphere Humanitarian guidelines are scheduled for an update in 2018. Readers are advised to visit the Sphere Project website for the updated guidelines.

The purpose of the Humanitarian Charter and the Minimum Standards in Disaster Response was to improve the effectiveness of humanitarian assistance initiatives, and to increase the accountability of international agencies, and arguably even the donors participating in humanitarian efforts. The charter and the standards are based on the belief that first, all possible steps should be taken to alleviate human suffering that arises out of conflict and calamity, and second, that those affected by a disaster have a right to life with dignity and therefore a right to assistance (The Sphere Project, 2011). There is a common belief that all possible measures should be taken to alleviate human suffering arising out of conflict or calamity. The principle of a right to a life with dignity is drawn from the UN Charter and the Universal Declaration of Human Rights. Life with dignity is a fundamental human right; however, individuals and cultures may have different perceptions of what this concept means. Nurses must therefore participate and collaborate with local representatives of the community to ensure understanding and cultural compliance.

The Humanitarian Charter is committed to achieving a quality service and encourages both agencies and governments to adopt such standards. Standards have been drawn up to ensure adequate supplies of water, to minimize the spread of disease, and to provide sanitation, vector control, management of waste, and promotion of hygiene. Additionally Sphere minimum standards arguably demonstrate the basic level of assistance required for all people at any time. Achievement of the minimum standards can, however, depend on a range of factors, sometimes beyond the control of the agencies (e.g., environmental factor). A need for such a strong focus on standards has been questioned when grave issues such as lack of access to populations or gross violation of protection persist. Sphere has argued that such standards were initiated for the purpose of improving quality and accountability of a humanitarian response.

Nurses are one of the largest groups in the frontline within the humanitarian community, especially in the healthcare arena. As highly skilled professionals, they have a vast contribution to make in relation to quality assurance in international disaster response, especially with respect to knowledgeable, effective, efficient use of resources, as well as being educators and promoters of health. Evaluation of the effectiveness and quality of any contribution is important for overall quality assurance and improvement in aid relief delivery worldwide. Continuous quality improvement and quality assurance are key to ensuring accountability for efficient and effective delivery of humanitarian aid. Nurses are ideally placed to influence and monitor these two processes.

COMMUNICATION AND TRANSPORT AS OBSTACLES TO AID RELIEF

It is common for a disaster to affect more than one country at a time, or to cross borders. Disasters that involve multiple nations create additional obstacles that must be effectively addressed in order for humanitarian efforts to be successful. The two primary obstacles faced by disaster relief professionals are those of communication and transport. The success or failure of the communication and transport systems in any disaster response will influence the overall outcome of the relief response effort. In the developed world, high-tech communications systems are often ineffective in disaster situations. Equally, in the developing world, communication and transport may not have existed in the first place. Irrespective of location, disasters will result in communication and transport difficulties. Those involved in disaster response must always have a well-thought-out and easy-to-use communication and transport plan.

The physical size, location, and geography of the countries affected by the disaster may also contribute to transportation hardship. Some types of disasters (e.g., floods, hurricanes, and earthquakes) physically disrupt roads, bridges, tunnels, and railway lines. Transportation needs include movement into the situation (human resources, supplies, and equipment) and movement out of the situation (moving victims away from chemical or radiation disasters). International environmental disasters occurring with nationalities at war pose even larger challenges as conflicting members of the society may limit transportation, making the safety of those involved an additional consideration. Natural disasters such as famine may result in thousands of people migrating from one area to another.

It is therefore essential that expertise be available and appropriately tasked to undertake a command and control role in ensuring that there is a coordinated and focused response. It is essential to ensure that those involved in the relief response effort are appropriately trained in the use of a wide variety of communications systems and can use with confidence accepted protocols for passing information accurately, for example the International Phonetic Alphabet. It should be noted that a few areas of the world do not have the capability to support the use of mobile or cell phones. Nevertheless, even in countries that do have established networks, these may be compromised during disasters. Effective communications are essential in that they are an adjunct to the ability to deploy an appropriate response in a timely fashion. Predeployment training and transportation planning are imperative for the success of any response. Technology such as the now highly developed Geographic Information Systems (GIS) has greatly enabled planners to have a real insight into the scale of the problem for which they are planning. This technology is proving its worth repeatedly in terms of responding to complex disasters. Additionally, of course, there is the easily accessible Google Earth system that can give planners a great deal of information about terrain and population density.

There are challenges to ensuring that an effective communications and transport plan is in place and operating to potential. A great deal of time and effort is required to ensure that this takes place. Poor communication and a less than timely arrival of transport carrying essential aid can seriously compromise the credibility of the organization involved.

The issue of personal safety when deployed in response to a disaster is highly important. It is evident from the numerous kidnappings over recent years that the symbols that once gave at least some semblance of protection are no longer respected as such and it could be argued to accentuate the risk to the wearer. Predeployment training must be given to address the issue of personal security that is country/region specific as there is clearly no one training package that fits all scenarios. Post 9/11, there has been a shift in the paradigm in which the military were seen as deploying to create the so-called humanitarian space within which humanitarian actors, that is, the NGO organizations could operate in some safety; now the risks are inherent in all regardless of philosophy, mandate, or mission. As Wheeler and Harmer (2006) point out, there is also the issue of private military firms (PMFs) to consider. It is clear that there is a proliferation of such organizations working to contract in areas such as Iraq. The use of PMFs is somewhat controversial. They may support military operations, they may be used to support infrastructure development, and they may also be employed to provide security to humanitarian organizations. This raises the question of neutrality (if one believes this is possible) and impartiality given that the PMFs operate under contract. In 2017, this still remains a major issue for all humanitarian workers including nurses. The best general advice on personal safety normally centers around IFRC's "Stay Safe" manual that emphasizes the Seven Pillars of Security (Tangen, Dyer, & Julisson, 2011). This is a must-read document for nurses who are considering deployment.

As road traffic collisions and vehicle accidents are a major threat to life, those who deploy must have good awareness and skill. An international driver's license is essential. Drivers must be able to adapt to the types of vehicles that may be locally procured in frequently remote areas. It is often necessary to drive heavy manual vehicles often without the benefit of power steering and many of the accessories that are standard in the developed world. The ability to maneuver such vehicles over difficult and sometimes hostile territory is an essential skill as is the ability to recover vehicles should they go off the "road" (which can be anything from a trail to a paved street). It is important to have a codriver who acts as navigator, even in vehicles following well behind, as the movements of the lead vehicle also have to be checked. Codrivers can assist the driver, help prevent mistakes when driving under pressure, and provide relief when battling fatigue. The temptation to fill a vehicle to the maximum capacity may well be laudable; however, other considerations need to be made in the use of available space. Vehicle modifications may be required depending on environmental conditions, for example adding snow chains or sand tracks, or using heating or air-conditioning (if available and fuel allows). Replacement automotive parts can prevent a roadside breakdown. Adequate amounts of fuels and lubricants, and at least two spare tires that are functional and in good order, should be brought along. The driver must have the capability to change them if required. This is often a major undertaking with large vehicles. Maps, compasses, flashlights, first aid kits, rations, water, and personal survival equipment are essential additional items.

CARE OF DISPLACED PERSONS AND REFUGEES

Individuals, families, and communities are often forced to leave their homes or country because of disaster or the threat of disaster (United Nations High Commission for Refugees [UNHCR], 2017). "IDP" is the term used to describe persons who are displaced within national boundaries. It is estimated that 65.6 million people are forcibly displaced across the world (UNHCR, 2017). The term "refugee" is used to describe an individual who is displaced and moves across a national boundary. This distinction is very important. Refugees have a right to receive international protection, whereas IDPs remain the responsibility of the home government. The UNHCR (www .unhcr.org) has legal responsibility for refugees but not IDPs (UNHCR, 2017). Aid organizations can help in situations where populations are displaced within national boundaries but this is often random and inadequate. Negotiations with host governments or sometimes local authorities can be more difficult in the absence of UNHCR. Nurses who work in aid organizations or indeed local nurses must be aware of the distinction between the terms "IDP" and "refugee." It is suggested that IDPs are more vulnerable due to the absence of international protection. UNHCR currently cares for 22.5 million people in all corners of the world and in all types of situations (UNHCR, 2017). Conversely, the fact that refugees have a legal right to assistance can cause discontent in the host population if they are seen (or perceived) to be gaining better treatment and facilities than the host population. This is a difficult balancing act for the aid delivery teams.

Since the end of the 1960s, most refugees have originated from countries in the southern hemisphere (Médicins Sans Frontièrs, 1997). The mass population movements often associated with Sub-Saharan Africa during the 1980s have also occurred in Eastern Europe during the Balkan conflict and more recently are being manifested once again in the Mediterranean. Images of large groups of displaced people—mostly women, children, and older people—walking on roads or traveling in heavily laden vehicles or makeshift boats are synonymous with disasters worldwide. Englund (1998) described the problems associated with being uprooted from one's community; losing family members; and, more often than not, experiencing intimidation, persecution, and rape, that result in most refugees being physically and mentally traumatized. This analysis still stands today.

The priorities for management of healthcare in relation to such groups should center on basic requirements such as water and sanitation, food and nutrition, shelter and safety, control of communicable diseases, and psychosocial recovery. Individuals and groups who are refugees may be disoriented and traumatized but have the ability to retain creativity and survival methods. Individuals and communities who experience disasters may have already established coping mechanisms and methods for survival. Working closely with community leaders is critical to any healthcare plan. Recent evidence confirms that nursing can do a lot in relation to meeting basic healthcare requirements. A deep appreciation and cultural understanding to deal effectively with loss of human dignity and feelings associated with traumatic memories are important (Al Qutob, 2016; Davenport, 2017; McBride, Russo, & Block, 2016; Pinehas, van Wyk, & Leech, 2016).

Placing the existing cultural sensitivity and empathy related to the experience of displacement at the center of care, nurses can provide expert and person-centered emergency public health support. Initial assessment and care that involves measles immunization, water and sanitation, food and nutrition, shelter and site planning, lifesaving interventions in the emergency phase, maintaining normal social structures required for feelings of security, and maintaining psychosocial well-being are all critical.

SUMMARY

An increasing world population, increased urbanization, increased hunger, and an increasing threat from climate change, mean that many communities throughout the world are at risk of disaster and/or catastrophe. As they lack the necessary resources to respond effectively, there is an urgent need for nurses worldwide to work collaboratively with communities and focus on risk reduction, resilience, and capacity building. The scale of disasters—slow and acute— that is threatening the developing world is outstripping the capability for response. This is despite the exponential growth in NGOs and international groups providing aid. Disasters are becoming more complex and in many cases highly volatile situations. Terms such as "catastrophe" and "complex humanitarian emergencies" are now used. There is a need for an acute awareness on the part of all who participate in disaster relief of the ethical underpinnings and cultural, political, vehicle transport, communication systems, and personal security issues associated with disasters. Although a significant nursing presence in disaster response exists worldwide, there continues to be a paucity of empirical evidence documenting the influence of nursing on health outcomes. Clearly, there is a need for robust preparation of nurses that is both theoretical and practical, and this should be underpinned by empirical evidence about nursing in disasters. Such preparation must equip nurses to meet the holistic needs of nations, communities, families, and individuals who fall victim to disaster and require support and education to recover and build community resilience to mitigate future disasters. In a multinational/multicultural setting, there is a defined need for cultural awareness to be at the forefront of any disaster response. A community focus as opposed to a medical focus is recommended if the key concepts of nursing in disasters and catastrophes are to be realized.

STUDY QUESTIONS

1. Identify the five most affected countries by natural and human-initiated disasters or catastrophes in the past year. Are there similarities?

2. Examine the perinatal mortality and gross domestic product (GDP) of these countries. Consider the level of capacity building and/or community resilience that exists. What are your conclusions?

3. Select a recent paper on the management of healthcare in disaster or catastrophic situations and determine how nurses contribute to the overall relief effort.

4. Reflect on how you would cope in a disaster situation as a healthcare professional. List the major difficulties and advantages associated with working in multinational teams in disaster situations. Consider your cultural background in this context.

5. Describe the purpose of the Humanitarian Charter and the Minimum Standards.

6. Explain the importance of cultural awareness and cultural considerations in planning care during a disaster response.

7. Identify an ethical issue that you are likely to encounter in a disaster relief situation.

8. Select a recent disaster in a country or group of countries. Write a short plan on how you would set about improving the resilience of the local community to mitigate against future disasters.

9. You quickly realize that the disaster is still in the acute or emergency phase. Go to the World Vision (www .worldvision.org.uk), CARE (www.care.org), or Islamic Aid (www.islamicaid.org.uk) website. Find out how you can assist. Concentrate on the transport and communication difficulties, cultural issues, and ethical issues.

10. When you arrive in the host country, you are faced with assisting the local nurses establish a healthcare facility for a large refugee camp. Outline how you would organize your team in the first 72 hours. Concentrate on achieving the minimum standards for humanitarian relief and remain focused on accountability for nursing, personal security, and the safety of your team.

REFERENCES

Al Qutob, M. F. (2016). WHO and the refugee crisis in Jordan and beyond. *The Lancet Global Health, 4*(5), e304. doi:10.1016/S2214-109X(16)00067-X

Asgary, R., & Lawrence, K. (2014). Characteristics, determinants and perspectives of experienced medical humanitarians: A qualitative approach. *British Medical Journal Open, 4*(12), 1–14. doi:10.1136/bmjopen-2014-006460

Bjerneld, M., Lindmark, G., McSpadden, L. A., & Garrett, M. J. (2006). Motivations, concerns and expectations of Scandinavian health professionals volunteering for humanitarian assignments. *Disaster Management and Response, 4*(2), 49–58. doi:10.1016/j.dmr.2006.01.002

Carbonnier, G. (2015). Reason, emotion, compassion: Can altruism survive professionalisation in the humanitarian sector? *Disasters, 39*(2), 189–207. doi:10.1111/disa.12096

Chan, M. (2017). *Ten years in public health 2010–2017.* Geneva, Switzerland: World Health Organization.

Davenport, L. A. (2017). Living with the choice: A grounded theory of Iraqi refugee resettlement to the U.S. *Issues in Mental Health Nursing, 38*(4), 352–360. doi:10.1080/01612840.2017.1286531

Davies, K., & Bricknell, M. C. M. (1997). After the battle. *Nursing Times, 3*(29), 35–37.

Davies, K., & Higginson, R. (2005). The human factors in a disaster. *Nursing Clinics of North America, 40*(3), 579–586. doi:10.1016/j.cnur.2005 .04.004

Deeny, P., & McFetridge, B. (2005). The impact of disaster on culture, self and identity: Increased awareness by healthcare professionals is needed. *Nursing Clinics of North America, 40*(3), 431–440. doi:10.1016/j.cnur.2005.04.012

Englund, H. (1998). Death, trauma and ritual: Mozambican refugees in Malawi. *Social Science Medicine, 46*(9), 1165–1174. doi:10.1016/s0277-9536(97)10044-2

Eshghi, K., & Larson, R. C. (2008). Disasters: Lessons from the past 105 years. *Disaster Prevention and Management, 17*(1), 62–82. doi:10.1108/09653560810855883

Hunt, M. R. (2009). Moral experience of Canadian healthcare professionals in humanitarian work. *Prehospital and Disaster Medicine, 24*(6), 518–524. doi:10.1017/s1049023x00007445

International Council of Nurses. (2000). *Code of ethics for nurses.* Geneva, Switzerland: Author.

International Council of Nurses. (2001). *Nurses and disaster preparedness: A position statement.* Geneva, Switzerland: Author.

International Federation of Red Cross and Red Crescent Societies. (2014). *World Disasters Report.* Geneva, Switzerland: Author.

International Federation of Red Cross and Red Crescent Societies. (2017). *World Disasters Report.* Geneva, Switzerland: Author. Retrieved from http://www.ifrc.org/en/publications-and-reports/world-disasters -report

International Federation of Red Cross and Red Crescent Societies, & International Committee of the Red Cross. (1994). *The code of conduct for the International Red Cross and Red Crescent Movement and non-governmental organisations (NGOs) in disaster relief.* Geneva, Switzerland: Authors.

Janz, M., & Slead, J. (Eds.). (2000). *Complex humanitarian emergencies; Lessons from practitioners.* Monrovia, CA: World Vision.

Katoch, A. (2006). The responder's cauldron: The uniqueness of international disaster response. *Journal of International Affairs, 369*(19), 1836–1842. Retrieved from https://www.questia.com/library/journal/1G1-146073423/the-responders

Lavin, R. P. (2006). HIPAA and disaster research: Preparing to conduct research. *Disaster Management and Response, 4*(2), 32–37. doi:10.1016/j.dmr.2006.01.003

Leaning, J., & Guha-Sapir, D. (2013). Natural disasters, armed conflict and public health. *New England Journal of Medicine, 370*(8), 783–784. doi:10.1056/NEJMc1315507

McBride, J., Russo, A., & Block, A. (2016). The Refugee Health Nurse Liaison: A nurse led initiative to improve healthcare for asylum seekers and refugees. *Contemporary Nurse, 52*(6), 710–721. doi:10.1080/10376178.2016.1238774

Médicins Sans Frontièrs. (1997). *Refugee health: An approach to emergency situations.* London, UK: Macmillan Education.

Nabarro, D. (2005, May 4–6). *Putting it together: Stronger public health capacity within disaster management systems.* Final presentation at the WHO Tsunami Health Conference, Phuket, Thailand. Retrieved from http://www.who.int/hac/events/tsunamiconf/final_presentation/en/

Nightingale, F. (1860). *Notes on nursing: What it is and what it is not.* New York, NY: Dover Publications.

Office for the Coordination of Humanitarian Affairs. (2017). Cluster coordination. Retrieved from https://www.unocha.org/legacy/what-we-do/coordination-tools/cluster-coordination.

Pinehas, L. N., van Wyk, N. C., & Leech, R. (2016). Healthcare needs of displaced women: Osire refugee camp, Namibia. *International Nursing Review, 63*(1), 139–147. doi:10.1111/inr.12241

Relief Web International. (2017). Disasters. Retrieved from http://reliefweb .int/disasters

Rosen, G. (2002). Problems of assistance and protection in modern conflict. In I. Taipale, P. Mäkelä, K. Java, et al. (Eds.), *War or health.* London, UK: Zed Books.

Ryan, J. M., & Lumley, J. S. P. (2000). And finally . . . Failed states and failing states. *Trauma, 2*, 231–236. doi:10.1177/146040860000200307

Shepherd, A., Mitchell, T., Lewis, K., Lenhardt, A., Jones, L., Scott, L., & Muir-Wood, R. (2013). *The geography of poverty, disasters and climate extremes in 2030*. London, UK: Overseas Development Institute.

Tandon, R. (2013). "Board Games" governance and accountability in NGOs. In M. Edwards & D. Hulme (Eds), *Nongovernmental organization— Performance and accountability beyond the magic bullet* (pp. 40–50). London, UK: Earthscan.

Tangen, L., Dyer, J., & Julisson, K. (2011). Stay safe Geneva: International Federation of Red Cross and Red Crescent Societies. Retrieved from http://www.ifrc.org/Global/Documents/Secretariat/201402/Stay-Safe -management-EN.pdf

The Sphere Project. (2011). *Humanitarian charter and minimum standards in disaster response*. London, UK: Practical Action Publishing.

United Nations High Commissioner for Refugees. (2017). Refugee figures. Retrieved from http://www.unhcr.org/uk

United Nations. (2015). *The Sendai Framework 2015–2030*. New York, NY: Author.

Wahlstrom, M. (2005, May 4–6). Address to the Tsunami Health Conference, Phuket, Thailand. By Margareta Wahlstrom, Deputy Emergency Relief Coordinator of the United Nations and Special Coordinator for the Response to the tsunami affected communities. Geneva, Switzerland: World Health Organization. Retrieved from http://www.who.int/hac/ events/tsunamiconf/presentations/1_1_opening_wahlstrom_doc.pdf

Walker, P. (2005) Cracking the code: the genesis, use and future of the Code of Conduct. *Disasters, 29*(4) 323–336. doi:10.1111/j.0361-3666.2005.00295.x

Wheeler, V., & Harmer, A. (Eds). (2006). *Resetting the rules of engagement; trends and issues in military–Humanitarian relations*. London, UK: Humanitarian Policy Group Overseas Development Institute.

World Health Organization. (2006). The contribution of nursing and midwifery in emergencies: Report of a WHO consultation. Retrieved from http:// www.who.int/hac/events/2006/nursing_consultation_report_sept07.pdf

World Health Organization. (2014). *Mental health atlas*. Geneva, Switzerland: Author.

World Health Organization. (2017a). Definitions: Emergencies. Retrieved from http://www.who.int/hac/about/definitions/en

World Health Organization. (2017b). South Asia earthquakes and tsunamis. Retrieved from http://www.who.int/hac/crises/international/asia_tsunami/en

World Health Organization and International Councils of Nurses. (2009). *ICN framework of disaster nursing competencies*. Geneva, Switzerland: Author.

World Population Clock. (2017). Current world population. Retrieved from http://www.worldometers.info/world-population

17

NATURAL DISASTERS

Tener Goodwin Veenema, Andrew Corley, and Clifton P. Thornton

LEARNING OBJECTIVES

When this chapter is completed, readers will be able to:

1. Identify the major types of natural/environmental disasters and their physical, social, and economic impact.
2. Describe the morbidity and mortality commonly associated with each type of naturally occurring disaster.
3. Propose preparedness, prevention, mitigation, and response activities for each type of disaster.
4. Understand the implications of advanced warning systems.
5. Define terms regarding severe weather watches and storm warnings.
6. Articulate lessons learned from historic natural disasters.

KEY MESSAGES

Natural disasters are occurring globally with increasing frequency and intensity.

Hazards vary greatly by country and region, with some areas experiencing frequent recurring natural disasters and persistent vulnerability.

Nurses should be familiar with the types and consequences of commonly occurring natural disasters to contribute to public health efforts to prepare, prevent, mitigate, and recover from these events.

Rapid assessment of health needs in populations affected by natural disasters is critical, enabling healthcare providers and emergency management officials to prioritize resources and make decisions about responding.

Understanding the way that people are killed or injured in natural disasters is a prerequisite to preventing or reducing deaths and injuries during future disasters.

Understanding why people fail to prepare for disasters can inform initiatives designed to enhance readiness.

Nurses need to be familiar with commonly used definitions for severe weather watches and storm warnings.

CHAPTER OVERVIEW

Disasters due to natural causes often result in human pain and suffering, injury and loss of life, the physical destruction of dwellings, and social and economic disruption. This chapter presents the reader with a broad overview of the most frequently occurring natural/environmental disasters, their impact on communities, and their associated morbidity and mortality. Disaster preparedness, prevention, and mitigation activities specific to each type of disaster are discussed. Case studies of naturally occurring disasters are presented as evidence of the scope of their impact and can be used to evaluate previous disaster response efforts and to predict future needs.

Since earliest prehistory, much of human life, technology, and culture have been defined by our constant struggle against the forces of nature. Because weather-related events are ubiquitous and can occur without warning, humans have had little recourse but to prepare to respond to the wrath of the environment in which they live. Environmental devastation caused by natural hazards of terrestrial origin (earthquakes, volcanic eruptions, landslides, tsunamis, hurricanes and other severe storms, tornadoes and high winds, floods, wildfires, and drought) and solar-terrestrial hazards (solar flares and geomagnetic storms) is inevitable.

In contrast, the impact of natural disasters on communities—lingering disruption, persisting long after the causative event itself and exceeding the communities' ability to recover unaided—is determined as much or more by societal behavior and practice as by nature per se. Certainly, some negative impacts of natural hazards, at a minimum, can be mitigated or prevented entirely. Nonetheless, natural disasters kill and inflict human suffering. In addition, they destroy property, economic productivity, natural resources, and they harm the environment. Disaster response can also divert assets from much-needed investments in our future through research, education, and economic development.

■ Disaster science, accompanied by major advances in technology and meteorology, has provided a better understanding of the hallmark characteristics of natural/environmental hazards and the disasters that they cause.[1] This information enables nurses, healthcare planners, and public health officials to prepare for these types of events and to develop advanced warning systems to minimize injuries and the loss of life. As with other types of disasters, advanced preparation for a major natural disaster can result in significant reductions in mortality later on (Bissell, Pinet, Nelson, & Levy, 2004; Mayhorn & McLaughlin, 2014).

─────────

[1] The NOAA's National Severe Storms Laboratory (NSSL) is working to improve the lead time and accuracy of severe weather warnings and forecasts to save lives and reduce property damage. NSSL scientists are committed to their mission to understand the causes of severe weather and explore new ways to use weather information to assist National Weather Service forecasters and federal, university, and private sector partners.

■ Repeated disaster impact upon a community can result in a vicious cycle of deforestation, poverty, urbanization, and increased vulnerability (Sodhi, 2016).

■ Postdisaster research has demonstrated that both access to care and health-seeking behaviors are affected by natural disasters (Rodriguez & Aguirre, 2006), particularly in rural areas (Jacquet, Kirsch, Durrani, Sauer, & Doocy, 2016).

■ The mere availability of response and recovery services will not limit the burden of natural disasters if the victims of these events are unwilling or unable to use the services (Stimpson, Fernando, & Jeffries, 2008). Rapid assessment of disaster-related injuries and outreach efforts to meet the identified physical, mental health, and behavioral needs are critical.

■ Understanding the way that people are killed or injured in disasters is a prerequisite to preventing or reducing deaths and injuries during future disasters (Blaikie, Cannon, Davis, & Wisner, 2014; Shultz, Espinola, Rechkemmer, Cohen, & Espinel, 2016; Wisner, Blaikie, Cannon, & Davis, 2004).

TYPES AND CONSEQUENCES OF NATURAL AND ENVIRONMENTAL DISASTERS

A review conducted over 20 years has revealed that 90% of disasters have been caused by floods, storms, heatwaves, and similar other weather-related events (Centre for Research on the Epidemiology of Disasters [CRED], 2016). Meteorological disasters over the past 20 years have cost the United States over $1.8 trillion in economic losses. Natural disasters can be categorized as "sudden" or "slow" in their onset (Wisner et al., 2004). They are predictable because they cluster in geographical areas. Natural hazards are unpreventable and, for the most part, uncontrollable. Even if quick recovery occurs, natural disasters can have long-term effects. Natural disasters with acute onsets include events such as avalanche, blizzard, or extreme cold; earthquake; fire; flood; heat wave; hurricane, cyclone, or typhoon; tornado; tsunami or storm surge; volcanic eruption; and wildfire. Natural hazards with a slow or gradual onset include deforestation, desertification, drought, and pest infestation. The most important natural disasters and examples of their environmental effects are listed in Table 17.1.

Severity of Damage

Worldwide, most natural disasters are similar; they are limited in scale and duration, and are usually managed by local, regional, or national resources. Exceptions exist, such as the Indian Ocean Tsunami, where the extent of devastation required a global response.

The severity of damage caused by natural/environmental disasters is affected by population density in disaster-prone areas, local building codes, community preparedness, sophistication of communication systems, and the use of public safety announcements and education on how to respond correctly to the first signs of danger. Recovery following a disaster varies according to the public's access to pertinent information (e.g., sources of governmental and private aid), preexisting conditions that increase or reduce vulnerability (e.g., economic

TABLE 17.1 Natural Disasters and Environmental Impact

Natural Disaster	Environmental Effects
Blizzard/heavy snowfall	Avalanche, erosion, snow melt
Cold (severe)	Loss of plants and animals, river ice jams (flooding)
Cyclone/hurricane	Storm surge, flooding, landslide, erosion, deforestation, loss of plant and animal life
Drought	Fire, depletion of water resources, water shortages, deterioration of soil, loss of plant and animal life
Earthquake	Landslide, liquefaction, tsunami, avalanche
Extreme heat	Fire, loss of plants and animals, depletion of water resources, deterioration of soil
Landslides/mudslides	Erosion, destruction of plant life, flooding
Lightning	Fire
Thunderstorm/heavy rainfall	Flooding, fire, landslide, erosion, destruction of plant life
Tornado	Loss of plant and animal life, erosion, water disturbance
Tsunami	Flooding, erosion, loss of plant and animal life
Volcanic eruption	Loss of plant and animal life, deterioration of soil, poor air and water quality
Wildfires	Destruction of ground cover, poor air quality, erosion

Source: Centers for Disease Control and Prevention. (2017). Natural disasters and severe weather. Retrieved from https://www.cdc.gov/disasters

or biological factors), prior experience with stressful situations (e.g., resiliency), and availability of sufficient savings and insurance (resources).

Trends in Natural Disaster

With growing population and infrastructures, the world's exposure to natural hazards is inevitably increasing. A review of international disaster statistics over the past 105 years reveals an exponential increase in disasters; other research suggests that the frequency and severity of natural disasters continue to increase (Eshghi & Larson, 2008; Intergovernmental Panel on Climate Change, 2014; see Figure 17.1). This raises several questions. Is the increase due to a significant improvement in access to information and, thus, more accurate reporting? What part does population growth and infrastructural development

play? Is climate change behind the increasing frequency of natural hazards? What are the health consequences of climate change? Population growth worldwide is now predominantly located in coastal areas (with greater exposure to floods, cyclones, and tidal waves). Remaining available land for urban growth is generally risk-prone; for instance, floodplains or steep slopes subject to landslides.

A large proportion of the American population is at risk from only three types of natural/environmental disasters: earthquakes, floods, and hurricanes. Approximately 50 million people live in floodplains that have been highly developed as working and residential communities. Another 110 million people live in coastal areas, including the Great Lakes region. Trends such as increasing population densities, the progressive movement of populations to disaster-prone floodplains, the risk of hurricanes in coastal regions, and the construction of communities in areas vulnerable to wildfires means that our potential for catastrophic disasters is increasing (Hanes, 2016; Neumann, Vafeidis, Zimmermann, & Nicholls, 2015). Economic losses associated with these types of disasters are substantial (see Figure 17.2) and rising for reasons that are likely to continue in the near term:

- A simple rise in the value of vulnerable assets, as a result of population increase and economic growth in high-risk areas (see Figure 17.3).
- Increasing use of hazardous lands (coastal zones, fault zones, floodplains, unstable slopes, fire-prone areas, etc.) in response to both population pressure and demographic preferences.
- A continuing failure to use best seismic, wind, fire, and flood mitigation and engineering practice. Nations and private enterprises are beginning to take steps to reduce vulnerability, especially in construction following Hurricanes Katrina in 2005 and Sandy in 2012. However, existing construction may not meet codes providing the most protection, may not be situated safely, or tested by a major hazard.
- A growing shift in the economic losses from property damage to associated business disruption. This shift occurs as both developed and developing societies become increasingly dependent on critical infrastructure that is introducing new vulnerabilities to hazards. The direct costs of repairing road damage, restoring power to regional electrical grids, and reinstating disrupted water supplies are often small compared with the losses that are due to business stoppages while these repairs are being made (U.S. Government Subcommittee on Natural Disaster Reduction, 2006).

The risk of a disaster is determined by a complex relationship between natural hazards, vulnerability, and exposure; as these variables increase, the risk of impact from a disaster also increases. "Natural hazards" are events that have the potential to initiate disasters (e.g., cyclones, floods, hurricanes, earthquakes). Events such as climate change increase the potential for these adverse weather events and natural disasters. "Vulnerability" is the characteristic of the population that makes it particularly susceptible to the disaster. Situations like poverty, living in environmentally degraded areas, low education, and few financial resources increase the population's vulnerability.

Number of disasters
per year

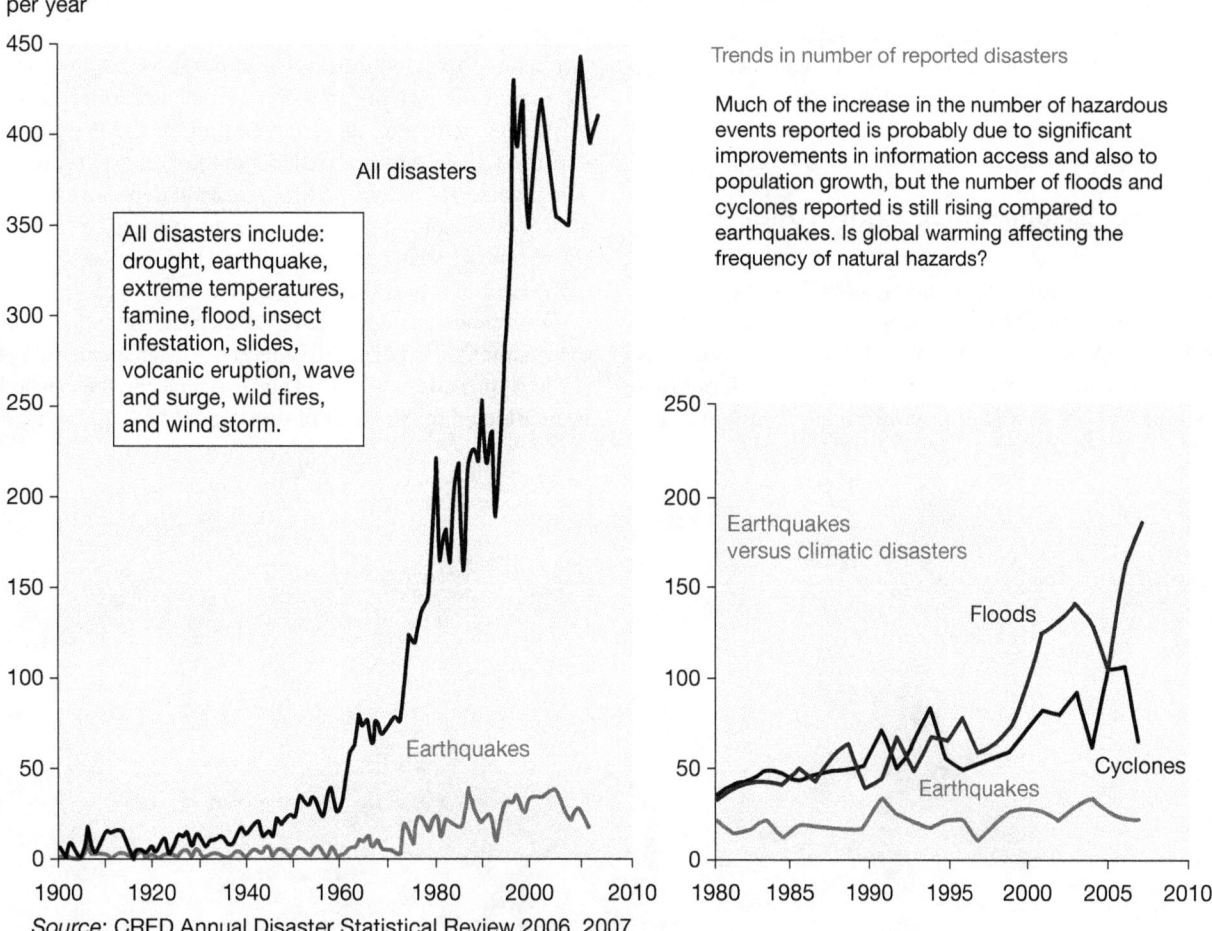

All disasters

All disasters include: drought, earthquake, extreme temperatures, famine, flood, insect infestation, slides, volcanic eruption, wave and surge, wild fires, and wind storm.

Earthquakes

Trends in number of reported disasters

Much of the increase in the number of hazardous events reported is probably due to significant improvements in information access and also to population growth, but the number of floods and cyclones reported is still rising compared to earthquakes. Is global warming affecting the frequency of natural hazards?

Earthquakes versus climatic disasters

Floods

Cyclones

Earthquakes

Source: CRED Annual Disaster Statistical Review 2006, 2007.

FIGURE 17.1 Trends in natural disasters.

Source: GRID-Arendal. (2009). Number of disasters per year. Retrieved from http://www.grida.no/resources/7324

Designer/author credit: Riccardo Pravettoni, UNEP/GRIDArendal.

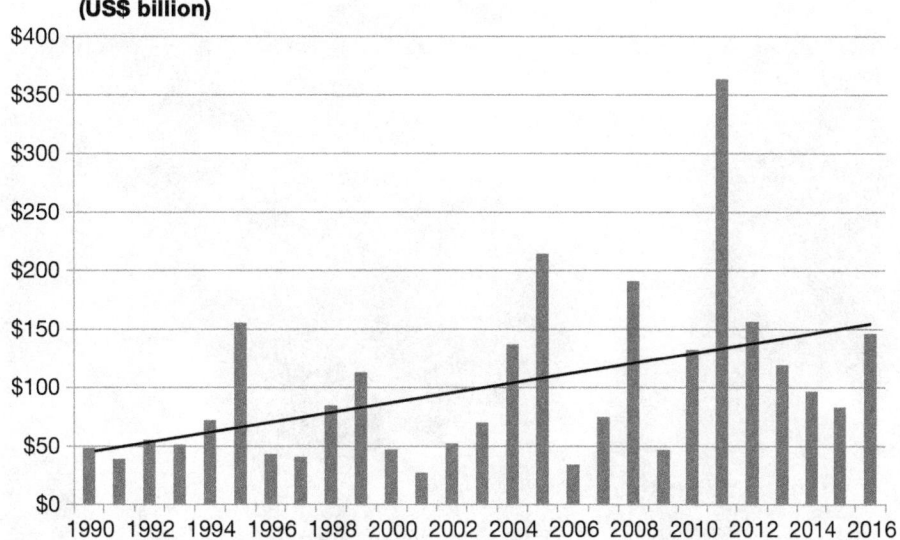

(US$ billion)

FIGURE 17.2 Global disaster losses from 1990 to 2016. Bars indicate annual disaster losses, while the line is a linear regression of disaster costs.

Source: Adapted from Centre for Research on the Epidemiology of Disasters. (2017). EM-DAT: The emergency events database. Retrieved from http://www.emdat.be

"Exposure" is the factor that describes a population's chance of being affected by disasters and is exacerbated by things like poorly planned developmental programs, regional threats, and prevention programs. The disaster's risk increases along with increases in natural hazards, vulnerability, and exposure (see Figure 17.3).

CYCLONES, HURRICANES, AND TYPHOONS

Cyclones are large-scale storms characterized by low pressure in the center surrounded by circular wind motion. The United States National Weather Service defines a tropical cyclone as "a rotating, organized system of clouds and thunderstorms that originates over tropical or subtropical waters and has a closed low-level circulation" (National Weather Service, 2013, p. 2). In practice, that circulation is a closed airflow at the earth's surface, going counterclockwise in the northern hemisphere and clockwise in the southern hemisphere. Severe storms arising in the Atlantic waters are known as hurricanes, whereas those developing in the Pacific Ocean and the China seas are called typhoons (see Figure 17.4). The precise classification (e.g., tropical depression, tropical storm, hurricane) depends on the wind force (measured on the Beaufort scale, introduced in 1805), wind speed, and manner of creation (see Box 17.1).

Hurricanes are devastating to the natural and man-made environment. The Federal Emergency Management Agency (FEMA) provides federal aid and assistance to those who have been affected by all types of disaster (FEMA, n.d.-a).

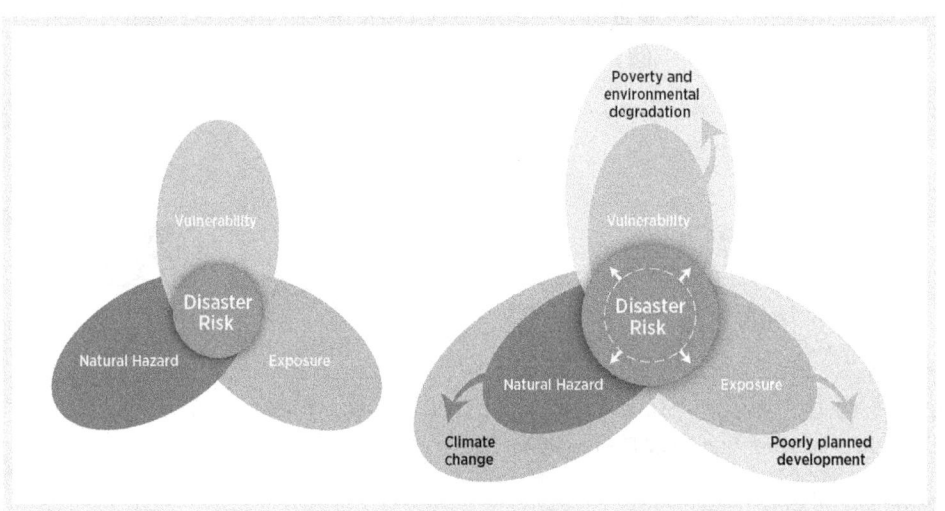

FIGURE 17.3 The interrelationship of natural hazards, exposures, and vulnerability in exposure to disaster risk.

Source: World Bank. (2013). *Building resilience: Integrating climate and disaster risk into development. Lessons from World Bank Group experience.* Washington, DC: Author.

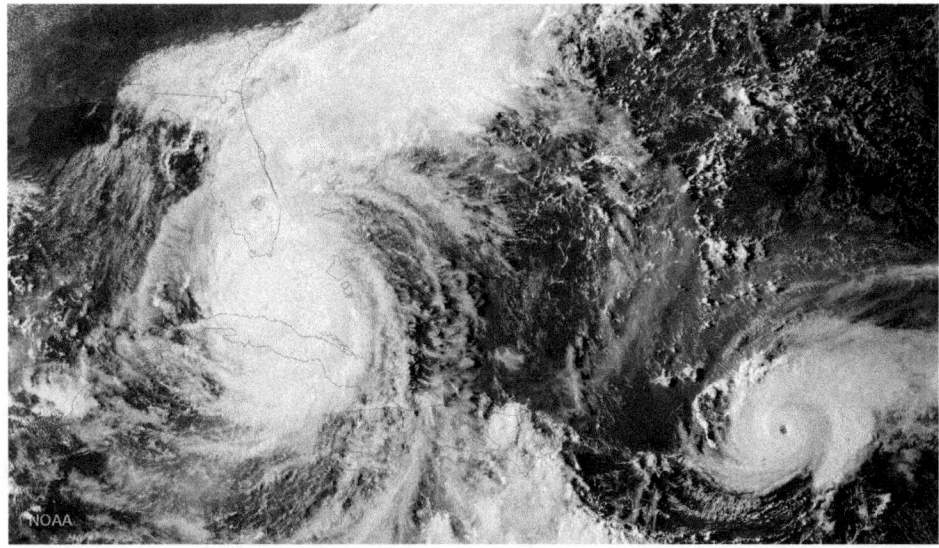

FIGURE 17.4 Hurricanes Irma and Jose in the Atlantic Ocean (September 9, 2017).

Source: National Oceanic and Atmospheric Administration. (2017). Saffir–Simpson Hurricane Wind Scale. Retrieved from http://www.nhc.noaa.gov/sshws_table.shtml.

Tropical Cyclone—A rotating, organized system of clouds and thunderstorms that originates over tropical or subtropical waters and has a closed low-level circulation. Tropical cyclones rotate counterclockwise in the northern hemisphere. They are classified as follows:

Tropical Depression—A tropical cyclone with maximum sustained winds of 38 mph (33 knots) or less.

Tropical Storm—A tropical cyclone with maximum sustained winds of 39 to 73 mph (34–63 knots).

Hurricane—A tropical cyclone with maximum sustained winds of 74 mph (64 knots) or higher. In the western north Pacific, hurricanes are called "typhoons"; similar storms in the Indian Ocean and south Pacific Ocean are called "cyclones."

Major Hurricane—A tropical cyclone with maximum sustained winds of 111 mph (96 knots) or higher, corresponding to Category 3, 4, or 5 on the Saffir–Simpson Hurricane Wind Scale.

Source: National Weather Service. (2017). *Tropical cyclones.* Retrieved from http://www.nws.noaa.gov/os/hurricane/resources/TropicalCyclones11.pdf

A hurricane is a tropical storm with winds that have reached a constant speed of 74 mph or more. Hurricane winds blow in a large spiral around a relatively calm center known as the "eye." The eye is generally 20 to 30 miles wide, and the storm may extend outward 400 miles. As a hurricane approaches, the skies will begin to darken, and winds will grow in strength.

As a hurricane nears land, it can bring torrential rains, high winds, and storm surges (see Figure 17.4). A single hurricane can last for more than 2 weeks over open waters and can run a path along the entire length of the eastern seaboard. August and September are peak months during the hurricane season, which lasts from June 1 through November 30. Satellites track hurricanes from the moment they begin to form, so warnings can be issued many days before a storm strikes. The greatest damage to life and property is not from the wind, however, but from tidal surges and flash flooding. Hurricanes are currently rated on a scale of 1 to 5, known as the Saffir–Simpson Hurricane Wind Scale (see Table 17.2). Category 3, 4, and 5 hurricanes are considered to be major storms (National Hurricane Center, 2017).

Owing to its violent nature, its potentially prolonged duration, and the extensive area that could be affected, the hurricane or cyclone is potentially the most devastating of all storms. Scientists at the National Hurricane Center have developed an excellent understanding of the nature of hurricanes through observation, radar, weather satellites, and computer models.

A distinctive characteristic of hurricanes is the increase in sea level, often referred to as "storm surge." This increase in sea level is the result of the low-pressure central area of the storm creating suction, the storm winds piling up water, and the tremendous speed of the storm. Rare storm surges have risen as much as approximately 46 feet above normal sea level. This phenomenon can be experienced as a large mass of seawater pushed along by the storm with great force. When it reaches land, the impact of the storm surge can be exacerbated by high tide, a low-lying coastal area with a gently sloping seabed, or a semi-enclosed bay facing the ocean (FEMA, n.d.-e).

TABLE 17.2 Saffir–Simpson Hurricane Wind Scale

Category	Winds	Effects
One	74–95 mph	No real damage to building structures. Damage primarily to unanchored mobile homes, shrubbery, and trees. Also, some coastal road flooding and minor pier damage.
Two	96–110 mph	Some roofing material, door, and window damage to buildings. Considerable damage to vegetation, mobile homes, and piers. Coastal and low-lying escape routes flood 2–4 hours before arrival of center. Small crafts in unprotected anchorages break moorings.
Three	111–130 mph	Some structural damage to small residences and utility buildings with a minor amount of curtainwall failures. Mobile homes are destroyed. Flooding near the coast destroys smaller structures with larger structures damaged by floating debris. Terrain continuously lower than 5 feet ASL may be flooded inland 8 miles or more.
Four	131–155 mph	More extensive curtainwall failures with some complete roof structure failure on small residences. Major erosion of beach. Major damage to lower floors of structures near the shore. Terrain continuously lower than 10 feet ASL may be flooded, requiring massive evacuation of residential areas inland as far as 6 miles.
Five	Greater than 155 mph	Complete roof failure on many residences and industrial buildings. Some complete building failures with small utility buildings blown over or away. Major damage to lower floors of all structures located less than 15 feet ASL and within 500 yards of the shoreline. Massive evacuation of residential areas on low ground within 5–10 miles of the shoreline may be required.

ASL, above sea level.

Source: National Oceanic and Atmospheric Administration. (2017). *Saffir–Simpson Hurricane Wind Scale.* Retrieved from http://www.nhc.noaa.gov/sshws _table.shtml.

The severity of a storm's impact on humans is exacerbated by deforestation, which often occurs as a result of population pressure. When trees disappear along coastlines, winds and storm surges can enter land with greater force. Deforestation on the slopes of hills and mountains increases the risk of violent flash floods and landslides caused by the heavy rain associated with tropical cyclones. At the same time, the beneficial effects of the rainfall—replenishment of the water resources—may be negated because of the inability of a deforested ecosystem to absorb and retain water.

In anticipation of a hurricane making landfall, disaster planners and healthcare providers should note that the Saffir–Simpson Hurricane Wind Scale does not address the potential for other hurricane-related impacts, such as storm surge, rainfall-induced floods, and tornadoes. It should also be noted that these general descriptions of wind-caused damage are to some degree dependent upon the local building codes in effect and how well and how long they have been enforced. For example, building codes enacted during the 2000s in Florida, North Carolina, and South Carolina are likely to reduce the damage to newer structures from that described further on. However, for a long time to come, the majority of the building stock in existence on the coast will not have been built to higher code. Hurricane wind damage is also very dependent upon other factors, such as duration of high winds, change in wind direction, and age of structures (National Weather Service, 2011).

Risk of Morbidity and Mortality

Deaths and injuries from hurricanes occur because victims fail to evacuate the affected area or take shelter, do not take precautions in securing their property, and do not follow guidelines on food and water safety or injury prevention during recovery (FEMA, n.d.-e). Nurses need to be familiar with the commonly used definitions for severe weather watches and storm warnings to assist with timely evacuation or to find shelter for affected populations (see Box 17.2).

Morbidity during and after the storm itself results from drowning, electrocution, lacerations, or punctures from flying debris, and blunt trauma or bone fractures from falling trees or other objects. Heart attacks and stress-related disorders can arise during the storm or its aftermath. Gastrointestinal, respiratory, vectorborne disease, and skin disease as well as accidental pediatric poisoning can all occur during the period immediately following a storm. Injuries from improper use of chain saws or other power equipment, disrupted wildlife (e.g., bites from animals, snakes, or insects) and fires are common. Fortunately, the ability to detect, track, and warn communities about cyclones, hurricanes, and tropical storms has helped reduce morbidity and mortality in many countries.

DROUGHT

Drought affects more people than any other environmental hazard, yet it is perhaps the most complex and least understood of this type of event. Drought is often seen as the result of too little rain and is often synonymous with famine. Fluctuation in rainfall alone does not cause a famine. Drought often triggers a crisis in arid and semiarid areas because rain is sparse and irregular. However, drought alone does not cause

BOX 17.2 Severe Weather Watches and Warnings Defined

Flood Watch: High flow or overflow of water from a river is possible in the given time period. It can also apply to heavy runoff or drainage of water into low-lying areas. These watches are generally issued for flooding that is expected to occur at least 6 hours after heavy rains have ended.
Flood Warning: Flooding conditions are actually occurring or are imminent in the warning area.
Flash Flood Watch: Flash flooding is possible in or close to the watch area. Flash flood watches are generally issued for flooding that is expected to occur within 6 hours after heavy rains have ended.
Flash Flood Warning: Flash flooding is actually occurring or imminent in the warning area. It can be issued as a result of torrential rains, a dam failure, or an ice jam.
Tornado Watch: Conditions are conducive to the development of tornadoes in and close to the watch area.
Tornado Warning: A tornado has actually been sighted by spotters or indicated on radar and is occurring or imminent in the warning area.
Severe Thunderstorm Watch: Conditions are conducive to the development of severe thunderstorms in and close to the watch area.
Severe Thunderstorm Warning: A severe thunderstorm has actually been observed by spotters or indicated on radar and is occurring or imminent in the warning area.
Tropical Storm Watch: Tropical storm conditions with sustained winds from 39 to 73 mph are possible in the watch area within the next 36 hours.
Tropical Storm Warning: Tropical storm conditions are expected in the warning area within the next 24 hours.
Hurricane Watch: Hurricane conditions (sustained winds greater than 73 mph) are possible in the watch area within 36 hours.
Hurricane Warning: Hurricane conditions are expected in the warning area in 24 hours or less.

Source: Federal Emergency Management Agency. (2012). *Severe weather watches and warnings definitions.* Washington, DC: Author. Retrieved from http://www.fema.gov

desertification. The ecosystem changes leading to desertification are all attributed to human activities, such as overcultivation, deforestation, overgrazing, and unskilled irrigation. Each of these activities is exacerbated by increasing human population size. The first three activities strip the soil of vegetation and deplete its organic and nutrient content. This leaves the soil exposed to the eroding forces of the sun and wind. The subsoil that is left can become so hard that it no longer absorbs rain. Water flows over its surface, carrying away the little topsoil that might have remained. Drought conditions can also trigger secondary natural disasters, such as wildfires. The public health implications of drought are extensive and include:

- Compromised quality and quantity of potable water
- Compromised food and nutrition

- Diminished living conditions (as they pertain to energy, air quality, and sanitation and hygiene)
- Recreational risks
- Mental and behavioral health
- Vulnerable populations
- Increased disease incidence (for infectious, chronic, and vectorborne/zoonotic diseases)

Risk of Morbidity and Mortality

Displaced populations suffer high rates of disease because of stress of migration, crowding, and unsanitary conditions of relocation sites. Morbidity and mortality can result from diarrheal disease, respiratory disease, and malnutrition. Mortality exceeding a baseline rate of 1 death per 10,000 people per day is the index of concern. Low weight-to-height is identified through the percentage of children two or more standard deviations (z-score) from the reference median compared with mean z-scores; children with edema are severely malnourished.

EARTHQUAKE

An earthquake, generally considered to be the most destructive and frightening of all forces of nature, is a sudden, rapid shaking of the earth caused by the breaking and shifting of rock beneath the earth's surface. This shaking can cause buildings and bridges to collapse; disrupt gas, electric, and phone service; and sometimes trigger landslides, avalanches, flash floods, fires, and huge, destructive ocean waves (tsunamis). Aftershocks of similar or lesser intensity can follow the main quake. Buildings with foundations resting on unconsolidated landfill, old waterways, or other unstable soil are most at risk. Buildings or trailers and manufactured homes not tied to a reinforced foundation anchored to the ground are also at risk because they can be shaken off their mountings during an earthquake. In April 2015, an earthquake in central Nepal killed nearly 9,000 people, injured another 22,000, and triggered an avalanche on Mount Everest, killing another 22 (Ovesen, 2016). The earthquake was the worst disaster to occur in the small country since an earlier earthquake in 1934 and was the world's deadliest natural disaster that year (CRED, 2016). Earthquakes can occur at any time of the year. Earthquake losses, like those of other disasters, tend to cause more financial losses in industrialized countries and more injuries and deaths in undeveloped countries (CRED, 2016; FEMA, n.d.-b).

The Richter scale, used as an indication of the force of an earthquake, measures the magnitude and intensity or energy released by the quake. This value is calculated based on data recordings from a single observation point for events anywhere on Earth, but it does not address the possible damaging effects of the earthquake. According to global observations, an average of two earthquakes of a Richter magnitude 8 or slightly more occur every year. A one-digit drop in magnitude equates with a 10-fold increase in frequency. In other words, earthquakes of magnitude 7 or more generally occur 20 times in a year, whereas those with a magnitude 6 or more occur approximately 200 times (FEMA, n.d.-b).

Earthquakes can result in a secondary disaster, catastrophic tsunami, discussed later in this chapter. Geologists have identified regions where earthquakes are likely to occur. With the increasing population worldwide and urban migration trends, higher death tolls and greater property losses are more likely in many areas prone to earthquakes. At least 70 million Americans face significant risk of death or injury from earthquakes because they live in the 39 states that are seismically active. In addition to the significant risks in California, the Pacific Northwest, Utah, and Idaho, six major cities with populations greater than 100,000 are located within the seismic area of the New Madrid fault (Missouri; FEMA, n.d.-b). Major low- and middle-income-country cities in which large numbers of people live on earthquake-prone land in structures unable to withstand damage include Lima, Peru; Santiago, Chile; Quito, Ecuador; and Caracas, Venezuela.

Risk of Morbidity and Mortality

Deaths and injuries from earthquakes vary according to the type of housing available, time of day of occurrence, and population density. Common injuries include cuts, broken bones, crush injuries, and dehydration from being trapped in rubble. Stress reactions are also common. Morbidity and mortality can occur during the actual quake, the delayed collapse of unsound structures, or cleanup activity. Disruption of the earth may release pathogens that when inhaled can lead to increased reports of infectious disease

Prevention/Mitigation

Mitigation involves developing and implementing strategies for reducing losses from earthquakes by incorporating principles of seismic safety into public and private decisions regarding the setting, design, and construction of structures (i.e., updating building and zoning codes and ordinances to enhance seismic safety), and regarding buildings' nonstructural elements, contents, and furnishings.

EPIDEMICS

An epidemic is an outbreak or occurrence of one specific disease from a single source in a group, population, community, or geographical area, in excess of the usual or expected level. An epidemic exists when new cases exceed the prevalence of a disease. Prevalence is the number of people within a population who have a certain disease or disorder at a given point in time. An acute outbreak—a sharp increase in new cases that affect a significant group—is generally considered an epidemic (Merrill & Timmereck, 2006). The spread of infectious disease depends on preexisting levels of the disease, ecological changes resulting from disaster, population displacement, changes in density of population, disruption of public utilities, interruption of basic public health services, and compromises to sanitation and hygiene. The risk that epidemics of infectious diseases will occur is proportional to population density and displacement. A true epidemic requires a susceptible population, the presence of a disease agent, and a mechanism that facilitates large-scale transmission (e.g., contaminated water supply or vector population).

All these conditions were met when in December 2013 a young boy in the small West African country of Guinea died of Ebola virus disease (EVD) and became the index case (the first case of an epidemic) of the world's largest-ever outbreak of the highly virulent hemorrhagic fever. By May 2016, a month before the declared end of the epidemic, the World Health Organization (WHO) and respective partner governments reported a total of 28,616 suspected cases of EVD and 11,310 deaths (WHO, 2016). While affecting primarily the West African countries of Sierra Leone, Guinea, and Liberia, cases were also reported in Nigeria, Mali, Senegal, the United States, the United Kingdom, Italy, and Spain, and highlighted the importance of establishing robust global infectious disease surveillance systems for today's world of global trade and travel. The outbreak also demonstrated the disparity in public and individual health resources available in high-income countries versus those in low- and middle-income ones (see Figure 17.5). However, because of increasing globalization, it has become clear that only through bolstering support for health systems in the most fragile states do more prosperous countries ensure their own health security (Heymann et al., 2015).

Quick response is essential because epidemics, resulting in human and economic losses and political difficulties, develop rapidly. An epidemic or threat of an epidemic can become an emergency when the following characteristics are present. Not every characteristic need be present and each must be assessed with regard to its relative importance locally:

- Risk of introduction to and spread of the disease in the population
- Large number of cases reasonably expected to occur
- Disease involved of such severity as to lead to serious disability or death
- Risk of social or economic disruption resulting from the presence of the disease
- Inability of authorities to cope adequately with the situation because of insufficient technical or professional personnel, organizational experience, and necessary supplies or equipment (e.g., drugs, vaccines, laboratory diagnostic materials, vector control materials)
- Risk of international transmission

The categorization of "emergency" differs from country to country, depending on two local factors: whether the disease is endemic and whether a means of transmitting the agent exists. Frequently, the introduction of a pathogen and the start of an epidemic may be through an animal vector; thus, veterinarians may be the first to identify a disease new to a community.

FLOOD

Prolonged rainfall over several days can cause a river or stream to overflow and flood surrounding areas. A flash flood from a broken dam or levee or after intense rainfall of 1 inch (or more) per hour often catches people unprepared.

Global statistics show that floods are the most frequently recorded destructive events, accounting for over 40% of the world's disasters each year. Since 1995, an estimated 2.3 billion people worldwide have been affected by such events. Floods are the most common type of disaster in the United States. The frequency of floods is increasing faster than any type of disaster. Much of this rise in incidence can be attributed to uncontrolled urbanization, deforestation, and the effects of climate change. Moreover, on the whole, adverse health outcomes are expected to dominate because of these climatic changes (Patz, Grabow, & Limaye, 2014). Floods may also accompany other natural disasters, such as sea surges during hurricanes and tsunamis following earthquakes (FEMA, n.d.-d).

Except for flash floods, flooding directly causes few deaths. Instead, widespread and long-lasting detrimental effects include damage to homes and mass homelessness, disruption of communications and healthcare systems, and heavy loss of business, livestock, crops, and grain, particularly in densely populated, low-lying areas. The frequent cyclic nature of flooding can mean a constant and ever-increasing drain on the economy of rural populations (Figure 17.6).

Risk of Morbidity and Mortality

Flood-related morbidity and mortality vary from country to country. Flash flooding, such as from excessive rainfall or sudden release of water from a dam, is the cause of most flood-related deaths. Many victims become trapped in their cars and drown when attempting

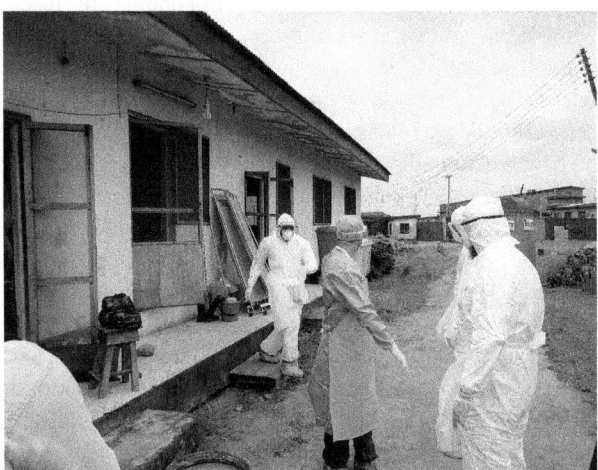

FIGURE 17.5 WHO workers donning personal protective equipment before entering an Ebola isolation ward in Lagos, Nigeria (2014).

Source: World Health Organization. (2017). Programmes: Ebola virus disease. Retrieved from http://www.who.int/ebola/en

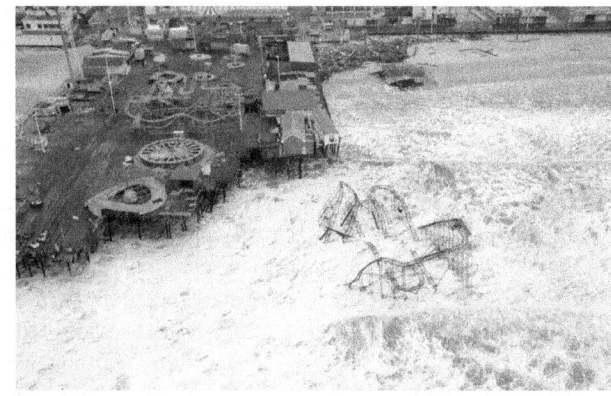

FIGURE 17.6 Hurricane Sandy floodwaters, New Jersey (2012).

Source: Dunphy, T. (2013). After sandy—The Jersey shore then and now. Retrieved from Restore the Shore Website: http://restoretheshore.com/after-sandy-the-jersey-shore-then-and-now-photos

to drive through rising or swiftly moving water. Other deaths have been caused by wading, bicycling, or other recreational activities in flooded areas. The health impacts of flooding include infectious disease morbidity exacerbated by crowded living conditions and compromised personal hygiene, contamination of water sources, disruption of sewage service and solid waste collection, and increased vector populations. Waterborne diseases (e.g., enterotoxigenic *Escherichia coli*, *Shigella*, hepatitis A, leptospirosis, or giardiasis) become a significant hazard, as do other vector-borne diseases and skin disorders. Injured and frightened animals, hazardous waste contamination, molds and mildew, and dislodging of graves pose additional risks in the period following a flood (FEMA, n.d.-d). Food shortages that are due to water-damaged stocks may occur because of flooding and sea surges.

The stress and exertion required for cleanup following a flood also cause significant morbidity (mental and physical) and mortality (e.g., myocardial infarction). Fires, explosions from gas leaks, downed live wires, and debris can all cause significant injury.

HEAT WAVE

Temperatures that hover 10°F or more above the average high temperature for the region and last for several weeks are defined as extreme heat. Humid or muggy conditions, which add to the discomfort of high temperatures, occur when a "dome" of high atmospheric pressure traps hazy, damp air near the ground. Excessively dry and hot conditions can provoke dust storms and low visibility. Droughts occur when a long period passes without substantial rainfall. A heat wave combined with a drought is a very dangerous situation (FEMA, n.d.-c).

Over time, populations can acclimate to hot weather. However, mortality and morbidity rise when daytime temperatures remain unusually high several days in a row and nighttime temperatures do not drop significantly. Because populations acclimate to summer temperatures, heat waves in June and July have more of an impact than those in August and September. There is often a delay between the onset of a heat wave and adverse health effects. Deaths occur more commonly during heat waves where there is little cooling at night, and taper off to baseline levels if a heat wave is sustained (FEMA, n.d.-c).

Risk of Morbidity and Mortality

Heat is the primary weather-related killer in the United States, resulting in hundreds of fatalities each year. In fact, on average, excessive heat claims more lives each year than floods, lightning, tornadoes, and hurricanes combined. In the disastrous heat wave of 1980, more than 1,500 people in the Midwestern United States and Southern Plains died. In the heat wave of 1995, more than 700 deaths in the Chicago area were attributed to heat. In August 2003, a record heat wave in Europe claimed an estimated 50,000 lives (National Weather Service, 2011).

Heat kills by pushing the human body beyond its limits. On average, about 175 Americans succumb to the taxing demands of heat every year. Our bodies dissipate heat by varying the rate and depth of blood circulation, by losing water through the skin and sweat glands, and, as a last resort, by panting, when blood is heated above 98.6°F. Sweating cools the body

through evaporation. However, high relative humidity retards evaporation, robbing the body of its ability to cool itself (National Weather Service, 2011). When heat gain exceeds the level the body can remove, body temperature begins to rise, and heat-related illnesses and disorders may develop.

The heat index (HI) published by the National Weather Service (weather.gov) is the temperature the body feels when heat and humidity are combined. Figure 17.7 shows the HI that corresponds to the actual air temperature and relative humidity. (This chart is based on shady, light wind conditions. Exposure to direct sunlight can increase the HI by up to 15°F.)

Most heat disorders occur because the victim has been overexposed to heat or has overexercised for his or her age and physical condition. Other conditions that can induce heat-related illnesses include stagnant atmospheric conditions and poor air quality (FEMA, n.d.-c).

Heat waves result in adverse health effects in cities more than in rural areas. During periods of sustained environmental heat—particularly during the summer—the numbers of deaths classified as heat related (e.g., heatstroke) and attributed to other causes (e.g., cardiovascular, cerebrovascular, and respiratory disease) increase substantially. Those at an increased risk for heat-related mortality are elderly persons, infants, persons with chronic conditions (including obesity), patients taking medications that predispose them to heatstroke (e.g., neuroleptics or anticholinergics), and persons confined to a bed or who otherwise are unable to care for themselves.

Adverse health outcomes associated with high environmental temperatures include heatstroke, heat exhaustion, heat syncope, and heat cramps. Heatstroke (i.e., core body temperature greater than or equal to 105°F/40.4°C) is the most serious of these conditions and is characterized by rapid progression of lethargy, confusion, and unconsciousness; it is often fatal despite medical

NOAA's National Weather Service

Heat index

Temperature (°F)

Relative humidity (%)	80	82	84	86	88	90	92	94	96	98	100	102	104	106	118	110
40	80	81	83	85	88	91	94	97	101	105	109	114	119	124	130	136
45	80	82	84	87	89	93	96	100	104	109	114	119	124	130	137	
50	81	83	85	88	91	95	99	103	108	113	118	124	131	137		
55	81	84	86	89	93	97	101	106	112	117	124	130	137			
60	82	84	88	91	95	100	105	110	116	123	129	137				
65	82	85	89	93	98	103	108	114	121	126	130					
70	83	86	90	95	100	105	112	119	126	134						
75	84	88	92	97	103	109	116	124	132							
80	84	89	94	100	106	113	121	129								
85	85	90	96	102	110	117	126	135								
90	86	91	98	105	113	122	131									
95	86	93	100	108	117	127										
100	87	95	103	112	121	132										

Likelihood of heat disorders with prolonged exposure of strenuous activity

☐ Caution   ☐ Extreme caution   ☐ Danger   ☐ External danger

FIGURE 17.7 Heat index (apparent temperature) chart.

Notes: Since heat index values were devised for shady, light wind conditions, **exposure to full sunshine can increase heat index values by up to 15°F**. Also, **strong winds**, particularly with very hot, dry air, can be extremely hazardous. The heat index chart shaded zone above 105°F shows a level that may cause increasingly severe heat disorders with continued exposure or physical activity.

NOAA, national oceanic and atmospheric administration.

Source: National Weather Service. (2017). Heat index (apparent temperature) chart. Retrieved from http://www.nws.noaa.gov/os/heat/index.shtml

care directed at lowering body temperature. Heat exhaustion is a milder syndrome that occurs following sustained exposure to hot temperatures and results from dehydration and electrolyte imbalance; manifestations include dizziness, weakness, or fatigue, and treatment is supportive. Heat syncope and heat cramps are usually related to physical exertion during hot weather.

Prevention

Basic behavioral and environmental measures are essential for preventing heat-related illness and death. Personal prevention strategies should include increasing time spent in air-conditioned environments, intake of nonalcoholic beverages, and incorporation of cool baths into a daily routine. When possible, activity requiring physical exertion should be conducted during cooler parts of the day (Box 17.3). Sun exposure should be minimized, and light, loose,

---

BOX 17.3 Adult Heat Wave Safety Tips

- **Slow down.** Reduce, eliminate, or reschedule strenuous activities until the coolest time of the day. Children, seniors, and anyone with health problems should stay in the coolest available place, not necessarily indoors.

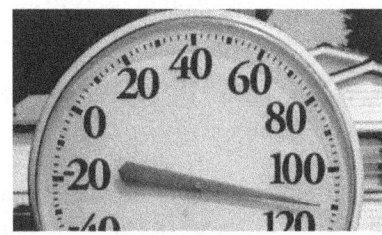

- **Dress for summer.** Wear lightweight, light-colored clothing to reflect heat and sunlight.
- **Put less fuel on your inner fires.** Foods like meat and other proteins that increase metabolic heat production also increase water loss.
- **Drink plenty of water, nonalcoholic and decaffeinated fluids.** Your body needs water to keep cool. Drink plenty of fluids even if you do not feel thirsty. Persons who have epilepsy or heart, kidney, or liver disease; are on fluid-restrictive diets; or have a problem with fluid retention should consult a physician before increasing their consumption of fluids. Do not drink alcoholic beverages and limit caffeinated beverages.
- **During excessive heat periods, spend more time in air-conditioned places.** Air-conditioning in homes and other buildings markedly reduces danger from the heat. If you cannot afford an air conditioner, go to a library, store, or other location with air-conditioning for part of the day.
- **Don't get too much sun.** Sunburn reduces your body's ability to dissipate heat.
- **Do not take salt tablets unless specified by a physician.**

Source: National Weather Service. (2017). Heat index (apparent temperature) chart. Retrieved from http://www.nws.noaa.gov/os/heat/index.shtml

---

cotton clothing should be worn. The risk for heat-induced illness is greatest before persons become acclimated to warm environments. Athletes and workers in occupations requiring exposure to either indoor or outdoor high temperatures should take special precautions, including allowing 10 to 14 days to acclimate to an environment of predictably high ambient temperature (FEMA, n.d.-c).

Nurses and other healthcare providers can assist in preventing heat-related illnesses and deaths by disseminating community prevention messages to persons at high risk (e.g., the elderly and persons with preexisting medical conditions) using a variety of communication techniques. They may also establish emergency plans that include provision of access to artificially cooled environments.

TORNADO

Tornadoes are rapidly whirling, funnel-shaped air spirals that emerge from a violent thunderstorm and reach the ground. Tornadoes can have a wind velocity of up to 200 mph and generate sufficient force to destroy even massive buildings. The average circumference of a tornado is several hundred feet, and it is usually exhausted before it has traveled as far as 20 km.

The following are facts about tornadoes:

- They may strike quickly, with little or no warning.
- They may appear nearly transparent until dust and debris are picked up or a cloud forms in the funnel.
- The average tornado moves southwest to northeast, but tornadoes have been known to move in any direction.
- The average forward speed of a tornado is 30 mph, but may vary from stationary to 70 mph.
- Tornadoes can accompany tropical storms and hurricanes as they move onto land.
- Waterspouts are tornadoes that form over water.
- Tornadoes are most frequently reported east of the Rocky Mountains during spring and summer months.
- Peak tornado season in the southern states is March through May; in the northern states, it is late spring through early summer.
- Tornadoes are most likely to occur between 3 p.m. and 9 p.m., but can occur at any time (FEMA, n.d.-g).

The severity of tornadoes is rated on the Fujita scale according to wind speed. The Fujita scale uses a scoring system of F0 (no damage) to F5 (total destruction). The extent of damage depends on updrafts within the tornado funnel, the tornado's atmospheric pressure (which is often lower than the surrounding barometric pressure), and the effects of flying debris. An enhanced Fujita scale was released in February 2007 and reflects updated metrics for existing wind based on damage occurring as a result of a tornado (see Table 17.3).

Risk of Morbidity and Mortality

Approximately 1,000 tornadoes occur annually in the United States, and none of the lower 48 states are immune. Certain geographical areas are at greater risk because of recurrent weather patterns; tornadoes most frequently occur in the midwestern and southeastern states. Although tornadoes often develop in

TABLE 17.3 Enhanced F Scale for Tornado Damage

	FUJITA SCALE		DERIVED EF SCALE		OPERATIONAL EF SCALE	
F No.	Fastest 1/4-Mile (MPH)	3-Sec Gust (MPH)	EF No.	3-Sec Gust (MPH)	EF No.	3-Sec Gust (MPH)
0	40–72	45–78	0	65–85	0	65–85
1	73–112	79–117	1	86–109	1	86–110
2	113–157	118–161	2	110–137	2	111–135
3	158–207	162–209	3	138–167	3	136–165
4	208–260	210–261	4	168–199	4	166–200
5	261–318	262–317	5	200–234	5	Over 200

Notes: The Enhanced F-scale still is a set of wind estimates (not measurements) based on damage. It uses 3-second gusts estimated at the point of damage based on a judgment of 8 levels of damage to the 28 indicators listed in Table 17.4. These estimates vary with height and exposure. **Important:** The 3-second gust is not the same wind as in standard surface observations. Standard measurements are taken by weather stations in open exposures, using a directly measured, "one minute mile" speed.

Source: National Oceanic and Atmospheric Administration. (2011). Enhanced F scale for tornado damage. Retrieved from http://www.spc.noaa.gov/faq/tornado/ef-scale.html

the late afternoon and more often from March through May, they can arise at any hour of the day and during any month of the year. Injuries from tornadoes occur from flying debris or people being thrown by the high winds (e.g., head injuries, soft tissue injury, or secondary wound infection; see Table 17.4).

Injury may result from the direct impact of a tornado, or it may occur afterward when people walk among debris and enter damaged buildings. A Centers for Disease Control and Prevention (CDC) study of injuries after a tornado in Marion, Illinois, showed that 50% of the tornado-related injuries were suffered during rescue attempts, cleanup, and other post-tornado activities. Nearly a third of the injuries resulted from stepping on nails. Other common causes of injury included falling objects and heavy, rolling objects. Because tornadoes often damage power lines, gas lines, or electrical systems, there is a risk of fire, electrocution, or an explosion. Injured victims need prompt treatment of injuries suffered during the storm. Responders need to exercise extreme care to avoid hazards. Stress-related disorders are common, as is disease related to loss of utilities, potable water, or shelter.

Prevention/Mitigation

Because tornadoes can occur so quickly, communities should develop redundant warning systems (e.g., media alerts and automated telephone warnings), establish protective shelters to reduce tornado-related injuries, and practice tornado shelter drills. In the event of a tornado, the residents should take shelter in a basement if possible, away from windows, while protecting their heads. Special outreach should be made to people with special needs, who should make a list of their limitations, capabilities, and medications and have ready an emergency box of needed supplies. People with special needs should have a "buddy" who has a copy of the list and who knows of the emergency box.

CDC HELMET AND TORNADO STATEMENT

The CDC continues to recommend, as its first recommendation, that people in the path of a tornado find a shelter or a tornado-safe room. The safest place in the home is the interior part of a basement. If possible, get under something sturdy such as a heavy table or workbench. If outdoors, lie down in a gully or ditch.

CDC understands that people are looking for any useful and effective ways to protect themselves. At this time there is no available research on the effectiveness of helmet use to prevent head injuries during a tornado, but we do know that head injuries are common causes of death during tornadoes. CDC has long made the recommendation that people try to protect their heads. Because the time to react may be very short, if people choose to use helmets they should know where they are and have them readily accessible. Looking for a helmet in the few seconds before a tornado hits may delay getting safely to shelter. If people choose to use helmets, these helmets should not be considered an alternative to seeking appropriate shelter. Rather, helmets should be considered just one part of their overall home tornado preparedness kit to avoid any delay.

Source: Centers for Disease Control and Prevention. (2017). Tornadoes. Retrieved from https://www.cdc.gov/disasters/tornadoes

THUNDERSTORMS

A thunderstorm is formed from a combination of moisture, rapidly rising warm air, and a force capable of lifting air such as a warm and cold front, a sea breeze, or a mountain range.

TABLE 17.4 Enhanced F Scale Damage Indicators

No.	Damage Indicator	Abbreviation
1	Small barns, farm outbuildings	SBO
2	One- or two-family residences	FR12
3	Single-wide mobile home	MHSW
4	Double-wide mobile home	MHDW
5	Apt., condo, townhouse (3 stories or less)	ACT
6	Motel	M
7	Masonry apt. or motel	MAM
8	Small retail bldg. (fast food)	SRB
9	Small professional bldg. (doctor office, branch bank)	SPB
10	Strip mall	SM
11	Large shopping mall	LSM
12	Large, isolated ("big box") retail bldg.	LIRB
13	Automobile showroom	ASR
14	Automotive service building	ASB
15	School—1-story elementary (interior or exterior halls)	ES
16	School—jr. or sr. high school	JHSH
17	Low-rise (1–4 stories) bldg.	LRB
18	Mid-rise (5–20 stories) bldg.	MRB
19	High-rise (over 20 stories)	HRB
20	Institutional bldg. (hospital, govt., or university)	IB
21	Metal building system	MBS
22	Service station canopy	SSC
23	Warehouse (tilt-up walls or heavy timber)	WHB
24	Transmission line tower	TLT
25	Free-standing tower	FST
26	Free-standing pole (light, flag, luminary)	FSP
27	Tree—hardwood	TH
28	Tree—softwood	TS

Note: An update to the *original F-scale,* by a team of meteorologists and wind engineers, was implemented in the United States on February 1, 2007.

Source: National Oceanic and Atmospheric Administration. (2011). Enhanced F scale for tornado damage. Retrieved from http://www.spc.noaa.gov/faq/tornado/ef-scale.html

All thunderstorms contain lightning. Thunderstorms may occur singly, in clusters, or in lines. Thus, it is possible for several thunderstorms to affect one location in the course of a few hours. Some of the most severe weather occurs when a single thunderstorm affects one location for an extended time. Thunderstorms can bring heavy rains (which can cause flash flooding), strong winds, hail, lightning, and tornadoes. Severe thunderstorms can cause extensive damage to homes and property (FEMA, n.d.-f).

Lightning is a major threat during a thunderstorm. Lightning is an electrical discharge that results from the buildup of positive and negative charges within a thunderstorm. When the buildup becomes strong enough, lightning appears as a "bolt." This flash of light usually occurs within the clouds or between the clouds and the ground. A bolt of lightning reaches a temperature approaching 50,000°F in a split second. The rapid heating and cooling of air near the lightning causes thunder.

Risk of Morbidity and Mortality

In the United States, between 75 and 100 Americans are hit and killed each year by lightning. Morbidity is reduced if, when caught outdoors, individuals avoid natural lightning rods such as tall, isolated trees in an open area, or on top of a hill, and metal objects such as wire fences, golf clubs, and metal tools. It is a myth that lightning never strikes twice in the same place. In fact, lightning will strike several times in the same place in the course of one discharge (FEMA, n.d.-f). Although thunderstorms and lightning can be found throughout the United States, they are most likely to occur in the central and southern states. The state with the highest number of thunderstorm days is Florida.

TSUNAMIS

Tsunamis, a series of waves usually generated by large earthquakes under or near the ocean, occur when a body of water is rapidly displaced on a massive scale. Submarine landslides and volcanic eruptions beneath the sea or on small islands can also be responsible for tsunamis, but their effects are usually limited to smaller areas. Tsunamis are often mistakenly referred to as tidal waves because they can resemble a violent tide rushing to shore. Powerful enough to move through any obstacle, damage from tsunamis results from both the destructive force of the initial wave and the rapid flooding that occurs as the water dissipates. Depending on the strength of the initiating event, underwater topology, and the distance from its epicenter to the shore, the effects of a tsunami can vary greatly, ranging from being barely noticeable to total destruction (FEMA, n.d.-h).

Tsunami waves can be described by their wavelength (measured in feet or miles), period (minutes or hours it takes one wavelength to pass a fixed point), speed (mph), and height. Tsunamis may travel long distances, increasing in height abruptly when they reach shallow water, causing great devastation far away from the source. In deep water, a person on the surface may not realize that a tsunami is forming while the wave increases to great heights as it approaches the coastline. Tsunamis are not preventable, nor predictable, but there are warning signs. Any of the following events may signal an approaching tsunami:

- A recent submarine earthquake occurs.
- The sea appears to be boiling, as large quantities of gas rise to the surface of the water.
- The water is hot, smells of rotten eggs, or stings the skin.
- There is an audible thunder or booming sound followed by a roaring or whistling sound.
- The water may recede a great distance from the coast.
- Red light might be visible near the horizon and, as the wave approaches, the top of the wave may glow red.

There are systems available and others being developed to provide alerts about impending tsunamis. Tsunami warning systems can detect tsunamis when the wave is still at sea. Some systems advise residents where to evacuate to in order to avoid an incoming tsunami. One of the earliest warnings comes from animals, which run to higher ground before the water arrives. Other mitigating actions include building high walls in front of populated coastal areas or redirecting the incoming water via floodgates and channels. However, the effectiveness of these strategies can be limited, as tsunamis can be higher than these barriers (FEMA, n.d.-h).

Risk of Morbidity and Mortality

In the immediate aftermath of a tsunami, the first health interventions are to rescue survivors and provide medical care for any injuries. For people caught in the waves, the force of the water pushes people into debris, resulting in the broadest range of injuries, such as broken limbs and head injuries. Drowning is the most common cause of death associated with a tsunami. Tsunami waves and the receding water are very destructive to structures in the run-up zone. Other hazards include flooding and fires from gas lines or ruptured tanks.

The floods that accompany a tsunami result in potential health risks from contaminated water and food supplies. Loss of shelter leaves people vulnerable to exposure to insects, heat, and other environmental hazards. Further, the lack of medical care may result in exacerbations of chronic disease. Tsunamis have long-lasting effects and recovery necessitates long-term surveillance of infectious and water- or insect-transmitted diseases, an infusion of medical supplies and medical personnel, and the provision of mental health and social support services.

Potential waterborne diseases that follow tsunamis include cholera; diarrheal or fecal–oral diseases, such as amebiasis, cryptosporidiosis, cyclosporiasis, giardiasis, hepatitis A and E, leptospirosis, parasitic infections, rotavirus, shigellosis, and typhoid fever; animal- or mosquitoborne illness, such as plague, rabies, malaria, Japanese encephalitis, and dengue fever (and the potentially fatal complication, dengue hemorrhagic shock syndrome); and wound-associated infections and diseases, such as tetanus. Mental health concerns are another consequence of tsunami events.

VOLCANIC ERUPTIONS

A volcano is a mountain that opens downward to a reservoir of molten rock below the surface of the earth. Unlike most mountains, which are pushed up from below, volcanoes are built up by an accumulation of their own eruptive products. When pressure from gases within the molten rock becomes too great, an eruption occurs. Extremely high temperature and pressure cause the mantle, located deep inside the earth between the molten iron core and the thin crust at the surface, to melt and become liquid rock or magma. When a large amount of magma is formed, it rises through the denser rock layers toward the earth's surface. Eruptions can be quiet or explosive. There may be lava flows, flattened landscapes, poisonous gases, and flying rock and ash (see Figure 17.8; FEMA, n.d.-i).

Because of their intense heat, lava flows are great fire hazards. Lava flows destroy everything in their path, but most move slowly enough that people can move out of the way.

Fresh volcanic ash, made of pulverized rock, can be abrasive, acidic, gritty, gassy, and odorous. While not immediately dangerous to most adults, the acidic gas and ash can cause lung damage to small infants, to older adults, and to those suffering from severe respiratory illnesses. Volcanic ash also can damage machinery, including engines and electrical equipment. Ash accumulations mixed with water become heavy and can collapse roofs. Volcanic ash can affect people hundreds of miles away from the cone of a volcano (Figure 17.8).

Sideways-directed volcanic explosions, known as "lateral blasts," can shoot large pieces of rock at very high speeds for several miles. These explosions can kill by impact, burial, or heat. They have been known to knock down entire forests (FEMA, n.d.-i).

Volcanic eruptions can be accompanied by other natural hazards, including earthquakes, mudflows and flash floods, rockfalls and landslides, acid rain, fire, and (under special conditions) tsunamis.

Active volcanoes in the United States are found mainly in Hawaii, Alaska, and the Pacific Northwest. Active volcanoes of the Cascade Mountain Range in California, Oregon, and

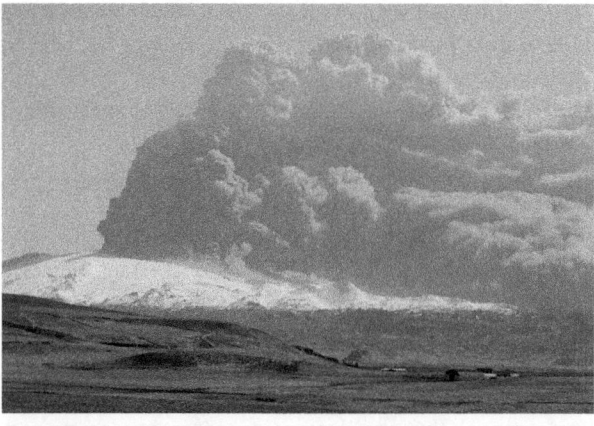

FIGURE 17.8 Eyjafjallajokull volcano plume, Iceland (April 2010).

Source: Photo Courtesy of Thorburn, H. (2010).

Washington have created problems recently. The danger area around a volcano covers approximately a 20-mile radius. Some danger may exist 100 miles or more from a volcano, leaving Montana and Wyoming at risk.

Risk of Morbidity and Mortality

Volcanic eruptions can endanger the lives of people and property located both near and far from a volcano. The range of adverse health effects on the population resulting from volcanic activity is quite broad and extensive. Immediate, acute, and nonspecific irritant effects have been reported in the eyes, nasal passages, and upper airways of persons exposed to volcanic ash. Victims can experience exacerbations of their asthma and chronic obstructive pulmonary disease (COPD) and can asphyxiate due to inhalation of ash or gases. Eruptions can result in blast injuries and lacerations from projectile rock fragments. Volcanic flow can cause fires and the destruction of buildings with victims experiencing trauma and thermal burns.

Activities for When a Volcano Erupts

- **Collaborate with emergency management specialists as needed.**
- **Follow the evacuation order** issued by authorities and evacuate immediately from the volcano area to avoid flying debris, hot gases, lateral blast, and lava flow.
- **Be aware of mudflows.** The danger from a mudflow increases near stream channels and with prolonged heavy rains. Mudflows can move faster than you can walk or run. Look upstream before crossing a bridge, and do not cross the bridge if a mudflow is approaching.
- **Avoid river valleys and low-lying areas.**

Protection From Falling Ash

- **Listen to a battery-powered radio or television for the latest emergency information.**
- **Individuals with a respiratory ailment should avoid contact with any amount of ash.**
- **Wear long-sleeved shirts and long pants.**
- **Use goggles and wear eyeglasses instead of contact lenses.**
- **Use a dust mask** or hold a damp cloth over your face to help with breathing.
- **Stay away from areas downwind** from the volcano to avoid volcanic ash.
- **Stay indoors until the ash has settled** unless there is a danger of the roof collapsing.
- **Close doors, windows, and all ventilation** in the house (chimney vents, furnaces, air conditioners, fans, and other vents).
- **Clear heavy ash from flat or low-pitched roofs and rain gutters.**
- **Avoid running car or truck engines.** Driving can stir up volcanic ash that can clog engines, damage moving parts, and stall vehicles.
- **Avoid driving in heavy ash fall** unless absolutely required. If you have to drive, keep speed down to 35 mph or slower.

WINTER/ICE STORMS

A major winter storm can be lethal. Winter storms bring ice, snow, cold temperatures, and often dangerous driving conditions. Even small amounts of snow and ice can cause severe problems for southern states where storms are infrequent (see Figure 17.9).

Nurses need to be familiar with winter storm warning messages, such as wind chill, winter storm watch, winter storm warning, and blizzard warning. "Wind chill" is a calculation of how cold it feels outside when the effects of temperature and wind speed are combined. On November 1, 2001, the National Weather Service implemented a replacement wind chill temperature index for the 2001/2002 winter season. The reason for the change was to improve on the existing index, which was based on the 1945 Siple and Passel Index. A "winter storm watch" indicates that severe winter weather may affect your area. A "winter storm warning" indicates that severe winter weather conditions are definitely on the way and emergency preparedness plans should be activated. A "blizzard warning" means that large amounts of falling or blowing snow and sustained winds of at least 35 mph are expected for several hours.

A new scale has been developed by the National Weather Service to classify snowstorms, similar to the Fujita and Saffir–Simpson scales that characterize tornadoes and hurricanes respectively. The Northeast Snow fall Impact Scale (NESIS) characterizes and ranks high-impact northeast snowstorms whose accumulations of snowfall total 10 inches or more. NESIS has five categories: Extreme, Crippling, Major, Significant, and Notable. The index differs from other meteorological indices in that it is interested in providing an indication of a storm's societal impacts, such as transportation, by assessing population data in addition to meteorological measurements. Snowstorms are tracked by the National Oceanic Atmospheric Administration's National Weather Service.

Risk of Morbidity and Mortality

Transportation accidents are the leading cause of death during winter storms. Preparing vehicles for the winter season and

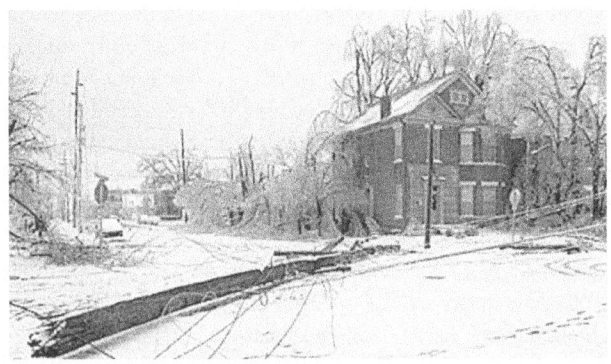

FIGURE 17.9 Ice storm damage in Paducah, Kentucky (2009). Ice covered much of the foliage in the region, weighing down trees and causing extensive damage to property.

Source: National Weather Service. (2009). Ice and snow storm of January 26–28, 2009. Retrieved from https://www.weather.gov/lmk/jan_2009_ice_and_snow

knowing how to react if stranded or lost on the road are the keys to safe winter driving. Morbidity and mortality associated with winter storms include frostbite and hypothermia, carbon monoxide poisoning, blunt trauma from falling objects, penetrating trauma from the use of mechanical snow blowers, and cardiovascular events usually associated with snow removal. Frostbite is a severe reaction to cold exposure that can permanently damage its victims. A loss of feeling and a light or pale appearance in fingers, toes, nose, or earlobes are symptoms of frostbite. Hypothermia is a condition brought on when the body temperature drops to less than 90°F. Symptoms of hypothermia include uncontrollable shivering, slow speech, memory lapses, frequent stumbling, drowsiness, and exhaustion (FEMA, n.d.-k).

Water has a unique property in that it expands as it freezes. This expansion puts tremendous pressure on whatever is containing it, including metal or plastic pipes. Regardless of the strength of a container, expanding water can cause pipes to break, causing flooding. Flooding creates a risk for drowning and electrocution. Pipes that freeze most frequently are those that are exposed to severe cold, like outdoor hose bibs, swimming pool supply lines, water sprinkler lines, and water supply pipes in unheated interior areas like basements and crawl spaces, attics, garages, or kitchen cabinets. Also, pipes that run against exterior walls that have little or no insulation are subject to freezing. Pipe freezing is a particular problem in warmer climates, where pipes often run through uninsulated or underinsulated attics or crawl spaces (FEMA, n.d.-k).

Prevention/Mitigation

Investing in preventive mitigation steps such as home winterization activities (insulating pipes, installing storm windows) will help reduce the impact of winter storms in the future. Winter storm preparation activities should include the following:

- Collecting winter clothing and supplies such as extra blankets, warm coats and clothes, water-resistant boots, hats, and mittens
- Assembling a disaster supplies kit containing a first aid kit, battery-powered weather radio, flashlight, and extra batteries
- Stocking canned food, a nonelectric can opener, and bottled water
- Winterizing vehicles, keeping gas tanks full, and assembling a disaster supply car kit
- Ensuring an adequate supply of any medications needed during and immediately following the storm

WILDFIRES

More and more people are making their homes in woodland settings in or near forests, rural areas, or remote mountain sites. As residential areas expand into relatively untouched wildlands, people living in these communities are increasingly threatened by forest fires. Protecting structures from fire in the wildland poses special problems, often stretching firefighting resources to the limit. Wildfires often begin unnoticed and spread quickly by igniting brush, trees, and homes (see Figure 17.10).

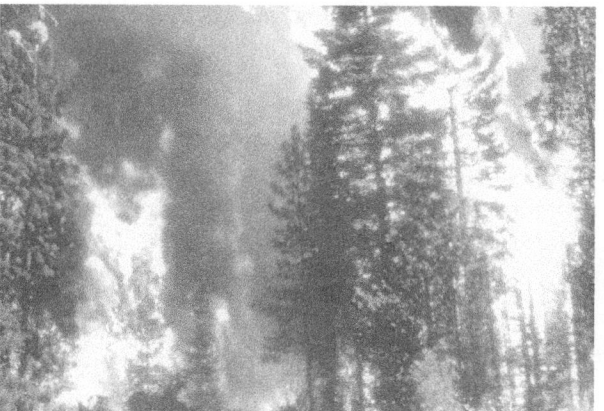

FIGURE 17.10 California wildfire.

Source: Bureau of Land Management. (2008). California wildfire. Retrieved from https://www.blm.gov/programs/public-safety-and-fire/fire-and-aviation

There are three different classes of wildfires. A "surface fire," the most common type, burns along the floor of a forest, moving slowly and killing or damaging trees. A "ground fire" is usually started by lightning and burns on or below the forest floor in the humus layer down to the mineral soil. "Crown fires" spread rapidly by wind and move quickly by jumping along the tops of trees. Depending on prevailing winds and the amount of water in the environment, wildfires can quickly spread out of control, causing extensive damage to personal property and human life. If heavy rains follow a fire, other natural disasters can occur, including landslides, mudflows, and floods. Once ground cover has been burned away, little is left to hold soil in place on steep slopes and hillsides. A major wildland fire can leave a large amount of scorched and barren land. These areas may not return to prefire conditions for decades. Danger zones include all wooded, brushy, and grassy areas—especially those in Kansas, Mississippi, Louisiana, Georgia, Florida, the Carolinas, Tennessee, California, Massachusetts, and the national forests of the western United States (FEMA, n.d.-j).

Risk of Morbidity and Mortality

Morbidity and mortality associated with wildfires include burns, inhalation injuries, respiratory complications, and stress-related cardiovascular events (exhaustion and myocardial infarction while fighting or fleeing the fire). Wildfire smoke is a mix of gases and fine particles from burning vegetation, building materials, and other materials. Inhaling wildfire smoke can cause serious lung damage, an exacerbation of existing lung disease, and lead to chronic lung disease.

Prevention/Mitigation

More than four out of every five wildfires are started by people. Negligent human behavior, such as smoking in forested areas or improperly extinguishing campfires, is the cause of many forest fires. Another cause of forest fires is lightning. Prevention efforts include encouraging people to do the following:

- Build fires away from nearby trees or bushes. Ash and cinders lighter than air float and may be blown into areas with heavy fuel load, starting wildfires.

- Be prepared to extinguish the fire quickly and completely. If the fire becomes threatening, someone will need to extinguish it immediately.
- Never leave a fire—even a cigarette—burning unattended. Fire can quickly spread out of control.
- Find out whether the area where people live is at risk of wildfire and develop a family wildfire evacuation plan (FEMA, n.d.-j).

SUMMARY

Natural and environmental disasters result in significant losses, physical destruction of dwellings, social and economic disruption, human pain and suffering, and significant injury and loss of life. Disaster preparedness activities including prevention efforts and advanced warning systems specific to each type of disaster can reduce or mitigate these effects.

All natural disasters are unique in that each affected region of the world has different social, economic, and health backgrounds. Some similarities exist, however, among the health effects of different natural disasters, which if recognized, can ensure that health and emergency medical relief and limited resources are well managed. (Noji, 2005)

Nurses should be familiar with the types and consequences of frequently occurring natural disasters to contribute to public health efforts to prevent, mitigate, and recover from these events. Nurses need to be familiar with commonly used definitions for severe weather watches and storm warnings. Careful review and evaluation of response efforts of previous naturally occurring disasters can be used to predict future needs. Scientifically valid information enables healthcare providers and emergency management officials to prioritize resources and make decisions about responding to natural disasters.

STUDY QUESTIONS

1. Is the risk of a major natural disaster occurring in the United States increasing or decreasing? Defend your position.

2. Hurricane Maria (2017) was a catastrophic natural disaster impacting the U.S. Virgin Islands and Puerto Rico. Describe the impact in terms of severity of damage and describe the health implications for the affected populations.

3. Describe the potential natural disasters that might occur in the greater New York City area and predict the resulting health impact upon the population.

4. Compare and contrast a drought disaster versus a flood disaster in terms of the health consequences on the affected population and its impact on the healthcare system.

5. Explain the meteorological relationship between thunderstorms and tornadoes. Design a public health educational campaign to reduce morbidity and mortality associated with severe thunderstorms and tornadoes.

6. Compare and contrast the adverse health outcomes resulting from extreme heat and winter/ice storms.

7. The 2017 Northern California wildfires destroyed a large geographical area across Napa, Sonoma, and Yuba counties and caused loss of life. Identify any advanced warning systems and preparedness activities that might help reduce morbidity and mortality in future wildfires.

INTERNET ACTIVITIES

Explore the following Internet resources.

1. **www.nhc.noaa.gov**

   This is the website for the National Weather Service's National Hurricane Center. What tropical storms are currently active in the Atlantic and Caribbean? In the Eastern Pacific? Where would you locate the sea surface temperature analysis charts? How do scientists use these measurements in predicting? Why is prediction of this storm important? Write an essay describing the health implications of hurricanes and describe strategies for mitigating these consequences.

2. **www.fema.gov**

   This is the website for FEMA. FEMA is charged with monitoring all types of natural/environmental disaster activity in the United States. You are the nurse assigned the task of compiling a notebook of factual information regarding "Protection Against Natural Disasters" to give to families in the following communities. Compile a list of fact sheets and information for all potential hazards for each of these communities:

   a. Fairfield, Connecticut
   b. Bald Head Island, North Carolina
   c. Webster, New York
   d. San Antonio, Texas
   e. San Francisco, California
   f. Santa Fe, New Mexico

3. **www.americanredcross.org**

   The American Red Cross website provides disaster preparedness and management advice for all types of naturally occurring disasters. What types of activities should nurses encourage people to do to prevent and mitigate the consequences of wildfires? What types of natural disasters are you and your family at risk for? Visit the American Red Cross website. Develop a personal family disaster preparedness plan based on what you find. Review it with each member of your family.

4. **www.fema.gov/disasters**

   You are working as an emergency manager for your county health department. Prepare a report documenting any and all *current* national situations for today's date. Compile a list of all state offices and emergency management agencies for the state in which you live. How would you locate current disease prevalence information for your community?

5. **www.nws.noaa.gov**

This is the website for the National Weather Service. Locate the 5-day forecast for your region.

REFERENCES

Bissell, R. A., Pinet, L., Nelson, M., & Levy, M. (2004). Evidence of the effectiveness of health sector preparedness in disaster response: The example of four earthquakes. *Family and Community Health, 27*(3), 193–203. doi:10.1097/00003727-200407000-00006

Blaikie, P., Cannon, T., Davis, I., & Wisner, B. (2014). *At risk: Natural hazards, people's vulnerability and disasters.* New York, NY: Routledge.

Bureau of Land Management. (2008). California wildfire. Retrieved from https://www.blm.gov/programs/public-safety-and-fire/fire-and-aviation

Centers for Disease Control and Prevention. (2017). Natural disasters and severe weather. Retrieved from https://www.cdc.gov/disasters

Centre for Research on the Epidemiology of Disasters. (2016). The human cost of weather-related disasters 1995–2015. Retrieved from http://reliefweb.int/sites/reliefweb.int/files/resources/COP21_WeatherDisastersReport_2015_FINAL.pdf

Centre for Research on the Epidemiology of Disasters. (2017). EM-DAT: The emergency events database. Retrieved from http://www.emdat.be

Dunphy, T. (2013). After sandy—The Jersey shore then and now. Retrieved from Restore the Shore Website: http://restoretheshore.com/after-sandy-the-jersey-shore-then-and-now-photos

Eshghi, K., & Larson, R. C. (2008). Disasters: Lessons from the past 105 years. *Disaster Prevention and Management, 17*(1), 62–82. doi:10.1108/09653560810855883

Federal Emergency Management Agency. (2012). *Severe weather watches and warnings definitions.* Washington, DC: Author. Retrieved from https://www.fema.gov

Federal Emergency Management Agency. (n.d.-a). About FEMA. Retrieved from https://www.fema.gov/about-agency

Federal Emergency Management Agency. (n.d.-b). Earthquakes. Retrieved from https://www.ready.gov/earthquakes

Federal Emergency Management Agency. (n.d.-c). Extreme hHeat. Retrieved from https://www.ready.gov/heat

Federal Emergency Management Agency. (n.d.-d). Floods. Retrieved from https://www.ready.gov/floods

Federal Emergency Management Agency. (n.d.-e). Hurricanes. Retrieved from https://www.ready.gov/hurricanes

Federal Emergency Management Agency. (n.d.-f). Thunderstorms & Lightning. Retrieved from https://www.ready.gov/thunderstorms-lightning

Federal Emergency Management Agency. (n.d.-g). Tornados. Retrieved from https://www.ready.gov/tornadoes

Federal Emergency Management Agency. (n.d.-h). Tsunamis. Retrieved from https://www.ready.gov/tsunamis

Federal Emergency Management Agency. (n.d.-i). Volcanoes. Retrieved from https://www.ready.gov/volcanoes

Federal Emergency Management Agency. (n.d.-j). Winter weather. Retrieved from https://www.ready.gov/winter-weather

Federal Emergency Management Agency. (n.d.-k). Wildfires. Retrieved from https://www.ready.gov/wildfires

GRID-Arendal. (2009). Number of disasters per year. Retrieved from http://www.grida.no/resources/7324

Hanes, P. F. (2016). Wildfire disasters and nursing. *The Nursing Clinics of North America, 51*(4), 625–645. doi:10.1016/j.cnur.2016.07.006

Heymann, D. L., Chen, L., Takemi, K., Fidler, D. P., Tappero, J. W., Thomas, M. J., . . . Rannan-Eliya, R. P. (2015). Global health security: The wider lessons from the west African Ebola virus disease epidemic. *The Lancet, 385*(9980), 1884–1901. doi:10.1016/S0140-6736(15)60858-3

Intergovernmental Panel on Climate Change. (2014). Summary for policymakers. In *Climate Change 2014: Impacts, adaptation, and vulnerability* (pp. 14, 23–31). Cambridge, UK: Cambridge University Press.

Jacquet, G. A., Kirsch, T., Durrani, A., Sauer, L., & Doocy, S. (2016). Health care access and utilization after the 2010 Pakistan floods. *Prehospital and Disaster Medicine, 31*(5), 485–491. doi:10.1017/S1049023X16000716

Mayhorn, C. B., & McLaughlin, A. C. (2014). Warning the world of extreme events: A global perspective on risk communication for natural and technological disaster. *Safety Science, 61*, 43–50. doi:10.1016/j.ssci.2012.04.014

Merrill, R. M., & Timmereck, T. C. (2006). *An introduction to epidemiology* (4th ed.). Boston, MA: Jones & Bartlett.

National Hurricane Center. (2017). Saffir-Simpson hurricane wind scale. National Hurricane Center Web site. Retrieved from https://www.nhc.noaa.gov/aboutsshws.php

National Oceanic and Atmospheric Administration. (2011). Enhanced F Scale for Tornado Damage. Retrieved from http://www.spc.noaa.gov/faq/tornado/ef-scale.html

National Oceanic and Atmospheric Administration. (2017). Saffir–Simpson Hurricane Wind Scale. Retrieved from http://www.nhc.noaa.gov/sshws_table.shtml.

National Weather Service. (2009). Ice and snow storm of January 26–28, 2009. Retrieved from https://www.weather.gov/lmk/jan_2009_ice_and_snow

National Weather Service. (2011). Hurricane preparedness—hazards. Retrieved from https://www.nhc.noaa.gov/prepare/hazards.php

National Weather Service. (2013). Tropical cyclones. A preparedness guide. National Oceanic and Atmospheric Administration Website. Retrieved from http://www.nws.noaa.gov/os/hurricane/resources/TropicalCyclones11.pdf

National Weather Service. (2017). Heat index (apparent temperature) chart. Retrieved from http://www.nws.noaa.gov/os/heat/index.shtml

Neumann, B., Vafeidis, A. T., Zimmermann, J., & Nicholls, R. J. (2015). Future coastal population growth and exposure to sea-level rise and coastal flooding—A global assessment. *PLOS ONE, 10*(3), e0118571. doi:10.1371/journal.pone.0118571

Noji, E. (2005). Public health issues in disasters. *Critical Care Medicine, 33* (1 Suppl), S29. doi:10.1097/01.CCM.0000151064.98207.9C

Ovesen, P. (2016). The humanitarian response to the 2015 Nepal earthquake. *UNChronicle, 53.* Retrieved from https://unchronicle.un.org/article/humanitarian-response-2015-nepal-earthquake

Patz, J. A., Grabow, M. L., & Limaye, V. S. (2014). When it rains, it pours: Future climate extremes and health. *Annals of Global Health, 80*(4), 332–344. doi:10.1016/j.aogh.2014.09.007

Rodriguez, H., & Aguirre, B. E. (2006). Hurricane Katrina and the healthcare infrastructure: A focus on disaster preparedness, response, and resiliency. *Frontiers of Health Services Management, 23*, 13–24. doi:10.1097/01974520-200607000-00003

Shultz, J. M., Espinola, M., Rechkemmer, A., Cohen, M. A., & Espinel, Z. (2016). *Prevention of disaster impact and outcome cascades.* Cambridge, UK: Cambridge University Press.

Sodhi, M. S. (2016). Natural disasters, the economy and population vulnerability as a vicious cycle with exogenous hazards. *Journal of Operations Management, 45*, 101–113. doi:10.1016/j.jom.2016.05.010

Stimpson, J. P., Fernando, A. W., & Jeffries, S. K. (2008). Seeking help for disaster services after a flood. *Disaster Medicine and Public Health Preparedness, 2*(3), 139–141. doi:10.1097/DMP.0b013e318183cfbb

U.S. Government Subcommittee on Natural Disaster Reduction. (2006, August). The challenge of disasters and our approach. Retrieved from https://pubs.usgs.gov/of/2003/ofr-03-211/NisquallyFinal.html#direct

Wisner, B., Blaikie, P., Cannon, T., & Davis, I. (2004). *At risk: Natural hazards, people's vulnerabilities and disasters* (2nd ed.). London, UK: Routledge.

World Bank. (2013). *Building resilience: Integrating climate and disaster risk into development. Lessons from World Bank Group experience.* Washington, DC: Author.

World Health Organization. (2016). Ebola data and statistics. Retrieved from http://apps.who.int/gho/data/view.ebola-sitrep.ebola-summary-latest?lang=en

World Health Organization. (2017). Programmes: Ebola virus disease. Retrieved from http://www.who.int/ebola/en

Hurricane Sandy—Lasting Impact on the Northeast United States

On October 29, 2012, Hurricane Sandy made landfall on the shores of New York, New Jersey, and Connecticut. These densely populated areas of the United States are rarely affected by hurricanes and severe water-related weather events and as such do not regularly prepare for hurricanes. Flooding of low-lying coastal areas occurs for a variety of reasons, such as tsunamis, intense local precipitation, river overflows, and storm surges. Severe cases of coastal storm surges oftentimes occur as a result of interplay of two or more of these flood mechanisms, as well as with other hazards such as human-induced alterations in coastal geography. Coastal areas the world over are characterized by expanding human populations and socioeconomic activities. This means that such floods can have severe impacts. Most casualties during tropical cyclones occur as the result of storm surges. Widespread efforts to mitigate coastal flood hazards are already apparent the world over, and this need will likely intensify throughout the coming years as the risks from climate change mount (Nicholls, 2006).

a result of the storm's 13-foot surge, which struck New York on October 29, flooding tunnels and subway lines and cutting power in and around the city (Figure 17.11). The East River overflowed its banks, flooding large sections of Lower Manhattan, including the Ground Zero construction site. The surge also caused tremendous damage to homes, buildings, roadways, boardwalks, and mass transit facilities in low-lying coastal areas in areas of Queens, Brooklyn, and Staten Island. Similar surges in South Florida were responsible for flooding and beach erosion. The events resulted in 43 deaths within New York and New Jersey (mostly from drowning in the home) and many additional injuries (CDC, 2014). After attacks on the World Trade Center (WTC) in 2001, the CDC enrolled 71,431 residents of New York City into the WTC Health Registry cohort study which provides the CDC with a pool of residents who were also affected by Hurricane Sandy. Approximately 10% of the 8,870 respondents enrolled in the WTC Health Registry reported they sustained injuries as a result of Hurricane Sandy. More than

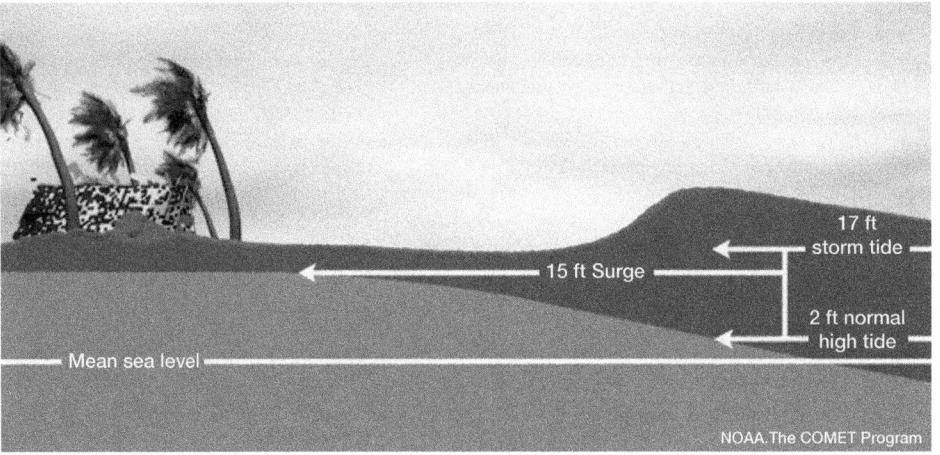

FIGURE 17.11 A storm surge is produced by an abnormal rise of water generated by a storm, above the predicted tidal level. A rise in water level can cause extreme flooding in coastal areas when storm surges coincide with normal high tide, creating a storm time capable of reaching up to 20 feet or more in some instances.

Hurricane Sandy was the most destructive hurricane of the 2012 Atlantic hurricane season. Worldwide, the storm was responsible for 233 deaths and $75 billion in damages. Twenty-four U.S. states were affected by the storm, including the entire eastern seaboard and as far west as Michigan and Wisconsin. Particularly severe damage was suffered in New Jersey and New York. Much of this damage was

70% of those had multiple injuries reported 1 week after Sandy hit land (CDC, 2014). Approximately 500 homes in New York City were destroyed, 26,000 homes and businesses required extensive repairs, and 319,575 buildings had some form of damage (FEMA, 2015). More than 42% of people in the area reported home flooding, 48.9% evacuated their homes, and 19.2% had intact homes not adequate for

(continued)

dwelling after the storm. Persons who did not evacuate their homes were more likely to report being injured and injuries were correlated with having at least 3 feet of flooding in the home; of those who had homes that were damaged or destroyed, nearly all injures were sustained during cleanup and repair (CDC, 2014). The storm has induced billions of dollars of damage due to need for repairs, lost tourism, and infrastructure reestablishment for several New England States (U.S. Department of Commerce, 2013).

LESSONS LEARNED

- Due to climate change, New York and New Jersey coastal sea levels have increased by over a foot in the last 100 years, thereby exacerbating Hurricane Sandy's storm surge. Experts have suggested that the hurricane's 13-foot surge is an example of what, by mid-century, will be considered a normal occurrence on the Eastern seaboard (Mason, 2012).
- While surges are only one aspect of a storm's mechanics, it is the most lethal, and surges have been responsible for millions of deaths over the last two centuries, primarily in low elevation coastal regions of Asia (Nichols, 2006).
- High death rates due to surges are correlated with high levels of human land claim and coastal modification. Coastal populations in low- and middle-income countries in which little consideration has been made for potential surges are at particularly high risk (Nichols, 2006).

- Hurricane preparation and precautionary messages emphasizing potential for injury hazards during evacuations and cleanup or repair after may mitigate the occurrence and severity of injury after a hurricane (CDC, 2014).
- High-impact, low-frequency events have potential for creating massive amounts of destruction due to infrequent planning and unfamiliarity of the region's inhabitants with the threat.

SOURCES

Centers for Disease Control and Prevention. (2014). Nonfatal injuries 1 week after hurricane Sandy—New York City metropolitan area, October 2012. *Morbidity and Mortality Weekly Report 63*(42), 950–954. Retrieved from https://www.cdc.gov/mmwr/preview/mmwrhtml/mm6342a4.htm?s_cid=mm6342a4_w

Federal Emergency Management Agency. (2015). FEMA MOTF Hurricane Sandy impact analysis. Retrieved from http://www.arcgis.com/home/item.html?id=307dd522499d4a44a33d7296a5da5ea0

Mason, E. (2012). *Hello again, climate change.* Retrieved from http://news.harvard.edu/gazette/story/2012/11/hello-again-climate-change

National Hurricane Center. (2015). Storm surge overview. Retrieved from http://www.nhc.noaa.gov/surge

Nicholls, R. J. (2006). Storm surges in coastal areas. In M. Arnold et al. (Eds.), *Disaster management series no. 6: Natural disaster hotspots case studies* (pp. 79–106). Washington, DC: World Bank.

United States Department of Commerce. (2013). Economic impact of Hurricane Sandy: Potential economic activity lost and gained in New Jersey and New York. Retrieved from https://www.esa.gov/sites/default/files/sandyfinal101713.pdf

Ebola Virus Disease—Exacerbation of Deadly Communicable Diseases by Environmental Disasters

The West African Ebola virus epidemic that spanned the years from 2013 to 2016 was the deadliest and most widespread Ebola outbreak in history. The epidemic began in December 2013 in Guinea and spread to involve patients in Liberia, Sierra Leone, Guinea, Nigeria, and Mali. Due to international travel and volunteer relief workers, deaths were also reported in the United States, Italy, United Kingdom, Senegal, and Spain. The outbreak was declared over on June 9, 2016 when the last known case tested negative 42 days earlier in Monrovia. During the time of the outbreak, a total of 28,616 cases were reported in Guinea, Sierra Leone, and Liberia with 11,310 deaths recorded as a result of Ebola. The outbreak created global concern and international panic as a massive threat to public health (WHO, 2017).

The response to Ebola required collaboration between multiple countries and within national, regional, and local

organizations. Community health workers, physicians, and nurses who were unfamiliar with the disease were called upon to aid in response. During this time, affected countries were also forced to deal with struggles of day-to-day life, including responding to national disasters. On September 15, 2015, heavy rainfall flooded the capital of Sierra Leone resulting in property destruction and displacing or injuring thousands of persons. Two days later, stadiums outside of the city were opened to provide shelter to those displaced by the floods while Ebola transmission was still occurring in the country. Over the course of two days, Ebola response organizations staffed the shelters, educated response workers on screening for Ebola, had ambulances on standby for transport of symptomatic patients to local hospitals, enacted isolation protocols for at-risk persons, and reallocated Ebola resources to the shelters. The area experienced increased

(continued)

CASE STUDY 17.2 (*continued*)

transport, bed usage, and Ebola testing compared to other areas of the country. As a result of the vigilant work of community health workers and first responders, there were no new reports of this highly virulent disease as a result of mass sheltering—a huge success for the response teams involved (CDC, 2016).

LESSONS LEARNED

- Natural disasters continue to present a threat to communities, even during other disasters and emergencies.
- The rapid implementation of Ebola screening and response plans played a key role in preventing further spread of a highly virulent disease within a high-risk population.

- Establishment and execution of an effective incident management system allowed for the mitigation of a serious environmental disaster and prevented this disaster from exacerbating an already-existing epidemic.

SOURCES

Centers for Disease Control and Prevention. (2016). Notes from the field: Ebola virus disease response activities during a mass displacement event after flooding—Freetown, Sierra Leone, September–November 2015. *Morbidity and Mortality Weekly Report, 65*(7), 188–189. Retrieved from https://www.cdc.gov/mmwr/volumes/65/wr/mm6507a4. htm?s_cid=mm6507a4_w

World Health Organization. (2017). Ebola outbreak 2014–2015. Retrieved from http://www.who.int/csr/disease/ebola/en

CASE STUDY 17.3

Climate Change and Heat Waves in India and Pakistan

In May 2015, India was struck by a severe heat wave, which, by early June, had killed at least 2,500 people in multiple regions. Then, beginning in June of that same year, an unrelated heat wave struck neighboring Pakistan, causing the death of another 2,000 people. Abnormally high temperatures in both countries were exacerbated by widespread failures of electrical grids, leaving many without working air-conditioners, fans, or water pumps. A third critical factor that served to augment the lethalness of Pakistan's heat wave was that it coincided with the month of Ramadan, an important month in the Islamic calendar that Muslims observe by fasting and not drinking from sunrise until sunset (Hindustan Times, 2015).

Meteorological analysis the following year confirmed what many had initially suspected: The chances of deadly heat waves, as had been experienced in India and Pakistan in 2015, have significantly increased over the past decade due to human-induced climate change. Furthermore, the chance of more frequent, intense heat wave activity is expected to grow as the planet continues to warm (Wehner, Stone, Krishnan, AchutaRao, & Castillo, 2016).

Researchers suggest that in the coming years, global human-induced climate change effects will not be limited to producing more extreme, frequent heat waves, but will likely intensify almost all natural disasters. Health is inextricably linked to climate change, making it vital for nurses to understand the issue and how it can affect their patient populations.

SOURCES

Hindustan Times. (2015, May 28). Melting asphalt at a crosswalk in Delhi, India during the country's 2015 heat wave [Photograph]. Retrieved from http://www.hindustantimes.com/india/heatwave -claims-over-1-100-across-country-temperatures-soaring/story -sbWxiVGj363u1wqorW2LVM.html

Wehner, M., Stone, D., Krishnan, H., AchutaRao, K., & Castillo, F. (2016). The deadly combination of heat and humidity in India and Pakistan in summer 2015. *Bulletin of the American Meteorological Society, 97*(12), S81–S86. doi:10.1175/BAMS-D-16-0149

18

ENVIRONMENTAL DISASTERS AND EMERGENCIES

Tener Goodwin Veenema, Clifton P. Thornton, and Andrew Corley

LEARNING OBJECTIVES

When this chapter is completed, readers will be able to:

1. Describe the importance of a safe, stable environment as a foundation for good health.
2. Discuss examples of environmental hazards and their impact on communities.
3. Identify the health outcomes associated with the most commonly occurring environmental emergencies/disasters.
4. Recognize the need for timely response and immediate removal of the environmental hazard.
5. Describe the role of the Occupational Safety and Health Administration (OSHA) and the Risk Management Program Rule with regard to chemical emergencies.
6. Identify strategies for the mitigation of environmental emergencies/disasters.
7. Explain the purpose of the National Environmental Tracking Network and its value to disaster planners.

KEY MESSAGES

Environmental challenges loom as the world population surpasses 7 billion.

An environmental emergency is a sudden threat to the public health or the well-being of the environment, arising from the release or potential release of oil, radioactive materials, or hazardous chemicals into the air, land, or water.

An environmental disaster is an environmental emergency whose scope and duration exceeds the local resources available to respond.

The health impact of an environmental disaster on a community may be immediate, ongoing, or delayed.

Collaboration with many types of governmental officials and community responders is critical to mitigate the damage that may occur from an environmental hazard.

Successful planning for potential environmental disasters/emergencies demands that nurses be knowledgeable of the environmental hazards endemic to the area, including the movement of hazardous substances through the area.

Working in conjunction with their public health colleagues and as members of an interdisciplinary disaster response team, nurses must be able to detect environmental changes that will create the potential for both immediate and long-term negative health outcomes.

CHAPTER OVERVIEW

Global climate change combined with a rapidly growing world population have advanced the probability of the occurrence of environmental disasters. This chapter provides information on the health consequences associated with large-scale environmental disasters and emergencies. Nurses responding to the needs of populations and communities affected by environmental disasters and/or emergencies require an understanding of (a) the immediate health effects related to the event, (b) the potential for long-term health effects resulting from the event, and (c) the federal agencies designated to respond to the event. In situations involving environmental hazards, nurses will be called on to work as members of interdisciplinary response teams comprising governmental officials, police, emergency medical services (EMS), firemen, and the U.S. military including the Coast Guard, Navy, Army, and Air Force.

ENVIRONMENTAL EMERGENCIES

In 2017, the world population surpassed 7.4 billion people (U.S. Census Bureau, *International program*, 2017), creating a taxing burden on our global environment whose impact will undoubtedly reveal itself in the decade ahead. Increases in world population translate into increased consumption of natural resources, a growing demand for the production of energy, the manufacture of large amounts of waste, and an ongoing strain on the sustainability of our environment. Coupled with an awareness of the ongoing and anticipated future impact of global climate change, it seems reasonable to state that our environment is changing dramatically—and not for the better. The combination of these factors will result in more frequent occurrences of disasters and environmental emergencies that threaten human health.

An environmental emergency is a sudden threat to the public health or to the well-being of the environment arising from the release or potential release of oil, radioactive materials, or hazardous chemicals into the air, land, or water. These emergencies may occur from transportation accidents, events at chemical facilities or other facilities using or manufacturing chemicals,

or as a result of natural or man-made disasters (Environmental Protection Agency [EPA], 2017a). Although there are multiple serious environmental problems with which public health and environmental safety officials are concerned, environmental emergencies and the activities that surround them are focused generally on sudden, immediate threats.

ENVIRONMENTAL DISASTERS

An "environmental disaster" is defined as an environmental emergency or ecologic disruption of a severity and magnitude resulting in deaths, injuries, illness, and/or property damage that cannot be effectively managed by the application of routine procedures or resources and results in a need for additional assistance. The consequences of the damage to the environment will vary based on the type of hazard, the mechanism of its release into the environment, the geographical location of the event, the determinants of human exposure (e.g., the weather conditions at the time of the event), and the length of time before the response. Whether the event is an acute one-time occurrence or a chronic, ongoing mechanism of disruption will also be a major determinant of the health consequences for the affected population.

As with natural disasters, health promotion and disease prevention activities must focus on the following:

1. The immediate removal of the hazard from the environment (or if this is not possible, the movement of the population away from the hazard)
2. Decontamination of exposed individuals
3. The restoration of services to meet the immediate physiological needs of the affected people
4. The prevention of further illness or injury as a result of exposure to the hazard

Disasters of a chronic or long-term nature (e.g., industrial contamination of soil and water supply) are more insidious and may be more difficult to address. The health outcomes of these types of environmental disasters may take years to manifest (e.g., certain cancers, endocrine disruption), and the scientific evidence that they will occur has been mounting for some time (Colburn, Dumanoski, & Myers, 1997; Schug, Janesick, Blumberg, & Heindel, 2011).

ENVIRONMENTAL PUBLIC HEALTH TRACKING: PROTECTING COMMUNITIES THROUGH INTEGRATED ENVIRONMENTAL PUBLIC HEALTH SURVEILLANCE

Environmental public health tracking is the ongoing collection, integration, analysis, and interpretation of data about the following factors:

- Environmental hazards
- Exposure to environmental hazards
- Health effects potentially related to exposure to environmental hazards

The goal of environmental public health tracking is to protect communities by providing information to federal, state, and local agencies. These agencies, in turn, will use this information to plan, apply, and evaluate public health actions to prevent and control environmentally related diseases (Centers for Disease Control and Prevention [CDC], 2017a). Public health tracking monitors known environmental hazards along with *the mechanism of action that may create the potential for disaster.* Some environmental hazards create the potential for a public health emergency because of regular exposure—*they are already present in the environment* in which the individual is living and working (e.g., lead, radon, asbestos). Other environmental hazards create the potential for a disaster or emergency by being *transferred from one location to another.* For example, it is the movement or transportation of hazardous chemicals, nuclear products, and petroleum products that creates the potential for exposure (e.g., oil spills, chemical spills, or radiation events).

ENVIRONMENTAL PROTECTION AGENCY

The U.S. EPA is the lead governmental agency responsible for monitoring the environment in the United States. The EPA's mission is to "protect human health and to safeguard the natural environment—air, water, and land—upon which life depends" (EPA, 2017b). Protecting human health is an integral part of the EPA's mission. The EPA conducts numerous research programs worldwide that study the effects of pollution on the human body. Research efforts include studies on how pollution affects children and people with asthma and other illnesses, and how water contaminants may affect swimmers and beachgoers. Monitoring environmental quality also plays an important role in protecting human health. The EPA works with state and local agencies, as well as with volunteer and other citizen groups, to monitor air and water quality and to reduce human exposure to contaminants in the air, land, and water.

The EPA provides leadership in the nation's environmental science, education, and assessment efforts, and works closely with other federal agencies, state and local governments, and Native American communities to develop and enforce regulations under existing environmental laws. The EPA is responsible for researching and setting national standards for a variety of environmental programs and delegates to states and tribes responsibility for issuing permits and monitoring and enforcing compliance. Where national standards are not met, the EPA can issue sanctions and take other steps to assist the states and tribes in reaching the desired levels of environmental quality. The EPA also works with industries and all levels of government in a wide variety of voluntary pollution prevention programs and energy conservation efforts.

CDC NATIONAL ENVIRONMENTAL PUBLIC HEALTH TRACKING NETWORK

Environmental public health tracking is a type of surveillance that is of great value to disaster planners as well as responders. Surveillance is a method to monitor trends by collecting, interpreting, and reporting data. The CDC's National Environmental Public Health Tracking Network brings together health and environmental data into one place, making it easier to compare hazards and environmental exposures with health outcomes at a local and national level. The Tracking Network collects health data and environmental data from national, state, and city sources, and provides supporting information to make the data available to planners. The Tracking Network has data and information on environments and hazards, health effects, and population health. The Tracking Network can be accessed at www.ephtracking.cdc.gov/showHome in order to:

- Use the query tool to view interactive maps, tables, and charts
- View info by location for county-level data snapshots
- Visit state and local tracking websites

EXAMPLES OF ENVIRONMENTAL HAZARDS AND THEIR IMPACT

Air Pollutants

Toxic air pollutants (also known as hazardous air pollutants) are those pollutants that cause or may cause serious health effects, such as cancer, severe respiratory disease, reproductive effects or birth defects, or adverse environmental and ecological effects (CDC, 2018). Examples of toxic air pollutants include benzene, which is found in gasoline; perchlorethlyene, which is emitted from some dry cleaning facilities; and methylene chloride, which is used as a solvent and paint stripper by a number of industries. Examples of other air toxics include dioxin, asbestos, toluene, and metals such as cadmium, mercury, chromium, and lead compounds. Most air toxics originate from human-made sources including those that are mobile (e.g., cars, trucks, buses) and stationary (e.g., factories, refineries, power plants), as well as indoor sources (e.g., building materials, cleaning chemicals, carbon monoxide, and mold). Some air toxics are also released from natural sources such as volcanic eruptions and forest fires

(EPA, 2017c). The World Trade Center disaster resulted in the release of multiple air pollutants causing significant disease (Reibman et al., 2016).

People exposed to toxic air pollutants at sufficient concentrations and durations may have an increased chance of getting cancer, pulmonary disease, or other serious health effects. These health effects can include damage to the immune system, as well as neurological, reproductive, developmental, respiratory, and other health problems. Acute and chronic exposure to some air pollutants can lead to immediate or prolonged death. In addition to exposure from breathing air toxics, risks are also associated with the deposition of toxic pollutants onto soils or surface waters where they are taken up by plants, ingested by animals, and eventually magnified up through the food chain. Humans and animals alike may experience health problems if exposed to sufficient quantities of air toxics over time (EPA, 2017d). For example, increases in ambient air ozone and air pollution can be linked to increased occurrences of asthma exacerbations because the exposure has been found to induce an increase in airway inflammation (Peden, 2002).

Urbanization and the ever-growing world population have introduced several challenges in air pollution. Emissions from electric utilities, vehicular exhaust, gasoline vapors, and chemical solvents are some of the largest contributors to production of low-level ozone (EPA, 2017i). Ozone is formed when these toxic substances react in sunlight close to the earth's surface and, unlike the ozone layer that protects from harmful ultraviolet (UV) radiation from the sun, exposure can lead to severe permanent respiratory disease (EPA, 2017i). Particle pollution, the suspension of particles of solids or liquids in the air from industrial or chemical products, has become exceptionally problematic (CDC, 2017b); in some cities, it can become severe enough to see, smell, and taste.

Research suggests that exposure to air pollutants affects the respiratory system to a greater extent and may introduce chronic systemic health problems (Kahle et al., 2015). Children, the elderly, those with existing pulmonary diseases, and those with chronic health conditions are particularly susceptible to adverse health outcomes from living in areas where particle pollution is more prominent. Living in urban areas and areas that receive more sunlight may correlate with increased exposure to air pollutants due to increases in exposure to industrial products and increased ozone productions. The EPA maintains an Air Quality Index (AQI) as a tool for the general public to monitor and avoid particle pollution, ozone, and smoke at www.airnow.gov. The EPA regulates air pollution under the Clean Air Act. The EPA is required to monitor and set strict limits for six criteria air pollutants in the United States (carbon monoxide, ground level ozone, lead, nitrogen oxides, particulate matter, and sulfur dioxide). The EPA helps states that are not meeting the requirements implement remediation plans containing measures needed to meet federal standards. The agency also conducts periodic reviews of the scientific literature on the health effects of criteria air pollutants. The reports are used to determine national standards. One weakness in the legislation is that the EPA does not regulate indoor air pollution levels (www.epa.gov/clean-air-act-overview/air-pollution-current-and-future-challenges).

Chemical Spills

The intentional release or accidental leakage or spill of certain chemical substances into the environment can have devastating consequences on human health. Nurses need to be aware of the environmental and safety hazards that exist in or near the communities in which they live and work. The Emergency Planning and Community Right-to-Know Act (EPCRA) was passed in 1986 in response to concerns regarding the environmental and safety hazards posed by the storage and handling of toxic chemicals (EPA, 2017e). These concerns were triggered by the disaster in Bhopal, India, in which more than 8,000 people suffered death or serious injury from the accidental release of methyl isocyanate. To reduce the likelihood of such a disaster in the United States, Congress imposed requirements on both states and regulated facilities (Speigel, 2014).

EPCRA establishes requirements for federal, state, and local governments; Native American tribes; and industry regarding emergency planning and community right-to-know reporting on hazardous and toxic chemicals. The community right-to-know provisions help increase the public's knowledge and access to information on chemicals at individual facilities, their uses, and releases into the environment. States and communities, working with facilities, can use the information to improve chemical safety and protect public health and the environment. There are four major provisions of the EPCRA:

- Emergency Planning (Sections 301–303)
- Emergency Release Notification (Section 304)
- Hazardous Chemical Storage Reporting (Sections 311 and 312)
- Toxic Chemical Release Inventory (Section 313)

For information on the management of a chemical emergency and decontamination guidelines, see Chapters 29 and 35. The World Health Organization (WHO) has published guidelines for the public health management of chemical incidents (www.who.int/environmental_health_emergencies/publications/Manual_Chemical_Incidents/en).

Risk Management Program Rule (40 CFR 68)

When Congress passed the Clean Air Act Amendments of 1990, it required the EPA to publish regulations and guidance for chemical accident prevention at facilities using extremely hazardous substances. The Risk Management Program Rule was written to implement Section 112(r) of these amendments. The rule, which built upon existing industry codes and standards, requires companies of all sizes that use certain flammable and toxic substances to develop a Risk Management Program that includes the following:

- Hazard assessment that details the potential effects of an accidental release, an accident history of the last 5 years, and an evaluation of worst-case and alternative accidental releases
- Prevention program that includes safety precautions and maintenance, monitoring, and employee training measures

- Emergency response program that spells out emergency healthcare, employee training measures, and procedures for informing the public and response agencies (e.g., the fire department) should an accident occur

Each company must submit to the EPA a risk management plan (RMP) that addresses these topics. The plans must be revised and resubmitted every 5 years (EPA, 2017f).

The purpose of the RMP is to reduce chemical risk at the local level. This information helps local fire, police, and emergency response personnel (who must prepare for and respond to chemical accidents) and is useful to individuals in understanding the chemical hazards in communities. Ideally, making the RMPs available to the public stimulates communication between industry and the public to improve accident prevention and emergency response practices at the local level.

Land, Waste, and Brownfields

Nearly everything we do creates waste products. Households generate ordinary garbage while industrial and manufacturing processes create solid and hazardous waste products. The EPA regulates all this waste under the Resource Conservation and Recovery Act (RCRA). Accidents, spills, leaks, and past improper disposal and handling of hazardous materials and wastes have resulted in tens of thousands of sites across our country that have contaminated our land, water (including groundwater and surface water), and air (both indoor and outdoor). The EPA has developed and maintains a Toxic Releases Inventory (TRI), a database containing information on disposal or release of over 600 toxic chemicals from thousands of U.S. facilities and information about how facilities manage those chemicals through recycling, energy recovery, and treatment. One of the TRI's primary purposes is to inform communities about toxic chemical releases into the environment (EPA, 2017g).

Brownfields are environmental disasters characterized by abandoned or underutilized industrial and commercial sites that are, or are perceived to be, chemically, physically, or biologically contaminated. With certain legal exclusions and additions, the term "Brownfield site" means real property, the expansion, redevelopment, or reuse of which may be complicated by the presence or potential presence of a hazardous substance, pollutant, or contaminant (EPA, 2017h). Manufacturing plants and military bases are not permanent establishments; they frequently close and relocate. New development on these Brownfield sites is the source of great debate among politicians, policy makers, and public health officials. The decisions regarding whether to build houses, schools, and new industry on these sites are often complicated by real or perceived environmental contamination. Grave concerns surround the reliability of Brownfield cleanup and subsequent protective measures (Greenberg, 2002; Meuser, 2013). Normally, cleanup involves removal of the top layer of soil and replacement with clean soil, then the application of an impervious cap to prevent any contamination left in the ground from reaching the surface. The future use of the property is often restricted (e.g., no digging, no fence posts, no food gardens). In reality, protection measures may be inadequate or improperly constructed, monitoring is difficult, and enforcement of deed restrictions is difficult. Given the inability to ensure that every renovated Brownfield site that becomes a house, school, or playground will be a safe and healthy environment, the potential for a public health emergency persists. Through the Economic Redevelopment Initiative, the EPA is responsible for assessing existing sites, preventing further contamination, safely cleaning up sites, and designing plans to reuse Brownfield sites.

Mold

Molds are a type of fungal growth that can be found in both indoor and outdoor environments. While the number of mold species currently remains unknown, at least 300,000 types of molds are known to exist. Molds are notoriously hardy organisms and can grow in nearly any environment including those that are harsh and do not typically support life. Molds thrive in warm, damp, and humid conditions and continuously reproduce through the production of spores. Natural disasters (especially those involving water and/or heat) often increase mold growth by altering the state of the natural environment.

Many people are sensitive to molds, and some have serious allergies that result in severe reactions, especially workers exposed to large amounts of molds in occupational settings, such as farmers working around moldy hay. Individuals with pulmonary disease, chronic lung disease, or immunocompromised states are more susceptible to the health effects of mold and may experience fevers, coughing fits, shortness of breath, respiratory compromise, and deadly infections.

In 2004, the Institute of Medicine (IOM) found there was sufficient evidence to link indoor exposure to mold with upper respiratory tract symptoms, coughing, and wheezing in otherwise healthy people; with asthma symptoms in people with asthma; and with hypersensitivity pneumonitis in individuals susceptible to the immune-mediated condition. The IOM also found limited or suggestive evidence linking indoor mold exposure and respiratory illness in otherwise healthy children. In 2009, the WHO issued additional guidance, the WHO Guidelines for Indoor Air Quality: Dampness and Mould (www.euro.who.int/document/E92645.pdf).

Oil Spills

The world continues its dependence on oil as an energy source. In the United States alone, citizens consume vast amounts of petroleum products—some 19.63 million barrels per day—to fuel the economy. Unlike many other oil-producing countries, the United States relies on private industry—not a state-owned or controlled enterprise—to supply oil, natural gas, and indeed all of its energy resources. This basic trait of the private enterprise system has major implications for how the U.S. government oversees and regulates offshore drilling (National Commission on the BP Deepwater Horizon Oil Spill and Offshore Drilling, 2011). It also fosters a competitive industry, which has led to worldwide advancement in technologies involved in finding and extracting oil and gas, but is encumbered with great risks. With billions of gallons of oil being constantly transported and stored throughout the world and moved across the seas, the potential for oil spills is significant, and the effects of spilled oil can pose serious threats to the environment.

The EPA works through its Spill Prevention, Control, and Countermeasures (SPCC) program,[1] at several hundred thousand oil storage facilities to prevent the discharge of all kinds of oil into the waters of the United States. As the lead agency responsible for prevention planning and enforcement measures, the EPA leads local and industrial responses to oil spills through extensive contingency planning, emergency training, and experience in containment and cleanup. In an attempt to prevent oil spills from reaching our nation's waters, the EPA requires that certain facilities develop and implement oil SPCC Plans. Unlike oil spill contingency plans that typically address spill cleanup measures after a spill has occurred, SPCC Plans are designed to ensure that facilities put in place containment and other countermeasures that would prevent oil spills that could reach navigable waters. A spill contingency plan is required as part of the SPCC Plan if a facility is unable to provide secondary containment, for example, berms surrounding the oil storage tank (EPA, 2017d).[2]

Despite the nation's best efforts to prevent spills, almost 14,000 oil spills are reported each year exceeding 1.3 million gallons of oil spilled annually. Major oil spills may easily increase that number by multiple factors. Oil spills require the mobilization of thousands of specially trained emergency response personnel and challenge the best-laid contingency plans. Although many spills are contained and cleaned up by the party responsible for the spill, some spills require assistance from local and state agencies and/or the federal government. Under the National Contingency Plan, the EPA is the lead federal response agency for oil spills occurring in inland waters, and the U.S. Coast Guard is the lead response agency for spills in coastal waters and deepwater ports. Despite a fast response, the damage to communities, wildlife (Bergeon Burns, Olin, Woltmann, Stouffer, & Taylor, 2014; Monson, Doak, Ballachey, Johnson, & Bodkin, 2002), and the physical and mental well-being of inhabitants can be extreme.

To date, the most significant major oil spill in the United States was the BP Deepwater Horizon spill in 2010. Concern for the impact on human health from the toxins released during the event was immediate. The CDC's National Center for Environmental Health (NCEH) initiated the agency's response on April 20. CDC activated its Emergency Operations Center (EOC), communicating with state and local health departments so that the agency could quickly support and respond to emerging health concerns in the region. The CDC's EOC was deactivated on August 20, after the leaking well was successfully capped. During the 4-month period of emergency activation, more than 450 CDC personnel monitored health effects, analyzed environmental data, communicated health recommendations,

and coordinated with response partners to mitigate immediate and short-term health threats in the Gulf States. The health impact upon workers assisting with the oil cleanup continues to be monitored.

Unconventional Gas and Oil Production

Unconventional gas and oil drilling (UGOD), namely hydraulic fracturing or "fracking," offers a means of releasing natural gas and oil from rock formations. Areas such as the Marcellus Shale in northeastern Pennsylvania; the Bakken Formation in North Dakota and Montana; and the Barnett, Permian, and Eagle Ford Formations in north, west, and south Texas are some of the large unconventional oil and gas plays that have made the United States the world's largest producer of shale formation oil and natural gas. In the past decade and a half, production from these unconventional formations has expanded tremendously and by 2015, domestic oil production from hydraulically fracked wells had reached 4.3 million barrels per day, accounting for over 50% of total U.S. oil output (U.S. Energy Information Administration [EIA], 2016a), and natural gas production by this same method was estimated to be 53 billion cubic feet per day, constituting 67% of total domestic U.S. natural gas extraction (U.S. EIA, 2016b).

Aside from the attendant effects of burning fossil fuels on population health and the environment, there is mounting evidence to suggest that the process of extracting oil and natural gas using UGOD techniques can have other, more immediate negative consequences on human health. Many of the hydraulic fracturing chemicals pumped into these formations in order to release their oil and gas, such as naturally occurring radioactive materials and volatile organic compounds (e.g., benzene and ethylbenzene), are known toxicants. These fracturing fluids, later present in flowback water, have been known to enter ground water reservoirs and nearby water wells. Surveys and reviews of electronic health records of patients have shown correlations between living within close proximity of UGOD sites and upper respiratory symptoms (Rabinowitz et al., 2015) as well as increased incidence rates of hospital admissions for cardiology, dermatology, neurology, oncology, and urology medical categories (Jemielita et al., 2015). Along with the toxic chemicals produced by UGOD, living near drilling sites has also been theorized to negatively impact public health through increased noise pollution, truck traffic, and psychosocial stress from community change (Jemielita et al., 2015).

While as of the writing of this book no large-scale human or environmental disasters have occurred due to UGOD, public health and environmental experts fear that, even with close federal and state oversight, populations living within proximity to this drilling could pay the price for this increased production of oil and gas through the deterioration of their long-term health.

Pesticides

Pesticides are frequently used to control insects, rodents, weeds, microbes, or fungi. In addition, they help farmers provide affordable and plentiful food supply. Pesticides are also used in other settings, such as homes and schools, to control pests as common as cockroaches, termites, and mice. Pesticides

---

[1] The SPCC rule includes requirements for oil spill prevention, preparedness, and response to prevent oil discharges to navigable waters and adjoining shorelines. The rule requires specific facilities to prepare, amend, and implement SPCC Plans. The SPCC rule is part of the Oil Pollution Prevention regulation, which also includes the Facility Response Plan (FRP) rule.

[2] On November 5, 2009, the EPA administrator signed a notice amending certain requirements of the SPCC rule in 40 CFR Part 112. The November 2009 amendments modify the December 2008 rule by removing the provisions to: exclude farms and oil production facilities from the loading/unloading rack requirements; exempt produced water containers at an oil production facility; and provide alternative qualified facilities eligibility criteria for an oil production facility.

pose significant risks to human health and the environment, when people do not follow directions on product labels or use products irresponsibly. For example, people might use pesticides when they are not really needed, apply too much, or apply or dispose of them in a manner that could contaminate water or harm wildlife. Even alternative or organic pesticides can have these unintended consequences if not used correctly (EPA, 2017h). There is abundant scientific evidence of the risks toxic pesticides pose to human health. More worrisome from a public health perspective are chronic health effects such as cancer, infertility, birth defects, miscarriage, and negative effects on the brain and nervous system.

For decades, stockpiles of obsolete, expired, and banned pesticides have posed significant health risks to people in developing countries. The United Nations Food and Agriculture Organization (FAO) estimates that 500,000 tons of obsolete pesticides no longer usable for their intended purposes are scattered throughout developing nations. Among the greatest concern are persistent organic pollutants, such as aldrin, chlordane, DDT, dieldrin, and endrin (United Nations FAO, 2001). These chemicals can cause nausea, convulsions, liver damage, and death. The global impact of accidental self-poisoning from pesticide ingestion was estimated in 2002 as 186,000 deaths, creating a disease burden equaling 4,420,000 disability-adjusted life years (DALYs; WHO, 2010).

End users in recipient countries may not be able to read contents, usage instructions, and precautions (where listed). Old pesticide containers may be used as containers for carrying drinking water or food. Governments may be aware of the threats that these chemicals pose, but they may be constrained by a lack of funds or absence of people with the knowledge as to how to properly dispose of them.

Radiation Release and Contamination

Radiological materials and unstable nuclear isotopes are present and nearly unavoidable in daily life. Background radiation, naturally occurring radiation from the environment, exists as unstable isotopes suspended in air, radon emitted from the earth's crust, cosmic radiation from outer space, isotopes within the human body (potassium and carbon), and infrequent radioactive elements from nature. This background radiation produces negligible low-level exposure of radiation to humans. Mankind has harnessed these sources of radiation and created nuclear and radiological technologies that greatly enhance human life through energy production, diagnostic tools (x-rays, CT scans, nuclear medicine tests), medical treatments (radiation therapy), nuclear industry, and commercial products. Nuclear materials have also been utilized in warfare as agents of nuclear terrorism and warfare with recent growing concern that more countries are producing nuclear weaponry.

As the production of nuclear materials continues to expand, the risk of environmental contamination from the transportation, storage, research, use, and disposal of nuclear materials increases. The U.S. Nuclear Regulatory Commission (NRC) is charged with the responsibility of protecting people and the environment from nuclear contamination (NRC, 2017). The NRC sets regulations for all acquisition, transport, use, and disposal of potentially radioactive materials. Nuclear material

exhibits health effects through the production of ionizing radiation that directly affects cell growth and development leading to burns, cancer, tissue damage, organ dysfunction, and death. Both acute exposure to high levels of radiation and chronic exposure to low levels of radiation can induce permanent effects. Nuclear material can emit radiation for years on end, leading to contamination of earth, air, and water for decades.

The International Nuclear and Radiological Event Scale (INES) was developed in 1990 by the International Atomic Energy Agency as a means to provide prompt communication of information related to nuclear accidents. The scale contains seven levels ranging from an anomaly (1) to a major accident (7). To date, there have been two events rated at a level 7—the Chernobyl disaster that occurred on April 26, 1986 and the Fukushima Daiichi nuclear disaster that began on March 11, 2011. Both events involved the release of massive amounts of radiation into the environment from nuclear plants. The events in Chernobyl resulted from a power surge during a test procedure that caused an explosion that produced updrafts lasting approximately 9 days and dispersed plumes of fission products into the atmosphere spreading across the Soviet Union and Western Europe. Fifty-six individuals died as a direct result of the explosion. To date, the WHO estimates that over 4,000 individuals have died from cancer caused by exposure to radiation from the Chernobyl incident (WHO, 2005). Epidemiological studies are ongoing to assess the impact of Chernobyl on human health and the environment. A 30-kilometer (19-mile) exclusion zone around Chernobyl has been established. Radioactivity is still present in the area and has altered the flora and fauna nearby. The groundwater, soil, and plants that grow in the area continue to contain lethal levels of radioactivity and make the region inhospitable to human life.

Water

Environmental emergencies involving water may originate from accidental or deliberate contamination of a water source with toxic chemicals. Hurricane Katrina (2005) provided an unforgettable example of the domino effect of a natural disaster (hurricane) creating a man-made disaster (the levees breaking and flooding occurring) to the third disaster event (an environmental disaster involving toxic contaminants and biological pathogen). Following Hurricane Harvey (2017), many Houston area neighborhoods received more than 40 inches (100 cm) of rain as the storm system slowly meandered over eastern Texas and adjacent waters, causing catastrophic flooding. With peak accumulations of 64.58 in (164.0 cm), Harvey is the wettest tropical cyclone on record in the United States. The resulting toxic floods inundated hundreds of thousands of homes, displaced more than 30,000 people, and prompted more than 17,000 rescues. Harvey floodwaters that were laboratory tested demonstrated the presence of sewage-related bacteria, chemicals and heavy metals, including arsenic, lead, mercury, cadmium, chromium, and silver (Scutti, 2017).

Pharmaceuticals

Pharmaceuticals are synthetic or natural chemicals that can be found in prescription medicines, over-the-counter therapeutic drugs, and veterinary drugs. Pharmaceuticals contain active ingredients that have been designed to have pharmacological effects and confer significant benefits to society. Pharmaceuticals can be introduced into water sources through sewage, which carries the excreta of individuals and patients who have used these chemicals, from uncontrolled drug disposal (e.g., discarding drugs into toilets), and from agricultural runoff containing livestock manure. They have become chemicals of emerging concern to the public because of their potential to reach drinking water and create an environmental emergency (WHO, 2011).

The ubiquitous use of pharmaceuticals (both prescribed and over-the-counter) has resulted in a relatively continuous discharge of pharmaceuticals and their metabolites into wastewater. In addition, pharmaceuticals may be released into water sources in the effluents from poorly controlled manufacturing or production facilities, primarily those associated with generic medicines (WHO, 2011).

The potential human health risk associated with exposure to very low concentrations of pharmaceuticals in drinking water is unknown, and the potential exists for these concentrations to increase. More research is needed to quantify the risks associated with various concentrations of exposure and the impact on health (WHO, 2011). On August 31, 2015, the U.S. EPA proposed a rule proposing a sector-specific set of regulations for the management and disposal of hazardous waste pharmaceuticals (www.epa.gov/hwgenerators/proposed-rule-management-standards-hazardous-waste-pharmaceuticals).

SUMMARY

Environmental emergencies involving the release, or threatened release, of oil, radioactive materials, or hazardous chemicals negatively affect the health of communities and the surrounding environment. Releases may be accidental, as in the case of a spill at a chemical plant, or may be deliberate. Releases may also be caused by natural disasters. Environmental emergencies may progress to become large-scale public health disasters. Climate change and increases in global population may increase the numbers of environmental disasters and emergencies.

Nurses must work to create an environment that promotes and sustains health for all its citizens. Increases in scientific knowledge regarding the development of toxic chemicals and advances in technology must be balanced by the wisdom restricting their transport and use. The impact on the health of a community resulting from an environmental emergency may be immediate, ongoing, or delayed for decades. Depending on the type of toxic agent and the duration of the exposure, populations may need to be closely monitored for years in order to evaluate the health impact of the event. Nurses must become educated regarding tracking environmental hazards in their communities, must become advocates for public policy limiting toxic agent use, and must become proponents of research into the health effects of these environmental agents.

STUDY QUESTIONS

1. What differentiates an environmental emergency from an environmental disaster?
2. What are the health implications of a massive chemical spill in a community?
3. Describe the multiple responsibilities of the EPA with regard to environmental health in the United States.
4. Identify and discuss the health impact of three environmental hazards that are readily found in the environment.
5. Why was the 2011 Japan tsunami and nuclear reactor disaster such a significant world event?
6. What are the legal, moral, and health implications of the redevelopment of Brownfield sites?
7. What are the health consequences of mold?
8. How should we prepare for environmental disasters in a world where the population exceeds 7 billion?

INTERNET ACTIVITIES

1. The individuals living in your neighborhood are growing increasingly concerned about the safety of the environment that surrounds their homes. You have been chosen by your neighbors as the person to investigate what is known about the area in which you live. Go to the U.S. EPA Tracking Network and search where you live using your zip code. Create a comprehensive report describing the following topics: air quality, water, land, and the potential of toxic elements in your environment.

2. You have been hired by the EPA to review the response to the five largest oil spills in U.S. history. You are charged with conducting the analysis and developing recommendations for the future prevention of, and response to, a major oil spill in U.S. territory (land and water). Start your research by identifying and reviewing the reports of each of these major oil spills at www.epa.gov/OILSPILL

REFERENCES

Bergeon Burns, C. M., Olin, J. A., Woltmann, S., Stouffer, P. C., & Taylor, S. S. (2014). Effects of oil on terrestrial vertebrates: Predicting impacts of the Macondo blowout. *BioScience, 64*(9), 820–828. doi:10.1093/biosci/biu124

Centers for Disease Control and Prevention. (2006). Health concerns associated with mold in water-damaged homes after Hurricanes Katrina and Rita—New Orleans area, Louisiana, October 2005. *Morbidity and Mortality Weekly Report, 55*(2), 41–44. Retrieved from https://www.cdc.gov/mmwr/preview/mmwrhtml/mm5502a6.htm

Centers for Disease Control and Prevention. (2017a). National environmental public health tracking. Retrieved from http://www.cdc.gov/nceh/tracking/default.htm

Centers for Disease Control and Prevention. (2017b). Particle pollution. Retrieved from https://www.cdc.gov/air/particulate_matter.html

Centers for Disease Control and Prevention. (2018). Air quality. Retrieved from https://www.cdc.gov/air/default.htm

Colburn, T., Dumanoski, D., & Myers, J. (1997). *Our stolen future.* New York, NY: Penguin.

Environmental Protection Agency. (2017a). Emergencies. Retrieved from https://www.epa.gov/emergency-response

Environmental Protection Agency. (2017b). About EPA. Retrieved from http://www.epa.gov/aboutepa

Environmental Protection Agency. (2017c). Fact sheet on air toxins. Retrieved from https://www.epa.gov/sites/production/files/2017-12/documents/monitoring_for_communities_fact_sheet_updated_171013_508.pdf

Environmental Protection Agency. (2017d). Air toxins. Retrieved from https://www.epa.gov/air-research/air-pollution-monitoring-communities-fact-sheet

Environmental Protection Agency. (2017e). Oil Pollution Act and Federal Facilities. Retrieved from https://www.epa.gov/enforcement/oil-pollution-act-opa-and-federal-facilities

Environmental Protection Agency. (2017f). Risk management program. Retrieved from http://www.epa.gov/rmp

Environmental Protection Agency. (2017g). Brownfields: Basic information. Retrieved from http://www.epa.gov/brownfields

Environmental Protection Agency. (2017h). Fact sheet on pesticides. Retrieved from http://www.epa.gov/pesticides

Environmental Protection Agency. (2017i). Ozone. Retrieved from http://www.airnow.gov/index.cfm?action=aqibasics.ozone

Greenberg, M. (2002). Should housing be built on former Brown-field sites? *American Journal of Public Health, 92*(5), 703–704. doi:10.2105/AJPH.92.5.703

Greenpeace. (1999). The Bhopal legacy. Retrieved from https://www.greenpeace.org/archive-international/en/publications/reports/the-bhopal-legacy-toxic-cont/

Jemielita, T., Gerton, G. L., Neidell, M., Chillrud, S., Yan, B., Stute, M., ... Panettieri, R. A., Jr. (2015). Correction: Unconventional gas and oil drilling is associated with increased hospital utilization rates. *PLOS ONE, 10*(8), e0137371. doi:10.1371/journal.pone.0137371

Kahle, J. J., Neas, L. M., Devlin, R. B., Case, M. W., Schmitt, M. T., Madden, M. C., & Diaz-Sanchez, D. (2015). Interaction effects of temperature and ozone on lung function and markers of systemic inflammation, coagulation, and fibrinolysis: A crossover study of healthy young volunteers. *Environmental Health Perspectives, 123*(4), 310–316. doi:10.1289/ehp.1307986

Meuser, H. (2013). *Soil remediation and rehabilitation: Treatment of contaminated and disturbed land* (23rd ed., pp. 127–162). Dordrecht, the Netherlands: Springer.

Monson, D., Doak, D., Ballachey, B., Johnson, A., & Bodkin, J. (2002). Long term impacts of the Exxon Valdez oil spill on sea offers, assessed through age dependent mortality patterns. *Proceedings of the National Academy of Sciences of the United States of America, 97*(12), 6562–6567. doi:10.1073/pnas.120163397

National Commission on the BP Deepwater Horizon Oil Spill and Offshore Drilling. (2011). *Deep water: The gulf oil disaster and the future of offshore drilling.* Retrieved from https://www.gpo.gov/fdsys/pkg/GPO-OILCOMMISSION/pdf/GPO-OILCOMMISSION.pdf

Peden, D. (2002). Pollutants and asthma: Role of air toxins. *Environmental Health Perspectives, 110*(Suppl. 4), 565–568. Retrieved from https://www.ncbi.nlm.nih.gov/pmc/articles/PMC1241207

Rabinowitz, P. M., Slizovskiy, I. B., Lamers, V., Trufan, S. J., Holford, T. R., Dziura, J. D., ... Stowe, M. H. (2015). Proximity to natural gas wells and reported health status: Results of a household survey in Washington county, Pennsylvania. *Environmental Health Perspectives, 123*(1), 21–26. doi:10.1289/ehp.1307732

Reibman, J., Levy-Carrick, N., Miles, T., Flynn, K., Hughes, C., Crane, M., & Lucchini, R. G. (2016). Destruction of the World Trade Center towers. Lessons learned from an environmental health disaster. *Annals of the American Thoracic Society, 13*(5), 577–583. doi:10.1513/AnnalsATS.201509-572PS

Schug, T. T., Janesick, A., Blumberg, B., & Heindel, J. J. (2011). Endocrine disrupting chemicals and disease susceptibility. *The Journal of Steroid Biochemistry and Molecular Biology, 127*(3–5), 204–215. doi:10.1016/j.jsbmb.2011.08.007

Scutti, S. (2017). Sewage, fecal bacteria in Hurricane Harvey floodwaters. *CNN.* Retrieved from http://www.cnn.com/2017/09/01/health/houston-flood-water-contamination/index.html

United Nations Food and Agriculture Organization. (2001). *Baseline study on the problem of obsolete pesticide stocks. FAO Pesticide Disposal Series 9.* Retrieved from http://www.fao.org/docrep/003/X8639E/X8639e00.htm

United States Nuclear Regulatory Commission. (2017). About NRT. Retrieved from https://www.nrc.gov/about-nrc.html

U.S. Census Bureau. (2017). International program: World population. Retrieved from http://www.census.gov/population/international

U.S. Energy Information Administration. (2016a). Hydraulic fracturing accounts for about half of current U.S. crude oil production. Retrieved from https://www.eia.gov/todayinenergy/detail.php?id=25372

U.S. Energy Information Administration. (2016b). Hydraulically fractured wells provide two-thirds of U.S. natural gas production. Retrieved from https://www.eia.gov/todayinenergy/detail.php?id=26112

World Health Organization. (2005). Chernobyl: The true scale of the accident. Retrieved from http://www.who.int/mediacentre/news/releases/2005/pr38/en

World Health Organization. (2010). Exposure to highly hazardous pesticides: A major public health concern. Retrieved from http://www.who.int/ipcs/features/hazardous_pesticides.pdf

World Health Organization. (2011). Water sanitation and health: Pharmaceuticals and drinking water. Retrieved from http://www.who.int/water_sanitation_health/emerging/info_sheet_pharmaceuticals/en/index.html

CASE STUDY 18.1

Bhopal

The release of toxic gases at Union Carbide's pesticide plant in Bhopal in 1984, the worst industrial disaster on record, killed 8,000 people and injured at least 150,000. Recent scientific investigations confirm that the victims of this environmental disaster are still suffering from its effects. A Greenpeace report published in 1999 found severe contamination of the factory site, surrounding land, and groundwater. Levels of mercury in some places were 6 million times higher than expected. Drinking water wells near the factory used by local people were heavily polluted with chemicals known to produce cancers and genetic defects (*Speigel*, 2014). A 2002 study by the Fact Finding Mission on Bhopal found lead, mercury, and organochlorines in the breast milk of nursing mothers (Agarwal & Nair, 2002). In 2010, *Time* magazine listed Bhopal as the worst industrial disaster in history.

The Bhopal disaster was a watershed in the area of environmental policy and legislation worldwide. Suddenly

(continued)

the horror of the industrial model of development became very stark and real. How and where industries were sited and how they dealt with the dangers that they posed to the communities around them became real questions. Bhopal was the one incident that led to worldwide regulation on chemicals and toxicity. Intertwined with all the information was the fact that communities need to be given information and be included as participants in industry decision making.

Devastating chemical environmental disasters are not exclusive to developing countries. A 1990 EPA analysis compared U.S. chemical incidents in the early to mid-1980s to the Bhopal incident. Of the 29 incidents considered, 17 U.S. incidents released sufficient volumes of chemicals with such toxicity that the potential consequences (depending on weather conditions and plant location) could have been more severe than in Bhopal. As a result of this, OSHA was asked to develop programs to prevent

chemical incidents, and the U.S. Congress authorized the EPA to promulgate the Risk Management Program Rule (40 CFR 68) for protection of the public, and OSHA to promulgate the Process Safety Management Standard (29 CFR 1910.119) to protect workers. The amendments also established the independent U.S. Chemical Safety and Hazard Investigation Board.

SOURCES

Agarwal, R., & Nair, A. (2002). Fact-finding mission on Bhopal. *Surviving Bhopal: Toxic present—Toxic future*. New Delhi, India: Srishti. Retrieved from http://cdn.cseindia.org/attachments/0.11729700_1505204490 _Surviving-Bhopal-2002.pdf

Backhaus, A., Salden, S. (2014). Bhopal's unending catrastrophe. *Speigel*. Retrieved from http://www.spiegel.de/international/world/disaster -persists-30-years-after-bhopal-gas-catastrophe-a-1006101.html

CASE STUDY 18.2

Environmental Lead Poisoning—Zambia, 2014

Lead is a naturally occurring toxic metal found in the earth's crust. Its variety of uses have made it a widespread resource used in countless industries. Mining, smelting, manufacturing, and recycling activities result in human exposure to lead. Ingestion and exposure lead to lead accumulation within the body, resulting in profound and permanent damage to development of the brain and nervous system, as well as kidney damage, stillbirths, miscarriages, and birth defects (WHO, 2017). Lead exposure has become a major and significant public health challenge across the globe but many industrialized nations have established regulations dictating the screening of children and workers for lead exposure and limiting the industrial use of lead which has greatly reduced the toxic effect of the substance. Lead poisoning is entirely preventable and can save the lives of thousands of children worldwide (WHO, 2017).

Unfortunately, many countries have not yet established regulations that guide the safe use of lead. Such an example lies within Zambia. Kabwe, the second largest city in Zambia, is home to several large mining and smelting operations (Caravanos, Fuller, & Robinson, 2014). Disruption of the earth's crust during these activities alters the natural composition of nearby soils. Aeration of dust particles and chemical processing of heavy metals have created toxic concentrations of lead in nearby soils; more than 98% of samples from communities near smelting plants tested

above the country's maximum limit for safe levels of lead. Blood lead levels taken from children in the area revealed an average blood lead level of 48.3 mcg/dL with the lowest reading at 13.6 mcg/dL (CDC, 2014). The upper value for the CDC reference range for blood lead level in children is 5 mcg/dL. The WHO recommends chelation treatment for anyone who tests above 45 mcg/dL (Caravanos et al., 2014; WHO, 2017).

Lead continues to be a threat to individuals, especially to children and pregnant women. Poor communities and unindustrialized nations are most at risk of lead poisoning. Older homes (especially those with lead pipes or lead paint), dwellings near smelting plants, and communities in areas where lead is naturally found continue to produce an increased risk of lead poisoning.

SOURCES

Caravanos, J., Fuller, R., & Robinson, S. (2014). Notes from the field: Severe environmental contamination and elevated blood lead levels among children—Zambia, 2014. *Morbidity and Mortality Weekly Report, 63*(44), 1013. Retrieved from https://www.cdc.gov/mmwr/ preview/mmwrhtml/mm6344a7.htm?s_cid=mm6344a7_w

World Health Organization. (2017). Lead poisoning and health. Retrieved from http://www.who.int/mediacentre/factsheets/fs379/en

BP Gulf Oil Spill Disaster

The BP *Deepwater Horizon* oil spill occurred on April 20, 2010, in the Gulf of Mexico. Oil flowed unabated for 3 months, making it the largest accidental marine oil spill in the history of the petroleum industry. The explosion that tore through the *Deepwater Horizon* drilling rig, as the rig's crew completed drilling the exploratory Macondo well deep under the waters of the Gulf of Mexico, began a human, economic, and environmental disaster. Eleven crew members died, and others were seriously injured, as fire engulfed and ultimately destroyed the rig. And, although the full scope of the disaster would not be known for several weeks, more than 4 million barrels of oil would gush uncontrolled into the Gulf waters—threatening livelihoods, precious ecosystems, and the health and well-being of those who lived on the shores. The landscape of the Gulf of Mexico, already battered and degraded from years of mismanagement, faced yet another blow as the oil spread and washed ashore. Five years after Hurricane Katrina, the nation was again transfixed, as this new tragedy unfolded in the Gulf (Figure 18.1). The costs from this industrial accident are not yet fully counted, but it is already clear that the impacts on the region's natural systems and people were enormous, and that economic losses total tens of billions of dollars (National Commission on the BP Deepwater Horizon Oil Spill and Offshore Drilling, 2011).

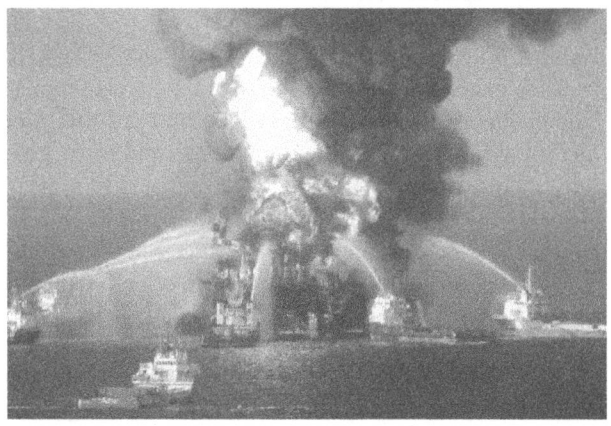

FIGURE 18.1 Fire boat response crews battle the blazing remnants of the offshore oil rig (Deepwater Horizon, April 21, 2010).

Source: U.S. Coast Guard (100421-G). Retrieved from http://coastguard.dodlive.mil/2011/03/coast-guard-aircrews-honored-for-excellence/100421-g-xxxxl-003-deepwater-horizon-fire

SOURCE

National Commission on the BP Deepwater Horizon Oil Spill and Offshore Drilling. (2011). *Deep water: The gulf oil disaster and the future of offshore drilling.* Retrieved from https://www.gpo.gov/fdsys/pkg/GPO-OILCOMMISSION/pdf/GPO-OILCOMMISSION.pdf

Aral Sea

The Aral Sea incident in Central Asia is one of the world's greatest environmental disasters. The 5 million people living in this neglected and virtually unknown part of the world are suffering not only from an environmental catastrophe that had no easy solutions but also from a litany of health problems (Small, van der Meer, & Upshur, 2001). The Aral Sea is a landlocked sea in Central Asia; it lies between Kazakhstan in the north and Karakalpakstan, an autonomous region of Uzbekistan, in the south. Formerly one of the four largest lakes in the world with an area of 68,000 sq km (26,300 sq mi), the Aral Sea has been shrinking since the 1960s, as the rivers that feed it (the Amu Darya and the Syr Darya) were diverted by the Soviet Union for irrigation. By 2007, it had declined to 10% of its original size, splitting into four lakes—the North Aral Sea and the eastern and western basins of the once far larger South Aral Sea and one smaller lake between the North and South Aral Sea. By 2009, the southeastern lake had disappeared and the southwestern lake retreated

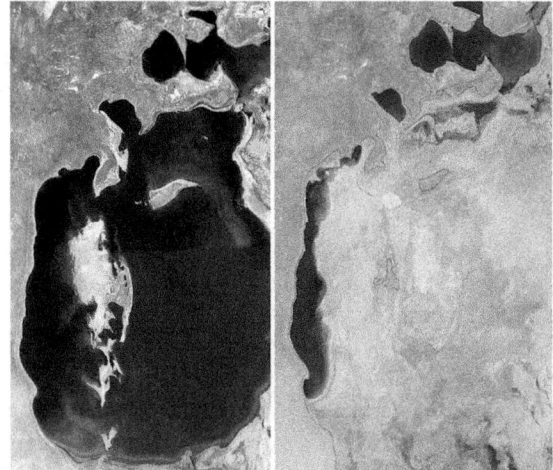

FIGURE 18.2 Aral Sea 1989 to 2014.

Source: NASA (2014). Retrieved from https://earthobservatory.nasa.gov/Features/WorldOfChange/aral_sea.php

(continued)

CASE STUDY 18.4 (continued)

to a thin strip at the extreme west of the former southern sea (Figure 18.2). By 2014, NASA imaging revealed that for the first time in history, the eastern basin has completely dried and is now known as the Aralkum Desert.

The Aral Sea is heavily polluted, largely as the result of weapons testing, industrial projects, and fertilizer runoff before and after the breakup of the Soviet Union. The region is often dismissed as a chronic problem where nothing positive can be achieved. Within this complicated context, Médecins Sans Frontières, winner of the Nobel Peace Prize in 1999, actively assessed the impact of the environmental disaster on human health to help the people who live in the Aral Sea area cope with their environment. Médecins Sans Frontières has combined a direct medical program to improve the health of the population while conducting operational research to gain a better understanding of the relationship between the environmental disaster and human health outcomes. In 2005, in an ongoing effort to save and replenish the North Aral Sea, a dam project was completed;

in 2008, the water level in the lake had risen by 24 m (79 ft) from its lowest level in 2007 (NASA, 2009). Salinity has dropped, and fish are again found in sufficient numbers for some fishing to be viable. However, the outlook for the remnants of the South Aral Sea remains bleak, and health problems plague those people living nearby (Cathcart, 2008).

SOURCES

Cathcart, R. B. (2008). Aral Sea refill: Seawater Importation Macroproject. Retrieved from www.daviddarling.info/encyclopedia/A/Aral_Sea _refill.html

National Aeronautics and Space Administration (2009). Image galleries. Retrieved from https://www.nasa.gov/multimedia/imagegallery/ index.html

Small, I., van der Meer, J., & Upshur, R. E. (2001, June). Acting on an environmental health disaster: The case of the Aral Sea. *Environmental Health Perspectives, 109*(6), 547–549. doi:10.2307/3455025

CASE STUDY 18.5

Japan Fukushima Nuclear Plant Disaster

At 2:46 a.m. Japan standard time on March 11, 2011, the Great East Japan Earthquake—rated at a magnitude of 9.0—occurred at a depth of approximately 25 km (15 miles), 130 km (81 miles) east of Sendai and 372 km (231 miles) northeast of Tokyo off the coast of Honshu Island. This earthquake resulted in the automatic shutdown of 11 nuclear power plants at four sites along the northeast coast of Japan. The earthquake precipitated a large tsunami that is estimated to have exceeded 14 m (45 ft) in height at the Fukushima Daiichi Nuclear Power Plant site. The earthquake and tsunami produced widespread devastation across northeastern Japan, resulting in approximately 25,000 people dead or missing, displacing many tens of thousands of people, and significantly impacting the infrastructure and industry in the northeastern coastal areas of Japan.

As a result of the earthquake, all of the operating units at Fukushima Daiichi automatically shut down, and offsite power was lost to the entire facility. The emergency diesel generators started at all six units providing alternating current (AC) electrical power to critical systems at each unit, and the facility response to the seismic event appears to have been normal. Approximately 40 minutes following the earthquake and shutdown of the operating units, the first large tsunami wave inundated the site followed by multiple additional

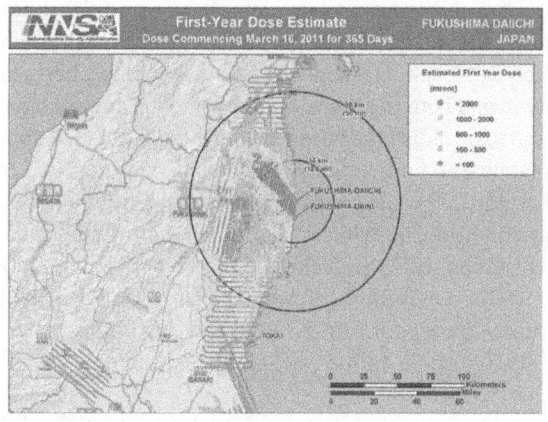

FIGURE 18.3 Fukushima Daiichi, first-year dose estimate (2011, April).

Source: Nuclear Incident Team, U.S. Department of Energy (2011). Retrieved from http://www.slideshare.net/energy/ radiation-monitoring-data-from-fukushima-area-04182011

waves. The estimated height of the tsunami exceeded the site design protection from tsunamis by approximately 8 m (27 ft). The tsunami resulted in extensive damage to site facilities and a complete loss of power.

(continued)

CASE STUDY 18.5 (*continued*)

The power plant operators were faced with a catastrophic, unprecedented emergency situation. They had to work in near total darkness with very limited instrumentation and control systems. Despite the actions of the operators following the earthquake and tsunami, cooling was lost to the fuel in the Unit 1 reactor after several hours, the Unit 2 reactor after about 71 hours, and the Unit 3 reactor after about 36 hours, resulting in damage to the nuclear fuel shortly after the loss of cooling. Without AC power, the plants were likely relying on batteries and turbine- and diesel-driven pumps. The operators were likely implementing their severe accident management program to maintain core cooling functions well beyond the normal capacity of the station batteries. Without the response of offsite assistance, which appears to have been hampered by the devastation in the area among other factors, each unit eventually lost the capability to further extend cooling of the reactor cores. The full toll of this incident and associated radiation release on the surrounding area is still being assessed (Figure 18.3).

CASE STUDY 18.6

Hurricane Katrina

On August 29, 2005, Hurricane Katrina made landfall on the Gulf Coast, leaving behind a trail of mass destruction in Louisiana, Mississippi, and Alabama. In Louisiana and Mississippi, the storm created an estimated 86 million cubic yards of debris; caused the spill of more than 7 million gallons of oil; produced floodwaters that deposited fuel oils, gasoline, bacteria, and metals in sediments; and passed over 18 Superfund National Priorities List (NPL) hazardous waste sites and more than 400 industrial facilities that store or manage hazardous materials. Because of flooding and hurricane storm surges, millions of hazardous products such as bleach, cleaners, oil, fuels, pesticides, herbicides, paint, and batteries were scattered into the environment. In Louisiana alone, the hurricane potentially affected approximately 850 underground storage tank facilities and more than 300,000 white goods (appliances, e.g., refrigerators and air conditioners, which may contain harmful substances, e.g., Freon; EPA, Office of the Inspector General, 2006).

Under the National Response Plan, the EPA is the lead federal agency for ESF 10—Oil and Hazardous Materials. ESF 10 responsibilities include the following:

- Addressing threats from actual or potential releases including oil spills, sediment contamination, and hazardous materials
- Managing hazardous household waste and other material releases that may pose a threat to public health or the environment, such as electronics or white goods

- Managing, overseeing, and assisting in the segregation of hazardous debris and waste

The EPA's postimpact activities included collecting and responding to information on the nature, magnitude, and timing of the hazardous materials releases. The EPA investigated and monitored sediment contamination following the recession of the floodwaters, contamination and release of Superfund sites and underground storage tank facilities, and multiple oil spills (EPA, Office of the Inspector General, 2006). Sediment samples (taken in September 2005 and February 2006) from the greater New Orleans area contained a variety of chemicals, including some metals, petroleum hydrocarbons, polycyclic aromatic hydrocarbons (PAHs), and pesticides, some in levels unacceptable to the EPA.

SOURCE

Environmental Protection Agency, Office of the Inspector General. (2006, May 2). Evaluation report: EPA provided quality and timely information on Hurricane Katrina hazardous materials releases and debris management (Report No. 2006-P-00023). Retrieved from https://www.epa.gov/sites/production/files/2015-10/documents/20060502-2006-p-00023.pdf

Mercury Spills—Small Incidents With Big Impacts

Exposure to elemental mercury vapor can cause adverse health effects, especially in children and fetuses. Governmental agencies and other organizations have tried numerous ways to educate the public about the hazards of elemental mercury and encourage the safe disposal of mercury-containing products. Despite measures to educate the public about the dangers of elemental mercury, spills continue to occur in homes, schools, healthcare facilities, and other settings, endangering the public's health and requiring costly cleanup. Mercury is most efficiently absorbed by the lungs, and exposure to high levels of mercury vapor after a release can cause cough, sore throat, shortness of breath, nausea, vomiting, diarrhea, headaches, and visual disturbances. To summarize key features of recent mercury spills and lessons learned, five state health departments involved in the cleanup (Iowa, Michigan, Missouri, North Carolina, and Wisconsin) compiled data from various sources on nonthermometer mercury spills from 2012 to 2015. The most common sites of contamination were residences, schools and school buses, healthcare facilities, and commercial and industrial facilities. Children under 18 years of age were present in about one-third of the spills, with approximately one in seven incidents resulting in symptoms consistent with acute mercury exposure. State and local health departments routinely evaluate the cleanup of homes and schools where mercury spills have occurred to ensure that mercury vapor concentrations are reduced to safe levels. Cleanup of elemental mercury is challenging because it is dense and breaks into tiny beads when spilled. Elemental mercury also adheres to surfaces such as shoes, which can promote the spread of contamination, further complicating collection and removal (Wozniak, Hirsch, Bush, Schmitz, & Wenzel, 2017).

Five cases that occurred during 2012 to 2014 illustrate the variety of mercury spills to which state health departments were asked to respond (Wozniak et al., 2017):

Armstrong, Iowa (2012). A person carried a jar containing approximately 12 pounds of mercury into a bar, where it accidentally spilled. Extensive mercury contamination was found in the bar and in the home of one of the bar patrons. Cleanup in the bar required removing the tile floor, sealing the subfloor, and superheating the indoor air with forced ventilation. Remediation of the home involved extensive cleaning and removal of contaminated items as hazardous waste, including a vacuum cleaner, washer, and clothes dryer. After cleanup of these locations by EPA contractors, mercury vapor monitoring was conducted under typical conditions to confirm that both locations were safe for reentry. Although the cleanup took 1 week to complete, no adverse health effects were reported because quick action by responders limited mercury vapor exposure.

Lenoir, North Carolina (2012). A student brought a test tube containing mercury to an elementary school. The test tube was dropped in a classroom, spilling approximately 0.5 pound of mercury. Five exposed students (aged 10–12 years) were taken to a hospital, decontaminated, and released. Multiple federal, state, and local agencies were involved in the response and assessment. Cleanup operations and environmental monitoring were conducted by an environmental contractor and EPA. The school was closed for 2 days before it was cleared for reoccupancy.

Kansas City, Missouri (2013). A resident hired a professional clock company to move his antique grandfather clock up a set of stairs. The clock had an estimated 15 pounds of mercury contained in the pendulum. During the move, nearly 2 pounds of mercury were spilled throughout the apartment building. Cleanup of this spill took approximately 2 weeks and resulted in the disposal of the pendulum and the mercury remaining inside it. No adverse health effects were reported among those living at the home.

Delton, Michigan (2014). A man attempted to extract gold from jewelry by combining it with elemental mercury and heating the mixture. He was severely poisoned from inhaling very high concentrations of mercury vapors. Multiple federal, state, and local agencies were involved in the cleanup of the home and the medical care of the patient, who survived, but required extensive medical treatment. The home was eventually demolished.

Bloomer, Wisconsin (2014). An old mercury-containing boiler was being removed from a home and approximately 3.5 pounds of mercury were released in the basement, garage, and driveway. The state health department provided cleanup guidance and a mercury vapor monitor to assist on-site agencies in overseeing cleanup of this large spill. Professional cleanup of the basement, garage, and driveway required the use of powdered sulfur and a specialized mercury vacuum. The washer and clothes dryer were also contaminated and were discarded as hazardous waste. No adverse health effects were reported by persons living in the home.

As health officials began to understand and appreciate the adverse health effects that exposure to mercury can cause in humans, state and federal agencies began to institute laws and regulations to reduce and control the use, release, and disposal of elemental mercury. These regulations have been effective at reducing environmental contamination from industrial and commercial sources;

(continued)

CASE STUDY 18.7 (*continued*)

however, numerous stores of elemental mercury still exist in smaller quantities in residences, schools, and healthcare facilities. Mercury spills can be expensive to clean up and bring to levels considered safe for long-term occupancy, with the cost varying based on the location and extent of contamination. During 2012 to 2015, EPA reported responding to 225 chemical-release incidents in which mercury was listed as the primary contaminant of concern; the average cost of cleanup to those incidents ranged from approximately $30,000 to $75,000 for each year from 2012 to 2015, and the highest cleanup cost during this time period was $913,915 in 2013. When mercury spills do occur, a quick and coordinated response is necessary to ensure the protection of public health and proper remediation. When a spill occurs, health departments, local or regional hazardous materials responders, state health and environmental agencies, regional EPA offices, poison control centers, and healthcare providers should be immediately informed.

SOURCE

Wozniak, R. J., Hirsch, A. E., Bush, C. R., Schmitz, S., & Wenzel, J. (2017). Mercury spill responses—Five states, 2012–2015. *Weekly Morbidity and Mortality Report, 66*(10), 274–277. Retrieved from https://www.cdc.gov/mmwr/volumes/66/wr/mm6610a3.htm?s_cid =mm6610a3_w

19

RESTORING PUBLIC HEALTH UNDER DISASTER CONDITIONS: BASIC SANITATION, WATER AND FOOD SUPPLY, AND SHELTER

Mary Pat Couig, Tener Goodwin Veenema, and Adam B. Rains

LEARNING OBJECTIVES

When this chapter is completed, readers will be able to:

1. Describe the 10 essential functions of public health as they relate to a disaster.
2. Describe the importance of a clean environment as a foundation for good health.
3. Appraise both risks and resources in the environment to meet the basic needs (food, water, shelter, and safety) for survival.
4. Discuss the major health risks in a population affected by a disaster and identify and prioritize according to prevention/control of disease, epidemics, and other hazards.
5. Describe rapid environmental assessment (REA) as a methodology for data collection in a disaster-affected community.
6. Discuss the Sphere Project humanitarian standards for disaster response.
7. Identify restoration of electricity as critical to protecting human health.

KEY MESSAGES

Populations affected by a disaster experience diminished environmental conditions that put them at risk of negative health outcomes.

Basic physiological needs must be met in a timely manner to ensure survival.

Sanitation is a cornerstone of the public health response.

Establishing, implementing, and continuously monitoring minimum standards for water and food safety, sanitation, shelter, personal hygiene, and vector control provide a firm foundation for health promotion.

Infectious disease outbreaks often occur in the postimpact and recovery phases of a disaster (not during the acute phase); nurses should be knowledgeable about diseases endemic to the affected area.

The risk of epidemics increases if drought, famine, and/or large displacements of people are involved.

The length of time that people spend in temporary shelters is an important determinant of the risk of disease transmission that might lead to major epidemics.

Working in conjunction with public health colleagues, and as members of an interdisciplinary disaster response team, nurses must be able to detect environmental changes that can increase the potential for the spread of infectious disease.

CHAPTER OVERVIEW

This chapter provides an overview of the basic concepts of health promotion and disease prevention for disaster nursing. It begins by introducing the three core functions of public health and the 10 Essential Public Health Services (Department of Health and Human Services [HHS], 2017b). Analysis of the fundamental public health functions during nondisaster circumstances provides a foundation for what concepts apply and what services must be mobilized should a major event occur. Nurses responding to the needs of populations and communities affected by disasters require an understanding of the basic tenets of environmental health, methods of health promotion, and disease-prevention strategies.

Rapid environmental assessment is introduced as a methodology for data collection in postimpact communities. Individuals affected by disasters must have their basic physiological needs met in a timely manner for survival. A framework for establishing public health priorities and minimum standards for water, food, sanitation and solid waste removal, shelter, and vector control is proposed. Response to public health emergencies such as outbreaks of food-borne illness is presented. The role of the public health nurse (PHN) in the response and recovery phases of any disaster becomes even more valuable, as these nurses have expertise in disease surveillance and optimization of population health outcomes.

Disasters destroy or disrupt the integrity of the physical environment, and the foundations of good health are temporarily and sometimes permanently lost. The consequences of this diminished environment will vary based on the geographical location of the disaster, the biological pathogens present, the susceptibility and health habits of the people living there, and the availability of resources and protective measures to compensate for the losses (Landesman, 2011). The earthquake in Mexico City (September 2017) and the U.S. Hurricanes Harvey,

Irma, and Maria (August & September 2017)—catastrophic events of epic proportion by any measure—provide evidence that, regardless of where a disaster may occur geographically, the basic physiological needs of each affected population will be fundamentally the same (Berger, 2006). Health promotion and disease prevention activities must focus on restoration of services to meet the immediate physiological needs of the affected people and to prevent the spread of infectious disease (Noji, 1996, 2000, 2007).

BASIC PUBLIC HEALTH FUNCTIONS

In its 1948 constitution, the World Health Organization (WHO) defined health as "a state of complete physical, mental and social well-being and not merely the absence of disease or infirmity" (WHO, 1948, p. 1). Public health is the profession, discipline, and system for providing healthcare to communities. Grounded in a multitude of sciences, public health's primary focus is prevention of illness, injury, and death (Merson, Black, & Mills, 2006). C.E.A. Winslow, frequently regarded as the founder of modern public health in the United States, defined public health as:

> ... the science and art of preventing disease, prolonging life and prompting physical health and efficiency through organized community efforts for the sanitation of the environment, the control of communicable infections, the education of the individual in personal hygiene, the organization of medical and nursing services for the early diagnosis and preventive treatment of disease, and the development of the social machinery which will ensure to every individual a standard of living adequate for the maintenance of health; organizing these benefits in such a fashion as to enable every citizen to realize his birthright of health and longevity. (Winslow, 1920, p. 184)

The current, public health infrastructure in the United States is a large, poorly defined, and loosely connected system of agencies and providers working to meet the healthcare needs in their communities. The fundamental obligation of these agencies responsible for population health is to:

1. Prevent epidemics and the spread of disease
2. Protect against environmental hazards
3. Prevent injuries
4. Promote and encourage healthy behaviors and mental health
5. Respond to disasters and assist communities in recovery
6. Ensure the quality and accessibility of health services

These responsibilities describe and define the function of public health in *ensuring* the availability of quality health services. In 1988, the Institute of Medicine (IOM) published a landmark report, *The Future of Public Health* (IOM, 1988). In addition to providing a comprehensive overview of public health in the United States, the report recommended that there be three core functions of public health—assessment, policy development, and assurance. Essential functions of public health were delineated in 1994 by an Essential Public Health Services Working Group of the Core Public Health Functions Steering Committee of the U.S. Public Health Service (see Figure 19.1; HHS, 2017b):

1. Monitor health status to identify and solve community health problems
2. Diagnose and investigate health problems and health hazards in the community
3. Inform, educate, and empower people about health issues
4. Mobilize community partnerships and action to identify and solve health problems
5. Develop policies and plans that support individual and community health efforts
6. Enforce laws and regulations that protect health and ensure safety
7. Link people to needed personal health services and assure the provision of healthcare when otherwise unavailable
8. Assure competent public and personal healthcare workforce
9. Evaluate effectiveness, accessibility, and quality of personal and population-based health services
10. Research for new insights and innovative solutions to health problems

Although the essential functions of the public health system provide a frame of reference for nurses and other healthcare providers responding to a major event, disasters compound the challenges for public health in numerous ways (see Appendix 19.1). The hurricanes of August and September 2017, Harvey, Irma, and Maria, are recent examples of the devastating effect that the forces of nature can have on health and social well-being. Potential hazards from hurricanes and floods include: vehicle- and nonvehicle-related drowning, carbon monoxide poisoning, electrocution, falls, lacerations, exposure to mold and industrial and household chemicals (Centers for Disease Control and Prevention [CDC], 2017b) and the potential for the spread of airborne or waterborne diseases (CDC, 2017a). Nurses responding to individuals, families, and communities affected by disasters are called on to provide much more than

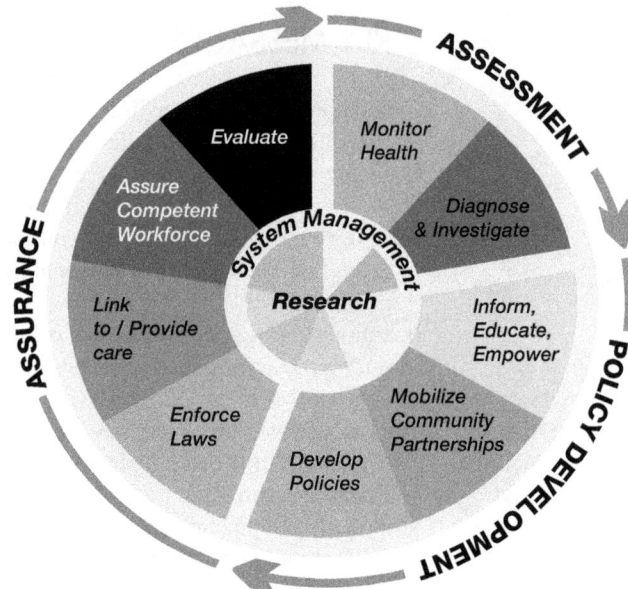

FIGURE 19.1 The three core functions and 10 essential public health services.

Source: Department of Health and Human Services. (2017b). The Public Health System and the 10 Essential Public Health Services. Retrieved from https://www.cdc.gov/stltpublichealth/publichealthservices/essentialhealthservices.html

just postimpact nursing care. Restoration of the environment and its resources to at least predisaster conditions is imperative to promote good health and prevent disease.

HEALTH PROMOTION

"Health promotion" is the process of enabling people to increase control over, and to improve, their health (WHO, 1986, 2009). Pender, Murdaugh, and Parsons (2010) describe health promotion as behavior motivated by the desire to increase well-being and actualize human health potential. In health promotion, empowerment is a process through which people gain greater control over decisions and actions affecting their health. Empowerment may be a social, cultural, psychological, or political process through which individuals and social groups are able to express their needs, present their concerns, devise strategies for involvement in decision making, and achieve political, social, and cultural action to meet those needs (WHO, 2009).

Historically, public health and nursing are the two primary disciplines concerned with the science and art of promoting health, preventing disease, and prolonging life through the organized efforts of society. In disaster situations, the use of organized efforts to eliminate hazards and restore the environment and its inhabitants to their optimal level of health becomes even more important.

The goals for health promotion in disaster nursing are as follows:

- To meet the immediate basic survival needs of populations affected by disasters (water, food, shelter, and security)
- To identify the potential for a secondary disaster

- To appraise both risks and resources in the environment
- To correct inequalities in access to healthcare or appropriate resources
- To empower survivors to participate in and advocate for their own health and well-being
- To respect cultural, lingual, and religious diversity in individuals and families and to apply this principle in all health promotion activities
- To promote the highest achievable quality of life for survivors

To achieve these goals, nurses must have a solid understanding of the basic principles of environmental health, methods of health promotion, and disease-prevention strategies. They must also maintain competencies in these areas in order to collaborate with other members of the team who provide healthcare.

It was Florence Nightingale who first illustrated for nurses the importance of understanding environmental principles. Nightingale, we should recall, waged a tireless campaign during the Crimean War to improve the health outcomes of soldiers in her care with fresh air, clean water, fresh bed linens, and a plentiful supply of healthy food. Because of her emphasis on health promotion efforts related to the environment, Nightingale was able to bring about substantial reform in the living standards of, and health services for, the armed services. Her work remains a shining example of how to apply the principles of public health and disaster nursing and thereby improve environmental conditions for affected populations (Nightingale, 1858).

MASLOW'S HIERARCHY OF NEEDS

Abraham Maslow is recognized for having established a theory of the hierarchy of human needs. He argued that humans are motivated by unmet needs and proposed that certain basic necessities (physiological, safety) must be satisfied for individuals to behave unselfishly and realize their full potential (Maslow, 1970). Based on this prioritization, Maslow grouped and ordered human needs into categories according to their primacy (Figure 19.2).

While the specifics of Maslow's theory are a focus of active debate, the hierarchy of needs provides a theoretical foundation for disaster response efforts. Even in circumstances of great upheaval, desolation, and despair, basic necessities of life must be met for individuals to recover and realize their inherent human potential.

Physiological needs are the basic essentials of life such as air, water, food, and sleep. When these needs are not satisfied, as frequently occurs in the postimpact period, individuals become ill and experience pain, suffering, and discomfort. These feelings motivate individuals to correct the imbalances in their environment to reachieve homeostasis. Once these needs are met, individuals become capable of attending to other needs in their lives.

Safety needs are concerned with establishing stability and consistency in a chaotic world. These needs are primarily psychological in nature, and again, are frequently disrupted by the effects of a disaster. Individuals who do not feel safe in the environment are incapable of addressing other prevailing life issues.

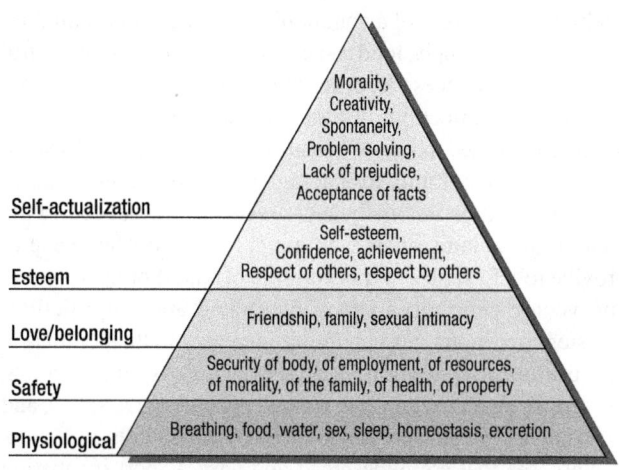

FIGURE 19.2 Maslow's hierarchy of needs.

The nature of the environment has a direct impact on a community's health and on the quality of life of its inhabitants. "Quality of life" is defined as an individual's perception of his or her position in life in the context of the culture and value system where that individual lives and in relation to personal goals, expectations, standards, and concerns. It is a broad-ranging concept that incorporates a person's physical health, psychological state, level of independence, social relationships, personal beliefs, and relationship to salient features of the environment (WHO, 2009). Restoration of these faculties and a collective reduction in fear and uncertainty must be accomplished as soon as possible. Disaster nursing practice also seeks to promote changes in behaviors that will compensate for disrupted physiological conditions. At the same time, health promotion and disease prevention activities must occur simultaneously in the immediate aftermath of a disaster.

RISK FACTORS FOR INFECTIOUS DISEASE OUTBREAKS FROM DISASTERS

Disasters destroy or destabilize the physical environment in which people work and live. Natural disasters that have a rapid onset and broad impact can produce many factors that work synergistically to increase the risk of illness and deaths resulting from infectious disease (Toole, 2008). Thus, in any disaster response, the first goal is to reestablish sanitary barriers as quickly as possible. Following this, efforts should be made to meet the basic physiological needs of the population. Therefore, strategies to accommodate population-based needs for water, food, waste removal, vector control, shelter, and safety should be planned for in advance. Following a disaster, continuous monitoring of the environment will allow nurses to immediately address potential hazards. In terms of epidemics, generally large-scale risks are low immediately following acute natural disasters, particularly in developed nations. Infectious disease outbreaks usually occur in the postimpact and recovery phases of the disaster.

The risks of epidemics increase when drought, famine, and large displacements of people are involved (Greenough, 2007). Any disaster that interrupts one or more levels of the public health infrastructure of a community, including the sanitation systems, water supply, food and nutrition sources, vector control programs, and access to primary care (e.g., immunizations) can trigger an infectious disease outbreak. Such interruptions produce increased modes of transmission of infectious diseases, increased susceptibility to endemic organisms among disaster survivors, and occasionally new organisms introduced to the area by those individuals who travel to the disaster scene to provide relief. Modes of transmission of waterborne, airborne, and vectorborne diseases are facilitated and amplified by disaster conditions. Susceptibility increases in the population because of the migration of large populations, malnutrition, overcrowding in shelters and camps, open wounds, stress, and exposure to extremes of hot and cold temperatures.

Diseases that are widespread and have a short incubation period will commonly appear first. Measles, diarrheal disease, and respiratory infections, all of which are preventable diseases, constitute the vast majority of deaths following a disaster (Merson, Black, & Mills, 2006). When a disease appears in a population following a disaster, investigation and full appraisal of the situation (data collection and risk assessment) must occur immediately.

RAPID ASSESSMENT OF POPULATION HEALTH NEEDS

Conducting a rapid, comprehensive assessment of population health requirements is one of the most important public health tasks in the immediate aftermath of a disaster. Responders should conduct a health assessment of the community as soon as possible within the first few days following the event (Connolly, 2005). This is a multifaceted process that consists of several key elements: (a) data collection for assessment of needs, (b) identification of available resources that match defined needs, and (c) prevention of further adverse health effects associated with the event.

The initial data collection as part of the rapid assessment should include the following:

1. An assessment of the current circumstances and quality of life of the victims—location, demographic data, routes of access, modes of transportation, communication systems, availability of basic services (water, electricity, communications, sanitation facilities, housing, and shelters), and availability of food
2. The scope of the damage—the number of deaths, the number of persons injured, the number who have disappeared, the number displaced and their location, the status and capacity of healthcare facilities, urgent needs, and human and material resources in the immediate area (Farmer, Jimenez, Rubinson, & Talmor, 2004)

Other data points for collection include the following:

1. The presence of an immediate or potential hazard (e.g., persistent toxic smoke or potential for chemical leak or spill)
2. The community's need for immediate outside assistance
3. The augmentation of existing public health surveillance for ongoing monitoring of healthcare needs

A team must be assembled, including public health officials, clinicians, epidemiologists, engineers, and local officials, if available. Frequently, members of the American Red Cross will also participate in this initial assessment. If the area affected is large, several teams may be needed to traverse the field site. All team members collecting data should use a standardized format. Advanced information on the status of the healthcare system (available beds, equipment) emergency medical services, and the availability of healthcare providers to respond is critical to assessing capacity. Accurate detailed maps should be obtained, delineating high-risk areas and the location of vulnerable populations. Baseline data on the population are critical prior to beginning the rapid assessment; for example, the use of preimpact epidemiologic data on frequencies and distributions of disease (e.g., incidence, prevalence, and mortality) will facilitate the analysis and planning for response (Connolly, 2005; Waring & Brown, 2005).

This rapid assessment is essential for successful interventions as it reveals where breakdowns in the public health infrastructure occurred and helps to identify and prioritize the health needs of the population. All immediate and potential health hazards must be identified.

The Role of the Public Health Nurse Following a Disaster

PHNs have a central function in the public health system and, as such, become invaluable resources both to the community and to other nurses during times of disaster (Atkins, Williams, Salinas, & Edwards, 2005). PHNs are experts in population health and routinely conduct disease surveillance, implement programs in health promotion, and are knowledgeable in healthy standards for food, water, and sanitation. Increased surveillance activities for disaster recovery add more responsibilities to the work of PHNs. In all types of disasters, *all responding nurses* will be empowered to exercise leadership and discerning judgment in the following:

- Assessing the affected community for the presence (or absence) of the fundamentals for health—clean water, safe food, sanitation, and shelter
- Reestablishing the sanitary barriers that protect communities from environmental hazards
- Detecting changes in the integrity of the environment and organizing activities designed to eliminate or mitigate existing health hazards
- Planning for continuous maintenance and monitoring of facilities basic to health regarding proper waste removal, adequate water and food supplies, shelter, and personal safety
- Responding aggressively to evidence of the transmission of disease to ameliorate the spread of an epidemic throughout the population
- Respecting and empowering affected individuals by giving them decision-making rights regarding all pertinent public health issues

As the experts in this field, PHNs are ideally suited for positions of responsibility and should be leading the teams of nurses.

THE SPHERE PROJECT

In 1997, an international initiative called the Sphere Project (The Sphere Project, n.d.-a, n.d.-b) was developed. The project published a set of minimum standards in core areas of humanitarian assistance. These standards can serve as a foundation for the disaster nursing prevention strategies previously described. The Sphere Project's primary goal is "to improve the quality of humanitarian assistance and the accountability of humanitarian actors to their constituents, donors and affected populations." (The Sphere Project, n.d.-a, n.d.-b). The cornerstone of the project was the establishment of the Humanitarian Charter. Based on the principles and provisions of international humanitarian law, international human rights law, refugee law, and the *Code of Conduct* for the International Red Cross and Red Crescent Movement, the Charter describes the core principles that govern humanitarian action and asserts the right of populations to protection and assistance (The Sphere Project, 2018). In 2018, the Sphere Project published revised and updated standards reflecting recent developments in humanitarian practice in water, sanitation, food, shelter, and health, based on feedback from practitioners in the field, research institutes and cross-cutting experts in protection, gender, children, older people, disabled people, HIV/AIDS, and the environment (The Sphere Project, 2018).

Vulnerabilities and Capacities of Disaster-Affected Populations

Women, children, older people, people with disabilities or chronic illness, people with mental health issues, and people living with HIV/AIDS constitute the groups most frequently at risk in disasters and public health emergencies. In certain contexts, people may also become vulnerable by reason of ethnic origin, religious or political affiliation, or displacement. This is not an exhaustive list, but it includes those groups most frequently identified. Specific vulnerabilities influence peoples' abilities to cope and survive in a disaster, and those most at risk should be identified in each context. When any one group is at risk, it is likely that others will also be threatened. Special care must be taken to protect and provide for all affected groups in a nondiscriminatory manner and according to individuals' specific needs. However, it should also be remembered that disaster-affected populations possess and acquire skills and capacities of their own to cope, and that these should be recognized and supported (The Sphere Project, 2018).

The Humanitarian Charter is concerned with the most basic requirements for sustaining the lives and dignity of those affected by disasters. The minimum standards aim to quantify these requirements with regard to a people's need for water, sanitation, nutrition, food, shelter, healthcare, and protection from hazards in the environment. Although designed to address international relief efforts, the Humanitarian Charter and Minimum Standards provide a useful operational framework for establishing public health priorities and accountability in any disaster response, regardless of location. In the event of a disaster within the geographical borders of the United States, the basic fundamental priorities for the health of a population remain the same.

Water

Too much or too little water is the leading cause of most of the world's disasters (WHO, 2017). However, international legal instruments recognize the right to water and sufficient, safe, acceptable, physically accessible, and affordable water for personal and domestic uses (The Sphere Project, 2018).

The Sphere Project proposes minimum standards for the water supply in disaster-relief efforts addressing access to the water supply, water quality, and water use facilities and goods.

Water Supply Standard 1: *Access and Water Quantity.* All people have safe and equitable access to a sufficient quantity of water for drinking, cooking, and personal and domestic hygiene. Public water points are sufficiently close to households to enable implementation of the minimum water requirement.

Key points
Average water use for drinking, cooking, and personal hygiene in any household is at least 15 liters (3.96 gallons) per person per day.
The maximum distance from any household to the nearest water point is 500 m (1640.42 ft).
Waiting time at a water source is no more than 15 minutes. It takes no more than 3 minutes to fill a 20-liter container.
Water sources and systems are maintained such that appropriate quantities of water are available consistently or on a regular basis. (The Sphere Project, 2018)

Nurses will need to work closely with public health officials and the agencies responsible for monitoring access to and quantity of the water supply in the postimpact phase of a disaster. The exact quantity of water needed for domestic use will vary according to the climate, religious and cultural habits of the affected population, and the amount of food they cook. Water consumption should be monitored and each family should be provided with its own water receptacle or bucket to reduce the spread of disease. In the immediate aftermath of a disaster, the first priority is to provide an adequate quantity of water, even if its safety cannot be guaranteed, and to protect water sources from contamination. A minimum of 15 liters per person per day should be provided as soon as possible, though in the immediate postimpact period, it may be necessary to limit treated water to a minimum of 7.5 liters per day per person. During emergencies, people may use an untreated water source for laundry, bathing, and so forth. Water quality improvements can be made over succeeding days or weeks (WHO, 2011).

A 5- to 6-day supply of water (5 gallons per person) should be stored for food preparation and personal hygiene, as part of essential disaster planning in communities at high risk of a natural disaster. Stored water should be changed every 6 months. Cloudy water or any water with a fetid odor should be discarded immediately.

In disaster situations, there may not be enough water available to meet the physiological needs of the affected population, and sources of potable water must be found. A satisfactory supply must be made available to every individual. Rainwater, surface water, and groundwater are sources of water. Rainwater is sporadic and generally unreliable as a water source. Surface water is found in lakes, ponds, streams, and rivers, and is generally the only type of water that is accessible and in large enough quantity to provide for a population following a major disaster. Although surface water is easy to collect, it is microbiologically unsafe and requires treatment before use. Attempts to access groundwater may be necessary in the event that surface water is unavailable or insufficient to meet demand. As with surface water, groundwater may harbor contaminants and must be evaluated for quality. Chlorine ("shock chlorination") can be used to treat sources of ground water, including wells. Every effort should be made to achieve a drinking water quality as high as possible. Protection of water supplies from contamination is the first and best line of defense, and ongoing monitoring of water quality must be conducted. Once water is collected, its quality will deteriorate over time. Source protection is almost invariably the best method of ensuring safe drinking water and is preferred to treating a contaminated water supply to render it suitable for consumption. Once a potentially hazardous situation has been recognized, however, the risk to health, the availability of alternative sources, and the availability of suitable remedial measures must be considered so that a decision can be made about the acceptability of the supply. A contaminated water source should not be closed to access unless another source has been identified. Providing people with more water is more protective against fecal–oral pathogens than providing people with *cleaner* water, according to studies conducted in developing countries (CDC, 1993a; Esrey, Potash, Roberts, & Shiff, 1991).

As far as possible, water sources must be protected from contamination by human and animal waste, which can contain a variety of bacterial, viral, and protozoan pathogens and parasites. Failure to provide adequate protection and effective treatment will expose the community to the risk of outbreaks of intestinal and other infectious diseases. To a great extent, the vulnerability of victims to waterborne illnesses depends on the preexisting levels of personal hygiene and sanitation (WHO, 1979). Those at greatest risk of waterborne disease are infants and young children, people who are debilitated or living under unsanitary conditions, the sick, and the elderly. For these people, infective doses are significantly lower than for the general adult population (WHO, 2011).

Water Supply Standard 2: *Water Quality.* Water is palatable and of sufficient quality to be drunk and used for personal and domestic hygiene without causing significant risk to health.

Key points
A sanitary survey indicates a low risk of fecal contamination.
There are no fecal coliforms per 100 mL at the point of delivery.
People drink water from a protected or treated source in preference to other readily available water sources.
Steps are taken to minimize postdelivery contamination.
For piped water supplies, or for all water supplies at times of risk or presence of diarrhea epidemic, water is treated with a disinfectant so that there is a free chlorine residual at the tap of 0.5 mg per liter and turbidity is below 5 NTU.
No negative health effect is detected that is due to short-term use of water contaminated by chemical (including carry-over of treatment chemicals) or radiological sources, and

assessment shows no significant probability of such an effect. (The Sphere Project, 2018)

Water quality is evaluated based on the presence of bacterial measures that indicate the presence of feces. Human feces contain millions of bacteria and even minute amounts of feces in water are often detectable via bacterial monitoring. WHO guidelines consider water with less than 10 fecal coliforms per 100 mL to be reasonably safe, whereas water with 100 or greater fecal coliforms per 100 mL is considered contaminated and unsafe for human consumption.

- The WHO recommends that social, economic, and environmental factors be taken into account through a risk-benefit approach when adapting the guideline values to international standards or during emergency situations.
- In the United States, the Environmental Protection Agency (EPA) enforces federal clean water and safe drinking water laws, provides support for municipal wastewater treatment plants, and takes part in pollution prevention efforts aimed at protecting watersheds and sources of drinking water. The Agency carries out both regulatory and voluntary programs to fulfill its mission to protect the nation's waters and has established standards for the microbial quality of water in the United States (EPA, 2017b).

Safe drinking water, even in the United States, cannot be taken for granted. There are a number of threats to drinking water: improperly disposed chemicals; human and animal waste; pesticides; wastes injected deep underground; and naturally occurring substances can all contaminate drinking water. Likewise, drinking water that is not properly treated or disinfected, or which travels through an improperly maintained distribution system, may also pose a health risk.

Disaster events disrupt the integrity of water containment and systems, and contamination can occur. Depending on the location of the disaster, nurses should use one or both of the WHO guidelines and the EPA standards to provide a foundation for assessment of risk and risk management for water-related infectious diseases following a disaster or major public health event. Much of this discussion addresses those parts of the world without an adequate infrastructure, whereas in the United States, nurses will most frequently encounter well-water contamination from flooding.

Drinking Water. Safe water for drinking and cooking includes bottled, boiled, or treated water. If possible, in the aftermath of a disaster, people should drink only bottled, boiled, or treated water until the water supply can be tested for safety. Health education of the public should include warning people not to use contaminated water to brush teeth, wash dishes, wash or cook food, or make ice. Water used for making edible ice should be subject to the same drinking water standard and should include specific sanitary requirements for equipment for making and storing ice. To kill harmful organisms, all members of the community should be instructed to boil their water in a *rapid boil for at least 1 to 2 minutes.* Water can also be treated to kill bacteria by adding chlorine or iodine tablets or 1/8 teaspoon of unscented Clorox bleach per gallon of water. The solution must be mixed thoroughly and allowed to sit for at least 30 minutes.

Water Supply Standard 3: *Water Use Facilities and Goods.* People have adequate facilities and supplies to collect, store, and use sufficient quantities of water for drinking, cooking, and personal hygiene, and to ensure that drinking water remains safe until it is consumed.

Key points
Each household has at least two clean-water-collecting containers of 10 to 20 liters (2.64 to 5.28 gallons), plus enough clean water storage containers to ensure there is always water in the household.

Water collection and storage containers have narrow necks and/or covers, or other safe means of storage, drawing, and handling, and are demonstrably used.

There is at least one standard bar of soap available for personal hygiene per person per month.

Where communal bathing facilities are necessary, there are sufficient bathing cubicles available, with separate cubicles for males and females, and they are used appropriately and equitably.

Where communal laundry facilities are necessary, there is at least one washing basin per 100 people, and private laundering areas are available for women to wash and dry undergarments and sanitary cloths.

The participation of all vulnerable groups is actively encouraged in the location and construction of bathing facilities and/or the production and distribution of soap, and/or the use and promotion of suitable alternatives. (The Sphere Project, 2018)

Water Security. In the decade since the terrorist attacks of September 11, 2001, the EPA has redoubled efforts to promote security at America's 168,000 public drinking water and 16,000 wastewater facilities. Through the National Drinking Water Advisory Council (NDWAC) and the Community-Based Water Resiliency initiative, the EPA partners with states and communities to help increase security of U.S. water systems (EPA, 2017a). One specific action the EPA has taken is to facilitate water supply vulnerability analysis. The EPA does this by assisting drinking water suppliers to assess infrastructure and address any weaknesses in its facilities, as well as to develop tools and technical assistance to assist utilities as they work to determine vulnerabilities to attack and prepare emergency response plans. In addition, they work to promote information sharing through a partnership to set up a secure Information Sharing and Analysis Center that will alert water utilities of potential terrorist intentional acts.

Sanitation

During a disaster or complex emergency, sewage systems (a complex network of pipes) may be damaged, plugged, or flooded, causing waste to spill into the environment and exposing people to a number of different hazards. The purpose of a sanitation system is to contain human excreta at the moment of defecation so that it is not free to spread through the environment, and thus to prevent the spread of diarrheal illness. Safe disposal of human excreta creates the first barrier to excreta-related disease, helping to reduce transmission through direct and indirect routes. Safe excreta disposal is therefore a major priority, and in most disaster situations should be addressed with as much speed and effort as the provision of safe water supply. The provision of appropriate facilities for defecation is one of a number of emergency responses essential for people's dignity, safety, health, and well-being. Reestablishing sanitation is the single most important protective measure that can be taken following a disaster (Landesman, 2005). The types of sanitation options in disaster response vary according to location and include latrines, flush toilets, and defecation fields (most frequently used in developing countries). The Sphere Project proposes the following minimum standards for excreta disposal in disaster relief efforts.

Access to Toilets

Excreta Disposal Standard 1: *Access to, and Numbers of, Toilets*
People have adequate numbers of toilets, sufficiently close to their dwellings, to allow them rapid, safe, and acceptable access at all times of the day and night.

Key points
A maximum of 20 people use each toilet.
Use of toilets is arranged by household(s) and/or segregated by sex.
Separate toilets for women and men are available in public places (markets, distribution centers, health centers, etc.).
Shared or public toilets are cleaned and maintained in such a way that they are used by all intended users.
Toilets are no more than 50 meters (164 ft) from dwellings.
Toilets are used in the most hygienic way and children's feces are disposed of immediately and hygienically. (The Sphere Project, 2018)

Emergency sanitation systems must also address the following issues:

- Communication must occur to notify people of the location of the facilities and to encourage their use.
- Paper, water, and soap must be located in or near the toilet facilities to ensure personal hygiene. Handwashing should be promoted.
- Women are provided a place with the necessary privacy for washing or disposing of sanitary protection products.
- Cleaning and maintenance routines for public toilets are established and function correctly and regularly.

Design of Toilets

Excreta Disposal Standard 2: *Design, Construction, and Use of Toilets*
Toilets are sited, designed, constructed, and maintained in such a way as to be comfortable, hygienic, and safe to use.

Key points
Users (especially women) have been consulted and approve of the location and design of the toilet.
Toilets are designed, built, and located to have the following features:

- *They are designed in such a way that they can be used by all sections of the population, including children, older people, pregnant women, and physically and mentally disabled people.*

- *They are located in such a way as to minimize threats to users, especially women and girls, throughout the day and night.*
- *They are sufficiently easy to keep clean to invite use and do not present a health hazard.*
- *They provide a degree of privacy in line with the norms of the users.*
- *They allow for the disposal of women's sanitary protection, or provide women with the necessary privacy for washing and drying sanitary protection cloths.*
- *They minimize fly and mosquito breeding.*
- *All toilets constructed that use water for flushing and/or a hygienic seal have an adequate and regular supply of water.*
- *Pit latrines are at least 30 meters (98.42 ft) from any ground-water source and the bottom of any latrine is at least 1.5 meters (4.92 ft) above the water table. Drainage or spillage from defecation systems must not run toward any surface water source or shallow groundwater source.*
- *People wash their hands after defecation and before eating and food preparation.*
- *People are provided with tools and materials for constructing, maintaining, and cleaning their own toilets if appropriate. (The Sphere Project, 2018)*

Mortality and morbidity rates among displaced populations in the first days and weeks following a disaster are often much higher than rates among the same population after the situation is stabilized. Thus, providing some sanitation facilities during the first days of the crisis is critical. Regardless of the type of facility used, it needs to be established before the population arrives at the site or soon after.

FOODBORNE ILLNESS

Foodborne illnesses are defined as diseases, usually either infectious or toxic in nature, caused by agents that enter the body through the ingestion of food. Every person is at risk of foodborne illness. Foodborne illness is usually classified in one of three ways: food infections, food poisoning, or chemical poisoning (Merrill & Timmreck, 2006).

"Food infections" are a result of the ingestion of disease-causing organisms (pathogens), such as bacteria and microscopic plants and animals. Examples of food infections are salmonellosis, giardiasis, amebiasis, shigellosis, brucellosis, diphtheria, tuberculosis, scarlet fever, typhoid fever, and tularemia. "Food poisoning" is the result of toxins formed in foods prior to consumption, often the waste products of bacteria. Staphylococcus food poisoning is a milder form of food poisoning, producing cramps and a short bout of diarrhea about 6 hours after consumption. The most serious and deadly form of food poisoning is that of botulism. "Chemical poisoning" is caused by poisonous chemicals from animals and plants that end up in the food.

Food Safety

Food safety is an increasingly important public health issue. Governments all over the world are intensifying their efforts to improve food safety (WHO, 2007). These efforts are in response to an increasing number of food safety problems and rising consumer concerns regarding contamination.

Magnitude of Foodborne Illness

Foodborne diseases are a widespread and growing public health problem, both in developed and developing countries. The global burden of foodborne disease is difficult to estimate; however, roughly 2.2 million people die each year as the result of diarrheal diseases (accounting for 5% of global mortality). A great proportion of these cases can be attributed to contamination of food and drinking water. Additionally, diarrhea is a major cause of malnutrition and the leading cause of death among children under 5 years of age.

In industrialized countries, the annual percentage of people suffering from foodborne diseases has been reported to be up to 30%. In the United States, the CDC estimates that 48 million people get sick from foodborne diseases, resulting in 128,000 hospitalizations and 3,000 deaths each year (CDC, 2016).

Although less documented, developing countries bear the brunt of the problem because of the presence of a wide range of foodborne diseases, including those caused by parasites. The high prevalence of diarrheal diseases in many developing countries may be associated with large population movements, but also suggests major underlying food safety problems.

Although most foodborne diseases are sporadic and often not reported, foodborne disease outbreaks may take on massive proportions. For example, in 1994, an outbreak of salmonellosis caused by contaminated ice cream occurred in the United States, affecting an estimated 224,000 persons (Hennessy et al., 1996; Vought & Tatini, 1998). In 1988, an outbreak of hepatitis A, resulting from the consumption of contaminated clams, affected some 300,000 individuals in China (Halliday et al., 1991).

Emergence of Foodborne Illness. New foodborne disease threats occur for a number of reasons. These include disaster conditions, an increase in international travel and trade, microbial adaptation, and changes in the food production system, as well as human demographics and behavior (such as complex emergencies).

- *The globalization of the food supply:* A large outbreak of cyclosporiasis occurred in North America in 1996 to 1997, linked to contaminated raspberries imported from South America (Herwaldt, Ackers, & Cyclospora Working Group, 1997).
- *The inadvertent introduction of pathogens into new geographical areas: Vibrio cholerae* was introduced into waters off the coast of the southern United States when a cargo ship discharged contaminated ballast water in 1991 (Cohen et al., 2012).
- *Travelers, refugees, and immigrants exposed to unfamiliar foodborne hazards while abroad:* International travelers and refugee populations may become infected by foodborne pathogens that are uncommon in their countries. It is estimated that about 90% of all cases of salmonellosis in Sweden are imported.
- *Changes in microorganisms:* Changes in microbial populations can lead to the evolution of new pathogens, development of new virulent strains in old pathogens, development of

antibiotic resistance that might make a disease more difficult to treat, or to changes in the ability to survive in adverse environmental conditions.

- *Change in the human population:* The population of highly susceptible persons is expanding worldwide because of aging, malnutrition, HIV infections, and other underlying medical conditions. Age is an important factor in susceptibility to foodborne infections. Those at the extremes of the age spectrum have either not developed or have partially lost protection from infection. In particular, for the elderly, foodborne infections are likely to invade the bloodstream and lead to severe illness with high mortality rates. People with a weakened immune system also become infected with foodborne pathogens at lower doses, which may not produce an adverse reaction in healthier persons. Seriously ill persons, suffering, for example, from cancer or AIDS, are more likely to succumb to infections with *Salmonella, Campylobacter, Listeria, Toxoplasma, Cryptosporidium,* and other foodborne pathogens. In developing countries, reduced immunity because of poor nutritional status renders people, particularly infants and children, more susceptible to foodborne infections.
- *Safety in food preparation:* Unhygienic preparation of food provides ample opportunities for contamination, growth, or survival of foodborne pathogens. Lack of handwashing and poor personal hygiene are associated with a number of foodborne illnesses including hepatitis A, shigellosis, giardiasis, and gastroenteritis. Improper food storage (caused by electricity failure), inadequate cooking, and poor personal hygiene are common causes of foodborne illnesses following a disaster.
- *Disaster conditions:* Lack of adequate storage facilities and refrigeration will threaten the integrity of a community's food supply.
- *Vulnerability of the nation's food supply:* The targeting of the nation's food supply by terrorist groups is currently a major concern for the U.S. government.

Major Foodborne Diseases From Microorganisms

Salmonellosis is a major problem in many countries. Salmonellosis is caused by the *Salmonella* bacteria and symptoms are fever, headache, nausea, vomiting, abdominal pain, and diarrhea. Examples of foods involved in outbreaks of salmonellosis are eggs, poultry and other meats, raw milk, and chocolate.

Campylobacteriosis is a widespread infection. It is caused by certain species of *Campylobacter* bacteria and in some countries, the reported number of cases surpasses the incidence of salmonellosis. Foodborne cases are caused mainly by foods such as raw milk, raw or undercooked poultry, and drinking water. Acute health effects of campylobacteriosis include severe abdominal pain, fever, nausea, and diarrhea. In 2% to 10% of cases, the infection may lead to chronic health problems, including reactive arthritis and neurological disorders.

Infections due to *enterohemorrhagic* (causing intestinal bleeding) *Escherichia coli,* for example, *E. coli* O157, and *listeriosis*, are important foodborne diseases that have emerged over the last decades. Although their incidence is relatively low,

they are severe infections with sometimes fatal health consequences, particularly among infants, children, and the elderly, making them among the most serious foodborne infections.

Pathogenic *E. coli* strains, such as *E. coli* O157, which produce a potent toxin, cause hemorrhagic infections in the colon resulting in bloody diarrhea or life-threatening complications such as kidney failure. *E. coli* O157 outbreaks have been related mainly to beef consumption; however, sprouts, lettuce, and juice have also been found to cause outbreaks.

Listeria monocytogenes is the cause of listeriosis, which has a fatality rate of up to 30%. The most frequent effects are meningitis and miscarriage or meningitis of the fetus or newborn. Many types of foods have been implicated in listeriosis cases. Often, a prolonged refrigeration period seems to have contributed to outbreaks.

Cholera is a major public health problem in developing countries and has caused enormous economic losses. The disease is caused by the bacterium *Vibrio cholerae.* In addition to water, contaminated foods can be the vehicle of infection. Different foods, including rice, vegetables, millet gruel, and various types of seafood have been implicated in outbreaks of cholera. Symptoms include abdominal pain, vomiting, and profuse watery diarrhea and may lead to severe dehydration and possibly death, unless fluid and salt are replaced.

Bovine spongiform encephalopathy (BSE), a fatal, transmissible, neurodegenerative disease of cattle, was first discovered in the United Kingdom in 1985. The cause of the disease was traced to an agent related to scrapie in sheep, which contaminated recycled bovine carcasses used to make meat and bone meal additives for cattle feed (www.aphis.usda.gov/animal_health/animal_diseases/scrapie). Recycling of the BSE agent led to a distributed common source epidemic of more than 180,000 diseased animals in the United Kingdom alone. The agent affects the brain and spinal cord of cattle, and lesions are characterized by sponge-like changes visible under a microscope. At this time, 19 countries have reported endemic BSE cases, and the disease is no longer confined to the European community; a case of BSE has been reported in a cattle herd of Japan.

In human populations, exposure to the BSE agent (probably in contaminated bovine-based food products) has been strongly linked to the 1996 appearance of a new transmissible spongiform encephalopathy of humans called "variant Creutzfeldt–Jakob disease" (vCJD).

Foodborne Illness Investigation

The 1993 Jack-in-the-Box epidemic caused by *E. coli,* which received widespread media attention, brought concern for food protection and preparation into the national limelight. Hamburger meat contaminated in meat processing plants was identified as the possible source of infection. Over 400 people became ill and four children died as a result of consuming the contaminated meat (CDC, 1993b).

Even if an epidemic of staphylococcal food poisoning is occurring (e.g., being acquired from a fast-food restaurant), most people simply take care of themselves at home. Hundreds of persons could be involved, but the medical and public health community might never know. The outbreak is short, individuals recover quickly, a physician is rarely seen, and the outbreak is not always reported to the public health department. In more serious foodborne and waterborne illnesses, such as salmonella, giardia, amoebic dysentery, and shigella, people do not recover so quickly; the symptoms are stronger, last longer, and medical intervention is usually needed. These diseases are serious and sometimes cause death; thus, they are more likely to be reported.

Investigation of a foodborne illness requires interviews, if possible, of all persons (ill and well) who were present at the time of the ingestion of suspect foods. Merrill and Timmreck (2006) describe those factors necessary to a good investigation as follows:

- Discovering who ate the food
- Discovering who did not eat the food
- For each food, calculating the attack rates among those who ate the food
- For each food, calculating the attack rates among those who did not eat the food
- Computing the relative risk—the ratio of the attack rate of those eating the food to those who did not eat the food

Steps in investigating a foodborne disease epidemic are listed in the following:

1. Obtain a diagnosis and disease determination.
2. Establish that an outbreak has taken or is taking place.
3. Determine which foods are contaminated and which are suspect.
4. Determine if toxigenic organisms, infectious organisms, or chemical toxins are involved.
5. Ascertain the source of contamination. How did the food become contaminated?
6. From determining the source of poison and contamination, ascertain how much growth or the extent of contamination that could occur.
7. Identify foods and people implicated in the containment and intervene to stop further spread of the disease.
8. Ensure medical treatment.
9. Exercise intervention, prevention, and control measures.
10. Develop and distribute reports to inform those who need to know—private citizens, appropriate leaders, and public officials (Merrill & Timmreck, 2006).

Challenges in Food Safety

Modern intensive agricultural practices contribute to the increase in the availability of affordable food and contribute to the use of food additives that can improve the quality, quantity, and safety of the food supply. Appropriate controls, however, are necessary to ensure their proper and safe use along the entire food chain. Other challenges that need to be addressed to help ensure food safety include the globalization of trade in food, urbanization, international travel, environmental pollution, deliberate contamination, and natural and man-made disasters. The food production chain has become more complex, providing greater opportunities for contamination (both intentional and nonintentional) and the growth of pathogens.

Food Safety Is Essential for Disease Prevention in the Aftermath of a Disaster

WHO has issued the following recommendations for ensuring the safety of food supplies following a disaster event (WHO, 2005):

KEY 1: Keep Clean (Prevent the Growth and Spread of Dangerous Microorganisms)

- Wash your hands with soap and water (or other means such as wood ashes, aloe extract, or diluted bleach) after toilet visits, before and after handling raw food, and before eating.
- Avoid preparing food directly in surroundings flooded with water.
- Wash/sanitize all surfaces and equipment—including hands—used for food preparation.
- Protect kitchen areas and food from insects, pests, and other animals.
- Keep persons with diarrhea or other symptoms of disease away from food preparation areas.
- Keep fecal material away from food preparation areas (separate kitchen and toilet areas).
- Avoid eating food (e.g., vegetables or fruits) raw if they may have been flooded (see also Key 5).

Dangerous microorganisms are widely found in the gut of animals and people and also in water and soil in areas with poor sanitation as well as in areas with flooding. These microorganisms can be transferred to food and can, even in low numbers, cause foodborne disease.

KEY 2: Separate Raw and Cooked Food (Prevent the Transfer of Microorganisms)

- Separate raw meat, poultry, and seafood from ready-to-eat foods.
- Separate animal slaughtering and food preparation areas.
- Treat utensils and equipment used for raw foods as contaminated—wash and sanitize before other use.
- Store separately raw (uncooked) and prepared foods.
- Avoid contamination with unsafe water—ensure water used in food preparation is potable or boiled.
- Peel fresh fruits before eating.

Raw food, especially meat, poultry, seafood, and their fluids may contain dangerous microorganisms that can be transferred onto other foods during food preparation and storage. Prevent the transfer of microorganisms by keeping raw and prepared food separate. Remember that cooked food can become contaminated through the slightest contact with raw food, unsafe water, or even with surfaces where raw food has been kept.

KEY 3: Cook Thoroughly (Kill Dangerous Microorganisms)

- Cook food thoroughly, especially meat, poultry, eggs, and seafood, until it is steaming hot throughout.

- For cooked meat and poultry to be safe, their juices must run clear and no parts of the meat should be red or pink.
- Bring foods like soups and stews to boiling and continue to boil for at least 15 minutes to make sure all parts of the food have reached at least 70°C (158°F).
- Although cooked food should generally be eaten immediately, if necessary, thoroughly reheat cooked food until it is steaming hot throughout.

Proper cooking kills dangerous microorganisms. The most important microorganisms are killed very quickly above 70°C (158°F), but some can survive up to 100°C (212°F) for minutes. Therefore, all cooked food should generally reach boiling temperatures and be cooked at such temperatures for extended periods. Remember that big pieces of meat will heat up only slowly. It is also important to remember that in emergency situations with the potential for significant contamination levels in food, the food should be cooked for longer periods.

KEY 4: Keep Food at Safe Temperatures (Prevent Growth of Microorganisms)

- Eat cooked food immediately and do not leave cooked food at room temperature longer than 2 hours.
- Keep cooked food steaming hot (more than 60°C or 140°F) prior to serving.
- Cooked and perishable food that cannot be kept refrigerated (below 5°C or 41°F) should be discarded.

Microorganisms multiply quickly if food is stored at ambient temperature—multiplication is quicker the higher the temperature and quickest at around 30°C to 40°C (86°F–104°F). The higher the number of microorganisms in the food, the higher the risk of foodborne disease. Most microorganisms cannot multiply in food that is too hot or too cold (higher than 60°C or lower than 5°C).

In the event of a power loss, refrigerators will keep food cold for approximately 4 to 5 hours, if unopened. Blocks of ice or dry ice can be used to extend the life of food. Only foods that have a normal color and odor should be consumed, and perishable foods should be discarded after 2 hours at room temperature regardless of their appearance or smell. Frozen food can be kept frozen with dry ice, but once thawed must be immediately cooked or discarded. As with refrigerated food, frozen food that thaws and has been at room temperature for 2 hours must be discarded.

Canned foods and unopened dry mixes will stay fresh for up to 2 years if stored in a cool, dry place away from any heat source. Cans that bulge or leak should be discarded. Flooded food supplies not in cans should be discarded. All stored food containers should be dated to monitor and rotate for maximum freshness.

KEY 5: Use Safe Water and Raw Materials (Prevent Contamination)

- Use safe water or treat it to make it safe through boiling or treatment with chlorine tablets (rapid boil for at least 1 or 2 minutes; treated to kill bacteria by adding chlorine or

iodine tablets or 1/8 teaspoon of unscented Clorox bleach per gallon of water; the solution must be mixed thoroughly and left sitting for at least 30 minutes).
- Wash or preferably cook vegetables and peel fruits that are eaten raw.
- Use clean containers to collect and store water and clean utensils to dispense stored water.
- Select fresh and wholesome foods; discard damaged, spoiled, or moldy food.
- Breastfeed infants and young children at least up to the age of 6 months.

Raw materials, including water, may be contaminated with microorganisms and dangerous chemicals, especially in areas hit by flooding. Likewise, the risk of vegetables and fruits being contaminated with water containing sewage is high under a flooding disaster. Toxic chemicals may be formed in spoiled and moldy foods. Safe water may be seriously contaminated with dangerous microorganisms through direct contact with hands or unclean surfaces. Breastfeeding protects infants against diarrhea through its anti-infective properties, and minimizes their exposure to dangerous foodborne microorganisms.

For more information, see the following website: www.who.int/foodsafety/consumer/5keys/en/index.html and www.who.int/foodsafety/foodborne_disease/en/.

The WHO Food Safety Program (see Figure 19.3) and other WHO programs work on strengthening food safety systems, promoting good manufacturing practices, and educating retailers and consumers about appropriate food handling. Education of consumers and training of food handlers in safe food handling is one of the most critical interventions in the prevention of foodborne illnesses (Figure 19.3).

Shelter From the Elements

When a disaster displaces individuals and families from their homes, finding safe shelter and protection from the elements becomes of paramount importance. Variability in climate, based on geographical location and the postdisaster meteorological conditions, creates health issues based on exposure to heat or cold. Exposure to cold in northern climates is directly associated with hypothermia, frostbite, and stress-related cardiovascular events. Additionally, living in cold conditions increases daily caloric demands to maintain the same activity level, regardless of sufficient and proper clothing. In general, approximately 1% more calories are needed for each degree below 20°C (68°F). Therefore, someone whose house temperature is 10°C (50°F) requires 10% greater food intake to sustain a normal activity level (Landesman, 2005).

Personal Hygiene

Health promotion during disasters or public health emergencies must address issues related to personal hygiene and in particular hand hygiene (CDC, 2017c). Personal hygiene is the single most important determinant of health and, at the same time, can be the most difficult behavior to change. Personal health habits are deeply rooted in cultural and religious beliefs and may vary significantly from population to population. Different languages often do not have comparable concepts or descriptions

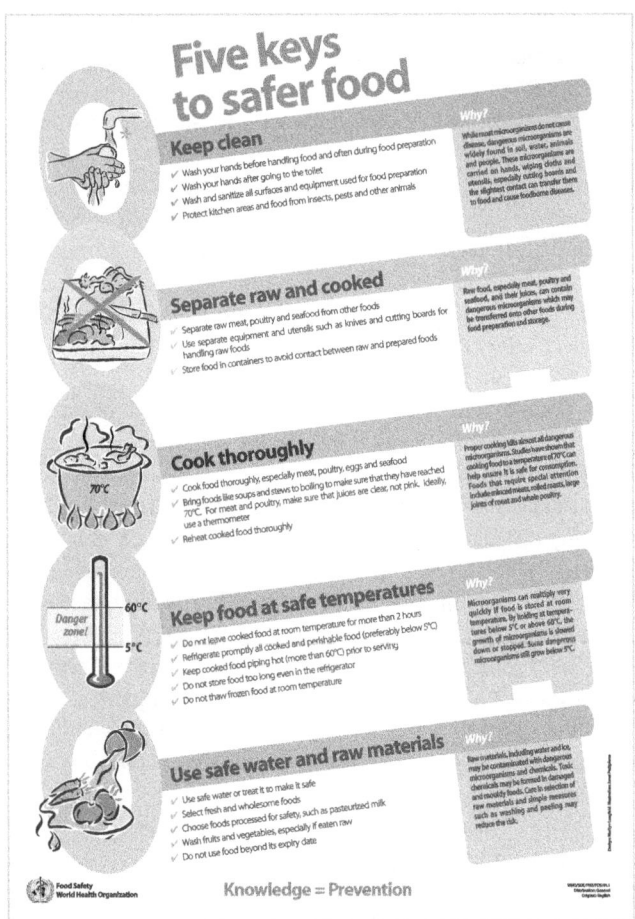

FIGURE 19.3 The WHO food safety program.

Source: World Health Organization. (n.d.) Five keys to safer food. WHO/SDE/PHE/FOS/01.1. Retrieved from http://www.who.int/foodsafety/publications/consumer/en/5keys_en.pdf

for "privacy" or "diarrheal illness." Personal hygiene habits will influence the overall health of the population regardless of the infrastructure and resources provided during a disaster response; the importance of soap and handwashing as a protection against fecal–oral illness cannot be overestimated. Soap provides protection against disease and, therefore, soap and water must be provided to all disaster victims and responders. Education, encouragement, and evaluation are also components of an effective health promotion campaign designed to improve personal hygiene practices. Education alone will not change behaviors, and nurses will find that they need to have the resources present (soap, water, basins, towels, alcohol-based hand purifiers) and be very persistent with insisting on their use.

Vector Control

Major environmental disasters such as tornadoes, floods, and earthquakes are known to displace many types of living organisms—human beings being but one of them. The disturbance of rats and many types of insects can create the potential spread of infectious disease following a disaster. Vectorborne diseases are a major cause of illness and death in many national and international situations. Depending on the location of the disaster, malaria is the vectorborne disease of greatest concern to public health. In the United States, monitoring of mosquito

infestations along with mosquito spraying is a routine part of posthurricane surveillance systems. Flies have been implicated in the transmission of diarrheal disease. Lice may carry typhus. Rats are known to destroy food stores, damage property and electrical wiring, and spread a number of diseases such as salmonella, plague, and leptospirosis. Nuisance pests such as bed bugs can cause physical discomfort and loss of sleep.

Vectorborne disease is a complex and challenging problem that often requires the interventions of professional experts in vector control. In the event of a situation where this expertise is not immediately available, there are simple and effective measures that nurses can take to reduce the spread of vectorborne disease. The Sphere Project establishes three standards for vector control:

1. *Individual and family protection.* All disaster-affected people have the knowledge and the means to protect themselves from disease and nuisance vectors that are likely to represent a significant risk to health or well-being.
2. *Physical, environmental, and chemical protection measures.* The numbers of disease vectors that pose a risk to people's health and nuisance vectors that pose a risk to people's well-being are kept to an acceptable level.
3. *Good practice in the use of chemical vector control methods.* Vector control measures that make use of pesticides are carried out in accordance with established international norms to ensure that staff, the people affected by the disaster, and the local environment are adequately protected, to avoid creating resistance to pesticides.

Methods of Vector Control

The control of vectorborne illness begins with making sure that people have access to shelters that are equipped with insect control. Site selection of the shelters is important, and people need to be settled away from a "malarial zone," if at all possible. Mosquito control is most important in geographical areas where malaria is a real health concern. Efforts may include drainage of standing water. Spraying to reduce breeding sites in stagnant water is a safe, simple, and effective way to reduce mosquito-related morbidity. Mosquito netting around beds may reduce exposure to these insects. Intensive fly control may be necessary in areas of high-density populations where there is a significant risk of diarrheal disease.

The purchase, transport, storage, use, and disposal of pesticides must be done according to international standards or those standards in accordance with the EPA. Basic environmental efforts can be taken to reduce the risk of vectorborne disease, such as establishing adequate shelters and a clean water supply and disposal of human and animal excreta and solid waste materials to reduce flies.

Disposal of Solid Waste Materials. Health promotion and disease prevention programs following a disaster must address the disposal of solid waste materials. If organic solid waste materials are not properly disposed, the major risks posed are fly infestation and rat breeding (see Vector Control) and contamination of surface water. Uncollected and accumulating solid waste and debris left after a natural or human-generated disaster may create a depressing and ugly environment, create discontent, and discourage efforts to improve other aspects of environmental health. Solid waste may clog waterways, leading to environmental health problems associated with stagnant and polluted surface water. Ultimately, disease outbreaks will increase.

The Sphere Project (2018) establishes the following minimum standards for solid waste management:

1. *Solid waste collection and disposal.* People have an environment that is acceptably uncontaminated by solid waste, including medical waste, and have the means to dispose of their domestic waste conveniently and effectively.
2. *Solid waste containers/pits.* People have the means to dispose of their domestic waste conveniently and effectively. Waste can be buried or in some cases burned.

Restoration of Electrical Power

The security of energy supply has become a major concern worldwide, given modern society's strong dependence on its adequate delivery. Not only does the functioning of industry, transportation, and communication and computer systems depend on a continuous energy supply, but our style and quality of living collapses when energy fails. Political conflicts, wars, and natural disasters directly threaten energy supply, and important policy concerns are being implemented as countries look at ways to protect themselves (Rudnick, 2011). The occurrence of natural disasters and their impact on electrical power system functioning has been of interest to countries worldwide, particularly in relation to earthquakes and hurricanes. Several countries such as Chile, China, Haiti, Japan, Mexico, the Philippines, Turkey, and the United States have experienced severe earthquakes that resulted in serious damage to their energy supply infrastructure, in addition to the loss of lives and property. The 2017 hurricanes destroyed the energy grid in Puerto Rico. For months, many communities across Puerto Rico had no electricity whatsoever. This secondary technical disaster caused significant morbidity and mortality, yet to be fully quantified. And not only earthquakes, tsunamis, and hurricanes menace electrical infrastructure; havoc can also be caused by severe weather conditions such as typhoons, tornadoes, floods and landslides, ice storms, volcanic eruptions, and even wildfires (Rudnick, 2011).

Restoration of electrical power to disaster-impacted communities is a critical step in restoring public health. For example, in the United States, over 2.5 million Medicare beneficiaries across the country rely on electricity-dependent medical and assistive equipment, such as ventilators and wheel chairs, and cardiac devices. Severe weather and disasters that cause power outages can be life-threatening for these individuals. Many will rapidly seek assistance from first responders, hospitals, and emergency shelters as their backup batteries and equipment begin to fail (HHS, 2017a). In an effort to assist community disaster planners, HHS developed the emPOWER MAP 2.0 (HHS, 2017a). Every hospital, first responder, electrical company, and community member can use the map to find the monthly total of Medicare beneficiaries with electricity-dependent equipment claims at the national, state, territory, county, and zip code level and turn on "real-time" natural hazard and National Oceanic and Atmospheric Administration (NOAA) severe weather tracking services to identify areas and populations that may be impacted and are at risk of prolonged power outages. Use of this tool helps emergency planners to develop emergency plans and response activities to restore and protect public health and assist at-risk community members prior to, during, and after an emergency. Visit empowermap.hhs.gov/ to learn more about the emPOWER MAP 2.0.

SUMMARY

Populations affected by a disaster may experience severely diminished environmental conditions that put them at risk of negative health outcomes. Health promotion and disease prevention initiatives must be implemented immediately to protect the health of all affected individuals, including meeting basic physiological needs in a timely manner to ensure survival. Infectious disease outbreaks will usually occur in the postimpact and recovery phases of a disaster (not during the acute phase), and the risks of epidemics increase if drought, famine, and/or large displacements of people are involved.

The establishment, implementation, and continuous monitoring of minimum standards for water safety, food safety, sanitation, shelter, and personal hygiene provide a firm foundation for health promotion. Successful planning for potential outbreaks demands that nurses be knowledgeable of the diseases endemic to the disaster area. Food safety is a particular concern, and not only during disaster conditions. Awareness of the emergence of foodborne illnesses is of importance to the health and well-being of the entire population. Restoration of electrical power as soon as possible following a disaster should be a priority. Working in conjunction with their public health colleagues, and as members of an interdisciplinary disaster response team, nurses must be able to detect environmental changes that will increase the potential for the spread of infectious disease.

STUDY QUESTIONS

1. What should health promotion and disease prevention activities focus on in the immediate aftermath of a disaster?

2. Describe health promotion and quality of life. Why are these important in disaster nursing?

3. Apply Maslow's hierarchy of needs theory to disaster nursing. How well can it be applied to disaster conditions? Defend your position. Research nursing theories of health promotion. Is there one that you would use in disaster situations?

4. What are the goals for health promotion in disaster nursing? Develop a response plan for the first 24 hours following a major disaster that works toward achieving these goals. What else should be included in this plan? How would you prioritize your actions?

5. What are the major risk factors for disease outbreaks from disasters?

6. Describe the factors that should be addressed in meeting the water needs of a population affected by disaster.

7. Describe the factors that should be addressed in meeting the sanitation needs of a population affected by disaster.

8. Identify the spectrum of foodborne illness. What is happening to the worldwide incidence of foodborne illness? Why?

9. What are some of the major microorganisms that cause foodborne illness?

10. Design an educational campaign for people who live in a place that is at high risk of a disaster to occur that will inform them of how to prepare food and water supplies.

11. Describe the protection of food supplies following a disaster.

12. Describe a plan for vector control following a disaster. Why is vector control important?

13. Discuss personal hygiene in terms of health promotion. What methods of health promotion would you employ to effect behavioral change in regard to personal hygiene?

14. What populations will be impacted most by loss of electrical power in a disaster?

ACKNOWLEDGMENT

The authors would like to recognize the contributions of a previous chapter author, Joy Reed, EdD, RN, FAAN.

REFERENCES

Atkins, R. B., Williams, J. R., Salinas, R., & Edwards, J. C. (2005). The role of public health nurses in bioterrorism preparedness. *Disaster Management and Response, 3*, 98–105. doi:10.1016/j.dmr.2005.07.004

Berger, E. (2006). Charity hospital and disaster preparedness. *Annals of Emergency Medicine, 47*, 53–56. doi:10.1016/j.annemergmed.2005.12.004

Centers for Disease Control and Prevention. (1993a). Mortality among newly arrived Mozambican refugees. *Morbidity and Mortality Weekly Report, 42*, 468–469, 475–477. Retrieved from https://www.cdc.gov/mmwr/preview/mmwrhtml/00020997.htm

Centers for Disease Control and Prevention. (1993b). Update: Multistate outbreak of Escherichia coli O157:H7 infections from hamburgers—Western United States, 1992–1993. *Morbidity and Mortality Weekly Report, 42*(14), 258–263. Retrieved from https://www.cdc.gov/mmwr/preview/mmwrhtml/00020219.htm

Centers for Disease Control and Prevention. (2016, August 19). Estimates of foodborne illness in the United States. Retrieved from https://www.cdc.gov/foodborneburden/index.html

Centers for Disease Control and Prevention. (2017a, October, 24). Advice for providers treating patients in or recently returned from hurricane-affected areas, including Puerto Rico and US Virgin Islands. CDC Health Advisory; CDCHAN-00408. Retrieved from https://emergency.cdc.gov/han/HAN00408.asp

Centers for Disease Control and Prevention. (2017b). Hurricane season public health preparedness, response, and recovery guidance for health care providers, response and recovery workers, and affected communities. *Morbidity and Mortality Weekly Report, 66*, 995–998. doi:10.15585/mmwr.mm6637e1

Centers for Disease Control and Prevention. (2017c, October 12). Personal hygiene and handwashing after a disaster or emergency. Retrieved from https://www.cdc.gov/disasters/floods/sanitation.html

Cohen, N. J., Slaten, D. D., Marano, N., Tappero, J. W., Wellman, M., Albert, R. J., ... Tauxe, R. V. (2012). Preventing maritime transfer of toxigenic *Vibrio cholerae. Emerging Infectious Diseases, 18*(10), 1680. doi:10.3201/eid1810.120676

Connolly, M. A. (2005). *Communicable disease control in emergencies: A field manual.* Geneva, Switzerland: World Health Organization.

Department of Health and Human Services. (2017a, December 01). HHS emPOWER 2.0 Shaping decisions to protect health in an emergency. Retrieved from https://empowermap.hhs.gov/HHSemPOWERMap2.0Factsheet_Final04072017.pdf

Department of Health and Human Services. (2017b, December 01). The public health system and the 10 essential public health services. Retrieved from https://www.cdc.gov/stltpublichealth/publichealthservices/essentialhealthservices.html

Environmental Protection Agency. (2017a). Drinking Water Advisory Council. Retrieved from https://www.epa.gov/ndwac

Environmental Protection Agency. (2017b). Summary of the safe drinking water act. Retrieved from https://www.epa.gov/sdwa

Esrey, S. A., Potash, J. B., Roberts, L., & Shiff, C. (1991). Effects of improved water supply and sanitation on ascariasis, diarrhoea, dracunculiasis, hookworm infection, schistosomiasis, and trachoma. *Bulletin of the World Health Organization, 69*, 609–621.

Farmer, J. C., Jimenez, E. J., Rubinson, L., & Talmor, D. S. (Eds.). (2004). *Fundamentals of disaster management.* Des Plaines, IL: Society for Critical Care Medicine.

Greenough, P. G. (2007). Infectious disease and disasters. In D. E. Hogan & J. L. Burstein (Eds.), *Disaster medicine* (pp. 44–55). Philadelphia, PA: Lippincott Williams & Wilkins.

Halliday, M. L., Kang, L. Y., Zhou, T. R., Hu, M. D., Pan, Q. C., Fu, T. Y., ... Hu, S. L. (1991). An epidemic of hepatitis A attributable to the ingestion of raw clams in Shanghai, China. *Journal of Infectious Disease, 164*, 852–859.

Hennessy, T. W., Hedberg, C. W., Slutsker, L., White, K. E., Besser-Wiek, J. M., Moen, M. E., ... Osterholm, M. T. (1996). A national outbreak of *Salmonella enteritidis* infections from ice cream. *New England Journal of Medicine, 334*(20), 1281–1286. doi:10.1056/NEJM199605163342001

Herwaldt, B. L., Ackers, M. L., & Cyclospora Working Group. (1997). An outbreak in 1996 of cyclosporiasis associated with imported raspberries. *New England Journal of Medicine, 336*(22), 1548–1556. doi:10.1056/NEJM199705293362202

Institute of Medicine. (1988). *The future of public health.* Washington, DC: National Academies Press. doi:10.17226/1091

Landesman, L.Y. (2005). *Public health management of disasters: The practice guide* (2nd ed.). Washington, DC: American Public Health Association.

Landesman, L. (2011). *Public health management of disasters: The practice guide* (3rd ed.). Washington, DC: American Public Health Association.

Maslow, A. (1970). *Motivation and personality* (2nd ed.). New York, NY: Harper & Row.

Merrill, R. M., & Timmreck, T. C. (2006). *An introduction to epidemiology* (4th ed.). Boston, MA: Jones & Bartlett.

Merson, H., Black, R. E., & Mills, A. J. (Eds.). (2006). Complex humanitarian emergencies. In *International public health: Diseases, programs, systems, and policies* (pp. 439–510). Gaithersburg, MD: Aspen.

Nightingale, F. (1858). *Notes on matters affecting the health, efficiency and hospital administration of the British army.* London, UK: Harrison and Sons.

Noji, E. K. (1996). Disaster epidemiology. *Emergency Medicine Clinics of North America, 14*, 289–300. doi:10.1016/S0733-8627(05)70252-2

Noji, E. K. (2000). The public health consequences of disasters. *Prehospital Disaster Medicine, 15*, 147–157. doi:10.1017/S1049023X00025255

Noji, E. K. (2007). Public health disasters. In D. E. Hogan & J. L. Burstein (Eds.). *Disaster medicine* (pp. 40–44). Philadelphia, PA: Lippincott Williams & Wilkins.

Pender, N., Murdaugh, C., & Parsons, M. A. (2010). *Health promotion in nursing practice* (6th ed.). Upper Saddle River, NJ: Prentice-Hall.

Rudnick, H. (2011). Impact of natural disasters on electricity supply [Guest Editorial]. *IEEE Power and Energy Magazine, 9*(2), 22–26. doi:10.1109/MPE.2010.939922

The Sphere Project. (n.d.-a). *Draft 2 of the Sphere Handbook now ready for review and feedback*. Retrieved from http://www.sphereproject.org/sphere/en/handbook/revision-sphere-handbook/draft-ready-for-feedback

The Sphere Project. (n.d.-b). *The Sphere Project in brief*. Retrieved from http://www.sphereproject.org/about

The Sphere Project. (2018). *The Sphere handbook*. Retrieved from http://www.sphereproject.org/handbook/revision-sphere-handbook

Toole, M. J. (2008). Communicable disease and disease control. In E. K. Noji (Ed.), *The public health consequences of disasters* (pp. 79–100). New York, NY: Oxford University Press.

Turncock, B. J. (2009). *Public health: What is it and how it works* (4th ed.). Sudbury, MA: Jones & Bartlett.

Vought, K. J., & Tatini, S. R. (1998). Salmonella enteritidis contamination of ice cream associated with a 1994 multistate outbreak. *Journal of Food Protection, 61*(1), 5–10. Retrieved from http://jfoodprotection.org/toc/food/61/1

Waring, S. C., & Brown, B. J. (2005). The threat of communicable diseases following natural disasters: A public health response. *Disaster Management and Response, 3*, 41–47. doi:10.1016/j.dmr.2005.02.003

Winslow, C. E. A. (1920). The untilled fields of public health. *Modern Medicine, 2*, 183–191.

World Health Organization. (1948). *Constitution of the World Health Organization*. Retrieved from http://apps.who.int/gb/bd/PDF/bd47/EN/constitution-en.pdf?ua=1

World Health Organization. (1979). The risk of disease outbreaks after natural disasters. *WHO Chronicle, 33*, 214–216.

World Health Organization. (1986). Ottawa Charter for Health Promotion. Retrieved from http://www.who.int/hpr/NPH/docs/ottawa_charter_hp.pdf

World Health Organization. (2005). Ensuring food safety in the aftermath of natural disasters: Annex: 5 Keys for safer food—In regions hit by disasters. Retrieved from http://www.searo.who.int/entity/emergencies/documents/guidelines_for_health_emergency_fsadvice_tsunami.pdf?ua=1

World Health Organization. (2007). Fact sheet: Food safety and foodborne illness. Retrieved from http://www.who.int/mediacentre/factsheets/fs399/en

World Health Organization. (2009). Milestones in health promotion: Statements from global conferences. Retrieved from http://www.who.int/healthpromotion/Milestones_Health_Promotion_05022010.pdf

World Health Organization. (2011). Environmental health in emergencies and disasters: Frequently asked questions in case of emergencies. Retrieved from http://www.who.int/water_sanitation_health/emergencies/qa/en

World Health Organization. (2017). Water—too much or too little—The foremost cause of natural disasters. Retrieved from http://www.who.int/features/archives/feature203/en

Appendix 19.1

Ten Essential Functions of Public Health

HOW PUBLIC HEALTH SERVES (THE PRACTICE OF PUBLIC HEALTH)

In nondisaster times, public health serves communities and individuals within them by providing an array of essential services. Many of these services are invisible to the public. Typically, the public becomes aware of the need for public health services only when a problem develops (e.g., an epidemic occurs). *The practice of public health becomes the list of essential services.* Both distinct from and encompassing clinical services, public health's role is to assure the conditions necessary for people to live healthy lives through communitywide prevention and protection programs.

Monitor Health Status to Identify and Solve Community Health Problems. This service includes accurate diagnosis of the community's health status; identification of threats to health and assessment of health service needs; timely collection, analysis, and publication of information pertaining to access, utilization, costs, and outcomes of personal health services; attention to the vital statistics and health status of specific groups that are at higher risk than the total population; and the management of integrated information systems in successful collaboration with private providers and health benefit plans.

Diagnose and Investigate Health Problems and Health Hazards in the Community. This service includes epidemiological identification of emerging health threats; public health laboratory capability equipped with modern technology to conduct rapid screening and high-volume testing; active infectious disease epidemiology programs; and technical capacity for epidemiological investigation of disease outbreaks and patterns of chronic disease and injury.

Inform, Educate, and Empower People About Health Issues. This service involves social marketing and targeted media public communication; the provision of accessible health information resources at the community level; active collaboration with personal healthcare providers to reinforce health promotion messages and programs; and joint health educational programs with schools, churches, and worksites.

Mobilize Community Partnerships and Action to Identify and Solve Health Problems. This service involves convening and facilitating community groups and associations—including those not typically considered to be health related—in undertaking defined preventative, screening, rehabilitation, and support programs, as well as skilled coalition-building ability to draw on the full range of potential human and material resources in the cause of community health.

Develop Policies and Plans That Support Individual and Community Health Efforts. This service requires leadership development at all levels of public health; systematic community- and state-level planning for health improvement in all jurisdictions; development and tracking of measurable health objectives as a part of continuous quality improvement strategies; joint evaluation with the medical system to define consistent policy regarding prevention and treatment services; and development of codes, regulations, and legislation to guide the practice of public health.

Enforce Laws and Regulations That Protect Health and Ensure Safety. This service involves full enforcement of sanitary codes, especially in the food industry; full protection of drinking water supplies; enforcement of clean air standards; timely follow-up of hazards, preventable injuries, and exposure-related diseases identified in occupational and community settings; monitoring quality of medical services (e.g., laboratory, nursing homes, and home healthcare); and timely review of new pharmacological, biological, and medical device applications.

Link People to Needed Personal Health Services and Ensure the Provision of Healthcare When Otherwise Unavailable. This service (often referred to as "outreach" or "enabling" services) includes assuring effective entry for socially disadvantaged people into a coordinated system of clinical care; culturally and linguistically appropriate materials and staff to ensure access to services by special population groups; ongoing *care management*; transportation services; targeted health information to high-risk population groups; and technical assistance for effective worksite health promotion and/or disease prevention programs.

Ensure a Competent Public and Personal Healthcare Workforce. This service includes education and training for personnel to meet the needs for public and personal health services; efficient processes for licensure of professionals and certification of facilities with regular verification and inspection follow-up; adoption of continuous quality improvement and lifelong learning within all licensure and certification programs; active partnerships with professional training programs to assure community-relevant learning experiences for all students; and continuing education in management and leadership developmental programs for those charged with administrative and executive roles.

Evaluate Effectiveness, Accessibility, and Quality of Personal and Population-Based Health Services. This service calls for ongoing evaluation of health programs, based on analysis of health status and service utilization data, to assess program effectiveness and provide information necessary for allocating resources and reshaping programs.

Research for New Insights and Innovative Solutions to Health Problems. This service includes continuous linkage with appropriate institutions of higher learning and research and an internal capacity to mount timely epidemiological and economic analyses and conduct needed health services research.

Source: From Turncock, B. J. (2009). *Public health: What it is and how it works* (3rd ed.). Sudbury, MA: Jones & Bartlett.

20

THE ROLE OF THE PUBLIC HEALTH NURSE IN DISASTER RESPONSE

Janice Springer

LEARNING OBJECTIVES

When this chapter is completed, readers will be able to:

1. Discuss the role of the public health nurse (PHN) within a multidisciplinary emergency response team.
2. Understand the basic tenets of public health nursing and their application to practice during a disaster.
3. Describe existing population-based resources the PHN can use to assist the victims of all-hazards incidents.
4. Acknowledge the importance of the PHN in the early detection of emerging infections resulting in rapid identification, containment, and response within the community.
5. Appreciate the importance of nursing leadership in preparing for large-scale public health emergencies.

KEY MESSAGES

PHNs practicing to the full extent of their education and licensure as clinical experts can assure the provision of high-quality, evidence-based care for populations affected by disasters.

The role of the PHN in a disaster event must be recognized and understood by all partners within a multidisciplinary emergency response team.

The role of the PHN must continue to evolve and expand to reflect the changing landscape of public health practice.

The guiding principles of public health nursing practice are well suited to the role of the PHN in a disaster.

PHN leaders should actively participate as full partners in disaster preparedness and mitigation activities.

CHAPTER OVERVIEW

The rich history of public health nursing illustrates the enduring contribution nurses have made in responding to disasters and aiding communities in their recovery process. Public health has always been about protecting and promoting the health of entire communities. From the time Florence Nightingale walked the halls of the wards at Scutari, PHNs have used their skills of assessment, intervention, and evaluation to improve health outcomes. Their influence has contributed to the development of local, regional, state, and national policies that have positively affected the lives of countless individuals. Today's public health nursing workforce continues in the tradition embodied by Nightingale, delivering services to assure that community members have access to preventive care, immunizations, safe food and water, and contact with needed services that may fall outside of medical needs. Public health nurses provide leadership in planning, preparing, and responding to disasters and public health emergencies.

Public health promotes and protects the health of people and the communities where they live, learn, work, and play. From conducting scientific research to educating about health, the public health workforce strives to assure the conditions in which people can be healthy and promotes wellness by encouraging healthy behaviors. Public health works to track disease outbreaks, prevent injuries, and shed light on why some of us are more likely to suffer from poor health than others.

The provision of comprehensive public health services is critical to the nation's health and well-being, and to homeland security and defense. While nurses from all specialties of practice may be called to participate in this response, PHNs in particular will need to make critical on-site decisions that will impact the victims and acute care institutions that must receive them. Global natural disasters and the emergence of new and virulent infectious diseases illustrate the importance for the PHN to continue to build expert knowledge and skill sets. The PHN is an integral part of a multidisciplinary disaster response team. PHNs play an integral role in meeting the National Preparedness Goal, part of the National Preparedness System defined as "A secure and resilient nation with the capabilities required across the whole community to prevent, protect against, mitigate, respond to and recover from the threats and hazards that pose the greatest risk (Association of Public Health Nurses, 2014; Federal Emergency Management Agency [FEMA], 2013). In 2011, the U.S. Department of Health and Human Services and the Centers for Disease Control and Prevention (CDC) published a fundamental document for planning in disaster for the Public Health System, *Public Health Preparedness Capabilities: National Standards for State and Local Planning.* PHNs and planners across the nation have focused on 15 critical areas of preparedness organized in alignment with the Public Health Domains of Biosurveillance, Community Resilience, Countermeasures and Mitigation,

Incident Management, Information Management, and Surge Management (CDC, 2011a, 2011b). The intent to create a national standard of readiness includes specific areas of public health responsibilities:

1. Community Preparedness
2. Community Recovery
3. Emergency Operations Coordination
4. Emergency Public Information and Warning
5. Fatality Management
6. Information Sharing
7. Mass Care
8. Medical Countermeasure Dispensing
9. Medical Material Management and Distribution
10. Medical Surge
11. Non-Pharmaceutical Interventions
12. Public Health Laboratory Testing
13. Public Health Surveillance and Epidemiological Investigation
14. Responder Safety and Health
15. Volunteer Management

In reviewing the key functions of each of these capabilities, public health must take leadership roles in determining risks, building partnerships, coordinating response, managing the response, communicating among partners, and assuring health and behavioral health resources are available to the public impacted by the events. PHNs are key to these contributions.

THE UNIQUE CONTRIBUTION OF THE PHN

In the years since the tragic events of 9/11, the United States has witnessed the increasing incidence of catastrophic events. Examples include: Hurricane Sandy in 2012, massive floods in Louisiana and Texas in 2016, the devastation of the 2017 hurricane season with consequences of flooding of Houston, evacuation of millions from Florida, devastation of Puerto Rico and the islands, and climate-influenced events such as wildfires in the west. Multilayered support systems and ongoing training are now standard procedure in local and state jurisdictions to better prepare nurses to respond to disasters and public health emergency events. Public health nursing draws on a wide variety of disciplines to adopt a population-based perspective on disease (Figure 20.1), and bring their expertise along with clinical skill sets designed to address natural disasters and the biological, chemical, and radiological threats that responders may encounter. In an emergency response effort, PHNs must continue their commitment to promote the broader health of the communities they serve.

The PHN is called on to "protect the health of populations using knowledge from nursing, social and the public health sciences" (American Public Health Association [APHA], 2013). Building partnerships within their community, the PHN assures ongoing access to the resources necessary to maintain the health of the public they serve.

The key characteristics of public health nursing practice include: (a) a focus on the health needs of an entire population, including the inequities and unique needs of subpopulations;

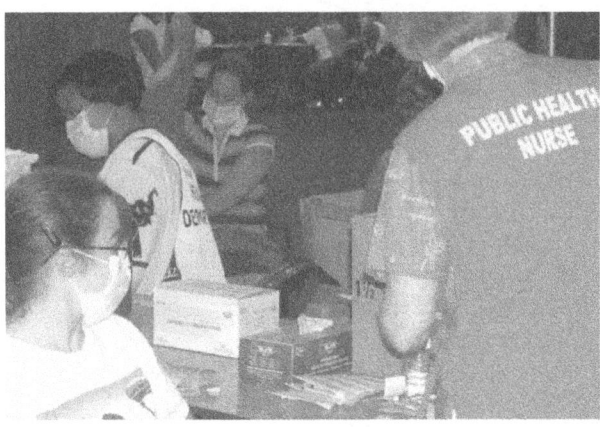

FIGURE 20.1 Public health nurse.

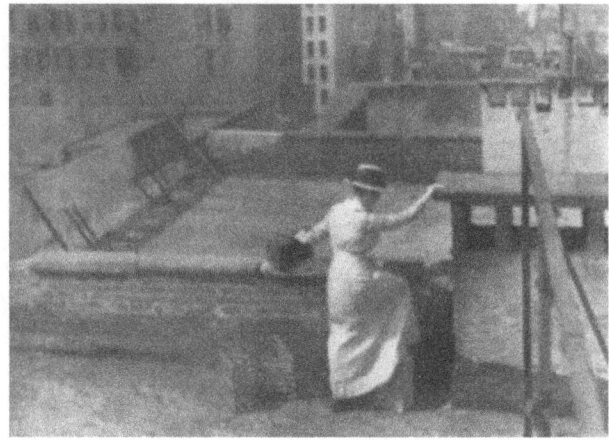

FIGURE 20.2 Early public health nurse.

(b) assessment of population health using a comprehensive, systematic approach; (c) attention to multiple determinants of health; (d) an emphasis on primary prevention; and (e) application of intervention at all levels—individuals, families, communities, and the systems that impact their health. PHNs use skills to advocate for their district by working with elected officials to institute change. These tenets of public health nursing practice make PHNs well suited to perform effectively in an emergency event.

Competencies for public health preparedness are described within the doctrine of several organizations: Public health nursing competencies (Quad Council of Public Health Nursing Organizations, 2012) and the Public Health Foundation (2010) promote the public health preparedness and response core competencies as a generic "all-hazards" guidance for planning training. Additionally, the International Council of Nurses (ICN, 2009) released their Framework of Disaster Nursing Competencies to build the capacity of nurses at all levels to better respond to a disaster. These competencies include skill sets that fall naturally within the realm of public health nursing's scope of practice.

The ICN framework for disaster nursing competencies includes:

1. Risk Reduction, Disease Prevention, and Health Promotion
2. Policy Development and Planning
3. Ethical Practice, Legal Practice, and Accountability
4. Communication and Information Sharing
5. Education and Preparedness
6. Care of Communities
7. Care of Individuals and Families
8. Psychological Care
9. Care of Vulnerable Populations (Special Needs Populations)
10. Long-Term Care Needs

Historical Perspective

Lillian Wald recognized public health nursing as a distinct discipline within the profession as early as 1915. Miss Wald first used the term "public health nurse" in 1893 to describe those nurses who practiced in the community. One can, however,

look further back to the years when Florence Nightingale used her skills of patient assessment to improve hospital care for Crimean War casualties. Drawing on observations of incidence and mortality, her written reports to the War Department in England resulted in meaningful hospital reform. Nightingale's commitment to evidence-based decision making and her understanding of the broader environmental context of health (Nightingale, 1859) helped cement the role of epidemiology in public health nursing practice (Figure 20.2).

McDonald (2001) notes that Florence Nightingale practiced evidence-based nursing 150 years ago. Her actions embodied the principles of *assessment, assurance*, and *policy development* and laid the groundwork for modern public health nursing. Nightingale's dedication was recognized by the establishment of a statistics department at a London college for the purpose of tracking disease patterns among hospital patients. Today, PHNs are challenged to learn and apply newly gained knowledge in a field that is rapidly expanding its scholarly framework. The clinical expertise of the PHN combined with a broad understanding of the community and its population is the basis of evidence-based nursing. Harkness (2011) states that evidence-based nursing is the integration of the best evidence on hand combined with the clinical competency the nurse brings to patient care. She goes on to explain that evidence-based public health draws upon research gleaned from the fields of science and the social sciences. Pairing this with the existing skill sets that the modern PHN brings to practice on a daily basis, it is fair to say that Miss Nightingale's foray into evidence-based nursing continues to this day.

Emerging Roles

PHNs are a recognized and appreciated part of their communities. Like all branches of nursing, they benefit from an established history of public trust. With their expertise in coordinating and implementing large-scale programs that address the needs of the community, PHNs are part of a public health leadership role in disaster response. This was evident between April 2009 and April 2010 when strategies to reach multiple at-risk populations were initiated in an effort to prevent the spread of H1N1 (Borse et al., 2013). In 2014, when Ebola virus disease broke out in west Africa, the U.S. public health system, including PHNs, was called upon to be prepared for their communities and to educate (Itano, Croker, Tormey, & Kim, 2014); in 2017, 180,000 people were evacuated due to an imminent dam breach in California, and PHNs were key to health support in shelters (E. Guzik, personal communication, April 2017). While the public health workforce has always prepared for and responded to community disasters, current threats to our communities necessitate training on a new and different level. The times in which we now live make it imperative that public health nursing keep pace with the demand for skills in the disaster and emergency response arenas.

ROLE OF THE PHN IN A DISASTER

Healthcare providers are often first responders and frequently first receivers of victims in times of disaster and public health emergencies. These events mandate that all healthcare providers have the appropriate education and training to deal with unusual challenges and use resources effectively. The PHN plays a vital role at the time of a disaster and it is critical that the PHN has a clear understanding of the close collaboration required among all types of health professionals—those involved with direct patient care, the emergency management system, and/or the public health system.

Employing the art and science of nursing with established public health sciences, that is, epidemiology, statistical analyses, and incident response and management, PHNs are prepared to do the following in an emergency response effort:

- Assess the needs of the whole community, including potentially at-risk populations, as the event unfolds based on the information available.
- Conduct surveillance activities within the health department as well as in cooperation with in-hospital infection control practitioners to control the spread of communicable disease.
- Assure the health and safety of themselves as well as their fellow responders.
- Maintain communication with local, state, or federal agencies, assuring the accurate dissemination of information to colleagues and the public-at-large.
- Operate points of distribution (POD) mass countermeasures centers as needed.
- Provide on-site triage of victims as needed.

In the United States, the National Response Framework authorizes certain critical functions to occur in a major disaster to maintain a civil and functional society. Immediately after the president declares a national disaster under the Stafford Act, 15 Emergency Support Functions (ESFs) are authorized to operate. Various federal agencies are responsible for the oversight and support of each of these functions (see Chapter 2, "Leadership and Coordination in Disaster Health Care Systems: The U.S. National Preparedness System" for more information). Healthcare providers are involved primarily in ESF 6 Mass Care, providing temporary sheltering and feeding of disaster victims; and ESF-8 Public Health and

Medical Services, providing emergency treatment for injuries related to the disaster.

The American Red Cross shares the support responsibility for providing Mass Care (housing in temporary shelters and meals) with the Department of Homeland Security and FEMA. When shelters are open, healthcare and mental healthcare are available to the clients who need access. It is often the statutory responsibility of the local government to plan for and manage care for its citizens in time of disaster. The language indicates that "Emergency Management *shall* coordinate state agency preparedness for and emergency response to emergencies and disasters; *shall* develop and maintain comprehensive state and local emergency operations plans and emergency management programs, and ensure that other state emergency plans that may be developed are coordinated and consistent with the comprehensive state emergency operations plan" (Minnesota Department of Health, 2016).

Although in approximately 60% of communities the American Red Cross does take a key role in operating shelters, local public health departments and PHNs should be in partnership and support of these operations. It is critical that all PHNs are prepared to establish and sustain operations for a community shelter and to understand how to interface with other response agencies with respect to the care and protection of shelter clients. If the disaster is small enough to be managed locally, the local or state health department may assume the responsibility for management of the event, in which case local PHNs play a major role in the disaster response and recovery operation. In catastrophic evacuations and environmental destruction, as occurred in 2017, the resources of all agencies are stretched, and the PHN roles require strategies to prioritize their expertise across substantial populations of sheltered persons, those impacted by contaminated surroundings, access to potable water, and targeted support of at-risk populations.

ESF-6 Mass Care

Many community shelter sites are predesignated, and the operations managed by the American Red Cross. Shelters must be able to accommodate cots and provide food service, so locations as schools, churches, or meeting halls are used. The local health department may provide PHNs to assist in the shelter and will certainly be responsible for the overall environmental conditions of the shelter. Nurses and other licensed health providers assist in meeting the disaster-related health needs of clients and disaster responders in the shelter environment through assessment, care, casework and data collection and surveillance (American Red Cross, 2017). In 2010, FEMA published a document to assist emergency managers and shelter operators in understanding and better preparing for the whole community, including persons with disabilities, access and functional needs, to be served in disaster shelters. Access and functional needs support services (FNSS) are services that enable individuals to maintain their independence in a general population shelter. Supportive services and equipment may involve obtaining replacement of durable medical equipment, consumable medical supplies, or other goods and services as needed. PHNs may be involved in these efforts and can play a major role in assisting Red Cross nurses with caring for these populations. FNSS are defined as services that enable individuals to maintain their independence in a general population shelter. FNSS includes:

- Reasonable modification to policies, practices, and procedures
- Durable medical equipment (DME)
- Consumable medical supplies (CMS)
- Personal assistance services (PAS)
- Other goods and services as needed

Children and adults requiring FNSS may have physical, sensory, mental health, and cognitive and/or intellectual disabilities affecting their ability to function independently without assistance.

Others who may benefit from FNSS include women in late stages of pregnancy, elders, and people needing bariatric equipment (FEMA, 2010).

The nursing care model for shelters is a relationship-based model of anticipatory care called Cot-to-Cot© (Springer & Casey-Lockyer, 2016). Nurses, their designees, and shelter workers make frequent rounds within the shelter and use a strategy called CMIST to do ongoing assessment of the client population and individuals over time. CMIST is an acronym to describe Communications, Maintaining Health, Independence, Supervision/Support/Self-Determination, and Transportation (Kailes & Enders, 2007). This assessment model moves away from a medical diagnosis framework to a more public health and independent-living model to support clients based on support needs for maintaining independence, and consequently, resiliency.

As described by Klaucke et al. (1988) in the *Morbidity and Mortality Weekly Report (MMWR)*, "Surveillance describes and monitors health events through ongoing and systematic collection, analysis, and interpretation of health data for the purpose of planning, implementing, and evaluating public health interventions" (pp. 1–18). Surveillance is a critical function within public health departments, and an essential skill for the PHN. A specific way to consider surveillance in a setting such as a disaster shelter is as a systematic way for early identification of acute illness patterns (e.g., fevers, diarrhea, respiratory illness) to be identified and reported; and/or how patterns and trends of illness and injuries that might be common to disaster shelter clients can be trended over time. Ideally this is done on an every 24-hour basis and the data are organized within the context of the daily shelter population demographics. In a setting such as a flood, the PHN might gather community data around exposure to hazardous materials (HAZMAT) from the flood waters as evidenced by symptoms, or after an explosion, changes in respiratory illness patterns in a neighborhood downwind from the plume.

ESF-8 Public Health and Medical Services

This ESF incorporates all of the services related to health during and after a disaster. It includes but is not limited to:

1. Assessment of health needs of the community
2. Surveillance of disease within the community
3. Potable water, waste water, and solid waste disposal
4. Drug and medical device safety
5. Rescue workers' health and safety
6. Mental healthcare
7. Vector control
8. Mortuary service
9. Veterinary service

Because the PHN knows the location and availability of community resources well and has worked with many of the agencies and individuals in the community, the PHN can play an important role in many of the activities related to ESF-8.

The PHN may be called upon to assist in a rapid needs assessment to determine the magnitude of the disaster and the impact on essential services, such as potable water supply, food supply, shelter, electricity, and sanitation capacity. The PHN must be prepared for disruption of routine health services—hospitals may be damaged; there may be environmental hazards and interruption of communication systems—all of which may lead to psychological stress within the population.

PHNs are population focused in their practice and can make significant contributions in community assessment, program planning, and minimizing the risk of communicable diseases. They can also recognize possible problematic responses to disaster situations and make referrals to the appropriate agencies. Surveillance is a critical skill in such times. The PHN must be capable of detecting unusual patterns of disease or injury, identifying persons at risk, implementing control measures, and informing the community of treatments and preventive measures. The CDC developed a now well-tested strategy for community surveillance called "CASPER"—the Community Assessment for Public Health Emergency Response (CDC, 2012). This tool enables public health practitioners and emergency management officials to determine rapidly the health status and basic needs of the community. PHNs are often community leaders in the management of the CASPER outreach process.

ROLE OF THE PHN IN PREVENTION AND HEALTH EDUCATION

PHNs will proclaim that prevention and health education make up the greatest portion of their work on a daily basis. Thus, prevention and education in preparation for disasters in the community should be a primary focus. The PHN may play a leadership role in the development of community disaster plans and in educating the public about disaster preparedness activities. The PHN must be sensitive to the variety of groups within the community and design the appropriate level of education and training for each of these target groups. Well-designed and delivered community disaster preparedness education may ensure that a greater number of lives are saved during a major disaster.

Families

- Families should be aware of the most common types of natural disasters for the geographical areas in which they live. Preparations should be made according to the probability of those kinds of emergency situations.
- Family members should know how to use a fire extinguisher and how to turn off utilities—gas, water, and electricity.
- The family should have a predesignated meeting place where they will gather if a disaster occurs when they can reunite, such as a church or school outside the immediate neighborhood.
- They should identify an out-of-town contact person and be sure that every member of the family has that telephone number. Sometimes it is easier to contact someone in another state than it is across town. This out-of-town contact person would receive telephone calls from members of the family to reunite them if they are separated during the disaster.
- Every family should assume that any assistance from response agencies will not be available immediately and they will be required to survive on their own for several days. Therefore, the home should contain the following emergency supplies:
  - Water: at least 0.5 gallon of drinking water per person per day
  - Food that does not require refrigeration or cooking, such as canned fruits, vegetables, and cereal, protein bars, and comfort food
  - Nonelectric (mechanical) can opener
  - Prescription and nonprescription medicines
  - First aid kit
  - At least one change of clothing for each family member
  - Blankets and bedding
  - Sanitation supplies such as soap, toilet paper, detergent, household bleach, personal hygiene items
  - Flashlights with extra batteries
  - Battery-powered radio and batteries
  - Approximately $500.00 in cash because ATMs may not be operable
  - Medicine dropper used to sanitize water—16 drops of chlorine bleach to 1 gallon of water
  - Duct tape
  - Important family documents—copies should be kept in a waterproof container, such as passports, wills, insurance policies, bank account numbers, motor vehicle records, social security cards, and copies of credit cards or identification cards
  - Pet supplies

Include items for the family pet, such as carriers, food, medicine, a photograph of the pet, as well as a list of veterinarians. Be sure that the pet has identification including phone numbers on a collar or embedded in a body microchip. Some people make arrangements for neighbors to take the pet if the family is away from the home at the time of the disaster. Many people will not evacuate their homes if they cannot take their pets with them. Some motels will take pets especially during an emergency and many communities have organized "pet-friendly" shelters. The American Red Cross works with community partners to assure that there are plans for persons with pets in times of sheltering.

Shelters must accommodate service animals, as interpreted through the Americans with Disabilities Act.

Community Groups

The PHN is one of a few healthcare professionals who interacts with many different groups in the community on a regular and established basis. When preparing a community for a disaster or public health emergency, the nurse must be available to assist a broad spectrum of groups such as schools, businesses, churches or other faith-based groups, other community organizations, and jails.

Primary and Secondary Schools

The American Red Cross has developed the Ready Rating Program which provides guidelines for schools to use when planning their disaster response (www.readyrating.org/Schools/ReadyRatingEssentials).

The 123-point Red Cross's Ready Rating 123 Assessment Tool and Ready Rating 123 Program Guide are the result of a comprehensive review of preparedness recommendations conducted by the American Red Cross National Office of Preparedness and Health and Safety Services, the national Ready Rating team, and the American Red Cross Scientific Advisory Council. All Ready Rating Program steps and recommendations are grounded in scientific research, best practices, and/or expert opinion from respected professionals representing multiple disciplines and perspectives.

Unfortunately, terrorist experts believe that schools may be targets for terrorism. Terrorists attempt to create fear and anxiety to achieve their goals. Every school should have a crisis management plan that includes partnering with the local emergency preparedness office, law enforcement, and fire and health departments. The plan should also address such emergencies as school shootings or man-made emergencies. There should be a command structure for those responding to a crisis. Key members must be familiar with their defined roles and how they relate to other responders. Every school is required to conduct fire drills each year, and since the event at Sandy Hook Elementary School in Newtown, CT, in December 2012, where 28 children and teachers were killed, school districts have implemented more comprehensive strategies for how to reduce violence, make schools safer, and increase access to mental health services (Cowan & Vaillancourt, 2013). Consideration must be given to physically or mentally challenged students who may have disabilities, mental health needs, or other access or functional support needs during these events. If the school has a school nurse, this individual is often part of the team charged with developing and maintaining the emergency response plan for the school. However, the PHN can raise the awareness of a need for such a plan and the PHN can review and assist in revising or expanding the plan. Many school districts no longer employ a nurse in each school and, as such, those responsibilities fall to the PHN in the community.

The U.S. Department of Education provides a website titled "Practical Information on Crisis Planning for Schools and Communities" (2017b; www2.ed.gov/admins/lead/safety/emergencyplan/crisisplanning.pdf).

They suggest some steps in planning for disasters in a school, such as the following:

1. Describe the types of crises the school plans to address.
2. How will the school operate during the crisis?
3. Develop methods for communicating with the staff, students, families, and the media.
4. Obtain necessary equipment and supplies.
5. Create maps and facilities information.
6. Provide accountability and student release procedures.
7. Prepare for immediate response—such as evacuation, lock down, or sheltering in place.

Many of the same recommendations apply to college campuses but considerations must be made for larger student bodies and a more open access to college campuses. The 2017 mass shooting in Las Vegas is an example of a type of community event that might engage the support of PHNs and the health department. The U.S. Department of Education offers an Action Guide for Emergency Management at Institutions of Higher Education (2017a; https://files.eric.ed.gov/fulltext/ED515949.pdf).

Faith-Based Groups

A significant number of people in the community can be found in congregational groups, such as churches, mosques, and synagogues. PHNs can present disaster preparedness classes to the social sections within these gatherings. Some of these faith-based groups have a parish or congregational nurse whose focus is the health of that community. The PHN can provide important emergency-related information to the congregational nurse and assist in reviewing disaster plans.

Correctional Institutions

If there is a jail or prison within the community, the PHN should be certain that its disaster plan is up to date and feasible. Security is always the highest priority in these facilities, but the PHN can also offer disaster-related information to the employees of the jail depending on the type of institution in the community. The National Institute for Corrections provides some guidelines in A Guide to Preparing and Responding to Jail Emergencies on their website (nicic.gov/guide-preparing-and-responding-jail-emergencies-self-audit-checklists-resource-materials-case).

Vulnerable Populations

The PHN should assist caregivers of persons living at home who might be considered vulnerable or at risk to be prepared for a disaster by ensuring that these individuals have critical information available at all times. This information might be consolidated in a "go-kit" or may be kept at their bedsides if they are bedridden.

Critical information may include:

- List of medicines and schedule for administration
- Names and telephone numbers of family members
- Eyeglasses and prescription
- Medical devices—hearing aids, prostheses
- Healthcare policies, credit cards, checkbook
- Insurance agent
- Driver's license
- Special dietary need
- A bag containing 72 hours of medicines, warm clothes, sturdy shoes, eyeglasses

If a disaster occurs, and evacuation is necessary, it is vitally important that this information be transported with the evacuee. Methods to store and transport critical data regarding patients in a hospital or long-term care facility in some type of device that the patients can wear on the wrist or around the neck should be considered (see Chapter 7, "Identifying and Accommodating High-Risk, High-Vulnerability Populations in Disasters" for an extensive discussion on Vulnerable Populations).

Post-Disaster Assistance

After Hurricane Katrina in 2005, an executive order was issued to simplify the process of applying for federal assistance. *Disasterassistance.gov* was created as a secure site to consolidate disaster assistance information in one location. Persons who are affected by a federally declared disaster can register online. Seventeen government agencies sponsoring almost 60 forms of assistance contribute to the website. *Disasterassistance.gov* simplifies the application process for applications for FEMA assistance and referral to the Small Business Administration for loans through online applications.

Care of the Caregiver

The PHN who is working with disaster survivors is subject to the same stressors as victims of the disaster. Often the nurse is suffering from personal losses while caring for disaster survivors. The PHN must be aware that any members of the response team may exhibit normal reactions to abnormal situations. Situations that cause stress for nurses may be: not being able to meet basic needs of survivors, inadequate work space and noise, and concern for one's own family. Communication is usually limited and the nurse may not have much information about his or her family. Other stressors for the PHN may be excessive physical demands in the temporary workplace, concern for personal safety, inadequate supplies, and the disorganization and chaos present in most disasters.

Suggestions for PHNs working in disaster response settings are: take frequent breaks, provide mutual support to coworkers, and follow the rules established for disaster workers, such as eating and sleeping schedules. A team approach is mandatory for a successful recovery effort.

Many veteran disaster workers describe delayed stress reactions after returning home from a disaster scene. Some volunteers describe feelings of disappointment with family members who may not be particularly interested in hearing about the details of the disaster. Mood swings are common but should subside within a few weeks after returning home. All of these symptoms are considered to be normal as long as they do not interfere with activities of daily living.

ROLE OF THE PHN IN A BIOLOGICAL EVENT

The CDC has categorized critical biological agents into classifications A, B, and C. Category A agents, anthrax, botulism, plague, tularemia, smallpox, and the viral hemorrhagic fevers, are seen as those agents with the greatest potential to cause mass casualties (see Chapter 30, "Biological Agents of Concern," for further discussion; CDC, 2017a). Categories B and C organisms are composed mainly of emerging infectious threats and existing and regularly occurring biological agents which, if weaponized, will result in widespread illness and deaths. These infectious agents would quickly disable a community and overwhelm the healthcare system (see Chapter 32, "Infectious Disease Emergencies," for further discussion). PHNs see many of these Categories B and C illnesses during day-to-day surveillance of their local area. Salmonella, shigella, *Escherichia coli* (0157; H7), cryptosporidium, and Hantavirus can be found in nature. PHNs who work in state and local health departments are familiar with all facets of planning, detecting, containing, and responding to an outbreak caused by a biological agent. Through an extensive reporting network, PHNs in every state report any unusual incidence of communicable diseases. Surveillance and monitoring efforts in pharmacies may report elevated sales of over-the-counter remedies such as cold preparations, antidiarrheal medications, and pain relievers. These reporting mechanisms serve as early warning systems, assisting public health practitioners to begin a local response based on up-to-date evidence (see Chapter 31, "Surveillance Systems for Detection of Biological Events," for further discussion).

Unlike some nurses who specialize in a defined area of direct patient care, the scope of the practice of PHNs can extend from community pre-event planning, surveillance and detection, delivering care during an event, to post disaster evaluation and recovery. This expanded scope of practice is what makes the PHN such a valued and integral member of an effective disaster response team. PHNs are accustomed to infectious disease management strategies, have pre-existing collaborative arrangements with other community agencies, are used to working with other healthcare professionals in primary and acute care systems, and may be familiar with local law enforcement personnel.

The specific role of each PHN during a biological event is a function of national competencies for public health preparedness, state and local regulations, and his or her home agency's preparedness plan specific to bioterrorism and emergency preparedness competencies (Columbia University School of Nursing Center for Health Policy, 2002). The overlap of these categories is in the areas of analytical assessment skills, basic public health, communications, and community-based practice; however, most of the competencies could apply in some measure to bioterrorism response. Levy and Sidel (2003) have described four overall roles for all health professionals in terrorism and public health. These are: (a) develop improved preparedness, (b) respond to the health consequences of terrorist attacks and threats, (c) take action to prevent terrorism, and (d) promote a balance between response to terrorism and other public health concerns. When aligned with the public health emergency preparedness competencies, these four roles create a framework for the public health nursing response to a biological event.

ROLE OF THE PHN IN INFECTIOUS DISEASE EMERGENCIES

In discussion of the importance of the PHN during a biological event, we have established that infection control is an integral part of public health nursing practice. PHNs are educators who consistently provide information to their communities to prevent or stop the transmission of infectious agents. Recent history supports the fact that new and reoccurring diseases—many of which are drug resistant—are making an impact on preparedness planning and subsequent response activities designed specifically for these novel microbes.

The 20th century saw several pandemics of varying impact. Avian strains of influenza previously not known to infect humans (CDC, 2016b), severe acute respiratory syndrome (SARS), a reemergence of H1N1, and particularly virulent strains of *E. coli, Listeria* and methicillin-resistant *Staphylococcus aureus* (MRSA) infections foretell the need for PHNs to be competent in their response to what will surely become an increase in foodborne, zoonotic, vector, and waterborne diseases as well as new strains of drug-resistant microbes. Modern-day travel can quickly bring an unfamiliar pathogen such as Ebola to the United States, demanding knowledge from the field of public health, and community education from PHNs (CDC, 2014).

Outbreak risk from vaccine-preventable diseases such as measles may be reduced through PHN community education and support—a daunting prospect, certainly, but one that PHNs are well equipped to handle. Determinants that influence the resurgence of both old and new infections include: the ability of the microbe to mutate and adapt to the prevailing treatment protocol; immune suppression of patients due to treatments or other immune compromise; climate and ecosystem changes; international travel, allowing for rapid transmission of existing illness or the introduction of specific microbes into a new environment; increasing numbers of citizens living at or below the poverty level; and the general lack of funding or breakdown of the public health system (Smolinski, Hamburg, & Lederberg, 2003). The PHN's consistent assessment of the district being served and the ongoing efforts to build community coalitions are valuable tools that can be used to identify at-risk or vulnerable populations residing within the district. PHNs who work in rural or medically underserved areas will have considered their demographics and the profile of their communities in their response plan. For instance, a POD location may be established within the geographical area affording the residents access to prophylaxis in the event of an outbreak. Public health is and should be an all-inclusive population-based art and science. The PHN's knowledge of the community served and the resources available places her or him in a position of leadership during the planning and response phases of an outbreak. A perceptive PHN may be the means by which a pattern of infection is first identified while taking a patient history or reviewing local disease reports.

ROLE OF THE PHN IN MEDICAL COUNTERMEASURE DISPENSING

PHNs will often be asked to participate in the implementation of local medical countermeasure dispensing POD plans. POD plans are activated (primarily under the direction of the local county medical director) when large numbers of the population will require vaccination or treatment within a short span of time. One example of this might be when the Strategic National Stockpile is activated, or surveillance activities reveal a community-wide outbreak of a communicable disease. To assist in understanding the PHN's role in a biological disaster, a prehospital model of practice must be defined:

- Follow agency protocol and report to disaster site or to POD center.
- Don appropriate personal protective equipment (PPE; if needed) before approaching site if appropriate. Assure that PHNs are familiar with the location and proper use of PPE as part of the planning process.
- Familiarize yourself with on-site nonclinical and clinical responders and establish yourself as a leader.
- Assess the status of patients at a POD and triage them accordingly.
- Establish a panel of PHNs who will be available to answer citizen questions about the situation at hand and what steps should be taken to stop the spread of communicable disease if appropriate. Prepare, in advance, fact sheets on the most common in communicable diseases, chemical, biological, radiological, nuclear, and explosive agents to distribute if needed.
- Identify a PHN as the liaison between the clinical operations of a response and the Public Information Officer (PIO) to assure accurate transmission of clinical information and the establishment of a go-to PHN on-site.

Triage, perhaps the most important part of the role of the PHN in a biological event, will differ significantly from basic hospital daily triage as practiced in an acute care setting. The symptomatic must be moved to a sick bay as soon as possible and transferred to the closest hospital; exposed persons can proceed through the POD to the dispensing station; the worried well may be seen by nonnursing personnel who will give them accurate information and instructions on how to remain informed. In a disaster, however, there are a few changes that need to be made. To maximize patient throughput for a POD or triage station when speed is of the essence, self-screening of citizens (with PHN review) may be used to lighten the burden.

As an expert in community resource management, a PHN may be assigned exclusively to assisting at-risk or vulnerable populations. For this reason, it is especially important to identify these populations when an emergency plan is being developed.

ROLE OF THE PHN IN A CHEMICAL DISASTER

A chemical emergency occurs when a hazardous chemical has been accidentally or intentionally released and has the potential to harm the health of people (CDC, 2016a). Unlike biological agents, which require an incubation period before symptoms appear, a chemical agent, when released, makes its presence known immediately by means of observation (explosion), self-admission (accidental release), or by the presence of rapidly emerging symptoms, such as burns, redness to the affected area, difficulty breathing, or convulsions. The CDC has classified chemical agents as nerve, incapacitating, pulmonary, blister/vesicant, blood agents, and biotoxins (see Chapter 29, "Chemical Agents of Concern," for further discussion).

In a chemical emergency, the PHN may be called on to do the following:

- Follow agency protocol and report to duty site.
- Don appropriate PPE before approaching disaster site.
- Establish the role of the PHN within the response team.
- Act quickly and assess the status of the victim's airway. Loosen any constrictive clothing and advise patient to sit upright if possible.

Emergency medical service squads may arrive on the scene with water to assist victims to irrigate their eyes as soon as possible. The PHN may assist in this effort until patients can be transferred to the hospital for treatment.

Gross decontamination may occur at the site of the chemical release (see Chapter 35, "Decontamination and Personal Protective Equipment," for further discussion). This involves the removal of the outer layer of clothing followed by washing with soap—or at least a water wash. While ambulatory victims may be able to walk through decontamination under their own power, the PHN may be called on to assist those people who are unable to move freely. Those debilitated most severely will be triaged by the PHN for hospital treatment immediately. The PHN will alert the acute care facility that patients needing decontamination are en route. Most hospitals are able to set up their own decontamination system outside the emergency room, assuring the safety of those patients and staff in-house.

The PHN manager should brief area hospitals to prepare them for walk-in patients not seen at the accident site. Limited nursing documentation needs to be maintained for this activity.

Health departments must prepare to disseminate shelter-in-place information to the residents of surrounding areas. A redundant communication system should also be in place so that citizens can be given an all-clear notification when the event has ended and it is safe to go outside.

PHNs must assure their own safety during a chemical event. After leaving the field, however, decontamination should be carried out before returning to the health department or home. In the event of an evacuation of residents, the PHN may be called on to staff a shelter where assessment of the population will be ongoing.

ROLE OF THE PHN IN A RADIOLOGICAL EVENT

When large doses of radiation are released accidentally (nuclear power plant) or deliberately (terrorist act), there is significant increased risk that adverse health conditions may develop

(CDC, 2017b). Every agency should develop protocols for implementation during a radiological emergency. The PHN should be aware of the following:

Being available to help others will not occur if you do not take steps to protect yourself first.

If by chance you are near the release site, move away from ground zero immediately.

In the event that you are in the area when the event unfolds, minimize your exposure by increasing your distance from the source of radiation and put a shield between you and the source, such as a nearby building.

PHNs working in a receiving station should assume that all victims have been exposed to or contaminated by radiation and should notify the HAZMAT team and don the appropriate level of PPE in advance of people arriving (see Chapter 35, "Decontamination and Personal Protective Equipment," for further discussion).

Once home, remove and bag (if possible) your clothing before entering your home and shower thoroughly using soap and water. Eyeglasses may be decontaminated by vigorously washing them with soap and water, but contact lenses should be thrown away.

ROLE OF THE PHN ON A MULTIDISCIPLINARY RESPONSE TEAM

The importance of the role of the PHN in disaster planning is demonstrated by her or his widespread inclusion on county, regional, and statewide planning committees, and as a key member of healthcare coalitions (Office of the Assistant Secretary for Preparedness and Response, 2012). These committees and coalitions provide opportunity for the PHN to share his or her unique abilities and experiences with the rest of the first responder team, to become a more familiar partner to the hospital team, and to contribute to the community response plan. It is also a chance for the PHN to learn more about what the role of other responders in the field will be. The PHN is well prepared to advise on community resources and make suggestions regarding program planning. By collaborating with other health and human service professionals, the PHN is accustomed to being part of a large interdisciplinary framework. Participation in a disaster response requires developing a better understanding of the duties of one's fellow responders and demonstrating knowledge of one's role.

The functionality of a disaster plan can be appreciated only once it has been tested. Drills and exercises are the best way to test a plan and for PHNs to "try on" their role as a team member. Tabletop exercises are valuable and convenient for in-house drills but a full-scale scenario-based drill involving all facets of the response plan, though expensive to run, offers the most rigorous way to ensure real-world success. Interagency cooperation and coordination are vital to planning, training, and response efforts. The PHN can participate with existing community partners—police, fire, hospital, school system personnel, and social service agencies—to provide support in all phases of emergency preparedness.

SUMMARY

PHNs have been promoting health through prevention, health education, and structured interventions in communities for well over a century. The population-based focus of public health practice has provided many initiatives that improve health and reduce the spread of infectious disease. Emergency preparedness and response for biological, emergent infectious diseases, chemical, and radiological events are part of the mission of public health. With their broad-based clinical knowledge, disease surveillance and management skills, and familiarity with community resources, the PHN is a critical member of the emergency response team.

STUDY QUESTIONS

1. What are the three key characteristics of public health nursing practice?

2. Discuss how public health nursing has had an impact on your community.

3. Describe the six activities in which a public health nurse might engage during disaster response activities.

4. There is a confirmed outbreak of influenza in four counties in your state. What will PHN responders do to protect the community?

5. Why would you do surveillance in a disaster shelter?

6. Describe ways in which your agency/institution can become an active part of disaster planning in your community.

7. Identify strategies to assist your local school nurses with emergency preparedness efforts. What resources might you access to locate guidelines for schools?

8. Identify the roles that a PHN could take as part of a multidisciplinary disaster response team.

REFERENCES

American Public Health Association/Public Health Nursing. (2013). The definition and practice of public health nursing. Retrieved from https://www.apha.org/~/media/files/pdf/membergroups/phn/nursingdefinition.ashx

American Red Cross. (2017). Preparedness essentials. Retrieved from https://www.readyrating.org/Schools/ReadyRatingEssentials

Association of Public Health Nurses. (2014). *The role of the public health nurse in disaster preparedness, response and recovery: A position paper.* Washington, DC: Author. Retrieved from http://www.achne.org/files/public/APHN_RoleOfPHNinDisasterPRR_FINALJan14.pdf

Borse, R. H., Shrestha, S. S., Fiore, A. E., Atkins, C. Y., Singleton, J. A., Furlow, C., & Meltzer, M. I. (2013). Effects of vaccine program against pandemic influenza A(H1N1) virus, United States, 2009–2010. *Emergency Infectious Diseases, 19*(3), 439–448. doi:10.3201/eid1903.120394

Centers for Disease Control and Prevention. (2011a). Notes from the field: Measles outbreak Hennepin County Minnesota, March 2011. *Morbidity and Mortality Weekly Report, 60*(13), 421. Retrieved from https://www.cdc.gov/mmwr/preview/mmwrhtml/mm6013a6.htm

Centers for Disease Control and Prevention. (2011b). *Public health preparedness capabilities: National standards for state and local planning.* Atlanta, GA: Author. Retrieved from https://www.cdc.gov/phpr/readiness/00_docs/DSLR_capabilities_July.pdf

Centers for Disease Control and Prevention. (2012). *Community assessment for public health emergency response (CASPER) toolkit* (2nd ed.). Atlanta, GA: Author.

Centers for Disease Control and Prevention. (2014). Cases of ebola diagnosed in the United States. Retrieved from https://www.cdc.gov/vhf/ebola/outbreaks/2014-west-africa/united-states-imported-case.html

Centers for Disease Control and Prevention. (2016a). Chemical emergencies. Retrieved from https://emergency.cdc.gov/chemical/index.asp

Centers for Disease Control and Prevention. (2016b). Pandemic resources avian influenza (H5N1). Retrieved from https://www.cdc.gov/flu/pandemic-resources/index.htm

Centers for Disease Control and Prevention. (2017a). Preparation and planning for bioterrorism emergencies. Retrieved from https://emergency.cdc.gov/bioterrorism/prep.asp

Centers for Disease Control and Prevention. (2017b). Radiation emergencies. Retrieved from https://emergency.cdc.gov/radiation/index.asp

Cowan, K., & Vaillancourt, K. (2013). Advocating for safe schools, positive school climate and comprehensive mental health series. *Communique, 41*(6), 1.

Federal Emergency Management Agency. (2010). *Guidance on planning for integration of functional needs support services in general population shelters.* Washington, DC: Department of Homeland Security. Retrieved from http://www.fema.gov/pdf/about/odic/fnss_guidance.pdf

Federal Emergency Management Agency. (2013). *Presidential policy directive (PPD) 8 components: Emergency readiness competencies for all public health workers.* Atlanta, GA: Centers for Disease Control and Prevention National preparedness goal, National Preparedness System, National Planning Frameworks. Retrieved from http://www.fema.gov/pdf/prepared/Npg.pdf

Harkness, G. A. (2011). Community and public health nursing: Present, past and future. In G. A. Harkness & R. F. DeMarco (Eds.), *Community and public health nursing evidence for practice* (p. 19). Philadelphia, PA: Wolters Kluwer/Lippincott Williams and Wilkins.

International Council of Nurses. (2009). *ICN framework for disaster nursing competencies.* Geneva, Switzerland: World Health Organization and International Council of Nurses.

Itano, A., Croker, C., Tormey, M., & Kim, M., (2014). *Monitoring West African travelers for Ebola virus disease in Los Angeles County: A three month review* (Acute Communicable Disease Control 2014 Special Studies Report). Los Angeles County, CA: Department of Public Health.

Kailes, J. I., & Enders, A. (2007). Moving beyond "special needs": A function-based framework for emergency management and planning. *Journal of Disability Policy Studies, 17*(4), 230–237. Retrieved from http://www.jik.com/KailesEndersbeyond.pdf

Klaucke, D. N., Buehler, J. W., Thacker, S. B., Parrish, R. G., Trowbridge, F. L., Berkelman, R. L, & Surveillance Coordination Group. (1988). Guidelines for evaluating surveillance systems. *Morbidity and Mortality Weekly Report, 37*(S-5), 1A. Retrieved from https://www.cdc.gov/mmwr/preview/mmwrhtml/00001769.htm

McDonald, L. (2001). Florence Nightingale and the early origins of evidence-based nursing. *Evidence-Based Nursing, 4*, 68–69. doi:10.1136/ebn.4.3.68

Minnesota Department of Health. (2016). Statutes and rules on emergency preparedness, disease outbreaks, and volunteer protections. MN Stat. 12.09, subd. 1, 2, 6, 7. St. Paul, MN: The Office of the Revisor of Statutes.

National Institute for Corrections. A guide to preparing for and responding to jail emergencies: Self-audit checklists, resource materials, case studies. Retrieved from https://nicic.gov/guide-preparing-and-responding-jail-emergencies-self-audit-checklists-resource-materials-case

Nightingale, F. (1859). *Notes on nursing: What it is and what it is not.* London, UK: Her Majesty's Stationery Office.

Office of the Assistant Secretary for Preparedness and Response. (2012). *Healthcare preparedness capabilities: National guidance for healthcare systems preparedness.* Washington, DC: U.S. Department of Health and Human Services. Retrieved from https://www.phe.gov/Preparedness/planning/hpp/reports/Documents/capabilities.pdf

Public Health Foundation. (2010). *Public health preparedness and response core competency model.* Washington, DC: Author.

Quad Council of Public Health Nursing Organizations. (2012). Core competencies for public health nurses, a project of the linkages between academia and public health practice funded by the Health Resources and Services Administration. Retrieved from http://www.achne.org/files/Quad%20Council/QuadCouncilCompetenciesforPublicHealthNurses.pdf

Smolinski, M. S., Hamburg, M. A., & Lederberg, J. (2003). *Microbial threats to health: Emergence, detection and response.* Washington, DC: Institute of Medicine/National Academies Press.

Springer, J., & Casey-Lockyer, M. (2016). Evolution of a nursing model for identifying client needs in a disaster shelter: A case study with the American Red Cross. *Nursing Clinics of North America, 51*(2016), 647–662. doi:10.1016/j.cnur.2016.07.009

U.S. Department of Education. (2017a). An action guide for emergency management of institutions of higher education. Retrieved from https://files.eric.ed.gov/fulltext/ED515949.pdf

U.S. Department of Education. (2017b). Practical information on crisis planning for schools and communities. Retrieved from http://www2.ed.gov/admins/lead/safety/emergencyplan/crisisplanning.pdf

21

CLIMATE CHANGE AND HEALTH: THE NURSE'S ROLE IN POLICY AND PRACTICE

Karen Levin and Thomas Chandler

LEARNING OBJECTIVES

When this chapter is completed, readers will be able to:

1. Describe the real and potential impacts of climate change on human health.
2. Appreciate the physical drivers of climate change.
3. Describe the nurse's role in mitigation and adaptation efforts to reduce climate change impacts on human health.
4. List vulnerable populations at most risk for poor health outcomes related to climate change.
5. Identify new studies that confirm observed climate changes and validate climate models.
6. Describe areas in practice and advocacy where nurses can contribute to addressing climate change and health risks, including how Green Teams can benefit an organization.

KEY MESSAGES

Widespread scientific consensus exists that the world's climate is changing. Some of these changes will likely include more variable weather, heat waves, heavy precipitation events, flooding, droughts, more intense storms, sea level rise, and air pollution. Each of these impacts could negatively affect population health.

While climate change is a global issue, the effects of climate change will vary across geographical regions and populations, with vulnerable populations at higher risk for adverse health consequences.

Healthcare professionals recognize that there is a direct and indirect connection between climate change and human health.

Knowledge of climate change drivers and their effects must be part of the nurse's assessment and decision making in the development of patient and community care plans.
The health of the public must be protected—nurses can play a vital role in the reduction of climate change–related impacts on human health.

CHAPTER OVERVIEW

Widespread scientific consensus exists that the world's climate is changing, with a majority of scientists in agreement that anthropogenic climate change is having increasingly adverse effects on human health (National Aeronautics and Space Administration [NASA] Global Climate Change, 2018; U.S. Global Change Research Program [USGCRP], 2017). Some of these changes include rising temperatures, more variable weather, heat waves, heavy precipitation events, flooding, droughts, more intense storms, sea level rise, and air pollution. Each of these impacts is currently or has the potential to negatively affect population health. While climate change is a global issue, the effects of climate change will vary across geographical regions and populations (Centers for Disease Control and Prevention [CDC], 2017a). The influence of climate change on human health appears in scientific, environmental, and public health literature, and, in more recent years, a growing discussion and advocacy for personal and professional response are present in the nursing literature. This chapter provides an overview of the influence of climate change on health, along with a selection of key findings from surveys exploring nurses' knowledge, beliefs, and challenges in responding to climate change. A wide range of ongoing activities at various practice settings offers resources for further study and action opportunities for nurses and their healthcare partners.

Climate change is widely considered one of the greatest public health threats currently facing humanity. Anthropogenic climate change, together with other natural and man-made health stressors, influences human health and disease in numerous ways (USGCRP, 2017). Some existing health threats will intensify and new health threats will emerge and not everyone is equally at risk. Important considerations of risk for climate change–related health impact include age, economic resources, and location (CDC, 2017a). In the United States, public health can be affected by disruptions of physical, biological, and ecological systems, including disturbances originating domestically and elsewhere. The impact of climate change on human health and the effects of these disruptions include increased respiratory and cardiovascular disease, injuries and premature deaths related to extreme weather events, changes in the prevalence and geographical distribution of food- and waterborne illnesses and other infectious diseases, and threats to mental health. Emphasizing this point, the 2015 Lancet Commission on Health and Climate Change argues that the response to climate change could be "the greatest global health

opportunity of the 21st century" (Watts et al., 2017). Evidence of the drivers of climate change and its impact on human health are further substantiated in USGCRP, 2017: *Climate Science Special Report: Fourth National Climate Assessment, Volume I.*

Built on the vast scientific body of global and climate change work to date, this chapter presents an overview of the basics of climate change. The perspective then shifts to the effects of climate change on human health consequences, what has been done, and what future work needs to be done. Since the days of Florence Nightingale, the practice of nursing has been rooted in "person, environment, and health" as the interrelated determinants of health (McDonald, 2001). Climate change's complex interaction and the social–physical determinants of health fit well into this framework. The nurse's role in mitigation measures to reduce the vulnerabilities of climate change's most negative effects on human health are presented. The illness, injury, death, displacement, and tremendous housing and economic losses as a result of climate change–related events such as the 2017 Atlantic hurricane season and the northern California wildfires reinforce the importance of this work.[1] The nurse's role in patient and community mitigation[2] and adaptation[3] measures to address climate change's most negative impacts on health requires a clear understanding of these interactions and health consequences.

PHYSICAL DRIVERS OF CLIMATE CHANGE

Despite often contentious public and political debate, the physical drivers of climate change are quite clear. Greenhouse gases such as carbon dioxide (CO_2) absorb heat (infrared radiation) emitted from the earth's surface. Since the mid-1800s when humans began to burn coal, gas, and oil, scientists have known that CO_2 is one of the main greenhouse gases of importance to Earth's energy balance. Other greenhouse gases (notably methane and nitrous oxide) are also increasing as a consequence of human activities. The observed global surface temperature rise since 1900 is consistent with detailed calculations of the impacts of the observed increase in atmospheric CO_2 (and other human-induced changes) on Earth's energy balance. Increases in the atmospheric concentrations of these gases cause the earth to warm by trapping more of this heat. Human (anthropogenic) activities—especially the burning of fossil fuels since the start

---

[1] Erdman, J. Atlantic Hurricane Season 2017 is Now Seventh Most Active in History. https://weather.com/en-CA/canada/news/news/2017-10-09-atlantic-hurricane-season-one-of-busiest-october.

[2] Actions being taken to reduce greenhouse gas emissions and to enhance the sinks or traps or remove carbon from the atmosphere.

[3] Actions being taken to lessen the impact on health and the environment due to changes that cannot be prevented through mitigation.

of the Industrial Revolution—have unquestionably increased atmospheric CO_2 concentrations by about 40%, with more than half the increase occurring since 1970 (National Academy of Science and Royal Society, 2015; USGCRP, 2017).

Since 1900, the global average surface temperature has increased by about 0.8°C (1.4°F). This has been accompanied by warming of the ocean, a rise in sea level, a strong decline in Arctic sea ice, and many other associated climate effects. Much of this warming has occurred in the last four decades and detailed analyses have shown that the warming during this period is mainly a result of the increased concentrations of CO_2 and other greenhouse gases. Continued emissions of these gases will cause further climate change, including substantial increases in global average surface temperature and important changes in regional climate. The magnitude and timing of these changes will depend on many factors, and slowdowns and accelerations in warming lasting a decade or more will continue to occur. However, long-term climate change over many decades will depend mainly on the total amount of CO_2 and other greenhouse gases emitted as a result of human activities (National Academy of Science and Building Royal Society, 2015).

There is overwhelming evidence that climate change has contributed to:

- Higher average global temperatures and sea levels
- Decreased sea and land use levels
- Changes in precipitation patterns
- Increased frequency of extreme weather events: heat waves, droughts, hurricanes, and wildfires
- Heavy pollution
- Shifts in animal and plant habitable ranges (Intergovernmental Panel on Climate Change [IPCC], 2014; National Academy of Science and Royal Society, 2015)

Addressing the genesis, impact, and prognosis for the future of climate change includes implementation of strategies designed to limit global energy consumption, reduce fossil fuel emissions, and slow the rate of warming (Department of Defense [DOD], 2014; Hansen et al., 2013; IPCC, 2014; Santer et al., 2017; USGCRP, 2014). Recent studies also emphasize the relationships between human health and climate change (Birnbaum, Balbus, & Tart, 2016; Ebi, Fawcett, Spiegel, & Tovalin, 2016; Marinucci, Luber, Uejio, Saha, & Hess, 2014; USGCRP, 2017).

Climate change connects to a wide range of health issues, ranging from cardiovascular deaths and respiratory illnesses related to heat extremes, to waterborne and vectorborne infectious diseases that are related to disruptions in mosquito, tick, and rodent habitats. Figure 21.1 shows the relationship between climate change and its impact on human health.

Although scientists recognize that some climate changes, such as lower cold-related mortality, will be beneficial, there is consensus that the majority of the changes will be highly detrimental (Bouzid, Hooper, & Hunter, 2013) for a wide range of health issues, with human morbidity rates varying according to geographical regions within the United States and globally (IPCC, 2014; Watts et al., 2017). The National Institute of Environmental Health Studies (NIEHS)-led Interagency Working

Group on Climate Change and Health identified major research areas that need to be further explored and understood (Portier et al., 2010). These include the following:

- Asthma, Respiratory Allergies, and Airway Diseases
- Cancer
- Cardiovascular Disease and Stroke
- Foodborne Diseases and Nutrition
- Heat-Related Morbidity and Mortality
- Human Developmental Effects
- Mental Health and Stress-Related Disorders
- Neurological Diseases and Disorders
- Vectorborne and Zoonotic Diseases
- Waterborne Diseases
- Weather-Created Morbidity and Mortality

The dynamics of climate change's regional weather changes and human exposures, direct or indirect, will be related most directly to extreme weather, flooding, and heat wave events as well as changes in geographical habitats of vectorborne diseases (Barna, Goodman, & Mortimer, 2012). Climate change–related water disasters have been associated with major environmental disruption resulting in exposures to toxins, molds, and infectious agents with resultant significant morbidity and mortality (Veenema et al., 2017). These health concerns represent cross-cutting issues for vulnerable and susceptible populations.

SELECTED HEALTH OUTCOMES

Extreme Weather Events

Wildfires, droughts, hurricanes, heavy rainfall, river flooding, landslides, mudslides, and soil erosion caused or exacerbated by climate change will result in injuries, fatalities, and illness that can result from postdisaster water quality and safety issues and waterborne diseases. Mass shelter care requires a coordinated multiagency response and surge capacity of healthcare personnel to assure adequate delivery of care, placing nurses in multiple roles at the front lines of care (Divakaran, Lembeck, Kerr, Calmus, & Potter, 2016).

Thermal Extremes (Heat and Cold)

Heat-related morbidity and mortality will increase (Schmeltz, Petkova, & Gamble, 2016). Research has demonstrated that the most severe impacts of extreme heat events—caused by air pollution as well as temperature—fall on children, the elderly, the chronically ill, the obese, people with hypertension (particularly if taking diuretics), and people taking psychiatric medications (Ebi, Fawcett, et al., 2016). In warm, dry regions already at risk of wildfires, the fire season could be extended and become more severe, increasing the risk to children and to adults with respiratory diseases who are particularly susceptible to particulates (soot) and carcinogens (D'Amato et al., 2015). Nurses can serve on local, state, and regional adaptation planning bodies for planning related to extreme heat and poor air quality events, identify those in their practices who are at

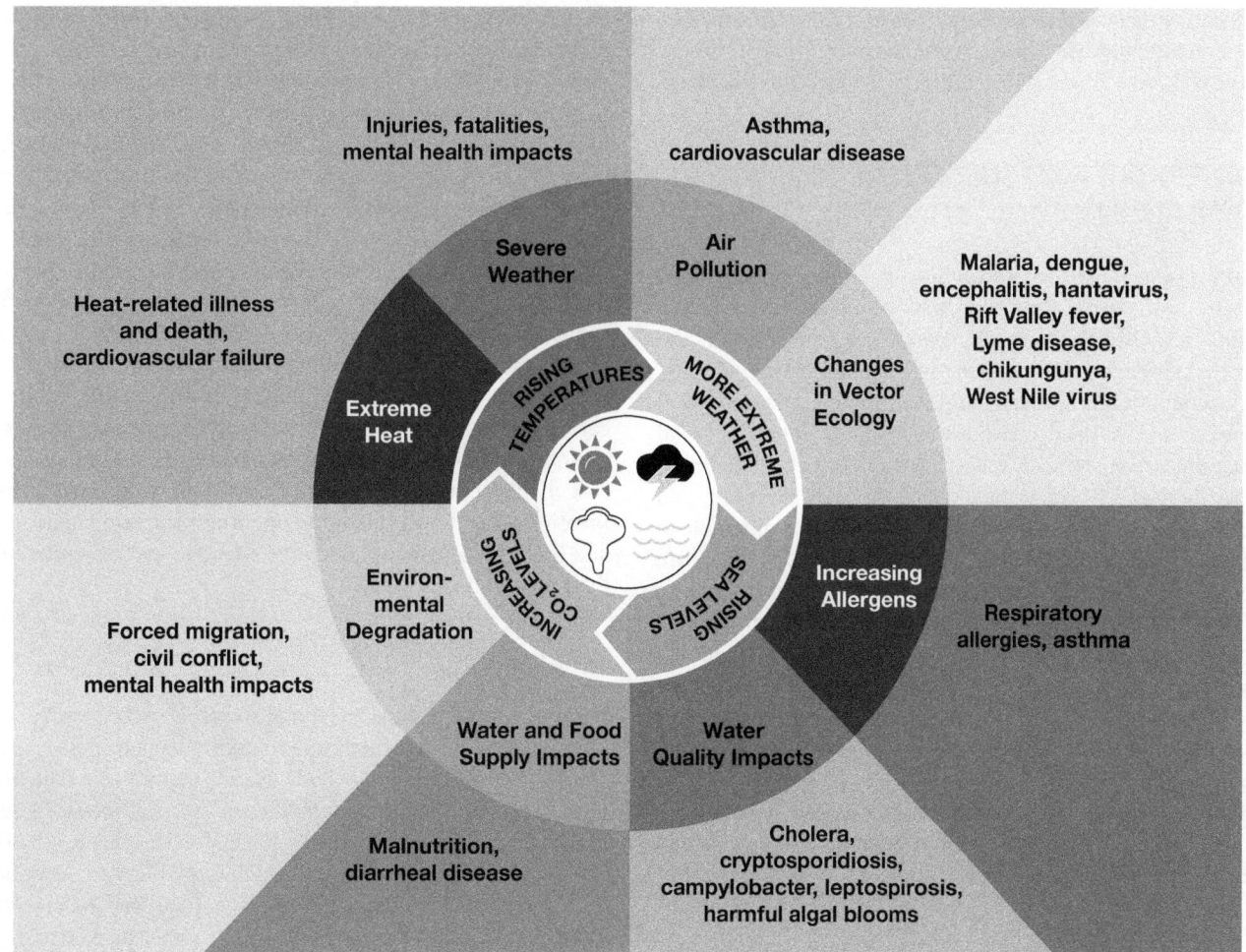

FIGURE 21.1 Impact of climate change on human health.

Source: Centers for Disease Control and Prevention. (2017a). Climate effects on health. Retrieved from https://www.cdc.gov/climateandhealth/effects/default.htm

most risk, including those who work outside in extreme heat, and provide targeted care plans to minimize the health consequences of extreme weather events (Prudent, Houghton, & Luber, 2016).

Vectorborne and Zoonotic Diseases

Climate change has and will continue to expand the habitats of climate-sensitive vectors, increase their reproduction rate, and thereby increase the prevalence of diseases transmitted by mosquitoes, ticks, and rodents[4] (Jia et al., 2017). Integrated vector management is essential to control vectorborne disease transmission. Health action alerts and social mobilization and communication at all levels are critical for ensuring appropriate and effective interagency and community communication between vector control staff and householders, and between partners within and outside the health sector where human-vector exposure occurs (i.e., schools, hospitals, and other workplaces). Nurses can and do provide essential roles in these communications: as collaborators for developing agency health alerts and

risk-prevention measures, and as public spokespeople during disease outbreaks. Nurses have been public spokespeople for health agencies and can collaborate on messaging community alerts, guidance on prevention measures and agency response to vector habitat changes and disease outbreaks. Additionally, nurses can coordinate when and how to use the mass media at national, regional, and local levels in collaboration with public information officers.

Food- and Waterborne Diseases

Climate change–related temperature fluctuations can also affect food- and waterborne infectious diseases[5] such as gastritis, which can be fatal in children (EPA, 2018), particularly those who already have other compromising vulnerabilities and/or illnesses. Lower-lying coastal regions could experience increased flooding, saltwater infiltration, severe and harmful algae blooms (HAB) such as Red Tides, thus increasing susceptibility to various other food- and waterborne diseases (Rossati, 2017). The expected continuation of global warming

---

[4] Malaria, West Nile virus, Eastern equine encephalitis, dengue [27], Rift Valley fever, and tickborne diseases such as Lyme disease.

[5] *Salmonella, Campylobacter, Vibrio spp., Leptospira, Giardia, and Cryptosporidium.*

will lead to increased risk of several food and waterborne diseases including those caused by *Salmonella, Campylobacter, Vibrio cholerae, Leptospirosis, Giardia*, and *Cryptosporidium*.

VULNERABLE AND SUSCEPTIBLE POPULATIONS

Health disparities exist in societies, creating subpopulations that are at higher risk of poor health outcomes. According to the U.S. Global Change Research Program Climate and Health Assessment,[6] key drivers of vulnerability include age, socioeconomic status, race, indigenous peoples, current level of health and regional variations such as floodplains, coastal zones, and urban areas, as well as the resilience of public health infrastructure. Children, the elderly, the sick, the poor, and some minority communities are among the most vulnerable to climate change–related health effects (CDC, 2017b). There are those in our communities who are more susceptible, such as children and the elderly, and those who are more vulnerable, such as people with medical issues, mental health and chronic diseases, and the urban poor who have an increased health risk from environmental exposures. Those who are both susceptible and vulnerable become subject to a magnified risk. Some, whose health will suffer the most, already feel they are at risk (Akerlof, Delamater, Boules, Upperman, & Mitchell, 2015).

Knowledge and awareness of climate change effects and their direct and indirect effects (Figure 21.2) must be part of

the nurse's assessment and decision making. It is critical that nurses have a solid understanding of climate change–sensitive diseases and those who are at risk of negative health outcomes to ensure that mitigation and risk communication strategies incorporate these elements. Nurses must identify those at higher risk of climate change's negative health consequences and ensure that they receive, understand, and can follow risk communications and guidance from all agency health alerts. Furthermore, it is essential that vulnerable communities have input into the planning processes of healthcare agencies and community practitioners to ensure effective risk communications. Nurses are in the best position to bridge and facilitate these connections (Marinucci et al., 2014). Nurses in direct client care, community-based healthcare workers, public health and/or home health nurses can leverage home visits to educate at-risk clients about climate change and health risk connections, identify mitigation, adaptation opportunities, and challenges and provide an action plan that is effective and responsive to their unique needs.

Children

For a variety of physiological and social reasons, children are more susceptible and vulnerable to environmental stresses than adults. They have a smaller body mass to surface area ratio and greater sensitivity to certain exposures such as heat waves (Miller, Marty, & Landrigan, 2016). Their immune and heating regulatory systems are not fully developed and thus are highly susceptible to extreme weather events, air pollution, food- and waterborne diseases, and vectorborne diseases (Ebi, Semenza, & Rocklöv, 2016). School nurses should be alert to children who have known

---

[6] http://nca2014.globalchange.gov/report/sectors/human-health#intro-section-2

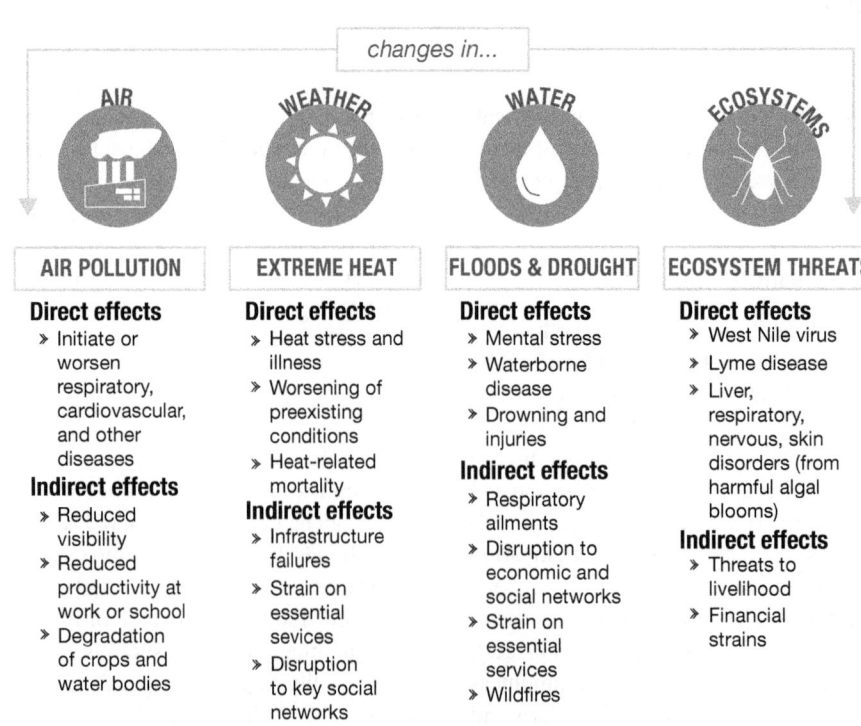

FIGURE 21.2 Direct and indirect health effects of climate change.
Permission granted by Minnesota Department of Health. (2017). Minnesota Climate and Health Program. Retrieved from http://www.health.state.mn.us/divs/climatechange

medical conditions and require intervention during environmental health alerts. In particular, school nurses are in a good position to contribute to policies that can "provide indoor alternatives" on bad air days for asthma-susceptible children[7] (Domrose, 2015).

Elderly

Elderly adults, who often live alone and may have preexisting heart or lung conditions, are especially susceptible to heat-related illnesses, hyperthermia, heat stress,[8] cardiovascular failure, and dehydration, which can lead to falls and other injuries. Nurses who practice in areas with a high elderly population can protect this population by identifying at-risk patients and providing them and their caregivers with guidance about staying well-hydrated, using home air conditioners, and visiting air-conditioned places and cooling centers.

Urban Poor

Poorer residents of high-density, heat-trapping urban environments often have less access to healthcare and "limited adaptive capacities, such as improved building materials, lack of air conditioning or ability to access cooling centers and their limited ability to relocate to a less stressed environment" (Ebi, Fawcett, et al., 2016a). Further, many of these vulnerable populations are located in flood-prone regions which are at risk of increased precipitation and sea level rise. Nurses must identify patients who live and work in these communities and ensure they are aware of their vulnerabilities and, together, create health-risk prevention plans.

Mental Health

Disasters, including climate- and weather-related ones, can induce in people with and without a history of mental illness alike, trauma, shock, anxiety, depression, complicated grief, posttraumatic stress disorder (PTSD), and strains on personal relationships (Trombley, Chalupka, & Anderko, 2017). They can also increase the incidence of alcohol and substance abuse, homicide, suicide, physical abuse, and spousal abuse. Research has further noted that climate change–oriented problems, such as mass migration from a coastal municipality, can induce psychological stressors not originally foreseen (Ziegler, Morelli, & Fawibe, 2017). Nurses should be aware of these potential stressors and be prepared to address them in collaboration with mental health professionals.

THE NURSE'S ROLE IN CLIMATE CHANGE

National studies show that nurses recognize the numerous ways that climate change affects health, yet many feel they are not well enough prepared to meet those challenges. In one study, nurses agreed that public health nursing had the responsibility to address health-related impacts of climate change,

yet some doubted that actions could decrease health-related impacts. Furthermore, most felt they were not prepared and that within their departments they did not have the ability to address health-related impacts of climate change due to limited resources and personnel allocated to this endeavor (Polivka, Chaudry, & Mac Crawford, 2012).

A study among hospital, primary care, and emergency room nurses in Sweden found that public health work was regarded as a health cobenefit of climate change mitigation and that nurses perceived a responsibility for individual and professional commitment to opportunities to positively influence the environment (Anåker, Nilsson, Holmner, & Elf, 2015). A similar study of Canadian nurses concurred with these studies in that nurses were only moderately knowledgeable about climate change and its specific health threats and felt this was an area for further development and training. They expressed interest in climate change as an important determinant of health and the need for integrating it into practice, in agreement with the Canadian Nurses Association's list of nurse actions to address climate change (Angelini, 2017; Laan, 2014).

Nursing is a clinical profession grounded in evidence. A nurse is a researcher and a consumer of research, identifying and translating new and emerging information to the practice setting. Integration of new findings often requires new ways of thinking and acting, engaging and incorporating a system-wide approach to meet healthcare needs both now and in the future. Nurses can apply mitigation and adaptation measures, personally and professionally, to address known and *emerging* health impacts in our changing climate (Angelini, 2017). As revealed in the aforementioned studies, many nurses believe there are negative health outcomes of climate change, believe there is a role for nurses, yet, they express a lack of preparedness for this role and a degree of uncertainty of the most appropriate tasks to carry out. For instance, consider the following description:

> A nurse midwife[9] noticed on days with elevated pollution levels that mothers-to-be with previously controlled asthma came into her office wheezing and struggling for breath, putting themselves and the fetuses they were carrying at risk. She adjusted medications and advised her patients to stay inside on bad air days, but many of them worked and didn't have cars or even air-conditioning. Staying out of the bad air wasn't a reasonable option. She asked herself, "What can I do to help?" (Domrose, 2015)

What Are Nurses Doing?

Collaboration and Practice

The scientific evidence for anthropogenic climate change has been established with increasing precision and as described earlier in this chapter, there are growing concerns about its potential to undermine the public health gains of the past century. There is also a growing consensus across private and public sector organizations at both the national and the

---

[7] Domrose, C. (2015, October 12). Quote from Laura Anderko, PhD, RN, Director of Mid-Atlantic Center for Children's Health and the Environment, School of Nursing and Health Studies, Georgetown University, DC.

[8] Advanced age represents one of the most significant risk factors for heat-related death in the United States (Health Implications of Climate Change Physicians for Social Responsibility) http://www.psr.org/assets/pdfs/heats-deadly-effects-1.pdf

---

[9] Domrose, C. (2015, October 12), Interview, quote from Katie Huffling, MS, RN, CNM, who later testified at an Environmental Protection Agency hearing in the matter of ozone levels and the relationship of air pollution and asthma and asthma and preterm pregnancy.

international levels that carbon reduction must be a policy aim. International nursing organizations have made strong position statements on the issue, arguing that nurses should be actively engaged as part of their roles in both clinical practice and health promotion. Nurses can work with the American Nurses Association (ANA) in the United States and other national and international nursing organizations to advocate for and develop public policies that address climate change at local and regional levels. The ANA has long partnered with environmental agencies and groups such as Healthcare Without Harm,[10] Practice Greenhealth (formerly Hospitals for a Healthy Environment), the U.S. Environmental Protection Agency and the University of Maryland, and collaborated on projects such as the Luminary Project[11] and RN no Harm.[12]

TABLE 21.1 Green Teams: Hospital Health Facilities, Health Clinics, Office-Based Practice

Waste reduction in the hospital	Ensure proper protocols are in place and followed. Can result in reduction in energy wastes and environmental toxicants released into the community.
Purchasing and materials management	Advocate for "environmentally preferable purchasing"; consider the cycle of products from management to disposal; examine products for toxins, i.e., mercury, polyvinyl chloride (PVC), carcinogens, endocrine disruptors
Unused pharmaceuticals	Improper handling of unused medications is one way pharmaceuticals can enter the water supply (Becker, Mendez-Quigley, & Phillips, 2010).
Cleaning products and hazards	Nurses and other employees are at risk of exposure to hazardous materials: housekeeping and sterilization chemicals, pharmaceutical residuals, and other toxins. Nurses and their teams can advocate for safer products, clear labeling, and following label and Occupational Safety and Health Administration (OSHA) directions for use and disposal.
Dietary services	Advocate for fresh and local purchasing, composting.

Source: McDermott-Levy, R. (2011). The nurse's role on green teams: an environmental health opportunity. *The Pennsylvania Nurse, 66*(1), 17–21. Retrieved from https://www1.villanova.edu/content/dam/villanova/sustainability/Faculty%20Research/McD-LNurseGreenTeam.pdf

Nurses can be involved in mitigation and adaptation in their healthcare practice settings through forming and participating on Green Teams.[13] Green Teams can be established in any practice setting, primary care, hospital or other healthcare facilities, skilled nursing facilities or hospice, wherever patient and healthcare supplies use recyclable product packaging, "red bag" receptacles for medical wastes, or where there is a policy for increasing corporate sustainability (Sayre, Rhazi, Carpenter, & Hughes, 2010). These collaborative teams provide nurses the opportunity to contribute their nursing knowledge, work across disciplines, and positively influence the communities they serve (McDermott-Levy, 2011; Table 21.1). Additionally, nurses can form "green committees" within their schools of nursing or be representatives on university committees (Powers & Kennedy, 2011).

Education and Policy

Nurses are responding to the urgent need to address climate change at multiple levels and in a variety of practice settings and through interdisciplinary collaborations with a wide range of healthcare delivery systems and partners. Nurses are currently engaged in climate change–related education, research, and interdisciplinary partnerships, alliances, policy, and advocacy. These efforts have expanded nurses' knowledge and perceptions through educational venues: classroom, guest lectures, seminars, partnership alliances, and participation in White House Climate Change and Health conferences, 2015 and 2016.[14,15]

2016 WHITE HOUSE ROUNDTABLE ON THE IMPACTS OF CLIMATE CHANGE ON PUBLIC HEALTH[16]

More than 30 deans of nursing (8), medical (8), and public health (15) schools took part in a White House roundtable on climate change and health with the commitment "to ensuring that we train the next generation of health professionals to effectively address the health impacts of climate change." The White House archives indicate 118 schools in the United States and other countries have signed *The Health Educators Climate Commitment*. A review of the Health Educators Climate Commitment Fact Sheet reveals that 71 U.S. medical and public health schools, and 13 U.S. schools of nursing signed the commitment pledge:

> to ensure that students, the next generation of health professionals, are prepared, through education and training, to effectively address the health impacts of climate change, and to ensure that the world has a cadre of climate change and health experts.

Schools proposed to review curricula for opportunities to address the effects of climate change on human health, and

---

[10] A U.S.–Canadian Collaboration, See "Consortiums Collaborations" section.
[11] The Luminary Project highlights nurses' efforts internationally. Shares best practices (see "Advocacy, Alliances and Interdisciplinary Partnerships").
[12] Nurses Work Group, Health Care Without Harm. https://noharm-uscanada.org/content/us-canada/nurses-workgroup

---

[13] Green Teams—multidisciplinary group of hospital-based nurses and employees who support and sustain institutional practices, e.g., in reduction of hospital wastes, energy, water consumption and overall carbon footprint.
[14] https://obamawhitehouse.archives.gov/the-press-office/2015/12/04/fact-sheet-health-educators-climate-commitment
[15] ANHE. https://envirn.org/anhe-white-house-climate-and-health-roundtable
[16] https://obamawhitehouse.archives.gov/realitycheck/the-press-office/2015/04/07/remarks-president-after-roundtable-impacts-climate-change-public-health

to work with academic colleagues and the White House on making a difference on a national scale.

GLOBAL CONSORTIUM IN CLIMATE CHANGE AND HEALTH EDUCATION

As of late fall 2017, more than 125 institutions of higher education have committed to ensuring that the health professionals of tomorrow are fully prepared to address all health risks—including those resulting from the health impacts of climate change. Representing an estimated 90,000 students from 15 countries on six continents, this global coalition has pledged to provide the next generation of health practitioners with the capacity to address the health needs of communities and patients, both now and into the foreseeable future. These learnings must be based on the best available science, and benefit from sharing best scientific and educational practices.

Advocacy, Alliances, and Interdisciplinary Partnerships

1. **Alliance of Nurses for Healthy Environments (ANHE)**[17]
   Founded and managed by nurses in multiple practices: hospital-based, public health, school-based, academics, and advanced practice settings, United States and global, the website offers current information, tools, and opportunities for nurses, in education, practice, research, and policy and advocacy. It includes a continuing education course.
   - **AHNE organized White House roundtable,** May 2016,[18] attended by national nursing organizations, to discuss the importance of addressing climate change and health to protect the public's health.
   - **Campaign for Action**[19] is working in every state to mobilize nurses, health providers, consumers, educators, and businesses to strengthen nursing on multiple fronts. Action goals are based on recommendations from the Institute of Medicine's *Future of Nursing* report.
   - **Climate Change, Health, and Nursing: A Call to Action,**[20] January 2017, is a review of the science and regional differences through case studies, concluding with opportunities for nurses to reduce harm by mitigating and adapting to these changes. **Nurses' voices are highlighted through short video stories** that describe the many ways nurses are leading the profession in addressing climate change. It is also possible for participants to include new stories.
2. **Green Initiatives in Schools (Powers & Kennedy, 2011)**[21]
   Examples of green initiatives provided by schools include providing first-year students with a stainless steel reusable coffee mug, encouraging car-pooling/mass transit, using green cleaning products, buying printers that print double sided by default, turning off computers when not in use, moderating temperatures in offices and classrooms, banning bottled water, encouraging electronic submission of assignments, using paper cups instead of plastic, donating used textbooks to other countries, encouraging telecommuting, using electronic calendars instead of paper ones, and storing student data electronically to save paper.
3. **Consortiums, Collaboratives**
   - **Climate Health Literacy Consortium (CHLC)**[22] CHLC is a collaboration of the leading organizations around the country working to educate the public about the health effects of climate change. This Consortium is committed to a concerted effort within the healthcare sector to educate healthcare professionals about the relationship between climate change and human health, thus leading to a deeper understanding of how climate change policy and consumption choices influence the health of our communities.
   - **Climate for Health** Five Major Nursing Organizations Commit to Climate Action: the Association of Public Health Nurses (APHN), National Association of Hispanic Nurses (NAHN), National Student Nurses Association (NSNA), Nurse Alliance of Services Employees International Union (SEIU) Healthcare, and the Public Health Nursing Section of the American Public Health Association (APHA) (see the Nursing Collaborative on Climate Change and Health to Catalyze Advocacy http://climateforhealth.org/five-major-nursing-organizations-commit-climate-action).
   - **Health Care Without Harm (HCWH)**[23] US-Canada NURSE'S TOOL KIT, Research collaboratives, Green healthcare initiatives, CleanMed conference, Community and Hospital Initiatives, Healthy Families and more.
   - **Conveying the Human Implications of Climate Change:**[24] A Climate Change Communication Primer for Public Health Professionals to support (a) educating the public and policy makers about climate change and associated health impacts and (b) being strong advocates in professional settings for mitigation and adaptation practices.
   - **Luminary Project** Collaboration network with the Nurses' Work Group of HCWH. It provides contact information to connect with nurses who develop environmental projects.[25]
   - **Nurses for Cool and Healthy Houses**[26] A collaboration of graduate students of the University of Michigan Public Health, Urban Planning and Natural Resources, the Fresno County Department of Public Health, and Fresno State University nursing students developed a Residential Climate Change Residential Intervention, "Nurses for Cool and Healthy Houses." The program includes a

[17] ANHE. https://envirn.org
[18] WH Conference. https://envirn.org/anhe-white-house-climate-and-health-roundtable
[19] Call to Action blog. https://campaignforaction.org/climate-change-health-nursing
[20] Call To Action. http://envirn.org/climate-change-health-and-nursing
[21] http://greenhealthcare.ca/wp-content/uploads/2016/02/CCGHC-DiscussionPaper-GreenNursing.pdf (p. 6)

[22] CHLC. https://noharm-uscanada.org/issues/us-canada/chlc-tools-and-resources
[23] HCWH. https://noharm-uscanada.org
[24] Conveying the Human Implications of Climate Change: A Climate Change Communication Primer for Public Health Professionals. https://www.climatechangecommunication.org/all/conveying-the-human-implications-of-climate-change/
[25] Luminary Project. https://noharm-uscanada.org/content/us-canada/luminary-project
[26] Collaborators were awarded funding from Health Care Without Harm to implement their ideas and to codirect "Nurses for Cool and Healthy Homes." https://www.phi.org/uploads/application/files/h7fjouo1i38v3tu427p9s9kcm-hs3oxsi7tsg1fovh3yesd5hxu.pdf

Home Heat Risk Assessment in the form of a short quickly administered checklist. See Nurses for Cool and Healthy Homes: www.youtube.com/watch?v=8TEAPFIO-00

FUTURE WORK TO BE DONE

What is missing is training for health workers to integrate this knowledge (climate and health) into daily practice, to enhance individuals' and communities' action to protect their own health while helping save the planet. (Carlos Dora, coordinator, Public Health and the Environment, World Health Organization and a member of the GCCHE Advisory Council.)

Although nursing associations' policies, position statements, and resolutions have long recognized climate change as a health threat, Divakaran et al. (2016) argue that climate change remains underrepresented in formal nursing curricula and practice. The authors observe that "although it is well known that health is influenced by social determinants, climate change is an underrepresented determinant of health within nursing and healthcare literature, curriculum, and practice. There is urgent need to recognize climate change as a current and future threat to human and environmental health" (Divakaran et al., 2016).

1. **Educate—Climate change integration in the curriculum**
   - *Undergraduate:* Integrate climate change and environmental health content into undergraduate nursing curricula with relevant impacts to human health.
     - *Course:* The most commonly cited class is the community health nursing course, but some schools have electives within nursing or science. Although some schools weave this content throughout the curriculum, other schools report integration only within the leadership or professional issues courses or a health and environment curriculum or a health promotion course (Powers & Kennedy, 2011).
   - *Scenario driven:* Make climate change real through clinically relevant scenarios in skill sessions: hands-on scenario-driven activities.
   - *Lecture:* Provide one lecture in the core curriculum explaining the links between health and climate, nested within a broader context of the links between health and the natural environment, with a focus on local health effects, inequity in health effects, and the opportunities for chronic disease prevention (Barna et al., 2012).
   - *Children-specific:* Increase healthcare provider training on human health impacts of climate change and educational programs that are children-specific.
   - *Continuing education (CE) courses:* Develop CE courses and increase distance learning webinar and courses with focus on climate change and health and nurse opportunities in education, mitigation, adaptation, and advocacy.
2. **Research:** Increase research to amplify current information and to model impacts of climate change and infectious diseases and to guide educational programs and governmental policy.
3. **Partnerships:** Increase relevant partnerships in the healthcare, private sector, research, and political sectors.

4. **Vulnerable Populations:**
   - Increase climate change–risk communications in vulnerable populations.
     - Design risk-communication messaging that targets high-risk populations.
     - Assure messages are culturally sensitive and address health risks and vulnerabilities.
   - Engage in Community-Wide Vulnerability Mapping. Nurses can contribute to the development of vulnerabilities and risk mapping by providing assessments and identification of vulnerable populations in their communities. See Denver's Department of Environmental Health, interactive heat mapping tool: climate and health equity vulnerability index at fourtwentyseven.maps.arcgis.com/apps/MapJournal/index.html?appid=64ef015257ad4ab7bc70363a33f24123.

SUMMARY

Research and increasing frequency of extreme weather events and changes in geographical areas of climate-sensitive infectious disease transmitters have served to revise considerably our understanding of climate-change impact on environments and human health. An important consequence of this understanding is the awareness that climate change's negative health effects are most severe for those who are most at risk and that these challenges to population health clearly demonstrate the imperative role of nurses (Goodman, 2016).

The skill set that nurses bring to mitigate against and adapt to climate change's influence on heath is essential. Effective solutions for protecting community health will depend on knowledgeable and competent nurses who can identify existing and anticipated emerging health threats in their regions. More schools are including climate change and health curricula in the coursework, yet this integration must increase to meet the challenges and the pledge by the Health Educators Commitment. Educators must also share their experience in teaching climate change to identify best practices. There are many resources and successful advocacy examples and tool kits for nurses to effectively adapt and mitigate the negative consequences. Furthermore, collaboration between nurses and their professional organizations can raise the volume of the professional collective voice in local, national, and international conversations. Through active roles as educators, research consumers, health messengers, client advocates, leaders, and change agents, nurses are vital partners in developing and implementing national and community strategies for protecting individual and overall community health. Nurses' advocacy extends to promoting public and policymaker awareness and preparedness for the fight against the negative health effects of climate change—bringing their knowledge, skills, and critical thinking to "the greatest global health opportunity of the 21st century."

STUDY QUESTIONS

1. Each region of the United States experiences, differently, real and potential climate change effects. How are the climate drivers in your practice community integrated into policies and practices? How are nurses involved?

2. How are most at risk vulnerable populations in your area of practice identified, who are those most susceptible and or vulnerable? And how are they integrated into the healthcare system, and what are the mitigation or adaptation plans in their nursing assessments?

3. How are nurses in your area of practice addressing climate change and health impacts or involved in other environmental/climate-sensitive practices or policies.

4. Where would climate change and health and the nurses role in practice and policy fit within the nursing curriculum, methodology and educational levels. How have other nursing programs incorporated climate change and health in their curriculum?

5. What are organizational support partners and how are they supporting Green Team development or promoting other environmental health and climate change health effects practices and policies?

USEFUL LINKS

Alliance for Nurses for Healthy Environments (ANHE)

- Climate Change, Health and Nursing: A Call to Action. Nurses' Personal Stories. http://envirn.org/climate-change-health-and-nursing
- Advancing Clean Air, Climate, and Health: Opportunity for Nurses. 3 Modules. https://envirn.org/advancing-clean-air-climate-health-opportunities-for-nurses

ANHE—Climate Action Network (CAN) International. www.climatenetwork.org/profile/member/alliance-nurses-healthy-environments-anhe

Centers for Disease Control and Prevention (CDC). www.cdc.gov/climateandhealth

CDC Climate Change and Health Fact Sheets

- Extreme Rainfall and Drought. www.cdc.gov/climateandhealth/pubs/precip-final_508.pdf
- Warmer Water and Flooding. www.cdc.gov/climateandhealth/pubs/warmer-water-final_508.pdf
- Climate Change Decreases the Quality of the Air We Breathe. www.cdc.gov/climateandhealth/pubs/air-quality-final_508.pdf
- Climate Change Increases Risk of Vectorborne Disease. www.cdc.gov/climateandhealth/pubs/vector-borne-disease-final_508.pdf

Climate Change Evidence and Causes. http://dels.nas.edu/resources/static-assets/exec-office-other/climate-change-full.pdf

Health Care Without Harm. https://noharm-uscanada.org

Nurses Work Group Within Health Care Without Harm. https://noharm-uscanada.org/content/us-canada/nurses-workgroup

National Academies of Science, Engineering and Medicine, Climate Communications Initiative. http://nas-sites.org/americasclimatechoices/cci

National Association of County and City Health Officers (NACCHO). www.naccho.org/programs/environmental-health/hazards/climate-change

National Institutes of Health Disaster Research Response (DR2). https://dr2.nlm.nih.gov

United Nations Framework Convention on Climate Change Paris Climate Accord. http://unfccc.int/paris_agreement/items/9485.php

U.S Global Change Research Program (USGCRP), 2017: Climate Science Special Report: Fourth National Climate Assessment, Volume I. https://science2017.globalchange.gov

REFERENCES

Akerlof, K. L., Delamater, P. L., Boules, C. R., Upperman, C. R., & Mitchell, C. S. (2015). Vulnerable populations perceive their health as at risk from climate change. *Journal of Environmental Research and Public Health, 12*(12), 15419–15433. doi:10.3390/ijerph121214994

Anåker, A., Nilsson, M., Holmner, Å., & Elf, M. (2015). Nurses' perceptions of climate and environmental issues: A qualitative study. *Journal of Advanced Nursing, 71*(8), 1883–1891. doi:10.1111/jan.12655

Angelini, K. (2017). Climate change, health, and the role of nurses. *Nursing for Women's Health, 21*(2), 79–83. doi:10.1016/j.nwh.2017.02.003

Barna, S., Goodman, B., & Mortimer, F. (2012). The health effects of climate change: What does a nurse need to know? *Nurse Education Today, 32*(7), 765–771. doi:10.1016/j.nedt.2012.05.012

Becker, J., Mendez-Quigley, T., & Phillips, M. (2010). Nursing role in the pharmaceutical life cycle. *Nursing Administration Quarterly, 34*(4):297–305. doi:10.1097/NAQ.0b013e3181f5640a

Birnbaum, L. S., Balbus, J. M., & Tart, K. T. (2016). Marking a new understanding of climate and health. *Environmental Health Perspectives, 124*(4), A59. doi:10.1289/ehp.1611410

Bouzid, M., Hooper, L., & Hunter, P. R. (2013). The effectiveness of public health interventions to reduce the health impact of climate change: A systematic review of systematic reviews. *PLoS One, 8*(4), e62041. doi:10.1371/journal.pone.0062041

Centers for Disease Control and Prevention. (2017a). Climate effects on health. Retrieved from https://www.cdc.gov/climateandhealth/effects/default.htm

Centers for Disease Control and Prevention (2017b). Climate and health: fact sheet. Retrieved from https://www.cdc.gov/climateandhealth/factsheet.htm

D'Amato, G., Holgate, S. T., Pawankar, R., Ledford, D. K., Cecchi, L., Al-Ahmad, M., ... Annesi-Maesano, I. (2015). Meteorological conditions, climate change, new emerging factors, and asthma and related allergic disorders. A statement of the World Allergy Organization. *World Allergy Organization Journal, 8*(1), 25. doi:10.1186/s40413-015-0073-0

Department of Defense. (2014). Executive summary, Secretary Chuck Hagel. In *Quadrennial Defense Review*. Retrieved from http://archive.defense.gov/pubs/2014_Quadrennial_Defense_Review.pdf

Divakaran, B., Lembeck, S., Kerr, R., Calmus, H., & Potter, T. (2016). Nurses see "The Big Picture": Addressing climate change as a social determinant of global health. *Creative Nursing, 22*(4), 243–248. doi:10.1891/1078-4535.22.4.243

Domrose, C. (2015). The climate connection: Nurses examine effects of climate change on public health. Retrieved from http://www.nurse.com

Ebi, K. L., Fawcett, S. B., Spiegel, J., & Tovalin, H. (2016). Carbon pollution increases health inequities: Lessons in resilience from the most vulnerable. *Revista Panamericana de Salud Pública, 40*(3), 181–185. Retrieved from http://iris.paho.org/xmlui/bitstream/handle/123456789/31234/v40n3a6-181-85.pdf?sequence=1

Ebi, K. L., Semenza, J. C., & Rocklöv, J. (2016). Current medical research funding and frameworks are insufficient to address the health risks of global environmental change. *Environmental Health, 15*(1), 108. doi:10.1186/s12940-016-0183-3

EPA: Climate Change Indicators. (2018). *Understanding the Connections between Climate Change and Human Health*. Retrieved from https://www.epa.gov/climate-indicators/understanding-connections-between-climate-change-and-human-health

Goodman, B. (2016). Developing the concept of sustainability in nursing. *Nursing Philosophy, 17*(4), 298–306. doi:10.1111/nup.12143

Hansen, J., Kharecha, P., Sato, M., Masson-Delmotte, V., Ackerman, F., Beerling, D. J., ... Zachos, J. C. (2013). Assessing "Dangerous Climate Change": Required reduction of carbon emissions to protect young people, future generations and nature. *PLoS One, 8*(12), e81648. doi:10.1371/journal.pone.0081648

Intergovernmental Panel on Climate Change. (2014). *Climate Change 2014: Synthesis report: Contribution of Working Groups I, II and III to the Fifth Assessment Report of the Intergovernmental Panel on Climate Change.* Geneva, Switzerland: Author.

Jia, P., Chen, X., Chen, J., Lu, L., Liu, Q., & Tan, X. (2017). How does the dengue vector mosquito *Aedes albopictus* respond to global warming? *Parasites & Vectors, 10*(1), 140. doi:10.1186/s13071-017-2071-2

Laan, M. S. (2014). *Analysing Ontario public health nurses knowledge, attitudes, and beliefs about roles and responsibilities in addressing climate change* (Dissertation). Queen's University, Kingston, ON, Canada. Database copyright ProQuest LLC.

Marinucci, G. D., Luber, G., Uejio, C. K., Saha, S., & Hess, J. J. (2014). Building resilience against climate effects—A novel framework to facilitate climate readiness in public health agencies. *International Journal of Environmental Research and Public Health, 11*(6), 6433–6458. doi:10.3390/ijerph110606433

McDermott-Levy, R. (2011). The nurse's role on green teams: An environmental health opportunity. *The Pennsylvania Nurse, 66*(1), 17–21. Retrieved from https://www1.villanova.edu/content/dam/villanova/sustainability/Faculty%20Research/McD-LNurseGreenTeam.pdf

McDonald, L. (2001). EBN Notebook, Florence Nightingale and the early origins of evidenced based nursing. *Evidence Based Nursing, 4*(3), 68–69. doi:10.1136/ebn.4.3.68

Miller, M. D., Marty, M. A., & Landrigan, P. J. (2016). Children's environmental health: Beyond national boundaries. *Pediatric Clinics of North America, 63*(1), 149–165. doi:10.1016/j.pcl.2015.08.008

Minnesota Department of Health. (2017). Minnesota climate and health program. Retrieved from http://www.health.state.mn.us/divs/climatechange

NASA Global Climate Change. (2018). Vital Signs of the Planet. Retrieved from https://climate.nasa.gov/evidence

National Academy of Science and Royal Society. (2015). Climate change evidence and causes. Retrieved from http://dels.nas.edu/resources/static-assets/exec-office-other/climate-change-full.pdf

Polivka, B. J., Chaudry, R. V., & Mac Crawford, J. (2012). Public health nurses' knowledge and attitudes regarding climate change. *Environmental Health Perspectives, 120*(3), 321–325. doi:10.1289/ehp.1104025

Portier, C. J., Thigpen Tart, K., Carter, S. R., Dilworth, C. H., Grambsch, A. E., Gohlke, J., ... Whung, P.-Y. (2010). A human health perspective on climate change: A report outlining the research needs on the human health effects of climate change. Research Triangle Park, NC: Environmental Health Perspectives/National Institute of Environmental Health Sciences. doi:10.1289/ehp.1002272.

Powers, P., & Kennedy, T. (2011). *Climate change content and Green initiatives in Canadian Schools of Nursing* (Discussion Paper #1). Branchton, ON, Canada: Canadian Coalition for Green Health Care.

Prudent, N., Houghton, A., & Luber, G. (2016). Assessing climate change and health vulnerability at the local level: Travis County, Texas. *Disasters, 40*(4), 740–752. doi:10.1111/disa.12177

Rossati, A. (2017). Global warming and its health impact. *The International Journal of Occupational and Environmental Medicine, 8*(1), 7–20. doi:10.15171/ijoem.2017.963

Santer, B. D., Solomon, S., Wentz, F. J., Fu, Q., Po-Chedley, S., Mears, C., ... Bonfils, C. (2017). Tropospheric warming over the past two decades. *Scientific Reports, 7*(1), 2336. doi:10.1038/s41598-017-02520-7

Sayre, L., Rhazi, N., Carpenter, H., & Hughes, N. L. (2010). Climate change and human health: The role of nurses in confronting the issue. *Nursing Administration Quarterly, 34*(4), 334–342. doi:10.1097/NAQ.0b013e3181f60df9

Schmeltz, M. T., Petkova, E. P., & Gamble, J. L. (2016). Economic burden of hospitalizations for heat-related illnesses in the United States, 2001–2010. *International Journal of Environmental Research and Public Health, 13*(9), 894. doi:10.3390/ijerph13090894

Trombley, J., Chalupka, S., & Anderko, L. (2017). Climate change and mental health. *American Journal of Nursing, 117*(4), 44–52. doi:10.1097/01.NAJ.0000515232.51795.fa

U.S. Global Change Research Program. (2017). In D. J. Wuebbles, D. W. Fahey, K. A. Hibbard, D. J. Dokken, B. C. Stewart, & T. K. Maycock (Eds.), *Climate science special report: Fourth national climate assessment* (Vol. I). Washington, DC: Author.

Veenema, T. G., Thornton, C. P., Lavin, R. P., Bender, A. K., Seal, S., & Corley, A. (2017). Climate change–related water disasters' impact on population health. *Journal of Nursing Scholarship, 49*(6), 625–634. doi:10.1111/jnu.12328

Watts, N., Adger, W. N., Ayeb-Karlsson, S., Bai, Y., Byass, P., Campbell-Lendrum, D., ... Costello, A. (2017). The Lancet countdown: Tracking progress on health and climate change. *The Lancet, 389*(10074), 1151–1164. doi:10.1016/S0140-6736(16)32124-9

Ziegler, C., Morelli, V., & Fawibe, O. (2017). Climate change and underserved communities. *Primary Care: Clinics in Office Practice, 44*(1), 171–184. doi:10.1016/j.pop.2016.09.017

Section IV

DISASTER RESPONSE

22

DISASTER TRIAGE

Lou E. Romig and E. Brooke Lerner

LEARNING OBJECTIVES

When this chapter is completed, readers will be able to:

1. Define triage.
2. Describe the differences between daily hospital triage, multiple or mass casualty incident (MCI)/disaster triage, and population-based triage.
3. Understand the situations in which each model of disaster triage is used.
4. Discuss how objective disaster triage tools are beneficial not only to the victims themselves but also to those tasked with performing triage.
5. Explain the criteria for each of the five basic primary disaster triage levels.
6. Discuss the differences between primary, secondary, and tertiary disaster triage.
7. Discuss the special situations presented during population-based triage.
8. Differentiate disaster triage tools and identify the tool used in your community/agency.
9. Identify the five key elements of triage tools.
10. Discuss how the presence of contaminated patients affects triage in the field and at the hospital.

KEY MESSAGES

Accurate triage provides responders with the opportunity to do the greatest good for the greatest number of casualties (with the least amount of harm), and is the cornerstone of good disaster medical resource management.

Disaster triage is employed when the types and/or amounts of available medical resources are inadequate to provide immediate comprehensive care to all victims.

Performing triage under disaster conditions requires a paradigm shift on the part of disaster response nurses and other first responders: The focus turns from doing the best for each patient to optimizing the outcome for all victims as a group, even if that means withholding resources from the most critically ill or injured patients.

Disaster triage is a dynamic process, with opportunities to retriage patients with each assessment and as additional resources become available.

Different models are available for disaster/mass casualty triage. Unfortunately, no primary disaster triage tool has been empirically validated in a prospective manner. However, a set of minimum core criteria that should be included in a triage system has been identified (Lerner, Cone, et al., 2011), and the Federal Interagency Committee on Emergency Medical Services (FICEMS) has started the implementation process for these criteria nationally (FICEMS, 2013). Nurses must be aware of the disaster triage tools and systems used by their local EMS system and hospital, as well as when it is appropriate to use them.

Primary triage is based on a rapid initial assessment and places patients into broad categories that prioritize them for treatment and/or transport.

Special circumstances may require unique triage procedures, including incidents involving hazardous materials (in which triage is severely limited until patients have been decontaminated) and community-wide events (in which population-based triage must focus on preventing further spread of the disease or risk of harm).

CHAPTER OVERVIEW

The United Nations defines a disaster as "a serious disruption of the functioning of a community or a society at any scale due to hazardous events interacting with conditions of exposure, vulnerability and capacity, leading to one or more of the following: human, material, economic and environmental losses and impacts" (United Nations International Strategy for Disaster Reduction, 2017). The emphasis on the (in)ability to cope with an incident using only native resources applies to many aspects of disaster preparedness and response but is particularly pertinent to a community's ability to respond to the acute medical needs generated by a disaster. When the ability to meet the demand for medical care is compromised by a lack of personnel, equipment, and supplies, special measures must be taken to ensure that the available medical resources are used in the most efficient, effective, responsible, and ethical manner possible. This process is called "triage," a familiar term to most urgent and acute medical care providers; however, "disaster triage" is different in practice and principle from the triage performed on a daily basis.

Emergency triage, whether done in the field by EMS providers or in hospital emergency departments (EDs) and alternative care centers, is a difficult and sometimes inconsistent process even on an average day. When disaster strikes and overwhelms the available medical resources, triage becomes, at the same time, more important and more difficult. Unlike everyday triage, where the choices affect primarily time to care, disaster triage is used to decide who will get the resources that are available and who will not. These choices are made to do the greatest good for the greatest number of people.

This chapter presents the fundamental concepts of disaster triage. Triage is the first medical action in any response for multiple or massive numbers of casualties. Decisions made during the triage process may have a significant impact not only on the individual victims, but also on the health outcomes of the entire affected population. Disaster triage is a difficult and intimidating task because it requires making rapid decisions in an often chaotic environment using minimal data, and places the job of making life-or-death decisions squarely on the shoulders of those performing triage.

There is a good chance that at least some of the healthcare providers called upon to perform the critical function of disaster triage will have never had the opportunity to perform the task in anything but a drill setting. Often with very little notice, providers must decide which patients need care, where they should receive it, in what order they should receive care, and, in situations of severely constrained resources, who should receive only palliative care or no care at all. In addition, some events, such as industrial incidents and intentional attacks involving chemical, biological, radiological, or nuclear agents, may require an alteration in the triage process due to the need to mitigate further injury by decontaminating patients before medical care can safely be provided.

BASIC PRINCIPLES OF DISASTER TRIAGE

"Triage is a process which places the right patient in the right place at the right time to receive the right level of care" (Rice & Abel, 1992). The word "triage" is derived from the French word *trier,* which means, "to sort out or choose." The Baron Dominique Jean Larrey, Napoleon's chief surgeon, is credited with organizing the first triage system (Robertson-Steele, 2006). The U.S. military first used triage to describe a sorting station where injured soldiers were distributed from the battlefield to distant support hospitals. Following World War II, triage came to mean the process used to identify those most likely to return to the battle after medical intervention. This process facilitated the provision of expeditious medical care to soldiers who could fight again. During the Korean and Vietnam conflicts, triage was further refined to resemble the process that is still used today in both military and civilian arenas.

Triage is the process of prioritizing which patients are to be treated first and is the cornerstone of good disaster management in terms of judicious use of medical resources (Auf der Heide, 2000). Accurate triage allows disaster nurses and other responders to do the greatest good for the greatest number of afflicted. Although the fundamentals of triage remain consistent wherever it is conducted, performing triage during a disaster presents unique challenges. Its overall success may be highly dependent on the competence, experience, and composure of the nurse, working in close concert with the rest of the emergency care team.

Disaster triage will always be a difficult and daunting task. Previous triage experience in an ED is excellent preparation for disaster triage. Burkle (1984) identified a variety of personal abilities that are essential to be an effective triage officer during a disaster:

- Clinically experienced
- Good judgment and leadership
- Calm and cool under stress
- Decisive
- Knowledgeable of available resources
- Sense of humor
- Creative problem solver
- Available
- Experienced and knowledgeable regarding anticipated casualties

To understand the subtle differences between the philosophies of different types of acute medical triage, it is important to know the most common terminology (Cone & MacMillan, 2005; Hogan & Lairet, 2002):

- *Daily triage* is performed by nurses on a routine basis in the ED, often utilizing a standardized approach, augmented by clinical judgment. The goal is to identify the sickest patients to assess and treat them first, before providing treatment to others who are less ill and whose outcome is unlikely to be affected by a longer wait. The highest intensity of care is provided to the most seriously ill or injured patients, even if those patients have a low probability of survival.
- *Incident triage* occurs when the ED is stressed by a large number of patients due to an acute incident or an ongoing medical crisis such as pandemic influenza, but is still able to provide care to all patients utilizing existing agency resources. Additional resources (on-call staff, alternative care areas) may be used, but disaster plans are not activated and treatment priorities are not changed. The highest intensity of care is still provided to the most critically ill patients. ED delays may be longer than usual, but eventually everyone who presents for care is attended to.
- *Disaster triage* is a general term employed when local EMS and hospital emergency services are overwhelmed to the point that immediate care cannot be provided to everyone who needs it because sufficient resources are not immediately available. The terms "multiple casualty/multicasualty" and "mass casualty" triage (both also known as "MCI triage") are often used interchangeably with "disaster triage." The distinction between "multiple" and "mass" casualties is principally in the number of victims and the degree of restriction of resources. There is no standardized threshold beyond which a multiple casualty incident becomes an MCI. Similarly, there is little consistency in number of patients that demand changing from everyday triage to true MCI triage because it is the capability of a system to respond that is more important than absolute patient numbers. For example, a bus crash with 15 to 20 victims might be called an MCI in a large EMS/healthcare system and MCI triage tools might be used, but all victims except those with injuries that are clearly incompatible with life will still be treated using all the normal resources of that system. The same crash might

overwhelm a much smaller system, requiring resources to be given to those most likely to survive while those who are unlikely to survive might have to wait to receive resources because there are not enough for everyone.

In true disaster triage, there is a paradigm shift in fundamental triage philosophy from "do the best for each patient, regardless of what it takes" to "do the greatest good for the greatest number" (Auf der Heide, 2000). Resource management becomes the linchpin driving the provision of care. The goal of triage shifts to identifying and prioritizing injured or ill patients who have a good chance of survival with immediate interventions that do not consume extraordinary resources (Auf der Heide, 2000). During a disaster, patients are usually sorted into one of the following categories (Lerner, Cone, et al., 2011):

- *Minimal or minor (designated with the color green)*: These are patients who are physiologically well compensated and likely to remain so for an extended period of time. These patients require only basic immediate care and can probably wait for a considerable period of time for definitive care with minimal risk of deterioration. Examples of minimal casualties might be those with minor lacerations, burns, or other soft tissue or orthopedic injuries without significant bleeding or neurovascular compromise. Victims with mild to moderate psychological stress reactions related to the incident can also often be triaged in the minimal category. In the event that hospital resources are overwhelmed, community emergency management plans might call for minimal-category patients to be directed to predesignated alternate care sites such as community clinics and urgent care centers.
- *Delayed (designated with the color yellow)*: These are patients with compensated physiology but a significant potential for deterioration or morbidity if there are long delays before definitive care can be provided. If sufficient resources are available, many of these patients can be temporarily treated and stabilized in the field. Examples include physiologically stable patients with possible spine or head injuries without acute neurological deficits, significant bleeding controlled with pressure dressings or tourniquets, and orthopedic injuries with signs of neurovascular compromise that improve after basic splinting.
- *Immediate (designated with the color red)*: These are patients with uncompensated physiology and injuries that are life-threatening but probably amenable to rapid interventions that do not require consumption of an inordinate amount of resources. These patients may die or sustain significant morbidity unless they receive rapid care in both the field and the hospital. Examples include patients with poorly controlled external bleeding, moderate burns, or penetrating trauma without other critical injuries, altered mental status, early shock, and respiratory distress (but not failure). These are the patients who, in general, should be transported first from the scene.
- *Deceased (designated with the color black):* These patients are those with no detectable vital signs, typically identified as victims not breathing on their own. In everyday practice settings, we would attempt resuscitation if there are no signs of obvious death, but in a disaster situation we simply

designate the victim as dead, since the resources required to revive a person in cardiac arrest are not available or are available but would be put to more effective use to attempt to save a greater number of other patients who have better chances of survival. Patients in the deceased category include those who are not breathing even after performing simple airway-opening maneuvers.

- *Expectant (designated with the color gray):* These patients are those who are still alive but due to their injuries and/or medical condition are unlikely to survive given the available resources. In everyday practice settings, providers would attempt to treat these patients even though their most likely outcome would ultimately be death. In a disaster, these patients would be assigned to wait for treatment until sufficient resources were available. To do the greatest good for the greatest number of people, the resources that would have been consumed by these patients are used to treat other patients who have a better chance of survival. Patients in the expectant category might include those with agonal respirations, massive head injuries, dismemberment, extensive burns, crush injuries, critical penetrating trauma, or multiple life-threatening injuries. In a mass radiation exposure event, patients with vomiting/diarrhea soon after exposure may be classified as expectant, as early gastrointestinal (GI) symptoms and signs are signals of lethal radiation poisoning. In a mass exposure to organophosphates/nerve agents, patients with seizures soon after exposure may also be classified as expectant, as they are a sign of likely lethal exposure. Patients designated as expectant should be reevaluated regularly. Once there are sufficient resources, these patients may be treated, provided with comfort care, or declared dead if there are no longer any signs of life.

It will never be easy to withhold care from a disaster victim who still has signs of life. It goes against our instincts and common practice. The need to recognize and accept futility becomes even harder when faced with a victim who is a child or sparks an unusually strong compassionate urge in responders (e.g., a fellow responder). It is possible that having an objective triage tool that dictates that patients meeting certain criteria be tagged as Deceased or Expectant may help protect triage officers from some of the emotional trauma inherent in the role because it is the tool that dictates the decision, not the responder himself or herself.

Special conditions during triage: Incidents involving chemical, biological, or radioactive agents may be intentional or unintentional (e.g., a truck crash involving the release of hazardous materials). These triage situations require personal protective equipment for all responders coming into contact with potentially contaminated patients and decontamination capabilities both in the field and at receiving facilities (Hogan & Lairet, 2002). During any disaster, triage personnel must ensure that they themselves do not become victims. One enters the scene for field triage only when scene safety has been assured (see Chapter 35 "Decontamination and Personal Protective Equipment," Mass Casualty Decontamination, for further information). Triage during special conditions does not change the sorting process so much as the circumstances in which it must be performed. The need to protect responders

and decontaminate victims often adds significantly to delays in triage and treatment. These delays may result in the deterioration of patients who might have been less seriously affected if more rapid care had been possible.

Population-based triage: The predominant disaster triage models taught in the United States are based on mass casualty scenarios that unfold in a single location at a single point in time. Emerging infectious diseases such as severe acute respiratory syndrome (SARS) and avian influenza, as well as the threat of bioterrorist events such as the deliberate dissemination of anthrax in 2001, serve to highlight the inadequacies of disaster triage systems for widespread, community-based events. SARS is a severe respiratory illness that is caused by a coronavirus and is transmitted especially by contact with infectious material (e.g., respiratory droplets or body fluids) and is characterized by fever, headache, body aches, a dry cough, hypoxia, and usually pneumonia. Other examples of events that might lead to large numbers of people who need assistance across a wide geographical area are natural disasters such as floods or hurricanes. It is important to note that regardless of the cause (man-made or natural), these events are managed medically in a similar fashion. Everyone in the population requires some intervention, ranging from timely and accurate medical information to vaccination and/or prophylaxis.

The main goal of population-based triage is to prevent secondary illness or injury such as disease transmission from infectious individuals or foodborne illness from contaminated or poorly refrigerated supplies. The messages and directions sent during population-based triage will depend on the type(s) of illness or injury that is trying to be contained. Depending on the severity, lethality, and/or transmissibility of the illness or injury being prevented, these events can be very serious and have a huge impact on a community.

Infectious disease containment strategies, such as social distancing, sheltering-in-place, isolation, and quarantine, are the first line of management under state public health law. In this model, everyone in the population falls into one of five population-based triage categories (SEIRV classifications), each requiring both generic and disease-specific interventions:

- *Susceptible individuals*—those individuals who are unexposed but susceptible.
- *Exposed individuals*—susceptible individuals who have been in contact with the disease and may be infected and incubating but still noncontagious.
- *Infectious individuals*—persons who are symptomatic and contagious.
- *Removed individuals*—persons who no longer can pass the disease to others because they have survived and developed immunity or died from the illness.
- *Vaccinated or on prophylactic antibiotics*—persons in this group are a critical resource for the essential workforce.

In such a situation, many people are being triaged simultaneously at multiple sites—triage and information centers, vaccination and/or other clinics, EDs, and hospitals. Triage nurses have a vital role in this process (whether triage is performed face-to-face or over telephone or Internet "hotlines"), classifying citizens and assigning them to levels and locations of care based on disease susceptibility, vulnerability, comorbid conditions, symptoms, infectiousness, and/or exposure. For example, in 2003, the Toronto Health System utilized their 1-800-telehealth hotline to disseminate pertinent information to the public through both recordings and live phone triage. Phone triage nurses fielded over 28,000 calls during the SARS outbreak and served as a major triage element, making triage decisions that prevented further mixing of patients and preventing unnecessary secondary cases (Svoboda et al., 2004). In an epidemic, those who are susceptible may be triaged to a vaccination area; those who are ill may be triaged to an acute care facility, an alternate care facility, or to remain at home. Those who are ill may also be triaged to isolation, whereas those who are exposed but not yet ill may need to be triaged to quarantine.

Population-based triage is in the early stages of development; there are currently no nationally accepted schemes. It is a concept that has only recently begun to be described and it is possible that, because there is such a wide spectrum of communicability, virulence, and available treatment for diseases that could rise to epidemic proportions, no single triage algorithm can be developed. However, it is essential that the triage nurse be prepared to utilize an event-specific triage algorithm when triaging during a population-based event. If such a situation were to occur, the algorithm to be used will likely be issued by state or territorial Departments of Health in concert with the U.S. Centers for Disease Control and Prevention (CDC).

PHASES OF DISASTER TRIAGE: FROM THE FIELD TO THE HOSPITAL

Prehospital care providers are trained and well practiced in triaging individual injured or ill patients to appropriate hospitals based on their needs for specialized care. Most EMS personnel have also been trained in disaster/MCI triage, although relatively few have ever had to perform true disaster triage in a large incident. They may employ MCI triage tools not only in MCIs that overtax local and regional EMS and hospital resources but also in smaller multicasualty incidents that primarily overwhelm the local field response resources. Field disaster triage protocols, aimed at maximizing the outcome for the greatest possible number of victims, are usually utilized only for the initial gross sorting of patients in the field. This phase is called "primary triage." The goal of primary triage is usually to sort patients into five triage categories: Immediate, Delayed, Minimal, Expectant, and Dead. Although there are many triage tools currently on the market and there are efforts to standardize the categories, it is important to be familiar with the tools that are used in and around your community since they may include slightly different categories and/or labels.

The primary triage phase is similar to the trauma primary survey, in which physiology is the focus rather than identification of specific injuries. The MCI triage tools used most commonly in the United States and around the world were developed to facilitate primary triage, not to act as the *only* point of patient assessment. Indeed, triage is a dynamic process. Each time a provider assesses a patient is an opportunity to reevaluate their triage prioritization. A victim may be upgraded (assigned a more

critical triage category) at any time in the ongoing assessment process. Likewise, a patient who becomes more stable during treatment in the field or hospital may be downgraded, although some authors disagree, stating that a patient should never be down-triaged (Hogan & Lairet, 2002). It is also important to recognize that errors may be made in the triage process and reassessment provides the opportunity to correct any errors.

A second patient assessment ("secondary triage") may be performed on-scene if transport is delayed for any reason or at the hospital itself. In secondary triage, additional information about each patient is obtained through a more thorough physical assessment and history (when available). This is similar to the traditional trauma secondary survey, in which physiology is reassessed and obvious injuries are identified. When secondary triage is done in the field, one of the goals is to determine which patients have conditions that can be temporarily but effectively treated on-scene using available personnel and resources (e.g., initial IV fluid resuscitation) and identify those whose immediate needs can be met only in a hospital setting (e.g., uncontrollable bleeding or other need for immediate surgical intervention). In this way, patients within the same triage category can be prioritized for transport when limited transport resources are available. For example, delayed patients requiring timely hospital-based interventions will be transported before other delayed patients who can be temporarily treated in the field. There is no uniformly adopted tool used in the United States for secondary triage. Some EMS agencies use their local trauma triage protocols or no standardized system at all. Other agencies use the Secondary Assessment of Victim Endpoint (SAVE) tool developed for use after earthquakes in California. SAVE combines standard trauma assessment techniques and a dynamic assessment of available resources to prioritize patients during prolonged delays to definitive care caused by severe resource constraints (Benson, Koenig, & Schultz, 1996).

Although it would make sense to transport the most critically ill patients from a disaster scene first, effective use of ground and air transport resources often requires that several patients be placed in each transport unit. In these cases, an Immediate patient may be transported with a Delayed or Minimal patient or patients to the same hospital instead of with another Immediate patient. In this way, multiple patients can be evacuated from the scene without overwhelming the capacity of the EMS personnel working in the transporting air or ground ambulances. Ideally, identified family members should also be transported to the same facility. This is especially true when there are injured children. Both injured and noninjured parents and other guardians may refuse to be separated from their children. This may result in the need to make difficult transport decisions, especially if an injured child requires specialty pediatric care available only at a distant facility. Parents have also been known to deny being injured or refuse care to remain with their child, only to request care once the child has been treated. In general, families should be transported to a facility capable of providing appropriate care for all family members; however, arranging to do so should not significantly delay the transport of the most critically injured patient.

Patients arriving at the hospital from an incident scene via EMS are then usually triaged again at the ED and sorted based on patient needs and the available resources at the hospital. Unless the hospital is or is likely to be overwhelmed by patients presenting for emergent care, the hospital staff may use their typical daily triage philosophy of doing the best for each patient. However, this is where communication between the scene and the area hospitals is very important, since a hospital may commit their resources to the patients at their facility only to find that many more patients may be arriving.

"Tertiary triage" may then become necessary if the hospitals' resources become overwhelmed. In this step, hospital personnel determine if the facility can provide appropriate care or if the patient will require stabilization and transfer to a facility capable of a higher level of care. In an MCI, hospitals may be required to accept patients they usually would not receive from EMS or would ordinarily have to transfer out for definitive care. This may occur because of the hospital's proximity to the incident or because the specialty facilities are also overwhelmed with disaster victims. The most common types of patients who might have to be stabilized and later transferred are children and those with multisystem trauma, burns, or spinal cord injuries. Freestanding pediatric hospitals might have to initially stabilize and then transfer adult patients, including parents who denied injuries or refused care until they were satisfied that their child was being cared for.

It is important to understand that it is possible that not all patients coming to a hospital from a disaster scene will be transported by EMS, especially if the hospital is close to the incident. In very large incidents, significant numbers of patients may be transported by private vehicle or even walk to the closest hospital. Children are portable; well-intentioned lay rescuers or family members may feel that children will receive care more quickly if they can get to a hospital without waiting for EMS to evaluate them. Most patients arriving at the hospital on their own have not yet been triaged at all. Every hospital must be prepared to perform the same primary triage sorting that is' done in the field, sometimes using the same tools. In these cases, the same flow of primary, secondary, and tertiary triage may be conducted at the hospital itself. Often while EMS is bringing patients in from the incident, other patients not associated with the disaster are also presenting for care in the ED as well as those who come from the incident by private vehicle. Hospital disaster triage policies and procedures sometimes fail to recognize and plan for the fact that regular ED patients will also present for care during a disaster. A hospital's obligations to these patients are not diminished by the fact that they are overwhelmed with disaster victims. This process of accommodating both disaster and nondisaster patients is often not addressed adequately, or at all, in hospital disaster plans and drills.

BASIC DIFFERENCES BETWEEN DAILY TRIAGE AND DISASTER TRIAGE AT THE HOSPITAL

Usual hospital triage is what is done every day during ordinary circumstances. Basic information is obtained that allows the triage nurse to make a judgment regarding the actual or potential severity of the problem and the degree of urgency for further evaluation and treatment. Box 22.1 lists the typical types of data that are gathered during hospital triage evaluation. High-volume EDs that frequently have longer delays for

---

BOX 22.1 Typical Data Elements Gathered at ED Triage During Normal Operations

Name
Age
Gender
Chief complaint (CC)
History of present illness (HPI)
Mechanism of injury (MOI)
Past medical or surgical history (PM/SHx.)
Allergies to food or medication (Allergies)
Current medications (Meds)
Date of last tetanus immunization
Last menstrual period (for females between the ages of 11 and 60) (LMP)
Vital signs: temperature, pulse, blood pressure, respiratory rate, oxygen saturation (VS)
Level of consciousness (LOC)
Skin vital signs (Skin vitals): temperature, color, moisture
Visual inspection for obvious injuries
Height and weight (pediatric patients) (Ht./Wt.)
Mode of arrival (MOA)
Private medical provider (PMD)
Other

ED, emergency department.

treatment tend to collect more information at the point of triage. Some may use the information gathered at triage to implement protocols allowing nursing staff to initiate testing and treatment before a physician or advanced practice provider (APP) sees the patient. Low-volume EDs rarely experience large volumes of patients or delays in detailed assessment and treatment, and tend to collect fewer data elements at triage, as other nursing and physician/APP staff see the patients rapidly. Detailed information is collected during initiation of treatment rather than in triage. During a disaster, in which a large number of patients arrive at the ED within a short time, the number of data elements collected during the initial triage encounter may need to be significantly reduced. Box 22.2 shows an abbreviated list of data elements commonly obtained when an ED is operating in disaster triage mode. This list represents elements that are essential to identify *emergent* cases. Depending on the nature and extent of the disaster as well as the volume of nondisaster patients, triage staff may have the time and resources to do a more complete assessment during the triage process and include additional elements from Box 22.1.

Daily Triage in the Hospital Setting

If EDs were able to handle each case as it arrived to the hospital, there would be no need for triage. Each patient would be treated immediately upon arrival to the ED. In 2013, there were over 130 million ED visits in the United States (CDC, 2013). The number of ED visits in the United States continues to grow each year. The demand for services frequently exceeds the capacity

ED, emergency department.

of the system at any given moment; therefore, a triage system has evolved in which the sickest patients are given priority. In the event of a multicasualty incident, additional staff and resources are sent to the ED and other acute care areas of the hospital but standard ED triage, often in an abbreviated form, is often still used. If a hospital's capacity is likely to be overwhelmed, patients being transported by EMS may be diverted to other institutions. It is only when the number and severity of casualties is greater than the hospital or available system can handle that true disaster triage is initiated in a hospital.

The main purpose of daily in-hospital triage is to identify those patients who have the highest degree of compromise for the purpose of providing rapid care to the sickest patients first. Patients with airway, breathing, circulation, or neurological emergencies are assigned the highest degree of urgency and receive care first. Individuals in extremis, even if they are expected to die or require an extraordinary amount of resources for their care, are provided with immediate treatment.

In-Hospital Triage Systems for Daily Operations

Most hospitals utilize a triage system that has three to five categories. The three main categories are *emergent* (Class 1), *urgent* (Class 2), and *nonurgent* (Class 3; Lanros & Barber, 1997). Where four or five levels are used, subcategories are added to either end of the spectrum. Table 22.1 illustrates the typical categories in three-, four-, and five-tier systems.

In a three-tier system, Emergent signifies a condition that requires treatment immediately or within 15 to 30 minutes.

Examples include cardiac arrest, airway obstruction, respiratory distress, uncontrolled acute bleeding, poor perfusion, acutely altered mental status, and acute pain. The Urgent category is assigned to patients with serious illness or injury that must be attended to as soon as possible, but for whom a wait of up to 2 hours would probably not add to morbidity or mortality. Examples include deformed long bone fractures, bleeding controlled with a pressure dressing, acute psychiatric problems (where the patient is in a safe environment), mild to moderate acute abdominal pain, and complicated open wounds. Nonurgent status is used for any patient who can wait more than 2 hours to be seen without the likelihood of deterioration. This includes problems or conditions such as simple fractures, minor lacerations, ear or throat pain, rash, or medication refill requests.

In a four-tier system, the Emergent category is usually subcategorized to identify those conditions that must be treated immediately (*STAT* or *1A*) versus rapidly (within a few minutes, *1B*). STAT conditions would include cardiac arrest, respiratory failure/arrest, airway obstruction, shock, and seizure. Conditions classified as 1B would include moderate to severe respiratory distress, cardiac dysrhythmia with adequate blood pressure, or heavy bleeding without hypotension or tachycardia.

In a five-tier system, the Nonurgent category is also subcategorized. Conditions that are nonacute, but require the technology of the ED to diagnose or treat, are categorized as *nonurgent ED* (Class 3). This would include conditions such as minor lacerations requiring sutures, or minor musculoskeletal trauma requiring x-rays for diagnosis. These types of conditions are frequently treated in an ED because there is a lack of access to these services on an emergency basis in the primary care setting. *Nonurgent Ambulatory Care* (Class 4) is used to classify those conditions that are nonurgent in nature and can routinely be provided in the ambulatory care setting. Examples of problems in this group are requests for medication refills, suture or staple removals, or chronic conditions that are stable such as preexisting skin rashes.

EDs that routinely experience significant overcrowding problems and long treatment delays often utilize a five-tier system, whereas those that rarely have delays tend to use a three-tier system. It has been suggested that EDs that usually use a three-tier system should be able to switch to a more detailed system (e.g., the five-tier system) during times of higher patient volumes to distinguish between sicker and less sick patients within the urgent and nonurgent groups. This is an adaptation that might be required in disasters and should be addressed in ongoing staff education and disaster drills.

TABLE 22.1 Hospital Triage Categories for a Three-, Four-, or Five-Tier System

Three-tier system	Emergent Class 1	Urgent Class 2	Nonurgent Class 3		
Four-tier system	Emergent Class 1A	Emergent Class 1B	Urgent Class 2	Nonurgent Class 3	
Five-tier system	Emergent Class 1A	Emergent Class 1B	Urgent Class 2	Nonurgent ED Care Class 3	Nonurgent Ambulatory Care Class 4

Disaster Triage in the Hospital Setting

True MCIs are uncommon in the United States. It is, therefore, very uncommon for hospitals in the United States to have to make decisions to withhold treatment from mortally injured disaster victims. Exceptions may include large disasters in rural areas with limited hospital and subspecialty (e.g., pediatric and burn care) capabilities and incidents such as Hurricane Katrina and the spring 2011 tornadoes in the midwestern and southern United States, in which hospitals were themselves compromised and sometimes rendered nearly inoperable but still faced with triaging and caring for both affected inpatients and incoming casualties.

Similar to EMS systems, what is deemed a disaster for one hospital may be seen as routine operations for another. For example, a large ED with an annual volume of more than 100,000 patients per year and full trauma care capabilities may not commence disaster operations for the arrival of even 10 trauma victims. Conversely, such a number of casualties may be overwhelming and require disaster resources in a smaller facility. Regardless of the size of the facility, each hospital must have in place a system to recognize when the available resources are likely to be inadequate and be able to implement disaster triage and operations at a moment's notice.

During a community-wide disaster, hospitals and their EDs usually activate their resources and prepare to receive an unusual influx of patients. Available non-ED staff report to a personnel pool for assignment, additional staff may be called in, and patients may be moved or procedures suspended to prepare for incoming casualties and their needs.

During normal operations, noncritical treatment and diagnostic interventions in the ED are sometimes delayed until the registration process is complete and medical record and account numbers are retrieved or generated. To eliminate this delay in disasters, previously made disaster or "STAT charts" should be prepared ahead of time, so that, as each patient enters the ED, a medical record number is immediately assigned. Using the STAT pack patient ID system, diagnostic testing can be performed without waiting for an actual registration in the hospital information system. Similar systems are used frequently in trauma centers, and they work well. These STAT charts contain a sequential STAT number or pseudonym ("Disaster 1" or "Disaster Orange") in the patient name section of the chart along with a predesignated medical record number. Preassembled STAT packets contain the STAT chart, a prestamped triage slip, identification band, and lab and x-ray requisition slips. Box 22.3 illustrates a typical STAT chart packet. As patients arrive at the ED disaster triage area(s), they are issued a STAT pack and the STAT chart numbers and/or pseudonyms are entered onto a disaster patient tracking log. The tracking log should also record the triage tag numbers of patients transported by EMS, as EMS officials often track patients by their tag numbers rather than patient name. Linking the triage tag number with other hospital-acquired patient identifiers can help in reuniting family members with their loved ones and help provide response partners with patient linkages for follow-up information important for after-action documentation and analyses. When time and resources permit, real names and other essential medical record information should be appended to the STAT chart record.

BOX 22.3 Contents of Typical Disaster STAT Pack Chart System

Preassigned STAT medical record number and STAT number or pseudonym
Prestamped:
    ED medical record
    Triage slip
    Laboratory slips
    X-ray requisitions
    Labels for blood tubes
    Patient identification band
Log form that contains preentered STAT medical record number and STAT number/name that can be used to track patients through the system

---

As EMS patients present to the ED, triage team staff should be stationed at the ambulance bay. Table 22.2 lists the staff required for a typical disaster triage team and their roles in the triage process. If there are a large number of casualties arriving simultaneously, two or more triage teams may be utilized. A triage team may need to be located at the ED walk-in entrance to assess patients arriving by personal vehicles and other forms of transportation that are not part of the EMS system. It is worth repeating that it is possible that not all disaster victims will arrive at the hospital having already been triaged, treated, or decontaminated prior to their arrival. The more patients presenting to the hospital, the more likely it is that ED staff will have to do disaster-style primary triage. More conventional triage may then be used as a form of secondary triage after patients are initially grossly sorted using field triage tools.

As the patient arrives, the triage team does a rapid triage evaluation, while a clerk applies a STAT record identification band, hands the corresponding triage slip to the triage officer, places the STAT chart on the gurney with the patient, and logs the STAT medical record number, STAT number/pseudonym, and, if possible, the patient name, as well as the ED area assignment. Ambulatory or wheelchair-bound patients may be asked to carry their own charts to their assigned treatment area. As a patient is stabilized and leaves the ED, the disposition is entered on the tracking log. If the patient name is not available at the time of triage, evaluation and treatment is initiated using the STAT medical record number and name.

After rapid assessment, the patient is triaged to a treatment location and team in the ED (or other designated area in the facility), where a more thorough evaluation and treatment will take place. It is also important to remember that during a disaster situation, nondisaster patients will continue to arrive at the ED. Provisions need to be made for these patients as well, as there is a risk of this group being ignored in the fray.

Note that many MCIs produce more Minor patients than any other triage category. It is not unusual that these patients are placed on a bus or other nonmedical transport vehicle(s) at the scene and transported in groups to one or more local hospitals for further evaluation. These Minor patients may present to the hospital early in the incident if the more seriously injured patients require extrication or experience other delays at the

TABLE 22.2 Staff Complement of a Typical Disaster Triage Team

Staff	Functional Role in Triage
Emergency physician*	Triage officer
Emergency nurse (1)	Evaluates patient and reports findings to officer, supervises clerk, nursing aid, and transporters
Emergency nurse (2)	Records all assessments
Nurse's aide/clerk	Applies prenumbered identification band
Transporter	Moves patient from triage area to assigned area in the ED

ED, emergency department.

Note: Depending on the size and nature of the disaster, and available staff, several triage teams may be assembled or different levels of staff may be used to perform these functional roles.

*In some facilities, a senior level ED registered nurse may be designated as the triage officer.

scene. It is important not to allow Minor patients to take up space and resources that may be needed for sicker patients just because they arrive first. It is sometimes useful to separate the minimal treatment area from the main part of the ED. For example, onsite clinics or urgent care areas may be used. These areas are then staffed with a mix of ED and other hospital personnel, and stocked with equipment and supplies for the care of minor wounds and musculoskeletal trauma. It is imperative to remember that an initial Minimal triage designation does not guarantee that a patient does not have a potentially dangerous injury. All Minor patients require a high index of suspicion and careful evaluation during secondary triage at the ED.

Several other complicating factors may affect triage and initial treatment operations at the hospital. Similar to what may occur in the field, injured adult caregivers accompanying injured children can interrupt patient flow if they refuse to be separated from their children. When this occurs, it is often best to triage each individual but then send the whole family to the treatment area designated for the triage category of the sickest individual. This may result in a child identified as being in the minimal category being sent to an area designated for those with delayed or immediate needs with their caregiver, who has been identified as needing more urgent care, or vice versa, but keeping them together may save time and effort later. Unaccompanied minors may require additional staff to stay with them, even if they do not require constant bedside nursing care. Nonclinical hospital staff can perform this function if they were recruited and trained as part of the disaster plan. Having a staff member with unaccompanied minors is a critical function that not only helps to ensure patient safety but also provides very important psychological support for the children.

Patients with acute emotional/psychological decompensation but otherwise minor injuries require not only medical care for their physical injuries but also assessment of their psychological

status. These patients often benefit from being placed in an area away from the noise and traffic of the main ED, attended not only by medical personnel but also by mental health professionals, social workers, or members of the clergy. It is also helpful to make these types of staff members available in areas where family members of the victims are coming to inquire about a loved one or are waiting while their relative receives treatment. One of many lessons that was shared from the 2016 Orlando nightclub shooting is the need to address the large numbers of friends, family members, and the media who will come to the hospital after an event looking for information (Heightman, 2017).

The need to deal with the psychological trauma of a disaster in the hospital-based acute care setting has only recently started to receive more attention. The concept of "Continuous Integrated Triage," proposed by Dr. Maurice Ramirez following his experience as a federal Disaster Medical Assistance Team member working with casualties at the Louis Armstrong International Airport in New Orleans after Hurricane Katrina, emphasizes the dynamic nature of disaster triage from the scene to the hospital and introduces the need to place an equal emphasis on the potential psychological impact of the disaster on victims, their loved ones, and field- and hospital-based responders (Shultz et al., 2007).

A final issue related to ED triage of disaster victims is the complexity of the real-time determination of a given ED's status and capacity at the time of an acute disaster. Many EDs work at or above capacity through much of the year. When a disaster occurs, EDs must often find ways to stretch their capacity even further to receive casualties. At the onset of a disaster, the local EMS system will often poll local hospitals to determine how many victims they can handle and of what level of acuity; a very quick assessment of the hospitals' status is often required. The determination is usually made by the ED nurse manager/charge nurse and ED attending physician(s), often in concert with the house nursing supervisor. Although it is the ED's capacity that is the foremost factor in the determination, the availability of operating rooms, intensive care unit beds, and onsite availability of clinicians and support staff is also important. The number, status, and acuity of ED patients already undergoing treatment as well as those waiting to be seen must be considered, along with the availability of treatment area beds for critical and less critical patients once the existing patients who can be moved to an alternate treatment area are physically relocated. Even the number of available stretchers can play a role, as patients transported on backboards with spinal motion restriction measures in place must be placed on the floor if stretchers are not available. What may seem like a simple request, to declare how many Immediate, Delayed, and Minimal patients an ED can receive, is in fact a complicated question that requires the consideration of many factors. Some hospitals use formulas to help make this determination but there is no easy way to give anything other than an estimate. In a prolonged or large-scale incident, hospitals may be repolled to determine their available capacity. Hospitals themselves should contact the coordinating center to change their status if they have more capacity than they originally estimated or if they have reached or exceeded their capacity. It is important to note that EMS agencies are not bound by the hospital capacity estimates. The need to juggle numbers and types of patients to clear the disaster scene efficiently sometimes results in a patient distribution that does not match declared capacities. Hospitals must remain as flexible as possible and expect to be challenged, but it is equally important that they be honest and report to EMS when there are patient safety issues and they can no longer take any or certain kinds of patients. This is possible only in systems with multiple hospitals. Once all hospitals have reached capacity, patients may need to be transported to more distant resources and/or the local hospitals may need to implement "real" disaster triage strategies and ration resources. The available resources in a community and the circumstances of the event will dictate when this point is reached; it will likely be sooner in more isolated areas.

PREHOSPITAL DISASTER TRIAGE

Although the military has been performing field triage for many years, specific prehospital MCI/disaster triage tools have been available in the United States only since the release of the Simple Triage and Rapid Treatment (START) tool in 1983. The majority of the tools used around the world for primary disaster triage are physiology-based and rely on a rapid assessment of respirations, perfusion, mental status and, often, the ability of victims to walk. See Box 22.4 for a list of the most commonly used prehospital MCI primary triage tools.

It is important to note that, although many tools are available, no primary MCI triage tool has been clinically validated prospectively (Kilner et al., 2011). Most of these tools were developed by clinicians based on clinical experience and, in some cases, utilizing components of trauma scores and tools that are used for everyday triage of trauma patients. A single tool, the Sacco Triage Method, was developed using a mathematical model-based analysis of retrospective outcome data from a statewide registry of trauma patients (Sacco et al., 2005). The body of literature on MCI triage tools consists primarily of analyses of drills, effectiveness of training, skills retention, and reproducibility (Deluhery, Lerner, Pirrallo, & Schwartz, 2011; Lerner, Schwartz, Coule, & Pirrallo, 2010; Navin & Waddell, 2004; Risavi, Salen, & Heller, 2001; Sanddal, Loyacano, & Sanddal, 2004; Sapp, Brice, Meyers, & Hinchey, 2010). There are limited reports of sensitivity and specificity of given tools in real incidents or nondisaster (ED/clinic) settings (Kahn, Schultz, Miller, & Anderson, 2009; Wallis & Carley, 2006). Clinical validation efforts are handicapped by the difficulty inherent in recording and collecting data in the chaos of disasters and the lack of standards by which to judge the clinical appropriateness of the triage decisions for individual victims. A recent publication has proposed a criterion standard definition for evaluating the accuracy of triage based on the diagnosis and the care that is ultimately provided that is likely to allow for more research to be conducted in the near future (Lerner, McKee, et al., 2015).

In 2008, a multidisciplinary committee funded by the CDC studied the existing MCI triage tools. Noting the lack of consistency and validation, the committee developed a primary triage tool, SALT Triage (see the next section), drawing from existing evidence and experience (Lerner, Schwartz, Coule, Weinstein, et al., 2008). Recognizing that designing a tool left little room for innovation, the committee was expanded and produced a set of evidence-based guidelines for common elements that should

be incorporated into all primary MCI triage tools in the United States. The guidelines are called the Model Uniform Core Criteria (Lerner, Cone, et al., 2011). A significant number of the pertinent professional associations in the United States endorsed these guidelines (Model uniform core criteria for mass casualty triage, 2011). An implementation plan for these guidelines was issued in 2013 by the FICEMS and these efforts are continuing to evolve (FICEMS, 2013). Research into population-based triage as well as secondary and tertiary triage is nonexistent and there are a limited number of papers written by topic experts in the field describing these practices. Additional research into the effectiveness of triage modalities and on triage as it relates to surge capacity is needed (Rothman, Hsu, Kahn, & Kelen, 2006).

Although the existing triage tools lack validation, a prevailing opinion is that it is better to use even a nonvalidated tool than no tool at all. Objective tools can help to bring some organization and standardization to a difficult process in a chaotic environment. Clinicians of different levels of training and experience can theoretically perform in a similar fashion by adhering to standardized guidelines and using tools to assist them in making a rapid triage decision for each patient. Perhaps as important as the effect of the triage process on the patients themselves is the effect on the providers performing triage. Primary triage may go against all the natural instincts of rescuers accustomed to trying to save each patient. Being responsible for making the call to withhold care and prioritize access to resources can be a heavy emotional burden that may adversely affect a provider both professionally and personally. By offering objective guidelines, the triage tool itself absorbs at least some of the responsibility of making those critical decisions.

It is important that ED-based clinicians know and understand the MCI triage tools and systems utilized by their local EMS agencies to be able to interpret their triage decisions and anticipate the resources needed by those patients based on their initial triage categorizations. Because SALT, START, and JumpSTART are commonly used primary triage tools in the United States, we will present them in some detail. Detailed information about other triage systems is widely available via Internet searches. Local EMS agencies may also be able to provide information about, and training for, hospital staff on the tools used in their jurisdictions.

There are several key aspects that are common to most triage systems. Death is usually defined by apnea. A pulse check is not performed because it is assumed that all nonobstructive adult apnea is accompanied by myocardial anoxia and pulselessness. Even if the victim were to have a pulse, it is unlikely it would continue long enough for sufficient additional resources to arrive to initiate resuscitation. If a victim is actively bleeding or unable to maintain an open airway, the responder performing triage may quickly attempt to control the bleeding and/or open the upper airway. However, the provider(s) assigned to conduct triage cannot stay with the victim. Most triage systems will allow the responder to apply a pressure dressing or tourniquet to control bleeding or open the airway with a jaw thrust maneuver and/or insertion of an oropharyngeal airway. If further interventions are needed, the provider may try to quickly obtain assistance from a bystander, minimally injured victim, or other first responder who will stay with the patient, but the responder(s) assigned to triage victims cannot stay to provide further treatment and must move to the next victim.

BOX 22.4 Prehospital MCI Triage Tools

All Ages
  The Sacco Triage Method
  SALT Triage
Adults Only
  Simple Triage and Rapid Treatment (START)
Pediatrics Only
  JumpSTART Pediatric MCI Triage
  The Pediatric Triage Tape
Age Not Specified
  Careflight Triage
  Triage Sieve

MCI, mass casualty incident; SALT, Sort-Assess-Lifesaving interventions-Treatment/transport.

SALT Triage

As described previously, a CDC-sponsored expert panel developed SALT Triage. It is nonproprietary and meets the model uniform core criteria for mass casualty triage. SALT stands for Sort-Assess-Lifesaving interventions-Treatment/transport, which describes the steps followed when performing SALT triage (Lerner, Schwartz, Coule, Weinstein, et al., 2008; Figure 22.1). It uses an all-hazards approach that is intended to be used for any age patient in any type of event.

The first step of SALT triage is global sorting. This step prioritizes patients for individual assessment using two voice commands. The first command directs patients to walk to a designated area, "If you can hear my voice and need help, please move to _____." Those who walk are the last priority for individual assessment; however, it is important to emphasize that these patients are not automatically triaged to the Minimal category; they need an individual assessment. These patients will be the last to be individually assessed, because they are the least likely to have a life-threatening condition (i.e., their brain and muscles are getting sufficient oxygen to process information and to move). The second command directs those who remain to wave, "If you can hear my voice and need help, please wave your arm or leg." The patients who do not move at all or those with obvious life threats (e.g., major bleeding) are prioritized first for individual assessment. Those who wave are the second group for individual assessment, and those who walked to the designated area are prioritized last for individual assessment. While the global sorting process will not be perfect, it will create some order to the scene. It is an initial attempt to organize numerous casualties into three groups, but every casualty still needs to be individually assessed.

The second step in SALT Triage is the individual assessment of each casualty. The individual assessment should begin with considering if the victim needs lifesaving interventions. These interventions include: (a) controlling major hemorrhage; (b) opening the airway with a basic airway maneuver (Two rescue breaths may also be delivered if a child is apneic after upper airway

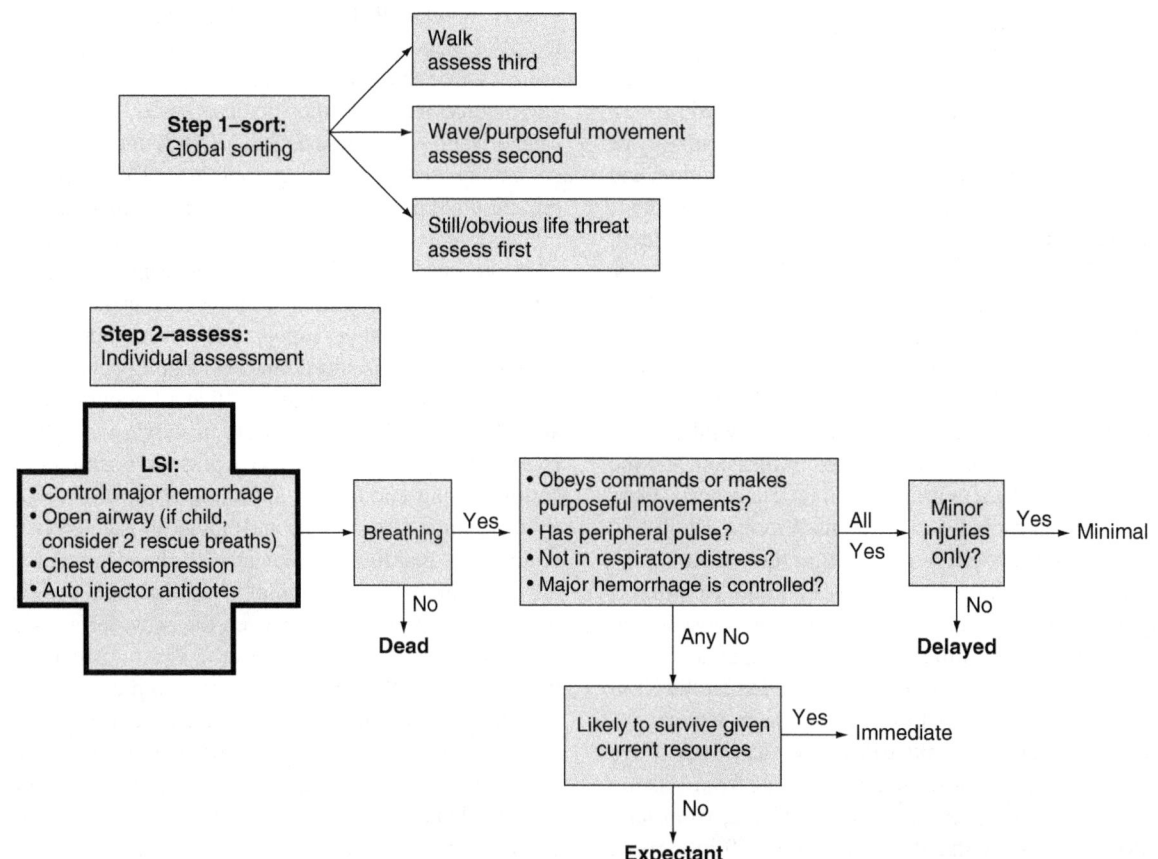

FIGURE 22.1 SALT Triage.

positioning; these breaths are given in an effort to help open the mid to lower airways.); (c) performing needle decompression for a possible tension pneumothorax; and (d) providing autoinjector antidotes. Each of these procedures should be provided quickly if the equipment is available and is within the provider's scope of practice. These specific interventions were selected because they can be done quickly and, with the exception of the lower airway opening ventilations, are known to improve the likelihood of survival.

Once any lifesaving interventions are performed, the responders should evaluate the patient and prioritize him or her for treatment and/or transport.

- **Dead:** those who are not breathing even after lifesaving interventions have been attempted.
- **Immediate:** those with difficulty breathing, uncontrolled hemorrhage, absence of peripheral pulses, and/or inability to follow commands; who are likely to survive given the available resources.
- **Expectant:** those with difficulty breathing, uncontrolled hemorrhage, absence of peripheral pulses, and/or inability to follow commands; who are unlikely to survive given the available resources.
- **Delayed:** those who are alert and follow commands, have palpable peripheral pulses, no signs of respiratory distress, and all bleeding is controlled, with injuries or an illness that in the opinion of the rescuer is more than minor.
- **Minimal:** those who are alert and follow commands, have palpable peripheral pulses, no signs of respiratory distress, and all bleeding is controlled, with injuries/condition that in the opinion of the rescuer are minor.

To learn more about using the SALT Triage method, there is an educational lecture available at www.Salttriage.org

Simple Triage and Rapid Treatment

The START triage tool is a commonly used adult MCI primary triage tool developed by the Newport Beach Fire and Marine Department and Hoag Hospital in California, first published in 1983 and revised in 1994 (Benson, Koenig, & Schultz, 1996). It was devised for use only for adults, with an arbitrary lower application limit of a patient weight of 100 pounds. The five basic parameters assessed with START are: (a) the ability to walk, (b) the presence or absence of spontaneous respirations, (c) the respiratory rate, (d) an assessment of perfusion, and (e) the ability to obey commands. These parameters are often referred to as respirations, perfusion, and mental status (RPM). The parameters are assessed in a sequential fashion for each patient, with the assessment being terminated immediately upon the identification of a critical threshold criterion.

The first action upon entering the scene (after identifying and starting mitigation of ongoing hazards) is to make an announcement stating:" Anyone who can hear my voice should get up and walk to a designated point, where they will be met by a rescuer at the first possible opportunity." All victims able to walk alone or with minimal assistance are designated as Minor. These patients are presumed to have well-compensated physiology, regardless of the nature of their injuries, because

all vital physiological functions must be adequate to coordinate and power the sophisticated task of hearing, interpreting, and obeying the command to walk. It is very important that a clinician assess all Minor patients as soon as possible in secondary triage or as part of any reassessment of primary triage. These victims might have deteriorated over time or have injuries or comorbid conditions that make them potentially unstable.

All of the victims who are unable to get up and walk are then assessed individually. Responders generally work from victim to victim in a grid pattern rather than trying to go to the obviously sickest patients first. For each victim the responder determines if he or she is breathing spontaneously. If an upper airway opening maneuver does not stimulate spontaneous respirations, the patient is triaged as Expectant without further assessment.

If the patient is breathing spontaneously on initial approach, the responder quickly estimates the respiratory rate. If the rate is faster than 30 breaths per minute, the patient is triaged as Emergent and the responder moves on to the next patient. If the patient is breathing at a rate of 30 breaths per minute or less, the responder assesses circulation by checking capillary refill or palpating for a pulse. In cool/cold weather, pulse palpation may be more accurate than capillary refill and is also easier to perform in poor lighting. Rescuers wearing multiple layers of gloves may find capillary refill to be easier than feeling a pulse. If the capillary refill (central or in the least-injured limb) is greater than 2 seconds or if there is no palpable pulse, the patient is triaged as Emergent. Remember that this patient is breathing, so the lack of a pulse is an indicator of shock but not cardiac arrest.

If the perfusion is adequate, as determined by capillary refill or pulse, the responder assesses mental status by asking the patient to follow a simple command such as "squeeze my hand." If the patient can presumably hear and interpret the simple command but cannot comply, he or she is tagged Emergent. If the patient can obey the command, he or she is tagged Urgent. To be triaged Urgent, a patient must be nonambulatory but have adequate respirations and circulation and, presumably, sufficient mental status to be able to guard his or her own airway.

TABLE 22.3 Using RPM to Classify Patients Using START

Category (Color)	RPM Indicators
Emergent (Red)	R = Respiratory rate > 30 P = Capillary refill > 2 sec or absent peripheral pulse M = Does not obey commands
Urgent (Yellow)	R < 30 P < 2 sec M = Obeys commands
Expectant: Dead or dying (Black)	R = Not breathing after jaw thrust
Minor (Green)	Able to walk

RPM, respirations, perfusion, and mental status; START, Simple Triage and Rapid Treatment.

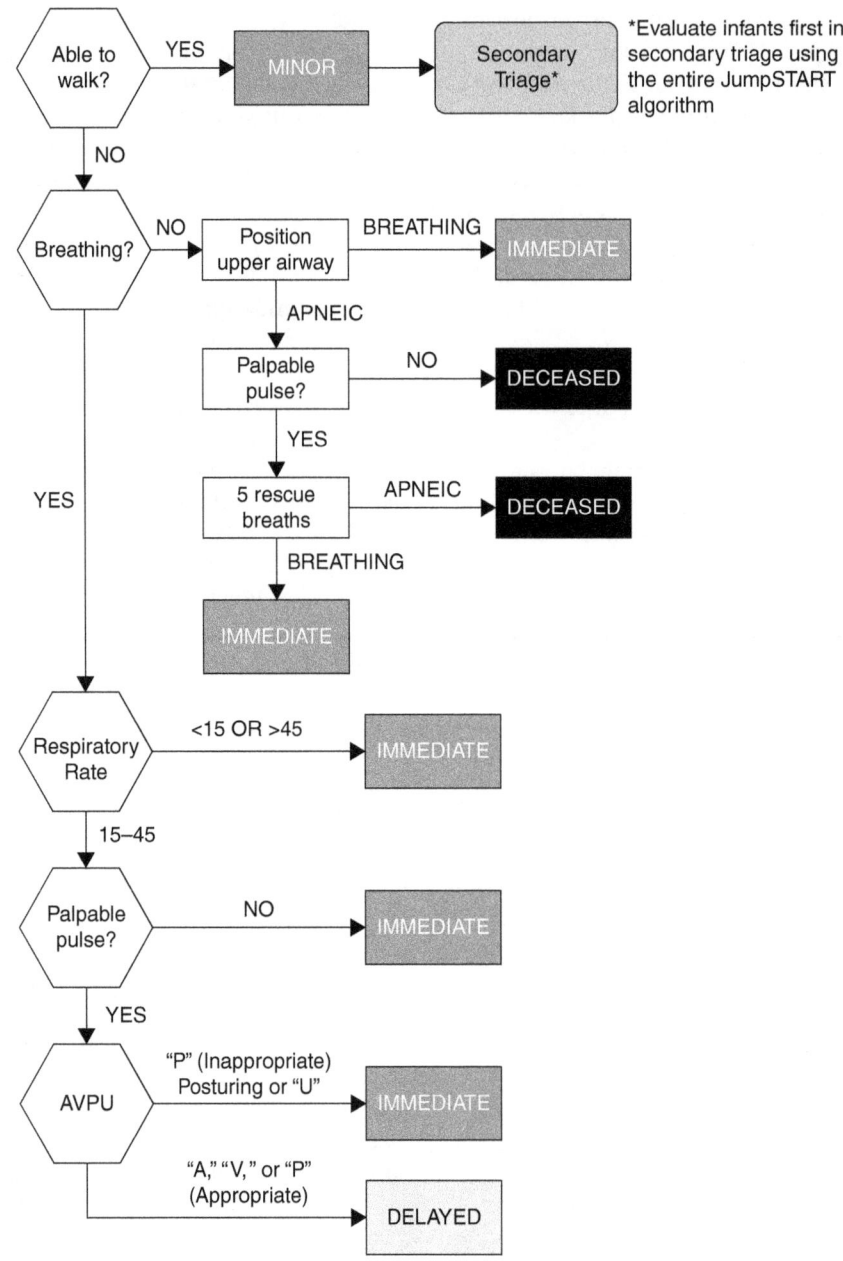

FIGURE 22.2 JumpSTART triage algorithm.

AVPU, alert, voice, pain, unresponsive; START, Simple Triage and Rapid Treatment.

Table 22.3 summarizes the critical decision thresholds utilized by START. The thresholds for Emergent and Urgent can be easily remembered by the mnemonic:

R (Respirations)	P (Pulse)	M (Mobility)
30	2	"Can do"

JumpSTART

The JumpSTART Pediatric MCI Triage Tool was the first objective tool developed specifically for the primary triage of children in the multicasualty/disaster setting. JumpSTART was developed in 1995 and modified in 2001 by Dr. Lou Romig, a pediatric emergency medicine physician with a background in both EMS and pediatric disaster preparedness and response.

Dr. Romig recognized that there were several decision thresholds for START that were not appropriate for pediatric physiology. JumpSTART addresses the unique physiology of children while paralleling the structure and procedures of START (Romig, 2002, 2007, 2011).

Figure 22.2 shows the JumpSTART algorithm. JumpSTART differs in several key ways from START:

1. JumpSTART should be used for "all victims who appear to be children" and START for "all victims who appear to be young adults or older." This means that START should be used for "tweens and teens" who have adult respiratory mechanics but may weigh less than START's stated lower limit of 100 pounds. A general guide for identifying those who "appear to be children" is the absence of secondary

sex characteristics such as breast development and growth of facial hair.

2. START's criterion for being tagged Minor is the ability to walk, but this may be inaccurate when triaging very young children and those with developmental or motor disabilities that prevent unassisted ambulation. All children who probably are not able to walk unassisted under normal circumstances should be assessed using JumpSTART. Any patient meeting an Emergent criterion is triaged as Emergent. For those patients who complete the algorithm and under JumpSTART would be considered Urgent, the responder performs a quick scan for external signs of significant injury (e.g., penetrating injuries, significant burns, tissue avulsions, amputations, crush injuries, abdominal distension, or vigorous active bleeding). If present, the patient remains Urgent and, if absent, the patient is triaged as Minor, even though they cannot walk.

3. Any child who is carried to the designated location when the walk command is given should be individually assessed first when sufficient personnel become available to attend to the patients in that area.

4. Because children primarily sustain respiratory failure/arrest before their hearts stop, there may be a short time period where a child may be apneic but still have detectable circulation. This is more likely to occur in a child because the heart does not stop functioning until it becomes anoxic and sustains significant damage. In adults, apnea more often follows cardiac arrest, while in children cardiac arrest more often follows hypoxia/apnea. It is theoretically possible that an apneic child who still has a perfusing rhythm may be salvageable if spontaneous ventilation can be reestablished (i.e., "window of salvageability"). Therefore, five rescue breaths should be provided to apneic children who have a detectable pulse.

5. Because a slow respiratory rate has more dire implications than tachypnea in a child, JumpSTART adds a low respiratory rate as a critical threshold.

6. Young children may be unable or unwilling to obey simple commands because they are not developmentally or behaviorally capable or are just scared. Therefore, the AVPU (alert, voice, pain, unresponsive) scale is used as an indicator of mental status rather than simply the ability to obey commands.

Although it is not unusual to find multicasualty scenes at which there are only adult patients, it is virtually guaranteed that when children are involved in an incident there will be adults to triage as well. The parallel structures of START and JumpSTART make it easier to switch back and forth between the algorithms depending on the apparent age of the victim being assessed. Figure 22.3 shows how START and Jump-START can be integrated.

When triaging a scene at which there are both adult and pediatric victims, the primary triage approach is the same as when dealing only with adults. The responder makes the announcement for ambulatory patients to proceed to a designated point and stay there. Any infant or child who is carried to the designated Minor area must be individually

assessed and triaged at the first possible opportunity. When the triaging responder finds an apneic child, he or she performs a jaw thrust. If the child starts to breathe, the child is triaged Emergent, just as in the START algorithm. If the child does not start to breathe, the responder checks for the pulse with which he or she is most comfortable assessing on a child. Note that this is different from START, and aims to detect children who may be in the "window of salvageability." It also acknowledges the innate imperative most clinicians feel to "go the extra mile" for a child. If no pulse is detectable, the child is presumed to be in full cardiopulmonary arrest and triaged as Dead. If a pulse is palpable, the responder quickly administers five breaths via a mouth-to-barrier device, attempting to open the lower airways and trigger spontaneous breathing. This is called the "ventilatory trial" and is the "jump start" that gives JumpSTART its name. Some agencies skip the pulse check and go directly to the ventilatory trial after upper airway opening fails to trigger respirations. If the child remains apneic after the five ventilations, he or she is triaged Expectant, regardless of the presence of a pulse, because there are insufficient resources to conduct a full resuscitation. If the child starts to breathe spontaneously, he or she is tagged Emergent.

JumpSTART's respiratory rate thresholds for spontaneously breathing children are 15 and 45 breaths per minute. Rates greater than 45 or less than 15 are triaged Emergent. When combined, the pediatric and adult critical respiratory rates then become easier to remember, as they are multiples of 15 (i.e., 15, 30, and 45). As with START, either capillary refill or pulse palpation is used to assess perfusion. The Emergent criteria of capillary refill greater than 2 seconds or failure to detect a pulse are the same as for START. Care should be taken not to spend more than 15 to 20 seconds trying to feel a pulse. The overall goal is to take a minute or less to triage each patient. If a pulse is that hard to find, err on the side of up-triaging, especially if the capillary refill is also prolonged.

The final assessment is that of mental status. Because obeying commands is dependent on both cognition and behavior, it is not a universally appropriate gauge of pediatric mental status. Pediatric patients are rated using AVPU instead (Jevon, Humphreys, & Ewens, 2008). If the patient is alert, responsive to voice, or localizes a painful stimulus, he or she is triaged Urgent. If the patient has only a generalized response to pain, exhibits posturing, or is truly unresponsive to all stimuli, he or she is triaged Emergent. As with START, an Urgent patient is one who presumably cannot walk due to the trauma but who has adequate respirations and circulation and sufficient mental status to protect his or her own airway.

TRIAGE TAGS

For the triage process to be effective, the findings from the triage process need to be communicated. This is typically done through triage tags that are attached to the patient. Triage tags can be a commercial product or as simple as using a marker to write the triage category directly on the patient or tying appropriately colored contractor's ribbon to the patient.

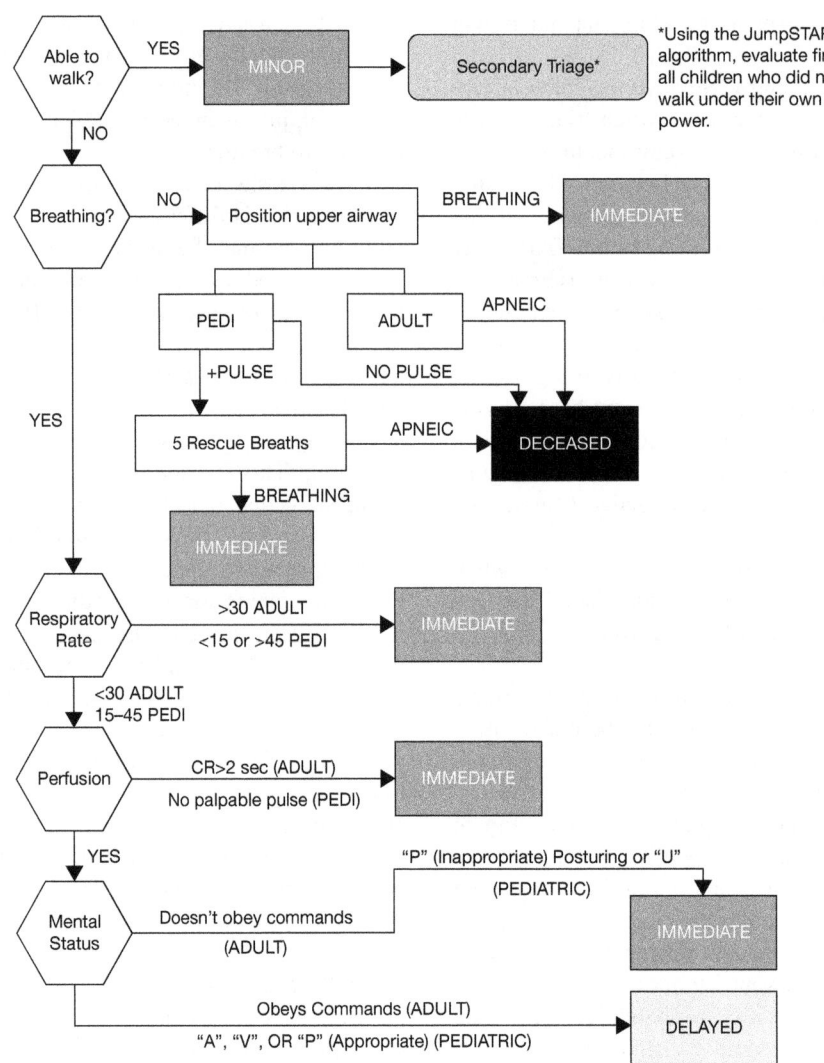

FIGURE 22.3 Combined START/JumpSTART triage algorithm.

RPM, respirations, perfusion, and mental status; START, Simple Triage and Rapid Treatment.

Source: Additional information about JumpSTART, including downloadable graphic files, drill materials, and educational presentations, is available at www.jumpstarttriage.com.

In some states or regions, common triage tags may be used to reduce costs and increase interoperability between agencies. Regardless of the type of tag used, there are some recommended features. Figures 22.4 and 22.5 show some typical features of triage tags. Patient tracking is very important, and using tags that include a unique identifier number can improve this process. Some tags may include bar-coded stickers or other features to simplify or automate the process for adding/communicating the unique identifying number to various patient-tracking logs and medical care records. Doing this can facilitate family reunification and other interagency information sharing. Another consideration is using triage tags that are waterproof and capable of being quickly and easily affixed directly to the patient—not to the patient's clothing. Tags should contain as much information as is available and should be easy to write on. Information to consider documenting on a triage tag includes the patient's name (when available), presenting injury or complaint, any interventions performed in the field or in triage at the hospital, and allergy and medication history. It is also extremely useful to add guardians' names and/or the guardian's own triage tag number to the tag of an injured child. In incidents in which EMS response is robust and patients are transported quickly, it may be impossible to add much information to the triage tag.

It is important for ED personnel to be familiar with the tags used by responders in their area, as well as with any tags that are used internally for casualties or in case of facility evacuation.

THE JOB OF THE TRIAGE OFFICER

The primary responsibility of the triage officer is to ensure that every victim has been found and triaged. Triage officers (meaning the person[s] in charge of triage, not implying a rank) and those responders assigned to perform triage do not

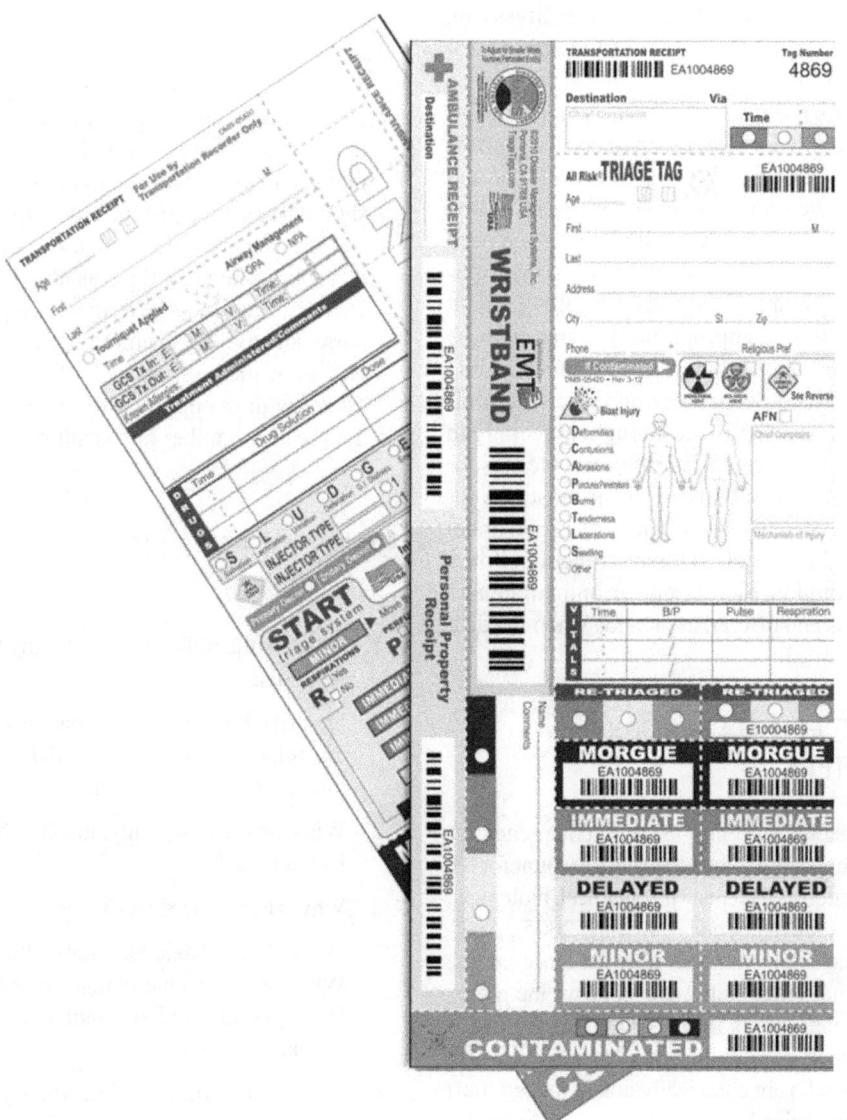

FIGURE 22.4 A typical disaster triage tag.

Source: Courtesy of Disaster Management Systems.

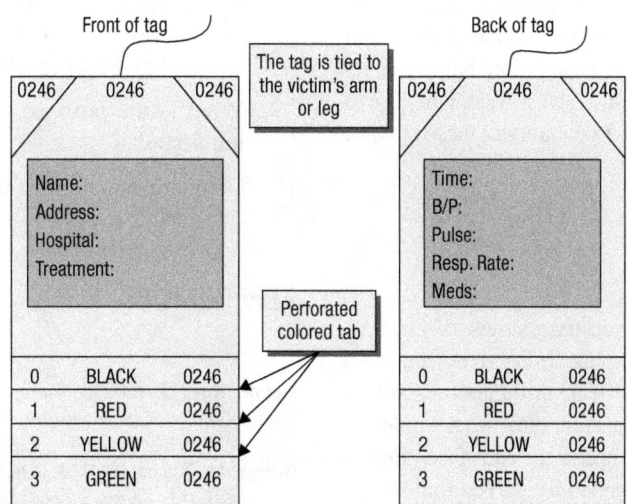

FIGURE 22.5 Example of a typical color-coded triage tag with perforated color bars.

provide immediate treatment other than to provide lifesaving interventions such as opening airways and trying to control active bleeding. In cases involving some chemical exposures, triage personnel may also administer medications via an autoinjector. In traditional MCI triage, the triage officer carries only supplies for performing lifesaving interventions and triage tags. The role of the triage officer is critical, as he/she is not only responsible for assuring that all victims have been identified and triaged but also for communicating the numbers of victims and the nature of their needs to the incident command supervisors so that appropriate resources can be requested and dispatched. The difficulty of being responsible for making possible life-and-death decisions based on minimal information cannot be emphasized enough, especially in the face of large numbers of casualties, pediatric victims, or victims who are fellow first responders. This is most true for responders in the field but may also be true for ED personnel who take on that role. Personnel who have functioned in a disaster triage role should be monitored for immediate and delayed stress reactions and offered assistance when needed.

DISASTER TRIAGE FOR HAZARDOUS MATERIAL DISASTERS

Field trauma triage systems currently used by emergency responders at MCIs and disasters do not adequately account for the possibility of contamination of patients with chemical, biological, radiological, or nuclear material (Cone & Koenig, 2005). Additionally, chemical or hazardous material disasters pose unique challenges in that hospital-based staff members have the potential to become victims themselves from exposure to the toxins or the physiological effects of working while wearing personal protective gear. Victims who are chemically contaminated must be decontaminated before being brought into the clean treatment area on scene or at the hospital (see Chapter 35 "Decontamination and Personal Protective Equipment," Mass Casualty Decontamination, for further information). Failure to do so may result in contamination of the staff, other patients, and the environment, and can potentially require evacuation and closure of the entire ED. Because some prehospital services may transport chemically exposed victims to the hospital prior to decontamination, and because other victims may leave the scene before being triaged and decontaminated, each hospital must have a system in place to employ special conditions triage and decontaminate these arrivals.

SUMMARY

Events may occur in which rapid assessment of large numbers of patients is required. The ability to correctly sort those patients may impact the health outcomes not only of individuals, but also of the community as a whole. Although empirical evidence to support the use of existing triage systems is lacking, it is generally agreed that the use of an objective triage system should help optimize

the allocation of scarce resources that defines a disaster. Successful use of a disaster-style triage system is a critical component of any hospital's acute surge capacity. Triage is the cornerstone of good disaster medical resource management in both the field and the hospital. Nurses should be aware of the different types of triage and triage systems used in and around their communities and when it is appropriate, use them as dictated by hospital policy. Disaster triage requires a significant paradigm shift for the nurse, and may be an emotionally distressing experience. However, the performance of accurate triage provides nurses with the opportunity to do the greatest good for the greatest number of casualties.

STUDY QUESTIONS

1. How are the philosophies of daily hospital triage different from disaster triage?
2. Describe how numbers of patients and available resources are related with regard to determining whether or not disaster triage must be used.
3. What are the basic daily hospital triage system categories? Explain each.
4. Why is there a need for disaster triage in the hospital setting?
5. Describe the basic elements of a disaster triage system. What do the triage categories of Immediate, Delayed, Minor, Dead, and Expectant mean? List types of problems for each category.
6. Discuss the differences between primary, secondary, and tertiary disaster triage.
7. During triage for mass casualty hazardous materials incidents, what are the differences in the triage activities in the hot, warm, and cold zones?
8. What are the five major cohort triage classifications during epidemic triage? To which area would each of these cohorts likely be triaged and what levels of care would they likely receive?
9. What is the purpose of triage tags and why are they important?
10. Compare and contrast triage for adults versus children.

REFERENCES

Auf der Heide, E. (2000). *Disaster response: Principles of preparation and coordination.* St. Louis, MO: CV Mosby. Retrieved from http://library.ndmctsgh.edu.tw/milmed/avitation/file-med/DisasterResponse.pdf

Benson, M., Koenig, K. L., & Schultz, C. H. (1996). Disaster triage: START then SAVE—A new method of dynamic triage for victims of a catastrophic earthquake. *Prehospital and Disaster Medicine, 11*(2), 117–124. doi:10.1017/S1049023X0004276X

Burkle, F. M. (1984). *Disaster medicine: Application for the immediate management and triage of civilian and military disaster victims.* New Hyde Park, NY: Medical Examination Publishing.

Centers for Disease Control and Prevention, National Center for Health Statistics. (2013). Emergency department visits. Retrieved from https://www.cdc.gov/nchs/fastats/emergency-department.htm

Cone, D., & Koenig K. L. (2005). Mass casualty triage in the chemical, biological, radiological, or nuclear environment. *European Journal of Emergency Medicine, 12,* 287–302. doi:10.1097/00063110-200512000-00009

Cone, D., & MacMillan, D. (2005). Mass-casualty triage systems: A hint of science. *Academic Emergency Medicine, 12,* 739–741. doi:10.1197/j.aem.2005.04.001

Deluhery, M., Lerner, E. B., Pirrallo, R. G., & Schwartz, R. B. (2011). Paramedic accuracy using SALT triage after a brief initial training. *Prehospital Emergency Care, 15,* 526–532. doi:10.3109/10903127.2011.569852

Federal Interagency Committee on Emergency Medical Services. (2013). *National implementation of the model uniform core criteria for mass casualty incident triage: A report of the FICEMS.* Retrieved from http://www.nhtsa.gov/staticfiles/nti/pdf/811891-Model_UCC_for_Mass_Casualty_Incident_Triage.pdf

Heightman, A. J. (2017). Lessons learned from EMS response to the Orlando Pulse Nightclub shooting. *Journal of Emergency Medical Services.* Retrieved from http://www.jems.com/articles/2017/01/lessons-learned-from-ems-response-to-the-orlando-pulse-nightclub-shooting.html

Hogan, D. E., & Lairet, J. (2002). Triage. In D. Hogan & J. Burrstein (Eds.), *Disaster medicine* (pp. 10–15). Philadelphia, PA: Lippincott Williams & Wilkins.

Jevon, P., Humphreys, M., & Ewans, B. (2008). *Nursing medical emergency patients.* Oxford, UK: Blackwell Publishing.

Kahn, C. A., Schultz, C. H., Miller, K. T., & Anderson, C. L. (2009). Does START triage work? An outcomes assessment after a disaster. *Annals of Emergency Medicine, 54*(3), 424–430. doi:10.1016/j.annemergmed.2008.12.035

Kilner, T. M., Brace, S. J., Cooke, M. W., Stallard, N., Bleetman, A., & Perkins G. D. (2011). In "big bang" major incidents do triage tools accurately predict clinical priority? *Injury, 42*(5), 460–468. doi:10.1016/j.injury.2010.11.005

Lanros, N., & Barber, J. (1997). *Emergency nursing* (4th ed.). Stamford, CT: Appleton Lange.

Lerner, E. B., Cone, D., Weinstein, E., Schwartz, R. B., Coule, P. L., Cronin, M., . . . Hunt, R. C. (2011). Mass casualty triage: An evaluation of the science and refinement of a national guideline. *Disaster Medicine and Public Health Preparedness, 5,* 129–137. doi:10.1001/dmp.2011.39

Lerner, E. B., McKee, C. H., Cady, C. E., Cone, D. C., Colella, M. R., Cooper, A., . . . Swienton, R. E. (2015). A consensus-based gold standard for the evaluation of mass casualty triage systems. *Prehospital Emergency Care, 19*(2), 267–271. doi:10.3109/10903127.2014.959222

Lerner, E. B., Schwartz, R. B., Coule, P. L., Weinstein, E. S., Cone, D. C., Hunt, R. C., . . . O'Connor, R. E. (2008). Mass casualty triage: An evaluation of the data and development of a proposed national guideline. *Disaster Medicine and Public Health Preparedness, 2*(Suppl 1), S25–S34. doi:10.1097/DMP.0b013e318182194e

Lerner, E. B., Schwartz, R. B., Coule, P. L., & Pirrallo, R. G. (2010). Use of SALT triage in a simulated mass-casualty incident. *Prehospital Emergency Care, 14*(1), 21–25. doi:10.3109/10903120903349812

Model uniform core criteria for mass casualty triage. (2011). *Disaster Medicine Public Health Preparedness, 5*(2), 125–128. doi:10.1001/dmp.2011.41

Navin, M., & Waddell, R. (2004). Triage is broken. *EMSWorld.* Retrieved from https://www.emsworld.com/article/10323785/triage-is-broken

Rice, M., & Abel, C. (1992). In S. B. Sheehy (Ed.), *Emergency nursing: Principles and practice* (p. 67). St. Louis, MO: Mosby Year Book.

Risavi, B. L., Salen, P. N., & Heller, M. B. (2001). A two-hour intervention using START improves prehospital triage of mass casualty incidents. *Prehospital Emergency Care, 5*(2), 197–199. doi:10.1080/10903120190940128

Robertson-Steel, I. (2006). Evolution of triage systems. *Emergency Medicine Journal, 23,* 154–155. doi:10.1136/emj.2005.030270

Romig, L. E. (2002). Pediatric triage. A system to JumpSTART your triage of young patients at MCIs. *Journal of Emergency Medicine Services, 27*(7), 52–58, 60–63.

Romig, L. E. (2007). Pediatric disaster triage: JumpSTART. In *Prehospital Trauma Life Support* (6th ed., pp. 373–377). New York, NY: Elsevier.

Romig, L. E. (2011). The JumpSTART pediatric MCI triage tool and other pediatric disaster and emergency medicine resources. Various citations. Retrieved from https://www.jumpstarttriage.com

Rothman, R. E., Hsu, E. B., Kahn, C. A., & Kelen, G. D. (2006). Research priorities for surge capacity. *Academic Emergency Medicine.* Retrieved from https://www.aemj.org/cgi/reprint/j.aem.2006.07.002v1

Sacco, W., Navin, D., Fielder, K., Waddell, R., Long, W., & Buckman, R. (2005). Precise formulation and evidence-based application of resource-constrained triage. *Academic Emergency Medicine, 12,* 759–770. doi:10.1197/j.aem.2005.04.003

Sanddal, T., Loyacono, T., & Sanddal, N. (2004). Effect of JumpSTART training on immediate and short-term pediatric triage performance. *Pediatric Emergency Care, 20,* 749–753. doi:10.1097/01.pec.0000144917.62877.8f

Sapp, R. F., Brice, J. H., Meyers, J. B., & Hinchey, P. (2010). Triage performance of first-year medical students using a multiple-casualty scenario, paper exercise. *Prehospital Disaster Medicine, 25*(3), 239–245. doi:10.1017/S1049023X00008104

Shultz, J., Espinel, Z., Galea, S., Hick, J. L., Shaw, J. A., & Miller, G. T. (2007). *Surge, sort, support: Disaster behavioral health for health care professionals.* Miami, FL: Center for Disaster & Extreme Even Preparedness.

Svoboda, T., Henry, B., Shulman, L., Kennedy, E., Rea, E., Ng, W., . . . Glazier, R. H. (2004). Public health measures to control the spread of the severe acute respiratory syndrome during the outbreak in Toronto. *The New England Journal of Medicine, 350,* 2352–2236. doi:10.1056/NEJMoa032111

United Nations International Strategy for Disaster Reduction. (2017). Terminology. Retrieved from https://www.unisdr.org/we/inform/terminology

Wallis, L. A., & Carley, S. (2006). Comparison of paediatric major incident primary triage tools. *Emergency Medicine Journal, 23*(6), 475–478. doi:10.1136/emj.2005.032672

23

DISASTER MANAGEMENT

Kristine M. Gebbie and Kristine Qureshi

LEARNING OBJECTIVES

When this chapter is completed, readers will be able to:

1. Describe the three types of disaster planning.
2. Explain the difference between an internal and external disaster.
3. Describe how an external disaster can create an internal disaster in a hospital.
4. Describe the different styles of disaster leadership and when to use each one.
5. Describe the five phases of disaster management.
6. Implement the Hospital Incident Command System during disaster management.
7. Discuss the role of interagency coordination and collaboration during disaster planning and response.
8. Discuss the impact of catastrophic events on the health system's capacity to maintain quality standards of care.

KEY MESSAGES

Planning is an essential element of any disaster management system in all health settings.

Effective disaster management requires system capacities, a competent staff, and a defined, executable, and practiced disaster response plan.

If not well-managed, external disasters can quickly become internal disasters for the organization involved.

The National Incident Management System (NIMS) provides guidance for the entire disaster response cycle. NIMS includes the Incident Command System (ICS), the management model designed to ensure coordinated command and control during disaster response.

Interagency cooperation and coordination are essential for effective disaster response.

After any disaster, an evaluation of the response must occur, with strengths and problems identified, and responsibility for needed change assigned.

Healthcare workers' ability and willingness to report to duty during catastrophic events will be facilitated when their needs and concerns are considered in planning.

During catastrophic events, many usual practices, including standards of care, may need to be adapted to meet the altered context.

CHAPTER OVERVIEW

The purpose of disaster preparedness and management in any community and in any healthcare facility is to maintain a safe environment and continue to provide essential services while responding to disruptions caused by an emergency. This is true whether the event is the result of something internal to the institution (e.g., fire, building collapse), external to the institution (e.g., flood, explosion, disease, power outage), or a combination. Disaster management includes preparedness/ risk assessment, prevention, mitigation, response, recovery, and evaluation. Effective planning is the first and arguably the most important element of disaster management. Strong leadership is required to mobilize and focus the organization's energy, and essential elements for success are system capacities that support the delivery of expected services; staff members and volunteers who are competent in their disaster response roles; a clearly defined, executable, and practiced disaster plan; and strong preexisting partnerships with collaborating organizations and agencies. In the United States, interagency collaboration and consistent terminology are required by the federal government through the NIMS (Department of Homeland Security [DHS], 2017; www.fema.gov/national-incident-management-system). This document and the associated National Response Framework (DHS, 2016) cover all phases of risk assessment, planning, prevention, response, recovery, and plan improvement. Within them, the ICS defines the table of organization and responsibilities required to manage any emergency or disaster response, particularly one that involves multiple agencies and levels of government.

In the world of healthcare, the Joint Commission (the major body accrediting hospitals and other health institutions in the United States) requires a comprehensive disaster plan that meets the requirements identified in NIMS (Joint Commission, 2016). As of 2017, the Centers for Medicare and Medicaid (CMS) expanded their emergency preparedness requirements for hospitals and healthcare facilities to maintain continuous eligibility to receive CMS funds (CMS, 2018). Most hospitals use the Hospital Incident Command System (HICS), which identifies the key components of managing the emergency within the hospital as well as coordination with other responding agencies (California Emergency Medical Services Authority, 2014). This system delineates a clear chain of command and authority and assigns specific disaster functional roles for staff members. After each disaster response, an evaluation must be done for the purpose of identifying what worked and what requires improvement. Afterward, follow-through activities must ensure that identified changes are implemented. Similar advance planning, practice, and evaluation should be done by all health and public health facilities, as they, too, are critical to any community's response to a disaster.

Contemporary thinking about disaster preparedness and response is grounded in the need to ensure a continuous process of building resilience for the institution and the community. "Resilience" is understood as "the ability of a system, community or society exposed to hazards to resist, absorb, accommodate to and recover from the effects of a hazard in a timely and efficient manner, including through the preservation and restoration of its essential basic structures and functions" (UN Office for Disaster Risk Reduction, 2015). While not a major component of this chapter, the reader is reminded to keep this concept in mind when considering any phase of disaster management.

Disaster management is a circular process, which begins with planning, moves through prevention and mitigation, is most visible during response, with evaluation and identification of areas for improvement leading back to planning and implementation of required changes. Some disasters may be prevented or avoided by thoughtful planning; strong leadership and sound disaster management can serve to mitigate the impact of many disasters. Advance planning that takes into account local geography, resources, and communications can facilitate the most effective response, including adapting care to meet the context in ways that will minimize injury and loss of life.

By now, with all of the media access we have, scarcely an hour passes after the landfall of a hurricane or the tremors of an earthquake before people around the globe are aware of and are following the unfolding disaster. Whether it is earthquakes in Nepal or Iran–Iraq, hurricanes in the United States and the Caribbean, or a volcanic eruption in Indonesia, there is an endless fascination with disasters and large-scale public health emergencies, even when there is no way for the remote watcher to make any difference in the course of the event. Disaster management of the 21st century goes beyond the original paradigm of incident response and postevent activities. It includes risk assessment, planning, prevention, mitigation, response, and recovery activities, all designed to strengthen resilience at all levels. In fact, a healthcare organization should spend more time on disaster preparedness planning and evaluation than on actual disaster response events. Focusing solely on actual response activities means that all resources may not be effectively used, and lessons learned in any one event may not be applied when making process improvements for future events. In any setting, the primary purpose of an emergency management plan is to maintain a safe environment during any type of emergency or disaster so that patient care or necessary public health services can continue to be delivered and staff are not exposed to undue risks. Important aspects of disaster management are *planning* and *practicing in advance* (Skryabina, Reedy, Amlot, Jaye, & Riley, 2017). Disaster planning requires the cooperative efforts of the health organization, other community agencies, and local governmental officials. Planning should focus on two levels: the planning necessary to ensure that the hospital, health department, or other health agency is appropriately coordinating with the overall community emergency plan, and internal planning to be sure that the organization is ready to manage its own internal operations during a disaster or emergency.

In a sentinel article, Cuny (1998) describes three types of advance planning activities: strategic, contingency, and forward planning. *Strategic planning* should be done to prepare the hospital, health department, or other health organization for any type of emergency or disaster, and includes planning for overall emergency management, staff training, and protection of the facility. *Contingency planning* is sometimes done in the form of appendices to the strategic (or all-hazards approach) plan. Contingency planning should provide actions that are consistent with the overall plan, to minimize the challenge to staff when a specific emergency or disaster requires a specialized activity. For organizations accredited by the Joint Commission, a hazard vulnerability assessment on which to base contingency planning is required. Finally, *forward planning* is done when the organization has been alerted to an impending disaster or event, as can occur following a severe weather warning, planning for a mass gathering in the community, projections of a disease outbreak, or communication about an overflow of casualties from an adjacent community. It focuses on plans for activation of the *existing* strategic and relevant contingency plans. Some forward planning is initiated years in advance, such as for Olympic sporting events; other planning begins only hours before the change in demand or circumstances may occur. Despite the fact that planning is critical to good disaster preparedness and response, it is frequently the step that receives the least attention. Auf der Heide (1989) attributes this to the "apathy factor." He reports that because disasters are low-probability events, disaster preparedness tends to get lost among the day-to-day events of our lives and in the workplace, community, and home settings. The public in general tends to be poorly informed about disaster preparedness and frequently either underestimates the risk for events or adopts an attitude of denial or fatalism. The government is more likely to earmark resources for programs that have a strong constituency, and frequently emergency preparedness planning is not on the priority list. In the United States, disaster planning and response have been a cross jurisdictional, interagency endeavor with poorly defined lines of authority and accountability. It is, therefore, difficult for a healthcare agency to make plans for interagency interface and coordination when the partners are difficult to identify.

However, beginning with the terrorism events on U.S. soil during 2001, the serious natural disasters of hurricanes in the Caribbean during 2017 that destroyed much of the infrastructure in Puerto Rico and the U.S. Virgin Islands, and the continuing threat of emerging and reemerging infectious diseases have resulted in continuing, heightened interest in the topic in the United States and the rest of the world. The passage of the Pandemic and All Hazards Preparedness Act (Public Law 109–417, 2006) strengthened the coordination of all preparedness activities and encouraged improved approaches at all levels of community. The value in planning is in its ability to anticipate problems that are likely to be encountered in a disaster and to develop practical, realistic, and cost-effective measures for response (Auf der Heide, 2002).

CLASSIFICATIONS OF DISASTERS

While the technical distinctions among types and levels of disasters may have little meaning to the individuals attempting to respond to a sudden surge in patients, the collapse of infrastructure, or the overlap of criminal behavior in a deliberately caused disaster, they may be very useful for thinking about strategic and contingency plans. The following concept descriptions are included to assist the reader to think broadly about the types of events that may necessitate use of an emergency management approach.

Internal Disaster

An internal disaster occurs when there is an event within an organization or facility that poses a threat to disrupt the environment of care. Such events are commonly related to the physical plant (e.g., loss of utilities or fire), but can arise from availability of personnel (e.g., a labor strike). Regardless of the cause, the management goal is to maintain a safe environment for the patients, continue to provide essential services, ameliorate the problem, and restore normal services. An all-hazards disaster plan provides an excellent template for response to such events.

External Disaster

An external disaster becomes a problem for a facility when the consequences of the event create a demand for services that tax or exceed the usual available resources. This could be the arrival within an hour of double the number of trauma patients usually seen over a 24-hour period, the arrival of victims of a chemical HAZMAT incident who need decontamination as well as medical attention, or a surge of ambulatory patient "walk-ins" associated with a reported communicable disease exposure in the community. A sudden unanticipated surge of patients can quickly overwhelm a hospital or healthcare facility, extending the impact of the disaster. To protect against large-scale influenza outbreaks in the community setting, an all-hazards disaster plan based on the ICS was used to support mass influenza vaccination–dispensing initiatives at a major university medical center (Swift et al., 2017). Influenza outbreaks that start in the community may rapidly spread to residents of nursing homes, placing a severe strain on day-to-day service delivery and operations (Lansbury, Brown, & Nguyen-vanTam, 2017).

Combined External/Internal Disaster

There are many circumstances that are external to the health organization that can trigger an internal disaster as well. A severe weather condition like a snowstorm or a geological event like an earthquake can create both conditions, by making it impossible for staff to travel safely to work, while leading multiple individuals who have experienced event-related trauma to seek care. An earthquake or nearby gas main explosion may cause structural damage to a hospital and surrounding buildings and roads, but also increase demand for care of mass casualties in the community. During Hurricane Sandy, three hospitals in New York City were evacuated and many of the nursing staff were redeployed to the receiving hospitals (VanDevanter, Kovner, Raveis, McCollum, & Keller, 2014). Such events require both a strong internal disaster management plan and close coordination of the health institution with the overall community disaster management system.

In addition to thinking through the needs for a disaster plan and disaster management for internal, external, or combined emergencies, the magnitude of the disaster in relation to the ability of the organization or community to respond is critical for health organizations or overall to a community. This approach is organized using three levels:

Level I: The organization, agency, or community is able to contain the event and respond effectively utilizing its own resources (each organization must ensure that each of its own employees is competent in basic emergency preparedness, and there is adequate surge capacity within its own organization to be prepared to respond to routine emergencies, some of which can be expected, such as power outages, weather events, or other limited events).

Level II: The disaster requires assistance from external sources, but these can be obtained from nearby agencies or adjacent communities (each organization must ensure that it has adequate linkages with other organizations and agencies in the surrounding community so when they are needed, the required local support and assets can be readily procured).

Level III: The disaster is of a magnitude that exceeds the overall capacity of the local community or region and requires assistance from state level or even federal resources (the community as a whole must ensure that it has adequate linkages with state- and federal-level organizations, has the ability to know when to request a higher level of assistance, and knows the communication chain of command for requesting state and or federal assistance). Figure 23.1 illustrates the complex flow of information required if all levels (community, state, federal government) are involved in an emergency response.

Depending on the severity of the disaster, recovery will usually occur on a continuum. The Federal Emergency Management Agency (FEMA) has outlined this continuum in the National Disaster Recovery Framework (2016b). This continuum begins with preparedness, then the disaster event, and considers

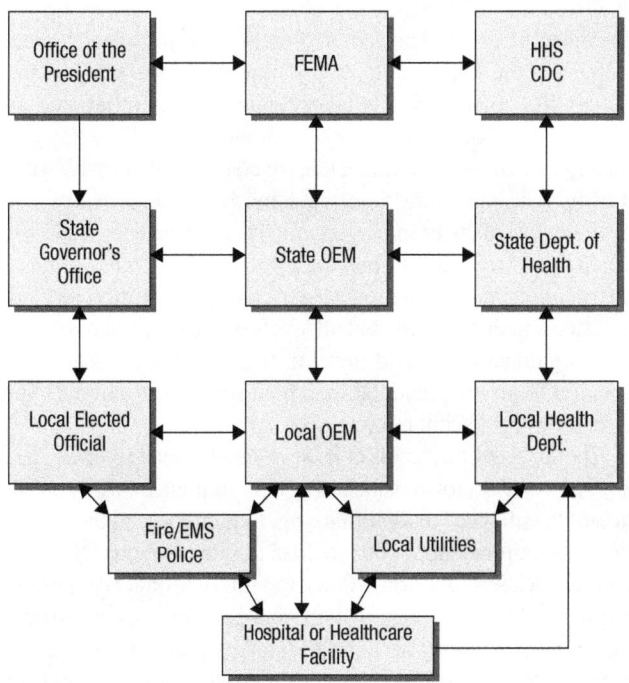

FIGURE 23.1 Flow of communication across levels of response in emergencies and disasters.

CDC, Centers for Disease Control and Prevention; EMS, emergency medical services; FEMA, Federal Emergency Management Agency; HHS, U.S. Department of Health and Human Services; OEM, Office of Emergency Management.

response in terms of short term (days), intermediate term (weeks–months) and long term (months–years). All-hazards plans need to consider all likely types and levels of disasters, and include these phases.

A disaster is not the time for senior management of a hospital, major health center, or local public health group and leaders of public agencies, utilities, and neighboring healthcare facilities to meet for the first time. It is essential to have a solid plan in place *a priori* for the most likely events, and that includes ongoing relationships with all likely partners, including public agencies (e.g., emergency medical services [EMS], fire, police departments) and utility companies (e.g., telecommunications, electric, water). Mutual aid agreements with similar types of facilities in the region should also be developed in advance of the need to use them should those in the immediate community be unavailable or at capacity. Commitment to disaster preparedness by the chief executive officer (CEO) and others in hospital leadership is critical to the success of the endeavor (Auf der Heide, 2002). Leadership at that level is essential to ensure that the needed resources of staff time, meeting space, investment in communications equipment, staff training, and exercises are built into the ongoing organizational budget. While the chief executive, except in very small organizations, is unlikely to be the planner or the emergency manager, the backing of the CEO is essential to making the work of everyone assigned to the planning and preparation task doable.

Within hospitals (and some other health facilities), the most common model for disaster response in the hospital sector is the HICS, developed by the California Emergency Medical Services Authority (2014). It is compatible with NIMS and the nationally required ICS, allowing the institution to be internally organized in the manner most compatible with the external groups with which coordination is so essential. Simply establishing HICS as the hospital's standard, however, does not remove the planning requirements. HICS is not a disaster plan, but a model or template on which a plan can be developed. The current version of HICS includes not only organizational guidance, but tools (e.g., forms, checklists) specific to some of the internal and external emergency situations that might confront the institution.

THE ROLE OF LEADERSHIP

Strong leadership is critical in disaster situations when "patient surge" challenges a hospital's capacity to respond and normally acceptable patterns of care are disrupted. Activation of the emergency operations plan triggers an ICS structure for leadership decision making. The importance of the CEO in the emergency planning and response process has been mentioned, but cannot be overstressed. It is actually the entire executive team that makes the difference, given the complexity of most health-related organizations. Implementation of the emergency operations plan and ICS protocols is ultimately subject to nursing and hospital leadership at the service and unit level. The results of these service-/unit-based leadership decisions have the potential to directly impact staff and patient safety, quality of care, and ultimately, patient outcomes

(Veenema, Deruggiero, Losinski, & Barnett, 2017). Whether it is the person responsible for daily operations, fiscal integrity, information processing, physical plant, or clinical care, or a senior staff person who has participated in assessing risk and developing the organizational plan, that person can then lead others during the stress of an actual emergency event, and will be ready to ensure that recovery is put in motion and that evaluation of the response leads to improvements for the next time.

Work to identify the critical competencies for leaders done at Columbia University developed the following list of actions that the leader should be able to do:

1. Describe the mission of the hospital during response to emergencies of all kinds, including the disaster response chain of command and emergency management system.
2. Demonstrate the ability to review, write, and revise as needed those portions of the hospital emergency plan applicable to your management responsibilities and participate in the hospital's hazard vulnerability analysis on a regular basis.
3. Manage and implement the hospital's emergency response plan during drills or actual emergencies within your assigned functional role and chain of command.
4. Describe the collaborative relationship of your hospital to other facilities or agencies in the local emergency response system and follow the planned system during drills and emergencies.
5. Describe the key elements of your hospital's emergency preparedness and response roles and polices to other agencies and community partners.
6. Initiate and maintain communication with other emergency response activities as appropriate to your management responsibilities.
7. Describe your responsibilities for communicating with other employees, patients and families, media, general public, or your own family and demonstrate them during drills or actual emergencies.
8. Demonstrate the use of any equipment (e.g., personal protective equipment or special communication equipment) required by your agency response.
9. Demonstrate flexible thinking and use of resources in responding to problems that arise carrying out your functional role during emergency situations or drills.
10. Evaluate the effectiveness of the response within your area of management responsibility in drills or actual emergencies and identify improvements needed.

Most leaders and managers have developed a leadership style which serves them well during times of nondisaster operations. Such styles usually span a spectrum of varying degrees of control—directive, supportive, participative, or achievement-oriented—and are often selected to match the needs of a particular circumstance, influenced by the preferences of the manager. To be effective, disaster managers need to be able to match the management style with the phase of disaster operations (Cuny, 2000). During the *noncrisis phases* such as risk assessment and planning, participative and achievement-oriented management styles work best.

Involvement of the staff during disaster planning activities allows experienced workers to identify what will work and what will not work and can readily identify vulnerabilities based on knowledge of routine operations as well as issues that have proven challenging in the past. In addition, staff who are involved in the planning will develop an interest in seeing the plan succeed and are more likely to follow it during times of crisis. Plans that are developed without the involvement of the staff all too often are merely compilations of procedures that are poorly understood by the staff, may lack critical information, and are not likely to be followed.

During the *response phase* of a disaster, a more directive style of leadership is required. At this time the leader must act quickly and decisively, and there is usually little time for extended consultation. For this reason, experienced managers who are confident in their knowledge of both the institution and the plan should be given leadership tasks. Staff members who have been involved in the planning process from the beginning will usually understand the need for this type of management during this time and follow orders and direction. The very specific lines of authority, responsibility, and communication embedded in the incident command structure are designed to facilitate this directive stage of response.

Finally, as the disaster winds down and the organization makes the transition to *recovery* and *evaluation,* leadership that is more collaborative and participatory will prove effective. Among other reasons, a less commanding approach will encourage honest assessment by participating staff, providing the essential information for future improvement. In addition, staff may have been traumatized by the event and require support from the leader.

Given that the leadership process is not the responsibility of a single CEO, it is important that multiple senior management staff have the opportunity to learn and practice key disaster leadership roles. It is also important to remember that an emergency or disaster may occur at any time of the day and on any day of the week. Healthcare staff members who work during evening, night, and weekend hours also need to be proficient in disaster management. This can be achieved only when the entire facility has the opportunity to participate in the planning and evaluation activities and preparation through practice and drills. Nurses at all levels of the hospital or healthcare organization should develop the knowledge, skills, and abilities to provide leadership in their respective unit during a disaster event (Veenema et al., 2016).

The collective awareness of those in the emergency preparedness and response sectors has been strongly influenced by the addition of "resilience" to their thinking. Beginning with the Hyogo Framework for Action, 2005 to 2015 (United Nations Office for Disaster Risk Reduction, 2005), the international community has worked to assist organizations and governments to consider the long-term ability of those affected by a disaster to resume their usual functioning, or even improve, as a basic part of all emergency planning. The most recent thinking about this perspective is found in the Sendai Framework for Disaster Risk Reduction 2015 to 2030 (United Nations Office for Disaster Risk Reduction, 2015). This chapter will not provide extensive discussion of resilience, but the reader is encouraged to explore the process further.

THE DISASTER MANAGEMENT PROCESS

Because it is so critical, the discussion so far has emphasized planning, which is only one of the five phases to any disaster management program (Kim & Proctor, 2002), and each phase has specific activities associated with it.

Preparedness/Risk Assessment

This requires the evaluation of the likelihood of emergencies or disasters for the specific institution. Issues to consider include weather patterns; geographical location; expectations related to public events and gatherings; age, condition, and location of the facility; and industries in close proximity to the hospital (e.g., nuclear power plant or chemical factory). All types of events need to be considered, including deliberate human-caused, technological, and natural events. Table 23.1 describes the types of disasters that commonly are included in a disaster management plan. Current literature often identifies this as the hazard vulnerability assessment: not only what are the likely hazards in the region or neighborhood, but what is the likelihood that the individual facility or organization will be harmed by or involved in the disaster.

The best disaster management plans are developed for an all-hazards approach and then have specific appendices for the events that are most likely to occur in the area. Each appendix will address those procedures that are unique for that incident. For instance, for a radiation incident, the appendix would include

reporting procedures, how to notify the Radiation Safety Officer, as well as procedures for decontamination of patients and disposal of contaminated clothing. The new FEMA Emergency Management Institute ICS Resource Center provides the most up-to-date HICS resource materials (FEMA ICS100). The Associated Center for HICS Education and Training includes the most up-to-date materials for hospital incident command. Each resource contains numerous sample appendices that can be utilized for different scenarios.

Risk assessment should also include an evaluation of staffing under various conditions. Depending on the nature and extent of the disaster and the demographics of the workforce, there may be variation in the employees' ability and/or willingness to report to work. During the past two decades many researchers have examined factors that influence a healthcare worker's ability and willingness to report to work during a disaster. Child care responsibilities and concern for one's own safety were the most likely factors that would influence an employee's decision not to report to work during a catastrophic disaster such as a chemical or biological attack (Shapira et al., 1991). Out of 50 New York City school health nurses responding to a survey, 49 reported at least one barrier that would impede their ability to report to work during an emergency situation, the most common barriers being child, elder, and pet care issues (Qureshi, Merrill, Gershon, & Calero-Breckheimer, 2002). In a larger study of more than 6,000 healthcare workers in all types of health facilities, it was found that employees who perceive greater potential to become ill or injured while working during

TABLE 23.1 Examples of Likely Events and Effect on the Hospital's Environment of Care

Type of Event	Examples	Potential Effect on the Organization's Environment of Care
Unintended Events	Transportation crash Industrial plant explosion Nuclear power plant failure	Patient census exceeding facility capacity Staff safety issue related to contamination
Biological	Epidemic: increase of communicable disease Bioterrorism	Staffing problems due to increase in sick time or fear Increase in patient census to exceed capacity of facility
Civil Disturbance	Riot Labor strike	Staffing problems due to fear Facility damage
Facility Infrastructure Failure	Water Electricity HVAC	Unsafe environment for the patients and staff
Geological	Earthquake Avalanche Volcanic eruption Tsunami	Staffing problems due to disruption of transportation system Increase in trauma volume that exceeds capacity of the facility Damage to facility Interruption of utilities and/or delivery of supplies
Warfare/Terrorist Attack	Mass casualty incidents	Staffing problems due to fear or disruption in transportation system
Weather	Snowstorm Heat emergency Hurricanes Tornadoes Floods	Staffing problems due to disruption in transportation system Increased patient census that exceeds facility capacity Damage to facility Interruption of utilities and/or delivery of supplies

HVAC, heating, ventilation, air-conditioning.

a disaster are less likely to be willing to report to work (Qureshi, Gershon, Gebbie, Straub, & Morse, 2005). Others (Lanzilotti, Galanis, Leoni, & Craig, 2002) found that health professionals' willingness to work in a field hospital during a mass casualty event as a result of a weapon of mass destruction (WMD) was influenced by their perceived ability to provide adequate care to the victims. Veenema, Walden, Feinstein, and Williams (2008) identified that nurses' willingness to respond to radiation events is affected by their own perceptions of personal safety and their clinical competence in caring for victims who have been exposed to radiation. In response to these concerns, the employer could make plans to open a child care center for employees' children, make arrangements for pet care through a local animal volunteer group, ensure the ready availability of personal protective equipment, and provide adequate safety training. In a study of over 1,300 essential employees in a Midwestern health network, Adams and Berry (2012) found that responsibilities related to child care are associated with the most significant barriers to reporting during a disaster. All healthcare facilities should include accommodations for staff who need to arrange for child care before they report to work during disasters. The requirement to educate staff about emergency operations, including response to WMD, is essential to improving employee willingness to report during an event. Hazard vulnerability risk assessments need to be reviewed at least on an annual basis, given the possibility that a new industry may have located to the area, or world events may have changed the potential for harm. The emergency management plan may have to be revised, and an appendix may have to be added for newly identified risks. This process then leads to the next phase of disaster management—mitigation.

Mitigation

Mitigation includes all steps that are taken to lessen the impact of a disaster should one occur and considered as prevention measures. For health facilities, examples of mitigation activities include installing and maintaining and testing backup generator power to mitigate the effects of a power failure or cross-training staff to perform other tasks to maintain services during a staffing crisis due to a weather emergency. Developing a plan that maintains the least variation from normal routines as possible with backup plans in the event the first response actions are not successful is critical. Plans for staffing can be used as an example. All disaster management plans need to include provisions to achieve adequate staffing to meet the needs of the existing as well as incoming patients. Notification protocols must be in place, and additional staff are called in as needed. However, what if the disaster disables the telephone (landline and cell) system? Having a backup plan is essential. Messaging over the Internet, via the radio or television, or even using human runners may be the means by which communication is made available. Not all disasters can be prevented. But mitigation activities can lessen the degree of the impact of the disaster. The critical components of a hospital disaster plan are identified in Box 23.1.

Response

The response phase is the actual implementation of the disaster plan. As discussed, the best response plans use an ICS, are relatively simple, are routinely practiced, and are modified

BOX 23.1 Critical Topics for a Healthcare Organization Emergency Response Plan (Additional Topics Must Be Added Based on the Facility Type, Mission, Size, and Location)

- Hazards vulnerability assessment (HVA) (frequency, response to findings identified)
- Drills and exercises schedule and types driven by the HVA
- Employee emergency response competencies (expected and methods for training/assessment)
- Incident recognition and reporting (procedure for reporting)
- Alerts and notifications for senior leadership, all levels of staff, and external agencies
- Specific triggers and authority for activation or deactivation of the emergency management plan
- Departmental and staff roles for each area/service within the organization
- Emergency response staffing plan
- Communication plan (internal and external including public, media, and local government)
- Identification and maintenance of essential services, and suspension of nonessential services
- Emergency credentialing procedures
- Volunteer management policies and procedures
- Health and medical operations for each clinical department of the facility
- Patient management (emergency victims and current patients/clients)
- Plan for altered standards of care for catastrophic disasters
- Fatality management (large scale and small scale)
- Decontamination plans and procedures
- Staff and responder safety
- Emergency housing for staff
- Logistics (supplies, equipment, and resources)
- Finance and emergency spending authorizations and tracking
- Resource management, including mutual aid agreements with local and out of state agencies/organizations
- Donations management (solicited and unsolicited)
- Infrastructure management and security (building, grounds, utilities, damage assessment)
- Evacuation procedures
- Safety and security of personnel, patients, and incoming victims
- Coordination with external agencies
- Family information
- Family reunification and unaccompanied minors

Source: Lewis, P., & Aghababian, R. (1996). Disaster planning, Part 1. *Emergency medicine clinics of North America, 14*(2), 439–451. doi:10.1016/s0733-8627(05)70261-3

when improvements are needed. Response activities need to be continually monitored and adjusted to the changing situation. If the health institution is to manage itself and its responsibilities through an emergency, it is essential to have in place infrastructure that can support the disaster response, which includes maintaining services for preexisting patients as well as the new arrivals; staff who are competent to perform their disaster response functional roles and able and willing to report to work during any sort of disaster. A clearly defined, executable, practiced emergency response plan and a strong foundation of preexisting relationships with partnering organizations and agencies that can be called on to provide mutual aid and support when needed is critical to an effective response.

The complexity of a health facility disaster plan will depend on the breadth of services and size of the organization. The Joint Commission Emergency Management Standards Support Collaboration Planning (2016) articulates key elements that must be addressed in a healthcare facility emergency plan. Among a range of resources, the American College of Emergency Physicians has also published a comprehensive sample plan (American College of Emergency Physicians, 2016).

Infrastructure

The capacity of the organization to respond to a disaster is a direct outcome of the established infrastructure. If the disaster is internal, the physical plant, utilities, staffing, supplies, and equipment or their emergency replacements must remain available and functional so that the environment of care remains safe and the essential services are provided to all patients. If the disaster is external, two types of operations need to take place simultaneously. Current patients need to be cared for or relocated elsewhere for ongoing care at the same time as the new arrivals are triaged and cared for. It is the disaster manager's responsibility to ensure that this is done. One method (covered in HICS) is to assign one individual the specific responsibility for directing the care to the preexisting patients and ensuring their safety. Organizations that utilize just-in-time processes for staffing or supply management need to take into account the possible sudden increases in demand imposed by an emergency or disaster. Making provisions for rapid procurement during these times can help to improve disaster response. Emergencies that are both internal and external may require the relocation of the entire health facility to an alternate location or to a neighboring institution with which there is a mutual aid agreement.

Staff Competency

Equally crucial to disaster management is ensuring that all levels of staff are competent to perform during disaster response. Emergency preparedness competencies refer to the ability of the staff to actually perform their functional roles for emergency response. Competencies are usually complex actions; therefore, the best method to evaluate competence is direct observation. This can be accomplished through drills or during actual response activities. The U.S. Disaster Information Management Research Center has published disaster-related competencies for 13 different groups of healthcare workers (National Library of Medicine, 2017). Groups have explicated competencies general to all hospital workers and ICN Framework of Disaster Nursing Competencies (ICN & WHO, 2009; Florida Department of Health, 2011); mid-level public health workers (Association of Schools of Public Health,

2010), and all medical/health workers in general (Subbarao et al., 2008; Walsh et al., 2012). There are interesting features in these competencies sets, primarily the commonality of the emphasis on having a personal and family disaster plan so that the worker can attend to the job needs, and attention to following role assignments and command structure that emerge from application of ICS to the event. Most of the individuals involved in response will be applying the skills and knowledge core to their own disciplines, but under different circumstances, following different leadership, or with different colleagues. Regular participation in drills and exercises is the established mechanism to ensure that the response will happen smoothly, with the least opportunity for harm to the responding worker.

The Plan

Staff in any healthcare organization should be fully conversant with the agency's emergency response plan. During the emergency response is not the time to begin to teach staff about the elements of the plan. Employees should know their most likely emergency response functional roles, and these should have been practiced beforehand by staff on all shifts. The planning (and the practice) should be realistic to the expectations of the institution, given the local risk assessment and the institution's capacity. For example, a hospital needs to plan for operating room capacity for mass casualty events; this would not be expected of a long-term care facility. In addition to the resource materials found in HICS, there are more detailed templates for emergency response plans available on state Departments of Health websites such as the Kansas State Department of Health at www.kdheks.gov/cphp/operating_guides.htm (2011).

Relationships and Partnerships

The geopolitical climate today makes it likely that the emergencies and disasters that any hospital can expect to encounter are likely to be more complex than simply knowing what ambulance services are likely to deliver patients, and of a higher magnitude of severity. With the decreased surge capacity of most hospitals (i.e., fewer staffed beds, little or no extra staff, etc.), the need to establish mutual aid agreements, plans to share resources, and ability and willingness to provide and receive support from local agencies are of paramount importance. The best method to establish such emergency response relationships is to plan a drill/exercise with other organizations and agencies. During such endeavors, managers and staff across the organizations get to know and trust one another and tend to develop plans that synchronize the partnering agencies. During a crisis they are then better able to work together. Every disaster manager needs to remember that *all disasters are local*. Each hospital or healthcare facility must have a plan in place that provides for procurement of local assistance or mutual aid, before reaching out to the state or federal agencies.

Although disaster managers spend the least amount of time in the response phase even in an actual emergency event, it is this phase that most employees remember. It is at this point that the disaster manager must change leadership styles. During disaster response, group decision making/consensus style management is replaced with structured and focused-direction style. Staff who have been involved in the planning process will recognize the need for this style of leadership and will cooperate. The most common framework to achieve this in the hospital setting is the HICS (www.hicscenter.org).

INTRODUCTION TO HOSPITAL INCIDENT COMMAND SYSTEM

The HICS is an incident management framework that can be used to organize a disaster plan and response. While it is specific to inpatient hospitals, the principles and system presented can be adapted for use in community health centers, long-term care facilities, and elsewhere. HICS reflects the same basic principles of command and control, chain of command, predefined positions, established reporting and communication relationships, use of common nomenclature, expandability and contractility of the scale of the operation, and span of control as does the national ICS embedded in NIMS (www.fema.gov/nationalincident-management -system). The fifth edition of the California Emergency Medical Services Authority HICS Guidebook (2014) can be accessed at hicscenter.org/Shared%20Documents/HICS_Guidebook_2014_7 .pdf. Readers are encouraged to visit the HICS website at hicscenter.org/SitePages/HomeNew.aspx to monitor for updates and identify opportunities for education and training.

The key features of an ICS, including HICS, are discussed briefly:

- *Predictable, responsibility-oriented chain of command*: In the HICS system there is *one* incident commander (IC) within the institution. This individual has overall responsibility for the management of the incident, and employees know who reports to them and to whom they report. Direction, requests for resources, and all information flow in a prescribed fashion up or down the chain of command. This person also has responsibility for ensuring that the institution collaborates properly through an overall IC, if there are multiple organizations involved in response.
- *Use of common nomenclature*: All agencies utilizing ICS and responding to the same event use the same titles and functional roles for the command staff positions. Use of common terminology assists different agencies with communicating with each other.
- *Modular, flexible organization*: Only those portions of the system that are needed for the response are activated. It can be expanded or scaled back according to the situation. This is efficient, conserves resources, and makes it applicable to both large and small events. Figure 23.2 illustrates this, showing the use of HICS for a small internal emergency, a larger trauma event, and a very large decontamination event.
- *Unified command structure*: This allows all agencies involved in the response to coordinate efforts by establishing a unified set of incident objectives and strategies.
- *Incident action plan (IAP)*: This is a plan for response to the event developed at the overall Incident Command Center when multiple agencies are involved in response to an emergency. It ensures that all agencies are working toward the same goal within the same time frames.

- *Facility action plan (FAP)*: A FAP describes the purpose, goals, and objectives for the hospital's response. All responders in the hospital then work toward the same goals and objectives. This plan would be developed for an internal event, when no other organizations are involved in the response.
- *Unity of command*: Each person reports to only one individual. Staff training will emphasize that this individual is filling an assigned role within the structure, and may not be the worker's day-to-day supervisor.
- *Manageable span of control*: Each manager has a defined number of human resources, limited to what experience has shown can realistically be managed. The ideal range is believed to be five to seven people per supervisor; however, where tasks are relatively simple, the personnel possess a high level of expertise, or the management team is in close proximity to those being supervised, this number of persons supervised can be higher than seven.
- *Use of job action sheets (JASs):* JASs define for each involved staff member the specific functional role to be carried out during the disaster response. These are particularly important for individuals assigned leadership roles within the ICS structure, as the areas of responsibility and lines of reporting may be quite different from the person's usual assignments. They provide quick reminders of start of shift and end of shift activities as well as the central part of each job, and can be annotated with necessary details on the event, location of assignment, or other details. They also facilitate improved documentation for better evaluation of response and for financial recovery after the event.

HICS Structure

HICS achieves command and control during disaster response through its chain of command, IAP, defined functional roles for each individual, and extensive use of incident response tracking forms. At the top of the organization tree are the command positions: IC, Safety, Liaison, and Public Information Officers (PIOs). Under the command positions are the staff positions that include the section chiefs and their reporting staff. As the disaster response evolves, sections are activated or deactivated. The only position that is always required for incident command is the IC. Figure 23.3 illustrates the HICS table of organization with examples of the typical hospital positions from which the assignees to these incident command positions might be drawn. It is important that the institution identify several individuals as the potential for each position, to have depth to cover multiple shifts, multiple days, and allow for the possibility that one or more people will be unavailable at the time of the emergency.

Each position to be filled has a specific functional role that is described on a JAS that includes the role to which the position reports; the mission of the position; and immediate, intermediate, and extended tasks. Figure 23.4 provides one example, the JAS for a medical technical expert in pediatric care. This is a position that might be filled by a pediatric nursing expert. This example was taken directly from the master HICS document; any institution making use of the JASs would have to review the details and be sure that they are edited to match the plan and resources of that institution.

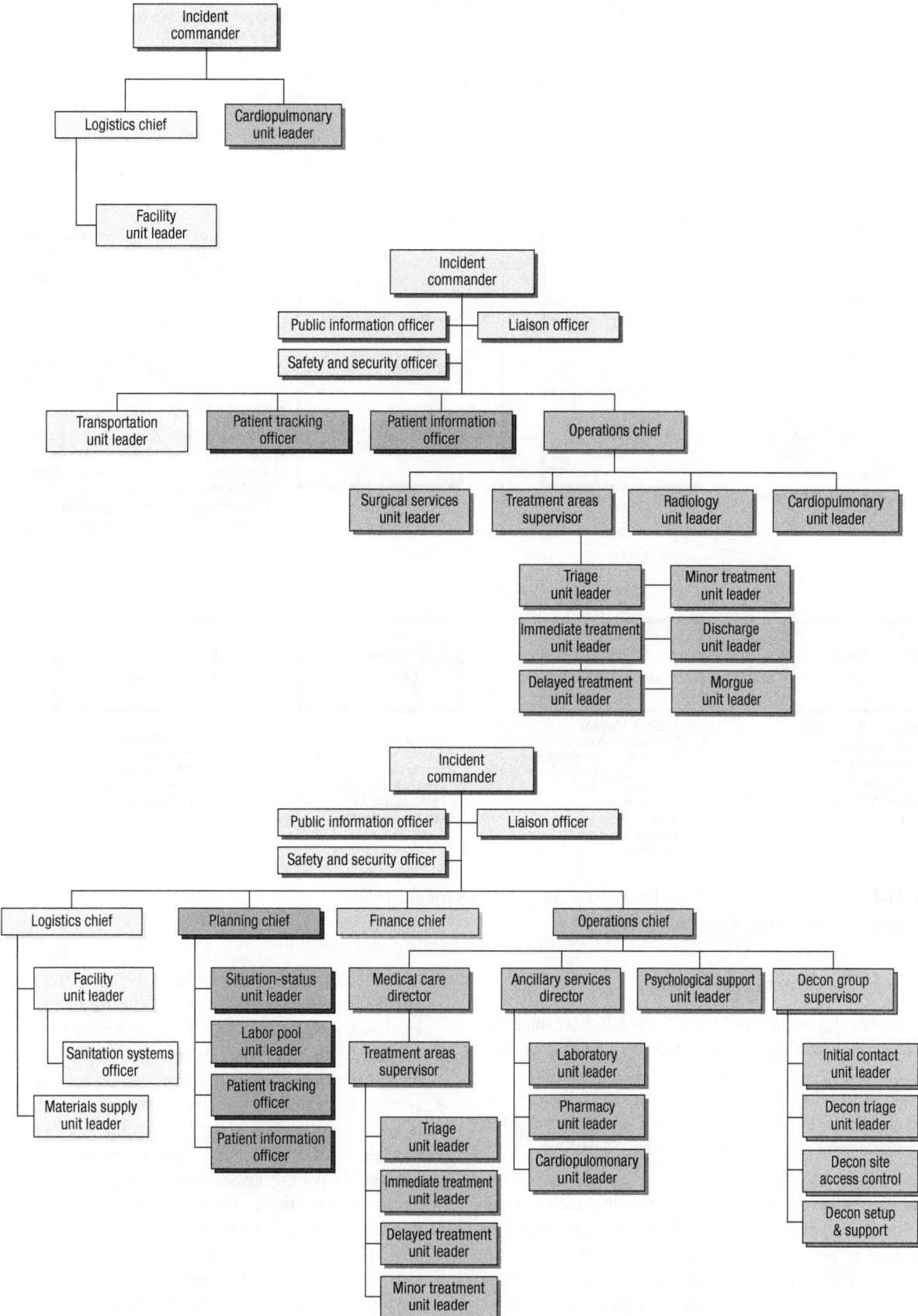

FIGURE 23.2 Expansion of HICS implementation when needed.

HICS, Hospital Incident Command System.

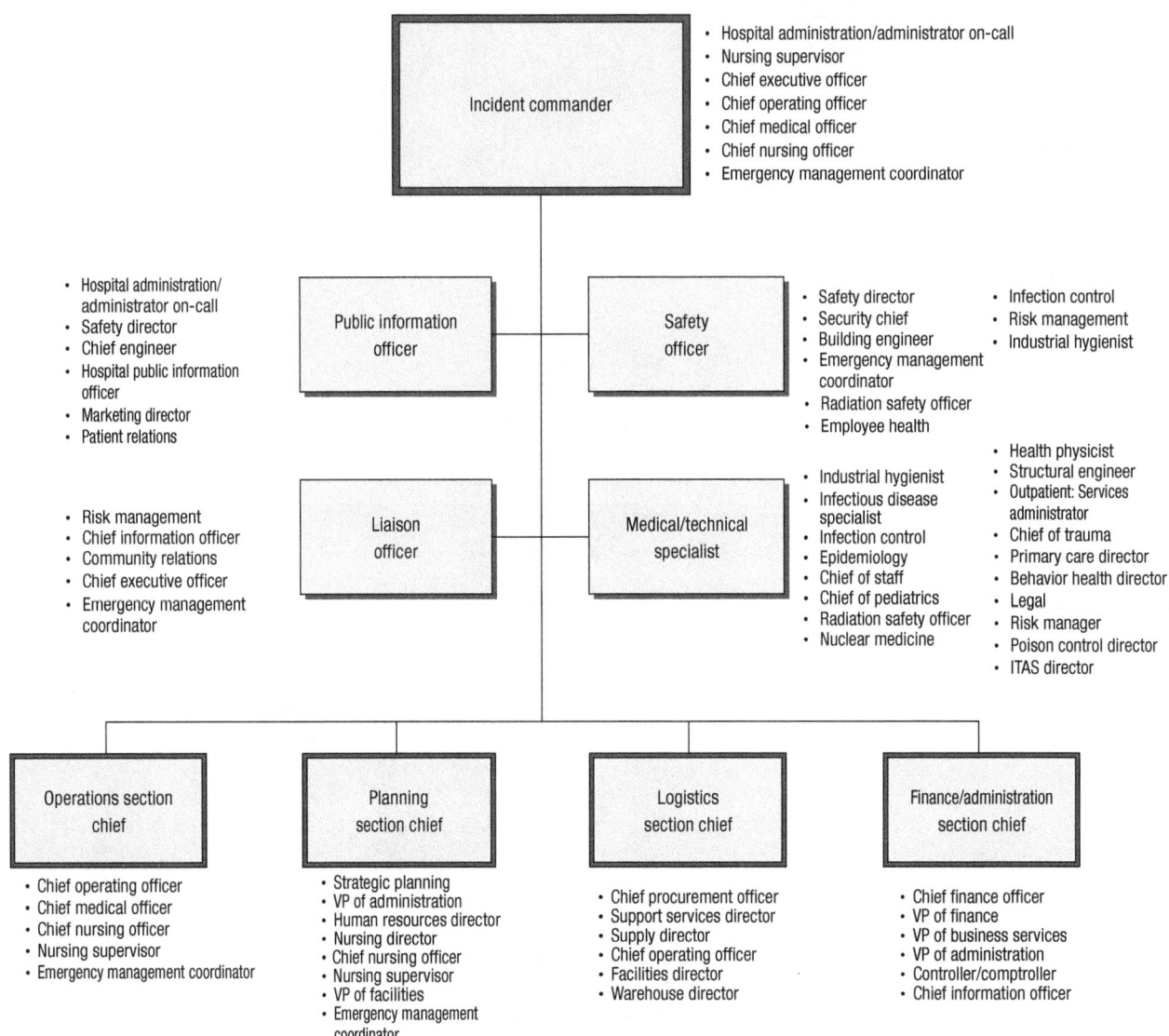

FIGURE 23.3 HICS organizational chart with potential assignees for each role.

HICS, Hospital Incident Command System.

Specific HICS Functional Roles

The command roles on the top of the ICS and HICS organization trees are the same, and apply across a variety of types of organizations. There are positions at the base of the tree related to the specifics of a hospital setting. The following brief descriptions of the command and top staff positions provide a sense of the hierarchy and span of control issues discussed earlier.

■ *Incident Commander*: The mission of the IC is to organize and direct the operations of the incident. The highest-ranking executive in the organization appoints the IC, based on experience in disaster management, knowledge of the organization, and the nature of the incident. From that point the IC directs the disaster response, immediately appointing the command staff (e.g., safety, liaison, and PIOs) and activates the sections (planning, operations, logistics, and finance) required by the event. The IC establishes an emergency operations center (EOC) and holds a meeting to develop the initial IAP. The IC manages on a macro level rather than a

micro level. At periodic intervals, the IAP is reviewed and updated as necessary. For instance, during an internal event such as a fire, the initial IAP may evacuate one floor of a hospital to the emergency department, but be followed by a revised plan to evacuate the entire hospital to other facilities.

■ *Safety and Security Officer*: The mission of the safety officer is to ensure the safety of the staff, facility, and the environment during the disaster operation. The safety officer has the final authority to make decisions as they relate to safety and hazardous conditions, and can overrule portions of an IAP if they are deemed too hazardous. A key goal is to ensure that no responding personnel become part of the injured needing care! With the threat of bioterrorism and chemical warfare, the role of the safety officer has taken on added importance.

■ *Liaison Officer*: The mission of the liaison officer is to function as a contact for external agencies, protecting the IC from requests from outside the organization. Any health facility is likely to interface with multiple local, state, or federal agencies. All communication from the hospital to these external agencies should go through the liaison officer to

Date: _____ Start: _____ End: _____ Position Assigned to: _____ Initial: ____

Position Reports to: _____ Signature: _____

Hospital Command Center (HCC) Location: _____ Telephone: _____

Fax: _____ Other Contact Info: _____ Radio Title: _____

Immediate (Operational Period 0–2 Hours)	Time	Initial
Receive appointment and briefing from the Incident Commander or Operations Section Chief, as assigned.		
Read this entire Job Action Sheet and review incident management team chart (HICS Form 207). Put on position identification.		
Notify your usual supervisor of your HICS assignment.		
Document all key activities, actions, and decisions in an Operational Log (HICS Form 214) on a continual basis.		
Meet with the Command staff, Operations and Logistics Section Chiefs and the Medical Care Branch Director to plan for and project pediatric patient care needs.		
Communicate with Operations Section Chief to obtain: • Type and location of incident • Number and condition of expected pediatric patients • Estimated arrival time to facility • Unusual or hazardous environmental exposure		
Request staffing assistance from the Labor Pool and Credentialing Unit Leader, as needed, to assist with rapid research as needed to determine hazard and safety information critical to treatment and decontamination concerns for the pediatric victims.		
Provide pediatric care guidance to Operation Section Chief and Medical Care Branch Director based on incident scenario and response needs		
Ensure pediatric patient identification and tracking practices are being followed.		
Communicate and coordinate with Logistics Section Chief to determine pediatric: • Medical care equipment and supply needs • Medications with pediatric dosing • Transportation availability and needs (carts, cribs, wheel chairs, etc.)		
Communicate with Planning Section Chief to determine pediatric: • Bed availability • Ventilators • Trained medical staff (MD, RN, PA, NP, etc.) • Additional short- and long-range pediatric response needs		
Ensure that appropriate pediatric standards of care are being followed in all clinical areas.		
Collaborate with the PIO to develop media and public information messages specific to pediatric care recommendations and treatment.		
Participate in briefings and meetings and contribute to the Incident Action Plan, as requested.		

FIGURE 23.4 Sample job action sheet: Medical/Technical Specialist—Pediatric Care. (*continued*)

HICS, Hospital Incident Command System.

Source: California Emergency Medical Services Authority. (2014).

	Time	Initial
Document all communications (internal and external) on an Incident Message Form (HICS Form 213). Provide a copy of the Incident Message Form to the Documentation Unit.		
Intermediate (Operational Period 2–12 Hours)	**Time**	**Initial**
Continue to communicate and coordinate with Logistics Section Chief the availability of pediatric equipment and supplies.		
Coordinate with Logistics and Planning Section Chiefs to expand/create a Pediatric Patient Care area, if needed.		
Continue to monitor pediatric care activities to ensure needs are being met.		
Meet regularly with Operations Section Chief and Medical Care Branch Director for updates on situation regarding hospital operations and pediatric needs.		
Extended (Operational Period Beyond 12 Hours)	**Time**	**Initial**
Ensure provision of resources for pediatric mental health and appropriate event education for children and families.		
Continue to ensure pediatric-related response issues are identified and effectively managed.		
Continue to meet regularly with the Operations Section Chief or Incident Commander, as appropriate, for situation status updates and to communicate critical pediatric care issues.		
Ensure your physical readiness through proper nutrition, water intake, rest, and stress management.		
Observe staff and volunteers for signs of stress and inappropriate behavior. Report concerns to Mental Health Unit Leader. Provide for staff rest periods and relief.		
Upon shift change, brief your replacement on the status of all ongoing operations, issues, and other relevant incident information.		
Demobilization/System Recovery	**Time**	**Initial**
Ensure return/retrieval of equipment and supplies and return all assigned incident command equipment.		
Upon deactivation of your position, ensure all documentation and Operational Logs (HICS Form 214) are submitted to the Operations Section Chief or Incident Commander, as appropriate.		
Upon deactivation of your position, brief Operations Section Chief or Incident Commander, as appropriate, on current problems, outstanding issues, and follow-up requirements.		
Submit comments to the Operations Section Chief or Incident Commander, as appropriate, for discussion and possible inclusion in the after-action report; topics include: • Review of pertinent position descriptions and operational checklists • Recommendations for procedure changes • Section accomplishments and issues		
Participate in stress management and after-action debriefings. Participate in other briefings and meetings as required.		
Documents/tools		
• Incident Action Plan • HICS Form 207–Incident Management Team Chart • HICS Form 213–Incident Message Form • HICS Form 214–Operational Log • Hospital emergency operations plan • Hospital organization chart • Hospital telephone directory • Radio/satellite phone • Local public health reporting forms		

FIGURE 23.4 (*continued*)

prevent duplicate requests or conflicting information. This may require a difficult change in behavior for those departments in the hospital that have preexisting working relationships and ongoing informal communication with others.

- *Public Information Officer*: As the title indicates, the individual in this role is responsible for providing information to the news media. When the media are handled appropriately, they can be an asset to the disaster response. The PIO is key to this process, and this position should be activated for any response that has the potential to involve the media. This individual would also be responsible for coordination with the interagency information process for any large event.
- *Medical/Technical Specialists*: These positions are activated as needed to provide guidance in the facility's EOC in a variety of special situations. Positions may include specialists in biological and infectious diseases, legal affairs, chemical exposure, radiological exposure, risk management, medical staff, pediatric care, clinic administration, hospital administration, and medical ethics.

In addition to the command positions just described, the EOC includes four sections, each headed by a staff chief. It is through these four sections that the remainder of the response participants receives information and directions.

- *Planning Section Chief*: The mission of the planning section chief is to collect and distribute any information available within the organization required for planning and the development of an IAP. The planning section chief ensures that the appropriate reports are being generated, and that the adopted facility IAP is communicated to the other section chiefs. This person in this position is responsible for planning activities to ensure adequate staffing, including oversight of any labor resource pools.
- *Operations Section Chief*: The mission of the operations section chief is to direct all patient care activities during disaster response. In a typical healthcare or hospital setting, this is the largest of the sections and engages the most personnel, with multiple branches and units within the section. This section includes clinical (medical and nursing) and ancillary services, and some possible configurations are illustrated in Figure 23.2. One branch within this section may be responsible for ongoing care of patients in the facility prior to the arrival of the casualty surge associated with the disaster.
- *Logistics Section Chief*: The logistics section chief has a mission to ensure that all resources and support required by the other sections are readily available. Responsibilities include maintenance of the environment and procurement of supplies, equipment, and food. Logistics ensures that the operations staff can focus on delivering services. For that to happen, the operations section chief must ensure that information about needed resources is directed to the Logistics Section in a timely manner.
- *Finance/Administrative Section Chief*: The mission of the finance section chief is to monitor the utilization of assets and authorize the acquisition of resources essential for the emergency response. This position is also frequently charged with ensuring that human resources policy and procedure consultation is available to the IC.

The shift in degrees of freedom, scope of responsibilities, and chain of command can be extremely difficult for many nurses, physicians, and others. For that reason, all of the clinical staff of a health facility need a working knowledge of this structure so that they are prepared to accept assignments within the operations section, follow the communication guidelines for their assigned jobs, and refrain from freelancing, that is, deciding independently where to go or for whom to care.

HICS Updates and Coalition Building

Throughout HICS guidelines, you will see the phrase Regional Hospital Coordination Centers (RHCC) or the equivalent used. Communities continue to develop regional approaches to coordinate hospital information sharing and medically related resource management during a crisis. The movement toward coalition building is supported by the CMS emergency preparedness requirements for participating providers and suppliers that became effective on November 15, 2016 and required implementation by November 15, 2017 (California Emergency Medical Services Authority, 2014).

COMMUNICATION DURING AN EMERGENCY EVENT

The organization's first need in communication is a mechanism (with a backup procedure) for contacting staff in the event a disaster response is activated. This includes alerting those in the facility at the time that the emergency plan has been activated, as well as a means of calling in off-duty staff to handle additional needs. Each departmental head in the organization needs to be able to contact all staff members. This most often involves use of mobile phones and text messaging, requiring a process to be sure that all staff phone numbers are kept up to date. While organizations are good at collecting this information at the time of employment, an organized approach to regular updating may be neglected and should be developed.

The most frequently cited failures in disaster response systems are in the areas of decision making and communication (Ingelsby, Grossman, & O'Toole, 2001; Townsend & Moss, 2005). Use of IC assists with decision making and maintaining order. However, in any type of agency, communication needs to be addressed on multiple levels: within the agency, between agencies, with the media and public, as well as with staff members and their families.

IC addresses interagency communication through the role of the liaison officer. The public's perception of how an agency performs during a disaster is largely influenced by media reports, and the work of the PIO becomes extremely important. All staff must know and follow the policy regarding release of information to any group—media, general public, or other responding agencies. Additionally, during emergency response activities, staff members who are at the facility providing care will need to be able to communicate with their families, whether they are on duty at the time of the event, or are called in as a part of surge requirements. It is most difficult to concentrate on any emergency response functional role while worrying about the safety of one's family. Making provisions for family communication will result in a more focused workforce for response activities, and may well increase the number of staff members who are willing and able to report when requested in a disaster situation.

Adapting Care to the Context

The occurrence of an emergency alters the context in which care is given. Contextual changes may include shortages of staff or supplies, provision of care in settings other than the usual patient care rooms, or numbers of patients far in excess of the usual capacity. Expected standards of care that can be followed during usual times may not be possible, requiring the facility to clarify expectations within the existing situation. This is another area in which management during the disastrous event requires thoughtful anticipation and planning. A key to the change is the shift from what is typical in any U.S. care setting, that of providing maximum care possible to each presenting patient before moving on to the next one, to an approach that ensures the greatest good for the largest possible number of patients. This may require a higher level of triage than is usually expected. The first step in this process is to acknowledge this as a real possibility, and engage staff in considering what changes might be made.

The Agency for Healthcare Research and Quality (AHRQ, 2005) has identified four levels of medical standards and provided guidelines that may be utilized by disaster managers when formulating such plans. The four levels include normal medical standards; near-normal medical standards (expanded scope of practice for some practitioners, use of alternate sites of care, and use of atypical devices, such as reusing disposable equipment after cleaning); key lifesaving care (many will receive only key lifesaving care and nonessential services will be delayed or eliminated); and, finally, total systems/standards alteration (severe rationing of care, with no treatment and only pain relief for some persons).

The guidelines are based on the following five principles:

1. During disaster planning, the goal should be to keep the system functioning to deliver the highest level of care possible to save as many lives as possible.
2. The planning must be comprehensive, community-based, include all types of agencies, and coordinated at the regional level.
3. There must be an adequate legal framework for providing care during a catastrophic event that has many casualties.
4. The rights of patients must be protected to the extent possible considering the circumstances.
5. Clear, effective communication with all is essential during all phases of a disaster, including before, during, and after an event.

A subsequent discussion among representatives of multiple health professions provided additional guidance on this most difficult process (American Nurses Association, 2008; Gebbie, Peterson, Subbarao, & White, 2009). These discussions emphasized the mutual responsibilities of every health organization to maintain a state of readiness for emergency or disaster response, and every health professional to maintain personal readiness for response. In further discussion, the priorities for care include maximizing worker and patient safety; maintaining airway and breathing, circulation and control of blood loss; and maintaining or establishing infection control (including continuity of medications for conditions such as tuberculosis). In developing this list, the participants identified activities typically done by a health professional that are of lower priority and that could be delayed or eliminated for some period of time (or provided by family members, nonlicensed assistants, or volunteers), such as routine care activities (e.g., blood pressure checks in nonacute patients, assisted ambulation), administration of oral medications, extensive documentation of care, maintenance of complete privacy and confidentiality, and elective procedures. The organizational activities to support the transition of care through the challenges of a disaster are outlined in Table 23.2.

TABLE 23.2 Facility Responsibilities Regarding Adapting Care

Timing	Actions
Pre-event	Develop descriptions of potential reconfigurations of clinician teams or physical resources
	Anticipate the inclusion of volunteers with varying levels of professional/technical training into care teams
	Ensure that emergency plans include capacity for just-in-time training specific to the event, including any needed changes in protocols
	Include opportunities for professional decision making about adapting standards of care in drills/exercises on a regular basis
During event	Distribute daily information on staffing expectations, including role of volunteers
	Communicate any legal changes, such as a governor's declaration of emergency, to staff
	Provide just-in-time training specific to the event, including any changes in expected protocols
Postevent	Return to pre-event status as quickly and smoothly as reasonable
	Participate in postevent evaluation
	Do a psychosocial needs assessment for those responding, and arrange assistance, if indicated

Source: Adapted from American Nurses Association. (2008). *Adapting standards of care under extreme conditions: Guidance for professionals during disasters, pandemics, and other extreme emergencies* (p. 19). Washington, DC: ANA Publications.

RECOVERY

During the recovery phase, the disaster is over and the facility attempts to return to usual operations. This may mean that all those injured during a major transportation crash have been admitted to the correct level of care, occupancy is back to usual level, and surge or volunteer staff are no longer needed. Recovery may be easier if, during the response, some of the staff have been assigned to maintain essential services while others were assigned to the disaster response. The timing and speed of recovery will be related to the overall scope of the disaster, and the degree to which it involved not only the specific health facility, but other resources in the community.

During this period of time, the disaster manager must be attuned not only to transitions in the operations of the organization, but to the staff as well. Plans should be in place to provide debriefing and any needed support for those staff members who were exposed to traumatic experiences or worked for prolonged periods of time and may be simply exhausted. It is during the recovery phase that a tally is made of the resources expended during the disaster response. This is important not only for restocking supplies but to provide documentation if there are external resources from which to recover some of the unusual costs. Usually the largest disaster response expenses to an organization are related to employee overtime costs. Tracking these costs as well as other additional expenses is essential as it can assist in recouping funds to aid in the financial recovery of the institution.

This documentation is also important for planning and justification of future budgets. For example, a hazard risk assessment that includes the experience of an average of three weather emergencies per year can use historical disaster response costs for forward budgeting.

EVALUATION AND FOLLOW-THROUGH

Every time an organization engages in a disaster response, whether as an exercise or in response to a real situation, an evaluation needs to be done, though it is often the phase that receives the least attention (Cosgrove et al., 2004). After any disaster, both employees and the community are anxious to return to usual operations. Before the details of the response fade from memory, it is essential that a formal evaluation be done to determine what went well (what really worked) and what problems arose. It is best if one person is designated to coordinate this effort.

The evaluation should be formal and include not only staff of the organization, but also those agencies with which the health facility interfaced during the response. Each unit or division should examine its own performance, making a list of what went well and what proved to be problematic. This information should be merged into an organization-wide evaluation that is prepared by representatives from each of the units or divisions, as well as senior management. As a final step, the organization should convene an evaluation meeting with all of the collaborating agencies to evaluate interagency performance. In each case, a detailed list of recommendations for changes to the emergency response plan should be compiled. The documentation from each of these sources should then be forwarded to the senior management and to the individual or committee responsible for the emergency plan, so that a list of recommendations for change can be developed. This list should take the form of an improvement plan, including who, what, and when as well as what resources are required to implement the changes. Although an individual should be assigned to follow the progress toward making the changes, ultimately the executive office of the organization needs to approve the resources needed to change the plan and hold staff accountable for meeting improvement deadlines. A final report that includes the critique and the improvement plan should be made available to all staff, as their continued investment in continuous improvement of emergency preparedness and response is key to the organization's performance. Following through with the changes identified demonstrates to the staff that emergency preparedness is valued and important.

SUMMARY

The ability of a healthcare organization to respond to emergencies or disasters is often reflective of the organization as a whole and the quality of its leadership. When provided with good disaster management leadership, staff will rise to the challenge and provide outstanding response during any disaster. The best way to ensure this is to engage staff in the planning process, provide decisive direction during the crisis, and then thoroughly evaluate the performance, making identified changes to improve the next response. Establishing relationships with agencies and other organizations in the community is essential for effective disaster management. The nature and complexity of disaster events require disaster managers to plan for the event where traditional standards of care may need to be adapted. Advance planning for such a catastrophic situation could save lives. Inclusion of resilience development will also enhance the opportunities for rapid recovery at the individual, organizational, or regional level.

As events unfold into the future, healthcare organizations and health professionals will face many new challenges, including the need to engage in disaster management on a more frequent basis. All disasters are local; therefore, the challenges and responsibilities for local hospital disaster managers are significant. However, these challenges can be met with adequate disaster planning and management, and better met when the health professionals in all communities meet the expectations of mastering key competencies and participating in training and exercising.

STUDY QUESTIONS

1. What are the different styles of disaster leadership? When and why would it be appropriate to use each style?

2. What are the phases of disaster management, and why is the planning phase so important?

3. What are the different levels of disasters, and how does planning differ for each level?

4. How can an external disaster contribute to the development of an internal disaster in a healthcare organization?

5. What do the terms "system capacity" and "employee emergency preparedness competency" mean? How are they different?

6. What are the basic principles of the HICS?

7. What is meant by the term "disaster response functional role"? Identify disaster response functional roles for nursing staff in your healthcare agency.

8. Why is postdisaster response evaluation and follow-through so important?

9. Discuss when and how the standards of care might change. What challenges would that likely pose for the staff?

10. Discuss how the concept of resilience is related to disaster/ emergency management.

USEFUL LINKS

- American Hospital Association: Disaster Readiness. www.hospitalconnect .com/aha/key_issues/disaster_readiness/resources/HospitalReady.html
- American Red Cross. www.redcross.org/services/nursing
- Center for Disaster Management. www.cendim.boun.edu.tr
- Centers for Disease Control and Prevention. www.cdc.gov
- Emergency Nurses Association. www.ena.org
- Federal Emergency Management Agency. www.fema.gov
- Hospital Emergency Incident Command System. https://emsa.ca.gov/ disaster-medical-services-division-hospital-incident-command-system -resources/
- Institute for Biosecurity. www.slu.edu/public-health-social-justice/ research/centers_institutes/institute_bsdp.php
- Internet Disaster Information Network. www.disaster.net
- Joint Commission on Accreditation of Healthcare Organizations. www.jacho.org/standard/faq/hos.html
- Natural Hazards Research and Applications Information Center. www .colorado.edu/hazards

REFERENCES

Adams, L., & Berry, D. (2012). Who will show up? Estimating ability and willingness of essential hospital personnel to report to work in response to disaster. *Online Journal of Issues in Nursing, 17*(2), 8. Retrieved from http://ojin.nursingworld.org/MainMenuCategories/ANAMarketplace/ ANAPeriodicals/OJIN/TableofContents/Vol-17-2012/No2-May-2012/ Articles-Previous-Topics-Essential-Hospital-Personnel-and-Response -to-Disaster.html

Agency for Healthcare Research and Quality. (2005). Bioterrorism and other public health emergencies: Altered standards of care in mass casualty events. Retrieved from https://archive.ahrq.gov/research/altstand

American College of Emergency Physicians. (2016). Hospital disaster resources. Retrieved from https://www.acep.org/search.aspx?searchtext=hospital disaster plan#sm.000033a67qv9bcoh10ce6pf48e7z0

American Nurses Association. (2008). *Adapting standards of care under extreme conditions: Guidance for professionals during disasters, pandemics, and other extreme emergencies.* Washington, DC: ANA Publications.

Association of Schools of Public Health. (2010). Public health emergency preparedness and response core competency model version 1.0. Retrieved from https://www.cdc.gov/phpr/documents/perlcpdfs/preparednesscom petencymodelworkforce-version1_0.pdf

Auf der Heide, E. (1989). *Disaster response: Principles of preparation and coordination.* St. Louis, MO: CV Mosby.

Auf der Heide, E. (2002). *Principles of hospital disaster planning.* In D. Hogan & J. Burstein (Eds.), *Disaster medicine* (pp. 57–89). Philadelphia, PA: Lippincott Williams & Wilkins.

California Emergency Medical Services Authority. (2014). Hospital incident command system. Retrieved from https://emsa.ca.gov/disaster-medical -services-division-hospital-incident-command-system-resources

Centers for Medicare and Medicaid Services. (2018). *Emergency preparedness rule.* Retrieved from https://www.cms.gov/Medicare/Provider-Enrollment -and-Certification/SurveyCertEmergPrep/Emergency-Prep-Rule.html

Cosgrove, S., Jenckes, M., Kohri, K., Hsu, E., Green, G., Feurestein, C., Catlett, C. L., … Bass, E. B. (2004). Evaluation of hospital disaster drills. Agency for Healthcare Research and Quality. Retrieved from https://archive.ahrq.gov/research/hospdrills

Cuny, F. (1998). Principles of disaster management: Introduction. *Prehospital and Disaster Medicine, 13*(1), 80–86. doi:10.1017/s1049023x00033082

Cuny, F. (2000). Principles of disaster management, management leadership styles and methods. *Prehospital and Disaster Medicine, 15*(1), 78–81. doi:10.1017/S1049023X0002495X

Department of Homeland Security. (2017). National incident management system (3rd ed.). Washington, DC: FEMA Publication. Retrieved from https://www.fema.gov/media-library-data/1466014682982-9bcf8245 ba4c60c120aa915abe74e15d/National_Response_Framework3rd.pdf

Department of Homeland Security. Federal Emergency Management Agency. (2016). National Disaster Recovery Framework. Washington, DC. Retrieved from https://www.fema.gov/media-library-data/1466014998123 -4bec8550930f774269e0c5968b120ba2/National_Disaster_Recovery _Framework2nd.pdf

Florida Department of Health. (2011). *Recommended core competencies for hospital personnel.* Retrieved from https://www.calhospitalprepare.org/ sites/main/files/file-attachments/corecompetenciesfloridadh2011.pdf

Gebbie, K. M., Peterson, C. A., Subbarao, I., & White, K. M. (2009). Adapting standards of care under extreme conditions. *Disaster Medicine and Public Health Preparedness, 3*, 111–116. doi:10.1097/DMP.0b013e31819b95dc

Ingelsby, T., Grossman, R., & O'Toole. (2001). A plague on your city: Observations from TOPOFF. *Clinical Infectious Diseases, 32*, 436–445. doi:10.1086/318513

International Council of Nurses and World Health Organization. (2009). *ICN framework for disaster nursing competencies.* Geneva Switzerland: Author.

Joint Commission. (2016). Emergency management standards supporting collaboration planning. Retrieved from https://www.jointcommission .org/assets/1/6/EM_Stds_Collaboration_2016.pdf

Kim, D., & Proctor, P. (2002). Disaster management and the emergency department: A framework for planning. *Nursing Clinics of North America, 37*(1), 171–188. doi:10.1016/s0029-6465(03)00091-4

Lansbury, L., Brown, C., & Nguyen-Van-Tam, J. (2017). Influenza in long term care facilities. *Influenza and Other Respiratory Viruses, 11*(5), 356–366. doi:10.1111/irv.12464

Lanzilotti, S., Galanis, D., Leoni, N., & Craig, B. (2002). Hawaii medical professionals assessment: A study of the availability of doctors and nurses to staff non-hospital, field medical facilities for mass casualty incidents. *Hawaii Medical Journal, 61*(8), 162–174. Retrieved from http://evols.library.manoa.hawaii.edu/bitstream/10524/53682/1/2002- 08p162-173.pdf

Lewis, P., & Aghababian, R. (1996). Disaster planning, Part 1. *Emergency medicine clinics of North America, 14*(2), 439–451.doi:10.1016/s0733-8627(05)70261-3

National Library of Medicine Disaster Information Management Research Center. (2017). Disaster competencies for healthcare workers. Retrieved from https://sis.nlm.nih.gov/dimrc/professionalcompetencies.html

Public Law 109-417. (2006). Pandemic and All Hazards Preparedness Act. Retrieved from http://frwebgate.access.gpo.gov/cgi-bin/getdoc .cgi?dbname=109_cong_public_laws&docid=f:publ417.109.pdf

Qureshi, K., Gershon, R., Gebbie, E., Straub, T., & Morse, S. (2005). Healthcare workers' ability and willingness to report to duty during a catastrophic disaster. *Journal of Urban Health, 82*(3), 378–388. doi:10.1093/jurban/jti086

Qureshi, K., Merrill, J., Gershon, R., & Calero-Breckheimer, A. (2002). Emergency preparedness training for public health nurses: A pilot study. *Journal of Urban Health, 79*(3), 413–416. doi:10.1093/jurban/79.3.413

Shapira, Z., Marganitt, B., Roziner, I., Schohet, T., Bar, Y., & Shemer, J. (1991). Willingness of staff to report to their hospital duties following an unconventional missile attack: A statewide survey. *Israel Journal of Medical Sciences, 27*(11–12), 704–711. Retrieved from https://www.ncbi.nlm.nih.gov/pubmed/1757251

Skryabina, E., Reedy, G., Amlot, R., Jaye, P., & Riley, P. (2017). What is the value of health emergency preparedness exercises: A scoping review study. *International Journal of Disaster Risk Reduction, 21*, 274–283. doi:10.1016/j.ijdrr.2016.12.010

Subbarao, I., Lyznicki, J. M., Hsu, E. B., Gebbie, K. M., Markenson, D., Barzansky, B., ... James, J. J. (2008). A consensus-based educational framework and competency set for the discipline of disaster medicine and public health preparedness. *Disaster Medicine and public health Preparedness, 2*(1), 57–68. doi:10.1097/dmp.0b013e31816564af

Swift, M., Aliyu, M., Byrne, D., Qian, K., McGown, P., Kinman, P. O., ... Yarbrough, M. (2017). Emergency preparedness in the workplace: The Flulapalooza model for mass vaccination. *American Journal of Public Health, 107*(S2), S168–S176. doi:10.2105/AJPH.2017.303953

Townsend, A. M., & Moss, M. L. (2005). Telecommunications infrastructure in disasters: Preparing cities for crisis communications. Center for Catastrophe Preparedness and Response and Robert F. Wagner Graduate School of Public Service at New York University. Retrieved from http://www .nyu.edu/ccpr/pubs/NYU-DisasterCommunications1-Final.pdf

United Nations Office for Disaster Risk Reduction. (2005). Hyogo framework for disaster risk reduction, 2005–2015. Retrieved from http://www .unisdr.org/we/coordinate/hfa

United Nations Office for Disaster Risk Reduction. (2015). Sendai framework for disaster risk reduction 2015–2030. Retrieved from https://www .unisdr.org/we/coordinate/sendai-framework

VanDevanter, N., Kovner, C., Raveis, V., McCollum, M., & Keller, R. (2014) Challenges of nurses deployment to other New York City hospitals in the aftermath of Hurricane Sandy. *Journal of Urban Health, 91*(14), 603–614. doi:10.1007/s11524-014-9889-0

Veenema, T. G., Walden, B., Feinstein, N., & Williams, J. P. (2008). Factors affecting hospital-based nurses' willingness to respond to a radiation emergency. *Disaster Medicine and Public Health Emergency Preparedness, 2*(4), 224–229. doi:10.1097/DMP.0b013e31818a2b7a

Veenema, T. G., Griffin, A., Gable, A. R., MacIntyre, L., Simons, R. A. D. M., Couig, M. P., ... Larson, E. (2016). Nurses as leaders in disaster preparedness and response—A call to action. *Journal of Nursing Scholarship, 48*(2), 187–200. doi:10.1111/jnu.12198

Veenema, T. G., Deruggiero, K., Losinski, S., & Barnett, D. (2017). Hospital administration and nursing leadership in disasters: An exploratory study using concept mapping. *Nursing Administration Quarterly, 41*(2), 151–163. doi:10.1097/NAQ.0000000000000224

Walsh L., Subbarao, I., Gebbie, K., Schor, K. W., Lyznicki, J., Strauss-Riggs, K., ... James, J. J. (2012). Core competencies for disaster medicine and public health. *Disaster Medicine and Public Health Preparedness, 6*(1), 44–52. doi:10.1001/dmp.2012.4

24

PUBLIC HEALTH EMERGENCIES INVOLVING COMMUNITY VIOLENCE AND CIVIL UNREST: TAKING PLANNED ACTION

Roberta Proffitt Lavin, Wilma J. Calvert, Sue Anne Bell, Sheila R. Grigsby, and Anne F. Fish

LEARNING OBJECTIVES

When this chapter is completed, readers will be able to:

1. Define civil unrest.
2. List the conditions in Ferguson, MO that contributed to civil unrest in 2014.
3. Describe the social issues that are foundational elements in civil unrest.
4. List the types of active shooters.
5. Discuss the types of preparedness activities in which a healthcare facility should engage for active shooters.
6. Describe the preparedness activities that will help a hospital or healthcare facility in relation to civil unrest.

KEY MESSAGES

Civil unrest is disharmony, expressive dissatisfaction, and/or disagreement between members of a community that leads to a situation of competitive aggression that may find expression as disruption of organization, conflicts, damage to property, and injuries.

Civil unrest peaked in the 1960 to 1970 era during the Vietnam War, but never returned to the infrequency prior to that period. Since 2010, the number of incidents has been increasing largely in response to police-involved deaths of unarmed Black men.

A myriad of social issues contributing to civil unrest include discriminatory housing policies that, although deemed illegal, continue to influence the economic status of those residing in such communities, perceived lack of power by community residents, limited education and economic opportunities and the resultant persistent and high levels of poverty in the community, and citizen mistrust of law enforcement.

Intentional killing of civilians or bystanders can fall into five different categories. These include active shooter, mass shooting, mass killings, terrorism, and active shooter in healthcare settings.

The Run-Hide-Fight Active Shooter protocol is a response for any individual involved in an active shooter incident. It involves a rapid assessment of whether there is a quick route of escape, a place to hide, and, if neither, then fighting back.

CHAPTER OVERVIEW

This chapter explores two distinct issues in the United States. The chapter begins with an overview of civil unrest in the United States with special attention given to the time period since 2010. An emphasis is placed on the preparedness and response necessary by healthcare systems. A brief review of the civil unrest and related social issues; a detailed overview of the incidents of Ferguson, MO; action steps for nurse administrators; types of active shooters; and actions to take during an active shooter incident are addressed. Definitions of civil unrest and active shooter are provided along with a discussion of each of the healthcare challenges they create. Nurses' skills that aid in preparedness and planning for both civil unrest and an active shooter incident are discussed. The chapter concludes with essentials for nursing leadership and suggestions for working in community health, an outpatient setting, or at the bedside for every setting.

There is no continent in the world safe from civil unrest and violence. One can debate the causes of societal discontent and the belief that the only way to address the underlying issues is through civil unrest and violence. What is not debatable is that both exist and historically have had periods of exacerbation. Most increases in civil unrest are related to racial and socioeconomic inequality and discontent with governmental policy. Mass shooting and active shooters, however, are more closely related to religious and political extremism and mental illness. The world appears to be in a period of discontent that has resulted both from an increase in civil unrest and from an increase in mass shootings.

Ideally, civil unrest and violence should be wholly distinct. Civil unrest, by design, is not violent, but designed to express discontent with social or political events. All too often it results in violence as it did in Ferguson, MO in 2014 and more recently in Charlottesville, VA in 2017. Mass shootings are a form of violent extremism, which is "the beliefs and actions of people who support or use violence to achieve ideological, religious, or political goals" (Australian Government, 2016, para. 1). Pinker (2011) famously argued that the level of violence in the world is decreasing. He speculates that the decline stems from

multiple factors, including a judiciary with a "monopoly on the legitimate use of force," commerce, feminization, the rise of literacy and mobility, and finally the rise of reason. He further speculates that the rise of mass media makes it less likely that we will return to more violent times and will continue to grow ever more intolerant of violence.

CIVIL UNREST

Inequalities in society, culture, and finance have resulted in community uprisings that are placing a greater burden on healthcare systems and nursing leaders to respond in a timely and appropriate manner. How we define civil unrest impacts how we prepare and the seriousness with which we prepare. Civil unrest is "disharmony, expressive dissatisfaction and/ or disagreement between members of a community, which leads to a situation of competitive aggression that may find expression as disruption of organization, conflicts, damage to property and injuries" (Ballantyne, 2006, p. 155). The level of civil unrest in the United States had been relatively consistent until the 1960s when there was a significant increase with the onset of the Vietnam War. After the end of the war the civil unrest declined, but has been steadily increasing since 1980 (see Figure 24.1).

The relatively recent events of civil unrest in cities across the United States have raised the awareness of injustice in our society and the need to recognize the human dignity of every person. While nursing has been acknowledged as more trusted than many other public services, nursing has largely failed to address the impact of civil unrest on both nurses, the organizations we lead, and the communities we represent. It is essential to recognize that while our roles will be similar to those we take during a disaster event, not all of the circumstances are the same. For example, because of heightened tension between police and the general population, the presence of police may not be possible and, even if possible, may not be desirable (Kotora et al., 2014).

If we approach civil unrest as another type of disaster, we must recognize that the efforts of many health professionals, especially nurses, are needed. During such times, it is likely that both hospitals and public health organizations will change their preparedness posture and may have increased staffing or ready call rosters for healthcare professionals. What is less clear is the extent to which healthcare organizations are working to recognize that the dynamics in civil unrest are more complex than a natural disaster and may be more like complex humanitarian emergencies in the sense that there is an internal breakdown at the local level that may require outside intervention to regain order.

The American Organization of Nurse Executives (AONE), in response to what they refer to as a "changing world" filled with "volatility, uncertainty, complexities, and ambiguities," convened a working group to address the role of the nurse leader in a crisis. The AONE gave much of its highest priority to good communication, projecting calm, understanding how people react, prioritizing the crisis plan, and being trusted patient advocates (Edmonson, Sumagaysay, Cueman, & Chappell, 2016). This is all consistent with what was seen on the ground during recent events in Ferguson, MO and Baltimore, MD.

FERGUSON, MO

On Saturday, August 8, 2014, Michael Brown was shot and killed in Ferguson, MO during an altercation with a police officer related to jaywalking. After being killed, his body laid out on the pavement for several hours in the sun, unattended without any processing by Ferguson officials. With the ability of people to communicate quickly through smartphones and social media, it provided the perfect medium for communities to share injustices in real time and unfiltered. In a matter of hours, the image of a young man's body lying in the street was shared around the world. Across the world including China, people were asking the question, "Where is Ferguson, MO?"

The history of the St. Louis region is clear in that systemic racism continues to be an active part of the culture. Dating back to the 1900s, citizens from this region have a history of being complacent when dealing with segregation and challenging the status quo. While there were some famous actions in the region like the Fairgrounds Park Riot of 1949 due to the integration of a public pool or the Jefferson Bank civil rights protests, it is not known for civil unrest. The practice of the press was not to provide any media coverage of such actions. This conscious effort to deny visibility of these occurrences was a systematic way of not recording history; therefore, not acknowledging the race problem in the region. White residents in the region did not understand nor did the public health infrastructure.

The historical context, as just outlined, provides a snapshot of why there are so many systemic problems in the area. This context helps to describe how public confidence in the Ferguson justice system had eroded to a critical level (Norwood, 2016). The movement in Ferguson was about more than the killing of an 18-year-old male for jaywalking. The movement was sparked by police force against Black people; excessive tickets for traffic, as well as quality of life–related issues and housing code violations that preyed on the most vulnerable; unemployment and underemployment; inadequate healthcare and public health concerns; inadequate housing; and substandard schools.

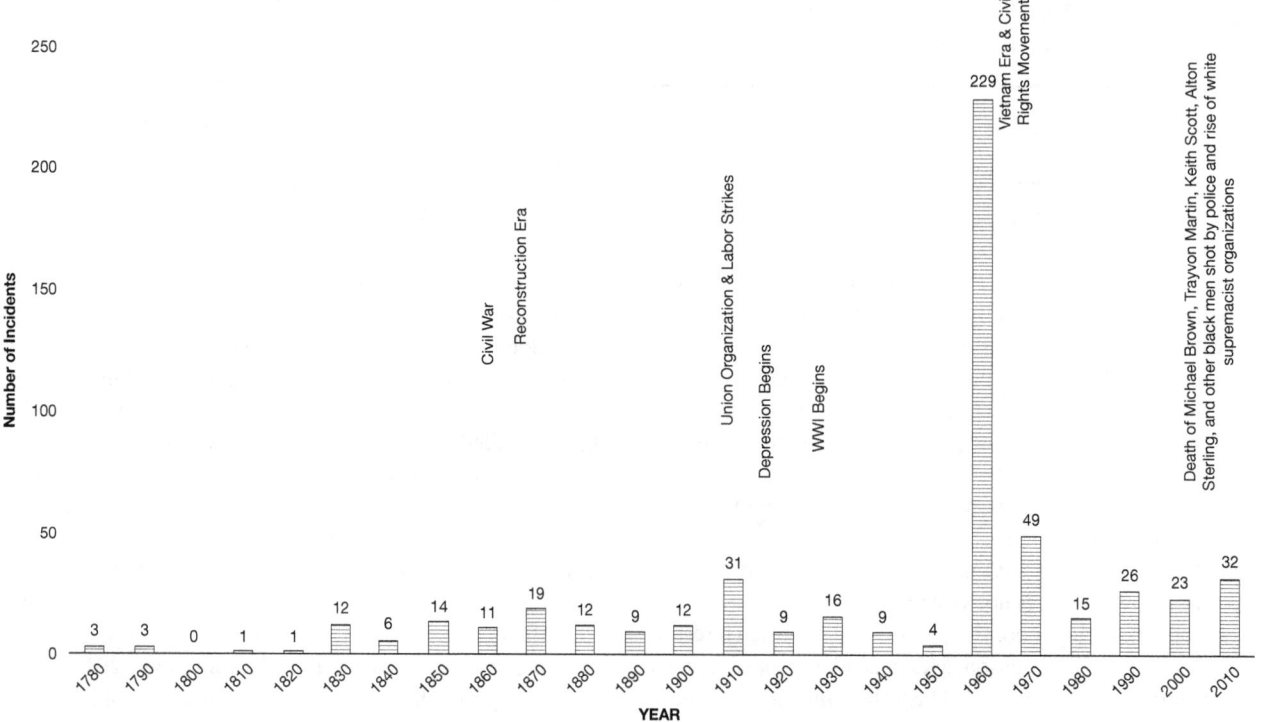

FIGURE 24.1 Civil unrest incidents in the United States.

Sources: Adapted from Armstrong Economics. (2017). Listing of US civil unrest incidents. Retrieved from https://www.armstrongeconomics.com/statistics/listing-of-us-civil-unrest-incidents; Wikipedia Contributors. (2017). List of incidents of civil unrest in the United States. Retrieved from https://en.wikipedia.org/wiki/List_of_incidents_of_civil_unrest_in_the_United_States

ococ nameosdfÍ

SOCIAL ISSUES AS FOUNDATIONAL ELEMENTS IN CIVIL UNREST

Civil unrest in response to oppressive conditions imposed upon the vulnerable in the United States is not a new phenomenon. The unrest was not uncommon during the civil rights movement of the 1960s. As someone who espoused nonviolence in response to the blatant oppression and segregation occurring in the United States during the 1960s, when interviewed by Mike Wallace during a particularly violent summer in 1966, the Reverend Dr. Martin Luther King, Jr. did not condemn the violence or the "Black Power" movement espoused by other civil rights leaders:

> I contend that the cry of "black power" is, at bottom, a reaction to the reluctance of white power to make the kind of changes necessary to make justice a reality for the Negro. I think that we've got to see that a riot is the language of the unheard. (King, M. L., Jr. (1966). Interview by M. Wallace. *60 Minutes Overtime*.)

The Rev. Dr. King used similar words in 1968, when asked to address the violence and looting that occurred, as well as escalation of instances of civil unrest throughout the United States, as Blacks and others fought for civil rights. This time, though, he elaborated on the issue, explaining that it would be inappropriate and "morally irresponsible" for him to condemn the riotous acts without "... condemning the contingent, intolerable conditions that exist.... These conditions ... cause individuals to feel that they have no other alternative.... And I must say tonight that a riot is the language of the unheard" (Farrell, 2011, para. 2). The 1960s provided a call to examine the social issues associated with civil unrest; similar conditions persist in the 21st century.

Too often in the United States, and most recently after the police-involved shootings of unarmed Black men such as Michael Brown and Freddie Gray, the protest led to acts by those participating that meet the definition of civil unrest (Ballantyne, 2006). Observers lay the blame for the events leading up to the civil unrest and any resultant negative effects of the unrest (e.g., burned-out businesses, an increased law enforcement presence, arrests) squarely on the shoulders of the demonstrators. It is easy, when civil unrest occurs, to attempt to solve the immediate unrest and even the long-term consequences solely through law enforcement efforts. This includes hiring additional law enforcement personnel, implementing trainings such as sensitivity, de-escalating, and deciding how to limit the use of excessive force and community policing (Rothstein, 2015). However, such a myopic perspective negates societal and governmental influences that had influenced and continue to influence the communities experiencing civil unrest. Contributing factors for civil unrest are frequently imposed upon economically disadvantaged groups through formal laws and practices steeped in tradition. With the advent of technology such as cell phone cameras, social media including Facebook and Twitter, YouTube videos, and 24-hour news cycles, some observers, instead of blaming the demonstrators, responded in shock and disbelief to the social issues that led to the demonstrations and incidents of civil unrest.

A myriad of social issues contributed to the unrest affecting predominantly Black urban areas such as St. Louis, MO (of which Ferguson, MO is an inner-ring suburb) and Baltimore, MD. July 1, 2016 population estimates for Blacks residing in Ferguson is 67% and 64% for Baltimore (U.S. Census Bureau, 2016). Many of the race-related governmental policies of segregation at the local, state, and federal levels that led to the civil unrest in Ferguson are like those in Baltimore (Rothstein, 2015). These issues include discriminatory housing policies that, although deemed illegal, continue to influence the economic status of those residing in such communities; perceived lack of power by community residents; limited educational and economic opportunities and the resultant persistent and high levels of poverty in the community; and citizen mistrust of law enforcement.

"White flight," known as the phenomenon of upper- and middle-class Whites relocating further and further away from the urban core into the suburbs, and other races (in this case Blacks) moving into urban neighborhoods, partially explains the racial makeup of Ferguson and Baltimore; but, the role of the government cannot be overlooked. Both cities have a history of segregated housing practices that effectively created racially segregated communities. Federal, state, and local laws, policies, and regulations were enacted to ensure that Blacks, including those in St. Louis and Baltimore, would be forced to live in communities separate from Whites (Rothstein, 2015). Such practices are now deemed illegal, but their deleterious effects persist in many urban communities. Closely related to the housing segregation is the economic segregation experienced by some of the Blacks residing in these communities. Often, those residing in these racially segregated cities work in low-paying jobs that limit their ability to relocate to neighborhoods that may have more resources and, as Rothstein (2015) describes, economic inequities prohibited some Blacks from relocating to single-family homes on large lots further out in the suburbs.

Racially segregated cities, such as St. Louis and Ferguson, not only experience the vestiges of legalized segregated housing, but also experience other disadvantages, such as limited political influence. Although Ferguson is approximately 67% Black (U.S. Census Bureau, 2016), the majority of the City Council members, including the mayor, were White; after the death of Michael Brown, half of the six elected City Council members were Black (City of Ferguson, n.d.; Ferguson Commission, 2015). Likewise, Black Ferguson residents had limited representation on the Ferguson-Florissant School Board, the primary public school district serving the area. In 2010, Dr. Art McCoy was elected superintendent of the Ferguson-Florissant School District, the first Black to occupy the position (FloValley News, 2017). However, in the latter part of 2013, the predominantly White school board placed Dr. McCoy on administrative leave for undisclosed reasons (Crouch, 2013); he ultimately resigned early in 2014, despite vocal community support (Lloyd & Singer, 2014). At the time of Michael Brown's death in 2014, only one of the seven elected school board members was Black (R. Perry, personal communication, July 4, 2017; St. Louis Post-Dispatch, n.d.). Positive changes are occurring in the leadership serving the Ferguson community: Three of the current seven elected school board members are Black (Ferguson-Florissant School District, 2017). This is important when considering emergency preparedness. Having trusted community members during times of civil unrest is essential.

If the elected officials do not represent the community, it will impact the ability to communicate with the public.

Housing segregation and limited economic opportunities, along with the resultant poverty, also served to ignite the Ferguson and Baltimore civil unrest. Segregated housing influences an individual's economic status through the availability of quality educational and employment opportunities. We earlier discussed the evolving nature of the once predominantly White composition of the Ferguson-Florissant school board to one that is more diverse, thus better representing the student population. Unlike Ferguson, the 2015 Baltimore School Board, whose members are appointed jointly by the governor of Maryland and the mayor of Baltimore, has five of 10 school board members who are Black (Baltimore City Board of School Commissioners, 2015). Both school districts serve predominantly Black students. Education is important to consider in any discussion on civil unrest because educational and economic opportunities are inextricably intertwined. Schools serving the most disadvantaged Black students, which describes many of the school-aged population in Ferguson and Baltimore, are often racially segregated and in economically disadvantaged communities.

Additional social factors contributing to civil unrest are high levels of unemployment and poverty, both of which are present in Ferguson and Baltimore. The national unemployment rate in May 2017 was 3.7%, compared to 7.5% for Blacks (U.S. Department of Labor Bureau of Labor Statistics, 2017). For White men, it was 3.4%, yet 6.5% for Black men (U.S. Department of Labor Bureau of Labor Statistics, 2017). The 2015 poverty rate (based on the U.S. Census Bureau's poverty threshold) for Blacks nationally was 24%, compared to 9% for Whites (Henry J. Kaiser Family Foundation, 2017). For Blacks in Maryland, the rate is 17% and 6% for Whites, and the poverty rate for Blacks in Missouri is 25%, compared to 7% for Whites (Henry J. Kaiser Family Foundation, 2017). Focusing specifically on households living below the U.S. poverty threshold, results from the *2011-2015 American Community Survey 5-Year Estimates* indicate that 28% of Blacks in Baltimore lived below the poverty threshold, compared to 14% of Whites (U.S. Census Bureau, n.d.). Results are even more disparate for Blacks and Whites in Ferguson living below the poverty threshold: 27% versus 7%, respectively (U.S. Census Bureau, n.d.). At $31,214, the median household income of Blacks in the St. Louis region was half the median household income for Whites, which was $61,254 (U.S. Census Bureau, n.d.). The economic-related disparities are stark for Blacks in the United States.

The strained relationship between the residents and law enforcement can also lead to civil unrest. The shooting of Michael Brown in Ferguson, MO and the death of Freddie Gray, who suffered a spinal injury while in the custody of the Baltimore, MD police department, were enough to fuel unrest in those communities. In 2014, the Ferguson police department had limited Black representation on its force; only three of the 53 officers were Black at the time of Michael Brown's death. St. Louis County is unique in that instead of being policed by one police department, it has more than 81 municipal courts and 60 independent municipal police departments (Ferguson Commission, 2015). With some of the small municipalities struggling financially because of a low tax base, police officers and municipal courts become revenue-generating bodies, bringing revenue to the municipalities (Better Together, 2014). Even though Ferguson has a large Black population, Blacks experience a disproportionate number of traffic stops. Police militarization, including armored vehicles, was brought into Ferguson to help quell the unrest. Without a doubt, the situation in Ferguson was volatile on both sides, but militarization did not lessen the volatility. In retrospect, some believe this militarization served to widen the gulf between the residents, protesters, and law enforcement.

The strained relationship is not unique to Ferguson: Baltimore has a history of tenuous relationships between residents and the local police department. One way it differs is the racial makeup of those in leadership positions in Baltimore. At the time of Freddie Gray's death in 2015, the mayor, president of the City Council, police commissioner, and almost half of the police department were Black. So, while race may have fueled the tensions in Ferguson, in Baltimore, residents believed police officers treated them harshly because of their socioeconomic status. Tim Lynch of the Cato Institute is quoted as saying Blacks residing in Baltimore's poorer neighborhoods believe the police treat them as second-class citizens, and are quick to resort to extreme policing to prevent criminal acts (Howell, 2015). Militarization of the Baltimore police department also occurred during the civil unrest after Gray's death (Cato Institute, 2015). As in Ferguson, the presence of a police department with military-type weapons, including an armored tank, reinforced preexisting tensions between residents and the police department, and shocked people observing the unrest on television or via social media.

Limited resources in economically challenged neighborhoods, including a lack of positive relationships with law enforcement and limited representation in governing bodies, foster a climate of hostility and mistrust between residents and societal institutions. Residents of these communities often feel marginalized and isolated. So, when a perceived insult or wrong occurs, sometimes residents harken to use the only "voice" they know: civil unrest.

According to *Forward Through Ferguson. A Path Toward Racial Equity* (Ferguson Commission, 2015), specific steps needed to move the region forward to lessen citizen mistrust of law enforcement include police and court reform, along with a consolidation of police departments and municipal courts. Among the changes cited in *Forward Through Ferguson* (2015) are eliminating incarceration for minor, nonviolent offenses, primarily driving offenses. There is certainly the need for hiring more Black police officers, especially in communities serving a largely Black population, and additional training focused on police tactics that help dispel negative images and perceptions of law enforcement. *Forward Through Ferguson* (2015) details priorities if Ferguson, Baltimore, and similar communities are to move forward, decreasing the likelihood of civil unrest.

Separately, the issues described in this chapter are disconcerting. The cumulative effect, though, makes conditions ripe for civil unrest, and it is the cumulative effects that helped to fuel the unrest in Ferguson, MO, Baltimore, MD, and other urban areas plagued by these social issues.

ACTIVE SHOOTER

Active shooter incidents cause devastating and long-lasting impact on communities, first responders, and the receiving healthcare facilities. These unpredictable events are on the rise in the United States. Between 2000 and 2013, the Federal Bureau of Investigation recorded 160 active shooter incidents, with an increase from 6.4 incidents per year between the years 2000 and 2006 to 16.4 per year between 2007 and 2013 (U.S. Department of Justice Federal Bureau of Investigation, 2013). Another study found that active shooter incidents increased from an average of 9 per year between 2000 and 2005 to an average of almost 17 shootings per year between 2006 and 2011 (Kelen, Catlett, Kubit, & Hsieh, 2012). Likewise, the number of mass shootings has increased (Figure 24.2). Nurses must be prepared to protect patient safety and provide nursing care in the event of an active shooter incident.

TYPES OF ACTIVE SHOOTERS

Intentional killing of civilians or bystanders can fall into several different categories. These include active shooter, mass shooting, mass killings, terrorism, and active shooter in healthcare settings.

Active Shooter

Multiple definitions for an "active shooter" exist. The most accepted one, and the one used by U.S. federal agencies, including the Department of Homeland Security, defines active shooter as "an individual actively engaged in killing or attempting to kill people in a confined and populated area" (U.S. Department of Justice Federal Bureau of Investigation, 2013). In most cases, active shooters use a firearm. In most circumstances, victims are targeted at random, as there is no pattern or reason for the selection of victims.

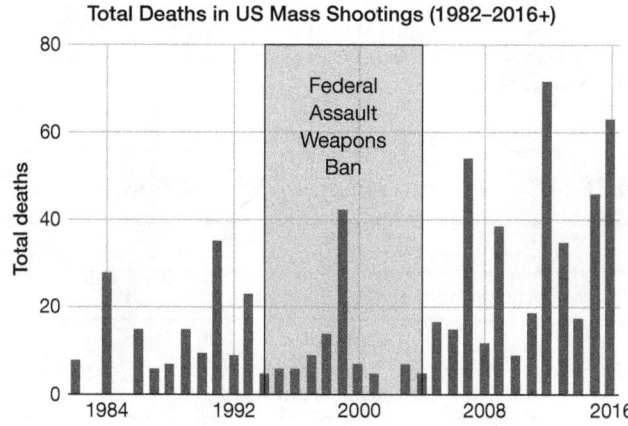

FIGURE 24.2 Total deaths in U.S. mass shootings by year (1982–2016).

Source: Data from Follman, M., Aronsen, G., & Pan, D. (2018). US mass shootings, 1982–2018: Data from Mother Jones' investigation. Retrieved from http://www.motherjones.com/politics/2012/12/mass-shootings-mother-jones-full-data.

Mass Shooting

Several definitions for "mass shooting" exist as consensus has not been reached. A mass shooting is defined as any incident in which four or more people are shot, whether injured or killed (Global Terrorism Database, 2017). Mass shootings can be carried out by an individual or a group.

In 2017, there have been 311 mass shootings in the first 10 months of the year. While all are horrible, two specific shootings drew national attention. The first occurred on October 1, 2017 in Las Vegas when a single gunman fired from the 32nd floor of the Mandalay Bay Hotel into a crowd of 22,000 concert goers killing 58 and injuring 546 (Bui, 2017). The second occurred on November 5, 2017 at the First Baptist Church in Sutherland Springs, TX. A single gunman killed 26 people and injured 20 others (Weill, 2017). In both cases the gunmen had high-powered assault rifles and other weapons. The victims were unable to escape and in both cases were in environments where they felt safe.

Mass Killings

The Investigative Assistance for Violent Crimes Act of 2012 defined a "mass killing" as three or more people killed in a single event (U.S. Department of Justice Federal Bureau of Investigation, 2013). It is important to note that this explanation is not limited to use of firearms, but also includes any non-gun–related killings. This definition is potentially flawed as it does not include persons who were injured but did not die as a result of the incident. It also does not include the death of the assailant in the event of being killed by the police or by his or her own hand.

Terrorism

Active shooter events differ from "terrorism." Although multiple definitions exist for terrorism, the Global Terrorism Database (2017) describes three criteria:

Criterion I: The act must be aimed at attaining a political, economic, religious, or social goal.
Criterion II: There must be evidence of an intention to coerce, intimidate, or convey some other message to a larger audience (or audiences) than the immediate victims.
Criterion III: The action must be outside the context of legitimate warfare activities.

Active Shooter Incidents in the Healthcare Setting

An "active shooter incident in the hospital setting" is not only a threat to personal and public safety but also a serious public health threat. The potential for violence in the healthcare setting is particularly high because it is a high-stress environment for patients who may have unstable mental health conditions and families coping with their medical needs (Kotora et al., 2014). While most hospital-based shooting incidents have involved the deaths of a small number of persons (Kelen et al., 2012), 67% of healthcare facility-based shootings occurred before police arrived and could engage the shooter (U.S. Department of Justice Federal Bureau of Investigation, 2013).

MITIGATION AND PREPAREDNESS

Preparedness activities for healthcare providers should focus on six key points (The Joint Commission, 2014):

- Involve local law enforcement in plans
- Develop and prepare a communication plan
- Assess and prepare the building
- Establish processes and procedures to ensure patient and employee safety
- Train and drill employees
- Plan for postevent activities

Many resources now exist to address active shooter preparedness, including law enforcement agencies, hospital associations, and healthcare systems. Ready-made drills and training materials are widely available.

An emergency action plan (EAP) is a systems-level approach to preparedness. A written EAP is mandated by the Occupational Safety and Health Administration for the purpose of defining and guiding actions during a workplace emergency (U.S. Department of Labor, n.d.). Understanding and being able to carry out the activities and plan in the EAP forms the basis of preparedness activities. Development of a comprehensive EAP requires careful and advanced coordination of healthcare systems alongside community partners, local emergency services, and law enforcement. An inclusive approach that involves planning, education, training, and preparation by all partners to maximize survival of staff and patients is the focus.

Conducting regular training exercises is another core component of preparedness for an active shooter incident (U.S. Department of Homeland Security, 2008). To be most effective, active shooter training activities should include a video or classroom component in addition to a hands-on community-based drill that involves both local law enforcement and emergency medical services. The drill should be an integral part of preparedness activities in all healthcare facilities, schools, and universities.

RESPONSE

The Run-Hide-Fight Active Shooter protocol (Table 24.1) is a well-known and advocated response for any individual involved in an active shooter incident (Houston Police Department, 2013). Run-Hide-Fight was originally produced by the City of Houston with the support of the Department of Homeland Security. It is based on the three central ideas to support users to immediately choose the best way to protect their lives by making the quickest and best assessment of what is occurring and which of the three options will have the safest and best outcome.

ACTIVE SHOOTER MANAGEMENT IN THE PREHOSPITAL SETTING

Most active shooter incidents are first managed in the prehospital setting, involving local law enforcement and emergency medical services as the first responders on the scene. Table 24.2 details the acronym THREAT, which stands for Threat suppression, Hemorrhage control, Rapid Extrication at the scene, Assessment by medical providers referring to triage, and then Transport to definitive care (Jacobs, 2014).

A rapid response can promote lifesaving interventions, provided the scene is safe. Remaining on the scene during dynamic events must be carefully evaluated. A recent National Academy of Medicine (NAM; Hick, et al., 2016) recommendation suggests that implementing mass casualty triage systems, such as START (Simple Triage and Rapid Treatment), along with staging and casualty collection points, may be detrimental as they may potentially delay the transport of injured patients to more definitive care. If patient transportation is in place, further assessment and usual trauma care, triage color coding, and interventions can safely be performed en route to a trauma center.

TABLE 24.1 Run, Hide, Fight—Active Shooter Protocol

Run	• Have an escape route and plan in mind • Leave your belongings behind • Keep your hands visible
Hide	• Hide in an area out of the shooter's view • Block entry to your hiding place and lock the doors • Silence your cell phone and/or pager
Fight	• As a last resort and only when your life is in imminent danger • Attempt to incapacitate the shooter • Act with physical aggression and throw items at the active shooter

Source: From U.S. Department of Homeland Security. (2017). Active Shooter Pocket Card. Retrieved from https://www.dhs.gov/publication/active-shooter-pocket-card

TABLE 24.2 Concept to Action—THREAT Acronym

T	Threat suppression
H	Hemorrhage control
RE	Rapid extrication to safety
A	Assessment by medical providers
T	Transport to definitive care

Source: Hick, J. L., Hanfling, D., Evans, B., Greenberg, S., Alson, R., McKinney, S., & Minson, M. (2016). Health and medical response to active shooter and bombing events. National Academy of Medicine. Retrieved from https://nam.edu/wp-content/uploads/2016/06/Health-and-Medical-Response-to-Active-Shooter-and-Bombing-Events.pdf

RECOVERY

Immediate after-action discussion (called a "hot wash") should be conducted after each training session and especially after an incident, to identify what went well and what needs to be improved. Best practices for planning for active shooter after-action planning are essential. Recommended resources may include:

- Planning and Response to an Active Shooter: An Interagency Security Committee Policy and Best Practice Guide available at www.dhs.gov/sites/default/files/publications/isc-planning-response-active-shooter-guide-non-fouo-nov-2015-508.pdf
- Homeland Security Exercise and Evaluation Program available at www.fema.gov/media-library-data/20130726-1914-25045-8890/hseep_apr13_.pdf
- Active Shooter Plan Template available at www.cdse.edu/documents/toolkits-physical/active-shooter-plan-template.docx

COMMUNITY RESILIENCE

Community resilience activities after an active shooter incident should focus on recovery. After an active shooter event, the effects on the community can be broad and profound. Efforts to promote "community recovery," defined as "the ability to collaborate with community partners to plan and advocate for the rebuilding of public health, medical and mental health systems" (Centers for Disease Control and Prevention, 2011), should be put in place through a collaborative process with all stakeholders involved. Because the impact of an active shooter incident extends well beyond the primary victims to encompass the bystanders, families, the healthcare facility, and the community, open communication postincident can build the foundation for community recovery.

MENTAL HEALTH SUPPORT

The mental health effects of an active shooter incident on both providers and victims cannot be underestimated (NAM, 2016). These events have both individual- and community-level effects. Immediate availability of mental health services is important for all involved in order to prevent psychological sequelae (American Psychological Association, 2016). For example, patients and employees should be referred to appropriate mental health resources offered by the hospital's Employee Assistance Program or other available services in the community.

Psychological first aid (PFA) is an evidence-based approach to supporting and assisting individuals across the life span after a traumatic event such as an active shooter incident. Intervening with PFA early postincident can promote adaptive coping through debriefing, calm reassurance, and community assistance so those impacted can feel safe and supported (U.S. Department of Health and Human Services, 2014).

ETHICS

Many ethical dilemmas exist surrounding any active shooter incident. As patient advocates, nurses may be placed in the difficult situation of choosing between protecting their own personal safety and protecting the life and health of their patients. One way to address this is through preparedness, by having open discussions during trainings and drills about these challenging and difficult decisions (U.S. Department of Health and Human Services, 2014). Nurses should carefully consider their personal values surrounding such situations as part of preparedness planning and be given the opportunity to process their experiences.

CONSIDERATIONS FOR NURSES IN MASS SHOOTINGS

With standardization and the establishment of best practices, nurses working in healthcare organizations can effectively mitigate how you will play during a crisis.

1. Can you respond?
2. Do you have family responsibilities that must take priority (dependent elder, young children)?
3. Will your job allow you time off?
4. Are you physically able to respond?
5. Are you psychologically prepared?
6. Are you trained?
7. Are you prepared for the possibility of being arrested?

CONSIDERATIONS FOR NURSES IN CIVIL UNREST

Disaster preparedness and response is a cycle that begins with planning and continues through recovery. As in disaster response, there is the initial desire of the public to respond. As the recovery drags on, the enthusiasm of the larger community and healthcare professionals diminishes long before the recovery is complete. Likewise, during civil unrest, there are many who want to go out and protest and support the protesters. As nurses, we must remember that long after the celebrities and the cameras have gone, the community and our nurses living in the community need our constant presence and assurance that we are there to support them through their recovery.

Whether you are in nursing leadership, working in community health, an outpatient setting, or at the beside, there are some essentials for every setting. All healthcare facilities and staff must be prepared. These are the 10 musts of preparedness for civil unrest.

1. Hospital security trained in crowd control during riots
2. Local leaders identified and trained in emergency management and as street medics
3. Local leaders and students included in drills that demonstrate how to stay safe during a riot

4. A communication plan established by local leaders, street medics, and hospitals (Kotora et al., 2014)
5. What is expected from other organizations modeled by nurse leaders (Kotora et al., 2014 [They are chosen for the role because they manage the largest workforce in the hospital and are trusted members of the community.])
6. The intersection of complex issues and the need to intervene with staff when there is a lack of understanding recognized by nurse managers
7. Orderly triage supported by previously trained local and prominent community leaders within the crowd (Kotora et al., 2014)
8. Mobile clinics used or home visits planned for and then provided during the crisis
9. Hospital and community partnerships designed to help heal young people impacted by violence with case management, mentorship, and evidence-based trauma interventions (Jacobs et al., 2014)
10. All nurses trained in trauma-informed care

SUMMARY

This chapter presented two all too common situations—civil unrest and active shooters. The frequency of both has shown a steady increase since the 1980s. In both civil unrest and active shooter situations there is both a role for community and for healthcare preparedness with the nurse taking a significant leadership position in both.

In civil unrest it is the community that is thrown into a state of disequilibrium and faces a situation that is perceived as threatening; the unrest disrupts the normal functioning of the community and infrastructure. Yet, the threat that resulted in the civil unrest is infrequently dealt with during the crisis period, but the underlying societal issues may impact the relationship between nurses, staff, and patients. Instead, authorities focus on crowd control preventing the loss of life or damage to property. Nurses must focus on interpersonal relationships and the provisions of services to the community during the crisis. Before and after the crisis, the focus should be on security training, building relationships, and understanding societal issues that impact people differently.

Like civil unrest, active shooters are becoming a frequent sight in the United States. An active shooter is any individual actively engaged in killing or attempting to kill people in a confined and populated area. Four primary types of active shooters were covered: mass shooters, mass killings, terrorism, and active shooters in a healthcare setting. Preparedness and active shooter drills can help individuals and facilities prepare. The most common training includes knowing when to run, hide, or fight. Unlike many facilities, hospitals are meant to have easy access to the public and, because nurses have a responsibility as the patients' advocates, the option to run and hide may cause an ethical conflict for nurses. Each person must know what he or she is willing to do and when personal safety must be considered.

Regardless of whether one is faced with civil unrest or an active shooter, there are helpful steps one can take to help ensure the safe functioning of the healthcare setting. Assessing one's own willingness to engage in civil discussions about underlying social issues and one's willingness to risk personal safety helps the nurse to be prepared. Each nurse can begin by evaluating his or her own priorities and beliefs. Evaluation of the safety plans of a facility and getting to know key community partners gives the nurse important data to assist in planning and response.

STUDY QUESTIONS

1. Consider your own community. If faced with the shooting of an unarmed teenager and rising tension within the community, what are the steps you as a nurse leader could take within a healthcare facility to prepare and who should be considered vital community partners?

2. A code is called indicating an active shooter is in the hospital. As the charge nurse on a unit during visiting hours, what are the actions that can be taken to protect both patients and visitors?

USEFUL LINKS

Active Shooter Plan Template. www.cdse.edu/documents/toolkits-physical/active-shooter-plan-template.docx
Better Together. www.bettertogetherstl.com
Forward Through Ferguson. forwardthroughferguson.org/report/executive-summary/clarifying-our-terms
Gun Violence Achieve. www.gunviolencearchive.org
Homeland Security Exercise and Evaluation Program. www.fema.gov/media-library-data/20130726-1914-25045-8890/hseep_apr13_.pdf
How to Prepare for and Respond During and After an Active Shooter Incident. www.fema.gov/media-library-data/1472672897352-d28bb197db538 9e4ddedcef335d3d867/FEMA_ActiveShooter_OnePagerv1d15_508 _FINAL.pdf
My Nursing Education. mynursingeducation.org/category/violence
Planning and Response to an Active Shooter: An Interagency Security Committee Policy and Best Practice Guide. www.dhs.gov/sites/default/files/publications/isc-planning-response-active-shooter-guide-non-fouo-nov-2015-508.pdf

REFERENCES

American Psychological Association. (2016). Managing your distress in the aftermath of shooting. Retrieved from http://www.apa.org/helpcenter/mass-shooting.aspx
Armstrong Economics. (2017). Listing of US civil unrest incidents. Retrieved from https://www.armstrongeconomics.com/statistics/listing-of-us-civil-unrest-incidents

Australian Government. (2016). What is violent extremism? Retrieved from https://www.livingsafetogether.gov.au/aboutus/Pages/what-is-violent-extremism.aspx

Ballantyne, B. (2006). Medical management of the traumatic consequences of civil unrest incidents: Causation, clinical approaches, needs and advanced planning criteria. *Toxicological Reviews, 25*(3), 155–197. doi:10.2165/00139709-200625030-00003

Baltimore City Board of School Commissioners. (2015, March 24). Public board meeting. Retrieved from http://www.baltimorecityschools.org/cms/lib/MD01001351/Centricity/Domain/8910/3_24_2015_Meeting_Minutes.pdf

Better Together. (2014). Public safety-municipal courts. Retrieved from http://www.bettertogetherstl.com/wp-content/uploads/2014/10/BT-Municipal-Courts-Report-Full-Report1.pdf

Bui, L., Zapotosky, M., Barrett, D., & Berman, M. (2017, October 2). At least 59 killed in Las Vegas shooting rampage, more than 500 others injured. *The Washington Post.* Retrieved from https://www.washingtonpost.com/news/morning-mix/wp/2017/10/02/police-shut-down-part-of-las-vegas-strip-due-to-shooting/?utm_term=.2f31beeba914

Cato Institute. (2015). *Cato Institute 2015 annual report.* Retrieved from https://object.cato.org/sites/cato.org/files/pubs/pdf/annual_report-2015.pdf

Centers for Disease Control and Prevention. (2011). *Public health preparedness capabilities: National standards for state and local planning.* Atlanta, GA: Author.

City of Ferguson. (n.d.). Council members. Retrieved from http://www.fergusoncity.com/171/Council-Members

Crouch, E. (2013, November 26). Ferguson-Florissant superintendent says he was given no grounds for suspension. *St. Louis Post-Dispatch.* Retrieved from http://www.stltoday.com/news/local/education/ferguson-florissant-superintendent-says-he-was-given-no-grounds-for/article_d1217bd8-b3bb-5a65-852e-f8cd4e255050.html

Edmonson, C., Sumagaysay, D., Cueman, M., & Chappell, S. (2016). The nurse leader role in crisis management. *Journal of Nurse Administration, 46*(9), 417–419. doi:10.1097/NNA.0000000000000367

Farrell, B. (2011, August 10). "Riot is the language of the unheard." What MLK would have said about the London riots. *Waging Nonviolence.* Retrieved from https://wagingnonviolence.org/feature/riot-is-the-language-of-the-unheard-what-mlk-would-have-said-about-the-london-riots

Ferguson Commission. (2015). Forward through Ferguson: A path toward racial equity. Retrieved from http://forwardthroughferguson.org

Ferguson-Florissant School District. (2017). Board of Education. Retrieved from https://www.fergflor.org/domain/73

FloValley News. (2017, July 17). Art McCoy named Ferguson-Florissant School District superintendent. Retrieved from http://www.flovalleynews.com/art-mccoy-named-ferguson-florissant-school-district-superintendent

Follman, M., Aronsen, G., & Pan, D. (2018). US mass shootings, 1982–2018: Data from Mother Jones' investigation. Retrieved from http://www.motherjones.com/politics/2012/12/mass-shootings-mother-jones-full-data

Global Terrorism Database. (2017). Frequently asked questions. Retrieved from http://www.start.umd.edu/gtd/faq

Henry J. Kaiser Family Foundation. (2017). State health facts. Poverty rate by race/ethnicity. Timeframe: 2015. Retrieved from http://www.kff.org/other/state-indicator/poverty-rate-by-raceethnicity/?currentTimeframe=0&sortModel=%7B%22colId%22:%22Location%22,%22sort%22:%22asc%22%7D

Hick, J. L., Hanfling, D., Evans, B., Greenberg, S., Alson, R., McKinney, S., & Minson, M. (2016). Health and medical response to active shooter and bombing events. National Academy of Medicine. Retrieved from https://nam.edu/wp-content/uploads/2016/06/Health-and-Medical-Response-to-Active-Shooter-and-Bombing-Events.pdf

Houston Police Department. (2013). Surviving an active shooter: Run–Hide–Fight. Retrieved from http://www.houstontx.gov/police/pdfs/brochures/english/Active_Shooter_Brochure_Main_Practice_2013.pdf

Howell, K. (2015, April 29). Baltimore riots sparked not by race but by class tensions between police, poor. *The Washington Times.* Retrieved from http://www.washingtontimes.com/news/2015/apr/29/baltimore-riots-sparked-not-by-race-but-by-class-t

Jacobs, L. (2014). The Hartford Consensus: How to maximize survivability in active shooter intentional mass casualty events. *World Journal of Surgery, 38*:1007. doi:10.1007/s00268-014-2481-7

Jacobs, L. M., Wade, D., McSwain, N. E., Butler, F. K., Fabbri, W., Eastman, A., … Burns, K. J. (2014). Hartford Consensus: A call to action for THREAT, a medical disaster preparedness concept. *Journal of the American College of Surgeons, 218*(3), 467–475. doi:10.1016/j.jamcollsurg.2013.12.009

Kelen, G. D., Catlett, C. L., Kubit, J. G., & Hsieh, Y. H. (2012). Hospital-based shootings in the United States: 2000 to 2011. *Annals of Emergency Medicine, 60*(6), 790–798. doi:10.1016/j.annemergmed.2012.08.012

Kotora, J. G., Clancy, T., Manzon, L., Malik, V., Louden, R. J., & Merlin, M. A. (2014). Active shooter in the emergency department: A scenario-based training approach for healthcare workers. *American Journal of Disaster Medicine, 9*(1), 39–51. doi:10.5055/ajdm.2014.0140

Lloyd, T., & Singer, D. (2014). McCoy resigns as Ferguson-Florissant superintendent. *St. Louis Public Radio.* Retrieved from http://news.stlpublicradio.org/post/mccoy-resigns-ferguson-florissant-superintendent#stream/0

Norwood, K. J. (2016). *Ferguson faultlines: The race quake that rocked a nation.* Chicago, IL: American Bar Association.

Pinker, S. (2011). *The better angels of our nature: Why violence has declined.* New York, NY: Viking.

Rothstein, R. (2015). From Ferguson to Baltimore: The fruits of government sponsored segregation. Retrieved from http://eprints.lse.ac.uk/61952/1/blogs.lse.ac.uk-From%20Ferguson%20to%20BaltimorenbspThe%20Fruits%20of%20Government-Sponsored%20Segregation.pdf

60 Minutes Overtime. (2013). MLK: A riot is the language of the unheard. Retrieved from http://www.cbsnews.com/news/mlk-a-riot-is-the-language-of-the-unheard

St. Louis Post-Dispatch. (n.d.). Voters' guide. Ferguson-Florissant school board. Retrieved from http://www.stltoday.com/news/local/crime-and-courts/what-s-the-fairest-way-to-elect-school-board-members/article_d79937dd-2dd4-59e9-8cce-3ac9525db2bb.html

The Joint Commission. (2014). Quick safety issue four: Preparing for active shooter situations. Oakbrook Terrace, IL. Retrieved from https://www.jointcommission.org/assets/1/23/Quick_Safety_Issue_Four_July_2014_Final.pdf

U.S. Census Bureau. (n.d.). Poverty status in the past 12 months. 2011-2015 American Community Survey 5-year estimates. *American FactFinder.* Retrieved from https://factfinder.census.gov/faces/tableservices/jsf/pages/productview.xhtml?src=bkmk

U.S. Census Bureau. (2016). QuickFacts. Baltimore city, Maryland; Ferguson city, Missouri. Retrieved from https://www.census.gov/quickfacts/fact/table/baltimorecitymaryland,fergusoncitymissouri/PST045216

U.S. Department of Health and Human Services. (2014). Incorporating active shooter incident planning into health care facility emergency operations plans. Retrieved from http://www.phe.gov/preparedness/planning/Documents/active-shooter-planning-eop2014.pdf

U.S. Department of Homeland Security. (2008). Active shooter: How to respond. Retrieved from https://www.dhs.gov/xlibrary/assets/active_shooter_booklet.pdf

U.S. Department of Homeland Security. (2017). Active shooter pocket card. Retrieved from https://www.dhs.gov/publication/active-shooter-pocket-card

U.S. Department of Justice Federal Bureau of Investigation. (2013). A study of active shooter incidents in the United States between 2000 and 2013. Retrieved from https://www.google.com/url?sa=t&rct=j&q=&esrc=s&source=web&cd=1&ved=0ahUKEwib1b7T_JvQAhWE7CYKHdvdDQwQFggdMAA&url=https%3A%2F%2Fwww.fbi.gov%2Ffile-repository%2Factive-shooter-study-2000-2013-1.pdf&usg=AFQjCNGeZ-z-W1DIBCrFizVuoxH0LRnu9g&sig2=K7-Xdzm7s7JbgG-HkckvLQ&cad=rja

U.S. Department of Labor. (n.d.). Occupational Safety and Health Administration: Evacuation plans and procedures eTool. Retrieved from https://www.osha.gov/SLTC/etools/evacuation/index.html

U.S. Department of Labor Bureau of Labor Statistics. (2017). Table A-2. Employment status of the civilian population by race, sex, and age. Retrieved from https://www.bls.gov/news.release/empsit.t02.htm

Weill, K. (2017, November 5). Deadliest church shooting in American history kills at least 26. *The Daily Beast.* Retrieved from https://www.thedailybeast.com/deadliest-church-shooting-in-american-history-strikes-sutherland-springs-texas

Wikipedia Contributors. (2017). List of incidents of civil unrest in the United States. Retrieved from https://en.wikipedia.org/wiki/List_of_incidents_of_civil_unrest_in_the_United_States

25

MANAGEMENT OF BURN MASS CASUALTY INCIDENTS

Lisa Puett

LEARNING OBJECTIVES

When this chapter is completed, readers will be able to:

1. Identify main components of a burn disaster plan.
2. Describe the etiology, basic pathophysiology, and initial management of burn injury.
3. Discuss the impact of a burn mass casualty incident on a healthcare system and differentiate between surge capacity and sustained surge capacity.
4. List the American Burn Association (ABA) criteria for referring a patient to a burn center.

KEY MESSAGES

Historically, traumatic mass casualty incidents (MCIs) are likely to involve burn injuries.

The ABA, U.S. burn centers, and governmental agencies have written a national response plan for burn MCIs and continue to prepare the nation's healthcare system.

It is essential that communities become familiar with the national plan and integrate this knowledge into their local response plans.

The U.S. National Bioterrorism Hospital Preparedness Program indicates that each care facility must have "a plan to care for at least 50 cases per million people for patients suffering burns or trauma" to receive national funding disaster preparedness. A major burn disaster is defined as any incident with 50 or more burn injuries and/or 30 or more burn-related deaths.

CHAPTER OVERVIEW

Thermal injury continues to be a major cause of morbidity and mortality in the United States. In 2013, fire killed more Americans than all natural disasters combined, with over 3,400 deaths and nearly 16,000 injured. Fire loss rates have been trending down over the last decade; however, the United States is still ranked as having the twelfth-highest fire death rate of the 28 industrialized countries examined by the World Fire Statistics Centre. Death rates vary from state to state based on climate differences as well as socioeconomic, educational, and other factors (United States Fire Administration [USFA], www.usfa.fema.gov).

According to the ABA, the definition of a "burn MCI" is any catastrophic event in which the number of burn victims exceeds the capacity of the local burn center to provide optimal care. Up to 30% of casualties from historic MCIs have required burn care, with 10% being burn-only injuries and the remaining 20% being a combination of burns and other trauma. The etiology of these incidents may be natural or man made, intentional or accidental. They can occur with industrial accidents, structural fires or collapses, terrorist attacks, mass transit accidents, earthquakes, wildfires, or other catastrophic events. Burn patients may constitute a small percentage of the total number of people injured, but this group consumes a disproportionately large amount of healthcare resources compared to a nonburned trauma patient. For example, of those injured at the World Trade Center on 9/11, massive traumatic injuries were associated with imminent mortality and the walking wounded were treated and released. Burn patients, however, remained hospitalized for several months after the event and exhausted the local healthcare system (American Burn Association Board of Trustees and the Committee on Organization and Delivery of Burn Care, 2005).

It does not take a nationally publicized event to seriously impact a healthcare system; even a local apartment fire can cause a regional hospital system to exceed its surge capacity. A burn center's capacity is determined by available burn beds, burn surgeons, burn nurses, support staff, operating rooms, equipment, supplies, and related resources; it is a dynamic number. "Surge capacity" is the ability to evaluate and treat up to 50% more patients than the normal burn patient census when there is an emergency. "Sustained surge capacity" is the ability of the burn center to care for these increased numbers of patients throughout their entire hospital course. There is a critical difference in these two numbers. Often a burn center can surge to meet the immediate patient needs after a disaster but lacks the personnel and other resources to sustain this surge. They may need to quickly off-load patients to other care facilities. It is important to note that surge capacity is different at each burn center and may vary day to day.

The disaster life cycle for a mass burn casualty incident is similar in structure to all other disasters. This chapter will discuss preparedness, mitigation, response, recovery, and evaluation. It is imperative that disaster planners, first responders, and clinicians understand principles of burn disasters to be able to plan and implement an effective management strategy. Also, an understanding of burn care is needed to be able to make decisions regarding triage, transport, and treatment. In addition to restoring damaged infrastructure and initiating psychiatric follow-up, the recovery phase should lead into a thorough evaluation of the response. The evaluation should generate recommendations for revision of the disaster plan for future use.

PREPAREDNESS/PLANNING

Effective planning for a burn MCI must occur at multiple levels. Plans should regularly be rehearsed and updated. At the most basic level, families and businesses should design and practice escape plans and evacuation drills. Community response plans can be complicated, as they require the integration of many disciplines such as fire services, public safety, emergency medical services (EMS), public health, and hospital systems. These organizations should collaborate to create a structured response to local events that may range in size from a house fire to a major structural fire (hospital, school, airport, etc.). A detailed community hazard vulnerability analysis should be conducted to determine potential causes or sites of a burn disaster. Oil rigs, railroads, chemical or industrial plants, and arid forests are all possible sources of major fires. Low-income housing can be a potential hazard, as the building material may be of low quality, the units may be built close together, and improvised heating sources are frequently used. Schools, hospitals, and other large, densely populated buildings may not inherently be likely to catch fire, but certainly should be included in planning because of the potential for major life and property loss. Burn centers and other tertiary care facilities should have evacuation plans as part of their hospital disaster plans for internal disasters (Wachtel, 2002).

In the case of an external disaster, hospitals should have the ability to discharge any patient who does not immediately require hospital care (e.g., elective preoperative patients) to make room for patients from an MCI. This can be a complicated process and should be drilled regularly. Surge capacity should be calculated as part of the planning process and include not only physical beds but staff and supplies (e.g., ventilators and pain medication). Written transfer agreements between burn centers and other hospitals/burn centers are a requirement for a disaster plan; these agreements should include stipulations about whether or not patients will be transferred back to the referring hospital when it has available beds.

At the state and national levels, governmental agencies are responsible for creating or delegating disaster-planning responsibilities. EMS systems, usually directed by state regulatory agencies or health departments, are often responsible for much of the state-planning activities, including communications, transportation, and drills. Burn disasters are specifically included in the National Disaster Medical System (NDMS). Further discussion of this topic in included in the following section.

MITIGATION

Mitigation activities relating to burn MCIs include prevention, early detection, and fire extinction. Fire is among the most preventable of all traumatic events and disasters (USFA, 2016).

The single most important element of prevention is education at the individual, community, and national levels. Beginning in elementary school, children should be learning the basics of fire safety and prevention, including electrical device and kitchen safety, smoke alarm use, and escape plans. Resources for school-age education are abundant; websites such as www.ameriburn.org and www.usfa.fema.gov/kids provide information and interactive ideas for educating children. Community prevention includes enforcing fire codes in private residences and public buildings. Publicizing the importance and proper use of fire death prevention technology has traditionally been the domain of health departments and fire services. Smoke alarms, carbon monoxide detectors, sprinkler systems, and other devices have been shown to decrease morbidity and mortality significantly when properly used (USFA, 2016). Legislators need to be made aware of fire-related issues to develop appropriate policies and allocate funding. Legislator education can be done by individuals, nonprofit organizations, or private companies. After much lobbying by the ABA, New York State adopted legislation mandating the sale of fire-safe/self-extinguishing cigarettes in 2004; this is significant because smoking is a leading cause of fatal house fires in the United States (USFA, 2016).

The ABA has partnered with the Department of Health and Human Services (HHS) to identify and track the availability of hospital burn beds in the continental United States. This is done through weekly updates of an HHS website that collect data from U.S. burn centers, including number of total burn beds, number of available burn beds, surge capability, and staffing. In the event of a mass burn casualty incident, available beds are readily identifiable and the necessary contact information is available on the website.

In the first 3 to 7 days following an incident, it is possible that nonburn centers will have to care for burn patients until they can be transferred to burn centers. Even if there is a local burn center, its surge capacity may be reached quickly and other hospitals would need to care for patients until transfer arrangements could be made with burn centers across the state or country. This is a problematic mitigation issue because burn care is highly specialized: education and experience are key to successful patient resuscitation within the first 24 hours after injury. It is the responsibility of state disaster-planning agencies and burn centers in the United States to prepare their communities for a burn disaster with educational programs designed to teach stabilization and treatment of a burn patient within the first few days of injury. Advanced burn life support (ABLS) is a standardized 8-hour course designed to teach healthcare providers to assess and stabilize serious burns during the first critical hours following injury. The course can be taught at nonburn centers to enhance a community's capacity to respond to a burn MCI. Education beyond that of ABLS may also be required to allow providers to safely care for burn patients through the first few days after injury. This should include information pertaining to fluid resuscitation, maintaining limb perfusion, preventing and managing infectious complications, nutrition, wound care, and outpatient management.

Local hospitals or burn centers may need additional support staff to care for patients and assist with secondary triage of burn patients to other burn centers. Disaster Medical Assistance Teams (DMATs) can be deployed with a stock of burn supplies. There may be specialized burn personnel within the DMAT, such as a burn surgeon and nursing staff experienced in burn care. Once activated, the members become federal employees for liability purposes, eliminating the need for state licensure. The DMATs arrive at the site of a disaster with equipment and supplies to sustain themselves for 72 hours (HHS, n.d.). If further support is needed, the U.S. Army may deploy a specialized team known as Special MEDCOM Response Capabilities-Burn (SMRC-Burn). This unit replaces the former Special Medical Augmentation Response Team-Burn (SMART-Burn). SMRC-Burn can deploy to stabilize and transport burn patients or provide on-site augmentation of healthcare resources. The unit is part of the U.S. Army Institute of Surgical Research at Brooke Army Medical Center (U.S. Army Institute of Surgical Research) and is housed at the San Antonio Military Medical Center. The U.S. Air Force and Air National Guard may also supplement resources with critical care air transport teams (CCATT). These teams can provide evacuation and transport of critically injured patients (U.S. Medicine—The Voice of Federal Medicine, 2011). When replenishment of supplies is needed, the U.S. Strategic National Stockpile (SNS) includes burn-specific dressing supplies and medications and can be delivered within 12 hours to any location in the United States in the event of a burn MCI (Centers for Disease Control and Prevention [CDC], 2018). Further federal response information, including the processes of declaring a burn MCI a federal disaster and requesting the SNS, is outlined in Chapter 2, "Leadership and Coordination in Disaster Healthcare Systems: The U.S. National Preparedness System."

RESPONSE

Certain events are blatantly catastrophic, and it is immediately clear that a MCI has occurred. Activation of the disaster plan occurs and a structured response is mobilized. Other events, such as an apartment building fire, may not immediately declare themselves as disasters; as casualties accumulate and local resources are dispensed, it will become more evident that the disaster plan should be activated. The incident commander is key in this decision making. This person may be a firefighter or other first responder, depending on the nature of the incident. Please see Chapter 23 for information regarding the structure and function of the Incident Command System.

Burn Triage in MCIs

Primary triage ideally occurs at the disaster site, or it can be at the hospital receiving patients from the scene. Those overseeing triage should be in communication with the nearest burn and trauma centers to assist in decision making. In a burn MCI, the number of casualties could create a situation where secondary triage is necessary. Secondary triage occurs at a hospital or burn center when it has reached capacity and must begin transferring patients to other burn centers. The ABA triage policy is that all burn patients should be transferred to a burn center within 24 hours of injury. If healthcare resources are overwhelmed by casualties and transfer possibilities are insufficient, resources should be allocated to where they will do the most good for the most people. The ABA has developed a triage decision table of benefit-to-resource ratio based on patient age and total burn size (Taylor et al., 2014). This table applies only to MCIs where there are absolutely not enough resources available and classifies patients as: outpatients; high, medium, or low benefit-to-resource ratio; and expectant (ABA Board of Trustees and the Committee on Organization and Delivery of Burn Care, 2005).

Pathophysiology of Burn Injury

All burns—thermal, chemical, radiological, or electrical—are classified as first, second, and third degree, depending on the extent of skin injury (Table 25.1). Although burns are cutaneous injuries, the effects can influence nearly all systems of the body. The overall morbidity associated with a burn injury will be determined by burn depth, percentage total body surface area (TBSA) involved, patient age, and presence of inhalation injury. Children and older adults have thinner skin and are more likely to sustain a deeper burn injury. Patients at the age extremes are also less likely to tolerate the stress of burn shock. The presence of an inhalation injury severely impacts survival in all age groups and is an important predictor of burn mortality (Lentz & Elaraj, 2005; Sabri, Dabbous, Dowli, & Barazi, 2017).

Extensive burn injuries produce a systemic response that pulls fluid from the vascular system into the injured tissues and interstitial space. The larger the burn size, the greater the fluid loss will be. Without proper treatment, hypovolemic burn shock will result. This is why immediate initiation of fluid resuscitation is essential. A successful fluid resuscitation maintains intravascular volume and organ perfusion until burn shock has resolved, approximately 24 to 48 hours after injury.

Management of a Mass Casualty Burn Patient

Note: This section is intended to give basic guidelines for initial clinical management of a burn patient in a MCI. For information about participating in an ABLS course, go to www.ameriburn.org

Initial burn patient management priorities include:

1. Stop the burning process
2. Manage airway, breathing, and circulation
3. Begin fluid resuscitation
4. Keep the patient warm
5. Evaluate for other life- or limb-threatening injuries

Primary Survey

Stop the Burning Process

To prevent further injury and establish safety for the healthcare provider, the first rescue action may need to be stopping the burning process. Smoldering clothing should be removed and chemicals should be brushed away or irrigated as indicated. The use of ice or ice water is contraindicated because it causes vasoconstriction and potentially ischemia in the burned skin, resulting in a deeper injury. If the patient is found unresponsive, the cervical spine should be immobilized until injury is ruled out.

Manage Airway, Breathing, and Circulation

As in all emergency care, airway is the initial priority. Assess for a patent airway and evaluate breathing. Immediate intubation is indicated in patients with severe respiratory distress, signs of inhalation injury, decreased level of consciousness, or other inability to protect the airway. It is critical for patients with inhalation injuries to be intubated as soon as possible due to the significant increase in airway edema with fluid resuscitation (ABA, 2016). Traumatic intubations and multiple attempts can

TABLE 25.1 Burn Classification

	FIRST-DEGREE BURN	SECOND-DEGREE BURN	THIRD-DEGREE BURN	FOURTH-DEGREE BURN
Also referred to as	Superficial	Partial thickness	Full thickness	Full thickness with deep tissue loss
Depth of injury	Epidermis	Epidermis, some dermis	Epidermis, all dermis	Subdermal fat; may involve fascia, muscle, and/or bone
Appearance	Redness, intact skin	Fluid-filled blisters, pink dermis	Charred, leathery	Charred, leathery, disfigurement
Moisture	Dry	Moist	Dry	Dry
Perfusion	Normal	Quick capillary refill	Markedly delayed or absent capillary refill	Absent
Sensation	Normal/hypersensitive	Painful, pinprick sensation intact	Pressure sensation only or no sensation	Pressure sensation only or no sensation

worsen airway edema; therefore, the most skilled personnel must manage the airway. Large burns and facial burns do not always need immediate intubation but may require it once fluid resuscitation begins, before edema creates a difficult airway. Endotracheal tubes should be secured with twill tape in patients with facial burns, as adhesive does not stick to burned skin.

Patients who have been in an enclosed burning building should be suspected of having smoke inhalation injury and carbon monoxide poisoning until proven otherwise. These patients should be treated with humidified 100% oxygen. Smoke inhalation is unlikely in patients injured outdoors since smoke dissipates quickly in open-air environments. Findings that may be associated with inhalation injury include hoarseness, wheezing, facial burns, singed facial hair, and carbon deposits in the oropharynx or carbonaceous sputum. A definitive diagnosis of inhalation injury can be made with bronchoscopy (Sabri et al., 2017).

Begin Fluid Resuscitation

Two large-bore peripheral intravenous (IV) catheters should be placed to begin fluid resuscitation, through nonburned tissue if possible. If the catheters must be placed through burned skin, they should be sutured in place. Again, adhesive does not stick to burned skin. There should be a low threshold for placing an intraosseous needle in the field when there is difficulty obtaining access in a severely injured patient.

Second- or third-degree burns greater than 20% TBSA and patients with significant smoke inhalation injury will require fluid resuscitation. Peripheral IV catheters can be used, but placement of a central venous catheter may be beneficial. Blood pressure and heart rate are misleading indicators of adequate fluid resuscitation due to physiological factors including progressive edema to burned extremities, cellular fluid shifts, vasoconstriction, and pain. Urine output is an effective indicator of organ perfusion; therefore, it is used to evaluate the effectiveness of fluid resuscitation and to guide rate titrations as needed. An indwelling urine catheter should be placed to accurately measure urine output; urine output should be measured at least hourly.

There are multiple formulas that can be used to fluid-resuscitate a burn patient. The Parkland formula is well established and commonly used. Before calculation can be done, it is necessary to determine the patient's weight (in kilograms) and correctly estimate the percentage TBSA burned. A good estimation tool for use in the field, for both children and adults, is the Rule of Nines (Figure 25.1). Because of their disproportionately large heads, children under 30 kg require an adjusted approximation of percentage TBSA. A child's entire head represents 18% of the TBSA, and each lower extremity represents 14% of the TBSA. Another good estimation tool for children and scattered burns is the palmar method: the size of the patient's hand, including the fingers, represents approximately 1% of his/her TBSA.

Warmed lactated Ringer's (LR) solution should be used in burn fluid resuscitation. The Parkland formula indicates that a volume of 2 to 4 mL/kg/% TBSA burned should be administered over the first 24 hours from the moment of injury, with half of the volume being administered over the first 8 hours and the second half infused over the next 16 hours. Although this is the classic teaching of the application

of the Parkland formula, it is not the ideal way to resuscitate a burn patient. It is best to use the formula to determine the *initial* hourly rate and then follow the patient's urine output to guide the rest of the fluid resuscitation. This is a more accurate reflection of the individual's true fluid needs. The titration should reflect the amount of urine the patient is producing with a goal of 0.5 mL/kg/hr of output in adults and 1 mL/kg/hr in children less than 30 kg. A good rule of thumb is to decrease the fluid rate by 10% every hour that the patient has made the goal for urine output. If at any point the patient is not meeting the hourly output goal, increase the fluid rate by 20% and observe over the next hour. Ideally, the fluid is titrated down to a maintenance rate by 24 hours after the injury. The adult maintenance fluid requirement is 30 mL/kg/d plus an estimation of insensible losses—1 mL/kg/% TBSA burned. Small children less than 30 kg require maintenance fluids *throughout* fluid resuscitation in addition to the calculated Parkland formula rate (Table 25.2). A maintenance solution with 5% dextrose is best to prevent rapid loss of the child's glycogen stores (ABA, 2016).

Some clinical situations may require a higher than predicted total volume for fluid resuscitation. Be aware of the following risk factors for extra fluid requirements: smoke inhalation injury, associated trauma, large TBSA burns (>50%), deep burns, electrical injury, delayed resuscitation, or alcohol/drug use (ABA, 2016; Table 25.3).

Keep the Patient Warm

The patient's entire body should be briefly exposed to assess for burn size and depth (see estimation rules) and any concomitant injuries. In skin loss, the body loses its ability to regulate body temperature. After the examination, it is important to keep the patient warm using rescue blankets or dry sheets at the scene and warmed IV fluids, warm blankets, and approved body warmers at the hospital.

Evaluate for Other Life- or Limb-Threatening Injuries

Burn patients are usually awake and alert after they have been injured. If there is an alteration in mental status, consider the following: associated traumatic injury, carbon monoxide poisoning, hypoxia, intoxication, or preexisting medical conditions.

Burned tissue can swell significantly, so all constricting clothing and jewelry should be removed immediately to prevent circulatory compromise. Finger rings should be removed as soon as possible, with a ring cutter if necessary. Hand and

TABLE 25.2 Pediatric Maintenance Fluids: The 4-2-1 Formula

4 mL/kg for the first 10 kg PLUS	*For example*, a 29 kg patient's maintenance fluids would be:
2 mL/kg for the second 10 kg PLUS	4 mL × 10 kg = 40 mL + 2 mL × 10 kg = 20 mL + 1 mL × 9 kg = 9 mL
1 mL/kg for each kg over 20	Total = 69 mL/hr of D5LR

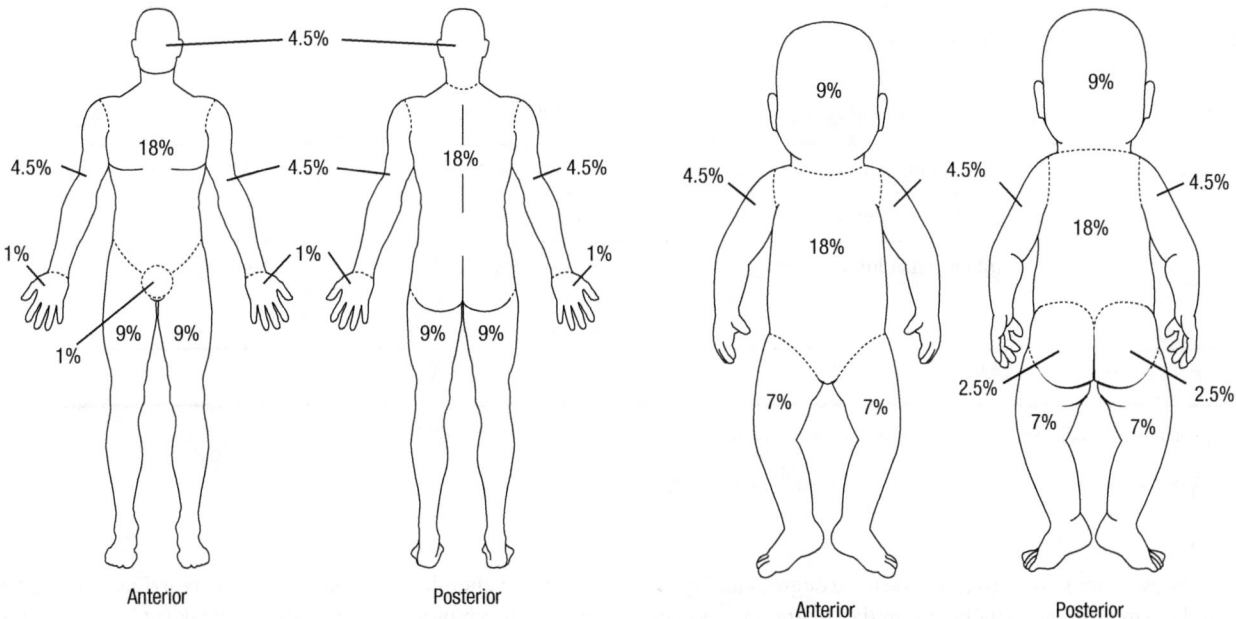

Anterior · Posterior · Anterior · Posterior

FIGURE 25.1 Burn size estimation. For irregularly distributed burns, the palm of the victim's hand represents approximately 1% of the total body surface area—Rule of Nines diagram.

finger swelling will make later removal very difficult. Earrings should also be removed as they can cause pressure necrosis in a swollen ear (Lentz & Elaraj, 2005).

Peripheral circulation should be monitored throughout resuscitation using an ultrasonic flow meter. Circumferential full-thickness extremity burns may compromise distal perfusion and require escharotomy. Digital vessels of each finger, radial, palmar arch, posterior tibial, and dorsalis pedis pulses should be checked hourly for progressive decrease in signal or total loss. If necessary, escharotomies should be done before loss of signal to avoid severe neurologic damage and tissue necrosis (ABA, 2016).

Secondary Survey

When the primary survey is complete, a thorough head-to-toe evaluation is conducted to assess for other injuries. The secondary survey should include an accurate history, the circumstances of the injury and medical history, and a complete examination to evaluate for other traumas such as fractures, contusions, shrapnel, or corneal injury.

Following is a patient pretransport checklist (before secondary triage to another healthcare facility):

- Primary and secondary surveys are complete.
- All urgent issues are addressed and the patient is hemodynamically stable.
- IV fluid resuscitation is initiated.
- Patient is warm and wrapped in sufficient clean, *dry* blankets.
- Endotracheal tube, IV catheters, urine catheter, nasogastric tube are secure and functioning.
- Documentation is complete and with the patient.

Burn Wound Care

The principles of burn wound care in a disaster are the same as any other time: keep the wound clean, moist, and covered. At the scene of a disaster, or when waiting for transport to the receiving facility, it is sufficient to cover the burn wound with a clean, *dry* sheet. Aggressive wound care should not begin until the patient has reached the receiving facility/burn center, as wounds will need to be assessed upon arrival. Judgment, of course, should be used: If the patient is going to be awaiting transport for more than 24 hours, initial wound care should be done (Wachtel, 2002).

The principles of burn care are essentially the same for thermal, chemical, electrical, and radiation burns. When the patient arrives at the receiving facility, the first step in burn wound care is to cleanse with mild soap and warm water. Remove any debris and loose, dead skin, and pat dry. A petrolatum-based ointment can be applied to wounds on the head and neck and be left uncovered. The ointment will need to be reapplied throughout the day to keep the wounds moist. Leaving the face uncovered allows better visual assessment and permits interaction with the patient. Mafenide acetate can be applied to nose and ear burns as it is more effective on cartilaginous tissue. Other burn wounds can be treated with a clear topical antibacterial ointment such as bacitracin, followed by a nonadherent mesh dressing and a gauze wrap to secure into place. Silver sulfadiazine should be avoided until the burns are evaluated by the burn center; this cream is thick and opaque, making it difficult to easily assess the burn wound (ABA, 2016).

Pain Control

Full-thickness burns tend to be less painful since the cutaneous nerves have been damaged or destroyed. Partial-thickness

TABLE 25.3 Fluid Resuscitation Formulas and Urine Output Goals

Burn Type	Age and Weight	Adjusted Fluid Rate	Urine Output Goal
Flame and Scald	Adults and children ≥14 years of age	2 mL/kg/% TBSA	0.5 mL/kg/hr
	Children <14 years of age and ≥30 kg	3 mL/kg/% TBSA	
	Infants and children <30 kg	3 mL/kg/% TBSA PLUS D5LR at maintenance rate	1 mL/kg/hr
Electrical Injury	All ages and weights	4 mL/kg/% TBSA	

D5LR, Lactated Ringers in 5% Dextrose; TBSA, total body surface area.

Source: American Burn Association. (2016). *Advanced burn life support provider manual.* Chicago, IL: Author.

burns, however, are known to cause variable degrees and types of pain. IV narcotics are usually required to maintain adequate pain control during wound care. Continuous infusions may be appropriate for those patients who are mechanically ventilated. Oral and subcutaneous routes should be avoided in burns greater than 20% TBSA because of decreased reliability of absorption secondary to burn shock.

Walking Wounded

Patients with first-degree burns or small nonlife-threatening deep burns can be treated as outpatients as long as they are able to care for themselves or have someone to help them. This population must be anticipated by the hospital staff and efficiently managed to avoid crowding and misdirection of resources. These patients often arrive early, before the critical patients, as they are able to self-extricate and transport. There should be a designated care area for the walking wounded, away from the arrival bays and high-acuity areas of the emergency department. The burns should be assessed, cleaned, and dressed. Before patients are sent home, they must have adequate pain control with oral medications and be able to meet their nutrition and hydration needs. Outpatient supply kits should ideally be assembled before an event occurs. The kits should include general wound care instructions, basic dressing supplies, and information about warning signs and follow-up care.

Special Topics

Chemical Burn Injury

Chemical agents fall into three categories: alkalis, acids, and organic compounds. Alkalis and acids may be found in home and commercial cleaning products, whereas organic compounds are usually found in petroleum products. The mechanisms of chemical injury are different, but the treatment remains the same. Acids injure by causing tissue coagulation, whereas alkalis cause liquefaction necrosis. Alkali burns can be potentially more destructive to tissues than acids because liquefaction enables the chemical to continue penetrating deeper into tissue (ABA, 2016).

Liquid chemicals should be copiously irrigated off the skin until pain symptoms subside; this may take at least 30 minutes. Neutralizing agents are *not* recommended. Powdered chemicals should be brushed off before skin irrigation begins. Chemical burns to the eye require continuous irrigation with clean water or normal saline for at least 15 minutes. When there is no access to running water, an improvised eyewash station can be made by spiking a bag of normal saline with IV tubing, cutting the tubing, and fitting the connector end of a new nasal cannula oxygen tubing over the IV tubing. The saline will flow from the nasal prongs in two streams, one for each eye.

In the event of a suspected chemical injury to a patient, first responders and clinicians must remember to wear appropriate personal protective equipment to prevent secondary exposure.

Electrical Injury

Electrical injuries account for approximately 4% of all burn center admissions and cause around 1,000 deaths per year (ABA, 2016). These injuries are usually work related. Appearance of electrical injuries can be deceiving: The surface injury may be small, but damage below the epidermis can be significant. This concept should be kept in mind during triage. Many factors will influence the degree of tissue damage, including type and voltage of electrical current, resistance, pathway of transmission in the body, and duration of contact (ABA, 2016). Deep conductive electrical burns, arc injuries, surface thermal burns, associated trauma (musculoskeletal, neurologic, etc.), cardiac arrhythmias, and compartment syndromes are all sequelae of electrical injuries. Arrhythmias occur with injury to the myocardium caused by the electric current at the moment of injury and the resulting ischemia. As with all traumatic injuries, management considerations include a primary survey and secondary survey, spine immobilization, proper fluid resuscitation, cardiac monitoring, maintenance of peripheral circulation, and ongoing wound care. Patients who sustain electrical conduction injuries are at risk for the development of compartment syndrome and may require a fasciotomy to decompress tissue compartments. Peripheral circulation should be continuously monitored. Electrical injuries often require more extensive IV fluid resuscitation than calculated by the Parkland formula because the visible cutaneous injury is not reflective of the extent of deep tissue involvement. Dark red pigment in the urine is usually a sign of myoglobin or muscle breakdown caused by deep tissue injury. An indicator of adequate fluid resuscitation is clearance of the pigment from the patient's urine.

Radiation Injury

The physical appearance of radiation burns and thermal burns may be the same. The difference between these two types of injuries lies not only in their etiology, but in the time it takes for the wound to appear. Thermal injury is visible almost instantaneously. Radiation injury can take days to weeks to appear, depending on the dose and length of exposure. A visible injury is an indication of a high localized dose of radiation. Although the patient's wound may be indicative of a large radiation exposure, the patient and the wound are *not* radioactive.

The use of radiation dispersal devices (RDD), commonly referred to as "dirty bombs," is particularly concerning for disaster-planning and emergency preparedness personnel. An RDD is an explosive device designed to spread radioactive material without a nuclear explosion (Briggs & Brinsfield, 2003). The initial blast from the explosion can kill or inflict mechanical trauma on those who are close in proximity to the explosion while the radioactive material is dispersed. Please refer to Chapter 34, "Radiological Incidents and Emergencies," for further information on decontamination, radiation sickness, and personal protective measures.

RECOVERY

The recovery phase of a burn MCI should aim to return the affected community to its predisaster state. Buildings and infrastructure that have been damaged by the incident should be repaired or removed if damage is too severe. The American Red Cross has traditionally reached out to those involved in fire-related disasters by helping them access available housing and resources to meet their needs. Psychological effects on those involved may persist years after the event. The mental health response is especially important in a burn MCI; those involved have experienced a potentially psychologically damaging event and can experience complicated emotional reactions. Please see Chapter 9, "Understanding the Psychosocial Impact of Disasters," for more information.

Burn patients consume many resources and have long lengths of stay. After the initial response to the disaster, these patients may remain hospitalized for months. A patient with 50% TBSA burns may be hospitalized for up to 50 days (ABA, 2016). Burn center staff may become exhausted, operating at or above capacity for this length of time. It is recommended that supervisors continually assess staff for signs of fatigue and stress.

EVALUATION

Each phase of the disaster, from planning though recovery, needs to be closely examined so that modifications can be made for future events. It is especially helpful to make any lessons learned available to the healthcare and disaster-planning communities at large through publications so that others can make use of the information. For example, the William Randolph Hearst Burn Center's experience following the World Trade Center disaster in 2001 was published in a prominent burn journal. One issue involved the NDMS nurses who were deployed to assist with patient care. Although the nurses were experienced in critical care and burn care, they were unfamiliar with the hospital and the computerized charting system. This increased frustration and decreased the efficiency of the nursing staff. The hospital solved this problem by creating a brief orientation class for these workers that allowed them to learn the necessary information quickly. This is certainly a problem that other institutions may encounter if NDMS workers are deployed to their aid and should be considered when developing a disaster plan (Yurt et al., 2005).

SUMMARY

Burns are unique injuries, and planning for a burn MCI may seem overwhelming. By following the basic principles of the disaster life cycle, an effective response plan can be created. For more information on your community or state plan for a burn MCI, contact your local and state health departments.

ACKNOWLEDGMENTS

The author gratefully acknowledges Christopher Lentz, Dixie Reid, and Brooke Primomo for their contributions to earlier versions of this chapter.

STUDY QUESTIONS

1. Discuss the role of a community hazard vulnerability analysis. Why is it important to incorporate this analysis into disaster planning and mitigation?

2. Explain the critical difference between surge capacity and sustained surge capacity. Discuss the determinants of a burn center's capacity and the challenges related to sustained surge capacity.

3. Although burns are cutaneous injuries, the physiologic response to a burn injury is systemic and can be further

complicated by concomitant trauma. List the five priorities of burn management and describe why each is important.

4. Name tools used by healthcare providers to estimate the percentage of body surface area burned. What is the tool most frequently used in the field by prehospital providers to estimate the percentage of body surface area burned.

5. You are caring for a 2-year-old (14-kg) patient who sustained second-degree flame burns to approximately 25% of her body 1 hour ago. She received 100 mL of lactated ringers en route to your hospital. Calculate the starting rate of her fluid resuscitation. Are maintenance IV fluids indicated? Why or why not? If maintenance fluids are indicated, what is the hourly rate?

REFERENCES

American Burn Association. (2016). *Advanced burn life support provider manual.* Chicago, IL: Author.

American Burn Association Board of Trustees and the Committee on Organization and Delivery of Burn Care. (2005). Disaster management and the ABA plan. *The Journal of Burn Care and Rehabilitation, 26*(2), 102–106. doi:10.1097/01.BCR.0000158926.52783.66

Briggs, S., & Brinsfield, K. G. (2003). *Advanced disaster medical response.* Boston, MA: Harvard Medical International Trauma and Disaster Institute.

Centers for Disease Control and Prevention. (2018). Strategic national stockpile. Retrieved from https://www.cdc.gov/phpr/stockpile

Harrington, D. T., Biffl, W. L., & Cioffi, W. G. (2005). The Station nightclub fire. *Journal of Burn Care and Rehabilitation, 26*(2), 141–143. doi: 10.1097/01.BCR.0000155537.60909.FC

Kennedy, P. J., Haertsch, P. A., & Maitz, P. K. (2005). The Bali burn disaster: Implications and lessons learned. *Journal of Burn Care and Rehabilitation, 2*(26), 125–131. doi:10.1097/01.BCR.0000155532.31639.0D

Lentz, C. W., & Elaraj, D. (2005). Treating thermal injury and smoke inhalation. In P. J. Papadakos & J. E. Szalados (Eds.), *Critical care: The requisites in anesthesiology* (pp. 349–351). St. Louis, MO: Mosby.

Rotondo, M. F., Cribari, C., & Smith, S. S. (Eds.). (2014). Guidelines for trauma centers caring for burn patients. In *Resources for the optimal care of the injured patient: 2014* (p. 100–106). Chicago, IL: Author.

Sabri, A., Dabbous, H., Dowlei, A., & Barazi, R. (2017). The airway in inhalational injury: Diagnosis and management. *Annals of Burns and Fire Disasters, 30*(1), 24–29.

Taylor, S., Jeng, J., Saffle, J. R., Sen, S., Greenhalgh, D. G., & Palmieri, T. L. (2014). Redefining the outcomes to resources ratio for burn patient triage in a mass casualty. *Journal of Burn Care and Research, 35*(1), 41–45. doi:10.1097/BCR.0000000000000034

U.S. Department of Health and Human Services. (n.d.). Disaster medical assistance teams. Retrieved from http://www.phe.gov/Preparedness/responders/ndms/ndms-teams/Pages/dmat.aspx

U.S. Fire Administration/National Fire Data Center. (2016). Fire in the United States 2004–2013 (17th ed.). Retrieved from https://www.usfa.fema.gov/downloads/pdf/publications/fius17th.pdf

U.S. Medicine—The Voice of Federal Medicine. (2011, February). Air Guard takes on CCATT mission. Retrieved from http://www.usmedicine.com/agencies/department-of-defense-dod/air-force/air-guard-takes-on-ccatt-mission

Wachtel, T. (2002). Burn disaster management. In D. Herndon (Ed.), *Total burn care.* New York, NY: Saunders.

Yurt, R. W., Bessey, P. Q., Gregory, J. B., Dembicki, R., Laznick, H., Alden, N., & Rabbits, A. (2005). A regional burn center's response to disaster: September 11, 2001, and the days beyond. *Journal of Burn Care and Rehabilitation, 26*(2), 117–124. doi:10.1097/01.BCR.0000155543.46107.E6

CASE STUDY 25.1

The Bali Burn Disaster

A deadly explosion and fire in a nightclub at the internationally renowned holiday resort of Bali, Indonesia, in 2002 was caused by terrorist attack. Bali, approximately 1,000 miles north of Australia, is a popular destination for Australian holidays. The attack resulted in the deaths of 200 people, 88 of whom were Australians. Three days after the initial disaster, 60 patients from Australia were flown home to receive ongoing medical care. Their burn injuries ranged from 15% to 85% TBSA, most of which were classified as full-thickness burns. In addition to the burn injury, primary and secondary blast injuries were associated with every patient. Initial first aid treatment was given at the disaster site and at local hospitals by Indonesian doctors and volunteers. Once initial triage was completed, 60 Australian and European burn patients were flown back to the northernmost city of Darwin for further evaluation, triage, and treatment. Of major concern was the transport of burn patients over the long distance. Transport makes monitoring of fluid resuscitation and temperature control difficult. Once landed, patients were triaged and then sent to hospitals throughout the country according to the availability of intensive care and burn unit beds. Mental health facilities with counseling were established at Australian airports. These services continued during the course of many weeks. During the course of this event, victims and a number of staff members presented with psychological problems and required counseling. Cases of survivor guilt also were noted in a number of patients, all of whom had lost family members or close friends.

The 3-day delay before receiving patients allowed Australian burn centers to prepare for the influx of these patients. Unlike many disasters, they were able to perform a thorough assessment of beds, ventilators, operating rooms, medical supplies, and staff. Considering that disasters with large numbers of burn injuries are commonly associated with the use of explosives, burn and trauma centers should create guidelines and training to address blast injuries and their management.

Source: Excerpted from Kennedy, P. J., Haertsch, P. A., & Maitz, P. K. (2005). The Bali burn disaster: Implications and lessons learned. *Journal of Burn Care and Rehabilitation, 2*(26), 125–131. doi:10.1097/01.BCR.0000155532.31639.0D

CASE STUDY 25.2

The Station Nightclub Fire

The Station nightclub fire was the fourth deadliest nightclub fire in U.S. history. It occurred in Warwick, Rhode Island, on February 20, 2003. Of the approximately 439 people inside The Station at the time of the blaze, 96 people died at the scene, and 4 more died in hospitals during the following weeks. Two hundred fifteen people were injured. The Station nightclub was a single-story wood frame building with an area of about 412 square meters (4,484 sq ft). The main entrance on the north side, with double doors, led to a short hallway with a single interior door. In addition to the main entrance, there were doors leading directly to the outside, adjacent to the platform on the west end of the building and at the side of the main bar at the east end of the building. The kitchen also had an exit door. There were windows along the north side of the building on both sides of the main entrance.

The fire began when pyrotechnics used during a rock concert ignited the polyurethane foam lining of the walls and ceiling of the stage, and spread quickly along the ceiling over the dance floor. Smoke was visible in the main entrance doorway in a little more than 1 minute after ignition, and flames were observed breaking through a portion of the roof in less than 5 minutes. Crowding at the main entrance to the building hampered egress from the nightclub. One hundred people lost their lives in the fire.

The 1950s-era building did not have a sprinkler system. Reports indicate that if the patrons of The Station were not out of the building within 3 minutes, they did not have a chance of survival. Within 30 minutes of the start of the fire, the building had completely collapsed.

A triage station run by Rhode Island's EMS was set up at the scene. Ambulances and helicopters ferried patients to 15 local and regional hospitals. Of concern was the communication during the disaster. Individual ambulance crews were given discretion as to which area hospitals to transport patients, resulting in some severely injured patients being transported to non-Level I centers. Communication among institutions was infrequent and it proved difficult to match patients with available resources in the community. Kent Hospital, which was the nearest to the nightclub, already had a full emergency department when the first burn patients began to arrive, some transported by ambulance, others driven by personal automobiles. Kent's emergency department stabilized and transported the sickest patients and admitted only patients with minor injuries.

Rhode Island Hospital (RIH), the state's only Level I trauma center, activated its disaster plan to mobilize staff and resources. The staff evaluated 64 patients during a 4-hour time block, with 47 patients being admitted and 18 being discharged from the emergency department. Of the 47 admitted patients, 33 patients had less than 20% TBSA burns, 12 patients had 21% to 40% TBSA burns, and 2 patients had 40% TBSA burns, and 28 patients had inhalation injury. During the next week, the team performed 23 operations and used two dedicated burn operating rooms. Twelve weeks after the admission of the first patient from The Station fire, the last patient was discharged to rehabilitation.

Source: Excerpted from Harrington, D. T., Biffl, W. L., & Cioffi, W. G. (2005). The Station nightclub fire. *Journal Burn Care and Rehabilitation,* *26*(2), 141–143. doi:10.1097/01.BCR.0000155537.60909.FC

CASE STUDY 25.3

Burn Center Referral Criteria

Burn centers are a unique national resource. According to the ABA, the United States currently has 132 burn care centers representing approximately 1,897 burn beds nationwide. A listing of these centers can be found at www.ameriburn.org. In comparison, there are as many as 1,000 trauma centers. In recognition of the complex nature of burn injuries, the HHS has incorporated burn centers into state and local disaster plans. They have also been recognized by the federal government in bioterrorism legislation. The ABA Burn Unit Referral Criteria are well published and followed in the medical community. Burn Unit Referral Criteria, as recognized by the ABA and the American College of Surgeons Committee on Trauma, include the following (Rotondo, Cribari, & Smith, 2014):

1. Partial-thickness burns greater than 10% TBSA.
2. Burns that involve the face, hands, feet, genitalia, perineum, or major joints.
3. Third-degree burns in any age group.
4. Electrical burns, including lightning injury.
5. Chemical burns.
6. Inhalation injury.

(continued)

CASE STUDY 25.3 (*continued*)

7. Burn injury in patients with preexisting medical disorders that could complicate management, prolong recovery, or affect mortality.
8. Any patients with burns and concomitant trauma (e.g., fractures) in which the burn injury poses the greatest risk of morbidity or mortality. In such cases, if the trauma poses the greater immediate risk, the patient may be initially stabilized in a trauma center before being transferred to a burn unit. Physician judgment will be necessary in such situations and should be in concert with the regional medical control plan and triage protocols.

9. Burned children in hospitals without qualified personnel or equipment for the care of children. In the absence of a regional pediatric burn center, an adult burn center may serve as a second option for the management of pediatric burns.
10. Burn injury in patients who will require special social, emotional, or long-term rehabilitative intervention.

Source: Excerpted from Rotondo, M. F., Cribari, C., & Smith, S. S. (Eds.). (2014). Guidelines for trauma centers caring for burn patients. In *Resources for the optimal care of the injured patient: 2014* (p. 100–106). Chicago, IL: Author.

26

TRAUMATIC INJURY DUE TO EXPLOSIVES AND BLAST EFFECTS

Tara L. Sacco

LEARNING OBJECTIVES

When this chapter is completed, readers will be able to:

1. Discuss the mechanisms of injury produced by explosions.
2. Identify injury patterns specific to explosions and blasts.
3. Discuss the clinical care of blast survivors with selected blast injuries.
4. Discuss the considerations related to injury patterns in military and civilian blast victims and those in the extremes of ages.

KEY MESSAGES

Blast victims present with injury patterns that are unique in their mechanism.

Penetrating and blunt injuries are commonly sustained following an explosion; however, there is a subset of injuries related to the mechanism of the blast wave.

Higher morbidity and mortality are associated with explosions occurring in confined areas and any related structural collapse.

Clinical guidelines and algorithms exist and should guide the care of blast victims.

Injuries sustained by military personnel will differ from those sustained by civilians.

CHAPTER OVERVIEW

The risk of injury from explosive devices affects both military and civilian populations. Occupational hazards, active military conflict, and terrorist activity are real threats nationally and abroad. These incidents have the potential to produce a large number of casualties, often overwhelming emergency medical systems. A clinical knowledge of the injury patterns specific to explosive devices is necessary for any practitioner caring for the traumatically injured. To fully understand these concepts, a basic knowledge of blast physics is required. This chapter reviews the mechanisms of injury produced from an explosion and the injury patterns healthcare providers can expect when caring for victims. Blast-specific injuries as well as their management are discussed. Differences in the risk and clinical presentation of civilian and military victims and those of the extremes of age are highlighted.

The National Consortium for the Study of Terrorism and Responses to Terrorism (2016) reported that there were over 11,700 terrorist attacks in 2015. These attacks, occurring in 92 countries, resulted in 35,300 wounded and 28,300 casualties. The overall number of terrorist attacks decreased by 13% in 2015 compared to 2014 and this is the first year attacks have decreased since 2012. However, the number of attacks increased in Afghanistan, Bangladesh, Egypt, the Philippines, Syria, and Turkey. Both civilian and military personnel have been targets of terrorist activity. Attacks against civilians are on the rise and groups are targeting transit systems, restaurants, night clubs, and other common meeting sites (Wolf, Bebarta, Bonnett, Pons, & Cantrill, 2009). Mass casualty incidents in which explosives were used against civilians have occurred in London, Madrid, Oklahoma City, and Boston, among other locations (Mathews & Koyfman, 2015). Regarding military injuries, 75% are related to blasts and explosions (Dougherty, MacGregor, Han, Heltemes, & Galarneau, 2011; Turegano-Fuentes, Perez-Diaz, Sanz-Sanchez, Alfici, & Ashkenazi, 2014). The devices deployed during combat are "... designed to cause massive bodily destruction by propelling large numbers of fragments toward the intended victim ... [which] initiates complex, multi-mechanistic forces on the body" (Champion et al., 2010, p. 1139). As compared to victims of other traumatic events, those injured in terrorist attacks are generally younger, suffer greater injury severity, have longer intensive care unit lengths of stay, require multiple surgical interventions, and have three times the mortality rate. The complex presentation of these patients leads to 28% higher hospital costs, and more than half of those injured will require inpatient rehabilitation (Bala et al., 2008). Although terror produces the majority of blast-related injuries, they may also result from known occupational, and in some cases, recreational hazards (Hoffer et al., 2010; Wolf et al., 2009).

Whether the result of an industrial accident or a terrorist attack, explosions produce victims who will present with blunt, penetrating, and burn injuries as well as those related to the blast wave itself (Jaffe & Peleg, 2010). Use of explosive devices in terrorist activity not only results in physical injury but leads to social, economic, and physical instability (Edwards, McMenemy, Stapley, Patel, & Clasper, 2016). Further, management of blast victims postevent can overwhelm medical facilities that will be functioning in a time of panic and chaos (Mathews & Koyfman, 2015). Patients presenting postblast experience polytrauma due to multiple mechanisms of injury (Boutillier, Deck, Magnan, Naz, & Willinger, 2016; Klein, Arieli, Sagiv, Peleg, & Ben-Galim, 2016). The unique challenges presented require that healthcare providers understand the mechanisms, injury patterns, and management of the blast-injured patient.

EXPLOSIVES: CLASSIFICATION AND PHYSICS

Explosives used in terrorist attacks can be classified into two categories: low-order explosives (LE) and high-order explosives (HEs). Explosions with LEs are of lower velocity (Wolf et al., 2009). Examples include gunpowder, pipe bombs, and petroleum-based explosives (e.g., Molotov cocktails). In contrast, the velocity of HE explosions result in supersonic blasts. Trinitrotoluene (TNT), Semtex, C-4, and ammonium nitrate fuel oil are examples of HEs (Mathews & Koyfman, 2015). These explosives can be further categorized as primary or secondary. Primary explosives are detonated by mechanical shock, friction, or heat, whereas secondary explosives need an initiating explosion to detonate (Wolf et al., 2009).

Military explosives often contain C-4 or Semtex whereas explosives used in terrorist activities may contain HEs or LEs. Historically, blast injuries in military personnel have been the result of mortar, grenade, and landmine explosion (Hoencamp et al., 2014). In recent conflicts, many attacks against both military and civilian populations have been related to the use of improvised explosive devices (IEDs) that contain fragments (shrapnel) that may also be contaminated with infectious materials (Mathews & Koyfman, 2015). These explosive devices reside in a container with a power source, a detonator, a switch, and a charge and may be remotely activated (Singh et al., 2016).

An explosion from an HE occurs when a solid or liquid is converted into gas following detonation. The gas produced expands from the epicenter of detonation and will displace the surrounding medium (air or water). A subsequent rise in atmospheric pressure, the positive pressure phase, creates a blast wave that generates a blast wind. The wind may have a velocity of several hundred kilometers per hour. Prior to returning to atmospheric pressure, a negative pressure phase occurs. The point of maximum atmospheric pressure during the positive pressure phase is termed the "peak blast overpressure." This, in combination with the blast wind, produces a wide range of injuries (Wolf et al., 2009). As the blast wind travels from the epicenter, it penetrates the surrounding media (buildings, humans, and other infrastructure). The wind is followed by fragments, and then the actual movement of the surrounding media (Owers, Morgan, & Garner, 2011). As the wave moves through a victim, implosion, spalling, and shearing occurs, producing injury from the wave itself (Falcone, 2013; Mathews & Koyfman, 2015). Figure 26.1 depicts the progression of a blast wave over time in an open space.

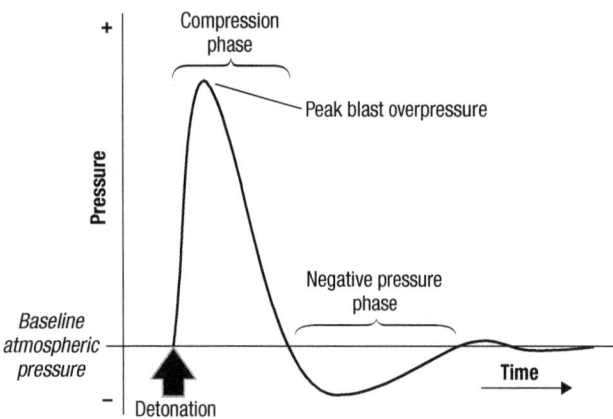

FIGURE 26.1 Progression of a blast wave over time.

Source: Adapted from Wolf, S. J., Bebarta, V. S., Bonnett, C. J., Pons, P. T., & Cantrill, S. V. (2009). Blast injuries. *Lancet, 374,* 405–415. doi:10.1016/S0140-6736(09)60257-9

Certain variants related to detonation will increase or decrease the likelihood of injury from a blast. As stated above, a blast that occurs in an open space or field has a positive and negative pressure phase (Wolf et al., 2009). Although the same principles apply when there is an explosion in an enclosed space, or within an area surrounded by many buildings, the blast wave is reflected and amplified (Mathews & Koyfman, 2015; Singh et al., 2016; Wolf et al., 2009). Additionally, in an enclosed space, the forces of detonation are contained, prolonging the duration of the positive pressure phase and increasing the peak overpressure. On comparison, victims of an enclosed space explosion have higher mean injury severity scores and mortality rates (Wolf et al., 2009). Also, when multiple IEDs are employed, they are not designed to detonate simultaneously. This will produce multiple blast waves that, if reflected off of surrounding structures, can merge into stronger waves. Taking all factors into consideration, the ideal blast wave depicted in Figure 26.1 is rarely the reality (Hicks, Fertig, Desrocher, Koroshetz, & Pancrazio, 2010).

An additional variation is an explosion occurring underwater. While air is a compressible medium, water is not. Therefore, the blast wave does not dissipate as quickly as those in open spaces (Nguyen, Hunt, Lindfors, & Grieffenstein, 2014). A blast wave underwater travels up to three times farther than one occurring in air. However, fragments do not travel as easily due to the density of water, diminishing secondary blast effects. Though there is not the typical blast wind produced in this medium, the explosion will cause the movement of water, increasing the risk of blunt injury (Owers et al., 2011). Despite the decrease in secondary mechanism, the other factors unique to underwater blast increase the risk for injury overall (Wolf et al., 2009).

Injury rates and patterns are affected by blast location, proximity to the blast epicenter, and amount of explosive used. Blasts may occur in open spaces, semiconfined spaces, or within a confined space (Edwards et al., 2016). IED explosions are classified as mounted or dismounted, based on target. Mounted IEDs target vehicles whereas dismounted IEDs target a crowd of people or individuals on foot (Taddeo, Devine, & McAlister, 2015). When a detonation occurs underneath a vehicle, it is considered an under body blast (Spurrier, Gibb, Masouros, &

Clasper, 2016). Victims' injury patterns will vary greatly related to the blast location and whether the IED is mounted or unmounted (Taddeo et al., 2015). Regarding proximity, the closer the victim is to the epicenter of the blast, the more severe the presenting injuries will be. Lastly, the blast force is positively correlated with the amount of explosive used; the greater the amount of explosive, the stronger the blast, thus resulting in greater injury consequences (Mathews & Koyfman, 2015).

MECHANISMS AND PATTERNS OF INJURY

The traditional injury classification following an explosion includes: primary, secondary, tertiary, and quaternary injury. Some authors also discuss a fifth (quinary) category in addition to the traditional classification. Injury patterns will vary based on the characteristics of the blast as previously discussed. Each type of blast injury may require different management and oftentimes victims will present with multiple injuries.

Primary blast injury (PBI) is a direct result of the change in atmospheric pressure and the blast wind. The mechanisms that cause injury include spalling, implosion, and shearing (Wolf et al., 2009). Air-filled organs are the most commonly injured by this mechanism, including the lungs, middle ear, and bowel (Singh et al., 2016). As the wave moves through tissues of different densities, particularly more dense to less dense, the denser medium is displaced and fragmented into the less dense, creating spalling. The gas in an air-filled space is compressed by the change in atmospheric pressure and creates implosion injuries as gas re-expands and releases energy. Finally, inertia creates shearing injury as tissues of different densities move at different speeds; the damage occurs at tissue interfaces. Although the tympanic membrane (TM), lungs, and bowel are most frequently injured, the central nervous, ophthalmic, musculoskeletal, and cardiac systems may endure injuries from the primary mechanism (Wolf et al., 2009).

The amount of force to produce PBI varies. For example, the pressure required for a TM rupture is 5 psi; however, pulmonary injury may occur around 40 psi (Singh et al., 2016). It is important to note that the closer a victim is to the epicenter, the more likely it is that he or she will sustain a PBI. Those sustaining blast lung or intestinal injuries are most likely to succumb to their injuries at the scene. Victims who survive a PBI are likely to have secondary, tertiary, and quaternary injuries (Garner et al., 2010; Ritenour et al., 2010). Primary injuries are also more likely to occur in an enclosed space explosion (Wolf et al., 2009).

Flying debris that is displaced by the blast wind is the mechanism behind secondary blast injury. Fragments from the explosive device will travel with the blast wind much farther than the overpressure that causes primary injury. Thus, secondary injury is much more common than primary injury. Blunt and, more likely, penetrating trauma will result (Wolf et al., 2009). Practitioners caring for secondary blast victims must be aware that these patients are at high risk for hemorrhage requiring fluid resuscitation (Garner et al., 2010). The injuries are further classified based on from where the fragments originate, either as primary fragments or secondary fragments. Primary fragment injuries are those from the explosive device shrapnel, whereas

TABLE 26.1 Mechanism of Blast Injury

Category	Characteristic Definition	Body Part Affected	Types of Injuries
Primary	• Unique to high-order explosives, occurs when the blast wave interacts with the body. The wave may be reflected as it interacts with tissues of different density.	• Air-filled structures are most susceptible: pulmonary, gastrointestinal, and auditory systems.	• Tympanic membrane rupture • Pulmonary barotrauma • Abdominal hemorrhage or perforation • Closed head injury • Ophthalmic injury
Secondary	• Ballistic wounds from debris and fragments. Primary fragments: from the weapon. Secondary fragments: from the environment.	• Any body system.	• Blunt and penetrating injury • Traumatic amputation • Lacerations • Closed head injury
Tertiary	• Victims being thrown into or onto structures by the blast wave. Structural collapse also included.	• Any body system.	• Blunt and penetrating injury • Fracture and traumatic amputation • Closed and open head injury • Crush and compartment syndromes
Quaternary	• Explosion-related injuries, illnesses or diseases not due to other mechanisms.	• Any body system. • May include exacerbation of preexisting disease.	• Burns • Inhalation injury • Exacerbation of preexisting disease • Environmental contamination
Quinary	• Result from additives to explosive devices and hyperinflammatory states postexplosion. Further investigation into this type is required.	• Any body system.	• Bacterial infection • Radiation exposure • Hyperinflammatory state

Sources: Adapted from Edwards, D. S., McMenemy, L., Stapley, S. A., Patel, H. D. L., & Clasper, J. C. (2016). 40 years of terrorist bombings—A meta-analysis of the casualty and injury profile. *Injury, 47*, 646–652. doi:10.1016/j.injury.2015.12.021; Falcone, R. (2013). Civilian blast injury. *Trauma Reports, 14*(5), 1–11; Mathews, Z. R., & Koyfman A. (2015). Blast injuries. *The Journal of Emergency Medicine, 49*, 573–587. doi:10.1016/j.jemermed.2015.03.013; Wolf, S. J., Bebarta, V. S., Bonnett, C. J., Pons, P. T., & Cantrill, S. V. (2009). Blast injuries. *Lancet, 374*, 405–415. doi:10.1016/S0140-6736(09)60257-9

secondary fragment injuries are environmental, typically from the destruction of infrastructure (Mathews & Koyfman, 2015). If the explosion is the result of a suicide bombing, bone fragments may also produce a secondary injury (Mathews & Koyfman, 2015; Singh et al., 2016). In this case, a heighted concern for infectious disease is warranted (Mathews & Koyfman, 2015).

Tertiary injury occurs as the body itself is displaced by the blast wind or from falling buildings and other infrastructure (Mathews & Koyfman, 2015) and may result in blunt or penetrating trauma as well (Singh et al., 2016). As compared to blasts in which buildings do not collapse, any blast with concomitant structural collapse raises the risk for more severe tertiary injuries and higher mortality rates. Most commonly victims will present with closed head injuries, abdominal trauma, contusions, fractures, and crush injury (Wolf et al., 2009). As with secondary injuries, there is a high risk for hemorrhage for which the clinician should be aware.

All other injury patterns are considered quaternary and quinary blast injuries. Burns, radiation exposure, inhalation injury, asphyxia, crush injuries, and psychosocial concerns are classified as quaternary injuries (Mathews & Koyfman, 2015; Wolf et al., 2009). Quinary injuries encompass a hyperinflammatory state in which patients present with hyperpyrexia, diaphoresis, decreased central venous pressure, and a positive fluid balance. This category is relatively new, and further research is required to fully understand this mechanism (Wolf et al., 2009). Examples of injuries, based on mechanism, are provided in Table 26.1.

BLAST INJURIES AND CLINICAL CARE OF SURVIVORS

Injuries from secondary, tertiary, and quaternary mechanisms will often mimic those from traditional traumatic mechanisms (e.g., motor vehicle accidents, penetrating trauma, falls from height, burns). Victims will present for care with multiple injuries from different mechanisms and, therefore, it is recommended that the clinical care of victims of blasts be guided by the Advanced Trauma Life Support algorithms (Falcone, 2013; Mathews & Koyfman, 2015). Further, burn injury is prevalent after blasts

TABLE 26.2 Veterans Affairs/Department of Defense Classification of TBI Severity

Criteria	Mild	Moderate	Severe
Structural imaging	Normal	Normal or abnormal	Normal or abnormal
Loss of consciousness	0–30 min	>30 min and <24 hr	>24 hr
Alteration of consciousness/mental state	Up to 24 hr	>24 hr	>24 hr; severity based on other criteria
Posttraumatic amnesia	0–1 d	>1 and <7 d	>7 d
Glasgow Coma Scale (best available score in first 24 hr)	13–15	9–12	<9

Source: Adapted from Veterans Affairs/Department of Defense. (2016). Clinical practice guideline for the management of concussion-mild traumatic brain injury. Retrieved from https://www.healthquality.va.gov/guidelines/Rehab/mtbi

(Wolf et al., 2009). More information on burn-related injury may be found in Chapter 25, "Management of Burn Mass Casualty Incidents" of this text. Although it is important to understand the latter four mechanisms of blast injury, primary injury presents as the most unique within this phenomenon. Following is a description of the PBIs that may be encountered.

Traumatic Brain Injury

During the conflicts in Iraq and Afghanistan, traumatic brain injury (TBI) has emerged as the signature wound. It has been estimated that half of those injured by blast serving in these areas present with a TBI (Hicks et al., 2010) and blasts have been responsible for greater than 85% of face, head, and neck injuries in the Iraqi theater (Dougherty et al., 2011). In PBI to the brain, the blast wave traverses the skull and brain parenchyma (Ling & Ecklund, 2011). The blast wave may result in diffuse axonal injury (Hicks et al., 2010; Mathews & Koyfman, 2015; Singh et al., 2016), intracranial hemorrhage (e.g., epidural, subdural, subarachnoid, and intracerebral; Mathews & Koyfman, 2015), cerebral edema (Hicks et al., 2010; Singh et al., 2016), vasospasm, and pseudoaneurysm formation (Singh et al., 2016). However, the majority of injuries are concussions and are considered mild TBI (Hicks et al., 2010). The Veteran Affairs/Department of Defense Classification of TBI Severity for details regarding mild, moderate, and severe TBI are presented in Table 26.2.

As compared to mild TBI of other mechanisms, blast-related mild TBI may result in more significant postconcussive syndrome (PCS) symptoms. Retrograde amnesia, compromised executive function, headache, confusion, difficulty concentrating, mood disturbance, changes in sleep patterns, and anxiety are all characteristic of PCS (Hicks et al., 2010). Survivors will often report vertigo and memory problems more frequently than their nonblast-injured counterparts (Wilk et al., 2010).

There is also a link between mild TBI and posttraumatic stress disorder (PTSD) in the blast-injured patient. The mechanism increasing the link between TBI and PTSD is thought to be damage to the prefrontal cortex, leading to increased susceptibility to emotional responses to a traumatic event. PCS symptoms may alter the blast victim's ability to adjust to the event, and may increase the likelihood of developing PTSD (French, 2010).

Management of the blast-injured patient with TBI is complex. Treatment should be guided by the Department of Defense's Clinical Practice Guideline for the Management of mTBI/Concussion, the Brain Trauma Foundation's Guidelines for Field Management of Combat Related Head Trauma, and the Brain Trauma Foundation's Guidelines for the Management of Severe TBI (Ling & Ecklund, 2011).

Ear Injury

TM rupture is the most common PBI reported in survivors. Depending on whether the blast occurs in an open or enclosed space, 2% to 32% of victims will experience a ruptured TM, and of those with other PBIs, 94% will also have a TM rupture (Wolf et al., 2009). Factors that increase the likelihood of TM rupture in blast victims include perpendicular orientation to blast epicenter, explosion within an enclosed space, prior injury or infection of the middle ear, and advanced age. The presence of cerumen may protect the TM or could act as a ramrod and increase the likelihood of injury. Ear plugs and headphones may interfere with the blast wave transduction to the middle ear, thus preventing injury (Ritenour et al., 2010).

Following a blast, patients with ear injuries may present with hearing loss, tinnitus, otalgia, dizziness, and imbalance. The latter signs and symptoms may also be indicative of TBI (Akin & Murnane, 2011). Because ongoing hearing loss and tinnitus are the second most common causes of disability claims for veterans, screening measures following a blast injury are important (Breeze, Cooper, Pearson, Henney, & Reid, 2011).

Screening for TM rupture in all blast-injured patients is recommended (Mathews & Koyfman, 2015). In the past it had been recommended that otoscopic examination be performed on all blast victims to screen for the risk of other PBIs. However, studies have demonstrated that some patients will present with these injuries and not also have TM rupture. Victims with intact TMs who are asymptomatic for other PBIs are unlikely to have occult injury (Wolf et al., 2009). Therefore, the use of otoscopic examination as a screening tool for PBIs other than TM rupture is not recommended. Breeze et al. (2011) have also recommended hearing assessment/audiometry as early as possible following blast injury.

Eye Injury

Though not often reported as a PBI, eye injury is very common in military conflict. PBIs to the eye are a result of the blast wave being amplified as it is reflected off of the orbital walls. Signs and symptoms of primary blast eye injuries are a hypotonic eye without globe rupture and traumatic cataracts. This injury typically resolves in approximately 10 days. Damage to the optic nerve, choroid, and retina may also be present (Scott, Blanch, & Morgan-Warren, 2015). Visual symptoms may also present following blast-related TBI (Dougherty et al., 2011). Screening recommendations for eye injury include routine ophthalmoscopy following a blast (Mathews & Koyfman, 2015).

Pulmonary Injury

Primary lung injury is common in those closest to the epicenter of the blast and is one of the most common causes of fatality at the blast scene (Falcone, 2013). As the blast wave moves through pulmonary tissues, disruption at the capillary–alveolar junctions occurs and shearing of the bronchovascular tree results. Injury to the lung may include hemorrhage, pneumothorax, air embolism, alveolovenous fistula, pulmonary contusion, and bronchopulmonary fistula (Wolf et al., 2009). Due to the mechanisms of implosion and spalling, the patient is at risk for pulmonary contusion and air embolus. Barotrauma may result in pneumothorax. The patient's presenting signs and symptoms include hypoxemia, respiratory distress, and hemoptysis following PBI to the thorax (Falcone, 2013).

Management of the patient with lung injury will depend on the severity of injury. Respiratory instability may necessitate the use of intubation and mechanical ventilation (Mathews & Koyfman, 2015). When considering the implementation of positive pressure ventilation, lung protective strategies, in addition to permissive hypercapnia, that should be implemented include low tidal volumes (5–6 mL/kg) and maintaining lower oxygen saturations (Wolf et al., 2009). Nontraditional ventilation methods, including high-frequency ventilation, jet ventilation, extracorporeal membrane oxygenation, and the use of nitric oxide, are also options. High peak airway pressures should be avoided (Mathews & Koyfman, 2015). Prophylactic thoracostomy in the setting of positive pressure ventilation, as well as thoracostomy to treat pneumothorax and hemothorax, is recommended. With all patients with blast lung injury, pain management is a great concern (Wolf et al., 2009).

Cardiovascular Injury

Blast injury to the cardiovascular system is also possible. Myocardial hemorrhage, cardiac contusion, and atrial rupture have been reported as primary injuries (Wolf et al., 2009). Subsequent to the blast, cardiac contusions can lead to vagal-induced bradycardia or other arrhythmias. The vagal stimulation may also result in hypotension. When this occurs, hemodynamic instability is refractory to fluid resuscitation. Compensatory mechanisms, such as vasoconstriction, may be ineffective in these blast victims (Mathews & Koyfman, 2015).

Abdominal Injury

PBI to the gastrointestinal system is rare, particularly in the absence of other PBIs (Turegano-Fuentes et al., 2014; Wolf et al., 2009). Those closest to the epicenter (Turegano-Fuentes et al., 2014) and victims of underwater blasts or blasts within an enclosed space are at the greatest risk for abdominal PBI (Mathews & Koyfman, 2015). The classic abdominal PBI is mural hematoma of the bowel. Shear force from the blast wave can also cause hemoperitoneum resulting from mesenteric vascular injury (Turegano-Fuentes et al., 2014). Intramural edema, hemorrhage, and microthrombosis in the intestine decreases tissue perfusion and places the victim at risk of delayed intestinal perforation. Shear injury may also immediately rupture the bowel wall, most commonly in the colon or ileocecal region (Wolf et al., 2009). In rare cases, hepatic, splenic, and renal injuries result from the blast wave. These solid organ injuries may present as infarction, ischemia, hemorrhage, or rupture (Turegano-Fuentes et al., 2014). The incidence of abdominal PBI is estimated at 3% of survivors. That being said, secondary and tertiary mechanisms of injury are much more likely to occur (Owers et al., 2011).

Presenting symptoms of blast-related gastrointestinal injury include melena, abdominal tenderness, nausea, vomiting, diarrhea, and absent bowel sounds (Mathews & Koyfman, 2015). Imagining studies typically used in this patient population include focused abdominal sonography for trauma (FAST) and abdominal computed tomography (CT). FAST may identify intraperitoneal fluid while CT is most specific for solid organ injury and intestinal perforation; contusion and mesenteric injury may be missed using these methods (Wolf et al., 2009). Patients presenting with peritonitis from perforation, free fluid on FAST or CT, or hemodynamic instability should be managed surgically with exploratory or decompressive laparotomy (Owers et al., 2011) and volume resuscitation (Wolf et al., 2009).

Musculoskeletal Injury

Traumatic amputation can result from primary, secondary, or tertiary mechanisms. As a PBI, the bone fractures from the blast wave, and the exposure to the sequelae of the blast wind results in amputation (Ramasamy et al., 2013; Singh et al., 2016). Many blast victims with traumatic amputation often succumb to other PBIs as the force required for amputation is great (Falcone, 2013; Mathews & Koyfman, 2015). In survivors with traumatic amputation, providers must be highly alert for other PBIs (Singh et al., 2016).

MILITARY AND CIVILIAN CASUALTIES

There are some important differences in injury pattern and severity between military and civilian victims of blast. Military personnel targeted by terrorist activity most often wear personal protective equipment that alters the way the blast wave affects the body. Examples of equipment utilized include helmets, goggles, and Kevlar body armor. This equipment may also protect the body from secondary injury from fragments (Champion et al., 2010). The use of body and vehicle armor, however, may actually result in an increase in PBI as soldiers may survive closer to the epicenter of a blast while utilizing protective gear. As previously stated, the closer one is to the blast, the higher the risk of primary injury. However, those who are close enough often will perish as a result of secondary injury (Owers, Morgan, & Garner, 2011).

Attacks on civilians are becoming more common throughout the world. Civilians, in contrast to military personnel, are not afforded the protection of helmets, vests, and body armor. Enclosed settings, including restaurants, buses, and subways, are being targeted. As the blast wave and wind is reflected off enclosed structures, the likelihood for PBI increases. In addition, those attacked in civilian bombings tend to be a more heterogeneous group, including pregnant women, children, and the elderly (Hicks et al., 2010). Finally, as many terrorists are targeting enclosed spaces for civilian attacks, there is often significant destruction to infrastructure (Garner et al., 2010). The damage to infrastructure and use of civilian emergency response has potential to delay treatment of victims in civilian bombings.

EXTREMES OF AGES AND PREGNANCY

There are unique considerations related to the care of blast victims who are pregnant or at the extremes of ages. Though uncommonly reported in the literature, civilian blast victims may be pregnant. Fetal demise may result from the mechanisms of the blast wave. The mother is at risk for all PBIs previously described and may be injured through secondary, tertiary, and quaternary mechanisms. Unfortunately, maternal death may be a reality. In such cases, postmortem cesarean sections for viable fetuses may be an option (Falcone, 2013).

Between 2002 and 2010, the most common blast-related injuries to children in Iraq and Afghanistan occurred to the head, neck, and soft tissue/skin (Edwards et al., 2012). Younger children may be at higher risk for more severe blast injuries in comparison to adolescents and adults. In the event of a suicide bombing, the perpetrator wears torso-level explosives. As detonation occurs, blasts may be directed toward the level of a child's head, explaining the higher risk for TBI in this age group (Jaffe & Peleg, 2010). Children injured by explosives in the Iraqi and Afghan theaters also have a higher reported mortality rate when compared to those hospitalized in U.S. pediatric hospitals and to U.S. military casualties in these areas. As with adults, proximity to the blast's epicenter and size of the blast itself influence patient outcomes. Further, and similar to adult civilians, the lack of protective gear and access to rapid evacuation from the blast site when compared to military personnel are contributory factors to injury pattern, severity, and survival in children (Edwards et al., 2012).

The physiological changes of aging will influence injury patterns in the geriatric population. Connective tissue thins, resulting in frailty and increased susceptibility to the consequences of implosion, spalling, and shearing. The TM tears more easily and globe rupture may be more likely. Osteoporosis will increase the risk of fracture from all mechanisms of blast injury. The ribs are less protective and lung tissue is more fragile, predisposing the geriatric blast victim to high risk for pulmonary injury. With aging, the brain naturally atrophies, leaving room within the skull. However, trauma to the head rocks the brain within the skull, increasing the risk for TBI. Lastly, comorbid conditions and polypharmacy in the geriatric population will complicate the medical management of survivors (Somes & Donatelli, 2014). As with all blast victims, Advanced Trauma Life Support recommendations, with considerations for pregnancy, children, and the elderly, should be followed.

EVENT MANAGEMENT

Managing the aftermath of an explosion is similar to managing any mass casualty incident. First responders and clinicians play an important role. Readers are directed to Chapters 23, "Disaster Management" and Chapter 22, "Disaster Triage," for more information on event management. In addition, the Centers for Disease Control and Prevention (CDC) has launched a blast injury smartphone and tablet mobile application for prehospital and hospital clinicians (Box 26.1; CDC, 2014). More information may be found in the Emergency Preparedness and Response section of the CDC's website.

BOX 26.1 CDC Blast Injury Mobile Application

This smartphone and tablet application supports prehospital and hospital healthcare providers and public health professionals in preparing for, and responding to, terrorist bombings and other mass casualty explosive events. Healthcare providers and public health professionals can use the application to:

- Quickly review critical steps to take from the moment an event happens;
- Learn blast injury patterns and treatment considerations;
- Scan information efficiently with minimal effort on the way to or at a scene and grasp clinical guidance to support key job functions;
- Access the full breadth of CDC's resources on blast injuries and mass casualty explosive events.

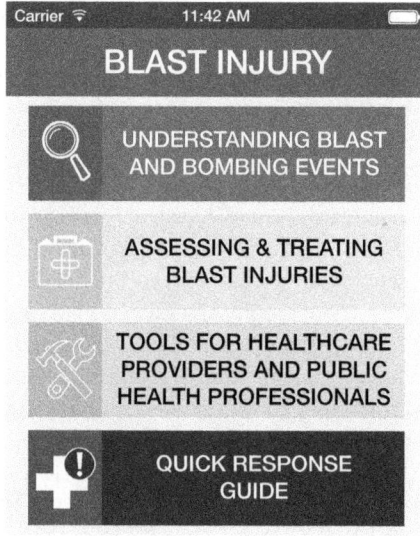

Retrieved from https://emergency.cdc.gov/masscasualties/blastinjury-mobile-app.asp

SUMMARY

Predicting timing, location, and severity of disasters, including terrorist attacks and explosions, is impossible. Clinicians in the military and civilian environments must be aware of the classic characteristics of trauma as well as the characteristics of blast injury. Emergency responders and clinicians in both civilian and military practice need to be astutely aware of blast mechanisms. Though injuries from secondary and tertiary mechanisms are most common, patients may present with TBI, TM rupture, pulmonary, cardiovascular, gastrointestinal, or musculoskeletal PBI. Victims at the extremes of ages may present with unique injury risks and patterns. Multiple injuries, from multiple mechanisms, are likely. As clinicians increase their knowledge of blast injuries, the care for blast victims will improve, both in the military and civilian populations.

STUDY QUESTIONS

1. What are the characteristics of high-order and low-order explosives? Provide examples of each.

2. Describe the pressure differences exhibited during a blast wave.

3. Discuss the difference between primary, secondary, tertiary, and quaternary blast injuries. Where do blunt and penetrating traumatic injuries fall in this classification system?

4. Discuss primary blast injuries in relation to the body system.

5. What clinical guidelines and tools are available to clinicians for the assessment and management of blast injuries?

6. What characteristics of the explosion will predict the severity of blast injury?

7. What are the differences in military and civilian casualties?

8. Discuss the considerations related to blast injury during pregnancy, in children, and in the elderly.

REFERENCES

Akin, F. W., & Murnane, O. D. (2011). Head injury and blast exposure: Vestibular consequences. *Otolaryngology Clinics of North America, 44*, 323–334. doi:10.1016/j.otc.2011.01.005

Bala, M., Rivkind, A. I., Zamir, G., Hadar, T., Gersenshtein, I., Mintz, Y., ... Almogy, G. (2008). Abdominal trauma after terrorist bombing attacks exhibits a unique pattern of injury. *Annals of Surgery, 248*(2), 303–309. doi:10.1097/SLA.0b013e318180a3f7

Boutillier, J., Deck, C., Magnan, P., Naz, P., & Willinger, R. (2016). A critical literature review on primary blast thorax injury and their outcomes.

Journal of Trauma and Acute Care Surgery, 81, 371–379. doi:10.1097/TA.0000000000001076

Breeze, J., Cooper, H., Pearson, C. R., Henney, S., & Reid, A. (2011). Ear injuries sustained by British service personnel subjected to blast trauma. *The Journal of Laryngology & Otology, 125*, 13–17. doi:10.1017/S0022215110002215

Centers for Disease Control and Prevention. (2014). CDC blast injury mobile application. Retrieved from https://emergency.cdc.gov/masscasualties/blastinjury-mobile-app.asp

Champion, H. R., Holcomb, J. B., Lawnick, M. M., Kelliher, T., Spott, M. A., Galarneau, M. R., ... Shair, E. K. (2010). Improved characterization of combat injury. *The Journal of Trauma: Injury, Infection, and Critical Care, 68*, 1139–1150. doi:10.1097/TA.0b013e3181d86a0d

Dougherty, A. L., MacGregor, A. J., Han, P. P., Heltemes, K. J., & Galarneau, M. R. (2011). Visual dysfunction following blast-related traumatic brain injury from the battlefield. *Brain Injury, 25*, 8–13. doi:10.3109/02699052.2010.536195

Edwards, D. S., McMenemy, L., Stapley, S. A., Patel, H. D. L., & Clasper, J. C. (2016). 40 years of terrorist bombings: A meta-analysis of the casualty and injury profile. *Injury, 47*, 646–652. doi:10.1016/j.injury.2015.12.021

Edwards, M. J., Lustik, M., Eichelberger, M. R., Elster, E., Azarow, K., & Coppola, C. (2012). Blast injury in children: An analysis from Afghanistan and Iraq, 2002–2010. *Journal of Trauma and Acute Care Surgery, 73*, 1278–1283. doi:10.1097/TA.0b013e318270d3ee

Falcone, R. (2013). Civilian blast injury. *Trauma Reports, 14*(5), 1–11.

French, L. M. (2010). Military traumatic brain injury: An examination of important differences. *Annals of the New York Academy of Sciences, 1208*, 38–45. doi:10.1111/j.1749-6632.2010.05696.x

Garner, J., Watts, S., Parry, C., Bird, J., Cooper, G., & Kirkman, E. (2010). Prolonged permissive hypotensive resuscitation is associated with poor outcome in primary blast injury with controlled hemorrhage. *Annals of Surgery, 251*, 1131–1139. doi:10.1097/SLA.0b013e3181e00fcb

Hicks, R. R., Fertig, S. J., Desrocher, R. E., Koroshetz, W. J., & Pancrazio, J. J. (2010). Neurologic effects of blast injury. *The Journal of Trauma: Injury, Infection, and Critical Care, 68*, 1257–1263. doi:10.1097/TA.0b013e3181d8956d

Hoencamp, R., Vermetten, E., Tan, E. C. T. H., Putter, H., Leenen, L. P. H., & Hamming, J. F. (2014). Systematic review of the prevalence and characteristics of battle casualties from NATO coalition forces in Iraq and Afghanistan. *Injury, 45*, 1028–1034. doi:10.1016/j.injury.2014.02.012

Hoffer, M. E., Balaban, C., Gottshall, K., Balough, B. J., Maddox, M. R., & Penta, J. R. (2010). Blast exposure: Vestibular consequences and associated characteristics. *Otology and Neurotology, 31*(2), 232–236. doi:10.1097/MAO.0b013e3181c993c3

Jaffe, D. H., & Peleg, K. (2010). Terror explosive injuries: A comparison of children, adolescents, and adults. *Annals of Surgery, 251*, 138–143. doi:10.1097/SLA.0b013e3181b5d7ab

Klein, Y., Arieli, I., Sagiv, S., Peleg, K., & Ben-Galim, P. (2016). Cervical spine injuries in civilian victims of explosions: Should cervical collars be used? *Journal of Trauma and Acute Care Surgery, 80*, 985–988. doi:10.1097/TA.0000000000001040

Ling, G. S. F., & Ecklund, J. M. (2011). Traumatic brain injury in modern war. *Current Opinion in Anesthesiology, 24*, 124–130. doi:10.1097/ACO.0b013e32834458da

Mathews, Z., & Koyfman, A. (2015). Blast injuries. *The Journal of Emergency Medicine, 49*, 573–587. doi:10.1016/j.jemermed.2015.03.013

National Consortium for the Study of Terrorism and Responses to Terrorism. (2016). Annex of statistical information. Country reports on terrorism 2015. Retrieved from https://www.state.gov/documents/organization/257738.pdf

Nguyen, N., Hunt, J. P., Lindfors, D., & Grieffenstein, P. (2014). Aerial fireworks can turn deadly underwater: Magnified blast causes severe pulmonary contusion. *Injury Extra, 45*, 32–34. doi:10.1016/j.injury.2014.02.021

Owers, C., Morgan, J. L., & Garner, J. P. (2011). Abdominal trauma in primary blast injury. *British Journal of Surgery, 98*, 168–179. doi:10.1002/bjs.7268

Ramasamy, A., Cooper, G. A., Sargeant, I. D., Evriviades, D., Porter, K., & Kendrew, J. M. (2013). An overview of the pathophysiology of blast injury with management guidelines. *Orthopaedics and Trauma, 27*(1), 1–8. doi:10.1016/j.mporth.2013.01.002

Ritenour, A. E., Blackbourne, L. H., Kelly, J. F., McLaughlin, D. F., Pearse, L. A., Holcomb, J. B., & Wade, C. E. (2010). Incidence of primary blast injury in US military overseas contingency operations: A retrospective study. *Annals of Surgery, 251*, 1140–1144. doi:10.1097/SLA.0b013e3181e01270

Scott, R. A. H., Blanch, R. J., & Morgan-Warren, P. J. (2015). Aspects of ocular war injuries. *Trauma, 17*, 83–92. doi:10.1177/1460408614539621

Singh, A. K., Ditkofsky, N. G., York, J. D., Abujudeh, H. H., Avery, L. A., Brunner, J. F., ... Lev, M. H. (2016). Blast injuries: From improvised explosive device blasts to the Boston marathon bombing. *RadioGraphics, 36*, 295–307. doi:10.1148/rg.2016150114

Somes, J., & Donatelli, N. S. (2014). Considerations when explosions involve geriatric patients. *Journal of Emergency Nursing, 40*, 78–81. doi:10.1016/j.jen.2013.09.005

Spurrier, E., Gibb, I., Masouros, S., & Clasper, J. (2016). Identifying spinal injury patterns in underbody blast to develop mechanistic hypotheses. *Spine, 41*, E268–E275. doi:10.1097/BRS.0000000000001213

Taddeo, J., Devine, M., & McAlister, V. C. (2015). Cervical spine injury in dismounted improvised explosive device trauma. *Journal of the Canadian Chiropractic Association, 58*, S104–S107. doi:10.1503/cjs.013114

Turegano-Fuentes, F., Perez-Diaz, D., Sanz-Sanchez, M., Alfici, R., & Ashkenazi, I. (2014). Abdominal blast injuries: Different patterns, severity, management, and prognosis according to the main mechanism of injury. *European Journal of Trauma and Emergency Surgery, 40*, 451–460. doi:10.1007/s00068-014-0397-4

Veterans Affairs/Department of Defense. (2016). Clinical practice guideline for the management of concussion-mild traumatic brain injury. Retrieved from https://www.healthquality.va.gov/guidelines/Rehab/mtbi

Wilk, J. E., Thomas, J. L., McGurk, D. M., Riviere, L. A., Castro, C. A., & Hoge, C. W. (2010). Mild traumatic brain injury (concussion) during combat: Lack of association of blast mechanism with persistent postconcussive symptoms. *Journal of Head Trauma Rehabilitation, 25*(1), 9–14. doi:10.1097/HTR.0b013e3181bd090f

Wolf, S. J., Bebarta, V. S., Bonnett, C. J., Pons, P. T., & Cantrill, S. V. (2009). Blast injuries. *The Lancet, 374*, 405–415. doi:10.1016/S0140-6736(09)60257-9

CASE STUDY 26.1

A propane tank has exploded at a family reunion. The reunion was taking place at an outdoor park with a pavilion approximately 30 feet from the grill where the tank exploded. The pavilion is the largest structure within the park. All other buildings are 1,000 feet away, surrounding the park. Attendees at the reunion are 6 months to 85 years of age. There was a 65-year-old and a 24-year-old father and son at the grill cooking when the tank exploded. The elderly relatives were sitting at tables in the pavilion when the explosion occurred. The majority of the children were on the playground which is approximately 250 feet away from the epicenter of the blast.

QUESTIONS

1. What injuries would you anticipate that the father and son closest to the epicenter would have?
2. What types of debris, if any, would you anticipate could cause secondary or tertiary injuries to the victims?
3. What are the special considerations for the elderly relatives who were injured?
4. What are the special considerations for the children who were injured?

CASE STUDY 26.2

There was an explosion at a local college campus occurring approximately 10 minutes after morning classes ended. The epicenter of the explosion was in the campus quad which is surrounded by large academic buildings. It has been reported that the explosive device was a pressure cooker with screws, nails, and glass fragments inside; the perpetrator detonated the device remotely. There are 2,500 students enrolled on this campus and approximately 300 faculty and staff, though it is unknown how many people were in the quad during the explosion versus those in buildings. There is significant structural damage to the surrounding buildings and multiple casualties. Victims range from 17 to 55 years of age.

QUESTIONS

1. For the victims in the quad, what injuries would you anticipate? Would you anticipate any injuries to those in the buildings?
2. What are the considerations for secondary and tertiary injuries for victims of this event?
3. How does the presence of the buildings influence the blast wave and therefore injury patterns?
4. In the event of building collapse, what types of injuries would you anticipate?

27

CARING FOR PATIENTS WITH HIV FOLLOWING A DISASTER

Susan Michaels-Strasser and Juliana Soares Linn

LEARNING OBJECTIVES

When this chapter is completed, readers will be able to:

1. Discuss disaster preparedness for health systems and HIV-positive persons in preventing and treating HIV infection.
2. Identify major reasons why HIV incidence may increase following a disaster.
3. Prepare for the needs of HIV-positive pregnant women and infants exposed to HIV.
4. Outline the key care and treatment issues for HIV-positive persons following a disaster.
5. Discuss palliative care needs of AIDS patients following a disaster.
6. Describe how nurses can keep themselves safe.

KEY MESSAGES

The needs of people with chronic illness are often overlooked in the immediate disaster aftermath as the focus is on emergency care and response.

Caring for patients with HIV and AIDS following a disaster is a complex but essential task.

To achieve epidemic control, reaching 90-90-90 is required.

Ensuring the continuity of care for HIV-infected individuals, maintaining antiretroviral (ARV) drug supply chains, and preventive measures such as prevention of mother-to-child transmission (PMTCT) and postexposure to HIV prophylaxis (PEP) should be planned and budgeted for.

People living with HIV and AIDS have ongoing needs which, if not met, can lead to severe negative health outcomes such as transmission from HIV-positive pregnant women to children, development of drug resistance, or increased morbidity and mortality.

Care of people living with HIV and AIDS includes identifying those in need and ensuring a continuous supply of ARV drugs as well as medicines to prevent or treat common opportunistic infections, especially tuberculosis (TB) and any other chronic needs.

CHAPTER OVERVIEW

We live in a world characterized by unexpected disruptive events. Political unrest and turmoil, warfare, and widespread social violence destroy the fabric of societies and lead to humanitarian crises. Increasingly, it is the growing number of natural disasters and conflicts and the public health emergencies that they create that contribute to undermine the physical and mental health of the affected populations. Such events result in increased morbidity and mortality in the affected population(s). In addition, immediate response efforts focus appropriately on rendering emergency healthcare and triage of victims. In this early phase, the goal for disaster response is to maximize benefits for the most people who uphold the ethical principle of utilitarianism (Persad, Wertheimer, & Emanuel, 2009). As the life cycle of the disaster progresses, other medical needs of victims can and should be addressed.

Large-scale events, such as the 2010 earthquake in Haiti, highlight the crisis that results for victims with underlying chronic illness (along with those suffering acute disaster-related injury) when a disaster destroys the healthcare system. More recently, the Syrian refugee crisis highlights both acute and long-term care needs amid war and displacement. People living with HIV must be prepared for unexpected events. Furthermore, this population's health needs should be incorporated into disaster preparedness activities and response plans to ensure significant gains in the HIV response are sustained. Whether the event is international or occurs on U.S. soil, it is critically important for nurses to possess the knowledge and skill set to respond in a timely and appropriate manner to both prevent and care for persons living with HIV.

Disasters can have a catastrophic impact on both acute and chronic health in the affected populations. Yet the needs of people with chronic conditions are often overlooked when patients with acute trauma overwhelm weakened health systems. Ensuring the continuum of chronic care should be seen as a priority in disaster preparation and planning. In the case of HIV care, the global community has moved toward a "test and treat" policy and therefore the number of people to be started on HIV treatment is due to increase (World Health Organization [WHO], 2016a). Secondly, science clearly shows that antiretroviral therapy (ART) is a highly effective prevention method both to drastically reduce mother-to-child transmission as well as transmission between partners with discordant HIV status (Cohen et al., 2011; Kuhn et al., 2010).

HIV is most prevalent in sub-Saharan Africa, a region with limited infrastructure and weak healthcare systems, which compounds abilities to respond to chronic care needs, such as HIV, following a disaster. Since a break in treatment for HIV-positive patients following a disaster can have a devastating impact on prevention, adherence, and HIV treatment outcomes, adequate preparation and planning are critical. Despite obstacles in low-resource settings and during times of upheaval, high quality, effective HIV service delivery is

possible where detailed planning, preparation, and strong partnerships exist. Although ambitious, the case studies in this chapter demonstrate that despite complex human emergencies, the 2020 goal of the Joint United Nations Programme on HIV and AIDS (UNAIDS, 2017) of reaching 90-90-90 whereby 90% of all people living with HIV will know their HIV status, 90% of all people with diagnosed HIV infection will receive sustained ART, and 90% of all people receiving ART will have viral suppression is not too ambitious.

This chapter thus reviews key issues, actions, and outcomes that are necessary to ensure a continuum of HIV services. The chapter draws on work in HIV services in southern Africa over two decades, work in international health and development programs as well as the Sphere Standards, and the Inter-Agency Standing Committee (IASC, 2010) Guidelines for Addressing HIV in Humanitarian Settings. These guidelines, due to be updated in 2018, are referenced and expanded on throughout the chapter.

THE SPHERE PROJECT AND MINIMUM STANDARDS

The Sphere Project and the development of a Humanitarian Charter and Minimum Standards in Disaster Response (begun in 1997 and updated several times since) is an effort to ensure quality and accountability among humanitarian agencies responding during times of disaster. These standards are compiled in the *Sphere Handbook* (The Sphere Project, 2011), which can be freely downloaded from the Sphere Project's website (www.sphereproject.org). It is available in multiple languages including, but not limited to, French, Arabic, and Spanish. The next edition of the Sphere Handbook is due in 2018.

Core and evidence-based minimum standards are described in the *Sphere Handbook* including minimum standards on:

1. Water supply, sanitation, and hygiene promotion (WASH)
2. Food security and nutrition
3. Shelter, settlement, and nonfood items
4. Health action, with HIV presented as a cross-cutting theme throughout the handbook (The Sphere Project, 2011)

REPRODUCTIVE HEALTH AND SEXUALLY TRANSMITTED DISEASES

Reproductive health and sexually transmitted infections (STIs), including HIV, may be overlooked or ignored during early disaster response activities (Collymore, 2001). While providing basic needs for survival (water, food, and shelter) and emergency treatment of injuries is critical, provisions should be made as soon as possible to support reproductive health needs and the prevention of sexually transmitted diseases. Alnuaimi, Kassab, Alia, Mohammed, and Shattnawi (2017) highlight the disparity in reproductive health outcomes between those affected by complex humanitarian crises and the general population. They note that in the current Syrian crisis, refugee mothers were significantly more likely to deliver by cesarean section and experience higher rates of anemia than their Jordanian counterparts. The 2014 West African

Ebola outbreak highlighted the fragility of maternal healthcare with a decrease in HIV testing during pregnancy and uptake of family planning services being noted (Brolin Ribacke, Saulnier, Eriksson, & von Schreeb, 2016). Propelled by the critical needs of adolescent girls and women during emergencies, the Eastern Europe and Central Asia (EECA) region has developed minimum standards in the Minimum Initial Service Package (MISP) for sexual and reproductive health (Lisam, 2014).

HIV-positive pregnant women represent a complex challenge for healthcare providers following a disaster. The goal to ensure a safe delivery and adequate care of the newborn may already be compromised by limited power supplies, lack of blood transfusion services, and disrupted access to emergency obstetric care and delivery by a trained health provider. Additionally, HIV-positive pregnant women require ongoing care for their HIV infection as well as prevention of transmission (vertical transmission) of HIV to their unborn child. If services are compromised, fewer women may seek care and those who do seek care may get compromised services due to breaks in supply chain or staffing. Basic care needs of HIV-positive pregnant women is discussed later in the chapter.

Disasters and Disruption of the Social Fabric of Communities

Disasters can cause the physical destruction of hospitals, clinics, homes, schools, governmental buildings, and businesses. Many businesses may choose to close their doors or limit hours of operation for fear of looting and lawlessness. Disasters can also result in the disruption of the family unit and unraveling of the social fabric of communities. People affected by disaster may struggle with depression, posttraumatic stress disorder (PTSD), and deteriorating socioeconomic conditions (Galea, Nandi, & Vlahov, 2005; National Institute of Mental Health, 2011). Shacham, Rosenburg, Önen, Donovan, and Turner Overton (2015), in a paper on the persistence of HIV-related stigma, explain that an individual assessment of patients' needs is important to understand the interplay between substance abuse, stigma, and psychological issues, which could all be exacerbated during times of acute stress and social upheaval.

Sexual and Gender-Based Violence

Populations affected by or displaced due to a disaster may experience a higher incidence of sexual or gender-based violence. Decreased social cohesion and decreased law enforcement result in increased vulnerability for many individuals. Children are particularly vulnerable due to their size, level of maturity, or physical separation from their parents or caregivers.

Internationally, victims of disasters may become victims of gender-based violence including rape and sexual assault. Women and children may be at risk of such violence as they carry out activities of daily living, such as collecting firewood or fetching water. When the rule of law is compromised, these daily tasks, which are common in many developing countries, may put people at increased risk of assault. The incidence of rape may increase when it is used as a weapon of war or when there is a breakdown in the rule of law (Benjamin, 2001). The IASC (2010) guidelines include principles for both minimum and expanded responses to protect populations from gender-based violence.

BOX 27.1 A Summary of *Sphere Handbook* Key Actions Related to HIV and AIDS

ESTABLISH

- Safety procedures and precautions for waste disposal
- Measures for rational use of blood and maintaining safe blood supplies
- Widespread access to quality condoms for both men and women
- Linkages between HIV and TB services

ENSURE

- Provision of syndromic management for STIs
- Provision of PEP is provided within 72 hours
- Access to prevention of PMTCT of HIV services
- Uninterrupted access to ART for persons on treatment as well as preventive services such as cotrimoxazole prophylaxis
- Prevention interventions for high-risk populations

PROVIDE

- Health education on HIV
- Treatment, care, and support for exposed infants (i.e., infants born to HIV-positive mothers)

ART, antiretroviral therapy; PEP, postexposure prophylaxis; PMTCT, prevention of mother-to-child transmission; STIs, sexually transmitted infections; TB, tuberculosis.

Source: Benjamin, J. A. (2001). Conflict, post-conflict, and HIV/AIDS—The gender connections. Women, war and HIV/AIDS: West Africa and the Great Lakes. Women's Commission for Refugee Women and Children (pp. 328–329). Retrieved from https://www.popline.org/node/234990

Minimum responses include completing a situation analysis of, and response plan for, victims of gender-based violence.

Key actions in sexual and reproductive health and HIV and AIDS are outlined in Box 27.1.

Reduced Access to Preventive Health Services

The increased occurrence in sexual and gender-based violence may occur simultaneously with decreased treatment of STIs and reductions in the implementation of basic HIV-prevention strategies such as PEP (postexposure prophylaxis) and treatment as prevention. Increasingly available for people at substantial risk of HIV infection, the use of pre-exposure prophylaxis (PrEP) with a consistent daily dose of tenofovir and emtricitabine is highly effective at preventing HIV transmission but consistent adherence is required for PrEP effectiveness (WHO, 2016a).

Reductions in prevention strategies may include: disrupted safe motherhood services including access to PMTCT of HIV services, lack of access to combination HIV-prevention approaches, and reduced access to family planning (including oral contraceptive pills, intrauterine devices [IUDs], and injectable contraceptives) as well as treatment of STIs. Access may be reduced or unobtainable to PEP for possible HIV exposure following incidents such as rape and health worker needlestick injuries. Preparing for such eventualities is critical for first responders and people affected by HIV and AIDS.

Sexually Transmitted Infections

Managing and preventing STIs should be seen as priorities following complex human emergencies where sexual and gender-based violence and breakdowns in the social fabric of society are noted. Preparing for and managing STIs should follow evidence-based practices and build on both local and international experiences and standard protocols currently available and recommended in the country or region affected. The syndromic management of STIs is a widely used primary healthcare and public health approach to treat people with symptoms of STIs in underresourced settings where laboratory testing is not routinely available. The syndromic management approach uses a set of standard criteria to determine the likelihood of a STI, which facilitates the initiation of the appropriate empiric treatment at the first visit. Treatment is based on symptoms using standardized treatment protocols. The WHO has developed a seven-module training program on syndromic management which is available in English, Spanish, and French (WHO, 2007).

In addition to syndromic management, point-of-care testing is increasing access to quality-assured diagnostics for STIs as well as same-day testing and treatment (STAT) in resource-limited settings and could be employed in disaster settings to increase diagnostic capabilities. One of the advantages of the point-of-care technology is to be accessible for both clinical and nonclinical staff (peers, expert patients, frontline workers) alike (Broeckaert & Challacombe, 2015). Point-of-care diagnostics can increase access to testing and treatment but at the same time quality assurance control mechanisms should be initiated and sustained. Recent studies have shown that use of point-of-care testing for syphilis alongside HIV in ongoing PMTCT services is acceptable, feasible, and cost-effective (Bitarakwate et al., 2011). A rapid diagnostic

test for hepatitis C, a global health threat associated with HIV in many settings, has recently had been approved by WHO to be used in low- and middle-income countries (WHO, 2016b). This represents an important opportunity to increase access to care and treatment to those who screen positive for hepatitis C, particularly in emergency settings. This is especially important as highly effective treatment with direct-acting antivirals become available worldwide (WHO, 2016b).

Disaster Preparedness Continuum

Figure 27.1 provides a sample continuum of care from disaster preparation through the initial response and rebuilding phase. The disaster preparedness continuum is helpful to depict issues requiring consideration before, during, and immediately after a complex human emergency. This diagram includes illustrative efforts in each phase of disaster preparation and response but many other responses can be planned and executed to ensure that prevention measures are in place and HIV-affected and infected populations receive the care, treatment, and support they need.

Community-based organizations (CBOs) and faith-based organizations (FBOs) work in development settings providing community or public health services.

It is important to ask the following questions when preparing for a disaster response:

1. Who is designated as in charge for the first 48 hours after disaster onset?
2. Who controls the release of funds to begin a response?
3. Who controls the supplies of essential drugs in the town, state, province, or country?
4. Is there a national disaster management unit? Is this unit functional and does it have plans from which it is working? Are these plans shared or available?
5. Is there a national body that typically coordinates HIV services? Is it involved in the disaster response?

The IASC (2010) has developed a very comprehensive matrix for addressing HIV in humanitarian settings. This matrix outlines

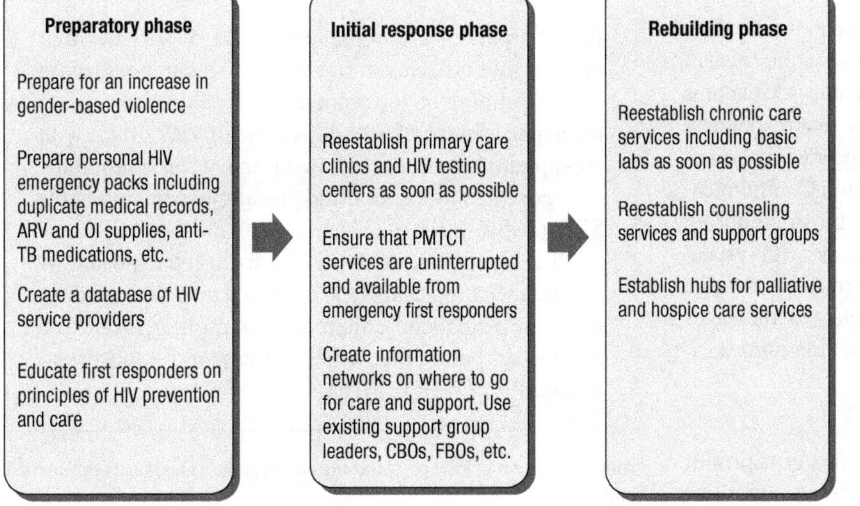

Preparatory phase

Prepare for an increase in gender-based violence

Prepare personal HIV emergency packs including duplicate medical records, ARV and OI supplies, anti-TB medications, etc.

Create a database of HIV service providers

Educate first responders on principles of HIV prevention and care

Initial response phase

Reestablish primary care clinics and HIV testing centers as soon as possible

Ensure that PMTCT services are uninterrupted and available from emergency first responders

Create information networks on where to go for care and support. Use existing support group leaders, CBOs, FBOs, etc.

Rebuilding phase

Reestablish chronic care services including basic labs as soon as possible

Reestablish counseling services and support groups

Establish hubs for palliative and hospice care services

FIGURE 27.1 Disaster preparedness continuum.

ARV, antiretroviral; CBOs, community-based organizations; FBOs, faith-based organizations; OI, opportunities infection; PMTCT, prevention of mother-to-child transmission; TB, tuberculosis.

activities during the preparatory phase, during the minimum initial response phase, as well as during the subsequent expanded response. Activities are presented according to sector including: HIV awareness-raising and community support; health; protection; food security, nutrition, and livelihood support; education; shelter; camp coordinator and management; water, sanitation and hygiene; and HIV in the workplace.

Primary Prevention

An HIV and AIDS emergency response package should be created and available for use in times of disaster. This emergency response package should include preventive measures such as information materials, condoms, contraceptives, and buffer stocks of essential drugs including, but not limited to, ARVs for PrEP, PEP, and ongoing treatment. Access to an uninterrupted supply of medicines including ARVs, anti-TB medicines, and opportunistic infection (OIs) medications are essential to prevent the emergence of HIV resistance, TB drug resistance, and emergence of OIs.

In addition to preventing HIV drug resistance through daily use of ARVs, treatment of patients with HIV is also seen as a key method of prevention, as ARVs reduce the viral load (VL) of HIV in the body and therefore decrease the risk of transmission from person to person and from mother to child (Cohen et al., 2011; Lima et al., 2008).

Global HIV treatment options have quickly evolved. Antiretroviral drugs are medicines that need to be taken daily to suppress HIV. There are currently six classes of antiretroviral drugs that work in different ways to interrupt viral replication. Each class of medicine targets different receptors or specific enzymes involved in the HIV life cycle. Drugs that focus on the enzyme protease are called "protease inhibitors" and those that focus on reverse transcriptase are known as "nucleoside," "nucleotide" or "non-nucleoside reverse transcriptase inhibitors." Drugs that target the HIV integrase enzyme are called the "HIV integrase strand transfer inhibitors." Drugs in this class include the second-generation *Dolutegravir*, a highly effective agent that is being considered as first-line therapy in many countries. Drugs that block the entry of HIV in the human cell can be divided in two classes, the "CCR5 coreceptor antagonist" and the "fusion inhibitors." While the first block the CCR5 coreceptor, the latter bind to the gp 41 protein.

As mentioned earlier, combination HIV prevention including male and female condom distribution and use is a key component of primary HIV prevention within disaster health services. Condoms should be a part of the essential supply list for first responders and relief agencies. Sex education, including peer education as well as the distribution of Information Education Communication (IEC) materials and condoms, should be provided during a disaster. Cultural considerations should be made with respect to the disaster-affected population to demonstrate respect and regard for its views and for insight into how prevention messages should be presented to best reach the affected communities.

Prevention of Disease Transmission

Medical, dental, and surgical materials and equipment should be disinfected and sterilized. The use of injections and injectables should be limited whenever possible and, when necessary, only sterile needles and equipment should be used. Medical waste and sharp instruments must be properly disposed of and sharps containers should be a standard part of any healthcare emergency response team. A plan to ensure adequate storage, removal, and destruction of sharps should be developed before a disaster and executed as soon as a disaster response is activated. Establishing needlestick injury prevention committees prior to a disaster, critically evaluating needlestick injuries, and conducting after-action reviews of all stick incidents should be prioritized as an important prevention strategy (Sharps Containers-etc, 2013). Performing short, rapid after-action reviews on each needlestick injury can help to identify environmental challenges and work conditions that are modifiable.

The reuse of sharps such as injection needles or surgical equipment after minimal or no sterilization procedures promotes the spread of bloodborne pathogens including HIV. Even in controlled settings with access to sterile and disposable equipment, accidental exposure can occur as in the case of needlestick injuries. Health service responders need to have access to PEP for themselves in case of an accidental exposure. Furthermore, PEP should be available as part of a disaster response to provide prevention medicine for victims of rape. Box 27.2 provides further explanation about PEP.

BOX 27.2 Post-Exposure Prophylaxis

WHAT IS PEP

PEP is the administration of ARV drugs to a known HIV-negative person who has had possible direct exposure to HIV-infected blood or body fluids. Some reasons why PEP may be needed include, but are not limited to, needlestick injuries in health workers and sexual assault/rape.

THE BASICS OF PEP

PEP "is part of a comprehensive set of services that include first aid, exposure risk assessment, counseling and, depending on the outcome of the exposure assessment, prescription of a 28-day course of ARV drugs, with appropriate support and follow-up and, when appropriate, emergency contraception and presumptive treatment for STI" (IASC, 2010, p. 22).

PEP is provided within 72 hours of the exposure. A regimen with three ARVs is preferred over the two-drug regimen. Enhanced adherence counseling should be included as part of the package of support for those who initiate PEP (WHO, 2016a).

ARV, antiretroviral; PEP, postexposure prophylaxis; STI, sexually transmitted infections.

Blood Donations and Transfusions

Careful consideration should be exercised regarding blood donations and transfusions. Blood safety standards must be upheld with regard to all blood donations and use of blood products. National Blood Transfusion services should be consulted and review of the safety of the blood supply should be secured before blood or blood products are used.

Secondary Prevention—Securing Essential Drugs for HIV-Positive People

In addition to ARV drugs just described, other drugs commonly used in HIV services include medicines to prevent or treat OIs such as cotrimoxazole (Bactrim), isoniazid preventive therapy (IPT), and anti-TB medications. Inconsistent use of these drugs can lead to drug resistance and/or emergence of OIs and should be avoided wherever possible. Stock outs due to inadequate supply chain and management system is a common barrier to implementation in resource-constrained settings. Adequate preparation and planning are needed to ensure that essential drugs are consistently available and patient adherence prioritized.

OIs are infections that are normally preventable or self-limiting in a person with a well-functioning immune system. HIV targets certain cells such as CD4 cells and leads to destruction of the immune response. Lowered counts of CD4 cells make a person vulnerable to infections such as candidiasis (thrush), herpes simplex virus, Pneumocystis pneumonia (PCP), and TB. While some OIs cause discomfort, others are serious and can be life-threatening. Besides the use to prevent OIs, studies have shown that cotrimoxazole helps reduce mortality among people with low CD4 counts (Suthar et al., 2015; Walker et al., 2007). IPT given to those with latent TB infection prevents the progression to active TB disease. Studies have demonstrated the benefit of combined use of IPT and ART to reduce mortality even in patients with high CD4 counts (Rangaka et al., 2014; TEMPRANO, 2015).

Practical Considerations for Nurse Safety

Nurses and other disaster relief workers should practice universal precautions and should be aware of the prevalence of HIV and AIDS in the population for which they are caring. Even in low prevalence areas, universal precautions remain essential prevention measures for both healthcare workers and the general population. During emergencies all necessary measures should be taken to ensure the safety of health workers and to maintain infection control procedures.

International disaster responders must be aware of the prevalence and distribution of HIV and AIDS in the population of the country in which they are working and should understand the drivers of the HIV epidemic in the affected area. Before responding, nurses should ensure that basic standards are in place to allow them, their coworkers, and staff to work as safely as possible to protect their patients and themselves. Adequate supplies of gloves, protective eyewear, garments, sharps boxes, and disposable syringes are essential.

Identifying Patients in Need

One of the biggest challenges in caring for individuals with HIV and AIDS following a disaster is identifying who they are. This may be challenging following the destruction or absence of any health records and in settings where stigma is high and people are fearful or concerned about disclosing their HIV status.

Consultation with local health providers, where available, can help to encourage HIV-positive people to seek care and treatment. Confidentiality should be maintained at the same time HIV-positive people are made aware of when and where services are available. Many countries use patient-held records which include HIV-specific information. These records provide vital information on patient history and can make the individual response during a disaster more efficient and effective.

Tracking HIV exposure in infants and identifying HIV-exposed and positive children in an emergency can be very difficult. Yet patient-held records can help to identify exposed and HIV-positive children in need of care. Many developing countries use an integrated child health card, commonly known as the "Road to Health" card which is kept by the family. This card includes basic well-child information (e.g., birth record, immunization status, growth, and development) as well as HIV exposure status and whether the mother and/or child received prevention of mother-to-child drug prophylaxis. New parents are given such a card to track their child's health during the first 5 years of life. These cards, commonly available in Africa, can provide health workers with a wealth of patient health information.

Figure 27.2 shows an example of such a card from the southern African country of Zimbabwe. Zimbabwe's Ministry of Health and Child Welfare explains the rationale behind the development of this card. "Given the scale of the HIV problem and the limited resources to deal with it, HIV prevention, care and treatment require to be integrated as far as possible into the existing health system if 'access for all' is truly to be approached ... Ensuring some form of simple communication within the health system to facilitate access to and provision of HIV related health services was thus identified as a specific need by the Ministry of Health and Child Welfare" (Miller et al., 2008, p. 5). Including HIV-related information on Zimbabwe's Road to Health Card will facilitate tracking of key information. Children who are born to HIV-positive women and therefore exposed to HIV will be noted and prevention and treatment services identified. Having access to such vital information during the chaos of a complex human emergency can be lifesaving.

Other methods to improve follow-up of HIV-positive individuals is (a) through the use of electronic medical records; (b) increased use of currently available records regarding care to AIDS patients through the AIDS Drug Assistance Program (ADAP) and other such programs; and (c) better coordination among state and federal emergency response agencies to ensure that care for chronic diseases, such as HIV and AIDS, is being provided effectively in the aftermath of a natural disaster (Federal Emergency Management Agency, 2009).

SALT AND SUGAR SOLUTION (SSS)
Give this SOLUTION as often as possible in case of DIARRHOEA and continue feeding and breastfeeding.

MVURA INE MUNYU NESUGAR
Ipa mwana MVURA IYI nguva dzose kana ane MANYOKA, moramba muchimupa zvokudya nekumuyamwisa.

AMANZI ALE TSHWAYI LETSHUKELA
Phana umntwana AMANZI LAWA sikhathi sonke uma EHUDA, njalo qhubeka umupha ukudla kanye lokumunyisa.

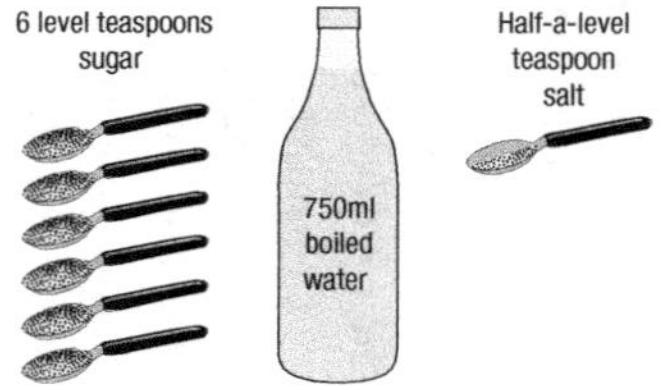

6 level teaspoons sugar

750ml boiled water

Half-a-level teaspoon salt

NOTES

MINISTRY OF HEALTH

CHILD HEALTH CARD

ZIMBABWE

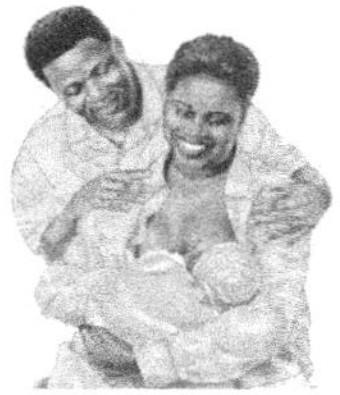

GOOD INFANT FEEDING PRACTICE
Give only breast milk for the first 6 months. Introduce solids and liquids from 6 months. Continue breastfeeding up to 24 months or beyond unless counseled otherwise by a health worker.

KUDYA KWAKANAKA KWEMWANA
Ipai mwana mukaka wezamu chete pamwedzi mitanhatu yekutanga.
Ipai kumwe kudya kana kunwa kudya pamwedzi mitanhatu. Rambai muchiyamwisa kusvika pamakore maviri kana kudarika kunze kwekuti makataurirwa mukadziviswa neve utano.

MUNYISA OKUNGABANGELI INGOZI
Munyisa ingane yakho okwenyanga eziyisithupha zakuqala.
Qala ukuyipha okunye okudliwayo lo kunathwayo uma isilenyanga eziyisithupha.
Qhubeka ukumunyisa ingane yakho ize ifike iminyaka emibili loba ukwedlula, ngaphandle uma uzetshisiwe ngabezempila kahle ukuba ungamunyisi.

For more information on infant feeding, contact-your nearest health worker.

IMMUNIZATIONS SCHEDULE

	AGE	IMMUNIZATION
PRIMARY COURSE	BIRTH/First Contact	BCG
	3 MONTHS	DPT1, HBV1, POLIO 1
	4 MONTHS	DPT2, HBV2, POLIO 2
	5 MONTHS	DPT3, HBV3, POLIO 3
	9 MONTHS	MEASLES
BOOSTERS	18 MONTHS	DPT AND POLIO
	5 YEARS	DT, POLIO

DPT: Diphtheria, Pertussis (Whooping cough) and Tetanus
HBV: Hepatitis B vaccine
BCG: To be repeated if there is no scar after 3 months

VACCINE		1	2	3	4	5
	DOSE					
	ENTER DATE GIVEN AND BATCH NUMBER					
BCG						
POLIO						
DPT						
HBV						
MEASLES						
DT						

VITAMIN A SCHEDULE

	YEAR	1	2	3	4	5	6
DOSE	ENTER DATE DATE GIVEN AND BATCH NUMBER						
1st							
2nd							

First dose at 6 months or earlier if not breastfeeding
Thereafter, dose is at every 6 months

INFANT FEEDING

	Birth	10D	6W	2M	3M	4M	5M
Follow-up time							
Infant feeding code							
Follow-up time	6M	7M	9M	12M	15M	18M	24M
Infant feeding code							

INFANT FEEDING CODES
1. Exclusive Breastfeeding
2. Exclusive Heat-Treated Breast Milk
3. Exclusive Commercial Infant Formula
4. Exclusive Modified Animal Milk
5. Mixed Feeding
6. Other Specify

CARE

NVP/Other ARVs given at birth?
(Circle Yes or No)   NO   YES

	6W	2M	3M	4M	5M
Follow-up time					
Cotrimoxazole (supplied)					

	6M	9M	12M	15M	18M
Follow-up time					
Cotrimoxazole (supplied)					

Parent/Caregiver pre-test counseled for
child test (Circle Yes or No)   NO   YES

Child tested date:

Test Number: _ _ _ _ _ Test Used (Specify)

Date Parent/Caregiver post-test
counseled for child's result:

Child's sample result (Circle)   0   1

Continue Cotrimoxazole? (Circle Yes or No)   NO   YES
If yes, refer to treatment card.

CARE COMMENTS:

NAME OF CHILD:

SURNAME OF CHILD:

SEX: DATE OF BIRTH:

NAME OF MOTHER:

PHYSICAL ADDRESS:

PLACE OF BIRTH:

HEALTH CENTER:

FIGURE 27.2 Zimbabwe Child Health Card, 2006. (*continued*)

Source: Miller, A., Madzima, R., Maruva, M., Mahomva, A., Keatinge, J., & Mbizvo, E. (2008). *Best practice. Revision of the Children Health Card in Zimbabwe: Modifying existing systems to improve general and HIV specific care of all children.* Harare, Zimbabwe: Ministry of Health and Child Welfare.

ARV, antiretroviral; BCG, bacillus Calmette-Guérin; DPT, diptheria, pertussis (whooping cough), and tetanus; DT, diphtheria and tetanus vaccine; HBV, hepatitis B vaccine; NVP, nevirapine.

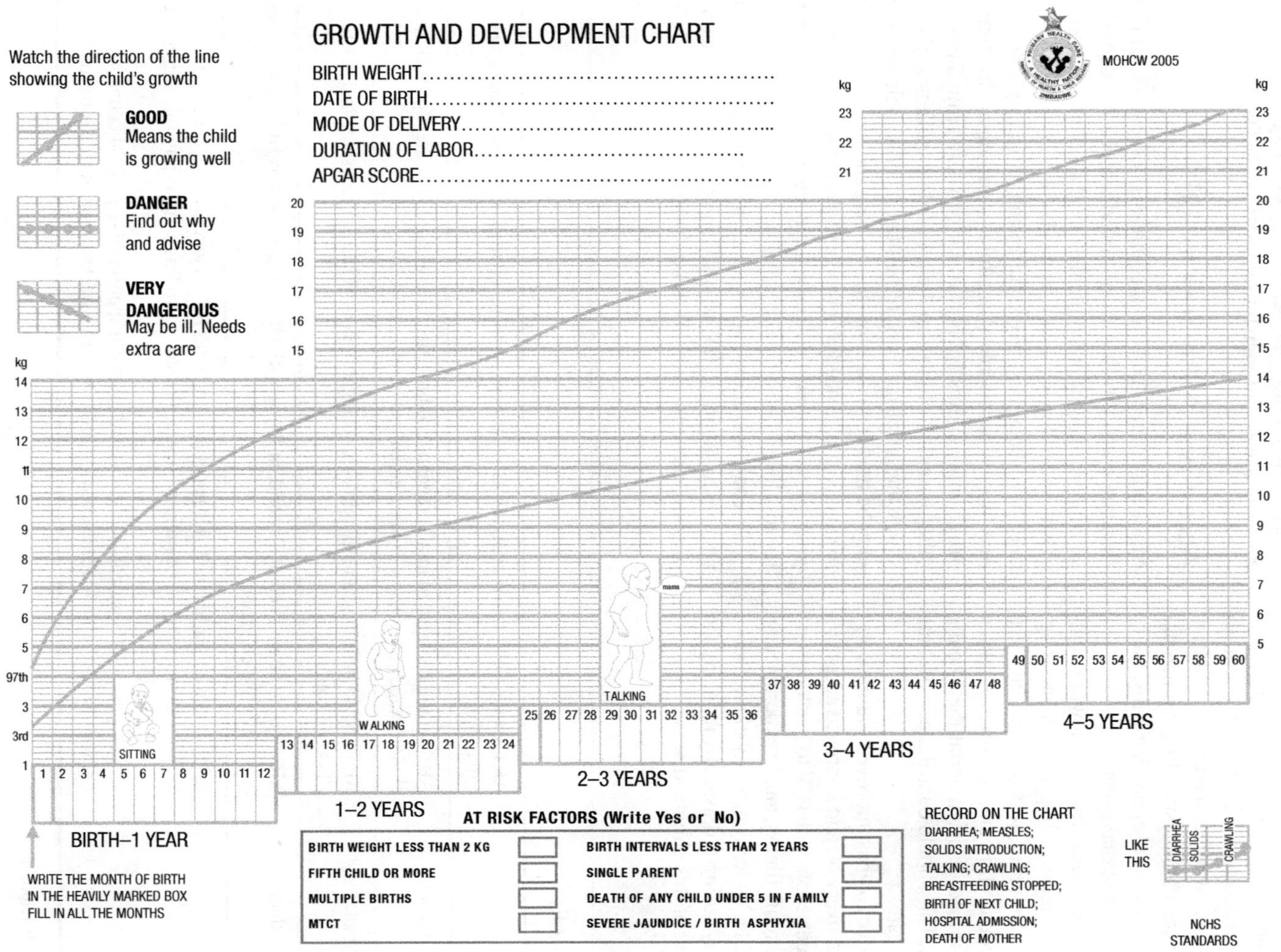

FIGURE 27.2 (*continued*)

Prevention of Mother-to-Child Transmission

Pregnant women who are HIV positive are at risk of transmitting the infection to their child either in utero, during labor, or postnatally through breastfeeding. Prevention of mother-to-children transmission or prevention of parent to child transmission (also referred to as vertical transmission) includes: (a) screening all pregnant women using an "opt out" policy, (b) initiation of lifelong ART and retention in care, and (c) ensuring safer infant feeding.

The second edition of the WHO Consolidated guidelines on the use of antiretroviral drugs for treating and preventing HIV infection released in 2016 moved away from the Options A, B, and B+ (WHO, 2016a). The WHO now advises that all pregnant and breastfeeding women who are HIV positive should initiate ART regardless of CD4 count and/or clinic stage (Table 27.1). Lifelong ART for pregnant and breastfeeding women has been adopted by most countries, including the 22 priority countries responsible for the majority of new infections among children. ART initiation for all pregnant and breastfeeding women has important benefits not only to the mother and her baby, but to prevent HIV transmission to her sexual partner.

This new guidance represents a critical step towards universal ART for pregnant and breastfeeding women and long-term sustainability of ART. However, it is as important that women receive adequate counselling and information about treatment and make an informed decision about their health even in emergency settings. This should contribute to lifelong adherence and retention in care.

The treatment of HIV infection has improved dramatically over the last decade. The discovery of, and improved access to, combination ART has enabled people with HIV to live longer, to see HIV as a manageable chronic illness, and to experience an overall improved quality of life. Wider availability of fixed-dose combinations and once-a-day dosing is drastically reducing the pill burden and management of this chronic disease.

Combination ARV medicine has demonstrated the ability to be highly effective at dramatically reducing the amount of circulating HIV. This is commonly referred to as the VL. The goal of treatment is to achieve an undetectable VL. This is achieved through strict treatment adherence to a combination of at least three ARV drugs. This is commonly referred to as HAART which stands for *h*ighly *a*ctive *a*ntiretroviral *t*reatment or *t*herapy.

Recommended ARVs are categorized by class of drug including:

- Nucleoside reverse transcriptase inhibitors (NRTIs)
- Nucleotide reverse transcriptase inhibitors (NtRTIs)
- Nonnucleoside reverse transcriptase inhibitors (NNRTIs)
- Protease inhibitors (PIs)
- Fusion inhibitors
- Entry inhibitors—CCR5 coreceptor antagonist
- Integrase strand transfer inhibitors (INSTIs)

Access and Adherence to ART

Strict adherence to ARV medicines is essential; HIV drug resistance can develop from nonadherence or inconsistent adherence. Yet, continuous uninterrupted adherence to medicines during and following a disaster can be very difficult. Medicines may have been destroyed, for example, during flooding or may not be accessible if a clinic is no longer functional or drug supply chains are not working to deliver medicines and other essential clinic supplies. People experiencing sudden shock and grief may not remember to take their medicines, may be unable to care for themselves, and may be struggling to survive. Basic needs for food and shelter may be competing priorities as would be caring for dependents and searching for lost loved ones.

Not only is continuous adherence important for HIV-positive patients to suppress HIV, so is adherence to anti-TB treatment, ongoing prevention of TB through the use of isoniazid (INH)

TABLE 27.1 When to Start ART

Adults (>19 years old)	ART should be initiated in all adults regardless of WHO clinical stage and at any CD4 cell count
Pregnant and breastfeeding women	ART should be initiated in all pregnant and breastfeeding women regardless of WHO clinical stage and at any CD4 cell count and continued lifelong
Adolescents (10–19 years of age)	ART should be initiated in all adolescents regardless of WHO clinical stage and at any CD4 cell count
Infants and children younger than 10 years of age	ART should be initiated in all children living with HIV, regardless of WHO clinical stage or at any CD4 cell count
Adults and children with TB	ART should be started in all TB patients living with HIV regardless of CD4 count: 1. TB treatment should be initiated first, followed by ART as soon as possible within the first 8 weeks of treatment 2. HIV-positive TB patients with profound immunosuppression (e.g., CD4 counts less than 50 cells/mm^3) should receive ART within the first 2 weeks of initiating TB treatment.

ART, antiretroviral therapy; TB, tuberculosis.

Source: World Health Organization. (2016a). *Consolidated guidelines on the use of antiretroviral drugs for treating and preventing HIV infection: Recommendations for a public health approach* (2nd ed.). Geneva, Switzerland: Author.

prophylaxis, and *Pneumocystis jirovecii* pneumonia prophylaxis through the use of cotrimoxazole.

Differentiated Service Delivery

Differentiated service delivery (DSD) is a patient-centered strategy to HIV service delivery. While keeping the public health approach, DSD considers alternative service delivery models for diverse groups of people living with HIV (PLHIV) such as patients with stable disease, unstable disease, or even displaced PLHIV (Duncombe et al., 2015). The aim of DSD is to enhance the quality and efficiency of services provided across the HIV care continuum, patient satisfaction, and utilization of resources. There are four main models of differentiated ART delivery (International AIDS Society, 2016):

- Facility-based individual models, which consider appointment spacing and "fast-track" ART refills
- Out-of-facility individual models where ART refills and appointments can be provided in the community or at home
- Healthcare worker–managed group models (facility- or community-based), where a healthcare worker provides refills to a group of patients
- Client-managed group models (community-based) where ART refill is managed by patients themselves

The community models are especially interesting to consider during humanitarian crises to avoid disruption of HIV services.

CLINICAL CONSIDERATIONS IN CARING FOR PATIENTS WITH HIV AND AIDS

Persons living with HIV and AIDS require periodic monitoring of their condition, current treatment regimen, and any adverse drug toxicities. Similar to management of other chronic conditions, establishment of a strong patient/provider relationship improves care and long-term management of the disease.

Following diagnosis and enrollment in a treatment program, patients on ARV medications receive chronic care services including adherence counseling and routine checkups to assess for drug side effects, drug toxicities, and ongoing response to treatment. Patients are also routinely assessed for signs and symptoms of OIs. In a disaster where HIV-positive people and people with AIDS experience overcrowding, poor sanitation, and inadequate nutrition, there may be a sudden increase in the incidence of OIs.

HIV services can begin without lab diagnostics through the use of a thorough history and physical examination and HIV clinical staging but in general, even in low-resource settings, access to HIV-related laboratory diagnostics is becoming increasingly common and a routine part of HIV care.

Examples of commonly run laboratory tests include:

- VL testing to assess a patient's response to ART and risk for clinical progression and treatment failure. WHO guidelines recommend VL testing as part of routine therapeutic monitoring for all HIV-infected children and adults on ART.

- CD4 cell count to monitor HIV patients, although VL testing is increasingly available and preferred. (WHO, 2016a).
- Basic chemistries with special emphasis on kidney (creatinine clearance) and liver function (e.g., serum glutamic oxaloacetic transaminase [SGOT], aspartate aminotransferase [AST]) as some ARV drugs can cause renal toxicity or liver inflammation.
- Assessing hemoglobin as some drugs can worsen anemia, for example, zidovudine (AZT).

SPECIAL CONSIDERATIONS IN CHILDREN AND PREGNANT WOMEN

In addition to the care outlined above, children need ongoing assessment of their growth and development, immunization status, and recalculation of their drug dosage requirement as they grow and gain weight. Adherence in children is equally important to adherence in adults. Yet, adherence challenges include ensuring infants and small children receive correct dosing as well as dealing with children who may not fully understand the importance of adherence. A child's status may be unknown if one's parent or primary caregiver is separated from the child or has died during a disaster. Regression and changes in behavior may also affect treatment adherence.

All HIV-positive women are eligible for immediate access to treatment under the policy of "test and treat." Ensuring access to pregnancy testing and ARVs should be prioritized for women of childbearing age. Special considerations during labor and delivery that may be interrupted during a disaster include access to ARVs and repeat HIV testing at labor for women previously testing negative.

Nursing Care Guidelines

As with other chronic conditions, nursing care of the HIV patient follows the continuum of care from pretreatment, ongoing treatment, and secondary prevention as well as end-of-life palliative care.

Prior to treatment, patients with HIV require counseling to ensure that once they start treatment, they are adherent. Pregnant women should be encouraged to test for HIV using an "opt out" approach. Pregnant women testing negative can be tested again later in pregnancy and during breastfeeding.

During the pretreatment phase in countries and context where eligibility is dependent on immunologic status, counseling is provided to promote positive living, facilitate disclosure to promote treatment support in the home or community, as well as discussion of the unique needs of discordant couples (where one partner is HIV negative and one is HIV positive). The pretreatment phase is being reduced or eliminated completely with the move to "test and start." This change requires strong nursing care and counseling at the time of diagnosis to support retention in care, disclosure, and drug adherence.

Once a person is on treatment, a primary objective is to preserve first-line treatment as long as possible. In poorly resourced settings, access to second- and third-line treatment is limited. Ensuring strict adherence is therefore essential. In addition, ongoing monitoring including routine laboratory assessment, VL testing, and review of signs of toxicity and mitigation of side effects are emphasized. Nursing care is especially important to assess treatment response, detect potential treatment failure, and monitor the need to switch to second-line regimens. Nursing care also includes psychosocial support and counseling on treatment fatigue, safe sex practices, and elements of positive living including good nutrition, limiting alcohol and smoking, and encouraging exercise and stress reduction.

Nutrition, Hygiene, and Sanitation

Access to clean, highly nutritious safe food is important for people with weakened immune systems. Food poisoning and waterborne illnesses, which may be self-limiting in a person without HIV, can have devastating consequences for an HIV-positive person. During disasters, not only can food be scarce, the ability to effectively clean and preserve food may be severely compromised. Clean water is also essential. There is an increased risk of poor outcomes if exposed to waterborne illnesses such as cholera. Undernutrition and food poisoning can be life-threatening to the HIV-positive and immunocompromised individual.

Children infected with HIV who suffer from chronic or acute malnutrition need access to energy (calorie)-dense, protein-rich foods. Therapeutic food, such as ready-to-use therapeutic foods (RUTF), is commonly used in emergency feeding settings that are established during disasters to treat severe malnutrition. The combination of malnutrition and HIV can be life-threatening for children and urgent specialized care is required to manage this comorbidity.

In most developing countries, exclusive breastfeeding for 6 months followed by ongoing breastfeeding is the most acceptable, feasible, affordable, safe, and sustainable way to feed both HIV-positive and HIV-negative infants. Areas where safe water is not routinely available and where the cost of infant formula is prohibitive will have high levels of breastfeeding. Therefore, targeting lactating mothers with nutritional support should be emphasized during the disaster response.

Nutrition key points:

- Ensure access to safe and highly nutritious food as well as clean water.
- Polluted water can have devastating consequences for immunocompromised people.
- Remember that HIV-positive patients (adults and children) generally have higher caloric requirements, especially if they are not yet on treatment. Young children should be encouraged to eat small, frequent (five) meals per day to ensure adequate caloric intake and adequate growth.
- Children's HIV medication is based on weight; therefore, if there has been a sudden change in weight, dose adjustments may be needed.

Drug Supplies and Drug Dumping

Drug supply chain needs to be assured during and after disaster. Emergency preparedness includes preparing for drug supply chain contingencies. Disaster preparation should anticipate environmental impacts on drug storage and distribution. Drug warehouses may be destroyed or flooded. Air-conditioning equipment and electricity may be damaged. The procurement of buffer stocks and backup generators should be secured.

Health promotion and anticipatory guidance with patients should encourage HIV-positive people to keep at least 1 month additional supply as a preventive, positive living measure.

Local, regional, and national leadership should ensure that drugs coming into disaster areas are not "dumped," are not expired, and meet national protocols and current treatment algorithms. Working with unknown drugs or formulas may lead to overdosing or underdosing, both of which can be devastating to the immunocompromised individual.

A nurse prepared to respond to a disaster should ask critical questions such as: Where are drug warehouses in the country or affected region? Are the drug warehouses still accessible? Are the drug stocks still viable? Who manages these warehouses and are they available and engaged in the disaster response?

In addition, ask if ARV drugs will be brought in from outside the country or region and will these drugs match national treatment guidelines? Will retraining of health workers be needed and if so, who will coordinate and manage this? These questions need to be answered efficiently so that disruption in treatment is minimized.

PSYCHOLOGICAL CONSIDERATIONS OF CARING FOR PATIENTS WITH HIV

The mental health needs of people during and after complex human emergencies are receiving greater emphasis and attention. Psychological considerations include understanding the incidence of PTSD and depression.

Psychological sequelae of a disaster can affect treatment adherence, influence safe sex practices, as well as one's ability to provide self-care and care for family members. Health workers should assess psychological needs as well as physical needs. The psychological needs of children must also be considered as children are tremendously dependent on adult caregivers and loss of a primary caregiver can have devastating effects on children.

SUMMARY

The needs of people with chronic illness are often overlooked in the immediate disaster aftermath as the focus is on emergency care and response. Caring for patients with HIV and AIDS following a disaster is a complex but essential task. Ensuring the continuity of care for HIV-infected individuals, maintaining ARV drug supply chains, and preventive measures such as PMTCT and PEP should be planned and budgeted for.

People living with HIV and AIDS have ongoing needs which, if not met, can lead to severe negative health outcomes. Without access to key HIV services such as PMTCT, vertical transmission of HIV will increase. If patients on HAART are unable to access their ARV medications, the development of drug resistance is a serious possibility. Care of HIV patients includes identifying those in need and ensuring a continuous supply of ARV drugs as well as medicines to prevent or treat common opportunistic infections, especially TB. Ensuring a continuum of HIV services should be prioritized when developing national, regional, and local disaster preparedness plans.

Guidelines exist to support healthcare workers, including the latest treatment guidelines from the WHO that are freely available on the WHO website (www.who.int) as well as the IASC Guidelines for Addressing HIV in Humanitarian Settings and the *Sphere Handbook*.

The case studies at the end of this chapter provide insight and lessons learned from providing HIV during complex humanitarian emergencies (Cases 27.1 and 27.2). A global health leader situated at Columbia University, ICAP has worked since 2003 with one central goal: to improve the health of families and communities (ICAP, 2018).

Working hand in hand with individuals at every level of the health system—from patients to healthcare providers to governmental officials—ICAP is dedicated to delivering high-performing health system strengthening initiatives that provide quality and affordable healthcare. The organization tackles the world's most pressing health threats and, in collaboration with partners around the world, implements transformative solutions to meet the health needs of individuals.

With its roots in comprehensive, family-focused HIV services, ICAP is known for capacity building and for its innovative, effective, and ethical programs that are implemented in the most challenging resource-limited settings. ICAP is also known for its collaborative and supportive approach to strengthening governmental health systems and local partners' capacity to deliver quality health services. To date, ICAP has worked to address major public health challenges and the needs of local health systems in more than 5,200 sites across 20 countries. Further information on ICAP's work in complex settings is available below and at the following website, icap.columbia.edu

REFERENCES

Alnuaimi, K., Kassab, M., Alia, R., Mohammed, K., & Shattnawi, K. (2017). Pregnancy outcomes among Syrian refugee and Jordanian women: A comparative study. *International Nursing Review, 64*(4), 584–592. doi:10.1111/inr.12382

Benjamin, J. A. (2001). Conflict, post-conflict, and HIV/AIDS—The gender connections. Women, war and HIV/AIDS: West Africa and the Great Lakes. Women's Commission for Refugee Women and Children. Retrieved from https://www.popline.org/node/234990

Bitarakwate, E., Strasser, S., Sripipatana, T., Shelley, K., Chintu, N., Musana, O., . . . Wilfert, C. (2011). *Introduction of rape syphilis testing*

within prevention of mother-to-child transmission of HIV programs in Uganda and Zambia: A field acceptability and feasibility study (Abstract No. TUPE470). 6th International AIDS Society (IAS) Conference on HIV Pathogenesis, Treatment and Prevention, Rome, Italy, July 17–20.

Broeckaert, L., & Challacombe, L. (2015). Rapid point-of-care HIV testing: A review of the evidence. *Prevention in Focus*. Retrieved from http://www.catie.ca/en/pif/spring-2015/rapid-point-care-hiv-testing-review-evidence

Brolin Ribacke, K. J., Saulnier, D. D., Eriksson, A., & von Schreeb, J. (2016). Effects of the West Africa Ebola virus disease on health-care utilization—A systematic review. *Front Public Health, 4*, 222. doi:10.3389/fpubh.2016.00222

Cohen, M. S., Chen, Y. Q., McCauley, M., Gamble, T., Hosseinipour, M. C., Kumarasamy, N., . . . Fleming, T. R.; HPTN 052 Study Team. (2011). Prevention of HIV-1 infection with early antiretroviral therapy. *The New England Journal of Medicine, 365*, 493–505. doi:10.1056/NEJMoa1105243

Collymore, Y. (2001). Uprooted people and HIV/AIDS in Africa: Responding to the risks. Population Reference Bureau (2011). Retrieved from https://www.prb.org/uprootedpeopleandhivaidsinafricarespondingtotherisks/

Duncombe, C., Rosenblum, S., Hellmann, N., Holmes, C., Wilkinson, L., Biot, M., . . . Garnett, G. (2015). Reframing HIV care: Putting people at the centre of antiretroviral delivery. *Tropical Medicine and International Health, 20*, 430–447. doi:10.1111/tmi.12460

Federal Emergency Management Agency. (2009, January 16). National Disaster Housing Strategy. Retrieved from https://www.fema.gov/media-library-data/20130726-1819-25045-9288/ndhs_core.pdf

Galea, S., Nandi, A., & Vlahov, D. (2005). The epidemiology of post-traumatic stress disorder after disasters. *Epidemiological Reviews, 27*, 78–91. doi:10.1093/epirev/mxi003

ICAP. (2018). Homepage. Retrieved from http://www.icap.columbia.edu/approach-and-impact/our-focus-areas

Inter-Agency Standing Committee. (2010). *Guidelines for addressing HIV in humanitarian settings*. Geneva, Switzerland: UNAIDS.

International AIDS Society. (2016). *Differentiated care for HIV: A decision framework for antiretroviral therapy delivery*. Geneva, Switzerland: Author.

Kuhn, L., Aldrovandi, G., Kinkala, M., Kanakas, C., Mwiyad, M., & Thea, D. (2010). Potential impact of new WHO criteria for antiretroviral treatment for prevention of mother to-child HIV transmission. *AIDS, 24*, 1371–1380.

Lima, V. D., Johnston, K., Hogg, R. S., Levy, A. R., Harrigan, R., & Anema, A. (2008). Expanded access to highly active antiretroviral therapy: A potentially powerful strategy to curb the growth of the HIV epidemic. *The Journal of Infectious Diseases, 198*, 59–67. doi:10.1086/588673

Lisam, S. (2014). Minimum initial service package (MISP) for sexual and reproductive health in disasters. *Journal of Evidence-Based Medicine, 7*, 245–248. doi:10.1111/jebm.12130

Miller, A., Madzima, R., Maruva, M., Mahomva, A., Keatinge, J., & Mbizvo, E. (2008). *Best practice. Revision of the Children Health Card in Zimbabwe: Modifying existing systems to improve general and HIV specific care of all children*. Harare, Zimbabwe: Ministry of Health and Child Welfare.

National Institute of Mental Health. (2011). *Post-traumatic stress disorder* (NIH Publication No. 08 6388). Bethesda, MD: Author.

Persad, G., Wertheimer, A., & Emanuel, E. J. (2009). Principles for allocation of scarce medical interventions. *The Lancet, 373*, 423–431. doi:10.1016/S0140-6736(09)60137-9

Rangaka, M. X., Wilkinson, R. J., Boulle, A., Glynn, J. R., Fielding, K., van Cutsem, G., . . . Maartens, G. (2014). Isoniazid plus antiretroviral therapy to prevent tuberculosis: A randomised double-blind, placebo-controlled trial. *The Lancet, 384*(9944), 682–690. doi:10.1016/S0140-6736(14)60162-8

Shacham, E., Rosenburg, N., Önen, N. F., Donovan, M., & Turner Overton, E. (2015). Persisting HIV-related stigma among an outpatient US clinic population. *International Journal of STD and AIDS, 26*(4), 243–250. doi:10.1177/0956462414533318

Sharps Containers-etc. (2013, July). Sharps safety for emergency medical responders. Retrieved from http://sharpscontainers-etc.com/sharps-safety-for-emergency-medical-responders

Suthar, A. B., Vitoria, M. A., Nagata, J. M., Anglaret, X., Mbori-Ngacha, D., Sued, O., . . . Doherty, M. (2015). Co-trimoxazole prophylaxis in adults, including pregnant women, with HIV: A systematic review and meta-analysis. *The Lancet HIV, 2*(4), e137–e150. doi:10.1016/S2352-3018(15)00005-3

The Sphere Project. (2011). *The Sphere Project: Humanitarian Charter and Minimum Standards in Humanitarian Response* (3rd ed.). Rugby, UK: Practical Action Publishing.

The TEMPRANO ANRS 12136 Study Group. (2015). A trial of early antiretrovirals and isoniazid preventive therapy in Africa. *New England Journal of Medicine, 373*, 808–822. doi:10.1056/NEJMoa1507198

UNAIDS. (2017). 90–90–90—An ambitious treatment target to help end the AIDS epidemic. Retrieved from http://www.unaids.org/en/resources/documents/2017/90-90-90

Walker, A. S., Mulenga, V., Ford, D., Kabamba, D., Sinyinza, F., Kankasa, C, . . . Gibb, D.; CHAP Team. (2007). The impact of daily cotrimoxazole

prophylaxis and antiretroviral therapy on mortality and hospital admissions in HIV-infected Zambian children. *Clinical Infectious Disease, 44*, 1361–1367. doi:10.1086/515396

World Health Organization. (2007). *Training modules for the syndromic management of sexually transmitted infections.* Geneva, Switzerland: Author.

World Health Organization. (2016a). *Consolidated guidelines on the use of antiretroviral drugs for treating and preventing HIV infection: Recommendations for a public health approach* (2nd ed.). Geneva, Switzerland: Author.

World Health Organization. (2016b). First WHO-prequalified hepatitis C rapid test opens door to expanded treatment. Retrieved from http://www.who.int/medicines/emp_newsletter_2016_q3_q4.pdf

CASE STUDY 27.1

Susan Michaels-Strasser, Shambal Aragaw, Juliana Soares Linn, Erica D'Aguila, Felix Ndagije, and Florence Bayoa

The Republic of South Sudan (RSS) has a generalized HIV epidemic with an estimated HIV prevalence among adults aged 15 to 49 years estimated at 2.5%, with 180,000 people living with HIV (PLHIV), and about 15,000 new infections in 2015.[1] Although the real magnitude of the epidemic is not fully known because of chronic conflicts that could not allow exhaustive studies, it is hypothesized that the HIV epidemic is geographically skewed within three Equatoria states, Eastern, Central, and Western Equatoria, accounting for 60% of new HIV infections.[2] While some progress in addressing HIV has been made, as of 2015 the national coverage for antiretroviral therapy (ART) was 10%, far below global targets for 90-90-90 and is due in part to the prevailing conflict.[3] In South Sudan's 2014 Global AIDS Response Country Progress Report, the government of South Sudan outlined national targets including increasing the number of PLHIV on ART from 10% to 80% (adults) and from 3% to 50% (children) by 2017 (South Sudan AIDS Commission and Ministry of Health).

RSS has a national strategic plan for HIV/AIDS known as the "National Strategic Plan" (NSP) for HIV and AIDS 2013 to 2017. The NSP is aligned to national and international frameworks, including the Sustainable Development Goals (SDGs) and specifically the health-related SDGs that target ending AIDS, tuberculosis, malaria and neglected tropical diseases, as well as combatting hepatitis and waterborne diseases.

The National HIV response is principally funded by the President's Emergency Fund for AIDS Relief (PEPFAR), the Global Fund to Fight AIDS TB and Malaria (GFATM), United Nations Agencies and Relief Agencies. The ongoing

humanitarian crisis, conflict, and the drop in oil prices have caused a severe fiscal crisis in South Sudan.

Despite the daunting challenges, with the support of implementing partners, the HIV treatment response has remained up to date with international guidelines, but at the same time contextualized to the country situation which is characterized by civil war, high number of returnees, and internally displaced persons (IDPs) facing humanitarian crisis. At the beginning of 2017, with support from ICAP, the WHO, and other implementing partners, the South Sudan Ministry of Health (MOH) started revising the HIV Care and Treatment guidelines to meet the WHO 2015 Test and Treat Guidelines. The guidelines in RSS provide context-specific recommendations for the delivery of HIV treatment services using a public health approach in a resource-constrained and conflict setting. The guidelines put into consideration that a large population including PLHIV face food insecurity and its potential impact on adherence to antiretroviral (ARVs) and opportunistic infections (OI) medications. The guidelines also provide direction on sustaining ART delivery during conflict, an essential minimum package of HIV services to be delivered during crises and conflict, a national HIV commodities supply chain standard operating procedures (SOP), and a remote site support strategy to ensure commodity management, staffing, and uninterrupted services to patients during times of unrest. Despite challenges, the country has managed to implement the use of VL testing, the gold standard for assessing treatment outcomes.

KEY CHANGES IN THE NEW RSS GUIDELINES

All newly diagnosed HIV-positive patients should be retested for HIV to verify their HIV-positive status prior to treatment initiation. This is being recommended as a measure to minimize "false-positive" test results considering the medical, psychological, social, and financial implications of lifelong

---

[1] Global AIDS Response Progress Reporting (GARPR), 2016.
[2] Republic of South Sudan. The President's Emergency Plan for AIDS Relief (PEPFAR) Country Operational Plan (COP), 2016. Strategic Direction Summary.
[3] South Sudan AIDS Commission and Ministry of Health (June 2015), South Sudan 2014 Global AIDS Response Country Progress Report. Republic of South Sudan.

(continued)

CASE STUDY 27.1 (*continued*)

ART treatment to an individual. The guidelines also advocate routinizing retesting for previously HIV-negative women who tested in the first trimester of pregnancy or first antenatal care (ANC) visit; who present in the third trimester during labor and/or delivery; and advocate for retesting every 3 months until 3 months after cessation of breastfeeding.

From a test and start approach, the guidelines stipulate that all HIV-positive adults and adolescents irrespective of CD4 counts or WHO stage should be started on ART (Treat All). Guidance is that a patient should be initiated on ART as soon as the patient is ready and preferably within 1 week of diagnosis. In adults and adolescents, the preferred first-line regimen is tenofovir + lamivudine (or emtricitabine) + efavirenz [TDF + 3TC (or FTC) + EFV] as a once-daily fixed dose combination (FDC) and should be prescribed for all population groups including adults, pregnant women, clients coinfected with HIV and TB or hepatitis B virus (HBV). With support from PEPFAR and Global Fund, RSS has introduced efavirenz 400 mg which has demonstrated fewer central nervous system–related side effects compared to the standard dose of 600 mg.

High quality integrated care is encouraged. For prevention of mother-to-child HIV transmission (PMTCT), the guidelines highlight that a complete set of fully integrated, routine antenatal care interventions should be offered where ART is initiated in all pregnant and breastfeeding women living with HIV, regardless of gestational age, WHO clinical stage and at any CD4 count, and continued lifelong. The guidelines underscore that for PMTCT, ART should be started, ideally, on the day of HIV diagnosis, and that an ongoing enhanced adherence support should be provided. PMTCT follow-up also emphasizes the role of VL monitoring.

The guidance also underscores that routine VL monitoring is recommended to facilitate state-of-the-art treatment monitoring but also to promptly and accurately detect treatment failure whenever it occurs. All patients started on ART are to have a routine VL test done at 6 and 12 months after beginning therapy and every 12 months for their lifetimes. In addition to this standard of care, VL tests are also to be conducted based on the clinical assessment for patients already on treatment who are showing evidence of immunologic and/or clinical failure.

As with previous guidelines, the new guidelines recommend that all PLHIV should be screened for TB including asking about TB exposure/contact history at each encounter with a health worker or visit to a health facility. Additionally, the new guidelines support that in PLHIV, isoniazid preventive therapy (IPT) will be administered for 6 months when patients have been screened "to have no symptoms or signs of TB; no history of active liver disease, liver insufficiency, or jaundice; no history of hypersensitivity to isoniazid; no history of exfoliative dermatitis and have been motivated for TB-IPT after being educated about the benefits, possible side-effects and risks."

In a country marred by unreliable early infant diagnosis (EID) testing and lengthy turnaround time (TAT) of results, rather than relying on a concrete positive result, the RSS guidelines have recommended that infant prophylaxis should be given based on *HIV risk stratification* until proven otherwise. High-risk infants are defined as: infants whose mothers have a high maternal VL >1,000 copies/mL during the last 4 weeks before delivery; born to an HIV-infected woman who has received less than 4 weeks of ART at the time of delivery; and born to a newly diagnosed HIV-infected woman during labor, delivery, and postpartum.

The guidelines indicate that health workers should offer high-risk infants dual ARV prophylaxis of AZT and Nevirapine (NVP) for 12 weeks after birth. The country has now recommended use of a PI-based regimen as the preferred first-line ART for children below 3 years of age. However, where LPV/r is not available mainly due to its requirement for cold chain conditions in a fragile situation marred by electricity blackouts, NVP-based regimens will be used for children under 3 years. For children above 3 years, EFV has been selected as the favored NNRTI backbone treatment. The national program anticipates that the heat-stable Kaletra pellets (LPV/r) will be introduced to replace the use of syrup with positive effect.

As underscored earlier on, differentiated service delivery models (DSDM) have been adopted as a preferred approach to ART delivery. DSDM is a novel approach that is client-centered, simplifies, and adapts HIV services across the cascade to reflect the healthcare needs, preferences, context, and expectations of various groups of people living with HIV (PLHIV). The guidelines recommend that stable clients who are doing well on treatment should be given five ARV pickup options, specifically: Fast-track ART Refill model; ART club refill model; ART Outreach model; Community ART Refill Groups; and, Family Member Refill model.

For HIV prevention in high-risk groups and key populations (KPs), ambitiously the RSS guidelines have adopted that PrEP will be offered to subpopulations at high risk of acquiring HIV such as commercial sex workers (CSW) and their clients, fishermen, long-distance truck drivers, men who have sex with men (MSM), uniformed forces, adolescents and young women engaged in transactional sex.

Whereas the RSS HIV program is relatively new and unstable due to chronic conflicts, with support of ICAP and other implementing partners, the program has kept pace with latest international guidelines and has been able to sustain ART services to patients in dire constraints. As conflicts change in form, predictability, and duration, it will be paramount for HIV programs, relief agencies and organizations, UN agencies and affected communities to partner to sustain services when conflicts, disasters, or calamities strike. Continued care is possible with strong preparation, planning, and partnerships.

Delivering HIV services in South Sudan

Susan Michaels-Strasser, Shambal Aragaw, Juliana Soares Linn, Erica D'Aguila, Felix Ndagije, and Florence Bayoa

ICAP began its partnership with South Sudan's Ministry of Health (MOH) in 2012. With support from the U.S. Presidents Emergency Plan for AIDS Relief (PEPFAR) through the Centers for Disease Control and Prevention (CDC), ICAP is providing technical assistance, training, and implementation support to South Sudan's MOH to strengthen fragile health systems impacted by decades of war. ICAP works closely with the MOH to improve the quality and reach of HIV testing and treatment across South Sudan.

In South Sudan, ICAP works at every level of the health system collaborating with national governments, district health management teams, and individual health facilities to strengthen the health system to support the national HIV response. Currently, ICAP supports 11 health facilities in five states across South Sudan. ICAP supports HIV testing services, quality assurance laboratory proficiency testing, EID and VL testing, and training and mentoring of healthcare workers. Guidelines, SOPs, patient information and education communication (IEC) resources and health worker job aids are also provided. In times of conflict, ICAP provides remote site support to enable continuity of care despite challenges.

While ICAP-South Sudan has faced inherent operational challenges due to the country's unstable political and economic context, strong outcomes have been achieved. In the last 6 months (October 2016 through March 2017), 13,783 individuals received HIV testing and counseling services and received their test results at ICAP-supported facilities. In addition, 1,701 pregnant women were tested for HIV and received their results; 131 pregnant women who tested positive for HIV were started on antiretroviral therapy (ART); 1,819 adults and children were newly enrolled on ART; 416 new and relapsed registered TB cases had documented HIV status; 33 ART patients were started on TB treatment; and 43 HIV-positive new and relapsed registered TB cases were initiated on ART during TB treatment.

A SUCCESS STORY: CREATING CONTINGENCY PLANS TO ENSURE CONTINUED HIV CARE IN EMERGENCIES AND PROTRACTED CONFLICT

South Sudan is the newest nation established after a protracted war that lasted for more than four decades. With less than 2 years as an independent country, South Sudan saw a civil war erupt again in December 2013, creating serious challenges for the continuation of HIV services and sustaining supply chains for people on lifelong ART. Based on the lessons learned from the 2013 crisis, ICAP collaborated with the MOH, WHO, the International Organization for Migration (IOM), and International Rescue Committee (IRC) to build the country's capacity and resiliency in the face of subsequent national crises.

Beginning in 2016, ICAP introduced a contingency plan to the national HIV/AIDS program during the annual HIV/AIDS review and planning workshop for states and the annual HIV/AIDS review and planning workshop for ART sites. ICAP also convened an HIV treatment and care contingency planning workshop for key national stakeholders and partners.

These ICAP-led collaborations revitalized an emergency TB/HIV technical working group and supported the development of a contingency plan for HIV services in crisis situations, SOPs for the continuation of HIV services in emergency situations, a minimum package of HIV services during crises, a national HIV commodities supply chain SOP (including a supply chain contingency plan for emergencies), training for facility- and state-level healthcare workers on continuation of services during emergency situations, and prepositioning of stock to nearby and key locations across the nation.

As a result of these efforts and preparatory activities led by ICAP, facilities were able to continue to provide services to patients, did not experience stock outs of antiretroviral drugs, and were able to dispense 3 months' worth of medication to patients so they could avoid needing to travel to facilities during an extended period of conflict.

Fortunately, plans and tools developed and disseminated during these workshops and trainings were available for implementation during the most recent crisis, which commenced in July 2016. During and in the immediate aftermath of the July 2016 crisis, which left over 300 people killed, ICAP was able to communicate with all 18 ICAP-supported ART clinics on a weekly basis as well as the central HIV commodities warehouse and humanitarian partners to ensure continued availability of ARVs.

> "We have some HIV patients who were in Juba during the July incident who lost everything," said a nurse at the Juba Teaching Hospital. "They were able to come back to the facility to get antiretroviral drugs and stay on treatment."

ICAP's interventions, together with the MOH, central warehouse, and health facilities before and during the July 2016 political crisis, enabled the continuation of HIV services and availability of ARVs and related commodities for the majority of PLHIV in South Sudan; this is a tremendous success that has not been achieved in previous crises.

Overall, these efforts enabled 937 patients to initiate ART during the crisis in 18 ICAP-supported health facilities. Facilities were able to retain 70% of adults and children on treatment 12 months after the initiation of ART, even during the political crisis.

Going forward, ICAP will continue supporting facilities and state and national MOHs to promote and implement the contingency planning exercise to sustain HIV care and treatment in case of emergencies and protracted war.

DISASTER CAUSED BY CHEMICAL, BIOLOGICAL, AND RADIOLOGICAL AGENTS

28

BIOLOGICAL AND CHEMICAL TERRORISM: A UNIQUE THREAT

Eric Croddy and Gary Ackerman

LEARNING OBJECTIVES

When this chapter is completed, readers will be able to:

1. Understand the difference between what might be possible versus probable in the case of terrorists using chemical and biological (CB) agents as weapons of mass destruction (WMD).
2. Distinguish between the features of a possible CB terrorist event.
3. Learn the basic categories of CB agents one might encounter in an unconventional attack.
4. Anticipate what challenges any hospital or clinic would face in the rush of casualties and "worried well" in the event of a real (or perceived) chemical or biological terrorist event.
5. Define the basic features of mass psychogenic illness and apply this to the public's reaction to real or perceived bioterrorist threats.

KEY MESSAGES

Historically, terrorists have used toxic compounds or pathogens in targeted attacks on civilians. Improvised chemical or biological weapons, although menacing to the general public, are likely to be limited in their ability to cause casualties. The effects of a chemical or biological terrorist event on society at large, however, may be greatly multiplied because of the mystique and fearsome images these weapons possess.

Because of the difficulties involved in using such unconventional weapons, it is more likely that terrorists will continue to use more conventional devices (explosives) or automatic weapons.

Chemical agents that could be used in terrorism are likely to cause casualties within an hour or more, whereas biological agents (as in bioterrorism) are not likely to be recognized at the very least until many hours or days after their release. Decontamination measures may be called for, especially in the case of chemical agents.

Nerve agents, cyanide, and a range of toxic industrial chemicals may be utilized against civilians in acts of terrorism. These are self-limiting events, however, and can be essentially regarded as hazardous materials (HAZMAT) incidents. In the event of bioterrorism, victims of exposure and subsequent infection are likely to be identified in healthcare settings, perhaps days or weeks following an event, constituting a public health issue with a potential for high numbers of casualties.

Finally, a significant challenge in a large incident involving chemical or biological agents are the numbers of sick, worried, and possibly panicked individuals showing up en masse at hospitals or clinics. Remaining calm and projecting confidence can ease the anxiety of such patients. This is just as important in cases of psychogenic illness, where an etiological agent is not found but in which victims present with any number of symptoms and require medical attention.

CHAPTER OVERVIEW

The prospect of chemical or biological terrorism, especially an event that causes mass casualties (i.e., a WMD) poses a great challenge to the U.S. healthcare system. The use of infectious organisms or toxic compounds by terrorists can have both immediate and long-term effects. But even if our understanding of terrorism is inchoate, it is also important to keep the real risks in perspective. The terrorist operates in a different world than a state-run military, and the contrast is especially important when it comes to developing chemical or biological weapons. Past experience, and the technically demanding nature of CB weapons suggest that terrorists will continue to rely mostly on conventional explosives and firearms. This is likely because, as one researcher put it, "although terrorists do innovate in various ways, groups have most often preferred to use weapons that have a proven track record" (Cronin, 2004). Since 2001, conventional weapons—in particular improvised explosive devices (IEDs)—have caused horrific numbers of deaths and injuries, notably in Iraq, Afghanistan, Syria, and elsewhere. By 2006, for example, IEDs were responsible for roughly half of all American casualties in Iraq and accounted for 30% of all deaths and injuries to U.S. military personnel in Afghanistan (Wilson, 2006). And even with the recent use of chemical weapons (chlorine and sarin nerve agent) by the Syrian regime against civilian targets (most recently in April 2018), it has been conventional bombs, artillery, and bullets that have been responsible for the vast majority (about 99 percent) of overall deaths and casualties in the Syrian conflict (approaching 511,000 as of April 2018).

In the event of mass casualty events, such as those that may result from an attack with large quantities of toxic nerve agents or biological pathogens, hospitals and other emergency healthcare facilities may be forced to make stark choices in triaging patients. Given the heightened awareness of the real or perceived threat of chemical or biological terrorism in today's society, it is also likely that mass psychogenic illness may present itself in a given population. Distinguishing such events involving mass anxiety from actual cases of biological and chemical terrorism may be quite difficult, at least early on.

During the Cold War (ca. 1945–1991), the United States and the former Soviet Union stockpiled massive CB weapons arsenals. Yet, in the years following the collapse of the Soviet Union, the threat of Warsaw Pact forces employing CB weapons against the Western NATO countries has all but vanished. Both the United States and Russia, between them once possessing some 70,000 tons of chemical weapons, are on their way to completely destroying these stocks. As for biological weapons, although suspicions remain, no conclusive evidence is available to indicate that these are currently possessed by Russia. The United States renounced offensive biological weapons research in 1969 and destroyed all remaining biological weapons in the early 1970s. Other nations, however, such as North Korea, are widely cited as having chemical and perhaps biological weapons capabilities (Bolton, 2002), and we have already seen that the Syrian regime of Bashar al-Assad has been responsible for killing thousands of its own people using chlorine gas and sarin—even after Syria had pledged to rid itself of chemical weapons in 2013.

Still, compared with the many instances of attacks using conventional explosives, the use of weapons employing toxic or infectious agents by terrorists has been relatively rare. Yet, particularly since the 1990s, much has been made (rightly or wrongly) of the threat from terrorists using CB agents. Although often referred to as WMDs, it is not clear that either chemical or biological weaponry can easily cause the thousands of casualties that one might expect from nuclear or even some conventional explosives. Nonetheless, the impact of a large CB terrorist event could be catastrophic for any populated city, presenting a unique and seemingly overwhelming challenge to the U.S. public healthcare system (Winslow, 1999). Although the list of CB threats in a war milieu is harrowing enough—nerve agents (e.g., sarin), anthrax, botulinum toxin, and so on—in the civilian context there are also other tools of unconventional warfare. These include the improvised use of toxic household products, the deliberate spread of foodborne pathogens, and the intentional release of industrial chemicals (Stern, 1999). In the fecund mind of a terrorist, there are doubtless many more possibilities.

Aside from the immediate care of those directly affected by CB agents, the psychological impact of this type of terrorism may prove just as challenging. To be sure, healthcare providers must be cognizant of the real dangers posed *by CB terrorism. But we also need to recognize the signs of mass anxiety, psychogenic illness, and other mental pathologies that may accompany real or perceived cases of CB terrorist attacks (Hyams, Murphy, & Wessely, 2002). How can one distinguish the true casualty from the "worried well"? How does the American healthcare system handle mass psychogenic illness in an age of CB terrorism? Are we prepared for long-term psychological sequelae such as PTSD? Some have even suggested that, indeed, in the case of bioterrorism, the psychological effect is a more prominent threat than its actual use (Moscrop, 2001).*

Regardless of how one views the threat of chemical or biological terrorism, it seems clear that the modern public health profession demands thorough knowledge and thoughtful approaches to the problem. Both past experience and current events suggest that, once thus committed, little can stop a determined terrorist from obtaining chemicals or biological pathogens/toxins and assembling these into some sort of delivery device. The immediate questions that should concern us are: How significant is the threat, and what should we do about it?

CHEMICAL TERRORISM AND BIOTERRORISM DEFINED

For the healthcare professional who is dealing with urgent casualties, it probably makes little difference as to what label one uses to describe a mass event involving CB weapons, whether it is the result of terrorism, criminal activity, or the work of a lone actor. However, to be reasonably consistent, a brief word is necessary to define terms. In this chapter, we will refer to terrorism as defined by Bruce Hoffman, who argues that it describes "the deliberate creation and exploitation of fear through violence or the threat of violence in the pursuit of political change" (Hoffman, 1998, p. 41). Thus, the use of chemical or biological agents as the main element of a terrorist attack or threat would be referred to as "chemical terrorism" and "bioterrorism," respectively.

When the use of CB weapons falls within the rubric of WMD, we are looking at acts of violence that involve large numbers of casualties. But what defines a "large number" of casualties (including dead and wounded)? Do we mean dozens, hundreds, or thousands?

To answer this question, let us look at an example of a terrorist WMD event in which a conventional explosive was used. The massive bomb (about 4,000 pounds) that destroyed the Murrah Building in Oklahoma City on April 19, 1995, killed 168 and injured hundreds more. Although no toxic chemicals or pathogens were involved, the scope and scale of destruction qualified this terrorist weapon as a WMD. (Timothy McVeigh and his coconspirator in the bombing, Terry Lynn Nichols, were later indicted on federal WMD-related charges.) At the risk of being arbitrary, we could use this example in terms of its numbers of casualties to define what we would consider to be a catastrophic event. Indeed, the

current definition of WMD used by the U.S. Department of Defense, while lengthy, covers these under a large rubric: to include "chemical, biological, radiological, or nuclear weapons or devices capable of a high order of destruction and/or causing mass casualties. This does not include the means of transporting or propelling the weapon where such a means is separable and divisible part of the weapon" (Burton, Burpo, & Garcia, 2014, p. 65).

But even a small number of casualties caused by either chemical or biological agents can have reverberating effects throughout our society. As an example, the letters containing anthrax spores mailed after September 11, 2001, resulted in the deaths of five people (Shane, 2002). While tragic, these numbers are far outweighed by various deaths that occur from shootings and other violence on a daily basis in the United States. Yet the anthrax attacks in fall 2001 shut down governmental buildings, post office facilities, while spurring a great number of individuals to take unwarranted steps, such as self-medicating (with antibiotics) and purchasing protective masks. The anthrax attacks clearly demonstrated the potential to cause large numbers of casualties, and we can therefore regard such as acts of bioterrorism.

Chemical and Biological Agents: Quick Definitions

"Chemical agents" include the many toxic chemicals that may be available to terrorists. Everything from chlorine gas to the highly potent nerve agents (e.g., toxic organophosphate compounds) are considered in this category. We can distill its essence in the following way: *Chemical weapons utilize the toxic nature of selected substances to cause death or injury. These chemical warfare (CW) agents may cause injury via the respiratory route, through the skin, or by ingestion.*

"Biological agents" are those pathogens used deliberately to infect persons, as well as toxins normally derived from plants or animals. As with naturally occurring infectious diseases, biological agents used in terrorism can infect through respiratory and ingestion routes. Vectors such as arthropods may also be involved, but are much less likely to be utilized in bioterrorism. Finally, save for trichothecene mycotoxins—the purported active ingredient in the now discounted "Yellow Rain" allegations of the 1980s (Desjardins, 2004)—none of the widely recognized biological warfare (BW) agent threats are dermally active (Wannemacher & Wiener, 1997).

WHY WOULD TERRORISTS USE CHEMICAL OR BIOLOGICAL AGENTS?

There are a number of reasons why terrorist groups or individuals might consider using CB agents. For someone intent on causing large-scale death and disruption, these agents, when used effectively, are theoretically capable of inflicting enormous casualties and causing massive disruption to society. Indeed, a lengthy 2003 treatise by a radical Saudi cleric took great pains to legitimize the use of WMD as a means to kill millions of civilians in the West (al-Fahd, 2003). Other terrorists may develop an inherent fascination with these rather exotic agents that for some evoke biblical or apocalyptic connotations.

Yet terrorists are most likely to be motivated to use chemical or biological agents for the following reason: By virtue of their novel and fearsome qualities, unconventional agents can be used as a "force multiplier" terror weapon against an unprotected population (Falkenrath, Newman, & Thayer, 1998). Because the primary goal of most terrorists is to strike fear and uncertainty, some authors have also suggested that

> the now routine journalistic association between chemical and biological weapons and the word terror confirms that the purpose of these weapons is to wreak destruction via psychological means—by inducing fear, confusion, and uncertainty in everyday life. These effects will take two forms, acute and long term. (Wessely, Hyams, & Bartholomew, 2001, p. 878)

Implicit in this statement is fear of the unknown, which can also be a powerful weapon for the terrorist. Especially for the general public, ignorance of the details concerning chemical or biological agents and their various means of delivery will be a source of acute apprehension. After all, the topic of CB warfare is relatively obscure, relegated mostly to military or scientific texts that have little bearing on what most people face from day to day. Furthermore, while the public may learn some details regarding CB agents from popular entertainment or superficial reading on the topic, this often only intensifies anxieties. When it comes to the topic of chemical or biological terrorism, people might ask themselves some very troubling questions: Will even low levels of toxic exposure mean painful death, long-term, debilitating illness, and birth defects? Will a bioterrorist release a pathogen that lays waste much of mankind, leaving only survivors who envy the dead? Even without the actual use of CB weapons, its mere suggestion can inject a powerful psychological element that is sometimes exacerbated by popular media and overactive imaginations. Terrorists are no doubt eager to capitalize on such vulnerabilities.

Another important consideration is that, to the extent that some terrorist groups may wish to acquire a nuclear weapon, designing an effective chemical or biological device would be relatively easier to build and deploy. Iranian President Rafsanjani's infamous statement in 1988 that chemical weapons were the "poor man's atomic bomb" seems appropriate here.

However, a better way of approaching this question might be to ask: Why *wouldn't* a terrorist choose a chemical or biological weapon? A number of researchers in terrorism have proposed a set of disincentives for a terrorist group to turn to such devices. One of the more often cited reasons is a traditional propensity among terrorists to use conventional weapons (bombs and bullets) that are a much more familiar technology for the average terrorist and more predictable in their effects. (We know now, for example, that Bruce Ivins, likely responsible for mailing anthrax in letters in 2001, was an experienced biodefense researcher with specialized expertise in processing anthrax bacteria.) Another argument is that because many terrorist groups usually rely on a political base for funding and other support, using chemical or biological agents might offend the moral sensibilities of their supporters (Gurr & Cole, 2000). (Usually left unexplained, however, is why such an audience would countenance the murder of civilians in the first place, including women and children.) Alternatively, some contend that terrorist organizations that do *not* rely on an outside constituency are *more* apt to employ CB weapons. This could include groups that are waning in influence and that, feeling they have nothing else to lose, may employ such weapons in a last desperate act (Hurwitz, 1982).

Disinformation or Hoaxes

The mere *threat* of an attack using dangerous chemical or biological materials can cause great anxiety and disorder, in any society. As a result of the attack using the nerve agent sarin on the Tokyo subway in 1995, for example, the numbers of psychosomatic victims and "worried well" far exceeded the actual number of victims. Subsequent to the attack, metropolitan Tokyo subways experienced a rash of false alarms, excited reports of unknown noxious odors in commuter subway trains, and other purported releases of irritating substances.

Prior to the few real cases of anthrax spores in letters in the fall of 2001, the United States had already experienced a rash of anthrax hoaxes; such incidents also occurred in other countries, including China. Most often these hoaxes involved mailed letters or parcels, sometimes containing a powder or other suspicious-looking substance, with a note saying that the victim had been exposed to anthrax. Before October 2001, none of these hoaxes contained any harmful substances, yet prudence dictated full security and decontamination procedures—often causing substantial disruption and incurring great financial costs in their response. During and subsequent to the appearance of the real anthrax letters, there were several hundred more hoaxes in both the United States and in other countries, perpetuating fear among the public, and requiring even more resource expenditure.

But it is also worth noting that "panic"—depending upon how one defines it—is less common than one may believe. In a cursory study of five cases: the 1995 sarin attack in Tokyo; September 11 (9/11); the anthrax letter attacks (2001); the July 7, 2005, London bombings; and chemical weapons use during World War I, "the evidence . . . suggests that in the immediate aftermath of an attack, the public is fairly resilient, calm, and rational in its reactions." The authors of this study suggest that "effective risk communication could mitigate the adverse behavioral reactions that could undermine a nation's response," and "to promote these desired behavioral responses, government can increase the public's understanding of [chemical, biological and radiological] terrorism without causing undue alarm" (Sheppard, Rubin, Wardman, & Wessely, 2006, p. 240).

How Might the Choice of CB Weapons Differ Between Military and Terrorist Use?

It is not just that CB agents are highly toxic or infectious. What is also common among CB agents that have been developed for warfare is their relative ease of dissemination. To be effective as weapons, they should also be reasonably stable in storage and maintain their potency until delivered to the target.

Another factor that has been considered of most importance to militaries—but not necessarily for terrorists—is the capacity of a given agent to cause large numbers of casualties (including dead and wounded). In the military context, for example, inflicting nonlethal injuries can create *more* logistical problems for the enemy. Chemical casualties that survive exposure, for example, generally require medical treatment, evacuation, and decontamination measures, resulting in serious logistical burdens. On the battlefield, forcing the enemy to care for the living—all the while having to conduct operations—makes chemical weaponry a significant "force multiplier."

Therefore, decades ago when the United States was still prepared to use offensive chemical weapons, reference tables were used to calculate the exact number of nerve agent shells required for a given target. U.S. Army manuals directed that only enough artillery shells were to be used to create incapacitating doses (not necessarily lethal ones) for the enemy. This was not done to be more humane, but rather to achieve the desired effect of causing mass casualties while conserving ammunition stores (United States, Department of the Army, Air Force, 1958).

Likewise, the United States and the former Soviet Union could choose among BW agents that were lethal or those that were mostly nonfatal, depending on the mission. Given that the inhaled route of anthrax infection is among the most lethal (more than 50% could die even with medical treatment), and a weapon delivering an aerosol of anthrax spores would mean large numbers of fatalities. In other situations, Venezuelan equine encephalitis (VEE) virus could be employed, in which case most of those infected with VEE would be incapacitated by the disease but relatively few would die (Smith et al., 1997).

The terrorist, however, will likely have very different criteria for choosing a CB agent for an attack. Unlike state-level militaries, terrorist organizations have much less flexibility, funds, or luxury of time and space to develop full-fledged CB weapon programs. (Some resourceful groups may pursue the acquisition of CB warfare agents developed by state programs, but most will be forced to improvise to some extent.) On the one hand, then, terrorists may be more likely than militaries to use lethal agents, as they do not necessarily share with the military the strategic goal of creating large numbers of wounded. Unlike most state-level military planners, terrorists will attempt to gain as much impact as possible from limited resources and are more likely to use more commonly found chemicals or pathogens—even if these are less toxic than modern warfare agents (e.g., nerve agents). Typical is an example in 2009, when a middle-aged Tucson, Arizona resident, Todd Russell Fries, built improvised chlorine gas devices that spread toxic vapors throughout a residential area. While no injuries were reported, the prosecuting attorney stated, "This defendant developed and executed a chlorine gas attack that impacted an entire neighborhood and had potential to cause tremendous harm and fear" (Gaynor, 2011). Lastly, unlike militaries facing well-equipped and well-trained troops, terrorists usually take aim at civilian populations who have no direct access to protective measures like gas masks or biosafety suits.

Terrorists, therefore, have a much wider scope in their choice of agents than do most militaries. After all, if creating havoc and fear among civilians is the primary goal, terrorists can choose from a wide range of lethal or irritating chemical compounds and pathogens. Foodborne pathogens and derived toxins could be utilized in some fashion, from the more deadly (e.g., botulinum toxin) to predominantly incapacitating (e.g., staphylococcal enterotoxins). Regardless of the agent employed, the psychological shock of such an event to a community, society, and polity may be more than sufficient for the purposes of CB terrorism.

Some Unique Aspects of a Chemical or Biological Terrorist Incident

Knowing beforehand that incoming patients are victims of a CB attack would, of course, be useful to anticipate and triage casualties, as well as to plan for long-term treatment modalities. But the fact that casualties were deliberately caused by a terrorist attack involving chemical or biological agents may go unrecognized for some time. Two examples illustrate this latter point.

In Matsumoto City, Japan, at almost midnight on June 27, 1994, the local police station was informed that patients were being rushed to the hospital and alerted to the fact that the nature of their injuries seemed most unusual. Further investigation discovered five deceased at an apartment complex. Two seriously affected individuals later died at the hospital, while another 270 victims were treated. Around the residential area, dead animals—dogs, birds, and large insects—were also discovered under foliage. Most of the casualties were located within about 150 m of a pond, in which dead fish and crustaceans were also found. Initial reports of casualties indicated that they were suffering from darkened vision, eye pain, miosis, nausea, and markedly lowered serum cholinesterase activity (Seto, Tsunoda, Kataoka, Tsuge, & Nagano, 2000). It took a week following the event to determine that sarin nerve agent was responsible. But the authorities (and aggressive news media) nonetheless spent the next several weeks hounding a local victim of sarin poisoning, Mr. Kono, now a leading suspect (albeit for spurious reasons). (Gamble & Watanabe, 2004). At long last, Japanese investigators finally suspected the Japanese apocalyptic millenarian cult, Aum Shinrikyo, was responsible. As it turned out, the aforementioned cult had, in fact, used sarin nerve agent in an attempt to assassinate local magistrates in Matsumoto City. None of these intended targets, however, were killed (Tu, 2002).

Likewise, the foodborne outbreak (salmonellosis) in The Dalles, Oregon, perpetrated by the Rajneeshees in September 1984, was not known to have been deliberately caused for almost a year. Were it not for a sudden and incriminating statement outburst by its leader that led to a full investigation by state and federal authorities, it is likely that the Oregon *Salmonella typhimurium* outbreak would have never been solved (Miller et al., 2001).

What Are the Real Risks of Chemical Terrorism/Bioterrorism?

Perhaps the greatest challenges presented by a large-scale CB terrorism attack are the logistical and psychological demands on the healthcare system. Not only is this a matter of staff resources, treatments, equipment, and decontamination measures, but also involves the very basic and challenging limitations of space. One can imagine the stress created by a mass casualty event when victims show up by the hundreds, maybe thousands, looking for beds. For the healthcare provider (and this is especially applicable in the military context), chemical or biological attacks may not only cause a significant number to die, but they will also create many more injured (or infected) requiring care. Hospital staff and other healthcare workers will be hard-pressed to cope with so many injured people of all ages, undoubtedly bringing enormous difficulties for any healthcare facility. Adding to the stressors already present, critical health support staff are also likely to be very concerned for their own safety and that of their families.

CHEMICAL TERRORISM

In nearly all respects, chemical terrorism is essentially a HAZMAT event. Unlike the effects of a contagious biological agent release (e.g., smallpox), chemical events are generally self-limiting. A chemical terrorist attack may include small or large numbers of casualties, and, depending on the agent used, victims may require special decontamination measures.

Delivery of Chemical Agents

In a military setting, the effectiveness of CW agents is optimized by producing contaminated areas with high concentrations of a toxic compound. Since World War I, the method of delivering chemicals has remained largely the same, such as filling artillery shells or bombs with a particular CW agent (e.g., xylyl bromide, mustard agent). Chemical compounds that are gaseous at room temperature (e.g., phosgene), or are extremely volatile (e.g., hydrogen cyanide or HCN), do not need much engineering to deliver. Because of their gaseous state, however, they also disperse rapidly, demanding a large quantity to be delivered to the target. Due to its high volatility, HCN attacks in military field situations have always been famously ineffective, as a classic treatise on chemical weapons remarked that "Because of its extreme volatility and the fact that its vapors are lighter than air, it is almost impossible to establish a lethal concentration of hydrocyanic acid [i.e., cyanide gas] in the field, and this is particularly true when the gas is put over in artillery shells" (Prentiss, 1937, p. 173).

For liquid or solid CW agents that do not produce vapors, creating large areas of contamination in the military context is accomplished by spraying from an aerial bomb or dispersing them from artillery (explosive) munitions. Maximizing the amount of CW agent in a given area is achieved by producing an aerosol, loosely defined here as a cloud of suspended liquid or solid particles. Although aerosols can increase the effectiveness and lethality of CW agents, some chemical compounds are versatile enough to deliver in other forms. Mustard, a blister agent, can produce contact injuries by contaminating surfaces, while its vapors also present a severe hazard to the upper respiratory system.

For a *terrorist* who is intent on causing chemical casualties, acquiring "higher end" agents such as military nerve agents (e.g., sarin) might be too difficult or even unnecessary. (The Japanese cult, Aum Shinrikyo, employed an organic chemist and had the requisite funding, laboratory equipment, and precursor chemicals.) Instead, the would-be chemical terrorist could utilize toxic chemicals procured from commercial suppliers, or even synthesize hazardous compounds for dissemination (Tour, 2000). By their very nature, improvised chemical weapons are also more likely to be crude and inefficient. For example, HCN would likely be effective only if utilized in a relatively small, confined space.

The list of potential chemical agents that could be used in terrorism is quite extensive. Full and detailed discussions on CW agents can be found in Chapter 29 "Chemical Agents of Concern" and in the literature (Marrs, Maynard, & Sidell, 1996). Rather than simply running through such a listing, it makes more sense to look at the most important physiological effects of different classes of chemicals that could be used in terrorism. These are:

- Nerve agents (e.g., sarin)
- Blood agents (e.g., cyanide)
- Lung irritants (e.g., chlorine gas)
- Vesicants (i.e., blister agents such as mustard gas or lewisite)
- Psychoincapacitants (e.g., BZ, LSD)
- Pesticides (more psychological than toxic in their effects)

Nerve Agents

Nerve agents include the chemicals tabun, sarin, soman, and VX. These toxic organophosphate compounds all operate on the same basic principle—they inhibit acetylcholinesterase (AChE), which normally break down acetylcholine, an essential neurotransmitter. The resulting abnormally high levels of acetylcholine in the body after exposure to nerve agents bring about respiratory and cardiovascular crises that can quickly lead to death. Terrorists should find little difficulty in learning about how to produce nerve agents. Information on the precursors and even synthesis steps for the production of toxic organophosphate compounds, including the military nerve agents (sarin, VX, etc.), are widely available in the open literature.

For the terrorist who operates in an improvised setting, other compounds, although less toxic than military nerve agents, may in some ways be easier to produce or acquire than the other classic war gases. Such substances may, in certain cases, also have legitimate medical or industrial uses and be available through specialty chemical suppliers.

International terrorists may also be pursuing the development of nerve agents for attacks on civilian targets. Persuasive (albeit controversial) evidence suggests that members of the Al-Qaeda terror network may have produced VX nerve agent while in Sudan with the connivance of Iraqi CW scientists (Croddy, 2002). However, with regard to the latter case, little or no evidence has been offered that provides convincing proof

(9/11 Commission, 2004). There are also reports that the Islamic State of Iraq and Syria (ISIS) has used the toxic industrial chemical phosphine (which has nerve agent-like effects) in at least three attacks in 2015 (Chivers, 2015). In any event, both Al-Qaeda and ISIS have expressed interest in conducting attacks using chemical and biological weapons (Warrick, 2015). There is also evidence that ISIS has produced its own sulfur mustard agent munitions in terrorist attacks in Syria, and may have also been pursuing acquisition of anthrax bacteria (McCormick, 2016).

In February 2017, the North Korean government assassinated Kim Jong-nam (half brother of the current dictator Kim Jong-un) using VX nerve agent, an extremely toxic compound that is also highly dermally active. In the incident, an operative in Malaysia wiped liquid VX on Kim Jong-nam's face, and he died on the way to the hospital. But here too, the use of this chemical agent was intended solely for one victim, and was most likely produced in a North Korean state laboratory.

Blood Agents

Another important category, the so-called blood agents, includes cyanide in its various forms. Cyanide blocks the enzyme cytochrome oxidase, shutting down the cellular energy transport system. In the form of its ingested salt (e.g., sodium cyanide), 200 to 300 mg of cyanide is necessary to cause death in most adults (Lovejoy & Linden, 1994). Solutions containing a cyanide salt can be made to produce HCN vapor, capable of causing death within minutes. (This is the operating principle of the gas chamber that has been used for capital executions in the United States.) Because of its widespread use in the mining and other industries, bulk supplies of potassium or sodium cyanide salts are ubiquitous. As an adulterant, cyanide salts could be employed to poison food or beverages.

Because of its ubiquity, perhaps it is only a matter of time before a terrorist group successfully uses cyanide in an attack. It should be borne in mind, however, that a substantial amount of HCN is required to cause death in most humans. For example, approximately 2,500 to 5,000 mg-min/m^3 is estimated to be the median lethal concentration (Baskin & Brewer, 1997), compared to 100 mg-min/m^3 for sarin nerve agent (Sidell, 1997). One should also expect that successful attacks employing HCN, like other volatile agents, demand large quantities of agent and enclosed spaces. Even under such conditions, it is difficult to conceive of more than several hundred casualties that would be due to cyanide-based devices.

Lung Irritants

Lung irritants attack the respiratory system, causing tightness in the airways, hypoxia, and in more severe cases, pulmonary edema (Urbanetti, 1997). Most known lung irritants require high volatilities or a gaseous form to cause injury to the alveolar spaces of the lungs. As previously seen in the case of cyanide, this also means that large concentrations or enclosed spaces are necessary to cause death or injury to many individuals. For a terrorist bent on using such compounds, the primary hurdles would be access to large enough quantities of agent and an effective delivery method to cause mass casualties.

One case in particular demonstrates the effects of a very toxic lung irritant, methyl isocyanate (MIC), on an unprotected and unsuspecting civilian population.

On December 3, 1984, a release of MIC—a chemical intermediate used in the synthesis of a pesticide—killed as many as 3,800 people in Bhopal, India. Not only is this tragedy significant in terms of the scope of the disaster, but there is persuasive evidence that the Bhopal catastrophe was the result of sabotage (Kalelkar, 1988). In the Bhopal case, a disgruntled employee decided to strike back at his employer by deliberately disrupting operations. Having deliberately introduced large quantities of water into a large tank holding MIC, the resultant heat and violent reaction caused a massive plume of MIC gas to float over populated areas of Bhopal. Local inhabitants, gathering around the plant to get a better look at the unfolding disaster, were among the first casualties.

Other common chemicals like chlorine could be deliberately released into the environment, putting wider populations at risk. This could occur within a facility or perhaps by sabotaging a container being transported via train or road. During the Atlanta 1996 Olympics, for example, U.S. federal authorities considered potential threats from improvised chemical devices, including the use of high explosives to puncture a train car loaded with toxic chemicals (U.S. Army Medical Command, 1999).

Lung irritants can be produced from commercially supplied compounds, or as by-products of chemical reactions. There have been recorded cases of bombers trying to include chemicals together with their explosives with the apparent intent to emit a poisonous gas. In Iraq in 2007, the progenitor of the Islamic State terrorist group launched a series of attacks involving chlorine tanks and explosives that caused hundreds of injuries, some as a result of exposure to chlorine gas (McNerney & Rhodes, 2009). Since having taken over large swathes of territory in Syria and Iraq since 2013, ISIS has dispersed chlorine on several occasions, using both traditional military delivery methods (artillery and mortars) and once again the incorporation of chlorine canisters into vehicle-borne IEDs.

Vesicants

The so-called vesicants or blister agents, such as mustard and lewisite, have less utility for terrorists wanting to kill lots of people. In a classic World War I combat setting, sulfur mustard was a highly effective casualty agent that caused (after about an hour delay) extreme irritation to eyes, skin, and the respiratory tract. Concentrations of 100 mg-min/m^3 create near-incapacitation of vision from the effects on the conjunctiva, whereas the lethal dosage of a blister agent like mustard gas is generally estimated to be between 1 and 2 g (topical or inhaled). Another irritating and vesicating agent, lewisite, possesses similar lethality, but its irritating effects are much more rapid (Sidell, 1997). The applications of a blister agent are more the purview of military operations (e.g., the Iran–Iraq War in the 1980s) than acts of chemical terrorism (Franke, 1967). However, there is evidence that ISIS has produced its own sulfur mustard agent munitions and used these in at least eight attacks in Syria and Iraq between July 2014 and August 2016 (Detusch, 2016; United Nations Security Council, 2016).

Psychoincapacitants

Psychotropic compounds such as the belladonna drug BZ (3-quinuclidinyl benzilate) or the hallucinogen LSD (lysergic acid diethylamide) have been viewed by militaries for use in combat, sabotage, and sometimes to be used against civilian uprisings. Their performance on the battlefield, however, are unpredictable and impractical (Compton, 1987). Largely because of its unknown effects on enemy soldiers, the United States destroyed its BZ stocks during the 1980s.

Because of its potency, BZ could present the terrorist with an agent for contaminating food or water. Aerosol dispersion is also possible, perhaps via solvent, but this may be technically problematic for improvised attacks. Effects on individuals would include delirium, hallucinations, and general mental confusion for at least 24 hours. Higher doses could be lethal, especially from complications that are due to its anticholinergic activity (e.g., hyperthermia). Other compounds may be extracted from plants of the belladonna variety and used as adulterants in food or beverages.

Pesticides

Pesticides refer to a group of agents used to kill a number of different "pests," such as weeds, insects, ticks, rats, and so forth. Pesticide compounds have also been used in various criminal and terrorist attacks. Modern pesticides have increasingly been developed and produced with low levels of toxicity in mammals, and their ultimate threat to humans is not great. However, many developing countries still make use of older varieties with greater toxicity, and controls on access to pesticides vary greatly, even across states within the United States. Numerous types of poisons have been used to kill mammals (mostly rodents), including cyanide, thallium, arsenic, sodium fluoroacetate, and the anticoagulant warfarin (most commonly used in developed countries). Because of their high toxicity, cyanide and fluoroacetate types of compounds are among the more menacing. Others such as herbicides and organophosphate insecticides, although toxic in large doses, are generally more of a concern to poison control centers (e.g., accidental ingestion) than for chemical terrorism. But what happens when a terrorist threatens (or accomplishes) a large-scale chemical attack by poisoning food or water with some pesticide compound? This will likely generate intense anxiety for the public, creating significant challenges for healthcare professionals.

Effects of Chemical Terrorism

The repercussions of a chemical terrorist event could be varied and far reaching. A large-scale attack using a nerve agent in a densely populated area would create havoc. In this instance one would expect to find many people disoriented, some with extreme rhinorrhea and bloody exudate from the nose, all the while twitching uncontrollably (fasciculations). In high concentrations, cyanide gas would kill its victims quickly unless treated early, whereas other exposed individuals may be relatively unaffected. Lung irritants may have immediate and long-term effects that, in more severe cases of inhalation, include pulmonary edema and the production of bloody and

frothy sputum. These signs, coupled with the necessity for respiratory assistance, are clearly ominous symptoms of a large dose exposure.

Some agents such as mustard (blister agent) and VX (among the most lethal nerve agent ever produced for weaponization) are also persistent, meaning they present severe, long-term contamination hazards. Because these can act topically, secondary contact exposure may continue to cause injury. It is of obvious concern to hospitals that such agents may be involved in future chemical terrorist attacks. Full decontamination procedures would be most appropriate in the case of a VX release, whereas other agents—such as cyanide or gases—will largely diffuse and become diluted in the environment. Persons exposed to highly volatile agents generally may require little or no special decontamination efforts. However, casualties caused by somewhat persistent CW agents such as sarin will often require a judgment call. In the open environment, sarin aerosol or vapors will not present a long-term contamination hazard. On the other hand, a casualty who has liquid sarin agent soaked in, say, his trouser cuffs will definitely require full removal of clothing and at least a water bath of skin surfaces.

Chemical Contamination of Water, Food, Beverages, and Consumer Products

Especially during the period of heightened security alerts following 9/11, the security of water has risen as a concern in developed societies, as was demonstrated in Wisconsin in 2002. In a June 14, 2002, press release from the governor's office, the following was reported:

> Janesville [Wisconsin] authorities and the FBI are investigating a break-in at a water facility reservoir. Earlier this week, it was discovered that barbed wire on a chain link fence was cut and a padlock on the reservoir had been forcefully removed. The Department of Natural Resources and the State Lab of Hygiene tested the water and so far all tests have been negative for any contaminants. Nonetheless, the decision was made by Janesville officials to isolate and drain the 5 million gallon reservoir and test the residue. (State of Wisconsin, 2002)

No toxic substances were found.

Although generally discounted as a threat because of dilution factors and chlorination, municipal water sources could nevertheless be targeted by terrorists using chemical agents. Given very large quantities of starting material, some highly toxic agents, such as organophosphates, may pose a threat to civilian water systems (Lohs, 1963).

That terrorists are interested in poisoning water for at least isolated attacks was demonstrated in February 2002. In an apparent plot on the U.S. embassy in Rome, foreign nationals were found with several pounds of potassium ferrocyanide and diagrams to the underground water pipes near the U.S. embassy. But if the intent to poison water was present, the means were not. The would-be terrorists might have looked at the name "ferrocyanide" and assumed it was toxic, but in actuality potassium (or sodium) ferrocyanide has low toxicity in mammals (World Health Organization, 1974). Had the perpetrators actually introduced the compound into the water system, it is unlikely that anyone would have noticed anything other than a strange flavor or color.

To be successful in an attack on a public water system, two major obstacles must be overcome by the terrorists: the very large volumes of water involved (dilution effect) and the redundant nature of modern water treatment systems (Croddy, 2001). Also, most water is not used for drinking or cooking but for other high-volume applications, such as watering lawns, washing clothes, washing dishes, bathing, and so forth. Furthermore, in today's world, fewer and fewer people drink directly from the tap but rather from bottled water sources. In sum, it is quite a challenge for a terrorist to conduct an operation against large public water supplies.

Large-scale contamination of food, beverages, or consumer products with a chemical agent presents many of the same challenges to the chemical terrorist as water, but perhaps to an even higher degree. The toxic compound would have to be introduced at a point where mass distribution would take place (without being detected), and then would have to survive processing or storage. Heightened awareness in food and product security will do much to prevent chemical terrorism or criminal acts of adulterating our food and beverage supply. However, terrorists may only need a few cases to produce great anxiety or possibly outright panic, as seen in cases of criminal extortion in the past.

Challenges Posed by a Chemical Terrorist Attack

If past experience is any indicator, confusion will reign during the early stages of a chemical terrorist event. For example, when patients were brought in from the Tokyo subway attack in 1995, the first bits of information were fragmentary at best, as will be described later. In a future chemical attack, one could expect similar delays in understanding what is really happening. Great anxiety among the public is to be expected, whether from dealing with the nature of the casualties themselves or loved ones who are looking for answers and updates "What is happening? Why is she sick?"

More critically, in cases of large numbers of serious chemical casualties, it may reach the point that limitations of personnel, time, equipment, and space do not permit the degree of medical intervention usually called for on any other given day. Most modern healthcare settings are not used to accommodating very difficult triage situations.

Furthermore, even without having been directly affected by a toxic or infectious agent, many persons will present themselves to emergency wards out of a justifiable concern for their health. Spurred by their own feelings or rumors of impending doom, many more individuals will also seek out medical consultations. Again, in the Tokyo sarin event of 1995, a thousand or so individuals probably were physiologically affected by the nerve agent release. However, a total of 5,510 people in Tokyo reported seeing a physician or emergency health professional as a consequence of the attack (Sidell, 1996). Arriving in ever-increasing numbers, these so-called "worried well" can overwhelm the capability of healthcare professionals to triage and treat casualties.

BIOTERRORISM

The act of biological terrorism (bioterrorism) involves the deliberate use of microbial pathogens or toxins. Unlike a chemical incident, the effects from bioterrorism may not be fully known until many hours or days after the event. In the case of biological casualties, except in specific instances such as an attack with anthrax spores, victims of a bioterrorist attack generally do not require special decontamination. Furthermore, while common perception is that a biological attack necessarily implies some sort of rapidly spreading epidemic—"the gift that keeps on giving"—most traditional BW agents are non-contagious. Containment measures are mandatory, however, in the event of a (most unlikely) smallpox outbreak, some hemorrhagic fevers, and pneumonic plague.

The notion of bioterrorism has a particularly frightening and intimidating aura for most people and may also possess an apocalyptic mystique for both terrorists and the public. Still, BW is essentially an *infectious disease* problem, or public health in reverse. In keeping with this theme of bioterrorism being the deliberate cause of infectious disease, bioterrorists may choose among the following categories of pathogens:

- Bacterial agents
- Viral agents
- Toxins (derived from plants or animals)
- Parasites (much less likely)

As in the case of the chemical agents mentioned earlier, the bioterrorist may choose pathogens or toxins that are very different from those developed by the militaries of the former Soviet Union and the United States (Sobel, Khan, & Swerdlow, 2002). For example, in the military setting, bacteria that cause dysentery (*Shigella dysenteriae*) or typhoid (*Salmonella typhi*) have little value in the modern battlefield, although their use has been suggested in the past as sabotage agents (Cohen, 2001). These same pathogens or toxins (e.g., botulinum) could be used as bioterrorist weapons, however, chiefly as contaminants in adulterated food or beverages (Wein and Liu, 2005).

Also, while much less likely, some parasitic microorganisms such as *Cryptosporidium parvum* or *Giardia lamblia* might be utilized by bioterrorists bent on infecting targets through drinking water or contaminated food. For healthy individuals receiving adequate medical attention, these organisms usually do not cause life-threatening diseases, but if delivered efficiently, they could incapacitate large numbers of people.

Bioterrorism and Delivery of BW Agents

Generally speaking, infectious agents and toxins are most efficiently delivered via aerosol, in particles ranging from about 1 micron to 10 microns. Somewhere around 5 microns is the sweet spot, where particles are more likely to deposit into alveolar spaces. It is at this point, as a U.S. expert in BW wrote during the late 1950s, that the "entrance and retention of infectious particles in the alveoli amounts almost to an intratissue inoculation" (Fothergill, 1958, p. 5).

The *exact* details of methods used to produce microbes or toxins, to prepare them for aerosolization, and to deliver these efficiently over a target are tightly guarded secrets. However, weaponization of a BW agent is largely a matter of engineering and materials science that can be accomplished with significant time, effort, and money.

As in chemical terrorism, a contrast should be made between the types of biological agent delivery devices developed for military use, and those weapons that could be employed in bioterrorism. In the military context, for example, BW agents such as anthrax spores (*Bacillus anthracis*) or tularemia bacteria (*Francisella tularensis*) are most efficiently aerosolized and disseminated over large, concentrated targets. However, as the United States experienced in September and October 2001, a bioterrorist could send pathogens—such as finely powdered anthrax spores—using a low-tech mode of delivery such as mailing them in an envelope. Although the results of the anthrax mailings were limited in terms of actual numbers of casualties (at least 17 became sick and 5 people died), the repercussions were serious enough to call into question the safety of millions of individuals. Concerns of secondary contamination led to shutting down a large part of the U.S. Postal Service system, while the U.S. Congress and the Supreme Court had to vacate their offices (Shane, 2011).

While in theory any disease-causing microbe or toxin could be used as a biological agent, only a relative few have been found to be practical for weaponization. In the military context, BW agents that have larger casualty-causing potential are those that form stable aerosols and are highly infectious. The only other possible routes available to the bioterrorist are attacks via ingestion (adulteration of foodstuffs) or injection (e.g., a needle or contaminated object that punctures the skin). For various reasons, these are not efficient methods to create large numbers of casualties.

What Agents Might the Bioterrorist Use?

We have already seen that chemical terrorists or bioterrorists can be resourceful and creative in choosing their agents. National military programs, such as those formerly operating in the United States and the former Soviet Union, typically chose BW agents among pathogens that are notoriously capable of infecting via aerosols and respiratory droplets. Not having access to the same financial largesse and technological base, terrorists will likely choose those BW agents that are more easily found, cultured, grown, and can be effectively disseminated.

One may also hypothesize that factors for terrorists choosing among possible agents include high lethality and name brand recognition. For example, militaries have long studied and developed *Coxiella burnetii*, the causative agent in Q fever, for use in biological weapons. Although its infectivity is extremely high (some have estimated its infectious dose being *one* inhaled organism), Q fever is a relatively mild disease and death is rare (Byrne, 1997). *Chlamydophila psittaci* (formerly *Chlamydia psittaci*), the causative agent in psittacosis (or ornithosis) is infectious via aerosol and also produces a moderately severe illness. Terrorists, in a quest to sow fear and wreak havoc,

could employ such nonlethal pathogens and still reap many of their intended effects.

Tularemia or rabbit fever, caused by the bacterium *F. tularensis*, is also highly infectious, requiring only 10 to 50 inhaled organisms to cause disease. It has wide variability in terms of morbidity and mortality. The more virulent North American serotype is approximately 30% fatal without treatment. Tularemia is also found among animals, particularly rabbits, and could be employed as an aerosolized weapon from crude preparations. For example, some cases of tularemia in which aerosols were formed during yard work or other activity (Teutsch et al., 1979). Still, although U.S. and Soviet militaries spent enormous amounts of effort weaponizing this BW agent, it is not clear that tularemia is what terrorists have in mind (Croddy & Krcalova, 2001).

Other potential bioterrorism threats are the causative agents of diseases like plague that can be spread via aerosol. But the isolation and culture of some organisms like *Yersinia pestis*, for example, presented problems even for large military programs. The development of a plague weapon stymied bio-weapons researchers in the United States (Henderson et al., 1998), whereas weaponizing Ebola virus presented problems for BW scientists in the former Soviet Union (Alibek, 1999). Pathogens such as Hantavirus are so difficult to grow in culture that it would not likely pose a BW threat (Franz et al., 2001).

However, *B. anthracis,* the causative agent in inhalation anthrax, still remains the premier bioterrorist threat today. The *B. anthracis* spore is nearly ubiquitous in nature and is not terribly difficult to isolate and grow. Being a spore former, the anthrax bacterium can withstand environmental stress while maintaining its virulence, as well as being hardy enough to withstand chemicals, ultraviolet (UV) light, and processes used in its weaponization. Finally, especially nowadays, the word "anthrax" alone strikes a fearsome chord in most people. Indeed, there have been recent unconfirmed reports that ISIS may have been pursuing acquisition of anthrax bacteria (McCormick, 2016).

Smallpox

There is also heightened concern that a bioterrorist could release smallpox, a disease that has been eradicated among the world's population since at least 1980. Officially, only two places on Earth still maintain viable smallpox virus in cold storage: Novosibirsk, Russia; and Atlanta, Georgia, at the Centers for Disease Control and Prevention (CDC). Some unconfirmed reports allege that other countries, however, including North Korea and perhaps others, still hold on to smallpox virus specimens. Could a terrorist release smallpox, and how would it affect a mostly immunologically naïve population?

Considering the extreme contagiousness of smallpox, and especially its ability to infect via respiratory droplets and aerosols, the mere thought of its recrudescence has been of enormous concern. Thus, in 2001 the United States began a massive stockpiling of enough smallpox vaccine for every person in the country (approximately 300 million doses) in the event of a smallpox outbreak (Gillis, 2001). By 2017, the National Strategic Stockpile had acquired enough smallpox vaccine to vaccinate any population at risk of infection in the United States.

It is also useful to remember where much of the concern began: in 1998, particularly after revelations were made concerning the Soviet Union having produced smallpox as a weapon, and with the series of attacks by Al-Qaeda (and other terrorist organizations) through 9/11, the general consensus was that a smallpox attack was not out of the question. And along with this heightened alert, there was some overreaction. The amount of attention given to the threat of smallpox—including a network television program (ER) having aired an episode involving a smallpox outbreak—likely contributed to the following false alarm (McKenna, 2002):

> On June 13, 2002, while aboard a domestic flight from San Francisco to Memphis, an off-hand remark by a passenger who said that he might have smallpox initiated an emergency response. In this particular incident, a nurse on board was asked to examine the person who reportedly had a rash. The flight crew also radioed ahead with the message that they might have an infectious disease–stricken passenger on board, and paramedics and emergency management officials were dispatched to meet the patient at the Memphis airport. An FBI supervisory agent concluded that the remark concerning smallpox, although unnerving, "was absolutely not intended to be disruptive to the flight. But everybody kind of got raised up over the possibility that somehow this might be a situation involving infectious disease. It was not." (Lee, 2002, p. A1)

Sabotage (Food and Water Contamination) Threats

Although it would likely be only effective on a small scale, a bioterrorist attack could include the contamination of food or beverages. For example, botulinum toxin could be an extremely potent food or beverage contaminant. Botulinum toxin is among the most toxic substances known, about 0.4 mcg being sufficient to kill most adults (Kime & Lowe, 1971). Still, poisoning a water reservoir using botulinum toxin or other agents is not a practical route for a bioterrorist, as the combined effects of water treatment, residual chlorine, and simple (charcoal) water filters eliminate most threats (Burrows & Renner, 1999). Smaller targets, such as water systems in buildings, may be vulnerable to BW agent attack, but the numbers of casualties here too would be limited.

We have already seen a case of large casualties that was due to food contamination with a bacterial agent. In this case, the 1984 attack by the Rajneeshee cult contaminated local salad bars with *S. typhimurium*, sickening some 751 people. No deaths were directly attributable to this bioterrorist attack. This type of assault—basically a crime of opportunity using foodborne bacteria—is the more likely type of bioterrorist event we may encounter in the future.

Challenges Posed by Bioterrorism

In the context of bioterrorism, one can separate the causes and effects of many disease processes into two basic categories: pathogenic microbes and toxins. Casualties from aerosolized biological toxins might present themselves within several hours, as compared with several days for most pathogenic microbes. Unlike chemical terrorism, where the effects of most agents are relatively quick and their detection relatively straightforward, the confirmation of a biological agent attack might come only many days after a release. Furthermore, the actual bioterrorist attack itself—say a release of an aerosolized cloud of anthrax spores over a large city—is unlikely to be noticed. The first sentinel victims will complain of vague ("flu-like") symptoms to their primary care physicians and perhaps only after some time will an epidemiological picture form. Where infection has occurred, several pathogens require rapid treatment or many to most victims will die.

In a biological event, one of the major concerns will be how to treat those who have been exposed, while managing others who are not at risk but are extremely concerned (the "worried well"). Just after the 9/11 attacks and the anxiety they caused, in early October 2001, even without evidence of a biological threat or attack, many worried people stockpiled antibiotics, including ciprofloxacin (Ricks, 2001). If thousands are suspected of being exposed, one can multiply this number many times for those who may believe they too are going to become sick. Furthermore, despite the fact that most of the classic BW agents are not contagious, this point may be lost on the public. All of these ramifications need to be considered when trying to deal with the real threat of a chemical or biological attack, be it terrorism or large-scale use by nation-states.

CASE EXAMPLES

Although there are many examples of terrorist plots and attempts to use CB agents, these case examples have been restricted to events that led to actual casualties. This allows a real-world appreciation of many of the concepts discussed earlier regarding the challenges facing the healthcare community in the event of a chemical or bioterrorist incident.

The Rajneeshees

As previously noted, in 1984, a cult called the Rajneeshees committed the only successful, large-scale biological attack in the United States. The Rajneeshee cult, followers of Bhagwan Shree Rajneesh, moved to rural Oregon from India in 1981 and soon developed hostile relations with the surrounding community. Within the cult, the person most involved in the acquisition and use of biological agents was Ma Anand Puja, a nurse who ran the Rajneeshee's medical facilities.

The Rajneeshees purchased samples of the bacterium *S. typhimurium* and grew these cultures in their laboratories. In August 1984, they distributed *Salmonella*-laced water to two local commissioners who opposed the cult. The cult leaders wanted to make voters sick to enable the group to win a local election. In September 1984, as part of a trial run, several members of the cult contaminated salad bars with *Salmonella* in 10 restaurants in the small town of The Dalles in Oregon. The leader of the group, Bhagwan, a professed pacifist, allegedly approved of this operation, reportedly saying that "it was best not to hurt people, but if a few died not to worry" (Carus, 2000). The result was that at least 751 people became ill with food poisoning. Local healthcare providers were overwhelmed by the number of patients, and, although no one died, several people became seriously ill. The Rajneeshees also made an unsuccessful attempt to contaminate local water supplies (Carus, 2000).

The Rajneeshees eventually abandoned their biological attacks when they realized that they could not win the elections. One of the most important lessons of the Rajneeshee case is that the *Salmonella* outbreak was initially identified by authorities as a natural outbreak. It was only some time later that it was discovered that the outbreak was intentional and had been perpetrated by the Rajneeshees. This case highlights the difficulties, in certain contexts, of distinguishing between a natural epidemic and bioterrorism.

Aum Shinrikyo

One event stands out as having brought to public attention the potential for terrorist use of chemical weapons—the Tokyo subway attack by the Japanese cult Aum Shinrikyo on March 20, 1995. The attackers used the nerve agent sarin, which Aum had manufactured in its own laboratories. The result of this chemical attack was 12 fatalities, 1,039 physiological injuries, and at least 4,000 people with psychogenic symptoms. The attack also highlighted some of the difficult issues that medical and emergency personnel will have to face in any future large-scale chemical attack.

Aum Shinrikyo was a religious cult dominated by Shoko Asahara, a leader who promulgated apocalyptic visions. Since the early 1990s the cult had been attempting to overthrow the Japanese government and impose a bizarre theocratic state. Asahara soon became fascinated by CB weapons and initiated a program to develop several warfare agents. It has been reported (Gurr & Cole, 2000) that Aum scientists also managed to synthesize sarin, tabun, soman, VX (nerve agents), and mustard agent.

The attack on the Tokyo subway in March 1995 brought to worldwide prominence the deadly designs of this apocalyptic organization. The attack was carried out simultaneously on five separate subway trains when Aum members punctured plastic bags containing a diluted solution of sarin using sharpened umbrella tips. As soon as the sarin vaporized, it began to affect passengers on the trains.

On arriving at various subway stations, emergency medical technicians (EMTs) were forced to deal with the chaos of hundreds of disoriented passengers exhibiting the classic symptoms of nerve agent exposure—difficulty breathing, impaired vision, vomiting, and convulsions. As the emergency responders lacked any protective clothing or equipment, some of them began to show symptoms of sarin exposure themselves. Adding to the confusion, responders also used different radio channels and were unable to communicate with various agencies.

Following the sarin attack around 8:00 a.m., between 8:40 and 9:40 a.m. more than 500 patients presented themselves at St. Luke's International Hospital (Okumura et al., 1998), located within 3 km of the affected subway stations. Hospital personnel were at first greeted with fragmentary and confusing information, initially having been told to prepare for victims of a gas explosion. Even the television news had more data than

did the emergency physicians on the scene. Further adding to the chaos was a preliminary, but incorrect, identification of the toxic chemical in question as acetonitrile, instead of what it really was—the toxic organophosphate sarin. Based on their training, medical personnel soon were able to identify sarin as the culprit. Not unexpectedly, given the large-scale nature of the attack, hospitals in the area did not have adequate supplies of atropine and 2-pyridine-aldoxime-methiodide (2PAM), the standard treatment for victims of nerve agent exposure. It did not help that many also suffered effects from secondary contamination in the healthcare setting (Smithson & Levy, 2000).

The final casualty figures were 1,039 victims, 17 of whom were identified as critical (requiring intensive care), 37 severely injured (gastrointestinal problems and muscular twitching), and 984 slightly injured (vision problems such as miosis). Ultimately, there were 12 fatalities (Woodall, 1997). However, more than 4,000 people who reported to hospitals (approximately 80% of the total number of patients) were actually psychogenic victims with no physiological signs of exposure (Smithson & Levy, 2000). The end result was that the main, central part of metropolitan Tokyo—one of the world's largest cities—was paralyzed for several hours. The attack also revealed serious shortcomings in the city's emergency response coordination and communication.

At first glance, the case of Aum Shinrikyo seems extremely alarming. Aum tried to kill thousands of people and came fairly close to succeeding. Even though the Tokyo subway attack caused limited fatalities, this was mostly because the sarin— hastily prepared just before the attack—was of low quality. But most critically, insofar as the real or perceived threat of WMD is concerned, the Tokyo incident changed the way the world viewed terrorism. It certainly caused the United States and other industrialized nations (among others) to review their domestic preparedness for terrorist attacks, including those involving chemical agents.

For example, following additional preparedness efforts that were originally spurred by the September 11, 2001 attacks, in the last several years the U.S. CDC has allocated "Chempack" nerve agent antidote containers, each containing enough pharmaceutical agents to treat up to 1,000 nerve agent casualties. Because of the need for fast therapeutic intervention in the event of a nerve agent attack, nearly 2,000 containers are forward deployed across the United States in 1,340 locations. These include Mark 1 Nerve Agent Antidote Kits (pralidoxime, atropine), diazepam (for convulsions) as well as formulations for children (pediatric doses). By 2018, following a procurement initiative under the Biomedical Advanced Research Development Authority (BARDA), a new anticonvulsive formulation midazolam (Pfizer) is expected to augment the nerve agent treatment regimen to better handle nerve agent (e.g., VX) casualties. And in light of recent chemical casualties in Syria, BARDA is also looking to fulfill requirements to better handle chlorine and mustard (vesicant) injuries under this program as well (U.S. CDC, 2017).

The 2001 Anthrax Attacks

Right on the heels of the events of September 11, 2001, the U.S. public was shocked by the first lethal terrorist attack in the United States using a BW agent (Aum Shinrikyo in Japan had made attempts to use biological agents in the mid-1990s but was unsuccessful). Letters containing the deadly bacterium *B. anthracis* were sent through mail to prominent politicians and media representatives. Despite hundreds of anthrax hoaxes over the preceding years in the United States, this was the first time that actual anthrax spores were used. In total, 22 people were diagnosed with the disease. Eleven were diagnosed with inhalation anthrax, five of whom died. Another 11 people were diagnosed with the cutaneous form of the disease (Frerichs, 2002). The victims of the attacks included workers in the media and the U.S. Postal Service who came into direct contact with the letters, as well as some cases resulting from cross-contamination.

Ultimately, after one of the largest law enforcement investigations in American history, the U.S. FBI concluded in 2008 that Dr. Bruce Ivins, a microbiologist working for the U.S. Army laboratory at Fort Detrick, Maryland, was responsible for these attacks. Ivins, who had worked on anthrax and vaccines for the U.S. biodefense program for decades (Pitt et al., 1999), committed suicide on July 29, 2008, by an overdose of acetaminophen (Tylenol). Although he made no confession, a preponderance of evidence points to Dr. Ivins and him alone for the anthrax letter attacks of September and October 2001 (Shane, 2011).

The 2001 anthrax attacks hold two main lessons for the medical profession. The first is the necessity of having some knowledge of the agents most likely to be used in bioterrorist events and maintaining a high index of suspicion when confronted by atypical clinical cases. The sooner a case is identified as the result of bioterrorism, the sooner measures can be taken to mitigate its effects. Prompt diagnosis can not only save the lives of patients, but it can also forestall a potential epidemic in the case of contagious organisms such as smallpox. The second lesson taught by the anthrax attacks is the degree of psychological stress such events place on the public. This stress can have repercussions for the medical system. Officials from U.S. federal health agencies reported that 32,000 Americans took antibiotics out of concern brought on by the anthrax mailings. During that time, a poll ($n \cong 1,015$) taken by the Harvard School of Public Health indicated that 25% of those surveyed were "very or somewhat worried" that they might become infected with anthrax from letters or at the workplace. Almost 15% said that they had taken one or more extreme cautionary measures, including the purchase of gas masks, firearms, or stockpiling antibiotics (LaSalandra, 2001).

MASS PSYCHOGENIC ILLNESS

In addition to the physiological injuries they may cause, attacks or even threats involving chemical or biological weapons will have certain negative effects on both those in the vicinity of the attacks and the general population. One possible effect is mass psychogenic illness.

Psychogenic illness describes a constellation of disease symptoms appearing in a group of individuals, yet the cause of their ailments cannot be determined. Usually this occurs within a group of people sharing a similar venue or experience who believe that their illness is caused by an environmental toxin or pathogen. Again, no etiological agents are ever identified in these incidents, although an unspecified odor is often reported that probably served as a trigger (Staudenmayer, 1999). Mass psychogenic illness tends to affect women and girls more than their male counterparts (Taylor & Werbicki, 1993). Heightened and repeated attention from 24/7 media news cycles (and nowadays, social media) usually causes more consternation among the most affected, and, ironically, a dedicated, professional response from emergency responders can make their psychogenic symptoms worse.

The psychological effects of bioterrorism in particular on the population at large—and even some trained professionals in emergency response—cannot be underestimated. Some authors note that the signs of a bioterrorist event may be very similar to mass psychogenic illness (Jones et al., 2000), thus complicating matters further. Similarly, heightened concerns over CB terrorism generally may be accompanied by an increased incidence of psychogenic illness.

Often for good reason, many people in modern developing and industrialized societies have heightened awareness of environmental hazards. This, coupled with high stress—including tension from current events involving terrorism—can contribute to instances of mass hysteria. Thus, although the effect of environmentalism has been largely salubrious, it has also sensitized many people to unwarranted fears involving chemicals and other unseen toxics (Petrie & Wessely, 2002). Especially when played up by the media, anxiety of toxic exposures can lead to mass psychogenic illness in a variety of situations, especially in school settings. Following the 9/11 terrorist attacks, for example, paint fumes sent 16 students and a teacher to a hospital (September 29, 2001), and more than a thousand students in the Philippines—complaining of general cold or flu-like symptoms—also sought medical attention because of unfounded rumors of bioterrorism (Wessely, Hyams, & Bartholomew, 2001).

In the context of chemical or biological terrorism, mass psychogenic illness presents two significant challenges for healthcare personnel. First, although justified when erring on the side of caution, emergency personnel need to be able to distinguish as quickly as possible between an actual chemical or biological attack, and instances of mass hysteria. This will prevent wasting valuable time and resources. It will also help lower public anxiety by foregoing unnecessary, costly, and potentially humiliating decontamination procedures and will allow healthcare workers to appropriately deal with the concerns of worried patients. Second, following an actual chemical or biological attack, emergency personnel need to be aware of the probability that many of those presenting themselves for treatment may not actually have been exposed to the agent. They must, therefore, be able to differentiate as quickly and accurately as possible between the physiological victims of the attack and the psychogenic victims, and deal with each accordingly. In the case of a nerve agent release, for example, one would obviously want to reserve the limited supply of antidotes on hand (e.g., atropine) for those who were actually exposed.

SUMMARY

A terrorist attack using chemical or biological weapons is an alarming prospect, all the more so after the tragedy of 9/11 and continuing terrorist campaigns worldwide. Although the likelihood of a large-scale chemical or biological terrorist attack is not as great as some media reports would have us believe, there are at least some terrorist groups and individuals who could attempt to attack civilians with CB agents. This makes preparing for such an event essential.

Chemical incidents are relatively quick-acting and limited, whereas biological incidents would take time— perhaps days—before they are recognized for what they are. In general, one can consider a chemical release or attack to be a "lights and sirens" affair, that is, rapid response and (hopefully) expeditious treatment of casualties. In many bioterrorist events, however, people would be unlikely to know that they were exposed to an infectious agent until the first symptoms appear, at the very least several hours (in the case of biological toxins) following the event.

Little can be said with certainty as to what would actually happen, or how the public at large would respond in the event of a major chemical or bioterrorist attack. There is general agreement, though, that should a chemical or biological agent be used in a violent act, the effects of this kind of terrorism will extend far beyond its immediate danger to the public. It is, therefore, incumbent on every healthcare provider to understand all aspects of this threat and to train and prepare for an event all hope will never occur.

STUDY QUESTIONS

1. A 33-year-old patient presents with a maculopapular rash of no discernible pattern, and he is very agitated and concerned. He says that he had chicken pox as a child, and the websites he has read indicate that it all leads to one conclusion: smallpox. What might you say to this individual to calm his fears?

2. Which groups appear to be interested in using CB agents? Why do you think they find these attractive?

3. If one were forced to choose between equipping ambulances with extra atropine auto-injectors in the event of a nerve agent release or instead equip these with cyanide antidote kits, which would you choose? Why?

4. In 2002, a spate of mysterious rashes appeared in school-children in the United States and Canada. According to the CDC's *Monthly Morbidity and Mortality Report* (June 21, 2002), "The sex distribution of cases varied among the schools, ranging from 33 percent to 100 percent female." An etiologic agent has yet to be found. Why did the CDC find it relevant to note the gender of the distributed cases?

5. Someone receives an envelope and on opening it discovers a white powder along with a letter that reads, "You have just been exposed to anthrax." What should that person do?

6. Working in the emergency room, you receive notification that there has been a confirmed attack on an office building using chlorine gas. For what type and number of casualties should you prepare?

7. Your neighbor tells you that he refuses to drink tap water because he fears that terrorists might contaminate it. Should you follow suit? Why?

REFERENCES

al-Fahd, N. H. (2003, May). A treatise on the legal status of using weapons of mass destruction against infidels. Retrieved from https://www.carnegieendowment.org/static/npp/fatwa.pdf

Alibek, K. (1999). *Biohazard.* New York: Random House.

Baskin, S. I., & Brewer, T. G. (1997). Cyanide poisoning. In F. R. Sidell, E. T. Takafuji, & D. R. Franz (Eds.), *Medical aspects of chemical and biological warfare* (pp. 271–286). Washington, DC: Borden Institute.

Bolton, J. R. (2002). Beyond the axis of evil: Additional threats from weapons of mass destruction. Heritage Lectures, 743, 3. Retrieved from https://www.heritage.org/defense/report/beyond-the-axis-evil-additional-threats-weapons-mass-destruction-0

Burrows, W. D., & Renner, S. E. (1999). Biological warfare agents as threats to potable water. *Environmental Health Perspectives, 107*(12), 980.

Burton, J. B., Burpo, F. J., & Garcia, K. (2014). 20th CBRNE Command. *Military Review, 96*(4), 64–65.

Byrne, W. R. (1997). Q fever. In F. R. Sidell, E. T. Takafuji, & D. R. Franz (Eds.), *Medical aspects of chemical and biological warfare* (pp. 523–537). Washington, DC: Borden Institute.

Carus, W. S. (2000). The Rajneeshees (1984). In J. B. Tucker (Ed.), *Toxic terror: Assessing terrorist use of chemical and biological weapons* (pp. 115–138). Cambridge, MA: MIT Press.

Chivers, C. J. (2015, July 17). ISIS has fired chemical mortar shells, evidence indicates. *New York Times.* Retrieved from https://www.nytimes.com/2015/07/18/world/middleeast/islamic-state-isis-chemical-weapons-iraq-syria.html

Cohen, A. (2001). Israel and chemical/biological weapons: History, deterrence, and arms control. *The Nonproliferation Review, 8*(3), 31.

Compton, J. A. F. (1987). *Military chemical and biological agents: Chemical and toxicological properties.* Caldwell, NJ: The Telford Press.

Croddy, E. (2001). *Chemical and biological warfare: A comprehensive survey for the concerned citizen.* New York: Copernicus Books.

Croddy, E. (2002). Dealing with Al Shifa: Intelligence and counterproliferation. *International Journal of Intelligence and Counterintelligence, 15*(1), 52–60. doi:10.1080/088506002753412874

Croddy, E., & Krcalova, S. (2001). Tularemia, biological warfare (BW), and the battle for Stalingrad (1942–1943). *Military Medicine, 166*(10), 837–838.

Cronin, A. K. (2004). Terrorist motivations for chemical and biological weapons use: Placing the threat in context. *Defense & Security Analysis, 20*(4), 313–320. doi:10.1080/1475179042000305778

Desjardins, A. E. (2004). Trichothecenes: From yellow rain to green wheat. *American Society for Microbiology News, 69*(4), 182–185.

Detusch, A. (2016, February 23). Exclusive: Samples confirm Islamic State used mustard gas in Iraq—diplomat. *Reuters.*

Falkenrath, R. A., Newman, R. D., & Thayer, B. A. (1998). *America's Achilles' heel: Nuclear, biological, and chemical terrorism and covert attack.* Cambridge, MA: The MIT Press.

Fothergill, L. D. (1958). Biological warfare and its defense. *Armed Forces Chemical Journal, 12*(5), 5–6.

Franke, S. (1967). *Manual of military chemistry* (Vol. 1). *Chemistry of Chemical Warfare* [*Lehrbuch der Militarchemie der Kampfstoffe*]. East Berlin, Germany: Deutscher Milita-rverlag.

Franz, D. R., Jarling, P. B., McClain, D. J., Hoover, D. L., Byrne, W. R., ... Eitzen, E. M. (2001). Clinical recognition and management of patients exposed to biological warfare agents. *Clinics in Laboratory Medicine* (*Laboratory Aspects of Biowarfare*), 21(3), 453.

Frerichs, R. (2002). American anthrax outbreak of 2001. UCLA Department of Epidemiology. Retrieved from http://www.ph.ucla.edu/epi/bioter/detect/antdetect_intro.html

Gamble, A., & Watanabe, T. (2004). *A public betrayed: An inside look at Japanese media atrocities and their warnings to the West.* Washington, DC: Regnery Publishing.

Gaynor, T. (2011, May 13). Arizona man arrested on chemical weapon charges. *Reuters* (online).

Gillis, J. (2001, December 3). Pledge for smallpox vaccine runs into tight-budget reality. *Washington Post,* p. A14.

Gurr, N., & Cole, B. (2000). *The new face of terrorism: Threats from weapons of mass destruction.* New York: I.B. Taurus.

Henderson, D. A., Inglesby, T. V., Bartlett, J. G., O'Toole, T. O., Russell, P. K. et al. (1998). *Plague: Civilian medical and public management following use of a biological weapon.* Unpublished manuscript.

Hoffman, B. (1998). *Inside terrorism.* New York: Columbia University Press.

Hurwitz, E. (1982). Terrorists and chemical/biological weapons. *Naval War College Review, 35*(3), 37–38.

Hyams, K. C., Murphy, F. M., & Wessely, S. (2002). Responding to chemical, biological, or nuclear terrorism: The indirect and long-term health effects may present the greatest challenge. *Journal of Health Politics, Policy, and Law, 27*(2), 273–291.

Jones, T. F., Craig, A. F., Hoy, D., Gunter, E. W., Ashley, D. L., Barr, D. B. et al. (2000). Mass psychogenic illness attributed to toxic exposure at a high school. *New England Journal of Medicine, 342*(2), 96–100. doi:10.1056/NEJM200001133420206

Kalelkar, A. S. (1988). *Investigation of large-magnitude incidents: Bhopal as a case study.* Paper presented at the Institution of Chemical Engineers Conference on Preventing Major Chemical Accidents, London, UK (May 1988). Retrieved from http://storage.dow.com.edgesuite.net/dow.com/Bhopal/casestdy.pdf

Kime, J. A., & Lowe, E. P. (1971). *Human oral dose for ten selected food- and waterborne diseases.* Frederick, MD: Department of the Army.

LaSalandra, M. (2001, November 9). Study finds little panic over bioterror. *The Boston Herald,* p. 16.

Lee, H. K. (2002, June 13). Airline passenger's rash sets off a smallpox scare. *San Francisco Chronicle,* p. A1.

Lohs, K. (1963). *Synthetic poisons* (2nd ed.). East Berlin: German Military Publishing House.

Lovejoy, F. H., & Linden, C. H. (1994). Acute poison and drug overdosage. In K. J. Isselbacher, E. Braunwald, J. Wilson, J. Martin, A. Fauci, & D. Kasper (Eds.), *Harrison's principles of internal medicine* (13th ed., pp. 2441–2461). New York, NY: McGraw-Hill.

McCormick, T. (2016). Foiled Kenya anthrax plot hints at Islamic State's scramble for Africa. *Foreign Policy.* Retrieved from http://foreignpolicy.com/2016/05/04/foiled-kenya-anthrax-plot-hints-at-islamic-states-scramble-for-africa/

McKenna, M. A. J. (2002, May 11). TV's smallpox drama unnerves health officials. *The Atlanta Journal and Constitution,* p. B1.

McNerney, E., & Rhodes, M. (2009). Al-Qaeda's WMD activities. In G. A. Ackerman & J. Tamsett (Eds.), *Jihadists and weapons of mass destruction* (pp. 405–432). Boca Raton, FL: CRC Press.

Marrs, T. C., Maynard, R. L., & Sidell, F. R. (1996). *Chemical warfare agents: Toxicology and treatment.* New York, NY: Wiley.

Miller, J., Engelberg, S., & Broad, W. (2001). *Germs: Biological weapons and America's secret war.* New York, NY: Simon & Schuster.

Moscrop, A. (2001). Mass hysteria is seen as main threat from bioweapons. *British Medical Journal, 323*(7320), 1023.

9/11 Commission. (2004). *The 9/11 Commission report: Final report of the national commission on terrorist attacks upon the United States.* New York, NY: W.W. Norton.

Okumura, T., Suzuki, K., Fukuda A., Kohama, A., Takasu, N., Ishimatsu S., & Hinohara S. (1998). The Tokyo subway sarin attack: Disaster management, Part 2: Hospital response. *Academic Emergency Medicine, 5,* 618–624.

Petrie, K. J., & Wessely, S. (2002). Modern worries, new technology, and medicine. *British Medical Journal, 324*(7339), 690–691.

Pitt, M. L. M., Little, S., Ivins, B. E., Fellows, P., Boles, J., Barth, J. ... Friedlander, A. M. (1999). *In vitro* correlate of immunity in an animal model of inhalational anthrax. *Journal of Applied Microbiology, 87,* 304. doi:10.1046/j.1365-2672.1999.00897.x

Prentiss, A. M. (1937). *Chemicals in war: A treatise on chemical warfare.* New York, NY: McGraw-Hill Book Company.

Ricks, D. (2001, October 3). Requests for medications on the rise. *Newsday,* p. A37.

Seto, Y., Tsunoda, N., Kataoka, M., Tsuge, K., & Nagano, T. (2000). *Toxicological analysis of victim's blood and crime scene evidence samples in the sarin gas attack caused by Aum Shinrikyo* (Unpublished manuscript). Chiba, Japan: National Research Institute of Police Science.

Shane, S. (2002, March 8). Anthrax toll could have been far worse, study finds. *The Baltimore Sun,* p. A7.

Shane, S. (2011, March 24). Panel of psychiatrists backs FBI's finding that scientist sent anthrax letters. *The New York Times,* p. 19.

Sheppard, B., Rubin, G. J., Wardman, J. K., & Wessely, S. (2006). Viewpoint: Terrorism and dispelling the myth of a panic prone public. *Journal of Public Health Policy, 27,* 219–245. doi:10.1057/palgrave.jphp.3200083

Sidell, F. R. (1996). Chemical agent terrorism. *Annals of Emergency Medicine, 28,* 223–4.

Sidell, F. R. (1997). Nerve agents. In F. R. Sidell, E. T. Takafuji, & D. R. Franz (Eds.), *Medical aspects of chemical and biological warfare* (pp. 129–179). Washington, DC: Borden Institute.

Smith, J. F., Davis, K., Hart, M. K., Ludwig, G. V., McClain, D. J. et al. (1997). Viral encephalitides. In F. R. Sidell, E. T. Takafuji, & D. R. Franz (Eds.), *Medical aspects of chemical and biological warfare.* Washington, DC: Borden Institute.

Smithson, A., & Levy, L. (2000). Ataxia: The chemical and biological terrorism threat and the U.S. response. *Stimson Center Report,* No. 35. Retrieved from https://www.stimson.org

Sobel, J., Khan, A. S., & Swerdlow, D. L. (2002). Threat of a biological terrorist attack on the U.S. food supply: The CDC perspective. *The Lancet, 359*(9309), 874–880. doi:10.1016/S0140-6736(02)07947-3

State of Wisconsin. (2002, June 14). Governor's office website. Retrieved from https://www.wisconsin.gov

Staudenmayer, H. (1999). *Environmental Illness: Myth and Reality.* Boca Raton, FL: Lewis Publishers.

Stern, J. (1999). *The ultimate terrorists.* Cambridge, MA: Harvard University Press.

Taylor, B. W., & Werbicki, J. E. (1993). Pseudodisaster: A case of mass hysteria involving 19 schoolchildren. *Pediatric Emergency Care, 9*(4), 216–217.

Teutsch, S. M., Martone, W. J., Brink, E. W., Potter, M. E., Eliot, G. et al. (1979). Pneumonic tularemia on Martha's Vineyard. *New England Journal of Medicine, 301,* 826–828. doi:10.1056/NEJM197910113011507

Tour, J. M. (2000). Do-it-yourself chemical weapons. *Chemical & Engineering News, 78*(28), 42–45. doi:10.1021/cen-v078n028.p042

United Nations Security Council. (2016). S/2016/738: Third report of the Organization for the Prohibition of Chemical Weapons-United Nations Joint Investigative Mechanism. Retrieved from https://www.un.org/ga/search/view_doc.asp?symbol=S/2016/738

U.S. Army Medical Command (1999). *Medical management of chemical casualties course, medical response to chemical warfare and terrorism* [Satellite broadcast]. Aberdeen Proving Ground, MD: U.S. Army Medical Research Institute for Chemical Defense and U.S. Federal Drug Administration.

U.S. Centers for Disease Control and Prevention. (2017). Strategic national stockpile: Chempack. Retrieved from https://www.cdc.gov/phpr/stockpile/chempack.htm

United States, Department of the Army, Air Force. (1958). *Capabilities and employment of toxic chemicals.* Washington, DC: Author.

Urbanetti, J. S. (1997). Toxic inhalational injury. In F. R. Sidell, E. T. Takafuji, & D. R. Franz (Eds.), *Medical aspects of chemical and biological warfare* (pp. 247–270). Washington, DC: Borden Institute.

Wannemacher, R. W., & Wiener, S. L. (1997). Trichothecene mycotoxins. In F. R. Sidell, E. T. Takafuji, & D. R. Franz (Eds.), *Medical aspects of chemical and biological warfare* (pp. 655–676). Washington, DC: Borden Institute.

Warrick, Joby. (2015). *Black Flags: The Rise of ISIS.* New York, NY: Doubleday.

Wein, L. M., & Liu Y. (2005). Analyzing a bioterror attack on the food supply: The case of botulinum toxin in milk. *Proceedings of the National Academy of Sciences of the United States of America, 102*(28), 9984–9989. doi:10.1073/pnas.0408526102

Wessely, S., Hyams, K. C., & Bartholomew, R. (2001). Psychological implications of chemical and biological weapons. *British Medical Journal, 323*(7318), 878–879. doi:10.1136/bmj.323.7318.878

Wilson, C. (2006). Improvised explosive devices (IEDs) in Iraq and Afghanistan: Effects and countermeasures. Congressional Research Service, Report for Congress, September 25, 2006.

Winslow, F. E. (1999). The first-responder's perspective. In S. D. Drell, A. D. Sofaer, & G. D. Wilson (Eds.), *The new terror: Facing the threat of biological and chemical weapons* (pp. 375–389). Stanford, CA: Hoover Institution Press.

Woodall, J. (1997). Tokyo subway gas attack [Letter]. *Lancet, 350*(9073), 296. doi:10.1016/S0140-6736(05)62271-4

World Health Organization. (1974). Seventeenth report of the Joint FAO/WHO Expert Committee on Food Additives (World Health Organization Technical Report Series, No. 539). Geneva, Switzerland: Author.

29

CHEMICAL AGENTS OF CONCERN

Justin K. Loden, Sean J. Kice, and John G. Benitez

CRITICAL INFORMATION

1. Notify local emergency responders by calling 911.
2. Call the Poison Center: 1-800-222-1222.
3. Centers for Disease Control Emergency Response Hotline: (770) 488-7100.
4. Do not wait for test results to begin immediate treatment.
5. Wear proper personal protective equipment (PPE) when handling hazardous materials (HAZMAT) and when treating exposed patients.
6. Protect the emergency department from secondary contamination.

LEARNING OBJECTIVES

When this chapter is completed, readers will be able to:

1. Identify the risk of exposure to chemical agents.
2. Describe the six major types of chemical agents used in chemical warfare.
3. List the five lifesaving procedures to perform before any needed decontamination.
4. Describe the primary assessment and resuscitation of HAZMAT victims.
5. Recognize the typical features (toxidrome) of each category of chemical agents.
6. Describe the need to conduct a focused health history to assess potential exposure to a chemical agent.
7. Describe the immediate psychological response of the individual, family, child, and community following a chemical incident.
8. Discuss the Centers for Disease Control and Prevention (CDC) Guidelines for the initial management of patients with acute toxic exposures.

KEY MESSAGES

HAZMAT incidents may result from accidental exposure, such as a transportation accident or an industrial accident, or an intentional terrorist act.

A large HAZMAT incident will create widespread social disruption and a surge of patients seeking care with the potential to overwhelm the healthcare system.

The ability to accurately identify chemical exposures in the field varies by geographical location and not all possible chemical exposures will be detected.

Chemical contamination may be recognized by odors emanating from victims, reports from first responders at the scene, or the victims' symptoms such as fainting, seizing, complaining of watering eyes, and dripping nose.

Chemical disasters may result in multiple ill individuals with similar complaints seeking care at the same time, usually from a common location.

Nurses need to be able to recognize and treat exposures to the chemical agents of concern, and a rapid decision must be made to protect the hospital from secondary contamination.

Managing the basics (airway, breathing, and circulation) is key to survival.

Storage of appropriate inventories of chemical antidotes, or quick access to such stores, is critical to the successful treatment of many chemical weapon victims.

CHAPTER OVERVIEW

Exposure to hazardous chemical agents can occur in the home, workplace, and in the community and may arise accidentally or through the intentional acts of terrorists. A variety of toxic chemicals may be used as chemical warfare agents (CWAs). These include nerve agents, vesicants, tissue (blood) agents, pulmonary agents, and riot control agents. Symptom onset may be immediate and occur in the field as is seen with nerve agent poisoning, or may be delayed for many hours as is seen after phosgene exposures. Treatment needs to be individualized depending on the class of chemical agents. Rapid administration of specific antidotes is critical to treat symptomatic cyanide or nerve agent poisoning. Other chemical exposures such as most choking or blistering agents do not have specific antidotes. Treatment in the latter cases is limited to decontamination and supportive care.

A major event involving the use of chemical weapons would potentially result in chaos and panic, widespread social disruption, and significant morbidity and mortality. Nurses need to have an awareness of the challenges that would be encountered in caring for victims of a chemical attack, and where to locate guidelines for patient care and event management.

Hazardous material (HAZMAT) is any substance with the potential to harm people, property, or the environment. This includes not only chemicals, but also biological, radiological, nuclear, and explosive substances. Outside of the United States, HAZMATs are often referred to as "dangerous goods." Specific HAZMATs that are intended or have the capability to cause death or serious bodily injury to a significant number

of people are typically referred to as "chemical, biological, radiological, nuclear" (CBRN) explosive agents or "weapons of mass destruction" (WMDs; 50 United States Code § 2302).

Modern industrialized society is dependent upon chemicals for manufacturing, agriculture, transportation, direct consumer use, water purification, and food preservation. The toxic and explosive properties of some chemicals make them a potentially significant burden to public health and safety either through accidental or intentional release. Many of these toxic chemicals (see Table 29.1) are produced, transported, and used in large quantities in urban and rural settings alike.

TABLE 29.1 Chemical Agents and Other Common Industrial Chemicals of Concern

Chemical Asphyxiants (Blood Agents)
- Arsine (SA)
- Azides (e.g., hydrogen azide)
- Carbon monoxide
- Cyanides and cyanogenic compounds
- Methemoglobin inducers (e.g., nitrates and nitrites)
- Sodium monofluoroacetate (compound 1080)
- Sulfides (e.g., hydrogen sulfide)

Incapacitating Agents
- 3-Quinuclidinyl benzilate (QNB/BZ)
- Fentanyl derivatives (e.g., kolokol-1, carfentanil, remifentanil)

Nerve Agents
- G-Series (e.g., sarin [GB], soman [GD], tabun [GA])
- V-Series (e.g., VX, VE, VG, VM, VR)
- Organophosphorus pesticides
- Carbamate pesticides

(continued)

TABLE 29.1 Chemical Agents and Other Common Industrial Chemicals of Concern (*continued*)

Pulmonary Irritants (Choking Agents)
- Ammonia
- Bromine (CA)
- Chlorine (CL)
- Hydrogen chloride
- Methyl bromide
- Methyl isocyanate
- Osmium tetroxide
- Diphosgene (DP)
- Phosgene (CG)
- Phosphine
- Phosphorus (elemental, white or yellow)
- Sulfuryl fluoride

Riot Control Agents (RCAs)
- Chloroacetophenone (CN)
- Chorobenzylidene-malonitrile (CS)
- Diphenylaminearsine (DM)
- Oleoresin-Capsaicin (OC)

Vesicants (Blister Agents)
- Mustards (e.g., mustard gas [H], nitrogen mustard [HN])
- Lewisites/chloroarsines (e.g., L-1, L-2, L-3)
- Mustard/lewisite (HL)
- Phosgene oxime (CX)

In 2012, approximately 2.58 billion tons of HAZMATs were produced and transported throughout the United States (U.S. Census Bureau, 2015).

HAZMAT INCIDENTS

A HAZMAT incident is an emergency response incident that involves the release of any HAZMAT. The release of hazardous chemicals may be overt, such as the result of an explosion or leak, or much more subtle, such as the intentional use of aerosol dispersal devices. In 1990, the Agency for Toxic Substances and Disease Registry (ATSDR) established the Hazardous Substances Emergency Events Surveillance (HSEES) system to collect and analyze information about HAZMAT incidents (excluding those involving only petroleum products) through June 2009 (see Case 29.1). Nineteen state health departments participated in the program while it was active. Several important principles were learned from HSEES (ARTSDR, 2012):

- Most incidents occurred at fixed facilities—not transportation accidents.
- The majority of incidents involved the release of only one chemical.
- The most commonly encountered chemicals at incidents vary by locale.
- Inhalation of airborne chemicals was the most common route of exposure.
- The vast majority of incidents did not generate victims.
- However, most victims came from multicasualty incidents.

- Employees and members of the general public accounted for most fatalities.
- Trauma followed by thermal burns produced the majority of fatalities.

According to *Recognizing and Identifying Hazardous Materials* (National Fire Academy and National Emergency Training Center, 1992), there are six primary clues that may signify the presence of HAZMATs:

- **Occupancy/Location:** The location of the HAZMAT incident or the victim's occupation can provide an indication as to the involved material.
- **Container Type:** The type of container typically provides a good indication as to the contents. The more substantial, durable, and fortified a container is, the more likely the material inside is dangerous. The Department of Transportation (DOT) regulations describe container specifications for the transport of HAZMATs.
- **Markings/Colors:** Facilities and vehicles must use special markings, including identification numbers and colors, to indicate the presence of HAZMATs (see the DOT Emergency Response Guidebook).
- **Placards/Labels:** Placards are used when HAZMATs are being stored in bulk, such as in cargo tanks. Labels designate HAZMATs kept in smaller containers.
- **Shipping Papers:** These should provide the shipping name, hazard class, identification number, and quantity, and may indicate whether the material is waste or poison. Shipping papers are required to accompany all shipments and list a 24-hour emergency information telephone number.
- **Senses:** Odor, vapor clouds, dead animals, and dermal/ocular irritation can indicate the presence of HAZMATs. However, some chemicals can impair an individual's sense of smell (e.g., hydrogen sulfide) while others have no odor, color, or taste at all (e.g., carbon monoxide).

CHEMICAL AGENTS IN THE ENVIRONMENT

The first challenge encountered in the event of a terrorist attack involving the use of CWAs is detection of the chemical in the environment. Because of their physical properties, the use of chemical agents in a domestic terrorist incident may not be associated with a high explosive event. Delivery of chemical agents may occur by spraying; contaminating water or air supplies; or delivery via missiles, artillery shells, or aerial bombing. Dispersal of a vapor hazard in a confined space may be particularly attractive to the terrorist.

In June 1994 and again in May 1995, the Japanese cult group Aum Shinrikyo created much havoc when they released the deadly nerve agent sarin in two Japanese cities. In the first attack in Matsumoto, Japan, sarin vapor was released in a residential area where judges unfriendly to the cult resided. Seven people died as a consequence of this nerve agent exposure, and 500 people were injured. The 1995 attack occurred in the Tokyo subway system. Several coordinated releases of this potentially deadly vapor, in a confined space, resulted in more than 5,000 visits to local emergency departments. Fortunately, the vast majority of exposed victims had few, if any, symptoms and there was only a handful of fatalities (Tucker, 2006; for further discussion, see Chapter 28 "Biological and Chemical Terrorism: A Unique Threat").

The type of incident that occurred in Tokyo is the classic example of the type of incident that can be anticipated as the result of a terrorist attack. The attack of sarin liquid was minimized, fortunately, because of the inefficient release of the liquid and its slow vaporization. The highest probability of detecting the presence of a CWA occurs in situations where there is a continuous source of vapor. By the time emergency medical responders arrive at the scene, significant dispersion of the agent can likely be expected, making detection difficult (Tucker, 2006). Once casualties of a vapor (gas) incident are removed from the scene of the attack and taken to medical care stations or facilities, the signs and symptoms of the patients may be the only clues to the detection of a chemical agent. Following the removal of victims from the source of the exposure, the threat of spreading the chemical agent to others remains but is relatively low. In the case of the Tokyo sarin gas attack, however, 9% of emergency medical services (EMS) workers and a significant number of hospital staff, including nurses, experienced acute symptoms of nerve toxicity from exposure to casualties in unventilated areas. This issue shows that liquid contamination of patients can cause contamination of other caretakers even away from the site of exposure. Typically, volatile gas–only contaminations do not cause problems with secondary contamination and the subsequent need for decontamination.

Emergency response systems and healthcare facilities will need to respond to terrorist chemical attacks in a manner similar to an incident involving HAZMATs. The same principles regarding triage, decontamination, and the allocation of resources in response to a HAZMAT incident will be needed during a terrorist chemical attack (Burda & Sigg, 2001).

HAZMAT EMERGENCY RESPONSE

The response to HAZMAT incidents is standardized by both the Occupational Safety and Health Administration (OSHA) at the federal level and industry wide by the National Fire Protection Association (NFPA), and following their guidance, specialized HAZMAT teams are called in to address these situations. Emergency responders arriving on the scene must be capable of determining that a HAZMAT incident has occurred and are responsible for determining whether the HAZMAT team should be called for assistance. Responders have different levels of training and preparedness (see Table 29.2) depending on their role in response. This training is required under OSHA and is reinforced through adoption by NFPA. Not all municipalities have a HAZMAT team, though one may be requested through mutual aid agreements from localities that do have them. Because of these specialized requirements, delays in response may occur and local fire departments may need to act independent of HAZMAT teams until additional resources can be mobilized.

Specific guidelines for indirect hospital response are laid out in OSHA Best Practices for Hospital-Based First Receivers of Victims from Mass Casualty Incidents Involving the Release of Hazardous Substances, January 2005. All hospital personnel who have a designated role in a HAZMAT response must be

TABLE 29.2 Hazardous Materials Training Levels

First Responder Awareness
Individuals who are likely to witness or discover a hazardous substance release and who have been trained to initiate an emergency response sequence by notifying the proper authorities.

First Responder Operations
Individuals who respond to releases or potential releases of hazardous substances as part of the initial response to the site. They are trained to respond in a defensive fashion without actually trying to stop the release. Their function is to contain the release from a safe distance, keep it from spreading, and prevent exposures. Requires First Responder Awareness and 8 hours of additional training.

Hazardous Materials Technician
Individuals who respond to releases or potential releases for the purpose of stopping the release. Requires First Responder Operations and 24 additional hours of training.

Hazardous Materials Specialist
Individuals who respond with and provide support to HAZMAT technicians. Requires Hazardous Materials Technician and 24 hours of additional training.

Source: Code of Federal Regulations Title 29, Part 1910.120.

TABLE 29.3 Levels of Personal Protective Equipment

Level A
Provides the highest level of dermal, respiratory, ocular, and mucus membrane protection. Equipment includes a fully encapsulated water/vapor-proof suit which contains a self-contained breathing apparatus (SCBA). The suit should contain a cooling and communication system.

Level B
Provides the highest level of respiratory protection, but dermal and ocular protection will suffice with splash-resistant gear. Equipment includes SCBA and splash-resistant clothing, hood, gloves, hard-hat, boots, booties, and a cooling and communication system.

Level C
Provides the same dermal and ocular protection as Level B, but uses an APR rather than SCBA. The APR filters the air rather than providing oxygen from an outside source.

Level D
Provides standard work protection from splashes with no respiratory and minimal dermal protection. The gear includes cover or standard work clothing, safety glasses, gloves, and face shield.

APR, air-purifying respirator.

Source: Code of Federal Regulations Title 29, Part 1910.120.

trained to the First Responder Awareness level. Staff must be comfortable with knowing how to locate and use PPE and be knowledgeable and practiced with the decontamination process. For victims of an unknown HAZMAT threat, powered air-purifying respirators (APRs) with high-efficiency particulate air (HEPA)/ organic vapor/acid filters, double gloves, chemical-resistant suits, hoods, and boots must be worn at the hospital decontamination zone, and additionally, all openings need to be sealed with tape. While a response to an unknown chemical requires stronger selection of PPE that what is normally worn, 29 CFR 1910.120 allows for PPE to be downgraded to the minimum needed to respond to a known hazard (see Table 29.3 and Chapter 35 "Decontamination and Personal Protective Equipment" for further discussion). Hospital personnel who are part of the decontamination team must also be trained to the First Responder Operations level, taking into account that they are acting out of the scene of the chemical release (Hick et al., 2003). Hospitals should also be prepared to

take care of pediatric and other victims with special needs and other unique-situations needs during a HAZMAT incident (Burke, Iverson, Goodhue, Neches, & Upperman, 2010).

Emergency services and healthcare facilities will need to respond to intentional chemical releases in a similar manner as an accidental HAZMAT incident. The same principles regarding triage, decontamination, and the allocation of resources will be needed (Russell, & Simpson, 2010). Intentional acts may be further complicated with the inclusion of law enforcement investigation. There are several Internet-based tools and applications available (see Table 29.4) to assist first responders and medical personnel as resources during a HAZMAT incident.

TABLE 29.4 Information Resources for HAZMAT Incidents

Agency for Toxic Substances and Disease Registry (ATSDR)	Provides 24-hour assistance to emergency responders in managing HAZMAT incidents. 1-770-488-7100 www.atsdr.cdc.gov/emergencyresponse.html
CHEMM Intelligent Syndromes Tool (CHEMM-IST)	Decision support tool to aid in toxidrome identification in HAZMAT victims. chemm.nlm.nih.gov/chemmist.htm
CHEMTREC	Provides 24-hour emergency contact for identification of HAZMAT and precautionary measures. 1-800-424-9300 www.chemtrec.com
First Responder Support Tools (FRST)	Provides critical map-based information to emergency responders in managing HAZMAT incidents. Available as a mobile web application. www.firstsupporttools.com
National Pesticide Information Center (NPIC)	Provides information about pesticides and pesticide-related topics. Available only weekdays from 8 a.m. to 12 p.m. Pacific time. 1-800-858-7378 npic.orst.edu
NIOSH Pocket Guide to Chemical Hazards	Provides general information and industrial hygiene information for workers, employers, and occupational health professionals. Available as a mobile web application. www.cdc.gov/niosh/npg/default.html
Regional Poison Control Center	Provides 24-hour assistance to emergency responders and healthcare personnel in managing HAZMAT victims. 1-800-222-1222
TOXMAP Environmental Health Maps	Provides information on previous HAZMAT incidents and location of HAZMAT. toxmap.nlm.nih.gov/toxmap
Toxicology Data Network (TOXNET)	Provides peer-reviewed information on toxicity, chemicals, medications, diseases, environmental health, occupational safety and health, risk assessment, and regulations. Available as a mobile web application. toxnet.nlm.nih.gov
U.S. Department of Transportation (DOT) Emergency Response Guidebook	Provides guidance to first responders on how to identify and respond to HAZMATs that may be involved in an incident. Available as a mobile web application. phmsa.dot.gov/hazmat/erg-mobile-app
Wireless Information System for Emergency Responders (WISER)	Provides assistance to emergency responders in managing HAZMAT incidents. Decision support tool to aid in chemical identification based on properties, symptoms, etc. Available as a mobile web application. wiser.nlm.nih.gov

HAZMAT, hazardous material.

DETECTION OF CHEMICAL AGENTS

HAZMAT teams are routinely equipped with a variety of chemical detectors and monitoring kits, primarily chemical-specific tests indicating only the presence or absence of a chemical. Remember that these are preliminary tests and are not conclusive and there are many false negatives and positives to these tests. The ability to detect and measure chemical agents in the field varies considerably by locale and may be severely limited or nonexistent. Some large metropolitan areas have adequate instrumentation, whereas other areas have no chemical detection capabilities at all. In those locations lacking adequate detection technology, and in most emergency departments, the signs and symptoms of the victims may be the only detection method available.

The goal of chemical weapons detectors and sensors is to alert to an imminent danger. Significant biotechnology research has been conducted and sponsored by the Department of Defense, as well as a large number of private biotechnology firms, on the development of portable specialized sensors. These scientists are attempting to develop new, lighter, and more portable detection tools and to refine the sensitivity and specificity of these types of instruments to greatly improve our detection capabilities. Handheld portable alarm detectors and alarm agent monitoring dose meter detectors are now used for control of contaminated and decontaminated areas, chemical disarmament, water contamination control, and medical sorting of casualties. Cutting-edge chemical techniques readily allow for the detection of single molecules; however, the use of these tools is limited to sophisticated research laboratories. Detectors for CWAs and chemical terrorist weapons must function in demanding, real-world environments where price, portability, and time are factors. Further complicating the situation is the possibility that a terrorist attack may involve the use of more than a single agent; therefore, the most challenging aspect for chemical agent identification is often extracting the agent of interest from the other chemicals in the environment.

CHEMICAL AGENTS OF CONCERN

Chemical agents vary widely and are categorized by their structure and/or physical effect on victims. Scientists often categorize hazardous chemicals by the type of chemical or by the effects a chemical would have on people exposed to it. The categories/types used by the CDC are as follows (CDC, 2016):

- Biotoxins
- Blister agents/vesicants
- Blood agents
- Caustics (acids)
- Choking/lung/pulmonary agents
- Incapacitating agents
- Long-acting anticoagulants
- Metals
- Nerve agents
- Organic solvents
- Riot control agents/tear gas

- Toxic alcohols
- Vomiting agents

CWAs are classified into groups: nerve agents, biotoxins (e.g., ricin), vesicants (blistering agents), tissue (blood) agents, pulmonary agents, and riot control agents. An important principle of chemical agents is the rapid onset of symptoms that often occurs within minutes of the initial exposure (Burda & Sigg, 2001). Therefore, to minimize casualties, there must be prompt initiation of rescue, decontamination, medical attention, and antidotal therapy. The National Response Center's Chemical and Biological Hotline (1-800-424-8802) based in Aberdeen, Maryland, serves as an emergency resource to all healthcare providers for technical assistance (Burda & Sigg, 2001).

Rapid diagnosis of patients who have been exposed to a chemical agent is critical to saving lives and preventing further injuries. The signs and symptoms of the patient provide the most important information on which to base treatment decisions. Frequently, clinicians cannot rapidly detect the presence of an agent within the body but must look for some by-product of the agent or a particular expression of symptoms (e.g., Diarrhea, Urination, Miosis, Bradycardia, Bronchorrhea, Bronchospasm, Emesis, Lacrimation, Salivation, Sweating [DUMBBBELSS], symptoms suggestive of cholinergic poisoning from nerve agents) that is suggestive that a chemical exposure has taken place. The specific nature of the biochemical reaction and the resultant clinical picture it produces will then lead clinicians to determine a course of therapy. Help can be obtained in putting the clinical picture together with the likely agent by contacting the nearest poison center and discussing the case with their specialist in poison information and medical toxicologist (1-800-222-1222) (Institute of Medicine & National Research Council, 1999).

MEDICAL COUNTERMEASURES

Treatment for exposures to most hazardous chemicals is limited to decontamination and supportive care. However, medical countermeasures do exist for some chemical agents (see Table 29.5), and it is important to recognize the opportunity to administer an antidote to the victim when one exists and if the right indications for it are present.

Some countermeasures have uses beyond toxicology (e.g., atropine) and will be readily available in large quantities, while others are used only to treat toxic exposures (e.g., dimercaprol) and unlikely to be available at most locations. Most hospitals will stock only a limited supply of these, typically enough to treat two to three patients for 24 hours based on the expected hazards in their area (Dart et al., 2009). Therefore, the hallmark of a successful management of a large-scale chemical attack involving mass casualties is based on a response plan that integrates local, state, and federal systems for the delivery and stockpiling of countermeasures for mass casualty events. The Strategic National Stockpile is the backbone for national-level medical countermeasure response. It comprises strategically positioned nerve agent kits called CHEMPACKs; the mass anthrax response kit called the 12 Hour Push Package, containerized for rapid air transportation; and mass warehoused material for selected responses called Managed Inventory. For

TABLE 29.5 Select Chemical Agents and Their Countermeasures

Chemical Agent	Countermeasure
Antimuscarinics	Physostigmine
Carbon monoxide	Normobaric oxygen, hyperbaric oxygen
Carbon tetrachloride	n-Acetylcysteine (NAC; for hepatic injury)
Cyanides	Hydroxocobalamin Sodium nitrite plus sodium thiosulfate
Fluoride compounds	Calcium Magnesium
Hydrazines	Pyridoxine (vitamin B6)
Hydrocarbons	Beta-blocker (for ventricular irritability)
Lewisites	Dimercaprol (BAL; topical)
Methemoglobinemia	Methylene blue
Mustards	Granulocyte colony-stimulating factor (for bone marrow suppression)
Nerve agents	Atropine Diazepam Pralidoxime (2-PAM)
Radioactive cesium	Prussian blue
Radioactive iodine	Potassium iodide
Radioactive thallium	Prussian blue
Opioids	Naloxone
Simple asphyxiants	Normobaric oxygen
Transuranic metals	Diethylenetriamene pentaacetate (DTPA)

BAL, British anti-Lewisite; NAC, n-Acetylcysteine.

more information, see www.bt.cdc.gov/stockpile. Even with this federal program, emphasis must be placed on which agents need to be available locally, how much is needed, and under whose authority they will be delivered and administered (see Chapter 33 "Medical Countermeasures Dispensing" for further discussion). Evidence supporting the efficacy of antidotes for CWAs/terrorism agents is weak for most categories. Ongoing research will likely yield changes in how existing ones are administered and how new countermeasures will be developed.

MEDICAL MANAGEMENT OF HAZMAT VICTIMS

Primary Assessment and Resuscitation

For victims exposed to liquid and solid chemicals, decontamination by healthcare providers wearing the appropriate PPE should precede resuscitation and primary assessment to prevent secondary contamination of unprotected healthcare providers (see Chapter 35 "Decontamination and Personal Protective Equipment," for

further discussion). All victims of a HAZMAT incident should be considered contaminated, regardless of on-site decontamination measures (Cox, 2016). The only procedures that should be performed prior to any needed skin decontamination are:

1. Opening and maintaining an open airway with spine stabilization and control, as needed;
2. Needle decompression of a tension pneumothorax;
3. Control of an exsanguinating external hemorrhage with a tourniquet; and
4. Administration of nerve agent antidotes via autoinjectors.

Resuscitation and primary assessment can be remembered using the mnemonic Airway, Breathing, Circulation, Disability, and Exposure (ABCDE). Circulation takes priority before airway and breathing (CAB) in victims with massive external hemorrhage or primary cardiac arrest, such as ventricular fibrillation or pulseless ventricular tachycardia (Ewy & Bobrow, 2016). In victims with exsanguinating hemorrhage, bleeding is controlled with direct pressure or a tourniquet on the affected extremity. Special attention should be given to HAZMAT victims with cardiac arrest. Primary cardiac arrest may occur after exposure to hydrocarbons (ventricular irritability) and hydrofluoric acid (hyperkalemia/hypocalcemia) and should be initially managed with minimally interrupted cardiac resuscitation (MICR) with passive oxygen insufflation. Most other HAZMATs would be expected to cause cardiac arrest secondary to respiratory arrest.

A = Airway (with spine stabilization and control, if needed)

Ensure an open and protected airway; suction as needed. Temporizing airway management with oropharyngeal/nasopharyngeal devices may be adequate during decontamination. Endotracheal intubation is the preferred airway management technique, when possible. Cricothyroidotomy may be required in victims with orofacial trauma or oropharyngeal/epiglottic/laryngeal edema.

B = Breathing

Ensure adequate ventilation and oxygenation. If victims are not breathing or not breathing adequately, assist with a bag-valve-mask and 100% oxygen, then intubate. If victims are able to protect their airway and breathing adequately, administer 100% oxygen to those with cardiopulmonary or neurological symptoms or potential exposure to chemical asphyxiants.

C = Circulation

Check for a pulse. If absent, begin cardiopulmonary resuscitation (CPR) or MICR, then check the rhythm and follow Advanced Cardiac Life Support (ACLS) guidelines. If the victim has a pulse, monitor the blood pressure and cardiac rhythm; follow ACLS guidelines. An IV of normal saline should be started on all victims with more than mild signs or symptoms. Monitor for shock and treat appropriately.

D = Disability (Nervous System)

Continually assess the victim's level of consciousness and neurological status. Victims with any neurological signs or symptoms should receive 100% oxygen. If seizures develop despite adequate oxygenation and normal glucose, treat with IV, IM, or IO benzodiazepines.

E = Exposure

The victim's clothing should have been removed during any needed decontamination. Careful attention should be paid to gas exposures as the victim's clothing could trap fumes and expose healthcare providers. Thoroughly assess the victim for signs of trauma, burns, and frostbite.

Secondary Assessment

Secondary assessment of HAZMAT victims includes history and physical examination. If possible, this should occur simultaneously with decontamination and/or during the primary assessment and resuscitation. This secondary assessment focuses on identifying a toxic syndrome (toxidrome), recognizing any preexistent illnesses, anticipating potential complications, and assessing for concurrent trauma. History can be remembered by using the mnemonic Allergies, Medications, Past Medical History, Last, and Events (AMPLE).

A = Allergies

Determine whether the victim is allergic to any substance or had an adverse event in the past.

M = Medications

Determine what medications the victim is prescribed. Current medications can give clues to the victim's preexistent illnesses and could also interact with resuscitative or antidotal therapies.

P = Past Medical History

Determine the victim's past medical history as preexistent illnesses can exacerbate reactions to various chemicals (e.g., asthmatics exposed to pulmonary irritants).

L = Last

Determine the last normal menstrual period in reproductive-age women to assess for potential fetal toxic exposures. Determine the last tetanus shot in victims with open wounds. Determine the victim's last meal to assess aspiration risk during endotracheal intubation.

E = Events

Determine the events surrounding the HAZMAT incident. Are there other victims who need to be rescued? When did the incident occur? Where did the incident occur? What HAZMAT was involved in the incident? What was the route(s) of exposure? How long was the victim exposed to the HAZMAT? What treatment(s) has already been administered?

Identification of the specific HAZMAT involved in the incident is critical to saving lives and preventing further injury. Because adequate chemical detection technology is often not readily available, and missing information and/or misinformation is the rule during the early phases of emergency response, the signs and symptoms of the victim provide the most important information on which to base treatment decisions. The concept of the toxidrome, a collection of signs and symptoms associated with a particular class of poison, is invaluable under such circumstances (see Table 29.6). Assistance can be obtained in putting the clinical picture together by contacting the nearest poison center and discussing the case with their specialist in poison information and medical toxicologist (1-800-222-1222) (Thompson, Theobald, Lu, & Erickson, 2014). Also, CHEMM-IST and WISER have algorithm tools that can help provide toxidrome and chemical identification based on the victim's signs and symptoms, particular odors, and so forth.

NERVE AGENTS

Nerve agents are among the most potent and deadly of the chemical weapons. They are rapidly lethal and hazardous by any route of exposure (Reutter, 1999; Tucker, 2006). First discovered accidentally during the 1930s by industrial chemists in Germany conducting pesticide research, the nerve agents tabun and sarin were developed into chemical weapons and stockpiled by the Nazi regime. Fortunately, Hitler did not order their use during World War II because German intelligence believed—incorrectly—that the United States and the Soviet Union had developed similar weapons. After the war, the victorious Allies competed among themselves for the secrets of the Nazi nerve agent program. In the early 1950s, British industrial scientists accidentally discovered a second

TABLE 29.6 HAZMAT Toxidromes

Asphyxiant	Chemical asphyxiants Methemoglobin inducers Pulmonary irritants	Dizziness, headache, confusion, weakness, syncope, coma, seizures, respiratory distress, lactic acidosis, cardiac arrhythmias/arrest Cyanides: erythema/flushed, although CO could be "normal" All others: cyanosis
Antimuscarinic	3-Quinuclidinyl benzilate	Mydriasis, blurred vision, erythema/flushed, anhidrosis, dry mucous membranes, urinary retention, tachycardia, hyperthermia, confusion, delirium, speech difficulty, visual hallucinations, seizures
Cholinergic	Nerve agents	Muscarinic Symptoms (DUMBBBELSS): diarrhea, diaphoresis, urinary incontinence, miosis, bradycardia, bronchorrhea, bronchospasm, emesis, lacrimation, salivation Nicotinic Symptoms (MTWHF): mydriasis, tachycardia, weakness, hypertension, hyperglycemia, fasciculations Central Symptoms (CCC): confusion, convulsions, coma
Hydrocarbon	Anesthetics Propellants Refrigerants Solvents	Skin irritation, defatting dermatitis, burns, sedation, coma, respiratory depression, bronchospasm, wheezing, pulmonary edema, premature ventricular contractions, ventricular tachycardia, cardiac arrest See Asphyxiant Toxidrome
Opioid	Fentanyl gas	Respiratory depression, coma, miosis
Pulmonary irritant	Pulmonary irritants Vesicants	Irritation of the eyes, nose, throat, trachea, and major bronchi. Bronchospasm, hemoptysis, wheezing, dyspnea, dysphonia/aphonia, stridor, hoarseness, laryngospasm, pulmonary edema. Noxious (nausea/vomiting). See Asphyxiant Toxidrome
Vesicant	Vesicants	Skin irritation, erythema, vesicles, bullae, debilitating pain. See Pulmonary Irritant Toxidrome

generation of nerve agents that were even more toxic than sarin and were dubbed "V agents" because of their venomous (skin-penetrating) properties. During the Cold War, the United States and the Soviet Union pursued a chemical arms race in which they produced and stockpiled various nerve agents in thousands of tons. These supertoxic poisons have no peaceful uses and when inhaled or absorbed through the skin, are lethal in tiny amounts by disrupting the operation of the nervous system (Tucker, 2006). Nerve agents are liquids at room temperatures with the capability of producing a vapor that may be well absorbed through the skin as well as the lungs and gastrointestinal (GI) tract. It is possible to disseminate the nerve gases in high enough concentrations that would cause one breath to be incapacitating or deadly. Detecting the presence of nerve agents is extremely difficult as freshly mixed they are clear and colorless liquids. Liquid agents are heavier than water and their vapor is heavier than air, allowing them to sink into low terrains and basements (Alibek et al., 2006; Weinstein & Alibek, 2003).

Nerve agents are classified in two groups: G and V (Reutter, 1999). The G agents include GA (tabun), GB (sarin), GD (soman), and GF. The V agents, which tend to be more pernicious, include VG (amigon), VS, and VX. These agents are all highly poisonous chemicals that act by binding to the enzyme acetylcholinesterase, thereby blocking its normal function of breaking down the neurotransmitter acetylcholine following its release at neuronal synapses and neuromuscular junctions throughout the peripheral and central nervous systems (CNS). As a result

of exposure to cholinesterase inhibitors, acetylcholine cannot be broken down, and accumulates at all cholinergic receptors. The result is continued receptor stimulation (Weinstein & Alibek, 2003). Organophosphate pesticides work in exactly the same way, and are recognized in the same fashion as nerve agents. Carbamate pesticides also act on the same enzyme, causing similar symptoms, but the pesticide breaks down over the next few hours and symptoms typically do not last as long as with nerve agents or organophosphate pesticides.

Recognizing Nerve Agents

Persons exposed to high concentrations of organophosphate nerve agents usually develop signs and symptoms within a matter of minutes after exposure. Clinical presentation of patients with gasping, miosis, copious secretions, sweating, and generalized twitching is very suggestive of nerve agent exposure (Weinstein & Alibek, 2003). The cholinergic toxidrome that results is characterized by muscarinic signs and symptoms (DUMBBBELSS) and nicotinic signs and symptoms: Mydriasis, Tachycardia, Weakness, Hypertension, and muscle Fasciculations (MTWHF). Severe diaphoresis and loss of other body fluids can lead to dehydration, systemic hypovolemia, and shock. Resultant respiratory muscle paralysis is a frequent cause of death. Agitation, seizures, and coma can also occur as a result of CNS effects (Sidell, 1997; Table 29.7).

Nicotinic symptoms may be observed initially, but muscarinic signs can be observed concurrently. Later in the course of

TABLE 29.7 Nerve Agents by Appearance and Odor

Agent	Appearance	Odor
Sarin	Clear, colorless	Odorless
Soman	Clear, colorless	Slight camphor odor (e.g., cough suppressant) or rotting fruit odor
Tabun	Clear, colorless	Faint fruity odor
VX	Clear, amber-colored	Odorless

poisoning, muscarinic signs predominate. Persistent depolarizing neuromuscular blockade may develop after initial resolution of the cholinergic crisis and can cause sudden respiratory failure and death (Reutter, 1999; Weinstein & Alibek, 2003). Initial patient diagnoses and treatments are likely to be based on observations of signs and symptoms by the paramedic or other healthcare professionals at the scene (Table 29.3). Rescuers and healthcare workers must prevent direct contact with victims through proper use of PPE and decontamination procedures.

Duration/Mortality

Recovery may take several months with nerve agents. Organophosphate agents result in recovery over several days to weeks, while carbamate poisoning recovery occurs within 1 day. Permanent damage to the CNS is possible after exposure to a high dose. G agents are lethal within 1 to 10 minutes and V agents are generally lethal within 4 to 18 hours, depending on the dose and route of entry.

Patient Assessment

Muscle fasciculations and eventual paralysis may occur. Symptoms usually occur within seconds of exposure to a nerve agent but may take several hours when exposure is only transdermal (see Figure 29.1). Effects and time of onset of a nerve agent are dependent on the concentration of the agent and the amount of time exposed, as well as the route of exposure.

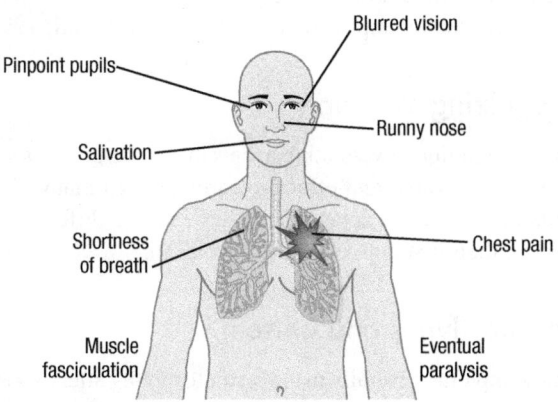

FIGURE 29.1 Nerve agents: Patient assessment.
Source: Rains Analytics (2007).

Mild inhalational exposure: Symptoms usually start at the site of exposure resulting in rapid onset of miosis, blurry vision, runny nose, chest tightness, dyspnea, and possible wheezing.
Severe inhalational exposure: Sudden coma, seizures, flaccid paralysis with apnea, miosis, diarrhea, and a victim who is "wet" (lacrimation, salivation, urination, sweating, copious upper and lower respiratory secretions).
Mild dermal exposure: Sweating and muscle fasciculations localized to the area of exposure, nausea, vomiting, diarrhea, and possible miosis.
Severe dermal exposure: Sudden coma, seizures, flaccid paralysis with apnea, miosis, diarrhea, and a victim who is "wet" (lacrimation, salivation, urination, sweating, copious upper and lower respiratory secretions). Onset of symptoms may be delayed by 30 minutes following exposure as the agents transit the skin.

Victims of a terrorist attack will usually have both inhalational and dermal exposures. Hours after treatment/decontamination, the agent, still in transit through the skin, may produce sudden and severe symptoms.

Clinical Diagnostic Tests

Red blood cell and serum cholinesterase levels are helpful to determine the extent of enzyme inhibition. Results will frequently take days to be delivered, except in some large hospitals where it may be done locally.

Patient Management

Do not approach contaminated victims unless wearing proper PPE. Provide supportive therapy and assisted ventilation as needed.

Treatment

The agents act rapidly and profoundly, and, therefore, poisoning from nerve agents is a serious medical emergency. Treatment consists of thorough decontamination and, once the path of exposure has been determined, appropriate emergency and supportive measures (see Table 29.8). Patients with respiratory failure and compromised airways require immediate endotracheal intubation and positive pressure ventilation. Suctioning may be needed to remove bronchial secretions. Treatment includes prophylactic anticonvulsants to prevent seizures, oximes to reactivate the inhibited acetylcholinesterase and reverse paralysis (only for nerve agents and organophosphate pesticides), and anticholinergics to antagonize the muscarinic effects (Evison, Hinsley, & Rice, 2002). Specific antidotes include atropine and pralidoxime. Atropine, an antimuscarinic agent, may be required in extremely large quantities, and routine hospital stocks can be quickly depleted. Atropine does not treat or reverse nicotinic effects such as fasciculations and paralysis. Pralidoxime (2-PAM, Protopam) acts to regenerate the enzyme activity at all affected sites, reverses paralysis, and is potentially curative if provided early enough and in sufficient doses for nerve agents and organophosphate pesticides. Patients may be put on atropine drips once initial symptoms stabilize. Seizures are treated with benzodiazepines (Alibek et al., 2006; Weinstein &

TABLE 29.8 Agent Treatment by Exposure Type

Exposure	Treatment
Inhalation	• If signs are severe, immediately administer, in rapid succession, all three Nerve Agent Antidote Kit(s), Mark I* injectors (or atropine if directed by a physician). • If signs and symptoms are progressing, use injectors at 5- to 20-minute intervals; use no more than three injections. • Atropine should be administered every 3–5 minutes to dry secretions. There is no benefit to using more than 3 injections of 2-PAM. • Give artificial respiration if breathing has stopped or is difficult; do not use mouth-to-mouth if face is contaminated.
Skin	• Decontaminate using soap and water.
Eyes	• Immediately flush eyes with water or saline for 10–15 minutes. • Don respiratory protective mask.
Ingestion	• Do not induce vomiting. • Immediately administer Nerve Agent Antidote Kit, Mark I.*

2-PAM, pralidoxime.

*Mark I kits contain atropine 2 mg and 2-PAMC1 600 mg in separate auto-injectors.

Source: Agency for Toxic Substances and Disease Registry. (2014). Toxic substances portal—Nerve agents (GA, GB, GD, VX). Retrieved from https://www.atsdr.cdc.gov/mmg/mmg.asp?id=523&tid=93

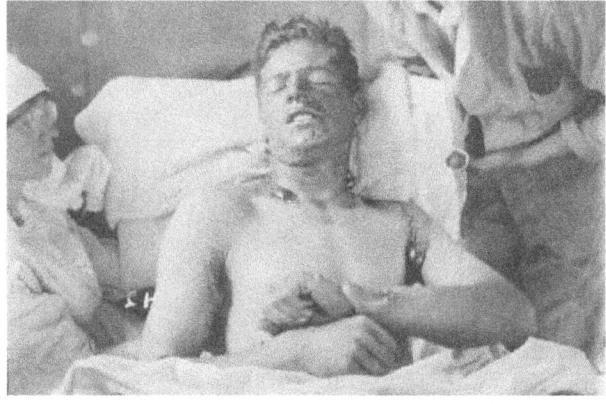

FIGURE 29.2 World War I soldier with mustard gas burns, ca. 1917–1918.
Source: Library and Archives Canada.

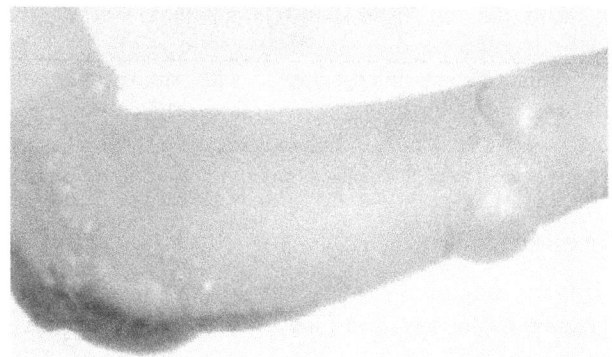

FIGURE 29.3 Bullae resulting from mustard gas exposure.
Source: Library and Archives Canada.

Alibek, 2003). Nerve agents serve no useful purpose to society and primary prevention through full chemical disarmament should be the goal (Tucker, 2006).

VESICATING/BLISTER AGENTS

Vesicants/blister agents are chemicals that severely blister the eyes, respiratory tract, and skin on contact. Possible substances included in this class are mustard agents, lewisites/chloro arsine agents, and phosgene oxime (Alibek et al., 2006).

Sulfur mustard has been used as a CWA in several wars (see Figure 29.2), most recently in the Iran–Iraq conflict. Thioglycol, an immediate precursor to sulfur mustard, has many industrial uses and is commercially available. At room temperature, sulfur mustard is an oily liquid that is only slightly soluble in water. At higher temperatures, it becomes a significant vapor hazard ("mustard gas"). It can permeate rubber and is readily absorbed through the skin, eyes, respiratory tract, and GI tract. Nitrogen and sulfur mustards and lewisite are cytotoxic alkylating agents. Sulfur mustard reacts within minutes with components of DNA, RNA, and proteins, and interrupts cell function. Mustard is the only one of the vesicants that does not cause immediate pain (Sidell, Urbanetti, Smith, & Hurst, 1997). Clinical signs and symptoms may develop within 2 to 12 hours but typically develop after 12 hours. The fluid-filled

bullae that eventually form do *not* contain mustard agent (see Figure 29.3). Ocular and pulmonary injuries also may occur, and respiratory involvement is the most common cause of mortality. Mortality ranges from 2% to 3%. Approximately 5 to 7 mL (100 mg/kg) of mustard spread over 25% of the body surface area is potentially lethal (Davis & Aspera, 2001). Lewisite liquid or vapor produces irritation and pain seconds after contact. Phosgene oxime in vapor or liquid form is highly corrosive and readily penetrates clothing and rubber. Exposure is characterized by immediate, severe pain and skin lesions similar to those caused by exposure to a strong acid (Sidell, 1997).

Recognizing Vesicants

Rapid recognition of vesicating agents in an emergency is a key step to ensure rapid and effective care. Though many blister agents are similar in appearance, they may be differentiated based on their distinctive odor (Table 29.9).

Exposure Types and Onsets

While symptoms generally manifest quite rapidly after exposure to a blister agent, the time course is a function of the route of exposure as well as the type and volume of vesicant involved (see Table 29.10).

TABLE 29.9 Identifying Vesicants by Appearance and Odor

Vesicant	Appearance	Odor
Nitrogen mustard	Colorless to yellow	Fishy, musty, soapy, or fruity
Sulfur mustard	Yellow or brown	Garlic, onions, or mustard*
Lewisite	Colorless	Geraniums
Phosgene oxime	Colorless	Irritating odor

*Sometimes has no odor.

TABLE 29.10 Vesicant Exposure Types and Onsets

Agent	Exposure	Onset
Nitrogen mustard	Inhalation Ingestion Skin/eye	Several hours Several hours 6–12 hours
Sulfur mustard	Inhalation Ingestion Skin/eye	Several hours Several hours 4–8 hours
Lewisite	Inhalation Ingestion Skin/eye	Rapid 15–20 minutes 15–30 minutes
Phosgene oxime	Inhalation Ingestion Skin/eye	Immediate No human data Immediate

Treatment

Blister/vesicant exposure is treated primarily as a thermal burn. Sulfur mustard decontamination is limited to immediate washing of exposed skin with water or soap and water, and flushing the eyes with copious amounts of water. Avoid 0.5% sodium hypochlorite solution or vigorous scrubbing as they may cause deeper tissue penetration. Typical burn therapy is accomplished with antibiotic ointment, sterile dressing, and other supportive therapy. Patients whose burns cover more than 20% to 25% of body surface area should be admitted to critical care units even though at presentation they may have relatively few signs and symptoms (Davis & Aspera, 2001). Lewisite ocular or dermal exposure can be treated with British anti-Lewisite (BAL) topical or ophthalmic preparations if available; however, they are not currently manufactured. Injectable BAL may help reduce systemic effects of lewisite, but it may not prevent dermal damage that has already occurred. Intubation and airway management may be required for patients with airway damage. Prevention of infection with careful cleaning and topical antibiotics and pain relief should be instituted as part of symptomatic and supportive care.

Duration/Mortality

The severity of the illness is dependent on the amount and route of exposure to the vesicant, the type of vesicant, and the medical condition of the person exposed. Exposure to high concentrations may be fatal.

Patient Assessment

All of these vesicant agents act by producing direct irritation and have similar clinical presentations (see Figure 29.4).

Ocular: Redness and burning of the eyes with lacrimation, blepharospasm, and lid edema
Upper airway: Nasal irritation and discharge, sinus burning, nose bleeds, sore throat, cough, and laryngitis
Pulmonary: Dyspnea, necrosis of large airway mucosa with sloughing, chemical pneumonitis, pulmonary edema, ARDS, respiratory failure
Skin: Irritation and redness with delayed production of wheals, vesicles, or bullae, followed later by areas of necrosis (see Table 29.11)

Clinical Diagnostic Tests

- CBC
- Glucose
- Serum electrolytes and renal function (blood urea nitrogen [BUN]/creatinine)
- Chest x-ray
- Pulse oximetry (or arterial blood gas [ABG] measurements).

Patient Management

Decontaminate patients before treating. Provide supportive therapy.

Therapy

There is no countermeasure; good supportive care is needed.

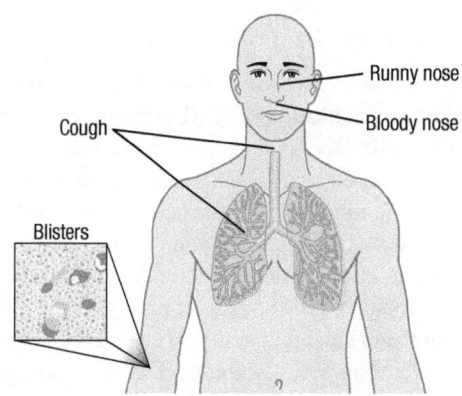

FIGURE 29.4 Vesicant agents: Patient assessment.
Source: Rains Analytics (2007).

TABLE 29.11 Agent-Specific Tips for Assessment

Agent	Assessment Tips
Sulfur mustard	Vesicles will have a "string of pearls" appearance and will then coalesce. A hoarse voice or barking cough is typically present or aphonia if the victim is exposed to a high concentration.
Lewisite	Single vesicle in erythematous area.
Phosgene oxime	Areas of dermal blanching with an erythematous ring within 30 seconds of exposure, progressing to a wheal within 30 minutes. Tissue necrosis after about 24 hours. NO vesicle!

TABLE 29.12 Identifying Tissue (Blood) Agents by Appearance and Odor

Agent	Appearance	Odor
Arsine	Colorless	Mild garlic or fishy
Carbon monoxide	Colorless	Odorless
Cyanides	Colorless or pale-blue	Bitter almond

BLOOD AGENTS

Blood or tissue agents are chemicals that affect the body by being absorbed into and distributed by the blood to the tissues. Substances include arsine, carbon monoxide, cyanide agents, and sodium monofluoroacetate. They may act on the blood itself or more distally in the critical tissues.

Arsine is formed when arsenic comes in contact with an acid. Arsine is a colorless, nonirritating toxic gas with a mild garlic odor (Table 29.12). Although arsine was investigated as a warfare agent during World War II, it was never used on the battlefield. Arsine is most commonly used in the semiconductor and metals refining industries. Inhalation is the primary route of exposure, causing red blood cell lysis and symptoms including weakness, shortness of breath, possible loss of consciousness, respiratory failure, paralysis, and death. Severely exposed patients are not likely to survive. If the initial exposure is survived, long-term effects may include kidney damage, neuropathy, and neuropsychological symptoms. Initial treatment includes fresh air, removal of contaminated clothing, washing contaminated skin, and symptomatic and supportive care. There is no specific countermeasure for treatment of arsine poisoning. Patients may need blood transfusions to replace damaged red blood cells (Walter, 2003; Weinstein & Alibek, 2003).

Recognizing Tissue (Blood) Agents

Cyanide in chemical weapons comes in four forms. These include cyanogen chloride (CK), hydrogen cyanide (AC), potassium cyanide (KCN), and sodium cyanide (NaCN). All forms may be released as a liquid, aerosol, or gas for inhalation; they may also be ingested or absorbed through the eyes and skin (Weinstein & Alibek, 2003). Sources of exposure include fumigants (rodenticides and insecticides), military poison gas, fire by-products, gold and silver ore extrication, mining, electroplating, and steel production. The cyanide anion, NC^-, whether delivered in hydrocyanic acid or in a cyanogen such as cyanide chloride, exerts its toxicity primarily by inhibiting mitochondrial cytochrome oxidase, which does not allow the tissues to utilize oxygen leading to lactic acidosis, hypoxia,

syncope, seizures, dysrhythmias, respiratory failure, and death within minutes after inhalation or ingestion of a sizable dose. There are three main laboratory findings indicative of cyanide exposure: (a) an elevated blood cyanide concentration (the most definitive); (b) metabolic acidosis with a high concentration of lactic acid; and (c) oxygen content of the venous blood greater than normal (although this is not specific to cyanide exposure). As with the nerve agents, however, the effects of cyanide exposure have such a rapid onset that treatment must begin long before any laboratory results are available (Hamel, 2011).

Patient Assessment

Cyanide Poisoning

The latency period for cyanides is 10 to 15 seconds up to several minutes. The signs and symptoms of mild cyanide poisoning are nonspecific and may be difficult to differentiate from other CWAs. The signs and symptoms of moderate-to-severe cyanide poisoning are profound and may appear similar to those of the nerve agents, but are most consistent with tissue hypoxia.

CK is an irritant and may produce lacrimation and upper airway irritation. When exposed to low concentrations of the other three forms of cyanide, victims will have 10 to 15 seconds of gasping, tachypnea, tachycardia, flushing, sweating, headache, giddiness, and dizziness, followed by nausea, vomiting, agitation, and confusion. At higher concentrations, the victim will have all these initial signs and symptoms, followed by bradycardia, apnea, seizures, shock, coma, and death. In all cases, death is caused by respiratory arrest and can be prevented by CPR. Cyanosis is a rare finding. Pupils may be unresponsive and dilated, but this is not specific to cyanide poisoning.

Arsine/Phosphine Poisoning

Upon inhalation, there may be a burning sensation in the chest followed by chest pain, but there may be no symptoms at all, leaving the victim unaware that he or she has been exposed. Symptoms of shortness of breath and weakness that is due to a sudden severe anemia may occur.

The length of time between exposure and exhibiting symptoms depends on the concentration and duration of exposure. A delay of 2 to 24 hours is typical before the onset of any symptoms.

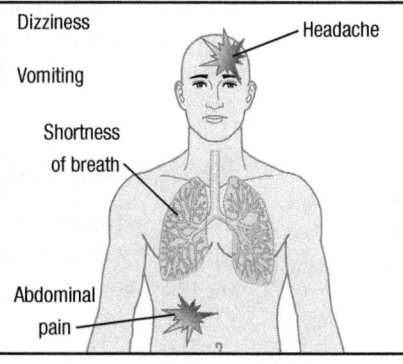

FIGURE 29.5 Cyanide and arsine: Patient assessment.

Source: Rains Analytics (2007).

Initial symptoms of arsine poisoning include nausea, vomiting, headache, malaise, weakness, dizziness, abdominal pain, dyspnea, and, occasionally, red-stained conjunctivae (see Figure 29.5). Symptoms progress to include hematuria and hemoglobinuria, jaundice, and possibly renal failure from the massive amounts of hemoglobin released into the blood and trapped in the kidneys. A slight odor of garlic may be detectable on the breath. Urine may appear bloody and patients may experience numbness, tingling, burning or prickling, memory loss, and disorientation. Severe anemia, low blood pressure, and an elevated serum potassium may be brought about by hemolysis 2 to 24 hours after exposure.

Later, look for enlargement of the liver, yellowing of the skin and whites of the eyes, or a bronze appearance to the skin.

Approximately 2 to 3 weeks after exposure to arsine, Mee's lines (horizontal white lines of the nails) may be observed.

Clinical Diagnostic Tests

- CBC
- Blood glucose
- Electrolyte determinations
- Urine for hemoglobinuria

Treatment

Treatment consists of proper circulatory and respiratory support until the antidote can be administered (Weinstein & Alibek, 2003). Contrary to what is popularly believed from movies and television, the effects of cyanide are not always irreversibly fatal, and victims may be successfully resuscitated by proper circulatory and respiratory support until the antidote can be administered. If the initial dose is not sufficient to kill the victim within minutes, treatment includes initial decontamination, administration of 100% oxygen, and utilization of a cyanide antidote kit (see Table 29.13) or hydroxocobalamin.

The cyanide antidote kit contains sodium nitrate and sodium thiosulfate. Nitrates convert hemoglobin to methemoglobin, which in turn binds cyanide, thus removing it from the mitochondrial oxidase complex. Sodium thiosulfate reacts with cyanide (attached to methemoglobin) to form nontoxic thiocyanate, which is then excreted into the urine. The kit is no longer manufactured, although the individual components are still made.

The current standard for cyanide is to treat with hydroxocobalamin, which has a high affinity for cyanide and forms the

---

TABLE 29.13 Blood Agent Treatment by Exposure Type

Exposure	Treatment
Inhalation	• Respiratory symptoms: Administer supplemental oxygen by mask. • Bronchospasms: Treat with aerosolized bronchodilators or cardiac sensitizing agents. (Arsine poisoning is not known to pose additional risk during the use of bronchial or cardiac sensitizing agents.) • Children with stridor: Administer racemic epinephrine aerosol. • Dose: 0.25–0.75 mL of 2.25% racemic epinephrine solution in 2.5 mL water. • Repeat every 20 minutes as needed, cautioning for myocardial variability. • If hemolysis develops, initiate urinary alkalinization. • Add 50 to 100 mEq of sodium bicarbonate to 1 L of 5% dextrose in 0.25 normal saline and administer intravenously at a rate that maintains urine output at 2 to 3 mL/kg/hr; maintain alkaline urine (i.e., pH > 7.5) until urine is hemoglobin free. • If anemia develops as a result of hemolysis, consider blood transfusions. • Renal failure: Consider hemodialysis.
Skin	• Irrigate with lukewarm (42°C) water.
Eyes	• Thoroughly irrigate with lukewarm (42°C) water or saline. • Examine the eyes for corneal damage and treat appropriately.

compound cyanocobalamin, which is vitamin B12. Vitamin B12 is water soluble and is excreted in the urine.

Exposure to carbon monoxide interferes with oxygen transport. As hypoxia progresses, more severe signs and symptoms of hypoxia may occur, including angina, seizures, respiratory depression, coma, and delayed neurological sequelae (DNS). Treatment with normobaric oxygen is critical to reverse tissue hypoxia early and prevent DNS. Hyperbaric oxygen (HBO) is controversial and not available at all locations; it may prevent the development of DNS.

Patient Management

Closely monitor serum electrolytes, calcium, BUN, creatinine, hemoglobin, and hematocrit. For victims of arsine poisoning, fluid administration amounts need to be monitored to avoid the onset of congestive heart failure symptoms.

Therapy

Cyanide Poisoning

Victims may be successfully resuscitated by proper circulatory and respiratory support while waiting for the antidote to be administered. Every effort should be made to administer the antidote as soon as possible.

PULMONARY/CHOKING AGENTS

Pulmonary/choking agents are chemicals that cause severe irritation or swelling of the respiratory tract, causing pulmonary damage and ultimately impairing oxygen delivery. Substances include ammonia, bromine, chlorine, hydrogen chloride, methyl bromide, methyl isocyanate, osmium tetroxide, phosgene, phosphine, phosphorus (elemental, white or yellow), and sulfuryl fluoride. Most are used in multiple industries, but some are easily found in the home (e.g., bleach, ammonia, and chlorine).

Recognizing Pulmonary Agents

While the process of identifying pulmonary agents is complicated by their sheer diversity, most may be distinguished on the basis of their characteristic appearance and odor (Table 29.14).

Exposure Type(s)/Onset

Exposure by inhalation, ingestion, or skin/eye contact typically leads to immediate onset of symptoms but, in some cases, onset may be delayed by as much as 48 hours. Irritant gases are classified according to their water solubility. Gases that are highly water soluble (e.g., ammonia, hydrogen chloride) react with moisture in the mucosal surfaces and cause irritation primarily in the upper airway. Prolonged or high-dose exposure may result in injury further into the bronchopulmonary system. Gases that are moderately water soluble (e.g., chlorine) cause injury to the upper airway to a lesser extent than those that are highly water soluble and also cause damage to the lower airway. Slightly water-soluble gases (e.g., phosgene) are less irritating to the upper airway and may result in prolonged exposure because victims do not immediately sense that they are being exposed to toxic gases. Injury to the lower airway with noncardiogenic pulmonary edema can be delayed. Therefore, appropriate observation and supportive care are imperative (Weinstein & Alibek, 2003).

Chlorine is a gas with intermediate water solubility, thereby causing injury to both the upper and lower airways. Exposure

TABLE 29.14 Identifying Pulmonary Agents by Appearance and Odor

Pulmonary Agent	Appearance	Odor
Ammonia	Colorless	Bleach
Bromine	Brownish	Bleach
Chlorine	Yellow-green	Pungent, irritating
Hydrogen chloride	Colorless, yellowish	Pungent
Methyl bromide	Colorless	Odorless or fruity/floral/sweet
Methyl isocyanate	Colorless	Pungent
Osmium tetroxide	Colorless, pale yellow	Pungent, chlorine-like
Phosgene	Colorless or white-to-pale-yellow cloud	Pleasant odor of newly mown hay or green corn
Phosphorus	"Smoking" or "luminescent"	Garlic
Sulfuryl fluoride	Colorless	Odorless

Note: Arsine/phosphine poisoning—There is no antidote for arsine or phosphine poisoning. Do *not* administer arsenic-chelating drugs. Patient may need blood transfusions.

to chlorine gas results in rapid onset of upper airway and pulmonary symptoms including choking, gasping, stridor, wheezing, shortness of breath, and respiratory compromise. Eye irritation and the development of a chemical conjunctivitis may also occur.

Phosgene is a gas with low water solubility. Exposure to this gas tends to affect predominantly the lower respiratory tree. An initially asymptomatic period for the first few hours after exposure is common. Onset of symptoms may first occur 24 hours after exposure. Typical symptoms include cough and shortness of breath. Noncardiogenic pulmonary edema may develop.

Duration/Mortality

The duration and risk of mortality depend on the amount of exposure and the patient's physical characteristics.

Patient Assessment

Initial symptoms include eye pain, redness, lacrimation, sore throat, runny nose, coughing, and headache.

After hours to several days, victims may develop nausea, hemoptysis, and the signs and symptoms of pulmonary edema including choking, dyspnea, rales, hemoconcentration, hypotension, and possible cyanosis (see Figure 29.6). Hypoxia and hypotension within 4 hours of exposure carries a poor prognosis.

Rarely, depending on concentration/time, pulmonary edema can occur within 30 minutes to 4 hours for chlorine and between 2 and 6 hours for phosgene. Most fatalities are within the first 24 hours and are due to respiratory failure.

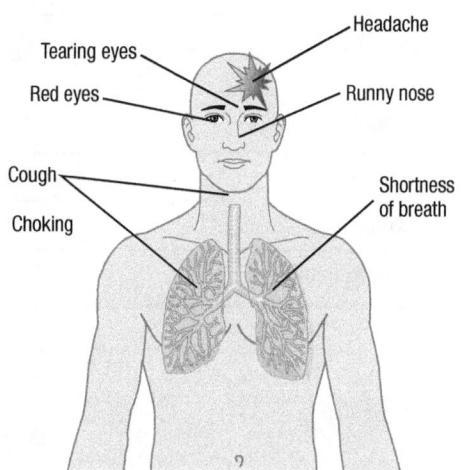

FIGURE 29.6 Pulmonary agents: Patient assessment.
Source: Rains Analytics (2007).

Clinical Diagnostic Tests

- CBC
- Glucose determinations
- Electrolyte determinations
- Chest radiography
- Pulse oximetry (if severe inhalation exposure is suspected)

Patient Management

Supportive Therapy

Systemic acidosis may occur with severe chlorine inhalation; monitor blood pH as appropriate.

TABLE 29.15 Pulmonary Agent Treatment by Exposure Type

Exposure	Treatment
Inhalation	• Respiratory symptoms: Administer supplemental oxygen by mask. • Bronchospasms: Treat with aerosolized bronchodilators or cardiac sensitizing agents. • Children with stridor: Administer racemic epinephrine aerosol. • Dose: 0.25–0.75 mL of 2.25% racemic epinephrine solution in 2.5 mL water. • Repeat every 20 minutes as needed, cautioning for myocardial variability. • Observe patients carefully for 6–12 hours for signs of upper airway obstruction. • Patients who have had a severe exposure may develop noncardiogenic pulmonary edema.
Skin	• Treat chemical burns like thermal burns. • If a victim has frostbite, treat by rewarming affected areas in a water bath at a temperature of 102°–108°F (40°–42°C) for 20–30 minutes and continue until a flush has returned to the affected area.
Eyes	• Continue irrigation for at least 15 minutes or until the pH of the conjunctival fluid has returned to normal. • Test visual acuity. • Examine the eyes for corneal damage and treat appropriately.
Ingestion	• Do not induce vomiting. • Do not administer activated charcoal. • Do not perform gastric lavage or attempt neutralization after ingestion. • If not given during decontamination, give 4–8 ounces of water by mouth to dilute stomach contents. • Consider endoscopy to evaluate the extent of GI tract injury.

TABLE 29.16 Identifying Riot Control Agents by Appearance and Odor

Riot Control Agent	Appearance	Odor
CN (Chloroacetophenone)	White	Fragrant (e.g., apple blossoms)
CS (Chlorobenzylidenemalonitrile)	White	Pungent (e.g., pepper)
DM (Diphenylaminearsine)	Yellow-green	Odorless

Therapy/Antidote

No antidote.

Treatment

Treatment for exposure to such respiratory agents is mainly supportive. Evaluation of respiratory function and oxygenation is critical. Pulse oximetry should be performed. High flow oxygen is required if hypoxemia is present. Patients with ventilatory failure or severe hypoxemia will need endotracheal intubation and mechanical ventilation (Table 29.15). No specific antidotes are available to reverse the effects of these chemicals. Supportive care may include beta-2 agonists to treat bronchospasm and pain and/or cough medications. Antibiotics and corticosteroids are not generally warranted unless the patient develops a bacterial superinfection or evidence of reactive airway disease.

RIOT CONTROL AGENTS

Riot control agents are chemical compounds that temporarily inhibit a person's ability to function by causing irritation to the eyes, mouth, throat, lungs, and skin. Sometimes known as "tear gas," riot agents are present in both liquid and solid forms and can be released in the air as fine droplets or particles. The purpose of their use is to incapacitate the victim. Riot control agents may be employed by police attempting to subdue an unruly crowd.

Several different compounds are considered to be riot control agents. The three major agents are:

- Chloroacetophenone (CN), also known as "mace"
- Chlorobenzylidenemalonitrile (CS)
- Diphenylaminearsine (DM)

Exposure to riot control agents is by inhalation or by contact with the skin and/or eyes and leads to rapid onset of symptoms.

Recognizing Riot Control Agents

Due to the circumstances of their typical use in the United States, identification of riot control agents may be simplified by communication with the police or other agency responsible for disseminating the agent. In the absence of additional information, appearance and odor may help reveal the agent's identity (Table 29.16).

Treatment

No specific treatment is required. Situation improves within 30 minutes after exposure ends (Weinstein & Alibek, 2003).

Duration/Mortality

Situation will improve 15 to 30 minutes after exposure ends. Death can be immediate when serious chemical burns are present in the throat and lungs.

Patient Assessment

Riot control agents affect primarily the eyes, causing temporary blindness that is due to lacrimation and blepharospasm. They also produce conjunctival redness; cough; chest tightness; sneezing; and mouth, nose, and throat irritation (see Figure 29.7). In raw or abraded skin, lacrimators can cause burning and erythema. Rarely, under conditions of high temperature, high humidity, and high concentration, vesicles may form hours later on exposed skin areas.

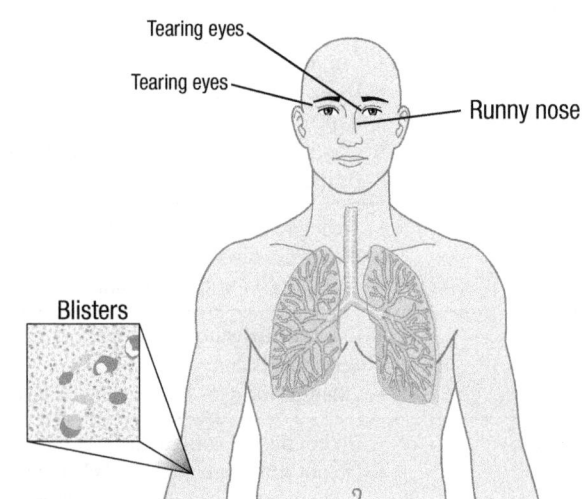

FIGURE 29.7 Riot control agents: Patient assessment.
Source: Rains Analytics (2007).

EMERGENCY DEPARTMENT PROCEDURES IN CHEMICAL HAZARD EMERGENCIES

Every hospital must prepare to treat victims of HAZMAT accidents before an event occurs. The hospital must provide appropriate HAZMAT training, provide PPE, and develop and disseminate policies and procedures necessary to quickly and efficiently treat contaminated patients (Hick et al., 2003; Levitin & Siegelson, 1996, 2002; OSHA, 2005; Pfaff, 1998). Guidelines for the initial management of patients with acute toxic exposures have been established by the CDC and OSHA and initial treatment protocols are agent-specific and are provided for review (see Box 29.1; CDC, 2010). At a minimum, nurses should be aware of the guidelines and how to access them quickly at the point of care (see Box 29.2).

BOX 29.1 Emergency Department Procedure in Chemical Hazard Emergencies

Preparations

1. Try to identify agent; call poison center for help (1-800-222-1222).
2. Break out personal protection equipment, decontamination supplies, antidotes, etc.
3. Is chemical hazard certain or very likely? If yes:
   - Don personal protective equipment.
   - Set up hot line.
4. Clear and secure all areas that could become contaminated.
5. Prepare and secure hospital entrances and grounds.
6. Notify local emergency management authorities if needed.
7. If chemical is a military agent and army has not been informed, call them.
8. If an organophosphate is involved, notify hospital pharmacy that large amounts of atropine and 2-PAM may be needed.

When Victim Arrives

(*Note:* A contaminated patient may present at an emergency room without prior warning.)

9. Does chemical hazard exist?
   - Known release/exposure (including late notification)
   - Liquid on victim's skin or clothing
   - Symptoms in victim, EMTs, others
   - Odor (H, L, phosgene, chlorine)
   - M-8 paper, if appropriate
   - If yes: Go to 10
   - If no: Handle victim routinely
10. Hold victim outside until preparations are completed (don PPE to assist EMTs as necessary).
11. If patient is grossly contaminated (liquid or skin, positive M-8 paper) OR if there is any suspicion of contamination, decontaminate patient before entry into building.

EMT, emergency medical technician; PPE, personal protective equipment.

Source: Centers for Disease Control and Prevention. (2010). Emergency room procedures in chemical hazard emergencies. Retrieved from https://www.cdc.gov/nceh/demil/articles/initialtreat.htm

---

BOX 29.2 Initial Treatment and Identification of the Chemical Agent

1. Establish airway if necessary.
2. Give artificial respiration if not breathing.
3. Control bleeding if hemorrhaging.
4. Check for symptoms of cholinesterase poisoning?

   - Pinpoint pupils
   - Difficulty breathing (wheezing, gasping, etc.)
   - Local or generalized sweating
   - Fasciculations
   - Copious secretions
   - Nausea, vomiting, diarrhea
   - Convulsions
   - Coma

   YES: Go to NERVE AGENT PROTOCOL.
5. Check for history of chlorine poisoning?

   YES: Go to CHLORINE PROTOCOL.
6. Burns that began within minutes of poisoning?

   NO: Go to 8.
7. Thermal burn?

   YES: Go to 9.
   NO: Go to LEWISITE PROTOCOL.

8. Burns or eye irritation beginning 2–12 hours after exposure?

   YES: Go to MUSTARD PROTOCOL.
   NO: Go to 9.
9. Is phosgene exposure possible?

   - Known exposure to phosgene
   - Known exposure to hot chlorinated hydrocarbons
   - Respiratory discomfort beginning a few hours after exposure

   YES: Go to PHOSGENE PROTOCOL.
10. Check other possible chemical exposures:

    - Known exposure
    - Decreased level of consciousness without head trauma
    - Odor on clothes or breath
    - Specific signs or symptoms

(continued)

BOX 29.2 Initial Treatment and Identification of the Chemical Agent (*continued*)

Phosgene Protocol

1. Restrict fluids, take chest x-ray, test blood gases. Results consistent with phosgene poisoning?
      YES: Go to 4.
2. Dyspnea?
      YES: OXYGEN, positive end-expiratory pressure.
3. Observe closely for at least 6 hours.
   - IF SEVERE DYSPNEA develops, go to 4.
   - IF MILD DYSPNEA develops after several hours, go to 1.
4. Severe dyspnea develops or x-ray or blood gases consistent with phosgene poisoning:
   - Admit to hospital
   - Give oxygen under positive end-expiratory pressure
   - Restrict fluids
   - Take chest x-ray
   - Test blood gases
   - May send to ICU

Mustard Protocol

1. Airway obstruction?
      YES: Tracheostomy.
2. If there are large burns:
   - Establish IV line—do not push fluids as for thermal burns.
   - Drain vesicles—unroof large blisters and irrigate area with topical antibiotics.
3. Treat other symptoms appropriately:
   - Antibiotic eye ointment
   - Sterile precautions PRN
   - Morphine PRN (generally not needed in emergency treatment; might be appropriate for inpatient treatment)

Lewisite Protocol

1. Survey extent of injury.
2. Treat affected skin with BAL solution (if available).
3. Treat affected eyes with BAL ophthalmic ointment (if available).
4. Treat pulmonary/severe effects:
   - BAL in oil, 0.5 mL/25 pounds body weight deep IM to max of 4.0 mL. Repeat q4h × 3 (at 4, 8, and 12 hours)
   - Morphine PRN
5. Severe poisoning?
      YES: Shorten interval for BAL injections to q 2 h.

Chlorine Protocol

1. Dyspnea?
   - Try bronchodilators.
   - Admit to hospital.
   - Give oxygen by mask.
   - Take chest x-ray.
2. Treat other problems and reevaluate (consider phosgene).
3. Respiratory system OK?
      YES: Go to 5.
4. Is phosgene poisoning possible?
      YES: Go to PHOSGENE PROTOCOL.
5. Give supportive therapy; treat other problems or discharge.

Nerve Agent Protocol

1. Severe respiratory distress?
      YES:
   - Intubate and ventilate
   - ATROPINE
     Adults: 6 mg IM or IV
     Infants/children: 0.05 mg/kg IV
   - 2-PAMC1
     Adults: 600–1,000 mg IM or slow IV
     Infants/children: 15 mg/kg slow IV
2. Major secondary symptoms?
      NO: Go to 6.
      YES:
   - ATROPINE
     Adults: 4 mg IM or IV
     Infants/children: 0.02–0.05 mg/kg IV
   - 2-PAMC1
     Adults: 600–1,000 mg IM or slow IV

Infants/children: 15 mg/kg
   - OPEN IV LINE
3. Repeat atropine as needed until secretions decrease and breathing is easier.
     Adults: 2 mg IV or IM
     Infants/children: 0.02–0.05 mg/kg IV
4. Repeat 2-PAMC1 as needed.
     Adults: 1.0 g IV over 20–30 minutes
     Repeat q 1 h × 3 PRN
     Infants/children: 15 mg/kg slow IV
5. Convulsions?
      NO: Go to 6.
      YES: DIAZEPAM 10 mg slow IV
     Infants/children: 0.2 mg/kg IV
6. Reevaluate q 3–5 minutes.
      If signs worsen, repeat from 3.

BAL, British anti-Lewisite; PRN, when necessary.

Note: Warn the hospital pharmacy that unusual amounts of atropine and 2-PAM (pralidoxime) may be needed.

SUMMARY

Toxic chemical exposures offer a variety of unique challenges to nurses, particularly emergency nurses and other first responders. Most HAZMAT accidents are small-scale events that happen at the workplace, involving only one or two patients. However, the current threat of chemical terrorism increases the likelihood that a large-scale event involving many casualties may occur. Many fire departments, EMS, and hospitals are not prepared to deal with these types of events. Furthermore, these agents, when mishandled, can turn a contained incident into a disaster involving the entire hospital and community. During a HAZMAT incident, victims often seek out the nearest hospital regardless of the institution's capability to handle a chemical event. Nurses and other providers need to be prepared in advance for this type of situation (adequate training and access to PPE), and be aware of the proper procedures for triage, decontamination, and initial management of an acute toxic exposure.

The large-scale use of chemical weapons has the potential to cause massive social disruption and significant morbidity and mortality. Nurses must support all efforts to advocate for chemical disarmament and the ultimate abolition of the use of nerve agents for any purpose.

STUDY QUESTIONS

1. Which chemical agent was used in the Tokyo subway system in 1995? How effective was this agent in causing physical injury?

2. List two antidotes used to treat sarin gas poisoning.

3. Describe the levels of training for HAZMAT exposure management. What should hospital personnel involved in HAZMAT response have as a minimal level of training?

4. True or false: Specific antidotes have been developed to treat poisonings from all the common types of CWAs.

5. True or false: Multiple ill individuals with similar complaints seeking care at the same time is suggestive of the use of chemical weapons.

6. True or false: Nerve agents are well absorbed through the skin.

7. A patient presents to the triage desk in your emergency department following exposure to some sort of gaseous substance in his office building while at work. He is 48 years old, appears anxious and agitated, and has rapid respirations.

Describe what should be done in terms of initial patient management.

8. The Joint Commission, which implements standards that must be met for hospitals to receive accreditation, has also established specific HAZMAT guidelines for hospitals. Locate a copy of these guidelines and identify the primary requirements they contain. Find out if your hospital or healthcare organization meets these guidelines.

INTERNET ACTIVITIES

1. How quickly can you locate the most current recommended protocols for emergency treatment of toxic chemical exposures? Locate the CDC website for the most current, valid, and reliable information.

2. What is the CDC's role in the transport and disposal of toxic chemical weapons?

3. Go to the website of the Federation of American Scientists on chemical weapons. Locate the CWAs section and find nerve agents. Describe what effect nerve agents have on the human body.

4. Locate the website for the United States Army Medical Research Institute for Chemical Defense. Locate the Triage of Chemical Casualties chapter. Describe each of the triage categories and how they would be used in a mass chemical exposure event.

5. How would you manage casualties with combined chemical exposures (more than one type of agent)?

6. What unique factors about children make them more susceptible to exposure to chemicals?

7. Go to the website of the Terrorism Research Center at www .terrorism.com/index.php. What types of resources are available at this site? Evaluate the benefit of these resources for nurses.

8. Go to the website of the Center for Nonproliferation Studies at cns.miis.edu/cns/index.htm. The Chemical and Biological Weapons Nonproliferation Program (CBWNP) monitors the global proliferation of chemical and biological weapons (CBWs) and develops strategies for halting and reversing their spread. What resources are available? What do they have to say about the use of chemical weapons? Identify readings that might help nurses understand the reality of the threat of chemical warfare.

REFERENCES

Agency for Toxic Substances and Disease Registry. (2012). *Hazardous substances emergency events surveillance (HSEES) annual report 2009.* Atlanta, GA: U. S. Department of Health and Human Services. Retrieved from https://www.atsdr.cdc.gov/HS/HSEES/annual2009.html

Agency for Toxic Substances and Disease Registry. (2014). Toxic substances portal—Nerve agents (GA, GB, GD, VX). Retrieved from https://www.atsdr.cdc.gov/mmg/mmg.asp?id=523&tid=93

Alibek, K., Dashiell, T., Dwyer, A., Lane, S., Patrick, W., Ponikvar, D., Rinard, J., & Sidell F. (2006). *Jane's chem-bio handbook* (3rd ed.). Alexandria, VA: Jane's Information Group.

Burda, A. M., & Sigg, T. (2001). Pharmacy preparedness for incidents involving weapons of mass destruction. *American Journal of Health-System Pharmacy, 58*(23), 2274–2281.

Burke, R. V., Iverson, E., Goodhue, C. J., Neches, R., & Upperman, J. S. (2010). Disaster and mass casualty events in the pediatric population. *Seminars in Pediatric Surgery, 19*(4), 265–270. doi:10.1053/j.sempedsurg.2010.06.003

Centers for Disease Control and Prevention. (2010). Emergency room procedure in chemical hazard emergencies. Retrieved from https://www.cdc.gov/nceh/demil/articles/initialtreat.htm

Centers for Disease Control and Prevention. (2016). Chemical categories. Retrieved from https://emergency.cdc.gov/agent/agentlistchem-category.asp

Cox, B. (2016). Hospital decontamination: What nurses need to know. *The Nursing Clinics of North America, 51*(4), 663–674. doi:10.1016/j.cnur.2016.07.010

Dart, R. C., Borron, S. W., Caravati, E. M., Cobaugh, D. J., Curry, S. C., Falk, J. L. … Zosel, A.; Antidote Summit Authorship Group. (2009). Expert consensus guidelines for stocking of antidotes in hospitals that provide emergency care. *Annals of Emergency Medicine, 54*(3), 386–394. doi:10.1016/j.annemergmed.2009.01.023

Davis, K. G., & Aspera, G. (2001). Exposure to liquid sulfur mustard. *Annals of Emergency Medicine, 37,* 653–656. doi:10.1067/mem.2001.114322

Defense Against Weapons of Mass Destruction, 50 USC § 2302.

Evison, D., Hinsley, D., & Rice, P. (2002). Chemical weapons. *British Medical Journal, 324*(7333), 332–335. doi:10.1136/bmj.324.7333.332

Ewy, G. A., Bobrow, B. J. (2016). Cardiocerebral resuscitation: An approach to improving survival of patients with primary cardiac arrest. *Journal of Intensive Care Medicine, 31*(1):24–33. doi:10.1177/0885066614544450

Hamel, J. (2011). A review of acute cyanide poisoning with a treatment update. *Critical Care Nurse, 31,* 72–82. doi:10.4037/ccn2011799

Hazardous Waste Operations and Emergency Response, Code of Federal Regulations Title 29, Part 1910.120.

Hick, J. L., Penn, P., Hanfling, D., Lapp, M. A., O'Laughlin, D., & Burstein, J. L. (2003). Establishing and training health care facility decontamination teams. *Annals of Emergency Medicine, 42,* 381–390. doi:10.1067/mem.2003.300

Institute of Medicine & National Research Council. (1999). *Chemical and biological terrorism: Research and development to improve civilian medical response.* Washington, DC: Authors.

Levitin, H. W., & Siegelson, H. J. (1996). Hazardous materials. Disaster medical planning and response. *Emergency Medicine Clinics of North America, 14*(2), 327–348. doi:10.1016/S0733-8627(05)70254-6

Levitin, H. W., & Siegelson, H. J. (2002). Hazardous materials disasters. In D. Hogan & J. L. Burstein (Eds.), *Disaster medicine* (pp. 258–273). Philadelphia, PA: Lippincott, Williams & Wilkins.

National Fire Academy and National Emergency Training Center. (1992). *Recognizing and identifying hazardous materials.* Capitol Heights, MD: National Audio-Visual Center.

Occupational Safety and Health Administration. (2005). OSHA best practices for hospital-based first receivers of victims from mass casualty incidents involving the release of hazardous substances. Retrieved from https://www.osha.gov/dts/osta/bestpractices/firstreceivers_hospital.pdf

Pfaff, B. L. (1998). Emergency department management of nerve agent exposure. *International Journal of Trauma Nursing, 4*(3), 71–78. doi:10.1016/S1075-4210(98)90072-4

Reutter, S. (1999). Hazards of chemical weapons release during war: New perspectives. *Environmental Health Perspectives, 107*(12), 985–990.

Russell, D., Simpson, J. (2010). Emergency planning and preparedness for the deliberate release of toxic industrial chemicals. *Clinical Toxicology, 48*(3), 171–176. doi:10.3109/15563651003698042

Sidell, F. R. (1997). Nerve agents. In F. R. Sidell, E. T. Takafuhi, & D. R. Franz (Eds.), *Medical aspects of chemical and biological warfare* (pp. 129–179). Washington, DC: Office of the Surgeon General.

Sidell, F. R., Urbanetti, J. S., Smith, W. J., & Hurst, C. G. (1997). Vesicants. In F. R. Sidell, E. T. Takafuhi, & D. R. Franz (Eds.), *Medical aspects of chemical and biological warfare* (pp. 197–228). Washington, DC: Office of the Surgeon General.

Thompson, T. M., Theobald, J., Lu, J., Erickson, T. B. (2014). The general approach to the poisoned patient. *Disease-a-Month, 60*(11), 509–524. doi:10.1016/j.disamonth.2014.10.002

Tucker, J. (2006). *War of nerves: Chemical warfare from World War I to Al-Qaeda.* New York, NY: Pantheon Books.

U. S. Census Bureau. (2015). *Transportation—Commodity flow survey: United States 2012.* Washington, DC: U. S. Census Bureau and U. S. Department of Commerce. Retrieved from http://www.census.gov/content/dam/Census/library/publications/2015/econ/ec12tcf-us.pdf

Walter, F. G. (2003). Semiconductor gases. *Advanced hazmat life support provider manual* (3rd ed., pp. 355–362). Tucson: University of Arizona.

Weinstein, R. S., & Alibek, K. (2003). *Biological and chemical terrorism: A guide for healthcare providers and first responders.* New York, NY: Thieme.

CASE STUDY 29.1

Hazardous Substances Emergency Events Surveillance System

OVERVIEW

The ATSDR, based in Atlanta, Georgia, is a federal public health agency of the U.S. Department of Health and Human Services. ATSDR serves the public by using the best science, taking responsive public health actions, and providing trusted health information to prevent harmful exposures and diseases related to toxic substances. In 1990, ATSDR established the Hazardous Substances Emergency Events Surveillance (HSEES) system to collect and analyze information about (a) sudden uncontrolled or illegal releases of hazardous substances that require cleanup or neutralization according to federal, state, or local law; and (b) threatened releases that result in public health action, such as evacuation. The HSEES system aims to reduce injury and death among first responders, employees, and the general public that result from releases of hazardous substances. It is the only federal database designed specifically to address the public health effects from releases of hazardous substances.

WHAT IS A HAZARDOUS SUBSTANCE EVENT?

A HSEES event is any release or threatened release of at least one hazardous substance (excluding releases involving only petroleum products). A substance is considered hazardous if it might reasonably be expected to cause adverse health effects to humans. Events are included in the system if the amount released, or threatened to be released, is required to be cleaned up according to federal, state, or local law. In addition, for threatened releases to be included in HSEES, they must cause an action to protect public health (i.e., evacuation).

WHO PROVIDES INFORMATION TO THE HSEES SYSTEM?

Fifteen state health departments participate in HSEES through cooperative agreements with ATSDR. These states are Colorado, Florida, Iowa, Louisiana, Michigan, Minnesota, Missouri, New Jersey, New York, North Carolina, Oregon, Texas, Utah, Washington, and Wisconsin. Participating states provide information about the release, such as time and place, circumstances, substances involved, persons affected, and public health action taken.

WHAT HSEES SYSTEM INFORMATION HAS SHOWN

- Approximately 9,000 hazardous substance releases occur annually in the 15 states reporting.
- Releases at facilities account for 70% to 75% of events, and transportation-associated releases account for 25% to 30% of reported events.
- Most releases occur on weekdays between 6 a.m. and 6 p.m.
- Releases tend to increase in spring and summer.
- Equipment failure and human error cause most releases at facilities.
- Human error and equipment failure cause most releases during transport.
- More than 90% of events involve the release or threatened release of only one hazardous substance.
- Releases of hazardous substances most often injure employees, followed by the general public and—less frequently—first responders and school children.
- Respiratory irritation and eye irritation are the most commonly reported symptoms or injuries.
- Approximately 50% of people who reported developing symptoms or injuries from a HSEES event are treated at a hospital and released.

Source: Centers for Disease Control and Prevention. (2005). *CDC fact sheet: Hazardous substances emergency events surveillance system.* Retrieved from https://www.atsdr.cdc.gov/hs/hsees/hsees_about-factsheet.pdf

CASE STUDY 29.2

Sheltering in Place Following a Chemical Release

WHAT "SHELTERING IN PLACE" MEANS

Some kinds of chemical accidents or attacks may make going outdoors dangerous. Leaving the area might take too long or put you in harm's way. In such a case, it may be safer for you to stay indoors than to go outside.

"Sheltering in place" means to make a shelter out of the place in which you are. It is a way for you to make the building as safe as possible to protect yourself until help arrives. Sheltering in place versus evacuation is a calculated decision where the cost benefit of staying in a semiprotected area is weighed against possible harm that could occur during evacuation. You should not try to shelter in a vehicle unless you have no other choice. Vehicles are not airtight enough to give you adequate protection from chemicals.

HOW TO PREPARE TO SHELTER IN PLACE

Choose a room in your house or apartment for the shelter. The best room to use for the shelter is a room with as few windows and doors as possible. A large room with a water supply is best—something like a master bedroom that is connected to a bathroom. For most chemical events, this room should be as high in the structure as possible to avoid vapors (gases) that sink. This guideline is different from the sheltering-in-place technique used in tornadoes and other severe weather and for nuclear or radiological events, when the shelter should be low in the home.

You might not be at home if the need to shelter in place ever arises, but if you are at home, the following items, many of which you may already have, would be good to have in your shelter room:

- First aid kit.
- Flashlight, battery-powered radio, and extra batteries for both.
- A working telephone.
- Food and bottled water. Store 1 gallon of water per person in plastic bottles as well as ready-to-eat foods that will keep without refrigeration in the shelter-in-place room. If you do not have bottled water, or if you run out, you can drink water from a toilet tank (not from a toilet bowl). Do not drink water from the tap.
- Duct tape and scissors.
- Towels and plastic sheeting. You may wish to cut your plastic sheeting to fit your windows and doors before any emergency occurs.

HOW TO KNOW IF YOU NEED TO SHELTER IN PLACE

Most likely you will need to shelter for only a few hours.

- If there is a "code red" or "severe" terror alert, you should pay attention to radio and television broadcasts to know right away whether a shelter-in-place alert is announced for your area.
- You will hear from the local police, emergency coordinators, or government on the radio and on television emergency broadcast system if you need to shelter in place.

WHAT TO DO

Act quickly and follow the instructions of your local emergency coordinators such as law enforcement personnel, fire departments, or local elected leaders. Every situation can be different, so local emergency coordinators might have special instructions for you to follow. In general, do the following:

- Go inside as quickly as possible. Bring any outdoor pets indoors.
- If there is time, shut and lock all outside doors and windows. Locking them may pull the door or window tighter and make a better seal against the chemical. Turn off the air conditioner or heater. Turn off all fans, too. Close the fireplace damper and any other place that air can come in from outside.
- Go in the shelter-in-place room and shut the door.
- Turn on the radio. Keep a telephone close at hand, but do not use it unless there is a serious emergency.
- Sink and toilet drain traps should have water in them (you can use the sink and toilet as you normally would). If it is necessary to drink water, drink stored water, not water from the tap.
- Tape plastic over any windows in the room. Use duct tape around the windows and doors and make an unbroken seal. Use the tape over any vents into the room and seal any electrical outlets or other openings.
- If you are away from your shelter-in-place location when a chemical event occurs, follow the instructions of emergency coordinators to find the nearest shelter. If your children are at school, they will be sheltered there. Unless you are instructed to do so, do not try to get to the school to bring your children home. Transporting them from the school will put them, and you, at increased risk.
- Listen to the radio for an announcement indicating that it is safe to leave the shelter.
- When you leave the shelter, follow instructions from local emergency coordinators to avoid any contaminants outside. After you come out of the shelter, emergency coordinators may have additional instructions on how to make the rest of the building safe again.

Source: Centers for Disease Control and Prevention. (2017). Chemical agents: Facts about sheltering in place. Retrieved from https://emergency.cdc.gov/planning/shelteringfacts.asp

30

BIOLOGICAL AGENTS OF CONCERN

David C. Pigott, Ziad N. Kazzi, and Sarah D. Nafziger

LEARNING OBJECTIVES

When this chapter is completed, readers will be able to:

1. Describe the Centers for Disease Control and Prevention (CDC) system for the categorization of biological agents of concern, with particular attention to Category A agents.
2. Identify the Category A biological agents and the diseases caused by these agents.
3. Describe the clinical presentation of patients infected with Category A agents.
4. Describe available therapies for these agents, including vaccines, if available, as well as the role of postexposure prophylaxis.
5. Describe the biosafety level (BSL) system, including the major elements of BSL-2, BSL-3, and BSL-4, as well as indications for personnel protective equipment and isolation.
6. Discuss the potential public health impact of an outbreak involving any Category A agent as well as the appropriate public health agencies involved in managing such an outbreak.

KEY MESSAGES

The CDC Category A biological agents present unique threats to public health as well as to healthcare professionals who may care for patients exposed to these diseases.

Attention to pertinent details of an exposed patient's history and physical condition may provide important diagnostic clues, allowing early institution of appropriate therapy and biosafety precautions.

Infection control issues raised by these biological agents of concern raise serious threats to healthcare professionals, including clinical and laboratory personnel who may encounter patients or clinical specimens suspected of harboring highly lethal bacteria or viruses.

CHAPTER OVERVIEW

Biological agents of concern are a group of highly patho-genic bacteria, viruses, and toxins with the potential to cause significant public health impact in terms of morbidity and mortality, as well as social disruption and public panic, par-ticularly when deployed as a biological weapon. The CDC developed a hierarchical classification system for biological agents, ranking specific agents in Categories A, B, and C, where Category A agents are the most virulent and pose the greatest public health threat. This chapter provides detailed descriptions of the Category A agents with special attention to epidemiology, pathogenesis, clinical diagnosis, treatment, and nursing care issues.

Biological agents with potential for causing significant human morbidity and mortality, particularly when used as a biological weapon, are introduced. When most of us hear the term "biological weapon," we think of anthrax-laden envelopes and vials of smallpox hermetically sealed in secret laboratories. While these two well-known examples are commonly referred to when discussing bioterrorism, other very real threats are much less exotic. Bioterrorism is generally referred to as the intentional use of a biological organism or one or more of its components to cause disease, social disruption, and panic. The intentional contamination of Oregon salad bars with Salmonella typhimurium in 1984 by followers of Bhagwan Shree Rajneesh was just as much an act of biological warfare as the anthrax attacks of late 2001 (Torok et al., 1997).

Potential agents of biological warfare range from the extremely rare to the very common, from Ebola virus to Esch-erichia coli. They vary widely in degree of infectivity, route of infection, and natural hosts. We pay special attention to those agents whose extreme pathogenicity, ease of use as a biological weapon, or potential for societal disruption place them in a distinct category in comparison with other causes of human disease. The CDC, one of the few centers in the world with the capability for research and containment of the more dangerous organisms such as smallpox, has created a hierarchy that ranks these biological agents in a system that considers their potential for causing life-threatening infection in humans, ease of dissemination or transmissibility, potential for public health impact, and requirement for special actions to facilitate public health preparedness (CDC, 2001b).

CLASSIFICATION OF BIOLOGICAL AGENTS OF CONCERN

In 1999, the CDC, in conjunction with selected civilian and military infection control and biological warfare experts, established a graded system of risk assessment and prioritization for potential biological warfare agents (Kahn & Sage, 2000; Rotz, Khan, Lillibridge, Ostroff, & Hughes, 2002). Biological Agent categories A, B, and C were created to classify these biological agents of concern. Agents were ranked based on sev-eral factors, including public health impact in terms of disease and mortality rates, dissemination potential, public perception, and the need for special public health preparations. The most dangerous are placed in Category A, followed by Categories B and C, whose potential for causing life-threatening disease, while still significant, is considered less of a public health risk than those in Category A.

Category A Agents

Category A agents are among the most deadly microbes known to man. They can be easily disseminated, or transmitted, from person to person, or they have high mortality rates as well as the potential for severe public health consequences, including public panic and social disruption. Their high infectivity poses a danger not only to those infected with the disease, but also to those who are treating the infected patients, including lab-oratory personnel who may come in contact with the infecting organism. Laboratory precautions for these agents are extremely strict, so much so that very few laboratories in the United States have the capability for working with these organisms. Until recently, the CDC and the United States Army Medical Institute of Infectious Diseases (USAMRIID) were the only two loca-tions in the United States approved to diagnose, contain, and conduct research into these Category A agents (USAMRIID, 2001). Recently, more BSL-3 and BSL-4 laboratories have been constructed throughout the United States.

Category A agents:

- Anthrax (*Bacillus anthracis*)
- Botulinum toxin (*Clostridium botulinum*)
- Plague (*Yersinia pestis*)
- Smallpox (*Variola major*)
- Tularemia (*Francisella tularensis*)
- Hemorrhagic fever (HF) viruses (including Arenaviruses, Bunyaviruses, Flaviviruses, and Filoviruses)

Category B Agents

Category B agents are the second highest priority risk agents as determined by the CDC. They share certain characteristics, such as the potential for moderate morbidity and lower mortality, compared with Category A agents. They are moderately easy to disseminate and require specific diagnostic capabilities as well as increased disease surveillance for detection. Several of these agents are extremely toxic but are not placed in Category A due to difficulties with dissemination or lower infectivity as compared to the Category A agents. All represent a significant public health risk if used as a biological weapon.

Category B agents:

- Brucellosis
- Epsilon toxin of *Clostridium perfringens*
- Food safety threats (e.g., Salmonella, Shigella, *E. coli*)
- Glanders
- Melioidosis
- Psittacosis
- Q fever
- Ricin toxin (from castor beans)
- Staphylococcal enterotoxin B

- Typhus fever
- Viral encephalitides
- Water safety threats (e.g., *Vibrio cholerae*, *Cryptosporidium parvum*)

Category C Agents

Category C agents represent "emerging" agents, that is, potential future infective threats, such as multidrug-resistant tuberculosis. Increased resources for research into the epidemiology and pathogenicity of these agents have been widely recommended.

These biological agents—although here separated into distinct groups—represent, as a whole, an array of infective organisms with significant potential for biological weaponization and damaging public health impact. The Category A agents, however, are particularly notable for their degree of lethality and potential for creating widespread morbidity and mortality among the general public. The remainder of this chapter examines each of the Category A agents in depth.

BIOSAFETY LABORATORY CLASSIFICATION

To provide guidance for laboratories handling samples of biological agents, the CDC has issued guidelines and a classification system for laboratories (CDC, 2009). This classification system categorizes laboratories from BSL-1 through BSL-4, with each successively higher numbered laboratory possessing a greater capability for biosafety hazard containment.

BSL-1 laboratories are equipped to work with biological samples that are not known to consistently cause disease in healthy adults and require only standard microbiological safety practices. BSL-2 laboratories may handle biological samples of agents that are associated with human disease and are transmitted either percutaneously or through ingestion or mucous membrane exposure. BSL-2 laboratories have more restricted access, require more strict containment precautions, and must have an autoclave available. BSL-3 laboratories handle exotic or indigenous agents that may cause serious or potentially lethal disease through the inhalation route of exposure. BSL-3 laboratories employ much stricter biosafety containment practices, including separation practices for laboratory space, negative pressure air handling, aggressive decontamination procedures, and strict control of laboratory access. BSL-4 laboratories may handle dangerous or exotic organisms that pose high risk of aerosol-transmitted laboratory infections that are frequently fatal and for which there are limited vaccines or treatments. BSL-4 laboratories employ the most careful containment procedures, including decontamination of every person or item that leaves the facility and dedicated supply and exhaust, vacuum, and decontamination systems.

ANTHRAX

History

Anthrax is a zoonotic disease, generally found in herbivores such as sheep, goats, and cattle that ingest spores from contaminated soil. The causative pathogen for anthrax is a spore-forming bacterium, *Bacillus anthracis* (see Figure 30.1). Human disease generally comes from contact with infected animals or animal products or, as evidenced by the events of late 2001, by intentional exposure (Inglesby et al., 2002). Anthrax has been present for centuries, and was previously identified as "wool sorters' disease" when detected among workers in woolen mills in 19th-century England (Cieslak & Eitzen, 1999). It was thought that inhalation of aerosolized anthrax spores from goat's wool was responsible. The spores are extremely resilient and can remain viable for decades. In 1942, British scientists tested an "anthrax bomb" on the Scottish island of Gruinard, rendering the island uninhabitable for over 40 years until government-sponsored cleanup efforts destroyed the still-infectious spores (Aldhous, 1990).

The potential use of anthrax as a biological weapon has been acknowledged for decades. An outbreak of inhalational anthrax in the area surrounding the Russian city of Sverdlovsk in 1979 was later attributed to Soviet efforts to create an anthrax-based biological weapon (Abramova, Grinberg, Yampolskaya, & Walker, 1993; Meselson et al., 1994; Sepkowitz, 2001). Iraq's biological weapons program, developed between 1985 and 1991, was known to include anthrax as well as other potent biological agents such as botulinum toxin (Zilinskas, 1997). The World Health Organization (WHO) estimated in 1970 that an airborne release of 50 kg of anthrax over an urban center of 5 million people would infect approximately 250,000 persons, causing 100,000 deaths, without adequate immediate treatment.

Epidemiology

Anthrax occurs in nearly every continent and in almost all countries. It predominantly presents as a cutaneous infection but may occur in gastrointestinal (GI), inhalational, meningeal, and injection form. Human disease occurs predominantly in two

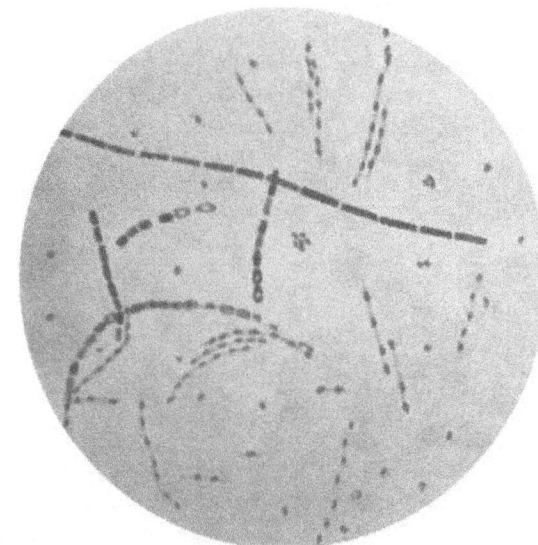

FIGURE 30.1 Photomicrograph of *Bacillus anthracis* from an agar culture demonstrating spores; Fuchsin-methylene blue spore stain.
Source: CDC.

settings: agricultural and industrial. In agriculturally derived cases of anthrax, patients contract the disease from contact with infected animals, typically sheep, goats, and cattle, although other animals can be affected. In industrial cases, contact with animal products such as contaminated wool, meat, or bonemeal has led to anthrax infection. Human-to-human transmission of anthrax has not been reported (Inglesby et al., 1999).

The worldwide incidence of anthrax is unknown but is estimated at several thousand cases per year. This number likely represents significant underreporting of the disease. In the United States, less than one case per year is typically reported. In 2006, one case of naturally occurring pulmonary anthrax was diagnosed in Pennsylvania in an African drum maker who was in contact with spores through mechanically scraping animal hides (CDC, 2006). Previously, the last case of naturally occurring inhalational anthrax had been reported in the United States in 1978 (Inglesby et al., 1999). The most recent acts of bioterrorism in the United States led to 23 identified cases of anthrax (11 inhalational, 12 cutaneous) between late 2001 and early 2002 (CDC, 2002b). Cases of injection anthrax were recently identified in heroin-injection drug users in northern Europe (National Health Service, 2011). Meningeal infection results from hematogenous spread and meningeal seeding and is seen as a complication of other forms of anthrax infection. Creation of an anthrax aerosol capable of dissemination and causing inhalational anthrax is likely confined to those entities with access to sophisticated biotechnology, making an anthrax attack by a lone individual or small group less probable.

Classification and Etiology

The causative pathogen for anthrax, *B. anthracis*, is an aerobic, gram-positive, spore-forming bacterium. The life cycle of *B. anthracis* has four major phases: the vegetative phase (from spores to replicating bacteria), an intense growth phase, a stationary phase, and the sporulation phase. Anthrax spores have a relatively high level of resistance to high temperatures and disinfectants (Hendricks et al., 2014). The anthrax bacterium also secretes powerful toxins: edema toxin and lethal toxin.

Diagnosis of anthrax is based on clinical presentation, laboratory analysis, and radiographic findings.

Anthrax occurs in four distinct forms: cutaneous, inhalational, GI, and meningeal. Although the cutaneous form represents the majority of anthrax cases, the inhalational and meningeal forms are historically responsible for most anthrax-related mortality (Hendricks et al., 2014). Cutaneous anthrax is typically contracted by contact with abraded skin by-products derived from infected herbivores, such as sheep, cattle, and goats. Inhalational anthrax has recently been associated with intentional aerosolization of anthrax spores but has historically been contracted by inhalation of spores from infected animals. The last case of naturally occurring inhalational anthrax occurred secondary to scraping animal hides in a poorly ventilated workspace. The worker did not use any personal protective equipment (PPE), and anthrax spores were detected in his workshop upon subsequent investigation. GI anthrax is presumably rare and is contracted via the consumption of meat from infected animals (Cieslak & Eitzen, 1999).

Pathogenesis

Inhalational Anthrax

Inhalation of anthrax spores represents the initial step in the pathogenesis of inhalational anthrax. Spores are phagocytosed in the lungs and then transported to the lymphoid tissue, particularly in the mediastinum, by macrophages. During a 1- to 6-day incubation period, the spores germinate and multiply dramatically, producing bacteremia. With worsening bacteremia, accumulation of the anthrax exotoxin progresses, resulting in severe edema and hemorrhagic mediastinitis (see Figure 30.2). Respiratory failure, septic shock, and death follow. Death from inhalational anthrax is essentially universal in untreated patients. Autopsy findings show evidence of multiple organ hemorrhage and necrosis as well as hemorrhagic meningitis in up to 50% of cases (Cieslak & Eitzen, 1999). Even with modern antimicrobial treatment and critical care support, inhalation anthrax has a 45% mortality rate (Jernigan et al., 2001).

Cutaneous Anthrax

Cutaneous anthrax occurs when anthrax spores enter the skin through cuts or abrasions. The affected area develops a small macule or papule that then ulcerates. A black painless eschar then follows, associated with extensive local edema and painful regional lymphadenopathy (see Figure 30.3). Systemic symptoms can follow.

Gastrointestinal Anthrax

GI anthrax is contracted by germination of ingested spores in the upper or lower GI tract. The GI forms of the disease are generally an upper GI form and a lower GI form. In the upper

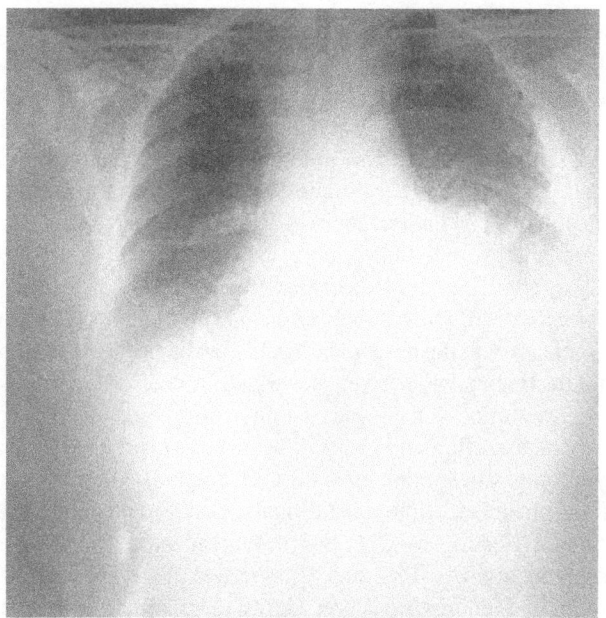

FIGURE 30.2 Chest radiograph showing widened mediastinum due to inhalation anthrax.

Source: CDC/Dr. P. S. Brachman.

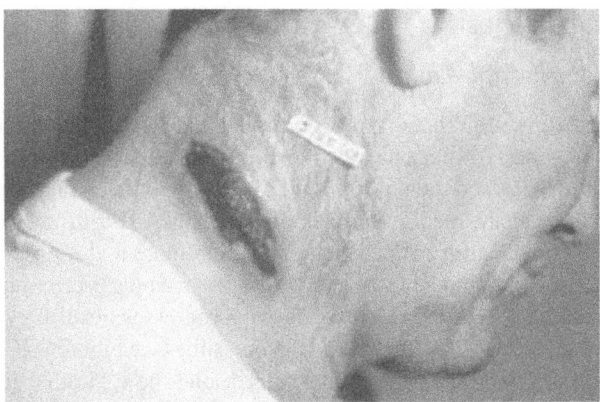

FIGURE 30.3 Cutaneous anthrax lesion on the neck.
Source: CDC.

GI form, oral or esophageal ulcers develop with associated edema, lymphadenopathy, and sepsis. In the lower GI form, partial necrosis of the GI tract can occur with symptoms including bloody diarrhea, acute abdomen, ascites, or sepsis.

Meningeal Anthrax

Meningeal anthrax results from hematogenous spread of other forms of anthrax. This form of anthrax is nearly always fatal, even with treatment (Sejvar, Tenover, & Stephens, 2005).

Injection Anthrax

Injection form of anthrax has been described in injection drug users (National Health Service, 2011).

Clinical Manifestations and Diagnosis

Diagnosis of inhalational anthrax in its early stages is very difficult as the patient's clinical presentation may be nonspecific (i.e., easily mistaken for viral upper respiratory illness or atypical pneumonia), such as nonproductive cough, chest pain, sore throat, myalgias, low-grade fever, and malaise (Mayer et al., 2001). Laboratory studies include gram stain, culture, and polymerase chain reaction (PCR) from accessible fluid, and serum anthrax lethal factor toxin assay (CDC, 2017). In later stages, after bacteremia becomes more pronounced, patients rapidly worsen with the development of respiratory failure, associated with the onset of bulky, hemorrhagic mediastinitis, manifesting as widened mediastinum on chest radiographs. Other causes of widened mediastinum must be excluded, such as thoracic aortic aneurysm or dissection or superior vena cava syndrome. Chest computerized tomography (CT) may also reveal pleural effusions, mediastinal widening, and pericardial effusion (Hendricks, 2014). Severe generalized edema, hemorrhagic pleural effusions, and hemorrhagic meningitis are also common. Meningitis has been shown to be uniformly fatal in a recent review of reported cases (Holty, 2006). Subarachnoid hemorrhage due to various causes should not be mistaken for the hemorrhagic meningitis seen in inhalational anthrax. Patients following this clinical course, particularly when presenting in temporal or geographical clusters, should raise suspicions of a biological weapon attack due to inhalational anthrax (Inglesby et al., 1999).

The diagnosis of cutaneous anthrax, likewise, is initially difficult. A history of skin contact with anthrax spores or potentially anthrax-contaminated animal products is helpful. In early stages, the skin lesion is very nonspecific, but the later presence of a painless black eschar accompanied by severe localized edema is essentially pathognomonic for the diagnosis. Other causes of painful lymphadenopathy such as staph, strep, plague, and tularemia may mimic cutaneous anthrax. Cutaneous anthrax lesions can also resemble the necrotic ulcerated lesions due to a brown recluse spider bite.

GI anthrax has never been reported in the United States. A history of eating contaminated meat or dairy products from infected animals, including abdominal pain, vomiting, diarrhea, development of acute abdomen, edema, or ascites, should suggest the diagnosis of GI anthrax. Other causes of abdominal pain, ascites, or GI symptoms should be entertained as well. Clusters of similarly affected patients who have also ingested anthrax-contaminated food items should also raise the suspicion of GI anthrax. The final diagnosis of anthrax is made by isolation and confirmation of the presence of *B. anthracis* from a clinical specimen such as from blood cultures or ulcer fluid, by immunofluorescent staining, or by confirmation of the presence of *B. anthracis* DNA in clinical specimens by PCR (Cieslak & Eitzen, 1999; Table 30.1).

Biosafety Issues, Protection, and Isolation

BSL-2 precautions are recommended for laboratory personnel who may come in contact with anthrax specimens, including handling of specimens in a laminar flow hood with protective eyewear, using gloves pulled over lab coats, and avoiding activities that may produce aerosol or droplet dispersal. BSL-3 precautions are recommended for personnel who work extensively with anthrax specimens, including producing quantities for research purposes. These include precautions similar to BSL-2 as well as respiratory protective equipment as needed, controlled access to the laboratory, decontamination of all waste, and a negative air pressure system in the laboratory. A case of laboratory-acquired cutaneous anthrax was confirmed in June 2002, involving a laboratory worker who contracted the disease by using ungloved hands to handle anthrax-containing vials (CDC, 2002b).

Healthcare workers who come in contact with patients in whom anthrax is suspected should use universal precautions at all times, including the use of rubber gloves, disposal of sharps, and frequent handwashing. No human-to-human transmission of anthrax has been reported, and respiratory isolation precautions are not needed. Patients with inhalational or cutaneous anthrax should be placed on contact isolation, due to the potential for contact with open wounds or wound drainage.

Public Health Implications

Even a single case of inhalational anthrax is a significant public health event because of its rarity and extreme pathogenicity. Given recent events, the presence of inhalational anthrax implies

TABLE 30.1 Clinical Manifestations of Anthrax Infection

Subjective Symptoms	Objective Findings (Physical Exam, Lab, Imaging Studies)	Notes
Inhalational anthrax Cough, chest pain, dyspnea, viral URI symptoms (sore throat, myalgias, mild fever) during prodrome	Lymphadenopathy, widened mediastinum on chest radiograph, pleural effusions	Signs/symptoms progress to respiratory failure, sepsis, and hemodynamic collapse in preterminal stages
Meningeal signs	Hemorrhagic meningitis (in up to 50%)	
Cutaneous anthrax Raised bump on face, hands, or arms, typically with black painless ulceration	Ulcer with black eschar, moderate to severe localized edema and lymphadenopathy	Time course is 1–7 days until appearance of typical ulcer
GI anthrax Vomiting, diarrhea, and abdominal pain	Diarrhea may be bloody. Acute abdomen may be present with or without ascites	Fluid volume loss may be severe

URI, upper respiratory infection.

an act of bioterrorism until proven otherwise. Notification of appropriate public health authorities is appropriate if any case of anthrax is suspected or confirmed. Initial steps should include notification of the hospital infection control officer and jurisdictional public health authorities. Laboratory personnel should alert state public health laboratories and also use the Laboratory Response Network for Bioterrorism to facilitate rapid, appropriate triage from the Rapid Response and Advanced Technology Laboratory at the CDC (Kahn & Sage, 2000). In light of relatively recent acts of bioterrorism involving anthrax, healthcare personnel should increase their vigilance for cases of suspected anthrax, especially among mail handlers.

Vaccination and Postexposure Prophylaxis

An anthrax vaccine is available but its use is currently reserved for pre-exposure prophylaxis in select high-risk populations such as some animal product handlers, select laboratory workers, and select military personnel. The vaccine can additionally be used for postexposure prophylaxis. The vaccine is a sterile, acellular vaccine known as AVA (anthrax vaccine adsorbed; Wright, Quinn, Shadomy, & Messonnier, 2010).

Postexposure prophylaxis is not recommended for contacts of patients infected with *B. anthracis,* or for healthcare workers who may treat anthrax patients. It is also not recommended for the prophylaxis of cutaneous anthrax. It is currently indicated only for persons who may have been exposed to airspace contaminated with aerosolized *B. anthracis* (Bell, Kozarsky, & Stephens, 2002). The duration of therapy is generally determined to be 60 days of either ciprofloxacin or doxycycline, with amoxicillin as an option for children and pregnant or lactating women. The U.S. Department of Health and Human Services has also announced additional options for prophylaxis of inhalational anthrax, especially for those in whom inhalational exposure may have been significant. These options include 60 or 100 days of prophylaxis, as well as 100 days of prophylaxis plus anthrax vaccine (CDC, 2001a; Hendricks et al., 2014; Nass, 2002).

Treatment

The treatment of anthrax depends on the type of anthrax and severity of illness. Cutaneous anthrax without systemic involvement can be treated with oral ciprofloxacin, doxycycline, levofloxacin, or moxifloxacin. The duration of treatment is 60 days for cases related to bioterrorism and 10 days for naturally acquired cases. Case fatality rates for cutaneous anthrax are less than 1% with treatment (Hendricks et al., 2014).

The recommended management of system anthrax, including inhalational, GI, and injection forms, involves an intravenous (IV) course of ciprofloxacin or clindamycin or linezolid. Total duration of recommended antimicrobial treatment is 60 days. If meningeal anthrax is suspected, then a multiple IV antibiotic regimen of ciprofloxacin plus meropenem plus linezolid is recommended. Several alternative antibiotics have also been recommended by the CDC to accommodate patients with allergies or drug shortage scenarios (Bower et al., 2015; Hendricks et al., 2014). Anthrax has traditionally been resistant to cephalosporins, including broad-spectrum cephalosporins such as ceftriaxone. Because of the rapid and recurrent accumulation of hemorrhagic pleural effusions, chest tube drainage of pleural fluid has produced dramatic improvement in clinical status. In the most recent outbreak of inhalation anthrax, 6 of 11 patients survived (Inglesby et al., 2002; Jernigan et al., 2001). In previous outbreaks of inhalational anthrax, case fatality rates have been as high as 86%, despite therapy (Meselson et al., 1994). A recent study has found that multidrug antibiotic regimens, pleural fluid drainage, and initiation of antibiotics in the prodromal phase significantly lowered mortality from inhalational anthrax (Holty, 2006).

Antitoxin treatments with raxibacumab and anthrax immune globulin are an area of ongoing research and interest in the treatment of systemic anthrax. Given the high mortality rate of systemic anthrax, addition of antitoxin treatment to an antimicrobial regimen for patients with systemic anthrax is recommended (Hendricks et al., 2014).

BOTULISM

History

Botulism is a neuroparalytic, primarily foodborne illness first described in 1897 (CDC, 1998). The disease is caused by a toxin produced by the anaerobic bacterium *C. botulinum*. Although botulism is rare, it can kill rapidly and foodborne botulism is a public health emergency carrying significant risk for widespread disease and death, as potentially preventable deaths may occur if the source of botulism is not discovered and eliminated. There are classically four major types of botulism: foodborne botulism, infantile botulism, wound botulism, and "other" botulism. This last category includes intestinal and iatrogenic botulism.

The botulinum toxin produced by *C. botulinum* is actually a group of distinct toxins with similar paralytic effects on the neurologic system. Botulinum toxin is the most poisonous substance known to mankind; less than 1 mcg is a fatal dose for an adult (Arnon et al., 2001).

The idea of a bioterrorist attack involving botulism stems largely from the extreme lethality of the botulinum toxin. Unsuccessful attempts have already been made to aerosolize botulinum toxin by a Japanese cult between 1990 and 1995. The United States Biological Weapons Program produced botulinum toxin during World War II. The former Soviet Union and Iraq have both admitted creating large stores of concentrated botulinum toxin. Much of Iraq's production of botulinum toxin, some 19,000 liters, remains unaccounted for. About 10% of persons within 0.5 km downwind of an aerosol release of botulinum toxin would be incapacitated or killed (Patrick, 1998, as cited in Arnon et al., 2001).

Recently, the extreme potency of botulinum toxin has led to multiple medical uses of this substance, including the treatment of cervical torticollis, strabismus, and other musculoskeletal disorders, as well as in cosmetic plastic surgery as "Botox" for the elimination of facial lines or wrinkles (Lemonick, 2002). The irreversible action of botulinum toxin on nerve transmission when used in minute amounts leads to prolonged therapeutic effects of greater than 3 months in duration. An iatrogenic form is also reported secondary to adverse effects of local injection of the toxin in cosmetic procedures or in patients with spasticity (Tugnoli et al., 2002).

Epidemiology

Foodborne botulism accounts for approximately 1,000 cases per year worldwide, of which approximately 30 occur in the United States. In 2015, the CDC received 199 confirmed botulism case reports, the majority of which were of the infant type (71%). Foodborne botulism accounted for 20% of cases, wound botulism for 8%, and 2% were classified in the "other" category (CDC, 2015a).

Home-processed foods account for 94% of U.S. foodborne botulism cases. Infantile botulism, a form of the disease in which *C. botulinum* spores are ingested by infants due to food contamination, occurs more commonly in California. Wound botulism, typically involving IV drug users who either inject drugs intravenously or in the subcutaneous tissue (a practice known as "skin-popping"), is reported one to three times per year in the United States. It can also occur in other types of contaminated wounds such as a severe crush injury or other areas of contaminated avascular tissue. Botulism due to intestinal colonization by *C. botulinum* is extremely rare; only seven cases have been reported in the literature (CDC, 1998).

Classification and Etiology

Botulism is caused by the neuroparalytic toxin produced by the bacterium *C. botulinum*, a common soil contaminant. This toxin has been divided into several groups. Types A, B, and E are the major types producing disease in humans, with Type A accounting for 44%, Type B, 36%, and Type E, 12.5% of cases. Type A botulism generally occurs in the western United States, while Type B is typically found in central and northeastern states. The majority of Type E botulism cases are found in Alaska. Types A and B are associated with the consumption of home-canned vegetables, fruits, and meat products, while Type E is seen with marine products.

Infantile botulism involves the ingestion of botulism spores. The most common identified vehicle for this ingestion in several case series was honey, involving approximately 20% of cases. In the majority of cases of infantile botulism, however, ingestion of honey was not reported. Other possible sources of botulism spores include foods and household dust. Because of the association between the ingestion of honey and infantile botulism, CDC recommends that honey not be fed to infants (CDC, 1998).

Pathogenesis

Clostridium botulinum is extremely widespread in soil, dust, and on the surfaces of many foods. The botulinum toxin is heat labile, and botulinum spores are killed by boiling at 100°C. The toxin, once ingested, blocks acetylcholine release from peripheral cholinergic nerve terminals. Adrenergic and sensory nerve endings are not affected. This neurotransmitter blockade is irreversible, requiring the growth of new nerve endings for nerve conduction to resume.

Clinical Manifestations and Diagnosis

Botulism presents as a progressive, descending, symmetric weakness or paralysis. It invariably begins with cranial nerve palsies, including dilated or nonreactive pupils (ophthalmoplegia) in 50% of cases. This paralysis progresses to involve the respiratory musculature causing respiratory failure and death if unrecognized and untreated. The need for often prolonged ventilatory support is common in botulism. Two-thirds of patients with Type A botulism need intubation and mechanical ventilation. The average duration of ventilatory support is 6 to 8 weeks but it may be as long as 7 months. Prolonged fatigue and exercise intolerance are common after botulism, lasting up to 2 years or more.

In foodborne botulism, complaints of nausea, vomiting, and diarrhea may accompany the initial neurologic symptoms. In later stages of the disease, constipation becomes more prominent. In infantile botulism, constipation is often the main symptom, along with characteristic flaccidity (the "floppy baby"), poor suck reflex, poor feeding, and poor head control.

Pitfalls in the diagnosis of botulism include failure to recognize the symptoms and to institute adequate ventilatory support. Botulism is likely underdiagnosed and can be mistaken for a number of neuromuscular and neurologic disorders. Diphtheria, encephalitis, poliomyelitis, Guillain–Barré syndrome, congenital neuropathies and myopathies, myasthenia gravis, and mushroom (muscarinic) poisoning are diagnoses potentially similar in presentation to botulism. The laboratory diagnosis of botulism is made by the identification of *C. botulinum* toxin in serum, stool, and gastric aspirate or food samples. *Clostridium botulinum*, *C. butyricum*, or *C. baratii* cultures can also be obtained from food, wounds, or stool.

Laboratory Issues, Protection, and Isolation

Botulinum toxin is extremely poisonous to humans. Coats, gloves, face shields, and protective cabinets are recommended for handling botulism specimens. Ideally, laboratory personnel should be vaccinated with *C. botulinum* antitoxin. Standard precautions should be used when caring for patients suspected of botulism. Respiratory isolation is not necessary.

Public Health Implications

Every case of foodborne botulism should be treated as a public health emergency. The potential for additional cases from a single contaminated food source is high. Every effort should be made to eliminate toxin-containing food items still available for public consumption to avoid additional morbidity and mortality.

Cases of botulism that appear in temporal or geographical groups should prompt rapid investigation into foodborne sources of illness as well as raise the possibility of bioterrorism in the form of inhalational botulism. Any suspected or confirmed case of botulism should prompt immediate contact with local and state health departments.

Vaccination and Postexposure Prophylaxis

A botulinum toxoid vaccine is made available as an investigational agent through CDC for laboratory workers who work regularly with botulinum toxin or *C. botulinum*. Postexposure prophylaxis is not recommended at this time for asymptomatic patients (Arnon et al., 2001).

Treatment

The mainstays of botulism therapy include ventilatory support as well as the administration of botulinum antitoxin. In the United States, the botulinum antitoxin is a heptavalent, equine antitoxin that provides antibodies to botulinum toxin Types A, B, C, D, E, F, and G. Other countries may use the trivalent antitoxin that provides antibodies to botulinum toxin Types A, B, and C. The antitoxin acts against only unbound toxin, and therefore its efficacy is greatest early in the patient's clinical course. It stops the progression of illness but does not reverse existing nerve dysfunction. Cathartics and enemas have also been recommended for elimination of botulinum toxin from the GI tract. Antibiotics are not recommended except for the treatment of wound botulism in conjunction with surgical debridement. Asymptomatic patients suspected of ingesting contaminated food items should be closely observed for any signs of illness. For infantile botulism, the human-derived botulism immune globulin (BIG) is effective. Administration of the equine-based antitoxin has not proven beneficial for infants (CDC, 1998).

PLAGUE

History

Plague is possibly the most feared infectious disease in the history of humankind. More than 200 million people have died from plague. In its most notorious manifestation, the so-called Black Death of the Middle Ages, plague was responsible for a pandemic that affected Europe between the 8th and 14th centuries, decimating nearly 40% of the population (McGovern & Friedlander, 1997).

The potential use of the bacterium responsible for plague, *Y. pestis*, as a bioweapon has been a subject of research both in the United States and the Soviet Union in the post–World War II era. A WHO study of a deliberate aerosolization of *Y. pestis* over an urban population estimated nearly 25% mortality among those infected with the pneumonic form of plague (WHO, 1970; see Figure 30.4).

Epidemiology

Plague is still present worldwide. The introduction of the disease to human populations occurs when plague-infected fleas, which typically infest rodent hosts, cause the death of these rodents in large numbers. Fleas then move from their natural hosts to humans, causing outbreaks of plague. In the United States, an average of 13 cases per year are reported, typically in western States. The WHO reported 2,861 cases in 1995 worldwide (Inglesby et al., 2000).

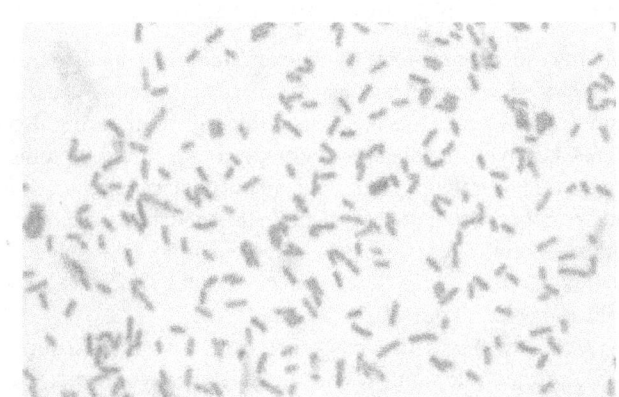

FIGURE 30.4 *Yersinia pestis*, gram-negative bacillus, 1,000× magnification.

Source: CDC/*Courtesy* of Lary Stauffer, Oregon State Public Health Laboratory.

Classification and Etiology

Plague is caused by *Y. pestis*, a nonmotile gram-negative bacterium. Transmission to humans is typically through the bite of an infected flea, although droplet spread from patients with pneumonic plague is another route of infection. Plague occurs in three forms: bubonic, pneumonic, and septicemic. The most common form of plague, and that responsible for the European pandemics, is bubonic plague. This form presents with painful, swollen lymph nodes, the "bubo" of bubonic plague, followed by generalized bacteremia. In septicemic plague, the infected fleabite vector is the same, but rather than developing buboes, patients develop sepsis followed by multiple organ failure. Pneumonic plague is spread by droplet dispersal from infected patients and severe pulmonary involvement is the cardinal sign.

Pathogenesis

The exact pathophysiology of plague is unknown. In bubonic plague, the patient is injected with *Y. pestis* via an infected fleabite. Bacteria then migrate to local lymph nodes and then multiply, causing development of a bubo, a large, swollen, extremely tender lymph node, usually in the groin, axilla, or neck. Plague bacteria continue to multiply, resisting phagocytosis by macrophages, leading to bacteremia, sepsis, shock, disseminated intravascular coagulation (DIC), and ultimately coma and death. In septicemic plague, patients, although bitten by infected fleas, do not develop the typical bubo, but instead progress to sepsis and DIC, often with gangrene and necrosis of fingers and toes.

Pneumonic plague, the most deadly form of the disease, occurs when *Y. pestis* infects the lungs, causing severe hemorrhagic, necrotizing bronchopneumonia; dyspnea; chest pain; cough; and hemoptysis. This process can either occur by hematogenous spread of the bacterium (secondary pneumonic plague) or by droplet spread from infected persons directly to the patient via inhalation (primary pneumonic plague). The most recent case fatality rates for pneumonic plague were 57%, despite therapy (Inglesby et al., 2000).

Clinical Manifestations and Diagnosis

Patients with plague present with fever, chills, and myalgias, as well as swollen, painful lymph nodes in bubonic plague. Nausea, vomiting, and cough productive of bloody sputum are also seen. Chest pain, dyspnea, and hemoptysis are later symptoms typical for pneumonic plague. A history of contact with infected rodents or fleas is important to elicit. In the United States, ground squirrels, prairie dogs, and rats have been reported as plague vectors, particularly in New Mexico, Arizona, Colorado, and California (see Figure 30.5; CDC, 2002a).

Other diagnoses that may present in a similar fashion to plague include adult respiratory distress syndrome, cat scratch disease, cellulitis, DIC, pneumonia, empyema and lung abscess, gangrene, and necrotizing fasciitis. Laboratory diagnosis of plague is confirmed by identification of plague bacterium on gram stain, or by culture of blood, sputum, or bubo aspirate.

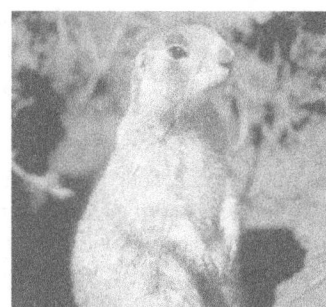

FIGURE 30.5 This burrowing rodent of the genus *Cynomys* can harbor fleas infected with *Yersinia pestis*, the bacterium that causes plague.
Source: CDC.

Biosafety Issues, Protection, and Isolation

BSL-2 precautions should be used for specimens from patients suspected of *Y. pestis* infection. BSL-3 precautions are needed only if extensive work with infected specimens is expected. Strict isolation should be maintained for all patients suspected of *Y. pestis* infection. Gowns, gloves, masks, and eye protection should be worn for at least the first 48 hours of treatment.

Public Health Implications

Plague is a nationally notifiable disease and represents a potential public health emergency due to the extreme infectivity of *Y. pestis* as well as mortality rates associated with plague. Local and state health departments should be notified if the presence of plague is suspected or confirmed.

Vaccination and Postexposure Prophylaxis

A plague vaccine was previously available in the United States, but production was discontinued in 1999. This vaccine protected against the bubonic form of the disease but did not provide protection against pneumonic plague. It was previously administered to military personnel working in plague-endemic areas, laboratory personnel working with *Y. pestis*, or researchers working with plague-infected animals or fleas. Research is ongoing into a vaccine against pneumonic plague (Titball & Williamson, 2001). Encouraging results have been obtained in mice (Elvin et al., 2005).

Antibiotic prophylaxis is recommended for contacts (including healthcare workers) of patients infected with plague as well as close surveillance of contacts refusing antibiotics. In May 2000, the Working Group on Civilian Biodefense, in their *Journal of the American Medical Association* review of plague as a potential agent of bioterrorism, recommended doxycycline and ciprofloxacin as postexposure prophylaxis for adults, children, and pregnant women.

Treatment

The historical antibiotic of choice for the treatment of plague has been streptomycin but may not be available in the United States where gentamycin or levofloxacin are first-line therapy choices. Alternative regimens include doxycycline, ciprofloxacin, moxifloxacin, and chloramphenicol. Patients with pneumonic plague may also require advanced medical supportive therapy in addition to antibiotics.

TULAREMIA

History

Tularemia is a highly infectious zoonotic disease caused by the bacterium, *F. tularensis*. It was first described in Tulare County, California, in 1911 (Francis, 1925). The first recognized human case of tularemia was reported in 1914. Tularemia can cause fever, skin or mucous membrane ulceration, lymphadenopathy, and occasionally life-threatening pneumonia. Its major threat (and its bioweapon potential) comes from its extreme infectivity; inhalation or inoculation of as few as 10 organisms is enough to cause disease (Dennis et al., 2001). In addition to its infectivity, *F. tularensis* can produce severe disease and death, if untreated.

Outbreaks of tularemia affected tens of thousands of soldiers on the eastern European front during World War II. It has been suggested that these epidemics may have been intentional in origin, part of an act of biological warfare (Alibek, 1999). Like other biological agents of concern, both the United States and the former Soviet Union stockpiled stores of tularemia bacteria for potential use during the 1960s and 1970s.

Epidemiology

Primarily a rural disease, tularemia has been reported in every state in the United States except Hawaii. It has also been reported worldwide, primarily in Eurasia, although its true incidence is likely underrecognized and underreported. Fewer than 200 cases are reported per year in the United States and the case fatality rate is less than 2%. Although males tend to be more often infected than females, this finding is probably related to the specific outdoor activities that may predispose individuals to contracting tularemia, such as farming, hunting, trapping, and butchering (Dennis et al., 2001).

Classification and Etiology

Tularemia, as previously noted, is caused by an aerobic, gram-negative bacterium, *F. tularensis*. It can present clinically in several different forms: ulceroglandular, glandular, oculoglandular, oropharyngeal, pneumonic, typhoidal, and septic forms. Tularemia is typically found in animals such as rabbits and rodents, and can be transmitted to humans in several ways. Contact with infected animal carcasses; ingestion of contaminated meat, soil, or water; inhalation of the bacterium (especially in laboratory workers); inoculation of the bacterium via cuts or abrasions as well as via the bite of infected arthropods such as ticks are among the ways tularemia can be contracted.

Pathogenesis

Francisella tularensis is a facultative intracellular bacterium that can infect humans via the skin, mucous membranes, GI tract, and lungs. The bacterium then multiplies inside macrophages, preferentially affecting lymph nodes, lungs and pleura, spleen, liver, and kidney. Inhalational exposures cause hemorrhagic airway involvement with bronchopneumonia. The absence of fulminant, rapid onset of respiratory failure, shock and death, despite antibiotic therapy, can distinguish inhalational tularemia from inhalational anthrax.

Clinical Manifestations and Diagnosis

Although tularemia can present in a myriad of ways—ulceroglandular, glandular, oculoglandular, oropharyngeal, pneumonic, typhoidal, and septic forms—the ulceroglandular and typhoidal forms make up the majority of tularemia patients. Ulceroglandular tularemia is the most common, comprising approximately 75% of cases (Edlow, 2001).

Tularemia initially presents with abrupt onset of high fever, headache, rigors, coryza, and sore throat. Dry cough, sweats, fever, and chills occur as the disease continues. The ulceroglandular form of tularemia presents with skin and mucous membrane ulcers, lymphadenopathy, or both. A cutaneous chancre-like ulcer is the most common finding (see Figure 30.6). The typhoidal form has less significant lymph node involvement, and skin lesions are absent. Pulmonary involvement is prominent, particularly with the typhoidal form. The differential diagnosis of tularemia also includes other diseases with prominent skin manifestations or pulmonary findings such as plague, diphtheria, psittacosis, Q fever, and other tick-borne diseases. The definitive diagnosis of tularemia is by culture, typically from sputum. ELISA, bacterial agglutination, and immunofluorescent techniques are also available.

Biosafety Issues, Protection, and Isolation

Tularemia is extremely infectious in aerosol form. Laboratory personnel have contracted inhalational tularemia simply by examining an open culture plate. BSL-2 precautions should be used for initial evaluation and then specimens should be forwarded to a BSL-3 laboratory for further testing (Dennis et al., 2001).

Despite its infectivity, human-to-human transmission of tularemia is not a risk, and therefore isolation is not needed. Universal precautions are recommended for patients suspected of tularemia infection.

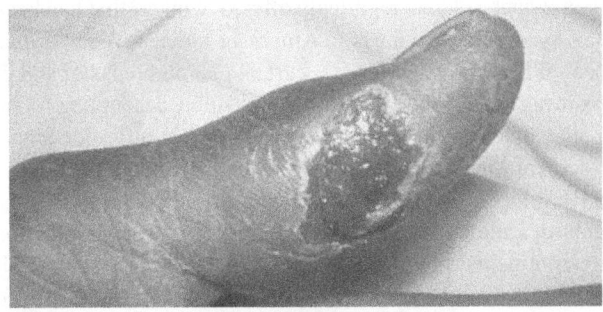

FIGURE 30.6 Thumb with skin ulcer of tularemia.
Source: CDC/Emory University; Dr. Sellers.

Public Health Implications

Tularemia is a nationally notifiable disease, and its significant infectivity via inhalation makes this agent a potential choice for bioterrorism. As for other Category A agents, any suspected or confirmed case of tularemia is an indication for immediate notifications of the hospital infection control officer, and local and state health departments.

Vaccination and Postexposure Prophylaxis

A live attenuated vaccine derived from a less virulent form of *F. tularensis* is available for laboratory personnel who routinely work with tularemia. Postexposure prophylaxis for contacts of tularemia patients is not recommended, as person-to-person transmission is not known to occur. For persons who may have been exposed to *F. tularensis*, for example, by an act of bioterrorism, a 14-day oral course of ciprofloxacin or doxycycline is indicated (Dennis et al., 2001).

Treatment

Streptomycin and gentamicin are the drugs of choice. Doxycycline and chloramphenicol have also been used, but more treatment failures have been reported with these regimens. Ciprofloxacin is another alternative therapy. For the first-line regimens as well as ciprofloxacin, a 10-day course of IV antibiotics is recommended. For second-line therapies, 14 days are recommended.

SMALLPOX

History

Smallpox is a disease that has been present for centuries. Epidemics of this viral disease, unique to humans, have been reported since ancient history. Once one of the most feared of all diseases, smallpox was declared eradicated worldwide by the WHO in 1980 (Henderson, 1980). The last case occurred in Somalia in 1977. A worldwide vaccination program against smallpox was responsible for the elimination of the disease. Routine vaccination of the general U.S. population against smallpox ended more than 25 years ago, leading to a population whose susceptibility to the disease is greater now than at any other time in recent history.

The first reported use of smallpox as a biological weapon probably originated during the French and Indian Wars (1754–1767), when British soldiers reportedly offered blankets that had been used by smallpox patients to American Indians. Whether this account is accurate or not, it is certain that outbreaks of smallpox ravaged the Native American population, accounting for up to 50% mortality in some tribes. Ken Alibek, a former Soviet biological weapons expert, reported that after 1980, the Soviets had developed the capability to produce smallpox virus in large quantities and were capable of adapting it for use in bombs and intercontinental ballistic missiles (Alibek, 1999). After smallpox was declared eradicated in 1980, the WHO recommended that all remaining stores of smallpox be either destroyed or transferred to one of two locations—CDC in Atlanta, Georgia, or the State Research Centre of Virology and Biotechnology in Novosibirsk, Russia (Breman & Arita, 1980). Later recommendations from the WHO in 1999 were that all stockpiles of smallpox be destroyed. After questions about further research into smallpox and smallpox vaccines were raised, the deadline for the destruction of remaining smallpox stores was delayed until 2002. In May 2002, the World Health Assembly decided to authorize the retention of existing Variola virus stockpiles for research purposes at the two locations named previously (World Health Assembly, 2002). The debate over whether or not to destroy remaining Variola samples continues. It is believed, however, that other laboratories within Russia, as well as in other countries, may still hold quantities of smallpox virus, raising the specter of unscrupulous scientists or groups selling stockpiles of smallpox for financial gain (Henderson et al., 1999).

Epidemiology

Smallpox occurs in two forms: variola major (the most dangerous and formerly widespread form of the disease) and variola minor. Case fatality rates among the unvaccinated from variola major were 30% or higher. Person-to-person transmission of the disease occurs by droplet spread from infected persons or by contact with contaminated clothing or bedding. Smallpox is highly contagious. The amount of virus sufficient to cause disease in 50% of susceptible persons is fewer than 10 viral particles. The virus is very hardy, remaining viable on clothing or other contaminated objects for months (Henderson et al., 1999).

Classification and Etiology

Smallpox, a DNA virus, is a member of the genus Orthopoxvirus, like monkey pox, vaccinia, or cow pox. It contains a large, complex viral genome and is the only Orthopoxvirus to be readily transmitted from person to person.

Pathogenesis

The main portal of entry is the respiratory tract. Skin, conjunctiva, and transplacental infection are less common. Once inoculation with the virus occurs, the smallpox virus survives and replicates successfully, despite the presence of an active host immune response. Infectivity rates are higher at the onset of the rash. The virus survives because of its ability to acquire and modulate host immune and inflammatory genes. Pox viruses are unique in their ability to replicate in the cytoplasm of infected cells.

Clinical Manifestations and Diagnosis

Variola major consists of three types. The classic form represents 90% of all cases. Flat and hemorrhagic smallpox occur in 7% and 2% of cases, respectively, and have a significantly worse prognosis (Moore, Seward, & Lane, 2006). Initially, persons who have been exposed to smallpox are asymptomatic during the incubation period. This typically lasts from 7 to 14 days, although estimates for an intentional smallpox exposure are from 1 to 5 days. After the incubation period, patients develop prodromal symptoms for 2 to 3 days, including high fever and nonspecific constitutional symptoms such as headache,

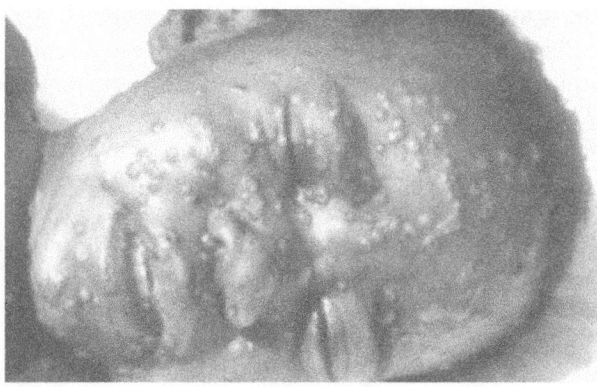

FIGURE 30.7 Face lesions on a boy with smallpox.
Source: CDC/Cheryl Tyron.

backache, fatigue, and malaise. As the fever subsides, the rash of smallpox appears.

The smallpox rash begins with a maculopapular rash on the face and then spreads to the extremities. The initial rash of smallpox is indistinguishable from that of varicella (chicken pox) but is later characteristic in appearance. Smallpox lesions become vesicular and then pustular, and are deeply embedded in the dermis. Although varicella lesions appear in "crops" in varying stages over the body, all smallpox lesions develop at the same pace. Smallpox lesions affect the face and extremities preferentially and also affect the palms and soles, unlike chicken pox, which involves primarily the trunk (see Figure 30.7). This manifestation stage lasts from 8 to 9 days.

Toxemia develops during this period due to circulating immune complexes and variola antigens, and is the primary cause of death. Secondary bacterial infection is uncommon. During the second week of illness, either death or recovery usually results (Henderson, 1999).

Biosafety Issues, Protection, and Isolation

Laboratory diagnosis of smallpox is essential and specimens should be obtained by people vaccinated against smallpox. Because of its aerosol infectivity, pathogenicity, and capability of person-to-person transmission, BSL-4 containment procedures, protective equipment, and facilities are necessary for evaluation of potential smallpox samples. These procedures include specially designed laboratory space secured with airlocks and decontamination rooms. Personnel working in these spaces must wear a one-piece positive pressure suit equipped with a HEPA-filtered life-support system. Multiple redundant backup systems and other safeguards are also in place with BSL-4 to prevent release of these extremely dangerous microbes (Department of Health and Human Services, 1999).

All patients in whom smallpox is suspected should be placed in strict respiratory isolation in negative pressure rooms. Contacts of the patient should be vaccinated and placed under surveillance. Isolated in-home or nonhospital facilities are preferable, due to the high risk of transmission of smallpox via aerosol within hospital environments (Henderson et al., 1999).

Public Health Implications

Any potential or confirmed case of smallpox represents an international public health emergency. Local and state public health officials should be notified immediately, with assurances that national public health officials will also be made aware. Strict quarantine with respiratory isolation for all contacts of the index patient is mandatory.

Vaccination and Postexposure Prophylaxis

Until 2002, smallpox vaccine was approved by the U.S. Food and Drug Administration for use only in persons in special-risk categories, including laboratory workers who work with smallpox or other related Orthopoxviruses. In July 2002, however, the Advisory Committee on Immunization Practices in preliminary recommendations recommended vaccinating roughly 500,000 healthcare and emergency workers against smallpox, given the possibility of terrorist attacks involving smallpox (Broad, 2002). From late 2002 through 2003, approximately 39,000 individuals received smallpox vaccination in the United States as part of this program. U.S. smallpox vaccination efforts were associated with a low rate of complications (~2%), although some serious reactions occurred, including myopericarditis and encephalitis (Casey et al., 2005). Under epidemic circumstances, the WHO recommends immediate and widespread vaccination of the general public. Smallpox vaccine is now offered to select individuals found to be at increased risk for exposure to variola (Petersen, Harms, Reynolds, & Harrison, 2016).

Smallpox vaccine is not recommended for use in certain groups who may be at risk for complications of the vaccine. In up to 0.2% or more of immunized populations, immunosuppressed individuals, pregnant women, and patients with atopic dermatitis may develop complications related to vaccinia, the Orthopoxvirus used in smallpox vaccine. Vaccinia immunoglobulin can be given to those at risk for these complications. Smallpox vaccine can also be given up to 4 days postexposure as postexposure prophylaxis with significant reduction in mortality.

Treatment

The treatment for smallpox is primarily supportive. Research is ongoing into antiviral therapies for smallpox but currently therapy for patients infected with smallpox remains supportive, with IV fluids, pain medications, and antibiotics as needed for secondary bacterial infections (Henderson, 1999). Cidofovir, an antiviral agent used primarily against cytomegalovirus infection, has shown some promise against Orthopoxviruses such as vaccinia and cow pox in animal studies (De Clercq, 2002). Currently it is approved in its IV form for use in the treatment of adverse effects of smallpox vaccination (CDC, 2003). Brincidofovir has fewer side effects than cidofovir and showed some promise for treatment of smallpox in limited studies. Tecovirimat is an investigational antiviral drug developed for the treatment of smallpox; however limited human data are available for this medication (CDC, 2016).

VIRAL HEMORRHAGIC FEVERS

Viral hemorrhagic fevers (VHF) are a group of febrile illnesses caused by RNA viruses from several viral families. They include the Filoviruses (Ebola and Marburg), the Arenaviruses (Lassa and New World Arenaviruses), Bunyaviruses such as Rift Valley fever, and the Flaviviruses (yellow fever, among others). These highly infectious viruses lead to a potentially lethal disease syndrome characterized by fever, malaise, vomiting, mucosal and GI bleeding, edema, and hypotension. The most notorious member of this group is Ebola, outbreaks of which have been associated with case fatality rates of up to 90%. These diseases are generally contracted via an infected animal or arthropod vector. Several fruit bat species have been shown to be natural reservoirs for certain VHF, such as Ebola and Marburg, although contact with infected animals or humans is not a prerequisite for transmission of infection (Leroy et al., 2005).

In 2002, the Working Group on Civilian Biodefense published an analysis of the potential of VHF for use as a bioterrorist weapon (Borio et al., 2002). They emphasize the great infectivity, ease of transmission, risk to public health, and high mortality associated with these infectious agents as reasons for their biological weapon potential. Early studies using nonhuman primates clearly proved that aerosol transmission of VHF is a known mechanism for infectivity (Johnson, Jaax, White, & Jahrling, 1995). A recent review of the potential for VHF agents to be used as weapons of bioterrorism concluded that although advanced laboratory systems and highly trained personnel would be needed to generate and safeguard a weaponized VHF agent, the deployment of such a weapon in the hands of terrorists is certainly within the realm of possibility (Cenciarelli et al., 2015). Even a "low-tech" use of human carriers of Ebola virus disease (EVD) or Marburg virus disease as a means to intentionally disperse the virus among at-risk populations has been a subject of discussion (See Figure 30.8).

Epidemiology

Cases of VHF in the United States are extremely rare and usually are found in patients who recently have visited endemic areas or among those with potential occupational exposure to HF viruses. A 1989 outbreak of an Ebola subtype in Reston, Virginia, popularized

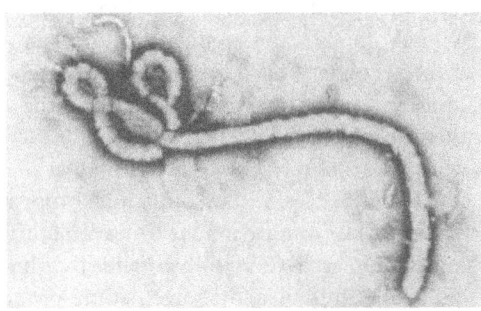

FIGURE 30.8 Transmission electron micrograph of Ebola virus.

Source: CDC/C. Goldsmith.

by Richard Preston in his 1994 novel, *The Hot Zone*, was noted to be lethal to nonhuman primates but caused only subclinical infection in humans (Preston, 1994). Sporadic outbreaks of Ebola and Marburg virus have been reported, mainly in central Africa. The largest Ebola outbreak to date occurred in West Africa from 2014 to 2016. This outbreak occurred primarily in Guinea, Sierra Leone, and Liberia, with more than 28,000 cases and more than 11,000 deaths. As a result of this outbreak, several sporadic cases of imported EVD also occurred in industrialized nations, including the United States, the United Kingdom, Spain, and Italy. During the recent West Africa Ebola outbreak, two imported cases were reported in the United States, including one death, and two locally acquired cases in healthcare workers (Chevalier et al., 2014). In late 2012, a Marburg virus outbreak in Uganda resulted in 26 confirmed and probable cases of Marburg virus infection, including 15 deaths (58%; Knust et al., 2015).

Lassa virus, an Arenavirus still very common in western Africa, is responsible for 100,000 to 300,000 cases of Lassa fever per year. Lassa fever has been reported in the United States in travelers from West Africa and was most recently reported in the United States in 2010 (Amorosa et al., 2010). The natural reservoir for Lassa virus is the *Mastomys* rodent. The South American Arenaviruses (e.g., Machupo, Sabia, Junin) are also spread by rodent contact, typically among farm workers. Rift Valley fever, caused by a Bunyavirus, is transmitted by the bite of an infected mosquito and is responsible for intermittent outbreaks in Africa. Also transmitted by infected mosquitoes, yellow fever continues to be a serious problem in tropical areas of South America and Africa, where vaccination is not widespread. 2013 WHO estimates suggest 84,000 to 170,000 cases per year occur in Africa (WHO Yellow Fever Fact Sheet). As of early 2017, an ongoing yellow fever outbreak in Brazil has led to more than 230 cases and 80 deaths (Paules and Fauci, 2017). Like yellow fever, Omsk HF and Kyasanur Forest disease are also caused by Flavivirus-carrying arthropods. In the case of these two diseases, transmission occurs via tick bite (Borio et al., 2002).

Classification and Etiology

The VHF agents are divided into four major viral families: Filovirus, Arenavirus, Bunyavirus, and Flavivirus. Table 30.2 categorizes these RNA viruses by viral family, disease, natural distribution, vector, and incubation period.

Aerosol transmission of certain VHF viruses has been theorized and has been seen in animal experiments. Case fatality rates for VHF infections vary widely, ranging from less than 1% for Omsk HF to up to 90% for Zaire ebolavirus (Borio et al., 2002). The case fatality rate for the 2014 to 2016 West Africa Ebola outbreak was approximately 40% (WHO, 2016).

Pathogenesis

The primary defect in patients with VHF is that of increased vascular permeability. HF viruses have an affinity for the vascular system, leading to mucous membrane hemorrhage with accompanying hypotension and shock. All of the viruses can also lead to thrombocytopenia and depletion of clotting factors, via either hepatic dysfunction or DIC. During extreme viremia, activation of multiple cytokines leads to increased vascular permeability,

TABLE 30.2 Viral Hemorrhagic Fevers

Virus Family	Disease (Virus)	Natural Distribution	Usual Source of Human Infection	Incubation (Days)
Filoviridae filovirus	Marburg and Ebola	Africa	Fruit bat	2–21
Arenaviridae arenavirus	Lassa fever	Africa	Rodent	5–16
	Argentine HF (Junin)	South America	Rodent	7–14
	Bolivian HF (Machupo)	South America	Rodent	9–15
	Brazilian HF (Sabia)	South America	Rodent	7–14
	Venezuelan HF (Guanarito)	South America	Rodent	7–14
Bunyaviridae Phlebovirus	Rift Valley fever	Africa	Mosquito	2–5
Flaviviridae Flavivirus	Yellow fever	Tropical Africa, South America	Mosquito	3–6
	Omsk hemorrhagic fever	Central Asia	Tick	2–9
	Kyasanur Forest disease	India	Tick	2–9

HF, hemorrhagic fever.

shock, and fatal circulatory collapse. On autopsy, frank necrosis of visceral organs (e.g., liver, spleen, and kidneys) has been seen in association with Ebola virus infection (CDC, 1995).

Clinical Manifestations and Diagnosis

The incubation period for HF viruses ranges from 2 to 21 days and initial symptoms may be variable, depending on the specific agent. These generally nonspecific early symptoms may include high fever, headache, myalgias, arthralgias, fatigue, flushing, and abdominal pain. Patients with Ebola infection often demonstrate a petechial rash by day 5 (Peters & LeDuc, 1999). Jaundice is common in patients with yellow fever and Rift Valley fever. Later symptoms include hematemesis, hematuria, bloody diarrhea, and generalized mucous membrane hemorrhage. The presence of altered mental status and cardiovascular collapse are preterminal events.

The differential diagnosis includes a number of viral and bacterial diseases, including influenza, meningococcemia, Rocky Mountain spotted fever, malaria, and others, as well as noninfectious causes such as idiopathic and thrombotic thrombocytopenic purpuras, hemolytic uremic syndrome, and DIC.

Clinical diagnosis is typically based on a history of travel to an endemic area, close contact with an infected person, or inadvertent contact with a VHF virus in a laboratory setting combined with clinical findings. In the event of a bioterrorist attack, geographical or temporal clusters of patients with similar clinical presentations are highly suggestive.

Laboratory verification is essential but potentially extremely hazardous. In 1994, a Yale virologist working with Sabia, a Brazilian HF virus, accidentally contracted the disease, and fortunately survived (Ryder & Gandsman, 1995). Clinical microbiology laboratories and public health laboratories are generally not equipped to diagnose or handle VHF specimens. Few laboratories in the United States have this capability, the most prominent of which are located at CDC, NIH, and the U.S. Army Medical Research Institute of Infectious Diseases (USAMRIID, 2001). Following the recent West Africa Ebola outbreak, there has been extensive discussion of laboratory safety measures designed to minimize risk for laboratory personnel charged with handling specimens from patients with suspected VHF, specifically Ebola (Iwen, 2015).

Methods of VHF laboratory diagnosis include ELISA, PCR, antibody assays, and viral isolation (see Figure 30.9).

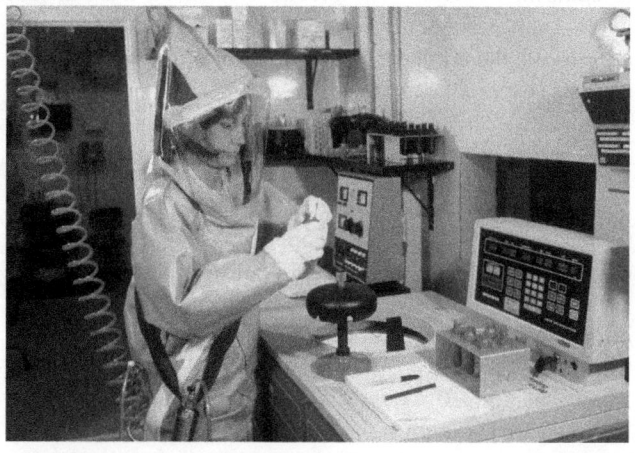

FIGURE 30.9 A CDC scientist wearing a protective suit with helmet and face mask is protected from agents as she conducts studies in the CDC BSL-4 laboratory.

BSL, biosafety level.

Source: CDC/Jim Gathany.

Biosafety Issues, Protection, and Isolation

BSL-4 precautions are necessary when handling specimens from patients suspected of VHF infection. Every effort should be made to ensure that specimens from these patients are secured and properly sealed for transportation to laboratories with the capability for VHF diagnosis. Following the recent West Africa Ebola outbreak, the CDC released specific management recommendations for patients suspected of having VHF infection, including the following:

- Place patients in a single patient room containing a private bathroom.
- Avoid entry of nonessential staff and visitors. Facilities should maintain a log of all people entering the patient's room.
- All staff entering the room should wear the following PPE:
  - Impermeable garment
  - Respiratory protection (N95 mask with single-use surgical hood or single-use full face shield OR powered air-purifying respirator [PAPR] with full face shield or hood)
  - Single-use examination gloves with extended cuffs
  - Single-use boot covers
  - Single-use apron (if patients have vomiting or diarrhea)
- A trained observer should read aloud to the healthcare worker each step in the procedure checklist and visually confirm and document that the step has been performed correctly.
- A separate area should be designated for donning and doffing of PPE. Ensure that space and layout allow for clear separation between clean and contaminated areas.

Note: These infection control recommendations were developed for use with patients with suspected or confirmed EVD, but may also be used for any patient with suspected VHF infection. For more details, see the CDC (2015b) Ebola Infection Control recommendations at cdc.gov/ebola.

Public Health Implications

Like the other diseases discussed previously, any suspected or confirmed case of VHF infection represents a significant public health emergency. Immediate notification of local and state health departments as well as of CDC is mandatory for patients suspected of VHF infection.

Vaccination and Postexposure Prophylaxis

Several experimental therapeutics and vaccines are in development for the treatment of EVD. ZMapp, a biopharmaceutical agent comprising three monoclonal antibodies against Ebola virus surface glycoproteins, was developed in a joint Canadian–U.S. effort in 2014 and has shown efficacy in nonhuman primate trials (Qiu et al., 2014). Although it was used experimentally in seven patients in 2014 (two of whom died), the utility of ZMapp in these patients was unclear. A multicenter randomized study of ZMapp versus standard therapy did not show clear efficacy, although there was a trend suggesting benefit in patients who received ZMapp (PREVAIL II Writing Group, 2016).

No approved vaccine exists for any of the VHF infections other than yellow fever. Development of a Lassa virus vaccine is continuing at the CDC. Yellow fever vaccine is readily available and is both safe and effective. Although there is no approved vaccine for either Ebola or Marburg virus, significant progress has been made in developing effective experimental Ebola vaccines using multiple viral vector strategies, including vesicular-stomatitis virus (VSV-EBOV) and chimpanzee adenovirus (cAd3-EBO-Z). Recent human trials in Africa and Europe have yielded safe, immunogenic vaccines against both Ebola and Marburg, based on postvaccine testing of antibody and T-cell response of trial participants (Agnandji et al., 2016; Kibuuka et al., 2015).

Ribavirin, a nucleoside analog, is recommended for postexposure prophylaxis for Lassa and possibly for other Arenaviruses, but only if signs of infection are present. Ribavirin has no efficacy against filovirus or Flavivirus infection (Borio et al., 2002).

Treatment

No Food and Drug Administration–approved antiviral therapy or vaccine is available for Ebola or Marburg virus infection. Supportive therapy should be the primary focus for clinicians treating patients with suspected or confirmed filovirus infection, including treatment for hypovolemia, electrolyte, metabolic and hematologic abnormalities, shock, multiple organ failure, and DIC. Large volumes of IV fluids have been used in resuscitation of patients with EVD evacuated from West Africa. Broad-spectrum antimicrobials have also been used in patients with evidence of septic shock (Mehta, Lyon, & Varkey, 2015). Care should be taken to avoid intramuscular injections and the use of aspirin or other nonsteroidal antiinflammatory drugs and anticoagulants.

For patients with Lassa and some other Arenavirus infections, mortality benefits have been obtained through the use of IV ribavirin, particularly when administered early in the patients' clinical course.

Studies evaluating the use of convalescent plasma, that is, plasma from previously infected, recovering VHF patients, following the recent West Africa Ebola outbreak have not shown a benefit (van Griensven et al., 2016).

SUMMARY

Clearly, the CDC Category A biological agents of concern—anthrax, botulism, plague, tularemia, smallpox, and VHF—represent grave public health risks, particularly if deployed as a biological weapon. This chapter provides the healthcare professional with a historical and epidemiologic background as well as a standardized, effective evaluation, and management approach for highly pathogenic viral and bacterial diseases. Key elements of the patient's history and physical, including a history of travel and animal or arthropod exposure, are essential to making the diagnosis. The principles of infection control that begin with universal precautions have been expanded upon in this chapter to enable the effective management of patients infected with even the most deadly infectious agents. Further research into the diagnosis and therapy of these agents is ongoing, and advances in this area will continue to provide safer and more effective management strategies for patients with these potentially lethal infections.

STUDY QUESTIONS

1. First-line therapy for Lassa fever infection includes which of the following?
   a. Gamma globulin
   b. Ribavirin
   c. Third-generation cephalosporins
   d. Plasmapheresis
   e. Convalescent serum

2. Which of the following Category A agents requires BSL-4 laboratory facilities?
   a. Smallpox and plague
   b. Anthrax and tularemia
   c. VHF and smallpox
   d. Botulism and plague
   e. Smallpox and anthrax

3. Which of the following is the most likely natural reservoir for Ebola virus?
   a. Small rodent
   b. Mosquito
   c. Green monkey
   d. Tick
   e. Fruit bat

4. Which of the following Category A diseases does not require contact isolation?
   a. Ebola
   b. Plague
   c. Anthrax
   d. Smallpox
   e. Tularemia

5. Which of the following Category A diseases is still endemic in the southwestern United States?
   a. Lassa fever
   b. Plague
   c. Anthrax
   d. Smallpox
   e. Tularemia

6. Which Category A agent classically causes a hemorrhagic mediastinitis, with rapid progression to respiratory failure?
   a. Botulinum toxin
   b. Plague
   c. Anthrax
   d. Smallpox
   e. Tularemia

REFERENCES

Abramova, F. A., Grinberg, L. M., Yampolskaya, O. V., & Walker, D. H. (1993). Pathology of inhalational anthrax in 42 cases from the Sverdlovsk outbreak of 1979. *Proceedings of the National Academy of Sciences of the United States of America, 90*, 2291–2294. doi:10.1073/pnas.90.6.2291

Agnandji, S. T., Huttner, A., Zinser, M. E., Njuguna, P., Dahlke, C., Fernandes, J. F., ... Siegrist, C.-A. (2016). Phase 1 trials of rVSV Ebola vaccine in Africa and Europe. *The New England Journal of Medicine, 374*(17), 1647–1660. doi:10.1056/NEJMoa1502924

Aldhous, P. (1990). Biological warfare: Gruinard Island handed back. *Nature, 344*, 801. doi:10.1038/344801b0

Alibek, K. (1999). *Biohazard* (pp. 29–38). New York, NY: Random House.

Amorosa, V., MacNeil, A., McConnell, R., Patel, A., Dillon, K. E., Hamilton, K., ... Nichol, S. T. (2010). Imported Lassa fever, Pennsylvania, USA, 2010. *Emerging Infectious Diseases, 16*(10), 1598–1600. doi:10.3201/eid1610.100774

Arnon, S. S., Schechter, R., Inglesby, T. V., Henderson, D. A., Bartlett, J. G., Ascher, M. S., ... Tonat, K.; Working Group on Civilian Biodefense. (2001). Botulinum toxin as a biological weapon: Medical and public health management. *Journal of the American Medical Association, 285*, 1059–1070. doi:10.1001/jama.285.8.1059

Bell, D. M., Kozarsky, P. E., & Stephens, D. S. (2002). Clinical issues in the prophylaxis, diagnosis, and treatment of anthrax. *Emerging Infectious Diseases, 8*, 222–225. doi:10.3201/eid0802.010521

Borio, L., Inglesby, T., Peters, C. J., Schmaljohn, A. L., Hughes, J. M., Jahrling, P. B., ... Tonat, K.; Working Group on Civilian Biodefense. (2002). Hemorrhagic fever viruses as biological weapons: Medical and public health management. *Journal of the American Medical Association, 287*, 2391–2405. doi:10.1001/jama.287.18.2391

Bower, W. A., Hendricks, K., Pillai, S., Guarnizo, J., & Meaney-Delman, D.; Centers for Disease Control and Prevention. (2015). Clinical framework and medical countermeasure use during an anthrax mass-casualty incident, 2015. *MMWR Morbidity and Mortality Weekly Report, 64*(4), 1–22. doi:10.15585/mmwr.rr6404a1

Breman, J. G., & Arita, I. (1980). The confirmation and maintenance of smallpox eradication. *New England Journal of Medicine, 303*, 1263–1273. doi:10.1056/NEJM198011273032204

Broad, W. J. (2002, July 7). U.S. to vaccinate 500,000 workers against smallpox. *The New York Times*, p. A1.

Casey, C. G., Iskander, J. K., Roper, M. H., Mast, E. E., Wen, X. J., Torok, T. J., ... Mootrey, G. (2005). Adverse events associated with smallpox vaccination in the United States, January–October 2003. *Journal of the American Medical Association, 294*(21), 2734–2743. doi:10.1001/jama.294.21.2734

Cenciarelli, O., Gabbarini, V., Pietropaoli, S., Malizia, A., Tamburrini, A., Ludovici, G. M., ... Gaudio, P. (2015). Viral bioterrorism: Learning the lesson of Ebola virus in West Africa 2013–2015. *Virus Research, 210*, 318–326. doi:10.1016/j.virusres.2015.09.002

Centers for Disease Control and Prevention. (1995). Update: Management of patients with suspected viral hemorrhagic fever—United States. *Morbidity and Mortality Weekly Report, 44*, 475–479.

Centers for Disease Control and Prevention. (1998). *Botulism in the United States, 1899–1996: Handbook for epidemiologists, clinicians, and laboratory workers*. Atlanta, GA: Author.

Centers for Disease Control and Prevention. (2001a). Additional options for preventive treatment for persons exposed to inhalational anthrax. *Morbidity and Mortality Weekly Report, 50*, 1142–1151.

Centers for Disease Control and Prevention. (2001b). Recognition of illness associated with the intentional release of a biologic agent. *Morbidity and Mortality Weekly Report, 50*, 893–897. Retrieved from https://www.cdc.gov/mmwr/preview/mmwrhtml/mm5041a2.htm

Centers for Disease Control and Prevention. (2002a). Summary of notifiable diseases—United States 2000. *Morbidity and Mortality Weekly Report, 49*, 1–102. Retrieved from https://www.cdc.gov/mmwr/preview/mmwrhtml/mm4953a1.htm

Centers for Disease Control and Prevention. (2002b). Update: Cutaneous anthrax in a laboratory worker—Texas, 2002. *Morbidity and Mortality Weekly Report, 51*, 482. Retrieved from https://www.cdc.gov/mmwr/preview/mmwrhtml/mm5122a4.htm

Centers for Disease Control and Prevention. (2003). Update: Cardiac related events during the civilian smallpox vaccination program—United States, 2003. *MMWR Morbidity and Mortality Weekly Report, 52*, 492–496. Retrieved from https://www.cdc.gov/Mmwr/preview/mmwrhtml/mm5221a2.htm

Centers for Disease Control and Prevention. (2006). Inhalation anthrax associated with dried animal hides—Pennsylvania and New York City, 2006. *MMWR Morbidity and Mortality Weekly Report, 55*(10), 280–282. Retrieved from https://www.cdc.gov/mmwr/preview/mmwrhtml/mm5510a4.htm

Centers for Disease Control and Prevention. (2009). *Biosafety in microbiological and biological laboratories* (5th ed.). Atlanta, GA: Author

Centers for Disease Control and Prevention. (2015a). Botulism annual summary, 2015. Retrieved from https://www.cdc.gov/nationalsurveillance/pdfs/botulism_cste_2015.pdf

Centers for Disease Control and Prevention. (2015b). Infection prevention and control recommendations for hospitalized patients under investigation (PUIs) for Ebola virus disease (EVD) in U.S. hospitals. Retrieved from https://www.cdc.gov/vhf/ebola/healthcare-us/hospitals/infection-control.html

Centers for Disease Control and Prevention. (2016). Medical management of adverse reactions. Retrieved from https://www.cdc.gov/smallpox/clinicians/vaccine-medical-management6.html

Centers for Disease Control and Prevention. (2017). Recommended specimens for microbiology and pathology for diagnosis of anthrax. Retrieved from https://www.cdc.gov/anthrax/specificgroups/lab-professionals/recommended-specimen.html

Chevalier, M. S., Chung, W., Smith, J., Weil, L. M., Hughes, S. M., Joyner, S. N., ... Lakey, D. L. (2014). Ebola virus disease cluster in the United States—Dallas County, Texas, 2014. *MMWR Morbidity Mortality Weekly Report, 21*;63(46), 1087–1088. Retrieved from https://www.cdc.gov/mmwr/preview/mmwrhtml/mm63e1114a5.htm

Cieslak, T. J., & Eitzen, E. M., Jr. (1999). Clinical and epidemiologic principles of anthrax. *Emerging Infectious Diseases, 5*, 552–555. doi:10.3201/eid0504.990418

De Clercq, E. (2002). Cidofovir in the treatment of poxvirus infections. *Antiviral Research, 55*, 1–13. doi:10.1016/S0166-3542(02)00008-6

Dennis, D. T., Inglesby, T. V., Henderson, D. A., Bartlett, J. G., Ascher, M. S., Eitzen, E., ... Tonat, K.; Working Group on Civilian Biodefense. (2001). Tularemia as a biological weapon: Medical and public health management. *Journal of the American Medical Association, 285*, 2763–2773. doi:10.1001/jama.285.21.2763

Department of Health and Human Services, Public Health Service, Centers for Disease Control and Prevention, National Institutes of Health. (1999). Laboratory biosafety level criteria. In L. Casey Chosewood & D. E. Wilson (Eds.), *Biosafety in microbiological and biomedical laboratories* (4th ed., pp. 30–59). Washington, DC: U.S. Government Printing Office.

Edlow, J. A. (2001). Tick-borne diseases, tularemia. *eMedicine Journal, 2*. Retrieved from http://www.emedicine.com/emerg/topic591.htm

Elvin, S. J., Eyles, J. E., Howard, K. A., Ravichandran, E., Somavarappu, S., Alpar, H. O., & Williamson, E. D. (2005). Protection against bubonic and pneumonic plague with a single dose microencapsulated sub-unit vaccine. *Vaccine, 24*(20), 4433–4439. doi:10.1016/j.vaccine.2005.12.016

Fifty-fifth World Health Assembly. (2002). *Smallpox eradication: Destruction of Variola virus stocks. Resolution WHA55.15*. Geneva, Switzerland: World Health Organization.

Francis, E. (1925). Tularemia. *Journal of the American Medical Association, 84*, 1243–1250. doi:10.1001/jama.1925.02660430001001

Henderson, D. A. (1980). *A victory for all mankind*. Geneva, Switzerland: World Health Organization.

Henderson, D. A. (1999). Smallpox: Clinical and epidemiologic features. *Emerging Infectious Diseases, 5*, 537–539. doi:10.3201/eid0504.990415

Henderson, D. A., Inglesby, T. V., Bartlett, J. G., Ascher, M. S., Eitzen, E., Jahrling, P. B., ... Tonat, K.; Working Group on Civilian Biodefense. (1999). Smallpox as a biological weapon: Medical and public health

management. *Journal of the American Medical Association, 281*, 2127–2137. doi:10.1001/jama.281.22.2127

Hendricks, K. A., Wright, M. E., Shadomy, S. V., Bradley, J. S., Morrow, M. G., Rubinstein, E., Bower, W. A.; Workgroup on Anthrax Clinical Guidelines. (2014). Centers for Disease Control and Prevention expert panel meetings on prevention and treatment of anthrax in adults. *Emerging Infectious Disease, 20*(2), e130687. doi:10.3201/eid2002.130687

Holty, J. E., Bravata, D. M., Liu, H., Olshen, R. A., McDonald, K. M., & Owens, D. K. (2006). Systematic review: A century of inhalational anthrax cases from 1900 to 2005. *Annals of Internal Medicine, 144*(4), 270–280. doi:10.7326/0003-4819-144-4-200602210-00009

Inglesby, T. V., Dennis, D. T., Henderson, D. A., Bartlett, J. G., Ascher, M. S., Eitzen, E., ... Tonat, K. (2000). Plague as a biological weapon: Medical and public health management. *Journal of the American Medical Association, 283*, 2281–2290. doi:10.1001/jama.283.17.2281

Inglesby, T. V., Henderson, D. A., Bartlett, J. G., Ascher, M. S., Eitzen, E., Friedlander, A. M., ... Tonat, K. (1999). Anthrax as a biological weapon: Medical and public health management. *Journal of the American Medical Association, 281*, 1735–1745. doi:10.1001/jama.281.18.1735

Inglesby, T. V., O'Toole, T., Henderson, D. A., Bartlett, J. G., Ascher, M. S., Eitzen, E., ... Tonat, K. (2002). Anthrax as a biological weapon, 2002: Updated recommendations for management. *Journal of the American Medical Association, 287*, 2236–2252. doi:10.1001/jama.287.17.2236

Iwen, P. C., Smith, P. W., Hewlett, A. L., Kratochvil, C. J., Lisco, S. J., Sullivan, J. N., ... Hinrichs, S. H. (2015). Safety considerations in the laboratory testing of specimens suspected or known to contain Ebola virus. *American Journal of Clinical Pathology, 143*(1), 4–5. doi:10.1309/AJCP26MIFUIETBPL

Jernigan, J. A., Stephens, D. S., Ashford, D. A., Omenaca, C., Topiel, M. S., Galbraith, M., ... Perkins, B. A.; Anthrax Bioterrorism Investigation Team. (2001). Bioterrorism-related inhalational anthrax: The first 10 cases reported in the United States. *Emerging Infectious Diseases, 7*, 933–944. doi:10.3201/eid0706.010604

Johnson, E., Jaax, N., White, J., Jahrling, P. (1995). Lethal experimental infections of rhesus monkeys by aerosolized Ebola virus. *International Journal of Experimental Pathology, 76*(4), 227–236.

Khan, A. S., & Sage, M. J. (2000). Biological and chemical terrorism: Strategic plan for preparedness and response. Recommendations of the CDC Strategic Planning Workgroup. *Morbidity and Mortality Weekly Report, 49*(RR-4), 1–14. Retrieved from https://www.cdc.gov/mmwr/preview/mmwrhtml/rr4904a1.htm#top

Kibuuka, H., Berkowitz, N. M., Millard, M., Enama, M. E., Tindikahwa, A., Sekiziyivu, A. B. ... Ledgerwood, J. E.; RV 247 Study Team. (2015). Safety and immunogenicity of Ebola virus and Marburg virus glycoprotein DNA vaccines assessed separately and concomitantly in healthy Ugandan adults: A phase 1b, randomised, double-blind, placebo-controlled clinical trial. *The Lancet, 385*(9977), 1545–1554. doi:10.1016/S0140-6736(14)62385-0

Knust, B., Schafer, I. J., Wamala, J., Nyakarahuka, L., Okot, C., Shoemaker, T., & Rollin, P. E. (2015). Multidistrict outbreak of Marburg virus disease—Uganda, 2012. *The Journal of Infectious Disease, 212*(Suppl 2), S119–S128. doi:10.1093/infdis/jiv351

Lemonick, M. D. (2002, April 29). The pros and cons of Botox. *Time, 159*, 77. Retrieved from http://content.time.com/time/magazine/article/0,9171,232593,00.html

Leroy, E. M., Kumulungui, B., Pourrut, X., Rouquet, P., Hassanin, A., Yaba P., ... Swanepoel, R. (2005). Fruit bats as reservoirs of Ebola virus. *Nature, 438*(7068), 575–576. doi:10.1038/438575a

Mayer, T. A., Bersoff-Matcha, S., Murphy, C., Earls, J., Harper, S., Pauze, D., ... Berman, E. L. (2001). Clinical presentation of inhalational anthrax following bioterrorism exposure: Report of 2 surviving patients. *Journal of the American Medical Association, 286*, 2549–2553. doi:10.1001/jama.286.20.2549

McGovern, T. W., & Friedlander, A. M. (1997). Plague. In R. Zajtchuk (Ed.), *Textbook of military medicine: Medical aspects of chemical and biological warfare* (pp. 479–502). Washington, DC: Office of the Surgeon General, Department of the Army.

Mehta, A. K., Lyon, G. M., Varkey, J. B. (2015). Treatment of Ebola. *The New England Journal of Medicine, 372*(17), 1674. doi:10.1056/NEJMc1500452#SA1

Meselson, M., Guillemin, J., Hugh-Jones, M., Langmuir, A., Popova, I., Shelokov, A., & Yampolskaya, O. (1994). The Sverdlovsk anthrax outbreak of 1979. *Science, 266,* 1202–1208. doi:10.1126/science.7973702

Moore, Z. S., Seward, J. F., & Lane, J. M. (2006). Smallpox. *Lancet, 367*(9508), 425–435. doi:10.1016/S0140-6736(06)68143-9

Nass, M. (2002). The anthrax vaccine program: An analysis of the CDC's recommendations for vaccine use. *American Journal of Public Health, 92,* 715–721. doi:10.2105/AJPH.92.5.715

National Health Service, National Services Scotland, Health Protection Scotland. (2011). An outbreak of anthrax among drug users in Scotland, December 2009 to December 2010: A report on behalf of the National Anthrax Outbreak Control Team. Glasgow, Scotland, UK: National Services Scotland. Retrieved from http://www.hps.scot.nhs.uk/resourcedocument.aspx?id=26

Paules, C. I., Fauci, A. S. (2017). Yellow fever—Once again on the radar screen in the Americas. *The New England Journal of Medicine, 376*(15), 1397–1399.

Peters, C. J., & LeDuc, J. W. (1999). Ebola: The virus and the disease. *Journal of Infectious Diseases, 179*(Suppl. 1), ix–xvi. doi:10.1086/514322

Petersen, B. W., Harms, T. J., Reynolds, M. G., Harrison, L. H. (2016). Use of Vaccinia virus smallpox vaccine in laboratory and health care personnel at risk for occupational exposure to Orthopoxviruses—Recommendations of the Advisory Committee on Immunization Practices (ACIP), 2015. *MMWR Morbidity Mortality Weekly Report, 65,* 257–262. doi:10.15585/mmwr.mm6510a2

Preston, R. (1994). *The hot zone.* New York: Random House.

PREVAIL II Writing Group; Multi-National PREVAIL II Study Team; Davey, R. T. Jr, Dodd, L., Proschan, M. A., Neaton, J., Neuhaus Nordwall, J., Koopmeiners, J. S., … Malvy, D. (2016). A randomized, controlled trial of ZMapp for Ebola virus infection. *New England Journal of Medicine, 375*(15), 1448–1456. doi:10.1056/NEJMoa1604330

Qiu, X., Wong, G., Audet, J., Bello, A., Fernando, L., Alimonti, J. B., & Kobinger, G. P. (2014). Reversion of advanced Ebola virus disease in nonhuman primates with ZMapp. *Nature, 514*(7520), 47–53. doi:10.1038/nature13777

Rotz, L. D., Khan, A. S., Lillibridge, S. R., Ostroff, S. M., & Hughes, J. M. (2002). Public health assessment of potential biological terrorism agents. *Emerging Infectious Diseases, 8,* 225–230. doi:10.3201/eid0802.010164

Ryder, R. W., & Gandsman, E. J. (1995). Laboratory-acquired Sabia virus infection. *The New England Journal of Medicine, 333,* 1716. doi:10.1056/NEJM199512213332516

Sejvar, J. J., Tenover, F. C., & Stephens, D. S. (2005). Management of anthrax meningitis. *The Lancet Infectious Diseases, 5,* 287–295. doi:10.1016/S1473-3099(05)70113-4

Sepkowitz, K. A. (2001). Anthrax and anthrax anxiety: Sverdlovsk revisited. *International Journal of Infectious Diseases, 5,* 178–179. doi:10.1016/S1201-9712(01)90066-9

Titball, R. W., & Williamson, E. D. (2001). Vaccination against bubonic and pneumonic plague. *Vaccine, 19,* 4175–4184. doi:10.1016/S0264-410X(01)00163-3

Torok, T. J., Tauxe, R. V., Wise, R. P., Livengood, J. R., Sokolow, R., Mauvais, S., … Foster, L. R. (1997). A large community outbreak of salmonellosis caused by intentional contamination of restaurant salad bars. *Journal of the American Medical Association, 278,* 389–395. doi:10.1001/jama.1997.03550050051033

Tugnoli, V., Eleopra, R., Quatrale, R., Capone, J. G., Sensi, M., & Gastaldo, E. (2002). Botulism-like syndrome after botulinum toxin type A injections for focal hyperhidrosis. *British Journal of Dermatology, 147*(4), 808–809. doi:10.1046/j.1365-2133.2002.49101.x

U.S. Army Medical Research Institute of Infectious Diseases. (2001). *USAMRIID's Medical management of biological casualties handbook* (4th ed.). Frederick, MD: Author.

van Griensven, J., Edwards, T., de Lamballerie, X., Semple, M. G., Gallian, P., Baize, S., et al.; Ebola-Tx Consortium. (2016, Jan 7). Evaluation of convalescent plasma for ebola virus disease in Guinea. *The New England Journal of Medicine, 374*(1), 33–42. doi:10.1056/NEJMoa1511812

World Health Assembly. (2002, May). Smallpox: Destruction of variola virus stocks. Resolution of the Fifty-Fifth World Health Assembly, Geneva. Geneva, Switzerland: Author

World Health Organization. (1970). *Health aspects of chemical and biological weapons* (pp. 98–109). Geneva, Switzerland: Author.

World Health Organization. (1980). *Resolution WHA 33.3.* Geneva, Switzerland: Author.

World Health Organization. (2016, May 11). *Ebola data and statistics.* Geneva, Switzerland: Author. Retrieved from http://apps.who.int/gho/data/view.ebola-sitrep.ebola-summary-20160511?lang=en

Wright, J. G., Quinn, C. P., Shadomy, S., & Messonnier, N. (2010). Use of anthrax vaccine in the United States: Recommendations of the Advisory Committee on Immunization Practices (ACIP), 2009. *MMWR Morbidity and Mortality Weekly Report, 59*(RR-6), 1–30. Retrieved from https://www.cdc.gov/mmwr/preview/mmwrhtml/rr5906a1.htm

Zilinskas, R. A. (1997). Iraq's biological weapons: The past as future? *Journal of the American Medical Association, 278,* 418–424. doi:10.1001/jama.1997.03550050080037

31

SURVEILLANCE SYSTEMS FOR DETECTION OF BIOLOGICAL EVENTS

Erica Rihl Pryor

LEARNING OBJECTIVES

When this chapter is completed, readers will be able to:

1. Describe the key activities of traditional public health surveillance.
2. Describe examples of current international and national infectious disease surveillance systems.
3. Discuss the use of Internet-based surveillance systems in detection of potential biological events.
4. Give examples of unusual patterns of disease occurrence that might indicate a deliberate release of a biological agent.
5. Describe mechanisms for early recognition by clinicians of infectious disease outbreaks.
6. Discuss key components of an integrated biosurveillance system for detection of biological events.

KEY MESSAGES

Current public health surveillance systems provide data for identifying patterns of disease occurrence associated with a biological event.

An effective public health response to a biological event requires early detection and recognition.

Early recognition and detection of biological events is crucial to maximize the opportunity for early initiation of effective treatment of exposed persons, and to minimize the opportunity for transmission of the agent.

Internet-based surveillance systems may enhance the timeliness of event detection.

Focusing on unusual patterns or clusters of illnesses can provide epidemiological clues to clinicians for the occurrence of a biological event.

Concepts related to early recognition and detection of Centers for Disease Control and Prevention (CDC) Category A agents can be applied to scenarios with other emerging or reemerging infectious disease threats.

The clinical laboratory is an important component of biosurveillance.

An emergency information system that facilitates rapid and timely exchange of data in a suspected outbreak is an essential component of a comprehensive biosurveillance system for biological events.

CHAPTER OVERVIEW

The focus of this chapter is on the systems of surveillance that will assist with recognition and detection of biological events, either naturally occurring disease outbreaks or deliberate bio-terror events. Key concepts related to traditional public health surveillance are presented. Several national and international surveillance systems are described in detail, along with the roles of state and local health departments in infectious disease surveillance. Real-time or near-real-time surveillance systems based on syndromic surveillance and Internet-based surveillance for event recognition are examined. Also highlighted is the need for emergency information systems that can facilitate rapid data collection and dissemination, and foster communication of key information among federal, state, and local response planners. The biological agents designated as Category A agents by the CDC are considered the highest priority for response planning because they pose the greatest potential threats if used in biological attacks. Attention is focused on the role nurses can play in recognizing and detecting potential biological events in their practice settings. Both epidemiological and clinical approaches to recognition are described. For clinical recognition, emphasis is placed on using a syndrome-based approach. Laboratory methods for detection also are discussed briefly. The final section of the chapter focuses on lessons learned from the 2014–2015 Ebola outbreak and future directions for development of global biosurveillance systems.

It is imperative that nurses understand the systems in place to assist in the detection and recognition of biological events, whether such events are naturally occurring outbreaks or a deliberate bioterror incident. How do health officials determine that a biological event is taking place? After determining that an outbreak is occurring, how do health officials monitor the event to determine the effectiveness of their response measures? An understanding of current national and international systems of infectious disease surveillance provides initial answers to these questions.

BACKGROUND

The need to improve surveillance infrastructure in the United States to address emerging and reemerging infectious disease threats, including the possibility of bioterrorist attacks, was

recognized more than 20 years ago (U.S. Department of Health and Human Services [HHS], 1998). In the ensuing decades, there has been a sustained effort by the CDC and other federal agencies to enhance the nation's surveillance infrastructure for detection of biological events by increasing surveillance personnel and laboratory-based surveillance capabilities at state and local health departments and by developing integrated health information networks (HHS; National Center for Emerging and Zoonotic Infectious Diseases [NCEZID], 2016). One ongoing program is the Emerging Infections Program (EIP), begun in 1995, which includes surveillance systems in selected states that specifically focus on emerging infections (NCEZID, 2017). Another ongoing program is the Laboratory Response Network (LRN), established in 1999 with the goal of improving public health laboratory capabilities for response to bioterror events (CDC, 2014c).

The CDC also developed a specific plan to address national preparedness and response to chemical or biological attacks (CDC, 2000). Key focal areas of that national preparedness plan were improving detection capabilities at local and state health departments through enhanced surveillance and improving response capabilities through updated communication systems. A CDC initiative in 2003 created a national-level syndromic surveillance system (BioSense) for early detection of bioterror events (Gould, Walker, & Yoon, 2017). This system evolved over the next decade into the National Syndromic Surveillance Program (NSSP; CDC, 2017j; Gould et al., 2017).

In 2007, HHS was charged in the Homeland Security Presidential Directive (HSPD) 21 to develop a broader approach to national surveillance, termed "biosurveillance" (HSPD, 2007). Biosurveillance encompasses traditional public health surveillance systems and also incorporates data from syndromic surveillance systems and unstructured data from nonpublic health sources (Sosin & Hopkins, 2010). Experiences with the 2009 pandemic of influenza A (H1N1), the 2012 emergence of Middle East respiratory syndrome (MERS) coronavirus (MERS-CoV), the 2014–2015 outbreak of Ebola virus disease in West Africa, and the emergence of Zika virus in North America all underscore the continuing need for development of surveillance systems that allow the rapid detection of novel, emerging, and reemerging pathogens.

HOW IS DISEASE OCCURRENCE MEASURED?

Epidemiologists use several terms to describe disease occurrence in a population. The level may be zero; there may be sporadic cases; or there may be a typical amount of disease present in a given area on an ongoing basis. A frequency of disease that is considered expected or baseline is referred to as the "endemic" level of a disease (Gordis, 2014). Several potential bioterror agents occur endemically in the United States, including CDC Category A agents such as tularemia and plague (Chang, Glynn, & Groseclose, 2003). When that expected level is clearly exceeded, the occurrence is considered to have reached an "epidemic" level, and public health officials may term that occurrence an epidemic or an outbreak (Gordis, 2014). An epidemic occurring on a global scale, such as the one that occurred with the novel influenza A (H1N1) strain in 2009, is termed a "pandemic." Public health surveillance data are used to determine endemic or baseline levels of disease occurrence, which allow detection of changes or unusual patterns that may indicate that an outbreak is occurring (CDC, 2004; Van Beneden & Lynfield, 2010).

WHAT IS PUBLIC HEALTH SURVEILLANCE?

In the field of public health, the term "surveillance" refers to "the ongoing, systematic collection, analysis, interpretation, and dissemination of health data" (CDC, 2001b, p. 2). The data collected and analyzed through surveillance systems provide information about patterns of disease occurrence in a population. In turn, this information forms the basis for action by public health officials in designing, implementing, and evaluating interventions to control or prevent disease (Birkhead & Maylahn, 2010).

Surveillance systems provide the structure to carry out this process. The first steps in establishing a surveillance system are to define the purpose of the system and to specify the desired objectives (CDC, 2001b; Teutsch, 2010). The purpose of a surveillance system for bioterror events would be the timely detection of such events. The objectives of the system would relate to using the data to implement an early and effective public health response to contain the impact of the attack (Sosin & Hopkins, 2010). The key activities carried out in a surveillance system are described briefly in the following sections.

Data Collection

Several types of data are routinely collected for traditional infectious disease surveillance, including morbidity, mortality, and health indicator data (Sosin & Hopkins, 2010). In the United States, each state has requirements for mandatory reporting by healthcare providers and facilities, including laboratories, of cases of notifiable infectious diseases (Birkhead & Maylahn, 2010). These notifiable disease reports are submitted to the health departments within each jurisdiction, and provide much of the available morbidity data for infectious diseases within the United States. There is a national notifiable disease list for which reporting is voluntary; these data are compiled through the National Notifiable Diseases Surveillance System (NNDSS; CDC, 2015b).

One essential component of the data collection procedure is a clear definition of what constitutes a case (CDC, 2012; Teutsch,

2010). Use of case definitions contributes to the consistency (reliability) and accuracy (validity) of data collection. For the diseases designated as notifiable in the United States, including potential bioterror agents, there are standard definitions for each of the diseases that specify the criteria for determining a confirmed case report (CDC, 2017a, 2017l). Other sources of data are often incorporated into surveillance systems (Teutsch, 2010). Examples of sources include vital records (e.g., death certificates that provide information on causes of mortality) and administrative databases (e.g., discharge diagnosis codes or billing information from healthcare organizations). All of these types of health indicator data may be useful in surveillance for biological events (Sosin & Hopkins, 2010). For example, a rise in the number of unexplained deaths or deaths due to influenza-like illness (ILI) or a sudden increase in the number of cases of a certain disease, such as botulism, could be an indicator of a naturally occurring outbreak or of a deliberate agent release (U.S. Army Medical Research Institute of Infectious Diseases [USAMRIID], 2014).

Data Analysis and Interpretation

After the raw surveillance data are compiled and organized, a first step is to perform analyses to describe the disease frequency in terms of person, place, and time (Teutsch, 2010). Current observed levels of disease occurrence are then compared with expected levels of occurrence for a given location and time to identify changes in disease patterns. Determination of whether there is an excess of cases in a given time and/ or place that is suggestive of a disease outbreak is based on these comparisons and consideration of alternate explanations for the observed data, such as a change in the case definition (CDC, 2012).

Interpretation of the analyses requires assessing the reliability and validity of the original data. Reliability has to do with the consistency of case reporting between providers, while validity depends on the completeness and accuracy of the case finding (Van Beneden & Lynfield, 2010). Clinicians can directly impact system validity based on the accuracy and completeness of their case reporting. The next question is to determine the possible explanations for the observed pattern if it is not as expected. For an apparent infectious disease outbreak, a key question is whether it is a naturally occurring increase or the result of a deliberate release of a biological agent (CDC, 2004).

Data Dissemination

The final step in the surveillance process is dissemination of information back to the original providers and to public health officials at various levels so that appropriate actions for control and prevention can be taken (Teutsch, 2010). The *Morbidity and Mortality Weekly Report* (MMWR), available online at www.cdc.gov/mmwr, is one of the principal methods used to disseminate such data in the United States at the national level. The Health Alert Network (HAN) is another system developed by the CDC to rapidly send information electronically to stakeholders (CDC, 2017f).

At the international level, official surveillance information is routinely disseminated by the World Health Organization

(WHO) through the *Weekly Epidemiological Record* (WER; WHO, 2017h). The WER is available online at www.who.int/wer/en/. The WHO also maintains the Disease Outbreak News (DON) website, with a listing of current, verified outbreaks (WHO, 2017a).

WHAT TYPES OF SYSTEMS ARE USED TO COLLECT SURVEILLANCE DATA?

The first indicator of a biological event may come from routine public health surveillance systems (Institute of Medicine [IOM] & National Research Council [NRC], 1999). Traditional public health surveillance systems are usually categorized as either "passive" or "active." The designation of passive or active refers to the role of the health department in the collection of the initial case reports (Teutsch, 2010; Van Beneden & Lynfield, 2010). With a *passive* system, case reports are initiated by healthcare providers. These reports are sent to the local health department where they are compiled and then relayed to the state and national, and sometimes international, levels. An example of a passive system is the NNDSS noted previously. Two well-recognized limitations of traditional passive systems are that reporting is often delayed and incomplete. Encouraging timely provider-based reporting is important because an outbreak may not become apparent until case reports from individual clinicians are compiled by the local health department.

With an "active" system, health department personnel initiate the search for cases through contacts with healthcare providers and facilities (Teutsch, 2010; Van Beneden & Lynfield, 2010). Active surveillance usually provides more complete case ascertainment, but due to the increased resource requirements, it is often done on a limited basis in the context of an outbreak investigation. For example, in 2017, an intense program of active surveillance, including case identification and contact tracing, resulted in the containment and resolution of an outbreak of Ebola virus disease in the Democratic Republic of the Congo (WHO, 2017b, 2017g).

Another type of surveillance system is a "sentinel" system (Birkhead & Maylahn, 2010). In contrast to a population-based system, in a *sentinel* surveillance system, data are collected from a sample of healthcare facilities or providers. An example of a sentinel system is the outpatient care provider network that supplies weekly information on influenza activity in the United States (CDC, 2016b). Another type of sentinel system involves periodic monitoring of specific animal or insect populations for evidence of certain infections. For example, currently there is sentinel surveillance of mosquitoes to track the geographical spread of Zika virus in vector species in the United States (CDC, 2017o).

A number of "special" systems have also been developed for specific types of surveillance data. For example, there are systems that use microbiologic data from laboratories to monitor trends in antimicrobial resistance for selected enteric pathogens (CDC, 2017i). Special systems may also be established for newly recognized or emerging diseases and may include a combination of several different types of surveillance systems. An example of a special system is the influenza surveillance system in the United States. The system includes passive, active, and sentinel surveillance components.

Public Health Surveillance System Example: Influenza in the United States

Influenza surveillance is of particular interest to public health officials because an increase in ILI may be an indicator of a bioterror event (USAMRIID, 2014). The surveillance system currently in place for influenza in the United States includes five main components (CDC, 2016b). One component is a laboratory-based reporting system that provides virologic surveillance on isolates submitted by public health and clinical laboratories throughout the United States. Data are provided by U.S. WHO Collaborating Laboratories and National Respiratory and Enteric Virus System (NREVSS) laboratories. A second component is the U.S. Outpatient Influenza-Like Illness Surveillance Network (ILINet), a sentinel system of over 2,900 outpatient care providers who report weekly on the percentage of clients in their practices presenting with flu-like illnesses. Another component of the system collects data on children and adults hospitalized with laboratory-confirmed influenza. A fourth component examines mortality from influenza. One source of data is through the National Center for Health Statistics (NCHS), which collects data on deaths from pneumonia and influenza. Another source of mortality data is case reporting of influenza-associated mortality in children under age 18. A final component of the influenza surveillance system are data collected from the State and Territorial Epidemiologists on the estimated level of flu activity in their given geographic area. Data from all of these surveillance components are compiled and disseminated weekly during the usual influenza season on a designated CDC website (https://www.cdc.gov/flu/weekly/; CDC, 2016b, 2017n).

Other Infectious Disease Surveillance Systems

There are many infectious disease surveillance systems currently in use, operating from the local to international levels. The discussion that follows is intended to highlight several surveillance systems and collaborative efforts that may be useful for detection of biological events.

In the United States, the CDC has the primary role in overseeing national-level surveillance and prevention/control activities related to infectious diseases (HHS, 1998). Among the most recognized national surveillance systems is the NNDSS (CDC, 2015b). The list of infectious diseases and conditions notifiable at the national level is reviewed annually by the CDC and the Council of State and Territorial Epidemiologists, and it includes most of the diseases identified as potential bioterror agents (CDC, 2015b, 2017a). State and territorial health departments provide summaries of notifiable disease cases to NNDSS, including the date, location, and basic demographic data on each case. These data were compiled and published in provisional form in the weekly MMWR until 2018, but now are posted on the NNDSS Data and Statistics webpage. Final data are published in an annual summary of notifiable diseases. The final data for 2014 were released in 2016, illustrating the time lag that can occur for finalized reporting and completion of data analysis and interpretation (CDC, 2016c). State-level NNDSS data are routinely collected and submitted to the CDC electronically (CDC, 2017g). State and territorial health departments are currently transitioning to the National Electronic Disease Surveillance System (NEDSS) Base System, an updated, standardized information system that facilitates automated clinical and laboratory case reporting (CDC, 2016a).

Several surveillance programs at CDC are part of the EIP. One of these programs is the population-based system that collects data on hospitalizations for influenza. Another EIP surveillance program is the Foodborne Diseases Active Surveillance Network (FoodNet), a collaborative program with the U.S. Department of Agriculture (USDA) and the Food and Drug Administration (FDA), that focuses on identifying cases of diarrheal illness resulting from foodborne pathogens (CDC, 2017d; NCEZID, 2017). An issue that may arise with potential bioterror events is that if more common pathogens are used, such as one of the agents producing gastrointestinal symptoms, it may be difficult to detect increases in occurrence above the usual endemic level (IOM & NRC, 1999; USAMRIID, 2014). The FoodNet system may be able to provide epidemiologic clues suggestive of outbreaks for the pathogens under surveillance, including outbreaks that are not naturally occurring (CDC, 2017d). Other CDC surveillance systems track infections in both human and animal populations. For example, the ArboNet system tracks not only human cases of infection with arboviruses, but also collects data from veterinary cases, and sentinel surveillance data from mosquitoes and other animals (CDC, 2015c).

The CDC is a collaborative partner in several international surveillance systems. One example of a collaborative effort is the Global Emerging Infections Sentinel Network (GeoSentinel). In the GeoSentinel system, the CDC partnered with the International Society of Travel Medicine (ISTM) to set up a provider-based, sentinel reporting network (CDC, 2015a; ISTM, 2016). This sentinel network functions through multiple clinics in the United States and abroad that specialize in tropical and travel medicine. Another example is the work of the CDC as one of the WHO Collaborating Centers for Influenza (CDC, 2017n).

The WHO plays a key role in collecting international surveillance data on infectious diseases, including disease outbreaks. Internationally notifiable diseases are specified by the International Health Regulations (IHR; WHO, 2017f). The 2005 revision of the IHR became effective in 2007. Under this document, there is a general requirement for member nations to notify the WHO of "an event that may constitute a public health emergency of international concern," and specific requirements are spelled out for reporting a single case of certain diseases (i.e., smallpox, severe acute respiratory syndrome [SARS], wild-type poliovirus, and any novel human influenza subtype; WHO, 2005). The updated regulations are also designed to strengthen surveillance and response capacities in individual countries (WHO, 2017f).

The Global Outbreak Alert and Response Network (GOARN) is the primary mechanism used by the WHO for global monitoring of disease outbreaks (Mackenzie et al., 2014; WHO, 2017e). The GOARN began in 2000 and provides electronic links between multiple institutions and networks in WHO member nations. These participants provide the expertise and skills for detection and response to outbreaks, including evaluation of unusual and/or dangerous pathogens. The system includes an outbreak verification team that routinely reviews reports to identify outbreaks with significant potential for international health impact (WHO, 2017d). Confirmed and rumored outbreaks are then relayed electronically to a large network of WHO member nations, health facilities and agencies, and disease experts (WHO, 2017e).

The GOARN systematically gathers intelligence on disease outbreaks from a variety of sources, including formal reports from WHO collaborating centers, and governmental health ministries and laboratories, as well as reports from academic institutions and other nongovernmental organizations (WHO, 2017c). An important informal source of outbreak reports is the Global Public Health Intelligence Network (GPHIN). This system was developed collaboratively by Health Canada and the WHO (Public Health Agency of Canada [PHAC], 2017). GPHIN uses a search engine to scan electronic media for rumors of outbreaks or other unusual health events. The GPHIN is an early example of the use of event-based information available on the Internet.

WHAT ARE THE ROLES OF STATE AND LOCAL HEALTH DEPARTMENTS IN DISEASE SURVEILLANCE SYSTEMS?

State and local health departments play important roles in infectious disease surveillance, as well as in prevention and control activities during outbreaks (Birkhead & Maylahn, 2010; CDC, 2004). State health regulations establish mandated reporting for specific infectious diseases and provide health officials with legal authority for certain prevention and control activities, for example, investigating outbreaks (Birkhead & Maylahn, 2010). The NNDSS represents a compilation of infectious disease surveillance data provided by the state and territorial health departments at the national level (CDC, 2015b). In addition, the CDC collaborates with selected state health departments for special systems, such as FoodNet (NCEZID, 2017).

It is at the local (county or city) health department level where most infectious disease surveillance activities occur (Birkhead & Maylahn, 2010). Local public health officials often interact directly with individual health providers and healthcare facilities for initial case reporting, follow-up investigation, and provision of feedback. Most prevention and control measures are also implemented at the local level, directed at specific individuals or groups or at the larger community. It is also at the local level that initial recognition and response to a bioterror event will likely occur (CDC, 2000; USAMRIID, 2014). That opportunity may be provided through a case report from an individual clinician.

WHAT IS THE ROLE OF CLINICIANS IN INFECTIOUS DISEASE SURVEILLANCE?

Case reporting by individual clinicians remains the principal component of many traditional infectious disease surveillance systems and an important mechanism for outbreak detection. However, as Giesecke (2017) has noted, a case report occurs at the endpoint of a chain of events. The infected person must be sufficiently ill to present for treatment. The health provider must include the agent on a differential diagnosis list and order appropriate diagnostic tests. Tests must be properly done to provide for confirmation of the organism. And finally, the health provider must submit the report to public health officials. All of these factors will affect the sensitivity of the surveillance system for detecting disease occurrence (Van Beneden & Lynfield, 2010).

Case reports from physicians and other healthcare providers are a key data capture method in traditional public health surveillance and will continue to be an important data source (CDC, 2004; IOM & NRC, 1999; Van Beneden & Lynfield, 2010). At the same time, given the importance of early detection to the effectiveness of the response plan, additional surveillance methods beyond the case-based approach have been developed to improve the timeliness and sensitivity of biological event detection. These newer approaches to surveillance are incorporated into the concept of biosurveillance.

WHAT IS BIOSURVEILLANCE?

"Biosurveillance" is defined as "active data-gathering with appropriate analysis and interpretation of biosphere data that might relate to disease activity and threats to human or animal health … to achieve early warning of health threats, early detection of health events, and overall situational awareness of disease activity" (HSPD, 2007, p. 1). Traditional, case-based systems and syndromic systems are important components of biosurveillance (Sosin & Hopkins, 2010). In addition, data from multiple Internet-based sources (e.g., news media reports and social network sites) have become an important source of event-based data regarding potential biological threats (Khan, Fleischauer, Casani, & Groseclose, 2010). The next sections provide information about syndromic surveillance and Internet-based surveillance systems.

Syndromic Surveillance

One definition of "syndromic surveillance" is "the ongoing, systematic collection, analysis, interpretation, and application of real-time (or near-real-time) indicators for diseases and outbreaks that allow for their detection before public health authorities would otherwise note them" (Sosin & Hopkins, 2010, p. 308). Initial development of syndromic surveillance

systems was focused on earlier and more complete detection of infectious disease outbreaks (CDC, 2004). The general process for early detection of biological events is shown in Figure 31.1. Data capture is essential for detection; methods that improve the timeliness of such capture allow a more rapid response to the event by public health officials.

The term "syndromic" in this context is something of a misnomer as it implies a focus solely on syndromes, that is, collections of clinical signs and symptoms or specific disease phenomena (Katz, May, Baker, & Test, 2011). Early syndromic systems used a variety of health indicator data other than clinical diagnoses and these types of data are still collected (CDC, 2004; Katz et al., 2011; Tokars, English, McMurray, & Rhodes, 2010). For example, some systems in clinical settings examine prediagnostic data such as chief complaints or laboratory test orders. Other systems examine early changes in health behavior before treatment is sought, such as work or school absenteeism or purchase of over-the-counter (OTC) medications (CDC, 2004; USAMRIID, 2014).

Syndromic surveillance systems developed in tandem with advances in information technology. A major component of many syndromic systems is the use of available electronic databases, including electronic health records, to capture prediagnostic and health indicator data. With such computerized data, automated search algorithms and advanced statistical analyses can be applied to detect unusual patterns that may signal an outbreak and often provide that signal earlier than is feasible using traditional surveillance methods (CDC, 2000; USAMRIID, 2014).

Because many bioterror agents may initially present with nonspecific symptoms, one limitation of a system based on presenting symptoms is the lack of *positive predictive value*; that is, the system will identify many potential cases that are unrelated to an event (i.e., false positives) along with the cases that may truly be related to an event (Sosin & Hopkins, 2010). This type of syndromic surveillance system is therefore most useful as a first step in identifying clusters of cases in need of further epidemiologic investigation rather than for identifying individual cases of a specific infectious disease (CDC, 2004).

The field of syndromic surveillance has evolved from the early focus on detection of bioterror events. At present, many different surveillance systems identified as syndromic systems are in operation in countries around the world, although there

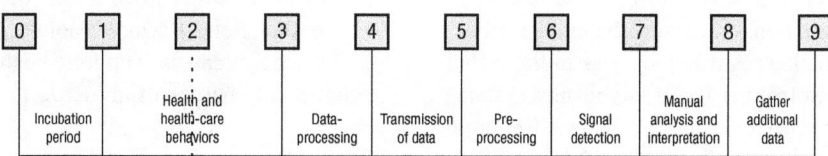

0. Onset of exposure
1. Onset of symptoms
2. Onset of behavior
3. Capture of data
4. Completion of data processing
5. Capture of data in surveillance system

6. Application of pattern recognition tools/algorithms
7. Generation of automated alert
8. Initiation of public health investigation
9. Initiation of public health intervention

FIGURE 31.1 Time line markers for early detection of biological events.

Source: From Centers for Disease Control and Prevention. (2004). Framework for evaluating public health surveillance systems for early detection of outbreaks: Recommendations from the CDC Working Group. *MMWR Morbidity and Mortality Weekly Report, 53*(RR-05), 6.

is no current consensus on the definition of what constitutes "syndromic surveillance" (Katz et al., 2011). Existing systems vary widely in scope and methodology. The systems collect different types of prediagnostic and health indicator data and vary in their reliance on technology for automated data collection and analysis. Some systems have a limited focus on specific diseases; other systems have a broader all-hazards focus (Gould et al., 2017; Katz et al., 2011). Some systems focus on data collection for initial event detection, while others collect data to assist with situational awareness and event monitoring. Despite the differences among systems, syndromic surveillance is recognized as an important component of global surveillance capacity (Katz et al., 2011).

One initial national syndromic system in the United States was BioSense, which focused on early detection of bioterror events (Gould et al., 2017). The system provided public health officials at all levels with secure, near-real-time access to aggregated health indicator data. BioSense was described as a system of systems in that data were aggregated from clinical and administrative databases from civilian, military, and veterans' healthcare facilities (Tokars et al., 2010). The original emphasis of the program has shifted from biological event detection to monitoring many different health events as the renamed NSSP (Gould et al., 2017). A current component of the NSSP is the BioSense Platform, a cloud-based system that allows exchange and analysis of syndromic data (CDC, 2017c, 2017j; Gould et al., 2017). The Electronic Surveillance System for the Early Notification of Community-based Epidemics, or ESSENCE, is one of the event-detection tools hosted on the platform (CDC, 2017c).

The use of syndromic surveillance systems has become common in the United States in the past decade. A 2014 survey of state public health authorities (PHAs) found that 80% of respondents routinely used syndromic surveillance systems (Reynolds et al., 2015). Of the 39 PHAs using syndromic systems, the most common system used was BioSense (30/39), either alone or in combination with another syndromic system. Of the respondents not solely using BioSense, all collected data on emergency department (ED) visits, underscoring the importance of acute care settings as data sources for syndromic surveillance.

Internet-Based Surveillance Systems

The Internet has the ability to provide instantaneous information to a substantial number of people throughout the world (Khan et al., 2010). In addition, major search engines collect large amounts of information regarding queries in the initial stages of an epidemic. New Internet-based surveillance systems have been developed in order to compile these unstructured *event-based* data sources (Choi, Cho, Shim, & Woo, 2016; Velasco, Agheneza, Denecke, Kirchner, & Eckmanns, 2014). Use of these informal sources of surveillance data is one factor that has contributed to increases in global capacity to detect biological events (Kluberg et al., 2016).

One forerunner of current Internet-based systems is the Program for Monitoring Emerging Diseases (ProMED-mail), first launched in 1994 and managed by the International Society for Infectious Diseases (ISID) since 1999 (ISID, 2014). The purpose of the system is to rapidly disseminate information about infectious diseases to subscribers. The system accepts information from various sources, including media reports and local observers, as well as official reports. Another early system is the GPHIN system used by the WHO (PHAC, 2017). A more recent system is HealthMap, first launched in 2006 (HealthMap, n.d.). This system reviews and compiles information from media and official reports, including data from GeoSentinel and the WHO, among other sources, and displays the information geographically. In the United States, program personnel in the CDC's Global Disease Detection Operations Center (GDDOC) review both official and unofficial data sources for potential disease events, in partnership with national and international agencies (CDC, 2017e). The CDC link to the WHO's GOARN is through the GDDOC.

Many Internet-based systems have been developed. Two recent reviews of more widely used Internet-based systems revealed similarities and differences among systems (Choi et al., 2016; Velasco et al., 2014). Together the two groups of reviewers examined 17 unique systems, seven of which were reviewed in both articles, including GPHIN, HealthMap, and ProMED-mail. A common goal across systems was enhancing early detection of events (Velasco et al., 2014). Many systems collected data from news/media reports, with some collecting data from social media or search engines. While some systems had public access, others were available by subscription only, while still others had restricted portal access. Some systems were moderated, with human analysts examining data for relevance, while others were fully automated (Choi et al., 2016; Velasco et al., 2014). The key benefits of Internet-based systems, including timeliness and the large data volume, enhance traditional public health surveillance systems; however, event-based systems have limitations (Choi et al., 2016). For example, the sheer volume of data may hinder rather than help public health officials (Velasco et al., 2014). Also, data from informal information sources are not always relevant or timely.

One novel approach to Internet-based surveillance is the Influenzanet system, a collaborative effort among multiple countries in the European Union (Influenzanet, 2017). Using standardized surveys, this online system collects self-reported data on symptoms of ILI from volunteers in the general population within each country, as well as demographic and health behavior information (Guerrisi et al., 2016). One advantage of this participatory surveillance system is that information is captured from individuals who have ILI symptoms but choose not to consult a healthcare provider (Peppa, Edmunds, & Funk, 2017; Perrotta, Bella, Rizzo, & Paolotti, 2017). Information from such individuals can assist public health officials in assessing the community burden of influenza for a given season (Peppa et al., 2017).

Internet-based surveillance systems have been shown to provide data that are consistent with traditional public health surveillance systems (Milinovich, Williams, Clements, & Hu, 2014). For example, researches in Italy reported that weekly incidence data from their component Influenzanet system (Influweb) correlated well with, and identified the peak incidence nearly a week earlier than, data from the existing sentinel physician system (Perrotta et al., 2017). The 2009 influenza A (H1N1) pandemic provided an opportunity for several groups of researchers to evaluate the event detection capabilities of specific Internet-based surveillance systems in comparison to traditional systems. Most researchers reported increased timeliness of event detection using the event-based system (Brownstein et al., 2010; Nelson, Brownstein, & Hartley, 2010; Nelson, Yang, Reilly, Hardin, & Hartley, 2012; Schirmer, Lucero, Oda, Lopez, & Holodniy, 2010); however, there were exceptions (CDC, 2011). These findings underscore the importance of ongoing evaluation of any surveillance system (Gajewski et al., 2014; Teutsch, 2010).

While some published studies have evaluated the performance of individual Internet-based surveillance systems, very few have compared performance among systems (Gajewski et al., 2014). In one such study, Barboza et al. (2014) examined the performance of six systems, including ProMED, GPHIN, and HealthMap, comparing the infectious disease event detection capabilities of each system with the gold standard data of official public health surveillance reports. They found that while the systems were similar in their early detection performance, those systems with human moderation performed better than fully automated systems. In addition, they noted that none of the Internet-based systems provided early detection for all of the events reported in the official public health system, underscoring the need to use systems in parallel (Barboza et al., 2014). Although timeliness of detection has been examined in several evaluation studies, there is a lack of information on how this information has been used by public health officials in their response to biological events (Gajewski et al., 2014).

Social networking sites, search engines, and event-based systems targeting electronic reports from multiple sources are uniquely positioned to gather and disseminate health information (Khan et al., 2010). Several advantages of this type of information exchange include earlier detection of outbreaks, no requirement for voluntary reporting, automation in the reporting cycle, and easy access to information. Along with the advantages, several disadvantages have been identified: information is sometimes erroneous or difficult to interpret, sensitivity and specificity are not always clear, public response to the information can be unpredictable, and health information privacy may not be protected (Khan et al., 2010; Velasco et al., 2014; Wilson & Brownstein, 2009). Future development of Internet-based systems should take these identified advantages and limitations into consideration.

Syndromic and Internet-based surveillance systems are counterparts to, not a replacement for, traditional public health surveillance (Choi et al., 2016; Milinovich et al., 2014). Integration of information collected from these different systems will be needed to enhance biosurveillance capabilities (Brownstein et al., 2010; Khan et al., 2010). Evaluation of the performance and impact of these new integrated biosurveillance systems will be an important component of their development (Gajewski et al., 2014).

Surveillance Partners

One component of the preparedness plan for bioterrorism at local health departments is to have a system of surveillance partners in place to assist with recognition of such events (HHS, 2001; USAMRIID, 2014). Potential partners include the medical examiner or coroner, emergency medical services and 911 dispatchers, laboratories, area pharmacists, poison control centers, and veterinarians, as well as organizations within the community. The use of surveillance partners is consistent with the concept of using data from multiple sources in a comprehensive biosurveillance system (Khan et al., 2010; USAMRIID, 2014).

WHAT IS THE ROLE OF ANIMAL SURVEILLANCE SYSTEMS?

Given the intrinsic link between human and animal health (Dixon, Dar, & Heymann, 2014), infectious disease surveillance in animal populations is another important component for detection of biological events (Jacobsen et al., 2016; USAMRIID, 2014). It has been estimated that 60% of emerging infectious diseases recognized since 1940 originated as diseases in animals (Jones et al., 2008). The periodic emergence of novel influenza viruses is an example of these interspecies connections (Dixon et al., 2014). In addition, many of the agents considered to have bioterror potential are diseases of animals (i.e., zoonoses), for example, anthrax and brucellosis (USAMRIID, 2014). There is a need for enhanced surveillance of animal pathogens as it is possible that a covert attack may be directed at animal populations directly or as an indirect route to impact human populations (Karlsson et al., 2013).

As with human infectious diseases, surveillance systems for infectious diseases in animals are in place (Jacobsen et al., 2016; USDA, 2017). The need for surveillance in both domesticated and wild populations adds complexity to the task (Dixon et al., 2014). In the United States, the CDC conducts surveillance related to multiple zoonotic and vectorborne diseases. A few examples include rabies, West Nile virus, and Zika virus (CDC, 2015c, 2017k, 2017o). The USDA (2017) maintains the National Animal Health Reporting System (NAHRS), which collects data on notifiable diseases for animal populations in agriculture and aquaculture. Another surveillance initiative is the Emerging Threats Program (ETP), overseen by the U.S. Agency for International Development (USAID). The ETP provides support for infrastructure development for animal surveillance in zoonotic disease hotspot areas of the world (Morse et al., 2012; USAID, 2016).

At the international level, the World Organisation for Animal Health, known by its historical acronym OIE, is a key source of global animal surveillance data. The OIE maintains the World Animal Health Information System (WAHIS), an Internet-based surveillance system to monitor diseases in animal populations (OIE, 2017a). OIE also maintains a list of notifiable diseases in animals (USDA, 2017). Another component of WAHIS is an alert system for member countries to provide early warning of events (OIE, 2017b).

HealthMap (n.d.) is an example of a global biosurveillance system that includes reports of outbreaks in both animal and human populations. This integrated approach to human and animal surveillance is an illustration of the information fusion that is critical in biosurveillance (Jacobsen et al., 2016; Khan et al., 2010). Another key element for biosurveillance is interdisciplinary collaboration (Dixon et al., 2014).

HOW DO EMERGENCY INFORMATION SYSTEMS FIT INTO A BIOSURVEILLANCE SYSTEM?

Whereas syndromic surveillance and Internet-based systems may enhance timely detection of outbreaks, the information generated is not of use unless it can be rapidly disseminated to the stakeholders responsible for implementing prevention and control efforts (Sosin & Hopkins, 2010). Such dissemination requires a communication infrastructure that facilitates the rapid (near-real-time) exchange of information (CDC, 2000; Department of Homeland Security [DHS], 2016b). The National Biosurveillance Integration Center at DHS provides daily summaries of biological incidents occurring in the United States and internationally to state and local health officials (DHS, 2016b). The CDC's Internet-based HAN is one initiative that was developed to provide rapid notification of health alerts and provide access to surveillance data by local and state health officials and other clinicians (CDC, 2017f). The CDC also established the Clinicians Outreach and Communication Activity (COCA) program to provide clinicians with information about emergency preparedness through a variety of methods, including email updates, conference calls, and webcasts (CDC, 2017b). Another strategy has been the establishment of designated websites for dissemination of information. The CDC has compiled an array of information for healthcare providers and the public on emergency and disaster planning for biological and other types of events. The entry page for this site is available at emergency.cdc.gov. At the international level, the WHO's DON website provides a listing of current outbreaks from all regions of the world (WHO, 2017a). The English language entry page for this site is available at www .who.int/csr/don/en/.

EARLY RECOGNITION AND DETECTION OF BIOLOGICAL EVENTS: ROLE OF THE CLINICIAN

As individuals with clinically apparent disease begin to seek medical care, it is likely that emergency room personnel or community-based healthcare providers will be the first individuals in a position to recognize and respond to a biological event, whether naturally occurring or the result of bioterrorism (CDC, 2000, 2001a; USAMRIID, 2014). Early recognition and detection of a biological event is important for two reasons. First, this will maximize the opportunity for early initiation of effective prophylactic treatment of exposed or potentially exposed persons. Second, early recognition leading to early control efforts will minimize the opportunity for transmission of the agent. Despite this, early detection of biological events may be difficult to achieve (CDC, 2000; IOM & NRC, 2011). Clinically apparent illness will occur several days to weeks after exposure, depending on the incubation period of the agent, and affected persons may be in widely dispersed locations and present to different healthcare providers (CDC, 2000, 2004; USAMRIID, 2014). Decisions made by clinicians in those facilities regarding what tests and treatments are ordered may

ultimately determine whether a case is correctly diagnosed and reported (IOM & NRC, 2011). Several methods to enhance clinical recognition of biological events are described in the following sections.

Enhancing Early Recognition in Clinical Settings

Acute Care Settings

The hospital ED is likely to be an initial setting in which persons affected by biological events first seek medical care. This was illustrated in the anthrax outbreak in October to November 2001. Of the 11 patients with inhalational anthrax, nine presented for initial care to a hospital ED, and the remaining two patients ultimately sought care in an ED as their symptoms worsened (Barakat et al., 2002; Jernigan et al., 2001). Clearly, healthcare providers in the ED and other acute healthcare settings are in a key position to help detect an outbreak, identify the pathogen, and alert PHAs.

How can early recognition be enhanced in the acute care setting? Three interrelated mechanisms facilitate early recognition. The first mechanism is to raise the awareness of clinicians of the potential threats posed by infectious diseases, whether because of a deliberate release of an agent or from a naturally occurring outbreak (Grundmann, 2014; Memish et al., 2014; USAMRIID, 2014). Clinicians must expand their frame of reference from a routine list of differential diagnoses to one that includes the possibility of deliberate exposures to infectious agents as the etiology for illnesses they see in their clinical areas (USAMRIID, 2014). This applies to practitioners working in various specialties within the hospital, including the ED, medical intensive care units, and infection control departments, among others. Hospital-based clinicians must also recognize that they may truly be the "first responders" in a biological attack and that their clinical decisions may ultimately affect the course of the outbreak (IOM & NRC, 2011; USAMRIID, 2014).

A second mechanism essential to early recognition of bioterrorist attacks is an increased attentiveness to unusual *patterns* of disease occurrence. Looking at patterns requires an epidemiological perspective, that is, an aggregate view of patients in a given clinical setting (USAMRIID, 2014). Clinicians must develop an eye for unusual patterns at this group level.

The third mechanism to facilitate early recognition is use of a syndrome-based approach in the clinical recognition of disease patterns. Using this approach, clinicians incorporate knowledge of typical clinical presentations of potential bioterror agents into their routine differential diagnosis lists and have a heightened attentiveness for these syndromes in their clinical settings (USAMRIID, 2014).

Early recognition is essential to enable early interventions in the event of a bioterrorist attack, but public health measures to investigate and contain the outbreak will not be implemented until public health officials are notified. Thus, an essential next step after identifying an unusual case or cases is reporting them to designated public health officials (CDC, 2001b; USAMRIID, 2014; Van Beneden & Lynfield, 2010). In addition, since individual clinicians may see only one or two patients, an outbreak may not be apparent until public health investigators combine these separate reports.

Community-Based Settings

Although hospitals are clearly part of the communities they serve, a distinction is often made between the hospital setting and healthcare provided in nonhospital settings. Examples of community-based settings where nurses practice include physician offices, ambulatory care centers, and mental health clinics. Clinicians in these settings must also perceive themselves as having a role in preparing for and responding to a biological event.

How can early recognition be enhanced in community-based settings? The approaches are essentially the same as for hospital-based clinicians. One component is a heightened awareness of potential bioterror agents by practitioners. A second component is increased attentiveness to unusual patterns of disease occurrence. A third component is use of a syndrome-based approach to clinical recognition of disease patterns. As with acute care clinicians, community-based clinicians must recognize that they may fill the role of first responders in a biological attack.

Community Health Settings

In contrast to community-based practice settings, which maintain a focus on individual clients or families, nurses practicing in community/public health settings provide healthcare in the context of "promoting and protecting the health of populations" (American Public Health Association [APHA], 2013, p. 2). While community health nurses may provide care to individuals and families, they maintain a population focus and perspective while doing so. As in acute or community-based practice settings, community health nurses must also consider their potential role as first responders should a biological event affect their community. They should also be familiar with the agents posing the greatest potential bioterror threats (i.e., CDC Category A agents) and the key syndromes associated with these agents. In contrast to practitioners in other settings, community health nurses typically have had educational preparation in considering disease from a population health viewpoint, including viewing disease patterns from an epidemiological perspective (APHA, 2013).

EPIDEMIOLOGICAL APPROACH TO BIOLOGICAL EVENT RECOGNITION

Epidemiological Clues to Recognition

In epidemiology, the term "pattern" "refers to the occurrence of health-related events by time, place, and person" (CDC, 2012, p. 15). Recognition of unusual patterns requires a population-based or epidemiological approach to data analysis and interpretation. What would constitute an unusual pattern of disease occurrence? Essentially, it is a group or cluster of cases that does not fit the expected pattern for a particular illness

or clinical syndrome based on time, location, or demographic characteristics (e.g., age or sex). Again, baseline information is needed for comparison to evaluate what is *unusual*. With awareness of the baseline data for their practice setting, nurses should be alert for unusual patterns of disease or health-related indicators.

Since many different agents could be used in a bioterrorist attack, and many of these agents have disease patterns that are initially nonspecific, it is important for clinicians to think from an epidemiological perspective and be able to recognize syndrome patterns suggestive of a deliberate agent release (USAMRIID, 2014). For example, one case of rapidly progressive febrile illness during the traditional influenza season may not be cause for suspicion, but a pattern of several such cases with the same clinical presentation over a short period of time should raise the index of suspicion for a bioterror event. Representative examples of unusual patterns of diseases that might suggest a deliberate bioterrorist act are presented in Box 31.1 (HHS, 2001; USAMRIID, 2014).

The value of spotting the unusual has been demonstrated by a number of infectious disease outbreaks in the United States. A classic example is the initial reports of the HIV epidemic. Alert clinicians in California and New York City noted clusters of rare illnesses, Kaposi's sarcoma, and *Pneumocystis carinii* pneumonia, among homosexual male clients in their practices (CDC, 1981a, 1981b). In the 1999 West Nile virus outbreak in New York City, a physician noted that patients with similar clinical signs had presented for treatment at the same hospital and alerted PHAs (Asnis, Conetta, Teixeira, Waldman, & Sampson, 2000; Fine & Layton, 2001). In both examples, it

---

BOX 31.1 Epidemiological Patterns Suggesting a Covert Biological Attack

1. A cluster of cases with similar clinical presentation and at a similar stage of illness
2. A cluster of unexplained illness in a defined population, such as that associated with a specific location or event
3. Unusually severe disease or higher mortality than expected for a given agent
4. A cluster of cases with an unusual or uncommon mode of transmission for a given agent
5. Multiple or serial outbreaks of different diseases in a defined population
6. A disease atypical for a given age category
7. A disease unusual for the region or season
8. Clusters of the same illness in dispersed locations
9. Clusters of illness or deaths in animals or livestock occurring in a similar time frame as human illness

Sources: From Army Medical Research Institute of Infectious Diseases. (2014). *USAMRIID's medical management of biological casualties handbook* (8th ed.). Frederick, MD: Author; U.S. Department of Health and Human Services & Centers for Disease Control and Prevention. (2001, July). The public health response to biological and chemical terrorism: Interim planning guidance for state public health officials. Retrieved from https://emergency.cdc.gov/documents/planning/planningguidance.pdf

was the recognition of an unusual pattern that prompted further investigation and the ultimate discovery of new or newly emerging pathogens.

SYNDROME-BASED APPROACH TO BIOLOGICAL EVENT RECOGNITION

Syndrome-based recognition relies on the clinical presentation of the patient, plus other clues to suggest specific agents. Laboratory or radiological tests can then assist with confirmation. Experience with the anthrax outbreak in 2001 suggests that, even in the early stage of illness, clues may be present to assist clinicians with their differential diagnosis (CDC, 2001a). Evaluation of the initial symptoms of the 11 patients with inhalational anthrax showed that rhinorrhea was uncommon, while shortness of breath and nausea and vomiting were common. This disease pattern is in contrast to the usual symptoms seen with influenza, where rhinorrhea is common and shortness of breath, nausea, and vomiting are uncommon. In addition, the anthrax cases all had abnormal chest radiographs, which are not typically seen with influenza (CDC, 2001a).

It is important to note that not all emerging pathogens will have a unique clinical presentation to aid in identification. Several published reports following the 2009 influenza A (H1N1) pandemic reported a lack of differences between the clinical presentations of patients with the pandemic H1N1 strain versus the seasonal influenza strains (Aguirre et al., 2011; Belongia et al., 2011; Crisinel et al., 2011). With a novel pathogen, the clinician must rely on laboratory identification of the organism and on epidemiological clues in the patient's history about the causative agent.

One important element of the patient's history may be travel to an area where an outbreak is occurring. In the 2009 pandemic of influenza A (H1N1), a travel history to Mexico was an early aid in identification of suspected patients in the United States (CDC, 2009). In the 2014–2015 Ebola outbreak, a travel history to an affected area was an important element in the screening protocol for suspected cases in the United States (CDC, 2014b).

Syndromes Associated With CDC Category A Agents

Most of the Category A agents, and many other potential bioterror agents, produce an initial prodrome of influenza-like or nonspecific symptoms before progressing to one or more syndrome patterns (USAMRIID, 2014). A detailed discussion of the diagnosis of each of the CDC Category A agents is presented in Chapter 30. The discussion below provides a brief description of syndrome patterns that can assist clinicians in recognizing these agents.

Botulism-Like Syndrome

Of the agents on the Category A list, only botulism toxin produces the unique pattern of proximal to distal descending paralysis, typically with a lack of sensory deficits (USAMRIID, 2014). Patients may initially present with symptoms such as

difficulty swallowing and double vision, with progressive flaccid paralysis that may lead to respiratory failure in severe cases. Any cluster of patients with this presentation is suggestive of a botulism outbreak, and if clinical histories rule out a potential common food source, this increases the suspicion of an inhalational exposure (CDC, 2001a; USAMRIID, 2014).

Hemorrhagic Illness

The viral hemorrhagic fevers (VHFs) include diseases caused by a number of different viruses. The clinical manifestations vary, but can be severe, including shock, disseminated intravascular coagulation (DIC), and other signs of increased vascular permeability. A petechial rash is also typical for many of the VHFs (USAMRIID, 2014).

Rash

Whereas fever is characteristic in many different infectious processes, the concomitant occurrence of a rash should provoke further clinical evaluation. In particular, clinicians should be familiar with the characteristic rash produced by smallpox and the features that distinguish it from the rash produced by varicella (USAMRIID, 2014).

Respiratory Syndrome

Several of the Category A agents produce rapidly progressive respiratory symptoms, including anthrax, plague, and tularemia (USAMRIID, 2014). Additional epidemiological clues can suggest a particular pathogen from the differential diagnosis list. Although naturally occurring respiratory infections can occur with all three agents, primary respiratory disease is an uncommon presentation with natural infections. Therefore, when any of these agents is suspected as the etiology for rapidly progressive pneumonia, a deliberate, aerosolized exposure should be suspected (USAMRIID, 2014).

Other Syndromes

The bacterial pathogens causing anthrax, plague, and tularemia produce different clinical manifestations depending on the mode of transmission. Lymphadenitis, with painful buboes in the groin, axilla, or neck is characteristic of the bubonic form of plague. Anthrax and tularemia may present with cutaneous forms of disease. Anthrax may also present with a gastrointestinal syndrome (USAMRIID, 2014).

Clinical Presentations for Other Potential Bioterror Agents

Although emphasis has been placed on CDC Category A agents because of their potential severe impact on public health, it is important to remember that other agents have the potential for use in deliberate acts of bioterror. As with the CDC Category A agents, several Category B agents, such as Q-fever, brucellosis, and glanders, may present with nonspecific influenza-like symptoms or respiratory symptoms (USAMRIID, 2014). Even common agents producing gastrointestinal symptoms may be used in a bioterror event, as was the case in 1984 when a restaurant-associated outbreak of *Salmonella typhimurium* occurred following deliberate food contamination (Török et al., 1997). Again, recognition of unusual patterns of disease, including clusters of patients with similar clinical presentations, can be the early indicator of a biological event, regardless of the etiologic agent (IOM & NRC, 2011).

Sosin and Hopkins (2010) note that reliance on known syndromes may be insufficient for clinical recognition. With a novel agent, the pattern of symptoms may not fit an established diagnosis. With a novel mode of transmission, the pattern of occurrence may not fit usual settings or demographic characteristics. In addition, the situation may develop rapidly and involve large numbers of individuals, resulting in overload of the healthcare system. Delays in laboratory identification of the organism may further delay an effective response.

The preceding discussion focuses on the ability of individual clinicians to detect and recognize infectious processes that may be related to a bioterror event or a novel infectious agent. To a certain extent, this relies on the art of clinicians—their expertise and clinical detective skills, which will clearly vary among practitioners. A key recommendation of the 2011 IOM and NRC report was development of decision support tools that are "clinically useful, bidirectional, and modifiable" for use by clinicians (IOM & NRC, 2011, p. 14). Development of new diagnostic decision support systems to assist clinicians in recognition and response to biological events is an area in need of further research.

LABORATORY DETECTION OF BIOLOGICAL EVENTS

The clinical laboratory is a critical component of biosurveillance (Olano & Walker, 2011; Sosin & Hopkins, 2010). Laboratory personnel are another category of healthcare providers who will need increased attentiveness to unusual patterns. They are in a position to detect changes in the number of culture requests or an increase in uncommon specimen types such as pulmonary aspirates (CDC, 2001a). In addition, laboratory records of culture patterns may show increases in unusual strains, or strains with resistance patterns not usually seen in a given facility or locality; or molecular diagnostics may indicate an unexpected degree of genetic homogeneity across specimens (HHS, 2001; Olano & Walker, 2011; USAMRIID, 2014). All of these patterns suggest occurrence of a biological event.

Laboratory Methods for Detection

Laboratory tests are critical to confirming the presence of suspected bioterror agents. The American Society of Microbiology (ASM) has published protocols for clinical laboratories to provide standard methods for use with such agents (ASM, 2016), and the ASM serves as an important resource for testing method protocols for many other infectious agents. A detailed discussion of laboratory methods is beyond the scope of this chapter. However, the common approaches for laboratory

identification for biological agents, including culture methods, nucleic acid-based techniques, and immunoassays, are described briefly (ASM, 2016; Karlsson et al., 2013; Olano & Walker, 2011).

For the CDC Category A bacterial pathogens of interest (*Bacillus anthracis*, *Yersinia pestis*, and *Francisella tularensis*), culture methods including initial staining and microscopy results are available rapidly and can assist clinicians with a differential diagnosis. In contrast to the bacterial pathogens, the Category A viral pathogens (i.e., smallpox and the VHFs) require the highest level of containment for culture procedures, and specimen collection and handling must be done with special precautions (ASM, 2016). Culture methods are an important tool for biological agent identification; however, these methods are not available for all organisms and may not be useful for novel pathogens (Karlsson et al., 2013).

Nurses are probably most familiar with molecular diagnostic (nucleic acid–based) techniques in the form of various types of DNA-based polymerase chain reaction (PCR) testing. The use of molecular diagnostic techniques in the clinical laboratory has grown tremendously in the past decade as a result of technological advances that have increased both timeliness and cost-effectiveness (Olano & Walker, 2011). More recently, the development of methods that allow direct gene sequencing has been an important tool in detecting novel agents in outbreak investigations. For example, a diagnostic PCR test was quickly developed following the identification of the first cases of MERS-CoV in Saudi Arabia in 2012 and was used as part of a subsequent active surveillance program of hospitalized suspected cases and contacts of confirmed cases (Memish et al., 2014).

Immunoassays rely on antigen–antibody reactions specific to a given agent (Kim et al., 2015; Rao, Mohan, & Atreya, 2010). Immunoassays can be less sensitive than culture or gene amplification approaches. Efforts are underway to develop improved immunodiagnostic tools for a variety of agents and toxins that will allow rapid diagnosis during the initial phases of illness.

Following the 2001 anthrax attack in the United States, there was considerable interest in development of biosensors for detection of biological agents in the environment and these efforts are continuing. Particular emphasis has been placed on development of detection methods for the causative agent of anthrax, *B. anthracis* (Kim et al., 2015; Rao et al., 2010). Air sampling detection systems to detect aerosolized bioterror agents are currently in use in the United States as part of the BioWatch program (DHS, 2016a). This early warning system has been in operation since 2003. The location of these monitoring systems remains undisclosed, with monitoring occurring continuously. Filters from the sampling system undergo frequent, nucleic acid–based testing at designated laboratories.

Future Directions for Laboratory Detection Methods

There is a continued need for improved laboratory methods for both medical and veterinary diagnostic tests (Jacobsen et al., 2016). User-friendly and cost-effective diagnostic tools for emerging and reemerging agents are needed that can provide rapid results in point-of-care settings (Jacobsen et al., 2016; Olano & Walker, 2011). One promising area of research is development of metagenomic detection methods (Karlsson et al., 2013). These methods will allow sequencing of the combined genomes of organisms in a clinical sample. Another area of research is the use of nanotechnology, which can contribute to miniaturization of diagnostic tools and biosensors (Kim et al., 2015; Olano & Walker, 2011).

Laboratory Response Network

The current LRN system is categorized into three levels: sentinel, reference, and national laboratories (CDC, 2014a). Sentinel laboratories have capabilities to perform microbiological testing for recognition of and ruling out potential bioterror agents. Their role is one of early detection and referral to an appropriate reference laboratory. Reference laboratories have additional capacities for confirmatory testing of specific agents. Their role is one of investigation and referral. In addition to laboratories at state and local health departments and several international reference facilities, the LRN also includes veterinary, agricultural, and environmental laboratories (CDC, 2017h). National laboratories have the specialized expertise and facilities needed to handle organisms, such as smallpox, that require the highest biosafety level. Their role is to provide definitive characterization of agents (CDC, 2014a). Nurses should be familiar with the laboratory capacities of the health facilities in which they work and understand the tiered response structure of support provided by the LRN in the event of a biological attack.

LESSONS LEARNED AND FUTURE DIRECTIONS

Lessons From the 2014–2015 Ebola Outbreak

The 2014–2015 Ebola virus disease outbreak in West Africa offers important lessons on the key role of surveillance systems in detection and response to a biological event. This outbreak was by far the largest Ebola outbreak on record, with nearly 29,000 cases and over 11,000 deaths, and was the first Ebola outbreak to spread internationally, resulting in a global public health threat (Coltart, Lindsey, Ghinai, Johnson, & Heymann, 2017). The three countries most impacted "had a shortage of public health surveillance capacities to detect, report, and respond rapidly to the outbreak" (p. 17). In addition, the lack of community engagement early in the outbreak negatively impacted "surveillance, contact tracing, [and] healthcare seeking behavior" (p. 15), all of which contributed to the continued propagation of the epidemic (Coltart et al., 2017).

A delayed global response to the outbreak also prolonged its course (Coltart et al., 2017; Jacobsen et al., 2016). As global resources were finally mobilized and deployed, control capacities increased in the affected countries (Coltart et al., 2017). This, coupled with improved community engagement, ultimately allowed healthcare and public health workers to effectively implement known control measures, including active surveillance and contact tracing, to bring the outbreak to an end. Another factor that contributed to the containment of the outbreak was the use of newly developed molecular diagnostic methods in the field, which allowed more rapid diagnosis of Ebola in suspected cases (Coltart et al., 2017).

The 2014–2015 Ebola outbreak offered many lessons for public health officials. The primary lesson learned regarding surveillance systems is the need for development of core public health surveillance capacity to meet the 2005 IHR standards (WHO, 2005) in all countries not currently meeting those standards (Coltart et al., 2017; Jacobsen et al., 2016). This surveillance capacity is needed for timely biological event detection and for effective outbreak containment. In addition, given the importance of the clinical laboratory in surveillance systems, there also is a concurrent need to develop core laboratory capacity to meet IHR standards (Jacobsen et al., 2016). While global capacity to detect biological events has increased (Kluberg et al., 2016), a recent estimate is that less than 20% of countries have met the IHR standards (Burkle, 2015). Providing resources to meet core capacity standards for surveillance and response will be key in enhancing preparedness for the next global public health threat.

Future Directions in Biosurveillance

The lessons learned from the 2014–2015 Ebola outbreak underscore the need for an integrated approach to infectious disease surveillance that incorporates human and animal populations in a transdisciplinary way (Jacobsen et al., 2016). Adoption of the One Health concept may facilitate system integration (Davis, Dar, & Heymann, 2014). According to the American Veterinary Medical Association (AVMA), "One Health is the integrative effort of multiple disciplines working locally, nationally, and globally to attain optimal health for people, animals, and the environment" (AVMA, 2017, para 1).

Integration will be needed at all steps in the biosurveillance process, from data collection to dissemination of information to inform public health response (Khan et al., 2010; Van Beneden & Lynfield, 2010). One example of such integration is the Surveillance Data Platform (SDP) with Shared Services, introduced by the CDC in 2016. The SDP uses cloud-based technology and is designed to improve the efficiency of data collection and usage, thereby accelerating decision making by public health officials (CDC, 2017m). As traditional public health surveillance and event-based surveillance systems are integrated, a key area for research will be to evaluate the effectiveness of these systems in biological event detection, their usefulness for outbreak investigation, including situational awareness, and their impact on public health decision making (Gajewski et al., 2014).

As noted earlier, work remains to achieve core surveillance capacities in many countries. This work is the first step toward the goal of a truly global surveillance infrastructure (Morse et al., 2012). Such global capacity will be essential in addressing future emerging infectious disease threats. New technologies offer the promise that current initiatives aimed at improving global surveillance capabilities for detection and response to biological events will evolve into systems that will allow future pandemics to be predicted and preempted (Morse et al., 2012).

SUMMARY

Public health surveillance is an essential process for detection of biological events. The traditional notifiable disease reporting system remains an important component of infectious diseases surveillance; however, the increasing availability of electronic health data and advances in information technologies provide opportunities for active, real-time surveillance systems (Khan et al., 2010; Sosin & Hopkins, 2010). Internet-based surveillance systems that rely on informal health event indicators and syndromic systems programmed for detection of unusual patterns in prediagnostic clinical data are approaches to providing earlier detection and monitoring of biological events, but such systems are an adjunct to, not a replacement for, traditional surveillance methods (Milinovich et al., 2014). Recent developments in Internet-based systems have provided access to large amounts of event-based data in near-real-time. The challenge for the future will be to develop the analysis methods and decision support tools to enhance detection and response to biological events within integrated, transdisciplinary biosurveillance systems (Jacobsen et al., 2016; Khan et al., 2010).

Nurses practicing in acute care, community-based, or community health settings have a potential role in detecting a bioterrorist attack or in identifying outbreaks of emerging or reemerging infections. Several mechanisms can assist clinicians in the early recognition and detection of these events. In evaluating individual patients, clinicians should consider potential bioterror agents on their differential diagnosis lists and be alert for syndrome patterns suggestive of a bioterrorist attack. In addition, nurses can use an epidemiological approach with their patient populations to look for unusual patterns of disease.

Laboratories play a major role in detection and confirmation of biological agents. In the United States, the LRN provides tiered capabilities for confirmatory testing (CDC, 2014a, 2017h). Current research projects hold the promise of rapid diagnostic and screening tests that can assist in timely, point-of-care response efforts to events. Even with the development of such technologies, it remains the responsibility of clinicians, including nurses, to think of themselves as potential first responders in a biological event and to acquire the knowledge necessary to assist with early detection, recognition, and reporting of such events. It will likely be the situational awareness of healthcare providers that is the key to detection.

STUDY QUESTIONS

1. What is public health surveillance?
2. Compare and contrast passive, active, and sentinel surveillance.

3. Why is it necessary to have baseline surveillance data to evaluate disease patterns?

4. For your community, identify the process that is used to report a notifiable disease to the local health department.

5. What are the advantages and disadvantages of data collection through Internet-based surveillance systems?

6. For your community, identify at least three potential surveillance partners.

7. What are three mechanisms that can facilitate early recognition of biological events by clinicians?

8. Which of the following case scenarios are suggestive of an intentional biological release? Provide a rationale for your response to each scenario.
   a. You are working in the ED of a large urban hospital. It is early winter. You have seen six patients this morning, ages 22 to 64, with a 1- to 4-day history of fever, chills, cough, and rhinorrhea. None report having received an influenza vaccination the previous fall.
   b. You are working in the ED of a medium-sized community hospital. During your shift today, you have seen four otherwise healthy young adults present with a history of fever and chills for 4 days, followed by rapidly progressive dyspnea and productive cough. Two of the patients were so hypoxic that they required endotracheal intubation and mechanical ventilation in the ED. The other two patients were admitted to the ICU, and were also intubated later in the day.
   c. In the local ED where you work, an emergency medical system call is received stating that five patients are being transported to your hospital. All five patients were found in the same building, and one of the patients is in respiratory distress. The other four are having blurred vision, difficulty swallowing, slurred speech, and difficulty walking. On examination, you find that all of the patients are afebrile and have flaccid paralysis.

INTERNET ACTIVITIES

1. This link leads to the summary reports of notifiable diseases in the United States from 1993 to 2014. Go to www.cdc.gov/mmwr/mmwr_nd/. Select the summary for 2014. Scroll down to "Part I: Summary of Notifiable Diseases in the United States, 2014." Use the data in Table 2j, which gives cases by geographic region, to make a list of states with reported cases of plague for that year. Similarly, make a list of states with reported cases of plague from 2010 to 2013.

   Using this information:
   - Identify states or region of the United States where a single case of plague might be a naturally occurring infection.

2. This link leads to the summary reports of notifiable diseases in the United States from 1993 to 2014. Go to www.cdc.gov/mmwr/mmwr_nd/. Select the summary for 2014. Scroll down to "Part I: Summary of Notifiable Diseases in the United States, 2014." Use the information in Tables 1

through 6 to compile information on the cases of tularemia that were reported that year.

Using this information:

- Prepare a one-paragraph summary of the person, place, and time characteristics of the 180 cases of tularemia that occurred in the United States in 2014.
- Discuss how a clinician might use this information to help distinguish between a cluster of naturally occurring infections and one that was the result of a deliberate release of the agent.

3. This is the link to the website on anthrax developed by the CDC. Go to www.cdc.gov/anthrax/. Review the material under "Basic Info," "Bioterrorism," and "Medical Care," and any other sections of interest.

Using this information:

- Construct a case-based scenario that would suggest inhalational anthrax resulting from a deliberate release of aerosolized spores.
- Construct a case-based scenario that would suggest a naturally occurring cutaneous anthrax infection.

(See Study Question number 8 for examples of case-based scenarios.)

REFERENCES

Aguirre, E., Papenburg, J., Ouakki, M., Fontela, P. S., Guimont, C., De Serres, G., & Bolvin, G. (2011). Comparison of pandemic and seasonal influenza in the pediatric emergency department. *Pediatric Infectious Diseases, 30*(8), 633–639. doi:10.1097/INF.0b013e3182103d54

American Public Health Association, Public Health Nursing Section. (2013). The definition and practice of public health nursing: A statement of the public health nursing section. Retrieved from https://www.apha.org/~/media/files/pdf/membergroups/phn/nursingdefinition.ashx

American Society of Microbiology. (2016). Sentinel level clinical laboratory protocols for suspected biological threat agents and emerging infectious diseases. Retrieved from https://www.asm.org/index.php/science-skills-in-the-lab/sentinel-guidelines

American Veterinary Medical Association. (2017). One Health: It's all connected. Retrieved from https://www.avma.org/KB/Resources/Reference/Pages/One-Health.aspx

Asnis, D. S., Conetta, R., Teixeira, A. A., Waldman, G., & Sampson, B. A. (2000). The West Nile virus outbreak of 1999 in New York: The Flushing Hospital experience. *Clinical Infectious Diseases, 30,* 413–418. doi:10.1086/313737

Barakat, L. A., Quentzel, H. L., Jernigan, J. A., Kirschke, D. L., Griffith, K., Spear, S. M., ... Hadler, J. L. (2002). Fatal inhalational anthrax in a 94-year-old Connecticut woman. *Journal of the American Medical Association, 287,* 863–868. doi:10.1001/jama.287.7.863

Barboza, P., Vaillant, L., Le Strat, Y., Hartley, D. M., Nelson, N. P., Mawudeka, A., ... Astagneau, P. (2014). Factors influencing performance of internet-based biosurveillance systems used in epidemic intelligence for early detection of infectious diseases outbreaks. *PLOS ONE, 9*(3), e90536. doi:10.1371/journal.pone.0090536

Belongia, E. A., Irving, S. A., Waring, S. C., Coleman, L. A., Meece, J. K., Vandermause, M., ... Shay, D. K. (2011). Clinical characteristics and 30-day outcomes for influenza A 2009 (H1N1), 2008–2009 (H1N1), and 2007–2008 (H3N2) infections. *Journal of the American Medical Association, 304*(10), 1091–1098. doi:10.1001/jama.2010.1277

Birkhead, G. S., & Maylahn, C. M. (2010). State and local public health surveillance in the United States. In L. M. Lee, S. M. Teutsch, S. B. Thacker, & M. E. St. Louis (Eds.), *Principles and practice of public health surveillance* (3rd ed., pp. 381–398). New York, NY: Oxford University Press.

Brownstein, J. S., Freifeld, C. C., Chan, E. H., Keller, M., Sonricker, A. L., Mekaru, S. R., & Buckeridge, D. L. (2010). Information technology and global surveillance of cases of 2009 H1N1 influenza. *The New England Journal of Medicine, 362*(18), 1731–1735. doi:10.1056/NEJMsr1002707

Burkle, F. M. (2015). Global health security demands a strong International Health Regulations Treaty and leadership from a highly resourced World Health Organization. *Disaster Medicine and Public Health Preparedness, 9*(5), 1–13. doi:10.1017/dmp.2015.26

Centers for Disease Control and Prevention. (1981a). Kaposi's sarcoma and *Pneumocystis pneumonia* among homosexual men—New York City and California. *MMWR Morbidity and Mortality Weekly Report, 30,* 305–308.

Centers for Disease Control and Prevention. (1981b). Pneumocystis pneumonia—Los Angeles. *MMWR Morbidity and Mortality Weekly Report, 30,* 250–252. doi:10.1016/S0196-6553(97)90061-4

Centers for Disease Control and Prevention. (2000). Biological and chemical terrorism: Strategic plan for preparedness and response. Recommendations of the CDC Strategic Planning Workgroup. *MMWR Morbidity and Mortality Weekly Report, 49*(RR-4), 1–14.

Centers for Disease Control and Prevention. (2001a). Recognition of illness associated with the intentional release of a biologic agent. *MMWR Morbidity and Mortality Weekly Report, 50,* 893–897.

Centers for Disease Control and Prevention. (2001b). Updated guidelines for evaluating public health surveillance systems: Recommendations from the Guidelines Working Group. *MMWR Morbidity and Mortality Weekly Report, 50*(RR-13), 1–35.

Centers for Disease Control and Prevention. (2004). Framework for evaluating public health surveillance systems for early detection of outbreaks: Recommendations from the CDC Working Group. *MMWR Morbidity and Mortality Weekly Report, 53*(RR-05), 1–11.

Centers for Disease Control and Prevention. (2009). Update: Swine influenza A (H1N1) infections—California and Texas, April 2009. *MMWR Morbidity and Mortality Weekly Report, 58*(16), 435-437.

Centers for Disease Control and Prevention. (2011). Assessment of ESSENCE performance for influenza-like illness surveillance after an influenza outbreak—U.S. Air Force Academy, Colorado, 2009. *MMWR Morbidity and Mortality Weekly Report, 60*(13), 406–409.

Centers for Disease Control and Prevention. (2012). *Principles of epidemiology in public health practice* (3rd ed. [Self-Study Course SS1978]). Retrieved from https://www.cdc.gov/ophss/csels/dsepd/ss1978/ss1978.pdf

Centers for Disease Control and Prevention. (2014a). Laboratory network for biological terrorism. Retrieved from https://emergency.cdc.gov/lrn/biological.asp

Centers for Disease Control and Prevention. (2014b). Surveillance and preparedness for Ebola virus disease—New York City, 2014. *MMWR Morbidity and Mortality Weekly Report, 63*(41), 934-936. doi: 10.1111/ajt.13114

Centers for Disease Control and Prevention. (2014c). The Laboratory Response Network partners in preparedness. Retrieved from https://emergency.cdc.gov/lrn/index.asp

Centers for Disease Control and Prevention. (2015a). GeoSentinel. Retrieved from https://wwwnc.cdc.gov/travel/page/geosentinel

Centers for Disease Control and Prevention. (2015b). National Notifiable Diseases Surveillance System (NNDSS). Retrieved from https://wwwn.cdc.gov/nndss/

Centers for Disease Control and Prevention. (2015c). West Nile virus: Surveillance resources. Retrieved from https://www.cdc.gov/westnile/resourcepages/survResources.html

Centers for Disease Control and Prevention. (2016a). National Electronic Disease Surveillance System (NEDSS) Base System (NBS): NBS overview. Retrieved from https://www.cdc.gov/nbs/overview/index.html#About

Centers for Disease Control and Prevention. (2016b). Overview of influenza surveillance in the United States. Retrieved from https://www.cdc.gov/flu/weekly/overview.htm

Centers for Disease Control and Prevention. (2016c). Summary of notifiable infectious diseases and conditions—United States, 2014. *MMWR Morbidity and Mortality Weekly Report, 63*(54);1-152. doi:10.15585/mmwr.mm6354a1

Centers for Disease Control and Prevention. (2017a). 2017 nationally notifiable conditions. Retrieved from https://wwwn.cdc.gov/nndss/conditions/notifiable/2017/

Centers for Disease Control and Prevention. (2017b). About COCA. Retrieved from https://emergency.cdc.gov/coca/about.asp

Centers for Disease Control and Prevention. (2017c). BioSense Platform. Retrieved from https://www.cdc.gov/nssp/biosense/index.html

Centers for Disease Control and Prevention. (2017d). Foodborne Diseases Active Surveillance Network (FoodNet). Retrieved from https://www.cdc.gov/foodnet/index.html

Centers for Disease Control and Prevention. (2017e). Global Disease Detection Operations Center: About us. Retrieved from https://www.cdc.gov/globalhealth/healthprotection/gdd/about.html

Centers for Disease Control and Prevention. (2017f) Health Alert Network (HAN). Retrieved from https://emergency.cdc.gov/han/index.asp

Centers for Disease Control and Prevention. (2017g). Integrated surveillance information systems/NEDSS. Retrieved from https://wwwn.cdc.gov/nndss/nedss.html

Centers for Disease Control and Prevention. (2017h). Laboratory response: On the front lines of America's health. Retrieved from https://www.cdc.gov/phpr/whatwedo/laboratory.htm

Centers for Disease Control and Prevention. (2017i). National Antimicrobial Resistance Monitoring System for Enteric Bacteria (NARMS). Retrieved from https://www.cdc.gov/narms/index.html

Centers for Disease Control and Prevention. (2017j). National Syndromic Surveillance Program (NSSP). Retrieved from https://www.cdc.gov/nssp/overview.html

Centers for Disease Control and Prevention. (2017k). Rabies: Is rabies in your state? Retrieved from https://www.cdc.gov/rabies/location/usa/surveillance/index.html

Centers for Disease Control and Prevention. (2017l). Surveillance case definitions. Retrieved from https://www.cdc.gov/nndss/case-definitions.html

Centers for Disease Control and Prevention. (2017m). Surveillance Data Platform (SDP) with Shared Services. Retrieved from https://www.cdc.gov/sdp/

Centers for Disease Control and Prevention. (2017n). Weekly U.S. influenza surveillance report: FluView. Retrieved from https://www.cdc.gov/flu/weekly

Centers for Disease Control and Prevention. (2017o). Zika virus: Reporting and surveillance. Retrieved from https://www.cdc.gov/zika/reporting/index.html

Chang, M., Glynn, M. K., & Groseclose, S. L. (2003). Endemic, notifiable bioterrorism-related diseases, United States, 1992–1999. *Emerging Infectious Diseases, 9*, 556–564. doi:10.3201/eid0905.020477

Choi, J., Cho, Y., Shim, E., & Woo, H. (2016). Web-based infectious disease surveillance systems and public health perspectives: A systematic review. *BMC Public Health, 16*, 1238. doi:10.1186/s12889-016-3893-0

Coltart, C. E. M., Lindsey, B., Ghinai, I., Johnson, A. M., & Heymann, D. L. (2017). The Ebola outbreak, 2013-2016: Old lessons for new epidemics. *Philosophical Transactions B, The Royal Society, 372*, 20160297. doi:10.1098/rstb.2016.0297

Crisinel, P. A., Barazzone, C., Kaiser, L., L'Huillier, A. G., Taguebue, J., Wagner, N., ... The H1N1 Pediatric Epidemiology Study Group. (2011). Comparison of clinical presentation of respiratory tract infections in H1N1/09-positive and H1N1/09-negative patients. *European Journal of Pediatrics, 171*(1), 159–166. doi:10.1007/s00431-011-1513-7

Department of Homeland Security. (2016a). The BioWatch program factsheet. Retrieved from https://www.dhs.gov/publication/biowatch-program-factsheet

Department of Homeland Security. (2016b). The National Biosurveillance Integration Center fact sheet. Retrieved from https://www.dhs.gov/publication/nbic-one-pager

Dixon, M. A., Dar, O. A., & Heymann, D. L. (2014). Emerging infectious diseases: Opportunities at the human-animal-environment interface. *Veterinary Record, 174*, 546–551. doi:10.1136/vr.g3263

Fine, A., & Layton, M. (2001). Lessons from the West Nile viral encephalitis outbreak in New York City, 1999: Implications for bioterrorism preparedness. *Clinical Infectious Diseases, 32*, 277–282. doi: 10.1086/318469

Gajewski, K. N., Peterson, A. E., Chitale, R. A., Pavlin, J. A., Russell, K. L., & Chretien, J. (2014). A review of evaluations of electronic event-based biosurveillance systems. *PLOS ONE, 9*(10), e111222. doi:10.1371/journal.pone.0111222

Giesecke, J. (2017). *Modern infectious disease epidemiology* (3rd ed.). Boca Raton, FL: CRC Press.

Gordis, L. (2014). *Epidemiology* (5th ed.). Philadelphia, PA: Elsevier.

Gould, D. W., Walker, D., & Yoon, P. W. (2017). The evolution of BioSense: Lessons learned and future directions. *Public Health Reports, 132*(Suppl. 1), 7S–11S. doi:10.1177/0033354917706954

Grundmann, O. (2014). The current state of bioterrorist attack surveillance and preparedness in the US. *Risk Management and Healthcare Policy, 7*, 177–187. doi:10.2147/RMHP.S56047

Guerrisi, C., Turbelin, C., Blanchon, T., Hanslik, T., Bonmarin, I., Levy-Bruhl, D., ... Colizza, V. (2016). Participatory syndromic surveillance of influenza in Europe. *The Journal of Infectious Diseases, 214* (Suppl. 4), S386–S392. doi:10.1093/infdis/jiw280

HealthMap. (n.d.). About HealthMap. Retrieved from http://www.healthmap.org/site/about

Homeland Security Presidential Directive 21. (2007). HSPD-21: Public health and medical preparedness. Retrieved from https://www.hsdl.org/?abstract&did=480002

Influenzanet. (2017). Influenzanet: A network of European citizens fighting against influenza. Retrieved from https://www.influenzanet.eu/en

Institute of Medicine and National Research Council. (1999). Recognizing a covert exposure in a population. In Institute of Medicine & National Research Council (Ed.), *Chemical and biological terrorism: Research and development to improve civilian medical response* (pp. 65–77). Washington, DC: National Academies Press.

Institute of Medicine and National Research Council. (2011). *BioWatch and public health surveillance: Evaluating systems for the early detection of biological threats* [abbreviated version]. Washington, DC: The National Academies Press. doi:10.17226/12688

International Society for Infectious Diseases. (2014). About ProMED-mail. Retrieved from https://www.promedmail.org/aboutus/

International Society of Travel Medicine. (2016). GeoSentinel. Retrieved from http://www.istm.org/geosentinel

Jacobsen, K. H., Aguirrre, A. A., Bailey, C. L., Baranova, A. V., Crooks, A. T., Croitoru, A., ... Agouris, P. (2016). Lessons learned from the Ebola outbreak: Action items for emerging infectious disease preparedness and response. *EcoHealth, 13*, 200–212. doi:10.1007/s10393-016-1100-5

Jernigan, J. A., Stephens, D. S., Ashford, D. A., Omenaca, C., Topiel, M. S., Galbraith, M.,... Anthrax Bioterrorism Investigation Team. (2001). Bioterrorism-related inhalational anthrax: The first 10 cases reported in the United States. *Emerging Infectious Diseases, 7*, 933–944. doi:10.3201/eid0706.010604

Jones, K. E., Patel, N. G., Levy, M. A., Storeygard, A., Balk, D., Gittleman, J. L., & Daszak, P. (2008). Global trends in emerging infectious diseases [Letter]. *Nature, 451*, 990-991. doi:10.1038/nature06536

Karlsson, O. E., Hansen, T., Knutsson, R., Löfström, C., Granberg, F., & Berg, M. (2013). Metagenomic detection methods in biopreparedness outbreak scenarios. *Biosecurity and Bioterrorism Biodefense: Strategy, Practice and Science, 11*(Suppl. 1), S146–S157. doi:10.1089/bsp2012.0077

Katz, R., May, L., Baker, J., & Test, E. (2011). Redefining syndromic surveillance. *Journal of Epidemiology and Public Health, 1*, 21–31. doi:10.1016/j.jegh.2011.06.003

Khan, A. S., Fleischauer, A., Casani, J., & Groseclose, S. L. (2010). The next public health revolution: Public health information fusion and social networks. *American Journal of Public Health, 100*, 1237–1242. doi:10.2105/AJPH.2009.180489

Kim, J., Gedi, V., Lee, S-C., Cho, J-H., Moon, J-Y., & Yoon, M-Y. (2015). Advances in anthrax detection: Overview of bioprobes and biosensors. *Applied Biochemistry and Biotechnology, 176*, 957–977. doi.:10.1007/s12010-1625-z

Kluberg, S. A., Mekaru, S. R., McIver, D. J., Madoff, L. C., Crawley, A. W., Smolinski, M. S., & Brownstein, J. S. (2016). Global capacity for emerging infectious disease detection, 1996-2014. *Emerging Infectious Diseases, 22*(10), e1–e9. doi:10.3201/eid2210.151956

Mackenzie, J. S., Drury, P., Arthur, R. R., Ryan, M. J., Grein, T., Slattery, R., ... Bejtullahu, A. (2014). The Global Outbreak Alert and Response Network. *Global Public Health, 9*, 1023–1039. doi:10.1080/17441692.2014.951870

Memish, Z. A., Al-Tawfiq, J. A., Makhdoom, H. Q., Al-Rabeeah, A. A., Assiri, A., Alhakeem, R. F., … Zumla, A. (2014). Screening for Middle East respiratory syndrome coronavirus infection in hospital patients and their healthcare worker and family contacts: A prospective descriptive study. *Clinical Microbiology and Infection, 20,* 469–474. doi:10.1111/1469-0691.12562

Milinovich, G., Williams, G. M., Clements, A. C. A., & Hu, W. (2014). Internet-based surveillance systems for monitoring emerging infectious diseases. *The Lancet Infectious Diseases, 14*(2), 160–168. doi:10.1016/S1473.3099(13)70244-5

Morse, S. S., Mazet, J. A. K., Woolhouse, M., Parrish, C. R., Carroll, D., Karesh, W. B., … Daszak, P. (2012). Prediction and prevention of the next pandemic zoonosis. *Lancet, 380*(9857), 1956-1965. doi:10.1016/S0140-6736(12)61684-5

National Center for Emerging and Zoonotic Infectious Diseases. (2016). Epidemiology and laboratory capacity for infectious diseases (ELC) cooperative agreement. Retrieved from https://www.cdc.gov/ncezid/dpei/epidemiology-laboratory-capacity.html

National Center for Emerging and Zoonotic Infectious Diseases. (2017). About the Emerging Infections Program. Retrieved from https://www.cdc.gov/ncezid/dpei/eip/index.html

Nelson, N. P., Brownstein, J. S., & Hartley, D. M. (2010). Event-based biosurveillance of respiratory disease in Mexico, 2007–2009: Connection to the 2009 influenza A (H1N1) pandemic? *Euro Surveillance, 15*(30). Retrieved from http://www.eurosurveillance.org/ViewArticle.aspx?ArticleId=19626

Nelson, N. P., Yang, L., Reilly, A. R., Hardin, J. E., & Hartley, D. M. (2012). Event-based internet biosurveillance: Relation to epidemiological observation. *Emerging Themes in Epidemiology, 9*(4).doi:10.1186/1742-7622-9-4

Olano, J. P., & Walker, D. H. (2011). Diagnosing emerging and reemerging infectious diseases: The pivotal role of the pathologist. *Archives of Pathology and Laboratory Medicine, 135,* 83–91. doi:10.1043/2010-0260-RAR.1

Peppa, M., Edmunds, W. J., & Funk, S. (2017). Disease severity determines health-seeking behaviour amongst individuals with influenza-like illness in an internet-based cohort. *BMC Infectious Diseases, 17,* 238. doi:10.1186/s12879-017-2337-5

Perrotta, D., Bella, A., Rizzo, C., & Paolotti, D. (2017). Participatory online surveillance as a supplementary tool to sentinel doctors for influenza-like illness surveillance in Italy. *PLOS ONE, 12*(1), e169801. doi:10.1371/journal.pone.0169801

Public Health Agency of Canada, Centre for Emergency Preparedness and Response. (2017). About GPHIN. Retrieved from https://gphin.canada.ca/cepr/aboutgphin-rmispenbref.jsp?language=en_CA

Rao, S. S., Mohan, K. V. K., & Atreya, C. D. (2010). Detection technologies for *Bacillus anthracis*: Prospects and challenges. *Journal of Microbial Methods, 82,* 1–10. doi:10.1016/j.mimet.2010.04.005

Reynolds, T., Gordon, S., Soper, P., Buehler, J., Hopkins, R., & Streichert, L. (2015). Syndromic surveillance practice in the United States 2014: Results from a nationwide survey [Abstract]. *Online Journal of Public Health Informatics, 7*(1), e90. doi:10.5210/ojphi.v7i1.5756

Schirmer P., Lucero, C., Oda, G., Lopez, J., & Holodniy, M. (2010). Effective detection of the 2009 H1N1 influenza pandemic in U.S. Veterans Affairs Medical Centers using a national electronic biosurveillance system. *PLOS ONE, 5,* e9533. doi:10.1371/journal.pone.0009533

Sosin, D. M., & Hopkins, R. S. (2010). Public health surveillance for preparedness and emergency response. In L. M. Lee, S. M. Teutsch, S. B. Thacker, & M. E. St. Louis (Eds.), *Principles and practice of public health surveillance* (3rd ed., pp. 306–320). New York, NY: Oxford University Press.

Teutsch, S. M. (2010). Considerations in planning a surveillance system. In L. M. Lee, S. M. Teutsch, S. B. Thacker, & M. E. St. Louis (Eds.), *Principles and practice of public health surveillance* (3rd ed., pp. 18–31). New York, NY: Oxford University Press.

Tokars, J., English, J., McMurray, P., & Rhodes, B. (2010). Summary of data reported to CDC's national automated biosurveillance system, 2008. *BMC Medical Informatics and Decision Making, 10,* 30. doi:10.1186/1472-6947-10-30

Török, T. J., Tauxe, R. V., Wise, R. P., Livengood, J. R., Sokolow, R., Mauvais, S.,… Foster, L. R. (1997). A large community outbreak of salmonellosis caused by intentional contamination of restaurant salad bars. *Journal of the American Medical Association, 278,* 389–395. doi:10.1001/jama.1997.03550050051033

U.S. Agency for International Development. (2016). Emerging pandemic threats. Retrieved from https://www.usaid.gov/news-information/fact-sheets/emerging-pandemic-threats-program

U.S. Army Medical Research Institute of Infectious Diseases. (2014). *USAMRIID's medical management of biological casualties handbook* (8th ed.). Frederick, MD: Author.

U.S. Department of Agriculture. (2017). National Animal Health Reporting System (NAHRS). Retrieved from https://www.aphis.usda.gov/aphis/ourfocus/animalhealth/monitoring-and-surveillance/SA_Disease_Reporting

U.S. Department of Health and Human Services & Centers for Disease Control and Prevention. (1998, October). *Preventing emerging infectious diseases: A strategy for the 21st century.* Reprinted February 2000. Atlanta, GA: Author.

U.S. Department of Health and Human Services & Centers for Disease Control and Prevention. (2001, July). *The public health response to biological and chemical terrorism: Interim planning guidance for state public health officials.* Retrieved from https://emergency.cdc.gov/documents/planning/planningguidance.pdf

Van Beneden, C. A., & Lynfield, R. (2010). Public health surveillance for infectious diseases. In L. M. Lee, S. M. Teutsch, S. B. Thacker, & M. E. St. Louis (Eds.), *Principles and practice of public health surveillance* (3rd ed., pp. 236–254). New York, NY: Oxford University Press.

Velasco, E., Agheneza, T., Denecke, K., Kirchner, G., & Eckmanns, T. (2014). Social media and internet-based data in global systems for public health: A systematic review. *The Milbank Quarterly, 92*(1), 7–33. doi:10.1111/1468-0009.12038

Wilson, K., & Brownstein, J. S. (2009). Early detection of disease outbreaks using the internet. *Canadian Medical Association Journal, 180*(8), 829–831. doi:10.150/cmaj.090215

World Health Organization. (2005). Notification and other reporting requirements under the IHR (2005). IHR Brief No. 2. Retrieved from http://www.who.int/ihr/ihr_brief_no_2_en.pdf

World Health Organization. (2017a). Disease Outbreak News (DONs). Retrieved from http://www.who.int/csr/don/en

World Health Organization. (2017b). Ebola outbreak Democratic Republic of the Congo 2017. Retrieved from http://www.who.int/emergencies/ebola-DRC-2017/en

World Health Organization. (2017c). Epidemic intelligence: Systematic event detection. Retrieved from http://www.who.int/csr/alertresponse/epidemicintelligence/en

World Health Organization. (2017d). Event verification. Retrieved from http://www.who.int/csr/alertresponse/verification/en

World Health Organization. (2017e). Global Outbreak Alert and Response Network (GOARN). Retrieved from http://www.who.int/ihr/alert_and_response/outbreak-network/en

World Health Organization. (2017f). International Health Regulations (IHR): About IHR. Retrieved from http://www.who.int/ihr/about/en

World Health Organization. (2017g). New technology allows for rapid diagnosis of Ebola in the Democratic Republic of the Congo. Retrieved from http://www.who.int/emergencies/ebola-DRC-2017/articles/rapid-diagnosis/en

World Health Organization. (2017h). The Weekly Epidemiological Record (WER). Retrieved from http://www.who.int/wer/en

World Organisation for Animal Health. (2017a). About us. Retrieved from http://www.oie.int/about-us

World Organisation for Animal Health. (2017b). The World Animal Health Information System. Retrieved from http://www.oie.int/animal-health-in-the-world/the-world-animal-health-information-system/the-oie-data-system

32

INFECTIOUS DISEASE EMERGENCIES

Kristine M. Gebbie and Kristine Qureshi

LEARNING OBJECTIVES

When this chapter is completed, readers will be able to:

1. Describe the relationships between emergencies and infectious diseases.
2. Identify factors contributing to emerging or resurgent infections.
3. Explain the epidemiological triangle.
4. List infectious diseases of high concern.
5. Describe key actions necessary to limit or end an infectious disease emergency.
6. Discuss future directions in the fight against infectious diseases.
7. Explain the potential roles of nurses in prevention, detection, and response to vectorborne epidemics.

KEY MESSAGES

Infectious disease is a major cause of global morbidity and mortality, often causing or associated with large-scale public health emergencies. Ninety percent of all infectious disease deaths are caused by only six diseases, of which half are due to three long-known infections (tuberculosis, malaria, and HIV).

The emergence or resurgence of an infectious disease requires the convergence of complex factors that can be genetic and biological, physical, ecological, social, political, or behavioral in nature.

Many emerging pathogens are *zoonotic* (communicated by animals to humans, or between humans or animals through an intermediary vector such as an insect).

Emergencies caused by infectious conditions may occur as the primary event, or a secondary challenge following or worsening another type of emergency.

Identifying and limiting any infectious disease is a constant challenge to public health systems and the communities they serve, especially so in emergency or disaster situations.

One Health recognizes that the health of people is connected to the health of animals and the environment. The goal of One Health is to encourage the collaborative efforts of multiple disciplines—working locally, nationally, and globally—to achieve the best health for people, animals, and our environment.

CHAPTER OVERVIEW

Despite the elimination of smallpox, the dramatic reduction in exposure to guinea worm in Africa and control of many vaccine-preventable diseases (e.g., polio), there is no indication that the challenge of epidemic infection has been eliminated. In fact, in 2017, the World Health Organization (WHO, 2017a) reported on Middle Eastern Respiratory Syndrome (MERS) in Saudi Arabia, human avian influenza A (H7N9) virus in China, Lassa fever in Nigeria, cholera in Syria, and vaccine-derived polio virus type 2 in the Democratic Republic of the Congo. Zika virus received a great deal of attention because of the secondary effects of what is usually a survivable infection (Centers for Disease Control and Prevention [CDC], 2017g).

Emerging infectious diseases (EIDs) are those that are newly evolved (e.g., severe acute respiratory syndrome [SARS]) or have altered their geographical range (e.g., West Nile virus; Morse, 1995). From the mid-20th century until the advent of AIDS in the 1980s, public health in the economically developed world had focused a majority of its efforts and resources on the prevention and mitigation of chronic diseases, believing that infectious diseases had been controlled to exist at an insignificant level. The global eradication of smallpox was seen as a key validation of this perspective (Institute of Medicine [IOM], 2005). This chapter provides both a context and specific information to assist nurses to identify and appropriately respond to infectious diseases in emergencies.

INFECTIOUS DISEASES AND EMERGENCIES

Infectious diseases that increase in incidence and prevalence, possibly to the point of epidemic, pandemic, or emergency, can be classified as being in one of three groups:

- *Emerging*—infections that have newly appeared in a human population and have not been previously known, such as SARS or new strains of avian influenza
- *Reemerging or resurging*—infections that have been known but demonstrate a marked increase in incidence or geographical range, such as the enormous surge of Ebola in West Africa or the reappearance of paralytic polio in countries that had stopped the condition

- *Deliberately emerging*—natural or bioengineered agents distributed by individuals as a criminal act of bioterrorism, such as the anthrax cases in the United States in the fall of 2001 or another agent that could be genetically modified to result in a greater impact (Morens, Folkers, & Fauci, 2004)

While the third category often receives the greatest attention from emergency and disaster response planners because of the anxiety associated with any deliberate attempt to harm the public, it is the least frequent of any infectious events. Any social disruption such as civil unrest or war can influence a sudden upswing in infections, as has happened in the three countries never certified as achieving the goal of over 99% reduction in paralytic polio (Pakistan, Nigeria, and Afghanistan). The disease in these countries also leads to increased risk and anxiety in border areas such as Eastern Europe (WHO, 2017a).

Any increase in the incidence and prevalence of a disease in a community is of concern, and public health agencies routinely monitor and require reporting of infectious diseases, watching for any indication of a developing emergency. Unlike the sudden, visible onset of an emergency associated with a hurricane, blizzard, transportation crash, earthquake, or explosion, infectious diseases may incubate in a community for hours or days, spread at varying rates, and not be identified immediately as an emergency until the number of diagnosed cases suddenly rises. Even when deliberately initiated, there may be no single "event" that initiates an emergency response. Likewise, unlike a fire that can be extinguished, or the removal of injured from a building collapse within a matter of hours or at most days, the spread of disease may continue for an extended period as treatment, prevention, and control measures are put in place. Nurses and other health professionals must remain alert to signs of infection, guided in part by subscriptions to local state or national public health alert systems. Finally, a public health emergency may be part of the aftermath of almost any other kind of emergency if proper steps to assure the public's health are not instituted when a disaster causes populations to be displaced or the community infrastructure to be disrupted.

From the public health perspective, any epidemic (a sudden increase above the expected number of cases in a specific period of time) or pandemic (worldwide spread) needs thoughtful attention and rapid implementation of control measures. The greatest concern is triggered by an epidemic or pandemic of a disease for which there is little or no immunity in the population, transmission from person to person is easy, and there is a high mortality rate in the absence of accessible definitive treatment. In addition to treatment of infected individuals when possible, actions may include isolation of the infected until no risks to others are posed or quarantine of those exposed until they are free of disease past the known incubation period. The West Africa Ebola epidemic of 2014–2016, which led to over 28,000 cases and over 11,000 deaths (WHO, 2017c), was magnified by the emergence of this known disease in areas that had long-standing population-supported cultural funeral practices that facilitated the rapid spread of the virus and very little health infrastructure. Clarifying not only the geographical extent of a disease, but also how it is measured in terms of ease of transmission, existing population immunity, availability of treatment, severity, and potential for prevention present a significant public communication problem. Announcing "a worldwide pandemic" of a transmissible, severe infection may be meaningful within the healthcare and public health community but is likely to cause confusion and anxiety within the broader population.

BRIEF HISTORY

In the late 1960s, testifying before Congress, U.S. Surgeon General William T. Stewart claimed "victory" in the war against infectious diseases. Stewart, along with other members of the medical and scientific communities, believed that there had been a transition in which burden of infectious disease had waned and chronic disease had become the dominant cause of morbidity and mortality in the modern age (Fauci, 2001). One comment from that period is:

> During his seminar on Drugs for Neglected Diseases Initiative and Product Development Partnerships, Dr. Philip Coyne noted that historically some scientists reported that in the near future all major infections would be eradicated. (Coyne, n.d.)

This perceived *epidemiological shift* from infectious to chronic disease had three stages:

- *The age of pestilence and famine*, characterized by high mortality rates and an inability to sustain population growth during a period when the science of microbiology had not developed
- *The age of receding pandemics*, with a decline in the mortality rate as epidemics became less frequent in a healthier population supported by improved science
- *The age of degenerative and man-made diseases*, continuing the decline in infectious disease mortality and emerging attention to conditions associated with gradual increases in life expectancy

In this final stage, Omran predicted that heart disease and cancer would become the greatest causes of morbidity and mortality, although the threat of infectious diseases was still very real (Omran, 2005). By 2016, obesity as a precursor to diabetes and other chronic conditions would be added to the list of noninfectious concerns, as dietary and lifestyle changes contribute to its increase, even in countries still experiencing malnutrition and starvation. However, in the 21st century, it is evident that while it is true that longer life spans associated with improved public health are associated with a global increase in degenerative and lifestyle-associated diseases, it is not possible to move away from simultaneous attention to infectious conditions.

THE BURDEN OF INFECTIOUS DISEASE

According to the WHO, in 2017, infectious diseases still accounted for approximately 15% of deaths globally, but 60% of deaths in Africa. The increase in noncommunicable disease deaths, and the development of health systems and treatment globally did reduce the proportion of communicable disease deaths to 10% (WHO, 2017f), but the numbers remain significant despite this statistical shift. Leading causes of infectious disease deaths are:

- Diarrheal disease
- HIV/AIDS
- Malaria
- Childhood diseases, primarily measles
- Pneumonia
- Tuberculosis
- Hepatitis B

These mortality figures do not take into account the burden of caring for infected individuals, both those who die and those who recover, nor the millions of cases of conditions secondary to infection, such as liver failure from hepatitis C, streptococcal rheumatic heart, or disability following paralytic polio. As with many problems, the burdens of infectious diseases are unequally distributed; areas with high levels of poverty, limited access to safe water or waste disposal, inadequate housing and nutrition carry the largest burdens (WHO, 2017f). It is these same factors that often follow a disaster, such as an earthquake, a widespread civil unrest, war, or failure of the health system, and make infectious disease emergencies possible.

While often discussed separately, vectorborne illnesses are another important group of infectious diseases that are implicated in serious outbreaks or epidemics. Each year there are 1 billion people affected by vectorborne diseases, and 1 million die from these illnesses (WHO, 2016b). Such diseases are transmitted primarily by vectors including mosquitos, flies, ticks, fleas, and snails. The epidemiological triangle composed of (a) agent (causative organism for the illness), (b) environment (factors that support the transmission, e.g., habitat for the vector, or surroundings of the host), and (c) host (a human who is susceptible to the disease) illustrates the factors that influence the spread of vectorborne illness. In vectorborne illness, an insect or animal carries the disease agent between an animal or another human to the susceptible host (Figure 32.1). Emergencies or disasters that markedly disrupt the environment can lead to conditions that support an increase in the vector population or reduce resistance and increase susceptibility of the host. Nurses need to be keenly aware of such conditions, as interventions aimed at the environment and or the host can markedly reduce the number of new cases.

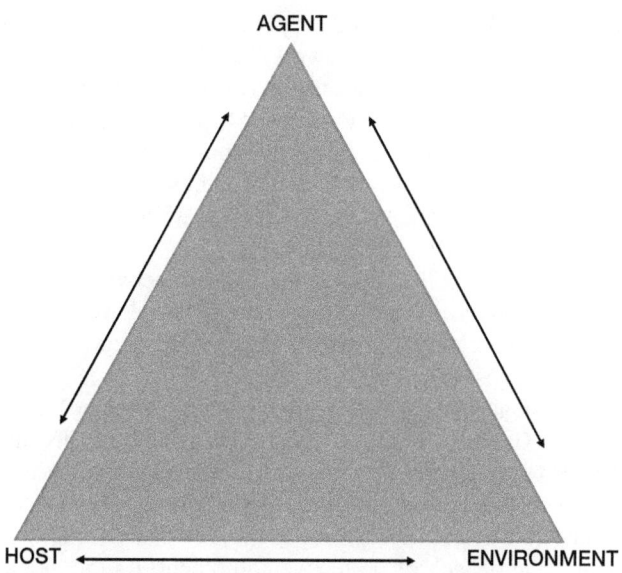

FIGURE 32.1 The epidemiological triangle.

FACTORS CONTRIBUTING TO THE SPREAD OF INFECTIOUS DISEASES

The emergence and spread of an epidemic requires the convergence of a diverse set of individual, social, and environmental factors (Table 32.1; IOM, 2003). Without an extensive analysis of all of these, the following discussion highlights some of the key issues.

Immune Status

Host susceptibility, the level of the ability of a human to ward off disease, is one of the most important factors in determining whether a microbe will successfully cause disease. The human immune system is a complex response to unfamiliar entities introduced into the body, and when functioning well is able to sustain health in the face of multiple challenges. The widespread use of vaccines has increased the proportion of the population that can successfully ward off many conditions such as measles that otherwise cause severe illness or death. One of the almost-defeated conditions, paralytic poliomyelitis, continues

to be a challenge as a 2011 outbreak in China revealed. The immunocompromised (e.g., those with HIV, on medication following an organ transplant, or undergoing cancer treatment) are much more susceptible to disease than those with healthy immune systems. The overuse of antibiotics that decrease the bacterial flora can also affect the immune systems of even immunocompetent hosts, and contributes to the emergence of organisms resistant to treatment. In addition, malnutrition, associated with approximately 45% of all child deaths worldwide annually, affects host resistance (WHO, 2016a). The complexity of maintaining immunity is illustrated by the annual reformulation of vaccine against influenza, as the viral agent undergoes rapid change from year to year. Appearance of a new form of influenza (or any other microbial agent) is likely to lead to an increase in disease burden.

Climate and Weather

Alternations in weather conditions, both short term and long term, have a strong influence on infectious conditions. For example, El Niño, a period of strong and prolonged warm weather, is associated with increased rates of death and disease associated with weather-related disasters such as floods and droughts. Increases in infectious, vectorborne diseases such as malaria, dengue, and Rift Valley fever can be attributed to El Niño because the standing pools of water created by increased rainfall become a rich breeding ground for mosquitos in wet weather (WHO, 2012).

Climate Change and the Changing Environment

Approximately 75% of emerging pathogens are *zoonotic*, or communicated by animals to humans. Climate change results in alteration of weather patterns and the earth's ecosystems. As temperatures rise and precipitation increases, the range of insect vectors (especially mosquitos) expands into new areas. This increases human contact with insect vectors and the likelihood of vectorborne outbreaks (National Institute of Environmental Health Sciences [NIEHS], 2017). In addition, as communities move or grow and intrude into surrounding ecosystems, pathogens have the opportunity to move from their long-standing animal hosts to humans, directly or through animal or arthropod vectors. Land development, deforestation, dam building, changes in farming techniques, and the

TABLE 32.1 Factors in Emergence of Infectious Diseases

• Microbial adaption and change	• International travel and commerce
• Human susceptibility to infection	• Technology and industry
• Climate and weather	• Breakdown of public health measures
• Changing ecosystems	• Poverty and social inequality
• Human demographics and behavior	• War and famine

Source: From Institute of Medicine (2003). *Microbial threats to health: Emergence, detection, and response.* Washington, DC: National Academies Press. Copyright 2007 by the National Academy of Sciences. Reprinted with permission.

consumption of natural resources all influence ecosystems as well. Rapid urbanization is associated with such disruptions, as new city residents often obtain housing in areas that have poor sanitation, crowded living conditions, and limited health and public health services. Megacities, those urban settings in which the population exceeds 10 million, including Manila, Calcutta, Cairo, San Paulo, London, and New York, are at increased risk for devastation resulting from postdisaster environmental hazards and infectious disease outbreaks (Khan & Pappas, 2011). Of the world's 31 megacities in 2016, 24 are located in the less developed regions of the world (United Nations, 2016), exacerbating their vulnerability to the impact of an infectious disease outbreak.

Risk Behaviors

Individual human behavior is also a part of many factors increasing conditions for the spread of infectious diseases. Two areas of human behavior that have received extensive attention in recent years are sexual and recreational drug use practices that facilitate the transmission of organisms in a population. Sexually transmitted infections (STIs), including HIV, gonorrhea, syphilis, and chlamydia, are spread among individuals who have multiple sexual partners and who do not routinely use condoms for at least partial protection. According to the WHO's 2016 estimate, over 1 million STIs (syphilis, gonorrhea, chlamydia, and trichomoniasis) are acquired every day (WHO, 2017e). The sharing of equipment for injecting substances such as heroin results in the sharing of bloodborne pathogens such as hepatitis C or HIV. As with the behavioral factors that contribute to chronic diseases (e.g., use of tobacco products; high-fat, high-calorie diets; limited physical activity), the human behavior and social dynamics associated with sexual activity and substance use/abuse must be taken into account in preventing or stopping an increase in infectious diseases (IOM, 2003).

International Travel and Commerce

The history of infectious disease spread is the history of population movement and travel. A population living in isolation may experience a spike in infections if a new pathogen is introduced, but that community will either be eliminated by the death of the entire population or will achieve symbiosis with the disease. Today, individuals travel to every corner of the globe quickly and easily, carrying their diseases along. While this has long been true (e.g., the history of disease and death in indigenous populations following European exploration and settlement, or the spread of plague following invading armies in the medieval period), the speed of modern travel has accented the risks. Travelers can bring diseases from "home" into a new area, or can be exposed to new pathogens in their destination. SARS was brought to Toronto from Hong Kong by a returning traveler, leading to an outbreak of 257 cases across Canada (2003). In addition to the 41 deaths (a 17% case fatality rate), there was substantial economic impact, as Toronto's tourism industry lost several million dollars because of a travel advisory that limited travel to Toronto (Conference Board of Canada, 2003). Fears of SARS disrupted travel plans for many, and led to marked increased requests for medical care or public health action in many other locations as well.

The globalization of food supply and the development of extensive food distribution networks have increased the risk of foodborne disease outbreaks that may occur far from the site of the pathogen's introduction into the food change. The CDC continues to monitor Maradol papayas imported from Mexico following outbreaks of two strains of salmonella. By August 2017, there were 109 cases in 16 states with 35 hospitalizations and one death (CDC, 2017c).

One example of the broad impact that an otherwise regional epidemic can have is the global response to the West Africa Ebola outbreak of 2014–2016. The Ebola epidemic was the first and largest epidemic of its kind, with widespread urban transmission and a massive death count of more than 11,300 people in Guinea, Liberia, and Sierra Leone. It quickly became clear that the impact of the disease on the already limited health system of the involved rural areas was devastating, with many healthcare workers succumbing to the disease due to lack of knowledge or lack of protective equipment. As the global community responded with health professionals traveling to become part of the response teams, some of those volunteers were exposed to the virus and were returned to their home countries for treatment. Cases of Ebola from the West Africa epidemic were diagnosed in healthcare workers and treated in Europe and the United States. The extremely high level of personal protective gear needed by caregivers caused fear on the part of the receiving countries' healthcare workers, though in some cases further exposure occurred because the recommended protective steps were not precisely followed. Further, at least one infectious individual was seen, returned home, and seen again before sufficient attention was paid to the combination of symptoms and recent travel to make an accurate diagnosis. Fortunately, this happened before multiple transmissions occurred and in a place where a high level of care was available. Nonetheless, the global cost of response was accentuated by these distant exposures secondary to the main epidemic.

DISEASES OF IMPORTANCE

Diseases of particular importance to address in disaster and emergency planning and response activities are those that are known to be (a) highly contagious, (b) have a high mortality rate, and (c) to which there is no or limited human immunity coupled with either no available treatment, or treatment to which the organism is resistant. In addition to the individual human burden, infectious diseases meeting these conditions have potential for serious economic impact locally or in a wider region. Given the criteria, almost any disease that can be traced to a viral or bacterial agent can become of importance if it becomes more virulent, migrates to a new geographical area, or is distributed differently by an animal or insect vector. For that reason, this chapter discusses in some detail six conditions of particular importance (cholera, dengue fever, HIV, influenza, Marburg hemorrhagic fever, and smallpox). Some of these diseases are more common than others and some are rare but harbor the potential to cause great illness. Considered together, these diseases serve to illustrate the challenges of responding to an infectious disease that is on the increase and is now or may one day become an emergency.

Cholera

Cholera is a disease that quickly may emerge into a public health emergency. Cholera spreads through drinking water or food contaminated by the bacterium *Vibrio cholerae*; large epidemics often stem from water supplies contaminated by fecal matter. Following the 2010 earthquake in Haiti, a major outbreak of cholera occurred, afflicting at least 770,000 Haitians and claiming over 9,200 lives. The Haitian epidemic alone resulted in an 85% increase in the number of cholera cases worldwide. According to the WHO, even prior to the earthquake, many Haitian households could have been at risk of a disease such as cholera due to a lack of safe water, sewage disposal or adequate housing and nutrition, even though there had been no reported cases for 100 years (WHO, 2011b). The earthquake aggravated the risk conditions, making apparent the lack of healthcare personnel and treatment resources (WHO, 2011a). Later analysis revealed that the postearthquake epidemic was confirmed to be a strain of the causal organism (*V. cholerae*) generally found in Southeast Asia, rather than the strains present elsewhere in Latin America (Chin et al., 2011). The Haitian outbreak is believed to have started near a UN camp hosting peacekeepers from Nepal who were in Haiti for relief efforts (*National Geographic News*, 2016).

Cholera infection can be a mild gastroenteritis, but about 5% of those infected develop severe diarrhea, and the high mortality rate associated with these severe cases is due to dehydration. Rehydration (with oral rehydration salts or intravenous fluids/electrolytes) can reduce the case fatality rate to below 1%. Introduction of the organism into an environment of healthy, well-nourished people with safe drinking water and modern sewage disposal might lead to a small number of cases, and possibly no deaths or hospitalizations. However, the Haitian experience vividly illustrates the burden of an infection imposed on an already stressed locale in which provision of basic sanitation has not been accomplished, and what might have been a stressful period of rebuilding the Port-au-Prince area has been further extended and complicated by the loss of life and the large number needing care. The traditional nursing interest in cleanliness and sanitation is essential for infection control (Table 32.2).

Dengue Fever

Dengue fever is a mosquitoborne viral infection that affects approximately 400 million humans each year (CDC, 2016a). The disease is on the rise worldwide and is endemic in tropical and subtropical areas of the globe. The WHO estimates that 40% of the world population is at risk of contracting the disease in more than 100 countries (WHO, 2017b). Dengue infection produces a flu-like illness that can range from mild to severe dengue illness. There are four subtypes of the dengue virus and it is thought that reinfection with the same subtype twice increases risk of a severe dengue reaction (CDC, 2016a). Currently, there is no available vaccine to prevent contracting dengue fever, and treatment includes supportive care. As the world's climate warms, it is expected that the range of the mosquito that carries dengue fever will expand, thus exposing more humans to the disease. Currently, the best method to control dengue fever is prevention. Key steps in prevention include: employ vector control (eliminate standing water breeding grounds for mosquitos and reduce mosquito population with environmental insecticide); reduce contact with mosquitos by covering skin with clothing and assuring screens on homes and use of approved mosquito nets impregnated with insecticide; reduce outdoor activities during the time of day the mosquito is most active (*Aedes aegypti* most active 2 hours after sunrise and 2 hours before sunset); and use insecticides on the skin. People who are infected with dengue fever can serve as a source for spread of the virus, as a mosquito bites one infected person and then serves as a vector to transmit the virus when it bites a second individual (Table 32.3).

Efforts that focus on environmental control coupled with good risk communication and extensive public education are required to control large-scale dengue fever outbreaks and prevent even larger epidemics. Community-based nurses have important roles to play in the prevention and response to dengue fever emergencies. Emergency nurses must be on the alert as they may be the first to notice a number of cases with suspicious signs and symptoms and should report any suspicion to their

TABLE 32.2 Clinical Profile of Cholera

Transmission	Clinical Symptoms	Diagnosis	Therapy
Exposure to drinking water or food contaminated by feces of an infected individual	Mild infection, little or mild gastrointestinal distress	Symptomatic, with definitive diagnosis based on laboratory examination of stool specimen	Immediate fluid and electrolyte replacement, with oral rehydration solution in large amounts
Direct person-to-person transmission unlikely	Severe disease (~5% of cases), profuse, watery diarrhea, vomiting, leg cramps		Intravenous fluid and electrolyte replacement may be needed in severe cases
	Death can occur within hours if severe disease not treated promptly		

TABLE 32.3 Dengue Fever

Transmission	Clinical Symptoms	Diagnosis	Therapy

Between people via mosquitos	• MILD: Principal symptoms are high fever and at least two of the following:
	  • Severe headache with pain behind the eyes
	  • Arthralgia
	  • Muscle and or bone pain
	  • Rash
	  • Mild bleeding (gums, petechiae)
	  • Low white blood cell count
	• SEVERE: Any of the following symptoms require emergency medical attention. Usually progresses after a 2–7-day febrile phase:
	  • Severe abdominal pain
	  • Red spots on the skin
	  • Bleeding from nose or gums (heavy)
	  • Vomiting blood or black, tarry stools
	  • Drowsiness or irritability
	  • Pale, cold, clammy skin
	  • Difficulty breathing
		• Clinical symptoms
		• Lab tests: early: 1–5 days (virus, viral nucleic acid, antigens)
		• Lab tests: later: after day 5 (antibodies)
		• Differential diagnosis: yellow fever, Japanese encephalitis, St. Louis encephalitis, Zika and West Nile virus
		• During a confirmed large-scale outbreak, diagnosis is made by clinical signs and symptoms
			• Fever management (acetaminophen only, NO ibuprofen or aspirin-containing medications)
			• Fluid management
			• Close monitoring for progression to warning signs which signal severe dengue

medical director and public health officials. Such actions can serve to avert a larger epidemic. Hospital nurses need to stay abreast of current techniques for fluid management, which is the mainstay of treatment for persons with severe dengue.

HIV/AIDS

HIV is spread through certain body fluids that attack the body's immune system, specifically the CD4 cells, often called "T cells," reducing the body's ability to fight off infections and disease. Left untreated, HIV reduces the number of CD4 cells (T cells) damaging the immune system and allowing for opportunistic infections and/or cancers. In the 1980s, HIV infection illustrated the challenges to the public health and medical care sectors when a new disease is identified and the public is highly fearful. This disease was likely endemic in some parts of Africa for an extended period before modern transportation and human behavior moved the disease into urban areas and into the western hemisphere. The disease was officially identified in 1981, though the causal organism was not known at that time (CDC, 2017b). The early clusters of U.S. cases in New York city and southern California were individuals with advanced stages of the disease and suffering from other opportunistic infections that could flourish in the absence of a good immune system. The lack of clarity on the full-life course of the disease presented a challenge to diagnosis, and the full extent of the epidemic, though the viral, bloodborne nature of the disease was hypothesized early, proved true. The public health response to the disease was complicated by multiple social factors, including the following:

■ The initial identification of the disease in men who had sex with men, a taboo subject in many parts of society
■ A high rate of infection in a group of migrant workers (Haitians working in the United States) that led to discriminatory actions against an entire nation

■ The association of the disease with multiple sexual partners and sex for money, another taboo topic
■ The spread of the disease in injecting drug users, a group that many considered beyond the pale of society and suffering from stigma and the perception of a deliberately induced problem

All of this led to an artificial separation of so-called "innocent victims" (newborns, boys with hemophilia, unsuspecting wives of closeted homosexual men) from others; hysterical fear of spread of the disease to the "general population" (which apparently does not include any of the above); and political activism on multiple fronts. The eventual isolation of the virus, development of diagnostic testing, availability of medications to treat opportunistic infections and control the virus itself, all place enormous strains on communities. HIV infection was associated with an increase in tuberculosis (among those infected, but also elsewhere in the community as resources were diverted to the new disease) and malaria, and in some countries, drastically reduced the life expectancy. A further challenge was the birth of infected babies to mothers with the virus.

This emergency did not occur overnight, and did not lead to the activation of community-wide emergency response systems, but presents an excellent example of an evolving public health emergency complicated by prejudice and resource constraints. The current availability of treatment has meant the marked reduction in neonatal HIV infection (77% of infected pregnant women receiving antiretroviral therapy), and an increase in life expectancy for those who can access and maintain treatment. Between 2000 and 2015, the death rate from the disease fell by 28%, even though only 60% of the infected know their status and only 46% were being treated (WHO, 2017d). There is no guarantee that there will not be some other new condition that emerges with similar challenges to communities (Table 32.4).

TABLE 32.4 Clinical Profile of HIV/AIDS

Transmission	Clinical Symptoms	Diagnosis	Therapy
• Exposure to causal agent (the HIV retrovirus) through blood or semen of infected individual (sexual activity or sharing injection equipment most common routes) • Maternal infection of fetus during pregnancy	• Shortly after initial infection, flu-like symptoms possible • Impaired immune response leads to vulnerability to opportunistic infections, which if untreated, may cause death	• Identification of antibodies through screening test confirmed through diagnostic laboratory test and assessment of viral load • Monitoring of viral load allows for adjustment of therapy	• Antiviral medication to keep viral load low and support immune function • Treatment guidelines are regularly updated by national and international health authorities • Prompt treatment of opportunistic infection, if it occurs • Use of prophylaxis during pregnancy/delivery or immediately after occupational exposure markedly reduces infection of newborn or worker

Nurses provided some of the best and worst examples of response to the emerging infection. This ranged from apparently fearless care of the terminally ill to fear of any personal contact including denial of assistance with eating. The latter fear-driven response was based more on panic and rumor than on science and nursing ethics.

Influenza

Influenza is a viral infection that is common around the globe, following a seasonal pattern of increase in winter and decrease in summer. The causal virus is one that undergoes genetic changes on a regular basis, making lifelong immunity impossible. The influenza vaccine developed annually incorporates strains expected to occur in the following flu season, and can markedly reduce the rate of infection when successfully deployed. There are three types of influenza viruses that infect humans worldwide—A, B, and C. Every year there are seasonal epidemics caused by the more common human influenza viruses A and B. In the winter of 2009–2010, a mutated version of the influenza A/H1N1 virus emerged and caused a significant pandemic. This virus is now referred to as the 2009 H1N1 virus, and has replaced H1N1 as a virus circulating in humans (CDC, 2016b). The WHO estimates that 284,000 people died worldwide after infection with this strain of the virus (Dawood et al., 2012). However, the most serious of pandemics was the influenza pandemic of 1918. The post–World War I outbreak was responsible for more than half a million deaths worldwide, and has been the benchmark used for influenza outbreak planning as a "worst-case" example. Other pandemics, such as those of 1957–1958 and 1968–1969, had a much smaller impact and are often overlooked when considering the parameters of potential outbreaks.

In recent years, avian influenza (commonly called "bird flu") has received worldwide attention. Although avian influenza A viruses usually do not cause infection in people, the disease can be transmitted from infected birds to people via direct contact with an infected bird or contaminated surfaces (CDC, 2017a). The most common avian influenza virus strains to infect humans are H5N1 and H7N9 (CDC, 2017f). Because these viruses do not commonly infect humans, there is little or no immune protection against them in the human population. Additionally, the CDC (2016c) reports that the influenza viruses that infect poultry have the potential to recombine with other human influenza A viruses. Should this occur, the result could be a worldwide pandemic with high mortality rates.

The issues that make a major influenza outbreak of concern to emergency preparedness are the potential overload on hospitals and other care facilities, exacerbated by worker illnesses. Not only might health facilities be understaffed, but some models predict large gaps in workers at other essential infrastructure jobs, causing breakdowns in community services. Emergency planners have developed pandemic plans (Department of Health and Human Services [HHS], 2017) and tools such as FluSurge, a spreadsheet that can assist in estimating demands for hospital-based services given estimates of length of outbreak and virulence of the virus (CDC, 2011).

The most important strategies to prevent infection with influenza virus include annual vaccination of populations for influenza, limiting contact with infected people or birds and bird feces in areas where bird flu is endemic, and observing frequent hand hygiene. Therapies for typical human influenza viruses should work in treating avian influenza infection in humans; however, influenza viruses can become resistant to drugs such as amantadine and rimantadine, decreasing their effectiveness. Currently, the U.S. government stockpiles candidate viruses for Asian H5N1 and Asian H7N9 viruses. In the event of a pandemic, these candidate viruses would be used to manufacture vaccines for these strains (CDC, 2017e). A substantial challenge in identifying and responding to influenza is the large number of conditions that present with "flu-like symptoms," coupled with the "work/don't work when ill" decisions of healthcare workers and others. Ongoing surveillance of the trends in influenza worldwide can inform early detection and prevention efforts (Table 32.5).

TABLE 32.5 Clinical Profile of Influenza

Transmission/Isolation	Clinical Presentation	Diagnosis	Therapy

• Transmission between persons is due to inhaled droplets from infected individual, once disease is in human population
• Hospitalized patients are isolated in negative pressure rooms to minimize transmission
	• "Influenza-like" symptoms:
	  • Fever
	  • Cough
	  • Sore throat
	  • Myalgia
	• Possibly:
	  • Pneumonia
	  • Severe respiratory disorder, viral pneumonia
	• A typical presentations:
	  • Nausea/vomiting
	  • Diarrhea
	  • Acute respiratory failure
		• Viral culture
		• IFA
		• Serologic studies
		• PCR
			• Oseltamivir and Zanamivir are both thought to be effective in treatment and prevention

IFA, immunofluorescence antibody; PCR, polymerase chain reaction.

TABLE 32.6 Clinical Profile of Marburg Hemorrhagic Fever

Transmission/Isolation	Clinical Presentation	Diagnosis	Therapy
• Human-to-human transmission is possible through bodily fluids, including those of the deceased • Natural reservoir of the disease remains uncertain • Isolate in negative pressure room • Universal precautions with N-95 or HEPA mask when giving care	• Fever • Cough • Headache • Conjunctivitis • Petechial rash (primarily truncal) • Shock • Liver failure • Hemorrhaging • Multisystem dysfunction	• ELISA • PCR • IgG capture ELISA if patient has recovered • Viral culture during the acute phase	• Supportive therapy

ELISA, enzyme-linked immunosorbent assay; HEPA, high-efficiency particulate air; IgG, immunoglobulin G; PCR, polymerase chain reaction.

Marburg Hemorrhagic Fever

Marburg hemorrhagic fever, a close relative of Ebola fever, is a very rare zoonotic disease of the *filovirus* family. Marburg was first identified in 1967 in Germany and the former Yugoslavia when 37 laboratory workers fell ill after exposure to monkeys imported from Uganda. All subsequent cases occurred in Africa where Marburg virus is indigenous. Incidence has been sporadic ever since with cases appearing in 1975, 1989, 1998–2000, 2004–2005, 2007, 2008, 2012, and 2014 (CDC, 2015a).

The largest known outbreak of Marburg began in March 2005 in the rural region of Uige in Angola. The disease spread particularly among people exposed to the virus during home care or at funerals, or through contact with bodily fluids of those who died from the disease. The dangerous use of home-based injections was also identified as a major cause of the outbreak's spread. By April 2005, the outbreak claimed 150 lives, including 12 healthcare workers. The outbreak had a 92% death rate, much higher than previous reports, suggesting that milder cases of the disease may have gone undetected. The outbreak was declared over in November 2005 by the Angola Ministry of Health (Toner, 2005).

Very little is known about how the Marburg virus is transmitted to a human from the animal host, though most initial victims have been in contact with nonhuman primates or their fluids or tissue. Once in a human population, however, the disease spreads easily among humans within close contact, especially in the hospital setting, and healthcare workers are at high risk for contracting the virus. Bodily fluids, contaminated equipment, blood, or tissues may all be sources of the disease. At present there is no vaccine for Marburg, nor is there treatment beyond supportive care (Table 32.6).

Because of the close contact necessary for transmission, an epidemic of Marburg is unlikely unless it is used as a bioterror agent (Fauci, 2006). Given that few clinicians have seen this disease, and only high-level containment laboratories work with it, it could become an agent of choice for a deliberately caused outbreak. For that reason, all clinicians including nurses are urged to remember the possibility of unusual conditions, to be familiar with public health systems and reporting wherever they practice, and the need to follow public health recommendations when issued.

Smallpox

Smallpox is the only disease considered to have been entirely eradicated from human populations (Barquet & Domingo, 1997). Formerly a major killer and disfigurer of humans

TABLE 32.7 Clinical Profile of Smallpox

Transmission/Isolation	Clinical Presentation	Diagnosis	Therapy

• Prolonged, face-to-face contact with the infected person throughout the symptomatic period until all scabs have fallen off
• Direct contact with bodily fluids or contaminated bedding/clothing
	• Initial symptoms (2–4 days):
	  • Fever (101–104 degrees)
	  • Malaise
	  • Head/body aches
	• Rash stages:
	  • Mouth and tongue (4 days)
	  • Pustular rash, Cover body within 24 hours
	• Distinguished by bumps in center of raised bumps (~10 days):
	  • Scabbing and resolution (~10 days)
		• Symptomatic, with careful attention to distribution and appearance of rash
		• Confirmation with PCR and viral isolation
			• No specific treatment:
			  • Supportive therapies only

PCR, polymerase chain reaction.

worldwide, the vaccine was available for many years before the international eradication effort coordinated through the WHO was mounted. Detailed historical review of cases and epidemics of smallpox dates back to the 17th century. In the late 18th century, Edward Jenner discovered that dairy maids who had contracted and recovered from the less serious cowpox were not susceptible to smallpox. He subsequently experimented with and eventually developed a technique of removing material from a human cowpox lesion and transferring it to another individual, thus creating the first vaccine against smallpox (Fenner, Henderson, Arita, Jezek, & Ladnyi, 1988). In 1958, the WHO initiated a program of global smallpox eradication which was intensified by 1967. The initiative involved surveillance and containment activities emphasizing identification of cases and rapid vaccination of all exposed contacts. Coordinated mass "ring" vaccination campaigns (advanced by the invention of the bifurcated needle allowing for improved and more efficient vaccination) resulted in the eradication of smallpox, officially acknowledged by the WHO in 1980 (Barquet & Domingo, 1997; IOM, 1999, 2005; Radetsky, 1999). The last endemic case of smallpox in the world occurred in 1977 in Somalia. Routine vaccination against the disease had been gradually limited to those traveling to endemic areas, and was discontinued, with only two laboratories (one in the United States and one in Russia) maintaining viral cultures for possible future research needs. Given the length of time since eradication, the world population is now considered extremely vulnerable to the deliberate introduction of smallpox into the population. For that reason, when bioterrorism became the focus of emergency preparedness planning in the public health sector, this disease received substantial attention, and vaccination of some health workers was urged, though the program came under considerable criticism (IOM, 2005). As with Marburg virus, the limited experience of physicians and nurses with this disease makes initial differentiation from other "pox" diseases critical. A U.S. outbreak of monkey pox (CDC, 2015b) was likely identified quickly and attended to just as quickly because of the initial concerns that an outbreak of smallpox might have been initiated (Table 32.7).

Public health and emergency response agencies have developed extensive plans for response to the identification of a case of smallpox, including isolation of cases, quarantine of exposed family members or others, and rapid institution of a vaccine program.

One Health

Although the term "One Health" is fairly new, the concept has long been recognized both nationally and globally. Since the 1800s, scientists have noted the similarity in disease processes among animals and humans, but human and animal medicine were practiced separately until the 20th century. In recent years, through the support of key individuals and vital events, the One Health concept has gained more recognition in the public health and animal health communities. The One Health concept recognizes that the health of people is connected to the health of animals and the environment. The CDC uses a One Health approach by working with physicians, veterinarians, ecologists, and many others to monitor and control public health threats and to learn about how diseases spread among people, animals, and the environment (CDC, 2017d).

One Health is defined as a collaborative, multisectoral, and transdisciplinary approach—working at the local, regional, national, and global levels—with the goal of achieving optimal health outcomes recognizing the interconnection between people, animals, plants, and their shared environment (CDC, 2017d).

FUTURE DIRECTIONS

Since the sudden increase in attention to emergency preparedness that was stimulated in the fall of 2001 by both the World Trade Center/Pentagon terrorism and the anthrax-by-mail attacks in the United States, there has been an enormous investment in developing an effective emergency response system that includes improved ability to detect and control infectious outbreaks. This has included expanded investment in electronic communication systems that link public health across the world, more laboratory resources for isolation and identification of organisms, investment in pharmaceutical agents to treat diagnosed disease, and integration of health into community-wide emergency response networks. While significant disasters such as extreme weather or geological events or mass casualty incidents (whether deliberate or accidental) can cause significant harm, they are self-limited in that the damage is localized to one region or area. Bioevents, such as epidemics, have the potential to spread rapidly and disrupt an entire country, global region, or the world. An understanding of key principles for early detection and reporting of unusual patterns of presenting cases, knowing where to obtain reliable information about prevention and treatment, and staying abreast of recent developments are essential to disaster nursing.

The Pandemic and All Hazards Preparedness Act of December 2006 (Public Law 109-417, 2006) has mandated consistency in training for all public health workers and created an interagency health emergency preparedness resource housed at the Uniformed Services University of the Health Sciences. More recently, the U.S. Federal Register posted regulations for core emergency preparedness and the Centers for Medicare and Medicaid Services (CMS, 2016) has developed a resource website for all hazards preparedness and specific events including pandemics and influenza.

Creatures invisible to the naked eye will continue to outsmart and outwit humans with the complexities of modern living presenting numerous opportunities for them to prove their strength and determination. The public health system must be prepared to identify new infectious disease threats and respond quickly, including collaboration with other elements of the emergency response system as appropriate. Nurses are not only the largest sector of the healthcare professions, but the single largest group of professionals working in public health. Whether practicing in public health, elsewhere in the community, or in an institutional setting, every nurse should be alert to the potential of new infections appearing and be prepared to participate as a full partner in the development and activation of a community response that is based in science and best practices. A holistic approach that considers the biological, environmental, societal, and behavioral underpinnings of EIDs is our best defense against this perpetual challenge.

STUDY QUESTIONS

1. Why are emerging infectious diseases (EIDs) of concern to those interested in emergencies and disasters? Select 10 diseases from the CDC website list of emerging diseases and research them at www.cdc.gov to determine if they are newly emerging, reemerging, or deliberately emerging.

2. In the last 5 years, what changes have occurred in your local environment that may contribute to an EID?

3. Individual behaviors play a significant role in disease transmission. What risk behaviors can you identify in addition to unsafe sex and drug use that could aid transmission of disease?

4. What competencies can each nurse achieve to be better prepared to address EIDs?

5. Why are EIDs a perpetual challenge?

6. What strategies can community-based nurses use to educate the public about prevention of vectorborne illness?

REFERENCES

Barquet, N., & Domingo, P. (1997). Smallpox: The triumph over the most terrible of the ministers of death. *Annals of Internal Medicine, 127,* 635–642. doi:10.7326/0003-4819-127-8_Part_1-199710150-00010

Centers for Disease Control and Prevention. (2011). FluSurge software. Retrieved from https://www.cdc.gov/flu/pandemic-resources/tools/flusurge.htm

Centers for Disease Control and Prevention. (2015a). Marburg hemorrhagic fever. Retrieved from https://www.cdc.gov/vhf/marburg/outbreaks/chronology.html

Centers for Disease Control and Prevention. (2015b). What you should know about monkeypox. Retrieved from http://www.cdc.gov/ncidod/monkeypox/factsheet2.htm

Centers for Disease Control and Prevention. (2016a). Dengue. Retrieved from https://www.cdc.gov/dengue/index.html

Centers for Disease Control and Prevention. (2016b). Types of influenza viruses. Retrieved from https://www.cdc.gov/flu/about/viruses/types.htm

Centers for Disease Control and Prevention. (2017a). Avian influenza A virus infections in humans. Retrieved from https://www.cdc.gov/flu/avianflu/avian-in-humans.htm

Centers for Disease Control and Prevention. (2017b). HIV/AIDS timeline. Retrieved from https://npin.cdc.gov/pages/hiv-and-aids-timeline#1980

Centers for Disease Control and Prevention. (2017c) Multistate outbreak of *Salmonella Kiambu* & *S. Thompson* limited to imported Marodol papayas. Retrieved from http://www.cdc.gov/salmonella/kiambu-07-017index

Centers for Disease Control and Prevention. (2017d). One health. Retrieved from https://www.cdc.gov/onehealth/basics/history/index.html

Centers for Disease Control and Prevention. (2017e). Prevention and treatment of avian influenza A viruses in people. Retrieved from https://www.cdc.gov/flu/avianflu/prevention.htm

Centers for Disease Control and Prevention. (2017f). Public health threat of highly pathogenic Asian avian influenza A (H5N1) virus. Retrieved from https://www.cdc.gov/flu/avianflu/h5n1-threat.htm

Centers for Disease Control and Prevention. (2017g). Zika virus. Retrieved from https://www.cdc.gov/zika/about/overview.html

Centers for Medicare and Medicaid Services. (2016). Core EP rule elements. Retrieved from https://www.cms.gov/Medicare/Provider-Enrollment-and-Certification/SurveyCertEmergPrep/Core-EP-Rule-Elements.html

Chin, C.-S., Sorenson, J., Harris, J. B., Robins, W. P., Charles, R. C., Jean-Charles, R. R., ... Waldor, M. K. (2011). The origin of the Haitian cholera outbreak strain. *New England Journal of Medicine, 364,* 33–42. doi:10.1056/NEJMoa1012928

Conference Board of Canada. (2003). Economic impact of SARS. Retrieved from http://www.conferenceboard.ca/e-library/abstract.aspx?did=539

Coyne, P. (n.d.). Seminar on drugs for neglected diseases initiative development partnerships. *The University of Notre Dame, Center for Rate and Neglected Diseases.* Retrieved from https://www3.nd.edu/~crnd/CTSS4Coyne.htm

Dawood, F., Iuliano, A., Reed, C., Meltzer, M. I., Shay, D. K., Cheng, P. Y., ... Widdowson, M. A. (2012). Estimated global mortality associated with the first 12 months of 2009 pandemic influenza A H1N1 virus circulation: A modelling study. *Lancet. Infectious Diseases, 12*(9), 687–695. doi:10.1016/S1473-3099(12)70121-4

Department of Health and Human Services. (2017). HHS pandemic influenza plan 2017 update. Retrieved from https://www.cdc.gov/flu/pandemic-resources/pdf/pan-flu-report-2017v2.pdf

Fauci, A. S. (2001). Infectious diseases: Considerations for the 21st century. *Clinical Infectious Diseases, 32*(5), 67–85. doi:10.1086/319235

Fauci, A. S. (2006). *Emerging and re-emerging infectious diseases: The perpetual challenge.* New York, NY: Milbank Memorial Fund.

Fenner, F., Henderson, D., Arita, A., Jezek, Z., & Ladnyi, I. (1988). *Smallpox and its eradication.* Geneva, Switzerland: World Health Organization.

Institute of Medicine. (1999). *Assessment of future scientific needs for live variola virus.* Washington, DC: National Academies Press.

Institute of Medicine. (2003). *Microbial threats to health: Emergence, detection, and response.* Washington, DC: National Academies Press.

Institute of Medicine. (2005). *The smallpox vaccination program: Public health in an age of terrorism.* Washington, DC: National Academies Press.

Khan, O., & Pappas, G. (2011). *Megacities and global health.* Washington, DC: American Public Health Association Press.

Morens, D. M., Folkers, G. K., & Fauci, A. S. (2004). The challenge of emerging and re-emerging infectious diseases. [Review]. *Nature, 430*(6996), 242–249. doi:10.1038/nature02759

Morse, S. S. (1995). Factors in the emergence of infectious diseases. [Review]. *Emerging Infectious Diseases, 1*(1), 7–15. doi:10.3201/eid0101.950102

National Geographic News. (2016). How cholera spread so quickly through Haiti. Retrieved from http://news.nationalgeographic.com/2016/08/haiti-cholera-crisis-united-nations-admission

National Institute of Environmental Health Sciences. (2017). Vectorborne and zoonotic diseases. Retrieved from https://www.niehs.nih.gov/research/programs/geh/climatechange/health_impacts/vectorborne/index.cfm

Omran, A. R. (2005). The epidemiologic transition: A theory of the epidemiology of population change. *Milbank Quarterly, 83*(4), 731–757. doi:10.1111/j.1468-0009.2005.00398.x

Public Law 109-417. 2006 Pandemic and All Hazards Preparedness Act. Retrieved from http://frwebgate.access.gpo.gov/cgi-bin/getdoc.cgi?dbname=109_cong_public_laws&docid=f:publ417.109.pdf

Radetsky, M. (1999). Smallpox: A history of its rise and fall. *Pediatric Infectious Disease Journal, 18*(2), 85–93. doi:10.1097/00006454-199902000-00002

Toner, E. (2005, April 6). Clinicians' Biosecurity Network: Airborne spread of SARS: Marburg outbreak. Retrieved from http://www.upmc-cbn.org

United Nations, Department of Economic and Social Affairs, Population Division. (2016). The world's cities in 2016—Data booklet (ST/ESA/SER.A/392). Retrieved from http://www.un.org/en/development/desa/population/publications/pdf/urbanization/the_worlds_cities_in_2016_data_booklet.pdf

World Health Organization. (2011a). Cholera country profile: Haiti. Retrieved from http://www.who.int/cholera/countries/HaitiCountryProfileMay2011.pdf

World Health Organization. (2011b). Fighting the rise in cholera cases in Haiti. Health action in crises monthly highlights-June 2011. Retrieved from http://www.who.int/hac/crises/hti/highlights/june2011/en/#

World Health Organization. (2012). 10 facts on climate change and health. Retrieved from http://www.who.int/features/factfiles/climate_change/en

World Health Organization. (2016a). Children: Reducing mortality. Retrieved from http://www.who.int/mediacentre/factsheets/fs178/en

World Health Organization. (2016b). Vector-borne diseases. Retrieved from http://www.who.int/mediacentre/factsheets/fs387/en

World Health Organization. (2017a). Communicable disease update. Retrieved from http://who.int/csr/don/en

World Health Organization. (2017b). Dengue and severe dengue. Retrieved from http://www.who.int/mediacentre/factsheets/fs117/en

World Health Organization. (2017c). Ebola virus fact sheet. Retrieved from http://who.int/mediacentre/factsheets/fs103/en

World Health Organization. (2017d). HIV/AIDS fact sheet. Retrieved from http://www.who.int/mediacentre/factsheets/fs360/en

World Health Organization. (2017e). Sexually transmitted infections. Retrieved from http://who.int/mediacentre/factsheets/fs110/en

World Health Organization. (2017f). World Health Statistics 2017. Retrieved from http://www.who.int/gho/publications/world_health_statistics/2017/EN_WHS2017_Part2.pdf?ua=1

33

MEDICAL COUNTERMEASURES DISPENSING

Susan Sullivan and Amanda Fuller Moore

LEARNING OBJECTIVES

When this chapter is completed, readers will be able to:

1. List essential planning elements for medical countermeasure (MCM) dispensing that an organization may need to consider.
2. Identify key stakeholders for the MCM dispensing planning process.
3. Describe models for MCM dispensing operations.
4. Discuss the Strategic National Stockpile (SNS).
5. Describe how to access current planning recommendations and resources for MCM dispensing.

KEY MESSAGES

The planning process for MCM dispensing must occur with key senior-level stakeholder input to ensure unity of purpose.

MCM dispensing plans need to integrate seamlessly with other organizational, local, state, and tribal emergency plans.

Medical countermeasure dispensing planning needs to be scalable and flexible, considering all hazards and threats.

The Centers for Disease Control and Prevention (CDC) Division of Strategic National Stockpile (DSNS) maintains a secure, password-protected website with extensive resources for planners.

CHAPTER OVERVIEW

Medical countermeasure (MCM) dispensing is the ability to provide vaccines, antiviral drugs, antibiotics, antitoxins, and other pharmaceuticals to an identified population in accordance with public health guidelines. This is an important public health function that often requires a community-based response. In an emergency, nurses and other healthcare practitioners are part of this effort. Through the CDC DSNS and the CHEMPACK Program, medical supplies and countermeasures, including nerve agent antidotes, are made available to facilities across the United States. These agencies not only have to deal with what specific pharmaceuticals to stockpile, but also must maintain them in multiple locations under prescribed storage conditions and shelf life. Requesting, managing, and using the array of MCMs require careful planning, organizing, equipment, and training among many organizations at various governmental and community levels. Written plans must be developed and maintained to clearly define each participating organization's roles and responsibilities in the requesting, receipt, staging, and distribution of pharmaceuticals as quickly as possible in an emergency situation. Various plans and organizations tasked with this responsibility are discussed.

Medical countermeasure (MCM) dispensing is the ability to provide MCMs (including vaccines, antiviral drugs, antibiotics, antitoxins, and other pharmaceuticals) in support of treatment or prophylaxis (oral or vaccination) to the identified population in accordance with public health guidelines and recommendations. CDC lists this function as one of 15 public health target capabilities in its March 2011 document on national standards for state and local planning (DSNS, 2011a).

This chapter is designed to inform nurses and other healthcare practitioners about the important public health function of MCM dispensing. Although this is a public health function, public health cannot do it alone. The speed, size, and scope of disasters and public health emergencies that demand such countermeasures require broad community-based response. Historically, smallpox eradication, polio elimination, the anthrax prophylaxis at the Capitol and U.S. Postal Service and, most recently, 2009 H1N1 influenza prevention efforts demonstrate that MCM delivery remains an essential tool for protecting public health and requires partner assistance to be performed successfully. In an emergency, we are all part of the public health workforce effort.

The intent of this chapter is to increase the reader's knowledge of the MCM planning guidance at the national level; the implementation at the state and local levels; and the resources available to assist individual organizational planning. Topics include discussion of the DSNS, 12-hour push pack, CHEMPACK, Cities Readiness Initiative (CRI), the Public Readiness and Emergency Preparedness (PREP) Act, resources such as the NACCHO (National Association of County and City Health Officials) Advanced Practice Center Toolkit, and the website of the DSNS.

THE DIVISION OF STRATEGIC NATIONAL STOCKPILE

To control costs and minimize waste, most healthcare organizations and retail pharmacies maintain an efficiently managed, standard inventory and rely on a robust delivery system to meet daily operational needs. In a major disaster or public health emergency, however, supply chains can be disrupted for prolonged periods, resulting in delay of lifesaving treatment. Planning by public health for MCM dispensing has been ongoing since 1999 when Congress tasked the U.S. Department of Health and Human Services (HHS) and the CDC with the responsibility for protecting the public's health during emergencies by delivering large quantities of essential medical material to states and communities within 12 hours of the federal decision to deploy.

Since that time, when concerns centered on bioterrorism, the CDC program has evolved to also address delivery of critical medical assets to sites of national emergencies resulting from natural disasters as well. The program is now referred to as the DSNS and is a division of the Office of Public Health Preparedness and Response (OPHPR), formerly the Coordinating Office of Terrorism Preparedness and Emergency Response, and resides within the CDC. Technical assistance for planning and the use of MCMs is provided by OPHPR's Division of State and Local Readiness (DSLR). The MCM group within DSLR provides technical assistance reviews, training, archived and ongoing webcasts, detailed planning guidance, and a password-protected file sharing, technical assistance and reporting site known as Online Technical Resource and Assistance Center (On-TRAC). The DSNS can provide either a broad spectrum of support for a poorly defined threat or substantial shipments of specific items when the threat is known. Surge buying capacity for emergencies or disasters is also available to the DSNS through the Veterans Administration system. It is important for a jurisdiction to know how to request SNS assets and use the asset request process that has been planned for by public health, jurisdictional authorities, and emergency management. The jurisdiction should be able to describe the emergency situation, articulate its response plan, and request what it specifically needs to respond to an event, rather than simply asking for "the SNS."

The SNS is a large quantity of medical supplies that may be requested by a state or in certain situations may be pushed out by the federal government during an emergency, as was the case with antiviral medications during the 2009 H1N1 pandemic. The stockpile includes the following:

- Medical supplies needed for intravenous (IV) administration, airway management, wound care, burn, and blast care
- Federal medical stations (FMSs), which provide inpatient nonacute care medical services and quarantine support and require local personnel for staffing
- MCMs such as radiation pharmaceuticals, antibiotics (oral and IV), nerve agent antidotes, vaccines (except pandemic influenza), antitoxins, and antivirals

It should be noted that the contents of the SNS are not fixed and may be updated based on the latest threat intelligence and countermeasure product development. To that end, the Biomedical Advanced Research and Development Authority (BARDA) is tasked with providing countermeasures for chemical, biological, radiological and nuclear threats, pandemic influenza, and emerging infectious diseases by establishing product, product development, stockpile acquisition, and product innovation requirements, and by enhancing manufacturing infrastructure.

BARDA (www.phe.gov/about/barda) is within the Office of the Assistant Secretary for Preparedness and Response (ASPR) in the HHS. BARDA manages Project BioShield, which includes the procurement and advanced development of MCMs for two groups of products: (a) chemical, biological, radiological, and nuclear agents; and (b) MCMs for pandemic influenza and other emerging infectious diseases that fall outside the scope of Project BioShield. BARDA also manages the Public Health Emergency Medical Countermeasures Enterprise (PHEMCE), an interagency effort that is responsible for defining, prioritizing, and focusing research on countermeasure requirements, as well as establishing deployment and usage strategies for MCMs in the SNS (www.cdc.gov/phpr/stockpile/stockpile.htm).

The DSNS responds to a large-scale public health emergency with three basic strategies:

1. Provide rapid delivery of a broad spectrum of drugs and other items in the initial hours of an event, to allow local authorities to begin responding to an ill-defined threat. An example is a 12-hour Push Package. With 12 locations across the country, a 12-hour Push Package can arrive anywhere in the United States within 12 hours of the federal decision to deploy. Each package weighs over 50 tons and, depending on the current formulary, consists of up to 130 containers. The 130 containers together fill a wide-body cargo aircraft. The receiving site needs to have *at least* 15,000 sq. ft. of warehouse space, although much more space is needed to accommodate the additional material that will likely arrive from a managed inventory (MI). Along with other critical medical supplies, each push package contains 500,000 10-day antibiotic regimens. Doxycycline, ciprofloxacin, and amoxicillin are the antibiotics most likely to be needed in a public health biological event. They are generally packaged in 10-day unit-of-use bottles. Limited quantities of pediatric suspension are available.
2. Provide continuous shipments of large amounts of supplies of specific items once a threat is known. This is generally arranged through the MI.
3. Provide technical assistance. This is accomplished with the SNS Services Advance Group (SSAG) that maintains a 90-minute recall posture to be able to conduct initial assessments of rapidly evolving situations. The SSAG can deploy to a site to work with state and local authorities to help them receive, distribute, and replenish SNS material.

The CHEMPACK Program

Another component of the DSNS is the CHEMPACK Program. In keeping with an all-hazard focus, this program has the mission to forward place a sustainable resource of nerve agent antidotes across the United States. Due to the need for immediate treatment in a nerve agent event, a traditional countermeasures response such as opening points of dispensing (PODs) would not be adequate. The CHEMPACK Program provides access to nerve agent countermeasures where it will be quickly available to state and local emergency first responders and acute care facilities to supplement their capabilities to manage a large-scale nerve agent exposure in a timely manner. The antidote contents include medications such as atropine to block excess acetylcholine, pralidoxime to break the nerve agent/cholinesterase bond, and diazepam to control acetylcholine-induced seizures. Packaged either in bulk or auto-injectors, these antidotes would be used by emergency medical services (EMS), fire and rescue, and any other on-scene responders as well as healthcare facilities. States have strategically placed CHEMPACK assets at locations where they have determined they will be most accessible in a response including hospitals, EMS bases, and fire stations. The CHEMPACK contents may be opened when the medical security of a community is threatened, multiple lives are at risk, local caches of antidotes are rapidly being used, and the amount needed will exceed local capacity. Security of the CHEMPACK assets are ensured through a surveillance system activated at the time of installation that is electronically triggered by any break of the container seal or loss of power. One container can treat approximately 400 patients depending on the severity of their symptoms.

The DSNS has established a secure website for authorized planners to obtain CHEMPACK information, share planning and training documents, and locate CHEMPACK points of contact. Designated CHEMPACK planners may request access by contacting their public health agency CHEMPACK representative.

RADIOLOGICAL COUNTERMEASURES

Evacuation as directed by local authorities from an affected area is the first and most important response in a radiological event, followed by decontamination (removal of contaminated clothing and showering) and screening at a designated community reception center. The process for screening for radiological contamination and countermeasure referral at these sites is explained in more detail through a virtual tour at emergency.cdc.gov/radiation/crc/vcrc.asp. There are MCMs available for those who may be exposed. The medications needed in a radiological event would depend on the type of radioactive material that was released. The SNS has potassium iodide (KI) for exposure to iodine radiation, which needs to be taken immediately before or after the exposure to be most effective. Communities with nuclear power plants usually preposition caches, often provided by the Nuclear Regulatory Commission (NRC), around a planned 10-mile area in schools and day-care settings, as well as in residences within the 10-mile area. Communities are educated on appropriate response actions through the nuclear power plant outreach programs and local governments. Any resident may also obtain KI over the counter at local U.S. pharmacies. However, an event not geographically related to a nuclear power plant would present a challenge, and require providing public information to a community that may not be aware of appropriate response actions and reception center locations for screening and countermeasure dispensing if indicated. In addition to KI, other SNS radiological countermeasures include Prussian blue for exposure to radioactive cesium or thallium, and calcium Diethylenetriamine pentaacetate (DTPA) followed by zinc DTPA for americium, curium, or plutonium radiation. DTPA is administered intravenously and would require medical monitoring in an appropriate level of care setting. Other drugs for hematopoietic support such as filgrastim are available in the SNS as well.

SHELF LIFE EXTENSION PROGRAM (SLEP)

To maximize the investment in MCM pharmaceuticals, the Food and Drug Administration (FDA) selectively samples lots of federally stockpiled medications for potency that have been stored under the prescribed environmental conditions. The SLEP is administered the U.S. Department of Defense. Such testing can save millions of dollars worth of medication that may be beyond the stated expiration date, yet is still of therapeutic quality. At this time, there is no SLEP for local or state caches of MCMs, although some jurisdictions have independently chosen to purchase and rotate limited stocks of select countermeasures for specific groups such as first responders or critical infrastructure personnel.

ORGANIZING TO RESPOND

Requesting, managing, and using the vast array of countermeasure resources available require careful planning, organizing, and exercising as well as equipment and training. Federal public health emergency preparedness (PHEP) grants to state, local, tribal, and territorial public health entities provide funding for these activities, guidance for planning, and help identifying specific preparedness deliverables that must be met by the recipients. The organization and management required to carry out MCM dispensing as well as any other preparedness target capability is described in the National Incident Management System (NIMS). NIMS is a comprehensive national approach to incident management, used at all jurisdictional levels and across functional disciplines, to improve the effectiveness of emergency response providers and incident management organizations across a wide variety of incidents. The two features of NIMS most useful to all levels of planners working on MCM dispensing are the Incident Command System (ICS) and the Homeland Security Exercise and Evaluation Program (HSEEP). The ICS is a management tool that uses a standardized way to organize any response, regardless of size or type. ICS provides accountability, interoperability, and organized authority.

At the jurisdictional level, written plans must be developed that clearly define each organization's roles and responsibilities in a MCM dispensing situation. Whether an organization is a freestanding clinic, urgent care center, community hospital, or academic health center, the impact of a public health event or emergency will strain the system. Healthcare organizations must collaboratively decide how best to support MCM dispensing in their communities while preserving the ability

of their resources to care for patients, protect staff, and serve the public (Joint Commission on Accreditation of Healthcare Organizations, 2003). These executive-level decisions are best made with input from a well-established, jurisdictional planning group, which may include

- Public health departments
- Jurisdictional Emergency Management/Office of Homeland Security
- Law enforcement
- Private businesses (including pharmacies)
- Emergency medical services (both public and private)
- Hospitals and clinics
- Medical professional organizations (including pharmacy boards and associations)
- Military installations
- Metropolitan Medical Response System participants
- Volunteer groups (e.g., Red Cross and Salvation Army)
- Radiation-specific groups (e.g., Radiation Control Programs, U.S. Environmental Protection Agency, or State Environmental Agency; the Conference of Radiation Control Program Directors provides a list of state radiation control programs at www.crcpd.org/mpage/Map)
- Private organizations such as retailers with supply chains and package delivery services (e.g., U.S. Postal Service, UPS, FedEx, and DHL)
- U.S. DHSS Regional Emergency Coordinators (DSNS, 2011a)

Plans need not start from scratch. Most existing jurisdictional and organizational plans for basic functions such as communications, materials management, and command and control can be adapted for MCM dispensing. While some jurisdictions have contracted for planning, outsourcing this task has not been found to consistently create the partnerships needed to achieve buy-in and sustain partnerships (Nelson et al., 2008).

From the outset, it is essential to have law enforcement involved in SNS planning. This national program represents $4 billion worth of MCM assets. It is the responsibility of the U.S. Marshals Service (USMS) to provide security for the program at the federal level. Within the USMS, the SNS Security Operations (SNSSO) performs this function. SNSSO was established in 2002 under a Memorandum of Agreement (MOA) between the USMS, the HHS, and the CDC. SNSSO has chief inspectors located in large metropolitan areas that have responsibility for senior inspectors across the country, who provide the DSNS with law enforcement protective services. The USMS has the broadest statutory authority of any law enforcement agency and is able to cross state lines to perform its security function regardless of where an incident occurs. The USMS protects the SSAG personnel and material, conveys any deployment concerns, and performs ongoing review of threats and vulnerabilities. Once assets are requested and deployment is approved, the USMS assures the arrival of assets to the designated receiving site locations. When the assets are signed over to the state or territory, they become the responsibility of that jurisdiction, which must then provide security. Upon receipt by the county, city, or tribal areas, the security responsibility also becomes local. Local jurisdictions must have a security plan for countermeasures distribution.

Assistance to state and local law enforcement can be enhanced through collaboration with the USMS, which can provide consultation on security surveys and vulnerability assessments. Local and state preparedness and response can benefit from an established relationship with the USMS.

STRUCTURING DISPENSING PROGRAMS

Public health agencies are tasked with planning to request, receive, stage, and immediately redistribute SNS assets to the community as quickly as possible. One method is through POD sites throughout a community. A POD is a location that employs a "pull" method to encourage the general public to come to identified common sites within the community to receive medications. These sites are a fundamental part of a MCM dispensing campaign. Persons come to a POD because they are exposed or potentially exposed to an agent of concern but are not having symptoms of illness and are there to receive preventive countermeasures or prophylaxis.

The CDC DSNS suggests the formula in Box 33.1 to identify the number of PODs that would be needed.

The CDC DSNS offers several resources for modeling clinic flow to assist planners with clinic operations. Nurse planners who are tasked with clinic operations planning should contact their local public health agency to obtain assistance in accessing the resources. Modeling can be useful for all planners, regardless of limited exercise/drill resources.

In addition, other large nonmedical employers such as businesses, universities, and agencies that are regarded as crucial infrastructure may also engage in focused MCM dispensing as a result of risk management and workforce protection planning with their health department preparedness programs. If an organization decides to partner with public health to provide MCMs to its employees, clients, and volunteers (referred to as "closed" point of dispensing), there are several key planning considerations.

Health departments and their partners should discuss and plan in accordance with their individual situation and needs. Based on a review of numerous state plans and national websites, these are the most common essential planning items for organizations partnering with their public health agency:

1. *Purpose/specific threat scenario:* The purpose of the plan should be stated and a brief explanation of the public health emergency situation and circumstances prompting the plan activation should be described.
2. *Contact information:* The plan should list the 24-hour emergency contact information for the health department and closed POD partner.
3. *Size/scope of closed POD (dispensing population characteristics):* Estimates of the number of persons to be served should be included along with descriptors of the population (e.g., staff only, staff and clients, staff families, volunteers). Consideration of special needs (English as a second language [ESL], handicapped access) among the dispensing population should be noted.
4. *Medical versus nonmedical screening:* The presence or absence of healthcare professionals will affect the number and type of personnel needed at the closed POD as well as the screening forms that will be completed. The plan should state the type of screening provided.
5. *Roles and responsibilities:* The plan should outline each partner's responsibilities (Table 33.1).
6. *Communication:* The plan should briefly describe how staff, clients, and other partners are kept informed in the event of an emergency and who is responsible for ongoing communication. Other communication plans may be referenced.
7. *Request, receipt, and storage:* The amount of medication a closed POD receives is based on the designated population. The response plans developed by public health state that each person will receive one 10-day supply (one bottle) of medication. The closed POD plan should describe the logistics for getting the medication, chain of custody procedures, storage, and resupply. Medications should be stored in a secure location (a locked room or locked cabinet where few individuals have access) and kept at controlled room temperature, as specified by the medication manufacturer (away from extreme heat or cold).
8. *Security:* Security measures should be taken to promote the safety of those working at and served by a closed POD. Partners should have discussions with their local law enforcement and/or security service early in the planning process to avoid security mistakes. The plan should briefly discuss how a security issue is handled during an event and this information should be included in staff training.
9. *Staffing and dispensing:* The number of staff needed for the operation should be listed and will depend on the number in the targeted dispensing population. The plan should outline a strategy and step-by-step process of dispensing operations most likely to occur at the closed POD such as a first come, first served strategy or a phased or tiered approach to dispensing by department or activity. If a partner has multiple sites, coordination of these locations should be briefly explained. Generally, a closed POD is not a clinic. Ill persons should be directed to seek appropriate medical care (e.g., personal healthcare provider, urgent care). The POD plan should describe

---

BOX 33.1 Number of PODs

$$TP \div (HPP - S) \div PPH = PODs$$

TP = Total population
HPP = Number of hours to provide prophylaxis to the population
S = Amount of hours needed to set up clinic
PPH = Number of persons per hour who are provided prophylaxis, also known as "throughput"
Assumptions for using this formula: PODs operate 24 hours a day; the population is equally distributed among all PODs; the PODs perform at 100% capacity at all times; a constant flow of people enter (and leave) each POD; and staffing is constant and adequate.

POD, points of dispensing.

how this situation will be managed since referrals may still need prophylaxis. The following five basic steps of dispensing should be included:

- Fill out form
- Show form
- Get prophylaxis
- Provide education
- Exit

10. *Documentation and demobilization:* The health department has a responsibility to provide reports to the state and federal governments regarding medication dispensing. It is important that all forms and reports are submitted back to the health department following the event. In addition to a closed POD partner final summary form, some inventory reports (number of people medicated and remaining inventory numbers) may be requested during the event. The plan should include basic reporting forms and list who is responsible for this function.

11. *Liability:* Homeland Security Presidential Directive 21 and, more recently, Presidential Preparedness Directive 8 emphasized the necessity of public health readiness. In addition, the CDC has identified the need for all communities to provide prophylaxis to 100% of their population within 48 hours. While no facility is protected against willful misconduct, certain legal provisions, such as the PREP Act, are put in place during public health emergencies. Partner agencies' risk managers and/or legal counsels need to be aware of these provisions as they review closed POD plans.

12. *Staff training and exercises:* The plan should translate key information into employee training programs to provide staff with as much information about dispensing site operations as possible. Much of this can be done pre-event. A well-trained staff will become essential to ensure the designated population receives medication in a timely manner, thereby promoting continuity of operations for an organization and meeting public health's dispensing time goal.

13. *Plan maintenance:* Initial plan development and revision should include human resource personnel, continuity managers, medical advisors, logistics specialists, security staff, and the local public health liaison. Frequency of plan revision should be clearly stated.

These "push" methods allow for dispensing by "pushing" MCMs to partner organizations such as private businesses, universities, or large organizations. These partner organizations, in turn, provide medication to their designated population in their "closed" POD site. These organizations would serve their defined, targeted population rather than the general public who would be "pulled" to come to an "open" public POD. The CDC DSNS provides many planning tools for PODs. Also, the NACCHO hosts an extensive "train the trainer" website www.closedpodpartners.org to enhance partnerships between public health and community organizations, in addition to other Advanced Practice Center (APC) tools available online (see Case Study 33.1).

Combinations of both "push" and "pull" methods can greatly increase the number of people who can receive countermeasures in a timely fashion. Examples of populations that may be considered for serving outside the open public POD include employees at large corporations, inmates of correctional facilities, governmental employees, residents of long-term care facilities, workers/students at universities, hospitalized patients, and homeless or undocumented people (DSNS, 2011b). In a large event, it is likely that multiple dispensing modalities will be used to quickly provide needed countermeasures.

In addition to traditional open and closed PODs, several types of alternate dispensing methods exist, including drive-through PODs (Carrico, 2002), direct deliveries to residences (Relucio, 2010), mobile dispensing sites, and the U.S. Postal Service (USPS) initiative (DSNS, 2011c). The postal initiative, a "push" method, is a collaborative effort between HHS, law enforcement, and the Letter Carriers Union and is being adopted in approved large metropolitan areas to provide a rapid delivery through the mail response in select zip codes that would buy time for traditional distribution methods to get underway. It is designed to augment rather than replace traditional POD methods and would be carried out only in targeted, predetermined zip code areas in response to an event.

Several essential POD functions can occur outside of the traditional POD location. Public information dissemination regarding the purpose of the dispensing effort, countermeasure precautions or contraindications, POD procedures such as head of household pickup for all family members, and tools for self-screening could save valuable staff time at traditional POD sites. If, for example, a jurisdiction is planning to use the

---

TABLE 33.1 Example of Responsibilities Breakdown

Local Health Department	Closed POD Partner
• Pre-event planning and technical assistance, including but not limited to policies, procedures, job aids such as POD layouts, fact sheets, dispensing algorithms, forms	• Designate staff to work with health department in planning
• Training/education to identified staff in partner organization	• Provide primary and secondary 24-hour emergency points of contact
• Supplying medication and forms	• Develop closed POD plan and provide a copy and periodic updates to health department
• Notifying closed POD partner of need to activate	• Identify closed POD location(s)
• Providing media guidance during event	• Maintain necessary supplies and equipment
• Collecting unused medications and copies of all medical documentation after dispensing process has been completed and closed POD has been deactivated	• Provide medications and collect data as directed
	• Participate in training and exercise opportunities in coordination with the health department

POD, point of dispensing.

postal option, all screening and triage messaging would occur through public information campaigns (e.g., media messages, fliers distributed with the medication; DSNS, 2011c).

CITIES READINESS INITIATIVE

Based on available evidence, the HHS determined that giving oral antibiotics within 48 hours of an anthrax exposure would likely prevent 95% or more of anthrax cases (DSNS, 2008). To prepare major U.S. cities and metropolitan areas to respond to a large-scale bioterrorism event and dispense to their entire community within 48 hours of the decision to do so, a federal grant program, the CRI, was established in 2004. This funding has improved communication, planning, and collaboration beyond jurisdictional borders and maximized shared resources. For example, CRI jurisdictions with an approved USPS Dispensing Plan may collaborate with local postal services to deliver antibiotics to select zip codes. CRI regions are selected based on population, geographical location, and potential vulnerability to a bioterrorism threat. A current list of CRI regions is available on the CDC website. While the prophylaxis of an entire population in 48 hours seems to be a lofty goal, planning toward that end simplifies more targeted, focused countermeasure delivery efforts, such as that which occurred in 2009 with the initially limited amount of pandemic influenza vaccine and the CDC-defined high-risk target groups.

MEDICAL COUNTERMEASURES PLANNING ELEMENTS

Timely notification and coordination with partners to identify roles and responsibilities consistent with the identified agent or exposure are important first steps in response planning for countermeasure distribution. Time, population size, and uncertainty influence planning. The CDC document, "Receiving, Distributing, and Dispensing Strategic National Stockpile Assets: A Guide for Preparedness" (DSNS, 2006), outlines guidance for public health planners for the 14 functions listed here:

1. *Developing an SNS Plan*
   A written plan is necessary for receiving, distributing, and dispensing SNS assets and should be incorporated into a state's emergency operations plan.
2. *Command and Control*
   Command and control describes how governmental authorities, emergency management, public health, law enforcement, and other groups coordinate their response to an event.
3. *Requesting SNS Assets*
   Requesting the deployment of SNS assets is a collaborative effort among all levels of officials, but begins at a local level when officials identify a potential or actual situation that they believe has the potential to overwhelm their resources. SNS assets are requested from CDC by the affected state's governor (or the governor's designee).
4. *Management of SNS Operations*
   Establishing an SNS Operations Management Team to help coordinate SNS assets and any additional assets already available.

5. *Tactical Communications*
   Redundant communication systems are required to effectively implement plans to distribute and dispense SNS assets.
6. *Public Information and Communication*
   Effective messages, methods, and materials to inform, educate, and mobilize the public to obtain prophylaxis in a short period of time is critical to a successful countermeasures distribution effort.
7. *Security Support*
   A comprehensive security plan for the receipt, distribution, and dispensing of SNS assets is critical to the safety of staff and the public during an emergency.
8. *Receiving, Staging, and Storing SNS Assets*
   The functionality of the receiving, staging, and storing (RSS) facility (the state-designated location for SNS assets) and the proficiency of the RSS team are factors in the speed with which countermeasures can be distributed.
9. *Controlling SNS Inventory*
   The configuration of countermeasures in appropriate, useful quantities for distribution to PODs and other sites is an important planning consideration.
10. *Repackaging*
    Most of the oral medications now come in prepackaged unit-of-use regimens. Only under rare circumstances will bulk items need to be repackaged.
11. *Distributing SNS Assets*
    This function is the delivery of SNS assets from the RSS facility to dispensing sites, treatment centers, and intermediate distribution points.
12. *Dispensing Medical Countermeasures*
    This function is the most important, complex, and resource-intensive of all of the SNS planning functions. Several methods of dispensing may be needed depending on the nature, size, and scope of the emergency.
13. *Treatment Center Coordination*
    Since a large event can quickly overwhelm the resources of a treatment center (hospitals and other providers of acute care), coordination is needed to better plan for adequate and timely reception of SNS assets that have been requested.
14. *Train, Exercise, Evaluate*
    Testing and refining a plan is accomplished through training, exercising, and evaluating (DSNS, 2006).

THE PUBLIC READINESS AND EMERGENCY PREPAREDNESS ACT

This federal legislation provides immunity from liability claims at the federal or state level arising from "administration and use of covered countermeasures to manufacturers, distributors, program planners and qualified persons involved in the administration and use of a covered countermeasure, as specified in a declaration by the Secretary of HHS (see *section 319F-3 of the Public Health Service Act (42 U.S.C. §247d-6d)*." The exception to this immunity is, as always, willful misconduct acts by the "covered persons."

A "covered countermeasure" may include vaccines, antidotes, medications, medical devices, or other FDA-regulated assets used to respond to pandemics, epidemics, or any biological, chemical, radiological, or nuclear threat.

"Covered persons" are manufacturers, distributors, program planners (including those who, e.g., provide consultation, generate policy, or provide a facility), "qualified persons" (e.g., licensed health professionals), the United States, officials, agents, and employees of any of the above.

This law was enacted in 2005 to alleviate liability concerns related primarily to pandemic influenza efforts. It authorizes the secretary of HHS to issue a declaration, which is published in the Federal Register, providing immunity from tort liability. A declaration from the secretary includes a determination of a threat or credible risk, a recommendation for some type of action (e.g., manufacture, testing, use), the category of diseases, health conditions, or health threats, and the effective time period, as well as the receiving population, geographical area of administration, and limitations (e.g., geographical area and means of distribution), and any additional "qualified persons." The types of medical items include covered countermeasures, qualified pandemic or epidemic products, security countermeasures, drugs, biological products, or devices authorized for emergency use (HHS, 2011). Such declarations have been issued in the past. For example, in 2008, there were PREP Act declarations for anthrax, botulism, pandemic antivirals, smallpox, and acute radiation syndrome countermeasures, as well as pandemic influenza diagnostics, personal respiratory protection equipment, and respiratory support devices. The PREP Act also provides for compensation for an eligible person determined to have been injured by a countermeasure. PREP Act information is available at the HHS website and organizations should always consult their public health legal counsel for advice specific to their planning situation.

Another federal tool with lifesaving potential for public health emergency response and countermeasure distribution is emergency use authorization (EUA). Issued by the FDA, EUA permits the use of an unapproved drug or medical product, or the use of an approved authorized drug or medical product in an unapproved manner, under certain emergency situations. The secretary must declare an emergency before an emergency use is authorized. For example, in November 2009, the secretary of the HHS declared the rapid and extensive incidence of 2009 H1N1 infection a public health emergency that justified the emergency use of certain drugs to treat 2009 H1N1 influenza. In response to this emergency, the FDA authorized the use of an *unapproved* IV antiviral drug, peramivir, to treat certain adult and pediatric patients with suspected or laboratory-confirmed 2009 H1N1 infection, or infection due to nonsubtypeable influenza A virus suspected to be 2009 H1N1 based on community epidemiology. The FDA also authorized the use of an *approved* drug, oseltamivir, for a pediatric age group (age ≤1 year) for which its use had not previously been approved.

New MCMs that may be used in a public health emergency are researched and developed through a clinical trial process that eventually results in an application submitted to the FDA. Before any drug or biological product is administered to people, an Investigational New Drug (IND) Application must be requested and such authorization must be received from the FDA. This authorization must be obtained prior to interstate shipment and administration of any new drug or biological product that is not the subject of an approved New Drug Application or Biologics/Product License Application.

Peramivir, for example, was an IND in phase III clinical trials when the 2009 pandemic began. It was used under EUA and the healthcare facilities and those who ordered, dispensed, and administered it appropriately were protected by the PREP Act. More recently, new diagnostic tests for Ebola and Zika virus detection have been used under EUA. The FDA maintains information on the use of MCMs under active EUAs on their website (www.fda.gov/emergencypreparedness/counterterrorism/ucm182568.htm). Full details on EUAs, including how to request and operationalize an EUA are available in the FDA document Emergency Use Authorization of Medical Products and Related Authorities (www.fda.gov/downloads/EmergencyPreparedness/Counterterrorism/MedicalCountermeasures/MCMLegalRegulatoryandPolicyFramework/UCM493627.pdf). In addition, this document contains information on the Emergency Use Instructions (EUI). An EUI allows CDC to prepare and disseminate information related to diseases or situations where an EUA may have been previously required. This information is often called a Fact Sheet and provides CDC a mechanism to efficiently provide pertinent information in a time of emergency that does not conflict with the Food Drug and Cosmetic Act.

Planners should be prepared for the additional written client information that must accompany the use of new countermeasures and the increased time for providers to offer counseling. These variables need to be factored into response efforts.

VACCINE STORAGE AND HANDLING

MCMs that rely on vaccines require additional planning. Vaccines are fragile and costly. Standards for vaccine storage and handling cannot be disregarded during an emergency. Power outages, equipment failure, and natural disasters can disrupt vaccine storage conditions leading to temperature excursions and nonviable vaccine. When vaccine is needed to manage an urgent public health situation, it is better to not vaccinate than to administer a dose of vaccine that has been mishandled. Preparedness coordinators and partners need to be aware that transportation of vaccines should be a rare occurrence and strict cold chain must be maintained.

CDC and state health department immunization programs have established procedures, processes, and training to assist facilities that administer vaccines with proper ordering, handling, and storage. These key elements can be thought of as the six Rights of Vaccine Management and are highlighted here. These six pillars of vaccine management must not be put by the wayside during an emergency.

Right equipment—Refrigerator and freezer units must be able to maintain required vaccine storage temperatures at all times and be spacious enough to hold the year's largest inventory including water bottles and freezer packs used for thermal balance without crowding. Vaccines can never be stored in dorm-style refrigerators/freezer units. Vaccines that must be stored frozen can never be placed in the freezer portion of household-type refrigerators. Vaccines can never be stored on the doors, floors, bins, or top shelves beneath the freezer unit vent. These types of units have demonstrated inability to hold the proper temperatures needed for vaccines, which is between 36°F and 46°F for vaccines requiring refrigeration, and between −58°F and +5°F for vaccines that must be stored frozen, according to the National Institute of Standards and Technology (NIST; www.nist.gov). Units must be protected from disruptions to the power supply such as inadvertent unplugging.

Right monitoring—Vaccine supplies require continuous monitoring with active display, alarms, and digital thermometers with a buffered probe in addition to digital data loggers. Thermometers should be placed centrally near the vaccine. Supply temperatures must be manually checked and recorded twice daily at the opening and close of the day. One backup thermometer with a current certificate of calibration must be on hand. Digital data loggers will soon be required for all Vaccines for Children (VFC) providers.

Right training—Vaccine personnel should include a primary and backup coordinator. All staff who handle vaccine must participate in documented training on proper vaccine storage and handling upon hire and annually, when new vaccines are added to the inventory, and when recommendations change. Hands-on training with the monitoring equipment and emergency packing supplies are best practices. CDC has web-based video training, "You Call the Shots," which covers the basics of vaccine storage and handling. In addition, there is a comprehensive 82-page CDC toolkit www.cdc.gov/vaccines/hcp/admin/storage/toolkit/index.html. Some state policies may differ from CDC, so both sources should be considered when planning for training.

Right Planning—The CDC requires that VFC providers have a written emergency vaccine storage and handling plan that is updated at least annually. The plan must be posted and include a designated backup storage location, contact information for persons responsible for preparing and transporting vaccine, packing instructions, and documentation steps during an emergency. The emergency plan is in addition to the routine vaccine management plan.

Right Response—Facilities must be able to quickly recognize temperature excursion, restore proper storage conditions, and label product as "do not use." Facilities must document time out of range, room temperature, and generate a data logger report. The state health department or manufacturer must be notified for guidance. Facilities must follow the instructions provided.

Right resources—In addition to the CDC website, www.cdc.gov/vaccines/hcp/admin/storage/index.html, state health department immunization programs and the American Academy of Pediatrics website www.aap.org/en-us/advocacy-and-policy/aap-health-initiatives/immunizations/Practice-Management/Pages/Vaccine-Storage-and-Handling.aspx have reliable information about vaccine management.

PEDIATRIC COUNTERMEASURES PLANNING

For all of the resources available, one glaring deficiency is in the pediatric population countermeasures planning. In addition, most hospital emergency departments (EDs) do not have sufficient quantities of pediatric equipment and supplies that meet national guidelines (American Academy of Pediatrics, American College of Emergency Physicians, & Emergency Nurses Association, 2009). As one example, the lack of vendors for surgical masks designed to fit children became apparent during the 2009 influenza pandemic. As another example, the formulary for pediatric autoinjectors for chemical antidotes is very limited. The 2010 report by the National Commission on Children and Disasters states that "the Strategic National Stockpile, intended to provide the public with medicine and medical supplies in the event of a public health emergency, is woefully understocked with MCMs for children" (National Commission on Children and Disasters [NCCD], 2010). For all the reasons discussed in Chapter 32, the pediatric population is more vulnerable to the adverse effects of chemical, biological, radiological, nuclear, and explosive (CBRNE) threats and are rarely, if ever, included in clinical trials for countermeasures. Also, antibiotics used for the Category A biological agents are primarily doxycycline and ciprofloxacin, which are infrequently used in the pediatric population. Limited quantities of these countermeasures are available in pediatric suspension formulation, resulting in the need for caregivers to crush, mix, and measure medication to assure proper dosing (Figure 33.1). The FDA has provided crushing instructions for doxycycline, but not ciprofloxacin due to the inability to make the taste palatable. Instructions are available in Spanish on the FDA website.

Recommendation 3.1 of the National Commission on Children and Disasters Report suggests that to correct this deficiency, Congress, HHS, and the Department of Homeland Security/Federal Emergency Management Agency should enhance availability of, and access to, pediatric MCMs at all levels for CBRNE threats. The report lists actions such as:

1. Funding and grant guidance for development, acquisition, and stockpiling of MCMs specifically for children for inclusion in the SNS and any other cache
2. Amending the Emergency Use Authorization to allow the FDA, at the direction of the HHS secretary, to authorize pediatric indications of MCMs for emergency use before an emergency is known or imminent
3. Forming a standing advisory body of federal partners and external experts to advise the HHS secretary and provide consensus on issues pertaining specifically to pediatric emergency MCMs
4. Designating a pediatric leader within HHS BARDA, and establishing a pediatric and obstetric working group to conduct gap analyses and make research recommendations
5. Including pediatric expertise on the HHS Enterprise Governance Board or its successor and all relevant committees and working groups addressing issues pertaining to MCMs
6. Establishing a partnership between the proposed MCM Development Leader and key pediatric stakeholders both within and outside government (NCCD, 2010)

Since this report, progress has been made. In 2014, an FDA review found "for most CBRN diseases for which there are MCMs in the SNS, there is parity between adult and pediatric preparedness." Gaps still exist in the areas of nerve agent antidote autoinjectors, regulatory approval of some products for pediatric use, and lack of scientific data on dosing, safety, and efficacy for other products.

The National Advisory Committee on Children and Disasters (NACCD) was also established in 2014 under the Pandemic and All-Hazards Preparedness Reauthorization Act of 2013 to

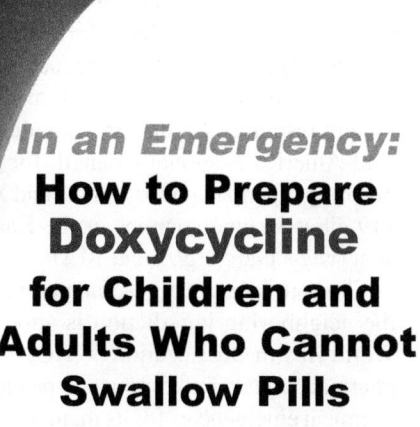

In an Emergency:
How to Prepare Doxycycline
for Children and Adults Who Cannot Swallow Pills

Mixing Doxycycline Hyclate 100mg Tablets with Food

Once you have been notified by your federal, state or local authorities that you need to take doxycycline for a public health emergency, it may be necessary to prepare emergency doses of doxycycline for children and adults who cannot swallow pills.

June 2008
Prepared by the U.S. Food and Drug Administration

 Supplies You Will Need
You will need these items to make doses of doxycycline for adults and children who cannot swallow pills:

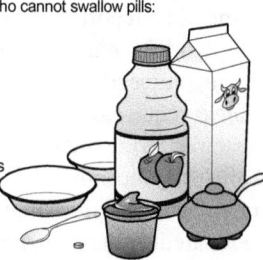

- 1 doxycycline pill (100 mg) *(Do not take doxycycline if you are allergic to tetracyclines)*
- a metal teaspoon
- 2 small bowls
- Water
- one of these foods or drinks to hide the bitter taste of crushed doxycycline:
  - milk or chocolate milk
  - chocolate pudding
  - apple juice and sugar

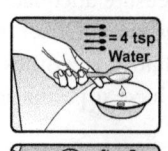

Crushing the Pill and Mixing with Water

1. Put 1 doxycycline pill in a small bowl.
2. Add 4 full teaspoons of water to the same bowl.
3. Let the pill soak in the water for 5 minutes so it will be soft.
4. Use the back of a metal teaspoon to crush the pill in the water. Crush the pill until no visible pieces remain.
5. Stir the pill and water so it is well mixed.

You have now made the Doxycycline and Water Mixture.

Child's weight: _____

 Adding Food to the Doxycycline and Water Mixture to Make It Taste Better

1. Weigh your child.
2. Find your child's weight on the left side of the chart below.
3. Next, look on the right side of the chart to find the amount of the Doxycycline and Water Mixture to mix with food. The chart shows you the amount to give your child for 1 dose. *(For a ½ teaspoon dose, fill the metal teaspoon half way. It is better to give a little more of the medicine than not enough).*

Child's Weight	Amount of Doxycycline and Water Mixture	Teaspoons
12 pounds or less	½ teaspoon	
13 to 25 pounds	1 teaspoon	
26 to 38 pounds	1½ teaspoons	
39 to 50 pounds	2 teaspoons	
51 to 63 pounds	2½ teaspoons	
64 to 75 pounds	3 teaspoons	
76 to 88 pounds	3½ teaspoons	
89 pounds or more and adults	Use the entire mixture	Entire Mixture

4. Add the right amount of the Doxycycline and Water Mixture from the chart above to the second bowl. For adults and children 89 pounds and more, use the entire mixture.
5. Add 3 teaspoons of milk **or** chocolate milk **or** chocolate pudding **or** apple juice to the second bowl. If you use apple juice, also add 4 teaspoons of sugar to the second bowl.
   - Stir well.

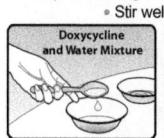 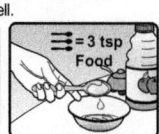 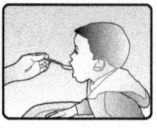
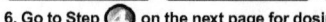

6. Go to Step 4 on the next page for dosing.

 Dosing the Doxycycline and Water Mixture Mixed With Food

1. Give all of the Doxycycline and Water and food mixture in the second bowl. This is one dose.
2. **Each child or adult should take 1 dose in the morning and 1 dose at night each day.**

 Storing the Doxycycline and Water Mixture (If There Is Enough for Another Dose)

- If you have enough leftover doxycycline and water mixture for another dose, you can keep it for the next dose.
- The doxycycline and water mixture can be stored in a covered bowl or cup. Label and date.
- Keep the mixture in a safe place out of the reach of children.
- Store the Doxycycline and Water Mixture at room temperature for up to 24 hours.
- Throw away any unused mixture after 24 hours and make a new Doxycycline and Water Mixture before the next dose.

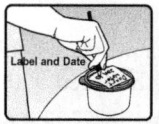 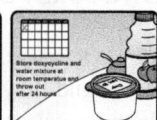

Do not take doxycycline if you have an allergy to tetracyclines

Get emergency help if you have any signs of an allergic reaction including hives, difficulty breathing, or swelling of your face, lips, tongue or throat.

Doxycycline may cause diarrhea, skin reaction to the sun, loss of appetite, nausea and vomiting. Birth control pills may not work as well if you take doxycycline.

Report any reaction to the medication to MedWatch at www.fda.gov/medwatch or 1-800-FDA-1088

FIGURE 33.1 Preparing doxycycline for children in an emergency.

provide expert advice and consultation to the secretary of the HHS and the ASPR on the medical and public health needs of children before, during, and after a disaster or public health emergency. In their 2015 report that focused on the areas of coalition building, workforce development, and MCM readiness, they made recommendations on the following MCM topics: (a) pediatric requirements for dosing, preparation, and delivery systems; (b) formulations; (c) uses of EUA/EUI/IND/Off-Label; (d) incentivizing industry for pediatric MCM development; (e) prepositioning; and (f) ethical issues (www.phe.gov/Preparedness/legal/boards/naccd/Documents/healthcare-prep-wg-20151311.pdf).

In addition to gaps in pediatric countermeasure adequacy, challenges are evident in pediatric disaster response. Of 4,146 EDs that answered the 2013 National Pediatric Readiness assessment, only 47% indicated that they have a pediatric disaster preparedness plan in place.

Despite these shortfalls, useful guidance does exist to improve pediatric disaster planning. Disaster planning needs to be family centered. For MCM dispensing, that concept translates into developing plans for keeping families together even though, for example, they may have different medication dosage requirements. One helpful resource is the Emergency Medical Services for Children (EMSC) website located at emscimprovement.center/resources/toolboxes. Their online guidance provides information on writing and implementing child-specific protocols; planning for children who are separated from their caregivers when disaster strikes; and most importantly for MCM dispensing, developing equipment and medication dosage forms and delivery systems appropriate for children. Additionally, the website offers online training for pediatric responders on topics such as psychological first aid. The American Academy of Pediatrics website also has many resources for families, facilities, and providers (www.aap.org/en-us/advocacy-and-policy/aap-health-initiatives/Children-and-Disasters/Pages/default.aspx). Much work remains to close the pediatric preparedness gap.

CROSS-JURISDICTIONAL PLANNING

On any given day, people travel for work, school, medical care, shopping, or leisure and may be faced with an emergency that prompts them to seek assistance in a jurisdiction that is unfamiliar to them. Countermeasure dispensing plans need to address how displaced populations will be accommodated. Developing informal or formal relationships with other neighboring preparedness planners fosters a collaborative environment prior to an event, helps prevent discordant policies and practices, and assists in maintaining situational awareness during an event. Working groups in locations such as the national capital region of Maryland, Virginia, and the District of Columbia also serve a similar purpose. For the past several years, some states have been holding annual meetings such as the Regional State Border Coordination Workshop. The workshop strives to build upon current planning efforts within the states of North Carolina, Virginia, Washington DC, Maryland, West Virginia, Pennsylvania, Delaware, New Jersey, and New York, and continue discussion of the various efforts,

challenges, and opportunities needed to achieve coordinated plans, as well as provide better support through integrated planning. Another benefit of cross border planning is surge capacity. Some states have formed mutual aid alliances to deal with public health emergencies that do not rise to the level of a federal- or governor-issued declaration but would require resources beyond an individual state's capacity. The Mid-America Regional Council, for example, is a regional planning organization for Kansas and Missouri encompassing 119 cities in nine counties of the Kansas City metropolitan area (www.marc.org/About-MARC).

Cross-jurisdictional planning is even more important when the neighboring jurisdiction is another country. While the World Health Organization (WHO) does maintain a cache of pharmaceuticals for response to pandemic, radiological, and chemical emergencies for its member countries, many governments with the resources to do so have worked to create their own stockpiles. For example, Canada has multiple locations of caches across its nation. Known as the National Emergency Stockpile System (NESS), these resources have been used to assist in national and international emergencies, such as wildfires, the Asian tsunami, and hurricane Katrina (www.phac-aspc.gc.ca). No single country, however, has the resources to support research, development, and acquisition of MCMs alone. A sustainable global MCM infrastructure requires developing collaborations. Initiated in 2001 by health ministers for Canada, France, Germany, Italy, Japan, Mexico, the United Kingdom, the United States, and European Commission, the Global Health Security Initiative (GHSI) strives to provide a forum for discussion of preparedness and response coordination among these countries. The WHO acts in an expert-advisor capacity. Through an annual ministerial-level summit and technical expert workgroups, the GHSI has been able to address issues that have impact worldwide. The 2009 influenza pandemic enabled the group to identify gaps and establish future priorities, including MCMs. Since that time, in light of increasing terrorist attacks on major cities worldwide and emerging global infections such as Zika, the GHSI has further committed to strengthening response capabilities to aid national and international coordination through tools such as the newly adopted, all-hazard GHSI Event Management Response Framework (www.ghsi.ca/english/statementBrussels2017.asp).

SUMMARY

The planning process of dispensing MCMs must include key stakeholders at a senior level to ensure unity of purpose. The final plan must integrate seamlessly with other plans at the organizational, local, state, and tribal levels. The plan must be scalable and flexible, considering all hazards and threats, including terrorism to natural disasters. The DSNS of the CDC maintains a secure website with extensive resources for planners at every level.

REFERENCES

American Academy of Pediatrics, American College of Emergency Physicians, and Emergency Nurses Association. (2009). Joint policy statement: Guidelines for care of children in the emergency department. Retrieved from http://pediatrics.aappublications.org/content/124/4/1233

Carrico, R. M. (2002). *Drive-thru flu shots: A model for mass immunization.* Louisville, KY: Chicago Press.

Department of Health and Human Services. (2011). Public Readiness and Emergency Preparedness Act (PREP Act) for Pandemic Influenza Medical Countermeasures Utilization Protocol & Decision Tools. Retrieved from https://www.phe.gov/Preparedness/legal/prepact/Pages/prepqa.aspx

Division of Strategic National Stockpile, Centers for Disease Control and Prevention. (2006). Receiving, distributing, and dispensing strategic national stockpile assets: A guide for preparedness. Retrieved from http://www.kdheks.gov/cphp/download/SNS_Planning_Guide_V10.02.pdf

Division of Strategic National Stockpile, Centers for Disease Control and Prevention. (2008, April). Point of dispensing standards. Retrieved from https://www.cdc.gov/phpr/documents/coopagreement-archive/fy2008/dispensingstandards.pdf

Division of Strategic National Stockpile, Centers for Disease Control and Prevention. (2011a). Public health preparedness capabilities: National standards for state and local planning. Retrieved from http://www.cdc.gov/phpr/capabilities

Division of Strategic National Stockpile, Centers for Disease Control and Prevention. (2011b). SNS functions: Dispensing medical countermeasures. Retrieved from https://www.cdc.gov/phpr/readiness/00_docs/capability8.pdf

Division of Strategic National Stockpile, Centers for Disease Control and Prevention. (2011c). Summary of postal model. Retrieved from https://www.phe.gov/preparedness/planning/postal/Pages/default.aspx

Joint Commission on Accreditation of Healthcare Organizations. (2003). *Health care at the crossroads: Strategies for creating and sustaining community-wide emergency preparedness systems.* Oakbrook Terrace, IL: Author.

National Commission on Children and Disasters. (2010). *Report to the president and Congress* [AHRQ Publication No. 10-M037]. Rockville, MD: Agency for Healthcare Research and Quality.

Nelson, C., Chan, E. W., Chandra, A., Sorensen, P., Willis, H. H., Comanor, K., . . . Hansell, L. (2008) *Recommended infrastructure standards for mass antibiotic dispensing.* Santa Monica, CA: RAND Corporation.

Relucio, K. (2010, July). *Door-to-door mass dispensing.* Conference poster presented at the Strategic National Stockpile Summit, Atlanta, GA.

CASE STUDY 33.1

The Advanced Practice Centers

Joan M. Fuchsman

The APCs were first established in 2003 by the CDC, through the NACCHO. APCs are exemplary local health departments (LHDs) that have been chosen to create innovative and practical resources to enhance the capability of LHDs and the public health system to prepare for, respond to, and recover from public health emergencies. All APC products are designed by LHD professionals for LHD practitioners. Since 2003, a total of 15 LHDs have served as APC sites, and developed 146 different products in use by LHDs throughout the country.

On the topic of medical countermeasures, APC sites have developed four products. More information about the APC can be found at toolbox.naccho.org/pages/index.html APC's Medical Countermeasure tools are:

1. *Clinic Planning Model Generator (website):* The Montgomery County, Maryland Advanced Practice Center, in collaboration with the Institute for Systems Research at the University of Maryland, has developed a Clinic Planning Model Generator. The software is intended to grant public health officials the ability to quickly create an accurate model that will provide immediate assistance with planning for a public health vaccination and/or dispensing clinic. It can be used either in the advance planning stages or for support during an actual event. In general, this computer model is designed to assist in planning a clinic with improved efficiency and performance while enlightening the planners on what to expect in the event of an outbreak. The computer model operates entirely in the Microsoft Excel environment, so some familiarity with this package is helpful.

2. *Emergency Dispensing Site Signage and Materials (CD):* In 2007, the Cambridge Advanced Practice Center for Emergency Preparedness developed a series of pictograms designed to promote universal access to emergency-dispensing site services. The signs were developed in collaboration with local and state public health professionals and experts in universal design and accessibility. The materials on this CD include a training series for dispensing site staff and volunteers and pictogram-based signs and pocket communicators. These tools are designed to facilitate communication and to promote universal access to dispensing sites and other mass care services. They were developed in collaboration with experts in universal design and accessibility, as well as local and state health professionals. The contents can be downloaded or provided to a print shop. These signs provide large, high contrast pictograms of station activities; simple, one-word descriptions in English and Spanish; and are available in 13 other languages.

3. *Mass Care Communication Tools (CD):* The Mass Care Communication Tools CD contains images, pocket communicators, and training materials to be used at alternate care sites and dispensing sites. The materials on this CD facilitate communication and promote universal

(continued)

CASE STUDY 33.1 (*continued*)

access. All the design files are appropriate for use with any commercial print shop. The CD includes:

- 11 alternate care site images with 13 translations
- 10 emergency dispensing site images with 13 translations, 13 screening and treatment images
- One dispensing site pocket communicator file
- Dispensing site training curriculum

4. *Plan to Be Safe—Training Modules for Emergency Operations of Dispensing and Vaccination Clinics (CD):* This public health clinic operations toolkit, developed

by the Montgomery County Advanced Practice Center, incorporates four training modules and comes with the following items:

- Instructor's guide
- Appendices of resources and templates
- CD-ROM containing PDF versions of all materials
- DVD with two training videos

Operation Caroline demonstrates a mock dispensing and vaccination clinic and Operation Dagwood demonstrates a mock smallpox vaccination clinic.

34

RADIOLOGICAL INCIDENTS AND EMERGENCIES

P. Andrew Karam

LEARNING OBJECTIVES

When this chapter is completed, readers will be able to:

1. Distinguish between radiation and radioactive contamination.
2. Describe the three basic types of radiation.
3. Recognize common types of radiological incidents and emergencies.
4. Describe the clinical signs of radiation exposure.
5. Understand the importance of treating significant medical problems in patients with radioactive contamination.
6. Explain basic radiological control methods.

KEY MESSAGES

Radiation is a part of our natural environment.

In large doses, radiation can cause a number of syndromes, including death.

In small doses, radiation is more likely to cause cancer later in life.

Radioactively contaminated patients (e.g., following a terrorist attack) pose relatively little risk to healthcare staff.

Contamination control measures when working with contaminated patients will help limit the spread of radioactive contamination to medical facilities.

CHAPTER OVERVIEW

Medical and nursing personnel may be called on to care for patients who have been exposed to high levels of radiation or who have been contaminated with radioactive material (often abbreviated as RAM). Some of these patients may be gravely ill with radiation sickness or may have radiation burns, whereas others may have no radiological problems other than minor skin contamination. It is essential that nurses and other medical and nursing personnel be able to recognize radiation injury and provide appropriate treatment. It is also essential that medical and nursing personnel understand that patients who are merely contaminated may be treated without risk of radiation injury to the medical staff, although contamination control measures are prudent if the patient's medical condition permits.

Radiation and radioactivity are used throughout society, and it is possible that, at some point, medical staff will have to deal with patients who are contaminated with radioactivity or who have been exposed to possibly damaging levels of radiation. At the same time, there is a decided lack of knowledge among medical staff about the effects of radiation, how to recognize radiation injury, and how to treat patients involved in radiological incidents. This lack of knowledge has resulted in medical staff delaying or denying treatment to mildly contaminated patients, recommending therapeutic abortions that are not medically necessary, failing to recognize radiation injury, and more.

A radiological incident may be as dramatic as a terrorist attack or as mundane as mild skin contamination from a small radioactive spill in a research laboratory. Radiological incidents have resulted in death from radiation sickness, but the vast majority of cases simply require decontamination and monitoring. With a very few, specific exceptions, patients involved in radiological incidents pose absolutely no risk to medical staff, who must treat the patient's medical conditions without regard to radiological risks. This chapter addresses these and other issues.

RADIATION BASICS

The word "radiation" usually refers to ionizing radiation—radiation with enough energy to create ion pairs in matter. Ultraviolet light can do this, as can x-rays, gamma rays, and other kinds of radiation. Visible light is also radiation, but it is not energetic enough to cause ionizations, so it cannot normally cause problems. By comparison, ionizing radiation can damage our DNA, causing health effects in sufficiently high doses.

It is important to distinguish between "radiation" and "radioactive contamination." Radiation is energy emitted by atoms that are unstable. Radiation travels through space with a range that depends on the kind of radiation—some kinds of radiation can travel only a few millimeters through air, whereas other types can travel for many meters. Radioactive contamination is the presence of radiation-emitting substances in a place where it is not desired. A patient may be contaminated with radionuclides, but that patient will not be inherently radioactive and can be decontaminated. RAM, by comparison, is inherently

radioactive—it is a physical property of that material in the same manner as mass or size—and they remain radioactive until they decay to stability.

Types of Radiation

There are three basic kinds of radiation that medical staff can expect to see: alpha, beta, and gamma radiation. These have distinct properties that are summarized in the following sections.

Alpha Radiation

Emitted by heavy atoms such as uranium, radium, radon, polonium, and plutonium (to name a few), alpha particles are helium nuclei, making them the most massive kind of radiation. Alpha radiation can cause a great deal of damage to the living cells it encounters, but has such a short range in tissue (only a few microns) that external alpha radiation cannot penetrate the dead cells of the epidermis to irradiate the living cells beneath. If inhaled, swallowed, or introduced into open wounds, however, alpha radiation can be very damaging. One example of this was the 2006 murder of Viktor Litvenenko in London that was accomplished by introducing less than 1 mcg of alpha-emitting polonium (Po-210) into his tea. In nature, alpha radiation is found in rocks and soils as part of the minerals, in air as radon gas, and dissolved in water as radium, uranium, or radon. Alpha emitters are also found in nuclear power plants, nuclear weapons, static eliminators, some luminous paints (radium may be used for this), smoke detectors, and some consumer products. Objects and patients exposed to alpha radiation may become contaminated, but they do not become radioactive.

Beta Radiation

Beta particles are electrons or positrons and are both lighter than alpha particles and possess a lower electrical charge. This means that they are not nearly as damaging, although they will penetrate up to a centimeter into tissue. Beta particles will give a radiation dose only to the skin, unless they are ingested or inhaled, or enter the body through open cuts or wounds. In nature, beta radiation is found as part of natural potassium, in rocks and soils, and in the atmosphere as naturally produced carbon 14 and tritium. Beta-emitting radionuclides are used in research, some luminous paints, and for both diagnostic and therapeutic medical purposes. Objects and patients exposed to beta radiation may become contaminated, but they do not become radioactive.

Gamma Radiation

Gamma rays are energetic photons, similar to x-rays. Gamma radiation is much less damaging than alpha radiation and is about as damaging as beta radiation. Unlike alpha and beta radiation, gamma radiation will penetrate the whole body (as x-rays will), so it will deliver radiation doses to internal organs as well as to the skin. In nature, gamma radiation is ubiquitous and is found in outer space and on the surface of the Earth. Gamma radioactivity is found in rocks and soils, as well as in naturally radioactive isotopes of potassium found in foods and our own bodies. Gamma radiation is used for many research, industrial, and medical purposes. Objects and patients exposed to gamma radiation may become contaminated, but they do not become radioactive.

Units of Radiation Dose

Radiation can cause two main kinds of damage to our bodies. The energy deposited in cells by radiation can directly damage the cells, breaking chemical bonds and interfering with a cell's ability to function properly or even killing the cell. If enough cells are incapacitated or killed in a short period of time, we will become sick or can die from this exposure. Exposure to relatively high doses of radiation in a short period of time (acute exposure) acts in this manner. The damage caused by acute radiation exposure is most strongly affected by the amount of energy that is absorbed by a cell. The unit that is used to measure the amount of energy deposition is the gray (Gy)—a unit of radiation absorbed dose that is equal to the deposition of 1 J of energy in 1 kg of material. The U.S. unit for absorbed dose is the rad, which results from the deposition of 100 ergs of energy per gram of absorber (1 Gy = 100 rad).

Radiation can also damage the DNA in a cell, ultimately leading to cancer years or decades later. Exposure to relatively low doses of radiation over a long period of time (chronic exposure) acts in this manner. Some kinds of radiation, such as alpha radiation, cause higher levels of DNA damage than other kinds of radiation, so they are more effective at causing cancer for the same absorbed dose. Such kinds of radiation have a high *quality factor* (also called *"relative biological effectiveness"*) because they cause more DNA damage and a higher risk of developing cancer than do other radiations that deposit the same amount of energy in the body. In essence, the *effective risk* from exposure to these types of radiation is higher than we would guess if we measured only the amount of energy deposited in the body. The unit sievert (Sv) is used to measure the amount of biological damage (and the cancer risk) from exposure to radiation. The U.S. unit for effective dose is the rem and 1 Sv = 100 rem.

Acute radiation exposure, which can cause radiation sickness, radiation burns, and so forth, is caused by the energy deposited in the body, and so it causes effects that will occur within hours, days, or weeks of the exposure. In the case of acute radiation exposure, then, we measure only the amount of energy deposited in the body, so we use units of Gy or rad.

When we are concerned about the long-term effects of radiation exposure, it is important to understand how much DNA damage is caused by the radiation, so the *quality* of the radiation must also be considered. Because of this, we measure radiation dose in units of Sv (or rem) when we are considering, for example, the risk that someone will develop cancer as a result of his or her radiation exposure. This is why regulations and radiation dosimeter reports use units of Sv or rem; they are concerned with protecting us against the risk of developing cancer several decades later in our lives.

In this chapter, we use units of Gy and rad when we are concerned about the short-term risk of skin burns, radiation sickness, or fatal radiation injury that results from acute radiation exposure and use units of Sv and rem when we discuss the risk of developing cancer many years or decades after the radiation exposure, or when we are discussing compliance with radiation safety regulations.

Background Radiation Exposure

We are all exposed to radiation on a daily basis from both natural and man-made sources. Background radiation levels vary widely depending on altitude, local geology, and latitude, but average background radiation dose in the United States and Canada is about 3.11 mSv or 311 millirem (mrem) annually from natural sources and an additional 3.16 mSv (316 mrem) from medical and other artificial sources (see Table 34.1).

There are trace amounts of radioactivity in rocks and soils, in our bodies, and in the air we breathe; and charged particles from the sun and our galaxy bombard our planet continually. This background radiation exposure is unavoidable, but our bodies are able to repair the resulting DNA damage. The average of all of these sources is about 3.11 mSv (311 mrem) each year but in some places (e.g., Ramsar, Iran and Kerala, India), the local geology and geochemistry are such that residents are exposed to radiation levels of up to 100 times as high, without apparent ill effects.

Man-made sources of radiation account for over 3 mSv/y (300 mrem/y) for U.S. residents, primarily from medical radiation. We are also exposed to variable amounts of radiation from consumer products, aviation, nuclear energy, and so forth. Some of these consumer products are smoke detectors, certain types of ceramic materials, some static eliminators, welding electrodes, and so forth.

In all, we receive slightly more than 6 mSv (600 mrem) annually from natural and artificial background sources of radiation; a dose that varies considerably in both directions depending on local geology, elevation, a person's access to (and need for) medical procedures, and other factors. It is worth noting that, even in areas with exceptionally high levels of natural radiation, inhabitants do not appear to suffer from any ill effects. This suggests that occupational exposure to moderately elevated radiation levels is not harmful.

TABLE 34.1 Common Sources of Radiation Exposure

Source	Annual Radiation Dose (mSv/y/mrem/y)
Radon	2.28/228
Biological radionuclides	0.29/29
Geologic materials	0.21/21
Cosmic radiation	0.33/33
Medical sources	3/300
Consumer products	0.13/13
Other	0.03/3
Total	6.27/627

TABLE 34.2 Effects of Acute Radiation Exposure

Dose Gy (rad)	Syndrome or Effect	Comments
~0.05 (5)	Chromosome changes	Increase in dicentric chromosomes and chromosome fragments noted
0.15–0.25 (15–25)	Blood cell changes	Begin to see depression in numbers of red and white blood cells
1 (100)	Radiation sickness	Mild at lower doses; severity and rapidity of onset increase rapidly with increasing dose
3–8 (300–800)	Hematopoietic syndrome	Changes in blood cell count from damage to crypt cells; severe radiation sickness, recovery possible with medical support
4 (400)	LD_{50}	With medical treatment, LD_{50} is about 8 Sv (800 rem)
10 (1,000)	Gastrointestinal syndrome, LD_{100}	Relatively rapid onset for vomiting
100 (10,000)	Cerebrovascular syndrome	Rapid incapacitation, death within a few days

LD_{50}, lethal dose 50 percent; LD_{100}, lethal dose 100 percent; rad, radiation absorbed dose.

HEALTH EFFECTS OF RADIATION EXPOSURE

Both patients and medical staff are understandably concerned about the health effects of exposure to radiation and radioactive contamination. There are two distinct types of radiation exposure, acute and chronic, and two primary exposure modes, radiation and radioactive contamination. Each exposure type and mode is slightly different and must be treated differently by medical staff (see Table 34.2). In addition, there are concerns about the reproductive effects of radiation exposure. In this section, these concerns are discussed.

Acute Exposure to High Doses of Radiation

Exposing the whole body to very high levels of radiation in a short period of time can be harmful or fatal to the patient.

Exposing parts of the whole body to very high radiation levels can also cause harm, but is usually not life-threatening. Acute radiation injury has been noted in the survivors of the Japanese atomic bombings, among surviving Chernobyl workers, in the wake of nuclear accidents, and among people who have found lost radioactive sources with high levels of activity. Acute radiation injury to limited parts of the body has also been noted in patients receiving excessive fluoroscopy, mineralogists, and materials scientists misusing x-ray diffraction equipment, industrial employees using linear accelerators, and radiation oncology patients. Perhaps the most common injuries in this category are severe radiation burns—usually to the hands—among people who have found and picked up abandoned radioactive sources.

Sunburn is a mild form of acute exposure to radiation, but it serves as a starting point to understanding acute radiation injury. At a skin dose of a few Sv (a few hundred rem), the patient will exhibit erythema and, at higher doses, blistering and peeling (dry and moist desquamation). Depending on

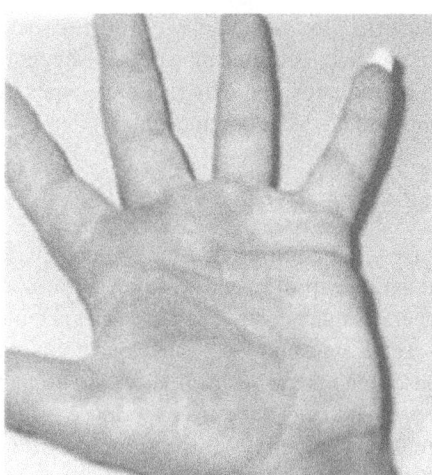

FIGURE 34.1 Ten days after exposure. Left hand of a patient who rubbed Cs powder on his palm. A diffuse secondary erythema is noted on the region proximal to fingers 2, 3, and 4. Delineation of bulla formation is barely visible.

Source: From Oliveira, A. R., Brandão-Mello, C. E., Valverde, N. J., Farina, R., & Curado, M. P. (1991). Localized lesions induced by Cs-137 during the Goiania accident. *Health Physics, 60*(1), 25–29. Reproduced with permission of the Health Physics Society.

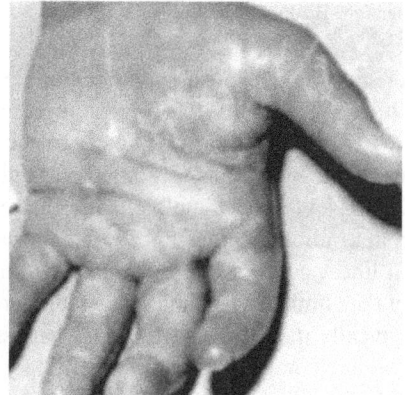

FIGURE 34.2 Fifteen days after exposure. A large, tense bulla associated with edema limited finger movement.

Source: From Oliveira, A. R., Brandão-Mello, C. E., Valverde, N. J., Farina, R., & Curado, M. P. (1991). Localized lesions induced by Cs-137 during the Goiania accident. *Health Physics, 60*(1), 25–29. Reproduced with permission of the Health Physics Society.

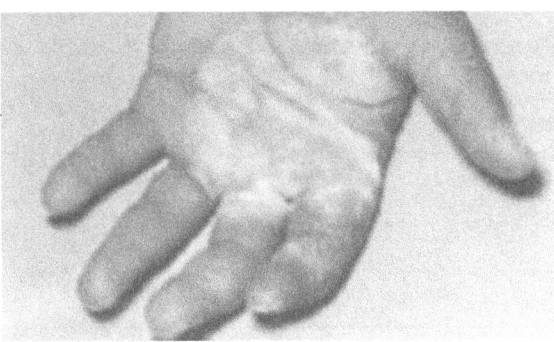

FIGURE 34.3 Twenty days after exposure. Note rupture of the bulla, with dead skin becoming whitish and the surrounding epidermis showing areas of dry desquamation.

Source: From Oliveira, A. R., Brandão-Mello, C. E., Valverde, N. J., Farina, R., & Curado, M. P. (1991). Localized lesions induced by Cs-137 during the Goiania accident. *Health Physics, 60*(1), 25–29. Reproduced with permission of the Health Physics Society.

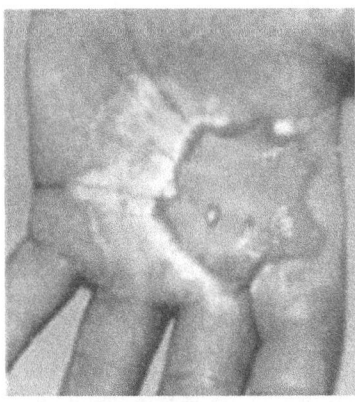

FIGURE 34.4 Fifty days after exposure. After debridement of necrotic epidermis, bright red denuded derma is covered with a thin layer of fibrous exudate. Note sparse islands of epithelialization and centripetal aspect of the healing process.

Source: From Oliveira, A. R., Brandão-Mello, C. E., Valverde, N. J., Farina, R., & Curado, M. P. (1991). Localized lesions induced by Cs-137 during the Goiania accident. *Health Physics, 60*(1), 25–29. Reproduced with permission of the Health Physics Society.

the characteristics of the exposure, one side of the body may be more affected—typically the side facing the radiation source. Very high radiation doses to parts of the body will produce these same symptoms to limited parts of the body. Figures 34.1 to 34.11 show the effects of radiation burns to the back (from a radiology procedure) and to the hands (from an industrial linear accelerator). Some patients may exhibit symptoms of both limited and whole-body radiation exposure. These are typically those who have come across abandoned radioactive sources and carry them home. Other effects of acute whole-body radiation exposure can include depilation, nausea, and a variety of radiation syndromes that are described in the following text. Some instances of radiation injury are illustrated in Figures 34.1 to 34.11.

Some cells are more sensitive to the effects of radiation than others. These cells typically share one or more of the following characteristics:

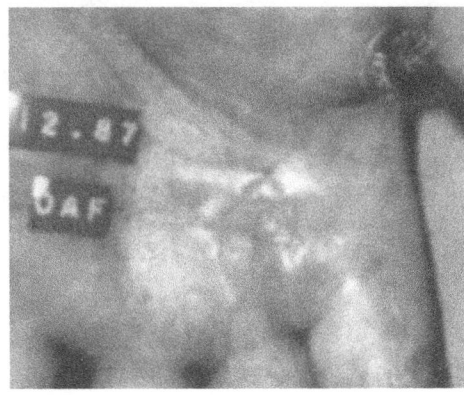

FIGURE 34.5 One hundred days after exposure. Resulting scar tissue is atrophic and retractile. Telangiectasis are observed under the translucent epidermis. A central, irregular, necrotic zone is evident in this unhealed injury.

Source: From Oliveira, A. R., Brandão-Mello, C. E., Valverde, N. J., Farina, R., & Curado, M. P. (1991). Localized lesions induced by Cs-137 during the Goiania accident. *Health Physics, 60*(1), 25–29. Reproduced with permission of the Health Physics Society.

- Less specialized cells (e.g., stem cells) are more sensitive to radiation than are highly specialized cells such as neurons because a higher number of genes are active in the cells.
- Rapidly dividing cells are more susceptible to radiation than cells that divide only rarely because there is less time for radiation damage to be repaired before the cell divides again.
- Cells with a long reproductive lifetime are more sensitive to radiation because they have a longer time to pass mutations on to progeny cells.
- Well-oxygenated cells are more sensitive to radiation as oxygen increases radiogenic DNA damage.

These factors help to explain why some tissues (e.g., the epithelial tissues and blood-forming organs) are more likely to be affected by radiation and why radiation exposure to these tissues is more likely to be carcinogenic.

Prodromal Syndrome

In some cases, radiation effects may appear within a few hours of radiation exposure and will persist for up to several days. In general, higher doses result in earlier and more severe symptoms. At lower levels of exposure, symptoms may include fatigue, nausea, and vomiting. At higher (and probably lethal) exposure levels, patients will also experience fever, diarrhea, and hypotension. Patients with prodromal syndrome have likely been exposed to at least 1 Sv (100 rem), but symptoms will appear at any higher level of exposure. Patients exhibiting symptoms (e.g., vomiting or bloody diarrhea) within 30 minutes of exposure have likely received a lethal dose of radiation.

Hematopoietic Syndrome

The blood-forming organs are among the most sensitive to the effects of radiation, so these organs are among the first to show

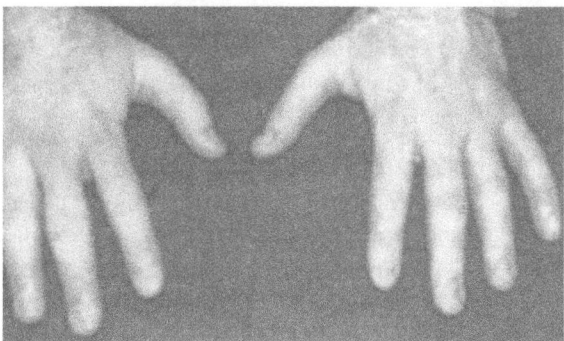

FIGURE 34.6 The victim's left and right hands on December 14, 1991 (3 days after the accident).

Source: From Schauer, D. A., Coursey, B. M., Dick, C. E., McLaughlin, W. L., Puhl, J. M., Desrosiers, M. F., & Jacobson, A. D. (1993). Radiation accident at an industrial accelerator facility. *Health Physics, 65*(2), 131–140. Reproduced with permission of the Health Physics Society.

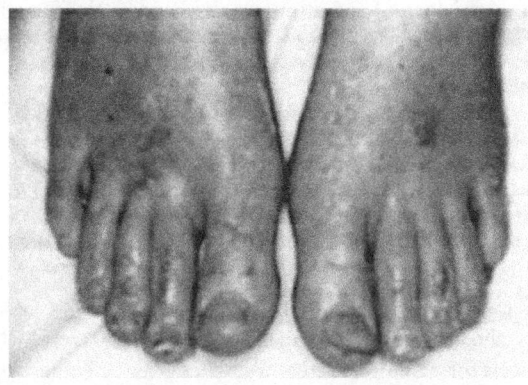

FIGURE 34.7 The victim's toes on February 11, 1992.

Source: From Schauer, D. A., Coursey, B. M., Dick, C. E., McLaughlin, W. L., Puhl, J. M., Desrosiers, M. F., & Jacobson, A. D. (1993). Radiation accident at an industrial accelerator facility. *Health Physics, 65*(2), 131–140. Reproduced with permission of the Health Physics Society.

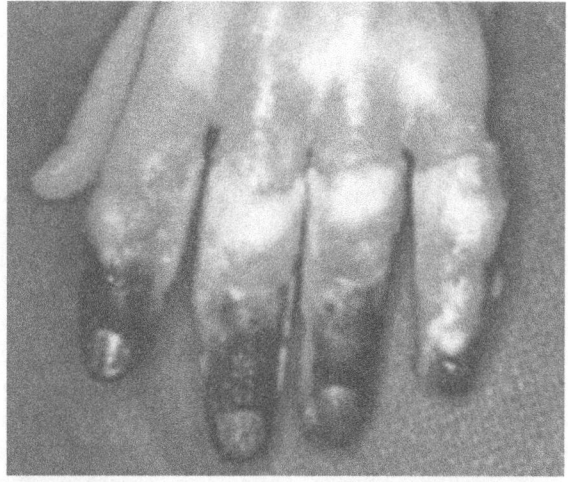

FIGURE 34.8 The victim's left hand on March 8, 1992.

Source: From Schauer, D. A., Coursey, B. M., Dick, C. E., McLaughlin, W. L., Puhl, J. M., Desrosiers, M. F., & Jacobson, A. D. (1993). Radiation accident at an industrial accelerator facility. *Health Physics, 65*(2), 131–140. Reproduced with permission of the Health Physics Society.

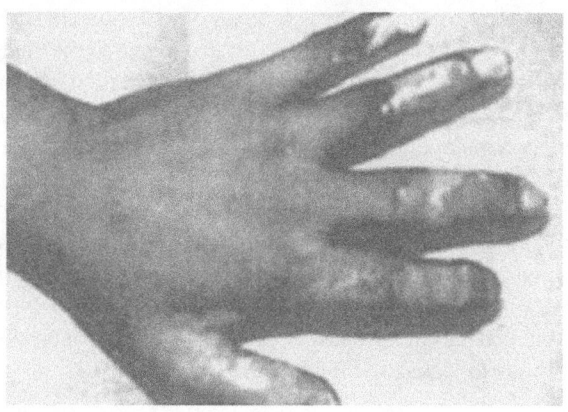

FIGURE 34.9 Left hand, dorsal surface.

Source: From Berger, M. E., Hurtado, R., Dunlap, J., Mutchinick, O., Valasco, M. G., Tostado, R. A., …, Ricks, R. C. (1997). Accidental radiation injury to the hand: Anatomical and physiological consideration. *Health Physics, 72*(3), 343–348. Reproduced with permission of the Health Physics Society.

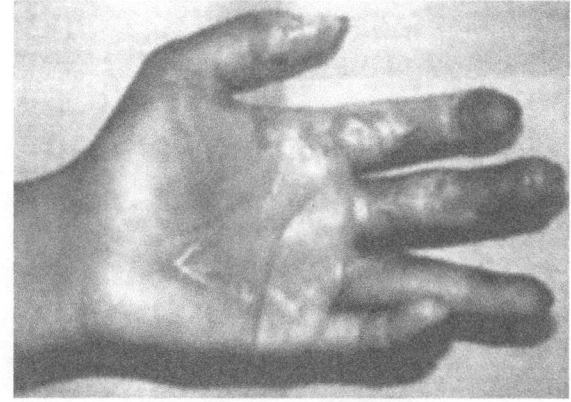

FIGURE 34.10 Left hand, palmar surface.

Source: From Berger, M. E., Hurtado, R., Dunlap, J., Mutchinick, O., Valasco, M. G., Tostado, R. A., …, Ricks, R. C. (1997). Accidental radiation injury to the hand: Anatomical and physiological consideration. *Health Physics, 72*(3), 343–348. Reproduced with permission of the Health Physics Society.

the results of high radiation exposure. Hematopoietic syndrome begins to appear at doses of 3 to 8 Sv (300 to 800 rem), when the precursor cells are sterilized or killed. This leads to a reduction in blood cell counts as older cells die and are not replaced, and it leaves the patient open to infection and other related problems. Following the initial prodromal syndrome, a patient may be relatively free of symptoms for some time, although a great deal is occurring. Patients with lower levels of exposure may recover from their exposure if the bone marrow can regenerate and if the patient receives medical support (typically antibiotic treatment). At higher levels of exposure, the patient will begin to exhibit chills, fatigue, hair loss, petechia, and ulceration of the mouth as well as infection, bleeding, immune system depression, and other symptoms resulting from the loss of blood cells. A dose of about 4 to 5 Sv (400 to 500 rem) is lethal to 50% of the exposed population without medical support. This is called the LD_{50} dose. With medical support, the LD_{50} dose is about 7 to 8 Sv (700 to 800 rem).

Treatment for patients suffering from hematopoietic syndromes includes replacing blood cells via transfusion, isolation from sources of infection, and antibiotic treatment.

Gastrointestinal Syndrome

Exposure to 10 Sv (1,000 rem) or more usually leads to gastrointestinal syndrome and death within 3 to 10 days of exposure. Radiation exposure in this range sterilizes dividing crypt cells, leading to loss of cells from the villi. Within a few days, the villi become almost totally flat as the outer surface sloughs off and is not replaced. In one particular case (a man exposed to between 11–20 Sv and 1,100–2,000 rem in 1946), the patient remained in relatively good condition for nearly a week, at which time he began suffering bloody diarrhea, circulatory collapse, and severe damage to the epithelial surfaces throughout the intestinal tract.

Treatments for patients suffering from gastrointestinal syndrome include antiemetics, sedatives, a bland diet, and fluid replacement. Antibiotic treatment and blood transfusions are sometimes helpful in keeping patients alive through the first few days or weeks. Unfortunately, however, this level of radiation dose is invariably fatal within a few weeks of exposure.

Cerebrovascular Syndrome

Exposure to exceptionally high doses of radiation (in excess of 100 Sv or 10,000 rem) will result in damage to the central nervous system, normally among the most radiation-resistant parts of the body. Cerebrovascular syndrome is accompanied by symptoms of all other radiation syndromes, and it usually results in death within several hours to a few days of exposure. Patients exposed to such high levels of radiation will experience almost immediate nausea, vomiting, disorientation, seizures, and other symptoms of neurological distress, followed by coma and death. Although the exact cause of death is not known, it is thought that part of the cause is the buildup of cranial pressure that is due to leakage of fluid from blood vessels.

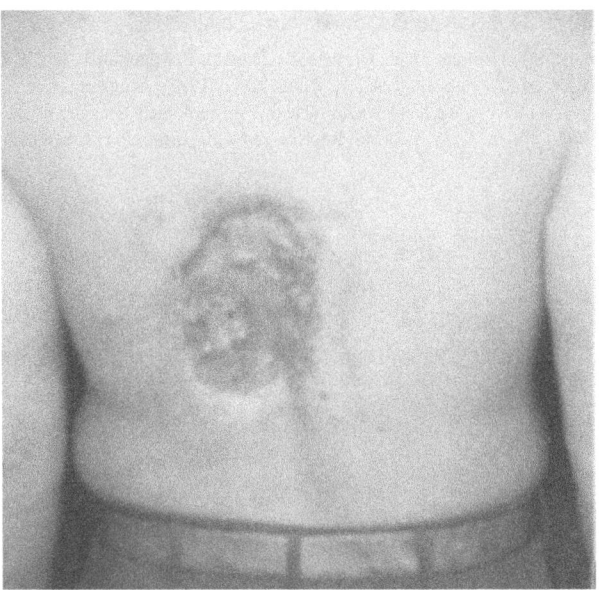

FIGURE 34.11 Radiation-induced skin injuries from fluoroscopy.

Source: Reprinted from Scientific Exhibit 060PH at the 81st Scientific Assembly and Annual Meeting of the Radiological Society of North America, November 26 to December 1, 1995. *Radiology, 197*(P), Suppl., 449.

Treatment for cerebrovascular syndrome is limited to providing pain relief and sedatives to control convulsions and anxiety because the syndrome is invariably fatal.

Chronic Exposure to Low Levels of Radiation

Everyone is chronically exposed to low levels of background radiation, and this exposure appears to have no adverse effects. There are many questions about the effects of exposure to low levels of radiation above background levels, however, and this is one of the most contentious areas in the radiation safety profession. There are currently two primary models, each of which will be discussed briefly. This section may be of interest to all medical staff because, even in the absence of radiological incidents, most medical personnel are exposed to low levels of radiation from x-rays, fluoroscopy, or computed tomography (CT) procedures.

The most serious concern is that long-term exposure to low levels of radiation may lead to cancer later in life. The two competing models describing the risk of cancer resulting from a given dose of radiation are the Linear, No-Threshold (LNT) model; and the threshold model. There are variations on both of these themes that will not be discussed.

LNT Model

The LNT model is the most conservative, meaning that it predicts the highest level of risk for any given radiation exposure. This model predicts that any exposure to radiation in excess of background levels is potentially harmful, and that the risk of getting cancer is directly proportional to the radiation dose received. LNT is the basis for radiation regulatory policies in the United States and, indeed, in virtually every nation on Earth. The LNT model predicts five additional cancer deaths for every person-Sv (100 person-rem of exposure). So, under this model, a single person with a lifetime radiation exposure of 0.1 Sv (10 rem) will have five chances in 1,000 (about 0.5%) of getting cancer from this exposure. Alternatively, this model also predicts that exposing 100 people to a dose of 10 mSv (1 rem) each will result in a total of five additional cancer deaths among the exposed population.

One problem with the LNT model is that it cannot be confirmed at low levels of exposure because of the statistical "noise" in the epidemiological studies performed. Because of this, the Health Physics Society has specifically advised against calculating risk for any exposure of less than 0.1 Sv (10 rem) to any person. In addition, the International Council on Radiation Protection (ICRP) has advised against the misuse of what is called "collective dose"—the second example given earlier. According to the ICRP, if the most-exposed individual receives an insignificant radiation dose, it is inappropriate to calculate the cancer risk to an entire population receiving that level of exposure or lower exposures. One analogy that comes to mind is with stones. One ton is equal to 1 million grams. There is no doubt that dropping a 1-ton rock on somebody's head will crush that person. The ICRP wants to avoid saying that throwing a million 1-g rocks at each of a million people will lead to one person being crushed to death. In reality, we will have a million irritated people, but nobody will be crushed. Similarly, exposing a million people to low doses of radiation probably will not affect the health of a single person, even if the collective dose is high.

Threshold Model

Another line of thinking suggests that there may be no adverse effects at all from exposure to low levels of radiation; that there may be a threshold, below which we see no risk. Under threshold models, there is a certain level of exposure that is completely safe, and it is only above that threshold that we begin to see an increase in cancer risk. Virtually all known harmful agents exhibit threshold effects.

One variation on the threshold model is the suggestion that exposure to low levels of radiation may produce beneficial effects. This is called "hormesis," and it is not as far-fetched as it might seem. We can all name substances that exhibit hormetic effects, including water, vitamin D, selenium, and aspirin. The thinking behind hormesis is that by providing a continuing challenge to our natural DNA damage repair mechanisms, these mechanisms are kept at their peak efficiencies and are better able to repair the spontaneous DNA damage that takes place all the time. Some studies of people living in high natural background radiation areas and those who are occupationally exposed to radiation suggest that one of these models may be more accurate than LNT in describing the risks from radiation exposure, but the evidence is not definitive and the debate will likely continue for some time to come.

Under LNT, the risks of developing cancer from occupational radiation exposure are about the same as the risks of any other occupational illness or injury—about one in 10,000. By comparison, the background cancer death rate is about 2,500 in 10,000 (25%), and about one person in 7,000 dies each year in traffic accidents (more than 40,000 in the year 2016). For the vast majority of radiation workers, the drive to work is far more hazardous than their occupational radiation exposure, even using the LNT model.

Reproductive Effects of Radiation Exposure

Radiation has been used for medical purposes for about a century, and in that time, innumerable men and women have been exposed to radiation. This includes tens or hundreds of thousands of pregnant women exposed to diagnostic radiation,

and many pregnant women were also exposed to radiation during the atomic bombings in Japan in 1945. *Among all of these women, prenatal radiation exposure of less than 50 mSv (5 rem) to the fetus has not been shown to have resulted in birth defects.* Higher levels of fetal radiation exposure have been known to lead to birth defects; primarily mental retardation, low birth weight, and low organ weight. Table 34.3 shows the medical recommendations (from Wagner, Lester, & Saldana, 1997) for several combinations of fetal radiation exposure and postconception age.

Radiology and the Pregnant Patient

Although every radiographic procedure is different, there are some general statements that can be made. One is that radiographic procedures (x-ray, CT, fluoroscopy) administered above the diaphragm (e.g., head, chest) or below the knees will not give a significant radiation dose to the fetus. It is also safe to say that the fetal radiation dose from a single CT scan or from several x-ray films is not high enough to cause birth defects or to call for a therapeutic abortion. Finally, medically necessary radiation should be administered if it is not possible to determine a patient's pregnancy status. If delaying a radiographic procedure may result in the patient's death or in serious complications, the procedure must be administered promptly, and the reproductive implications discussed after the patient is stable and awake.

The exact fetal radiation dose must be calculated for every case of exposure, based on information on file at each hospital. As a rule of thumb, until accurate dose calculations can be performed, one may make the following assumptions:

1. One x-ray that images the uterus will give a fetal dose of about 1 mSv (100 mrem).
2. One CT that images the uterus will give a fetal radiation dose of 20 to 50 mSv (2 to 5 rem).
3. Fetal dose from fluoroscopy in which the uterus is in the field of view is about 10 to 20 mSv (1 to 2 rem) for 1 minute of machine "on" time.

TABLE 34.3 Medical Recommendations for Fetal Radiation Exposure

Postconception Age	Fetal Dose (rem)	Recommendations
0–2 weeks	Any dose	No action necessary
2–15 weeks	<50 mSv (5 rem)	No action necessary
	50–150 mSv (5–15 rem)	May consider terminating pregnancy, depending on presence of other risk factors
15+ weeks	Greater than 50 mSv (5 rem)	No action necessary
	50–150 mSv (5–15 rem)	No action necessary
	>150 mSv (15 rem)	May consider terminating pregnancy, depending on presence of other risk factors

Source: Adapted with permission from Wagner, L. K., Lester, R. G., & Saldana, L. R. (1997). *Exposure of the pregnant patient to diagnostic radiations—A guide to management* (2nd ed.). Milwaukee, WI: Medical Physics Publishing.

These are only approximations, and the actual dose to the fetus must be calculated by a qualified and competent medical physicist or health physicist. They are reasonable estimates, however, and, for most equipment, are likely to be high rather than low estimates.

RADIOLOGICAL INCIDENTS AND EMERGENCIES

Radiological incidents and emergencies are any such events involving exposure of patients and/or emergency workers to radiation or radioactivity. A radiological incident is any instance in which people or the environment are exposed to radiation or radioactivity through accident or misuse (including deliberate misuse). A radiological emergency is any radiological incident in which there is the risk of injury or death, even if that risk is not from the radiation itself. For example, exploding a radiological dispersal device (RDD; colloquially called a "dirty bomb") might not cause radiation injury, but the blast will certainly place lives at risk. An attack with an RDD, then, is a radiological emergency, even though one may not actually

see any patients with radiation-caused injuries. Some examples of radiological incidents and emergencies are the following:

- Traffic accident involving a truck carrying research or medical radioactive isotopes
- Terrorist attack with an RDD (or "dirty bomb")
- Fire in a hospital or university radioactive waste storage facility
- Unplanned radioactive release from a commercial nuclear power station
- Detonation of a nuclear weapon
- Loss of a radioactive soil-density gauge or well-logging gauge
- Accidental exposure of a maintenance technician to radiation from an industrial linear accelerator
- Radiation burns to the fingers from the beam of an x-ray diffractometer in a soil science laboratory
- Accidental overexposure to an angiography patient from excessive fluoroscopy, resulting in radiation burns to the skin
- Spill of radioactive liquids in a research laboratory

The public, emergency responders, and medical personnel often respond inappropriately to radiological incidents and

TABLE 34.4 Obtaining Samples to Confirm Radiation Exposure

Sample	Reason	How Collected
All Radiation Injury Cases		
Complete blood count and differential immediately, followed by absolute lymphocyte counts every 6 hours for 48 hours if whole-body irradiation possible.	Radiation dose assessment; establish baseline (initial counts) for comparison with later counts to assess degree of injury.	Draw blood from noncontaminated area, cover puncture site afterward.
Routine urinalysis.	Determine kidney function and establish baseline for later comparison—most important if external contamination is a possibility.	Try not to contaminate sample during collection. Label samples with sequential numbers, date, and time.
When External Contamination Is Suspected		
Swab body orifices.	Assess potential for internal contamination.	Use separate saline- or water-moistened swabs to wipe inside of each nostril, mouth, and each ear.
Wound dressings or swabs from wounds.	Determine whether wounds are contaminated.	Save dressings in plastic bags. Use moist or dry swabs to sample secretions from each wound or use syringe or dropper to collect a few drops from each wound. Remove visible debris with tweezers, applicators, or forceps. Place all samples into individual containers, labeled with location, date, and time.
When Internal Contamination Is Suspected		
Urine—24-hour specimen times 4 days. Feces—24-hour specimen times 4 days.	Excreta may contain excreted radionuclides if there was an uptake.	Use 24-hour urine collection container.

Source: Reprinted with permission from Radiation Emergency Assistance Center/Training Site (REAC/TS). (n.d.). *The medical aspects of radiation accidents* (4th ed.). Oak Ridge, TN: Oak Ridge Associated University. Retrieved from https://orise.orau.gov/reacts/documents/medical-aspects-of-radiation-incidents.pdf

emergencies, usually owing to widespread misunderstanding of the risks posed by radiation and radioactivity. In particular, members of the public often panic and tend to attribute all real and perceived health problems to the effects of radiation. Emergency response personnel sometimes hesitate to approach the scene of radiological incidents, and medical personnel frequently delay or deny treatment to contaminated or irradiated patients. In addition, there are many instances in which medical personnel have failed to diagnose exposure to radiation, providing inappropriate medical care. In the case of Alexander Litvenenko (a former Russian spy killed with radioactive polonium in 2006), medical personnel failed to recognize the radiological nature of his affliction for almost 3 weeks. *Medical personnel must be able to recognize radiation injury and to provide appropriate medical assistance to personnel at the scene and in the hospital to all patients involved in radiological incidents and emergencies.*

Samples

Virtually all radiological cases will require some sampling to confirm the level of exposure and to help determine a treatment plan (see Table 34.4). Samples must be treated as potentially radioactive until proven otherwise. In addition, analytical equipment and areas may become contaminated, precluding their use for nonradiological patients until decontaminated. Blood samples must be obtained from uncontaminated (or decontaminated) areas to reduce the chance of inadvertent sample contamination and to prevent introducing contamination into a patient's blood. Samples collected by the patient (e.g., urine or stool) may be inadvertently contaminated by the patient. The patient should wear gloves to reduce this possibility.

On-Scene Medical Assistance

Medical personnel at the incident scene may be called on to treat or triage patients suffering from the effects of exposure to high levels of radiation or to treat or triage patients contaminated with radioactivity. Medical personnel should take all possible precautions to avoid accidental uptake of RAM. These include not eating, drinking, or smoking in contamination zones; promptly irrigating and covering open wounds; and thoroughly swabbing patients' skin before giving injections, drawing blood, or suturing. All persons entering a contaminated area should take standard precautions; they should wear protective gloves, shoe covers, outer protective clothing, and eye covering when working with radiologically contaminated patients or in contaminated areas. All persons leaving a contamination area should remove their protective clothing (including gloves and shoe covers) prior to exiting the area. Whenever possible (i.e., when patient care will not be compromised) all personnel—patients included—should be surveyed for contamination prior to exiting any contamination area. All equipment exiting the area should also be surveyed prior to release or should be sealed in plastic bags for later survey, possible decontamination, and release.

Caring for Patients Exposed to High Levels of Radiation

Life-threatening injuries and medical conditions must take priority over radiological injury and contamination. Medical injuries can be fatal within minutes or hours while radiological injuries manifest themselves over periods of days to months. Keeping patients alive in the short term must take precedence over worrying about long-term dangers. The National Council on Radiation Protection and Measurements (NCRP; Figure 34.12) has developed a flowchart to help medical practitioners sort out these competing priorities.

Patients exposed to moderately high levels of radiation (1 Sv = 100 rem or less) will likely exhibit no symptoms of radiation sickness while at the scene. Laboratory work will show a depression in red and white blood cells, but this may not appear for several days after the exposure. About 10% of patients exposed to 1 Sv (100 rem) will exhibit mild radiation sickness, but may not attribute it to radiation exposure.

The most critical range of exposures for medical intervention is that between 2 and 8 Sv (200 and 800 rem). Patients with exposures in this range may experience nausea, vomiting, fatigue, physical weakness, and/or psychological distress.

Patients exposed to higher levels of radiation will experience more severe radiation sickness that will appear more rapidly. A patient receiving a dose of about 4 Sv (400 rem) has a 50% chance of death without medical intervention, primarily from radiation-induced immune system suppression and subsequent infectious disease.

With medical support, such patients are likely to survive exposure. These patients will also experience radiation sickness. However, if the prodromal stage of radiation sickness appears within 30 to 60 minutes after exposure, the patient has likely received a fatal dose of radiation. Such patients should be made as comfortable as possible.

Some patients may be exposed to high levels of radiation that affect only a part of their bodies. In the aftermath of the Fukushima nuclear reactor meltdowns, for example, two workers whose leaky boots filled with radioactive water received second-degree radiation burns from beta-emitting radionuclides over their lower extremities. The physician who treated these men reported (personal conversation) that both men received standard care for second-degree burns, that both were released upon recovery, and that no sequelae were anticipated. In this case, since beta radiation has a range of only about 1 cm in tissue, the radiation burns extended only to that depth. In the case of radiation burns, it might be necessary to perform decontamination (if the patient's medical condition permits) prior to dressing the burns; in more severe cases, skin grafts might be necessary.

Differentiating between radiation burns and thermal burns can be difficult, and it is not always possible to make this distinction based solely on clinical evidence. Most radiation burns will lead to erythema, blistering, and other tissue damage, but so do many thermal burns and serious sunburn (see Table 34.5). In some cases, the patient will be able to provide

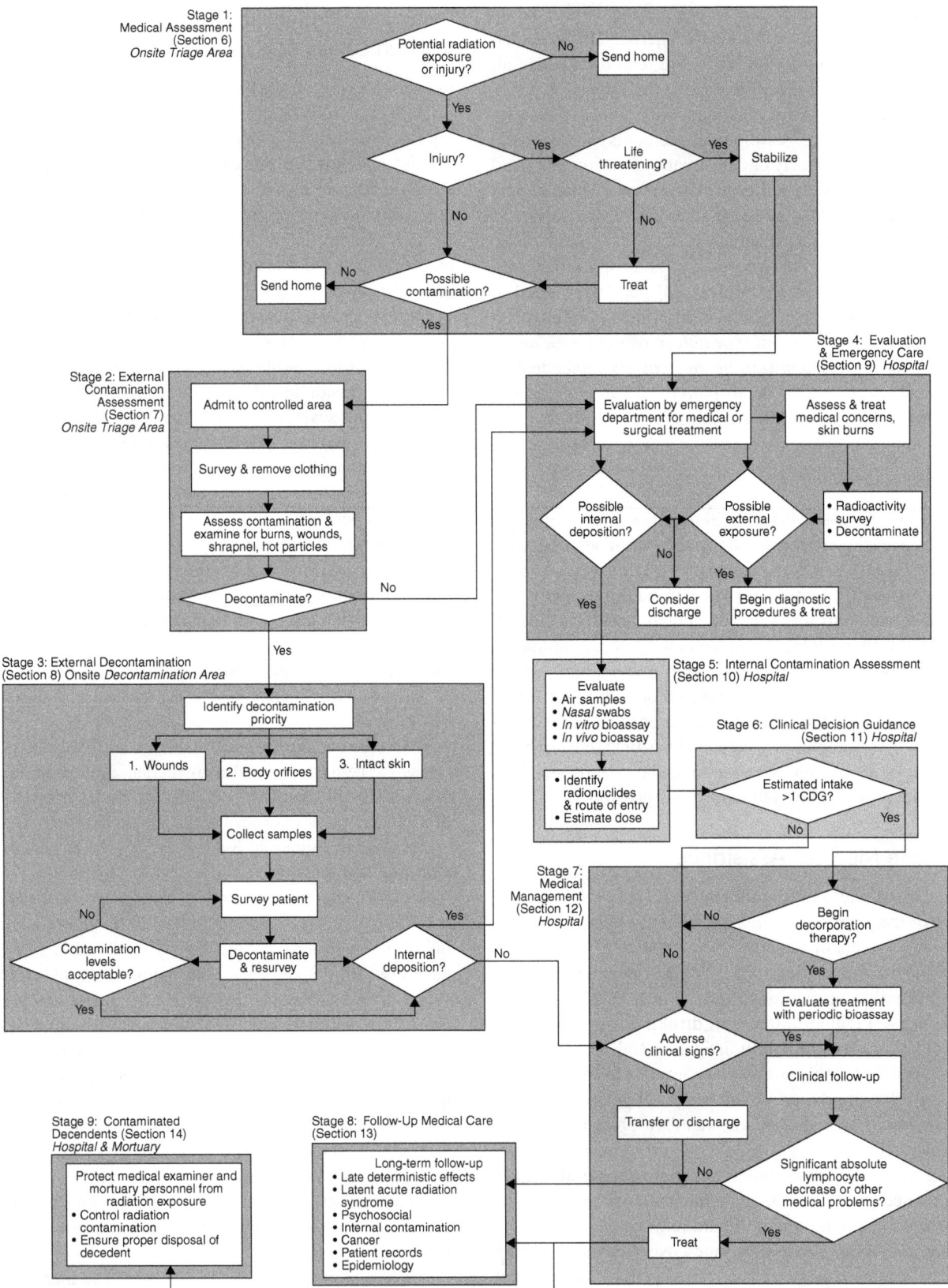

FIGURE 34.12 Decision tree for management of exposed persons.

Source: National Council on Radiation Protection and Measurements. (2009). *Report #161—Management of persons contaminated with radioactivity: Handbook* (Vol. 1). Bethesda, MD: Author.

TABLE 34.5 Symptoms of Radiation Exposure on the Skin

Condition	Skin Dose Sv (rem)
Erythema	6 (600)
Dry desquamation	10 (1,000)
Ulceration	20 (2,000)
Dermatitis (radiation-induced)	25 (2,500)
Epilation	3 (300)

Note: Patients exposed to large doses of beta radiation can have a very high dose to the skin with no corresponding whole-body exposure. Similarly, skin burns may affect only a part of the body. In other words, patients receiving a sublethal radiation dose may exhibit some of these symptoms.

Source: Reprinted with permission from Radiation Emergency Assistance Center/Training Site (REAC/TS). (n.d.). *The medical aspects of radiation accidents* (4th ed.). Oak Ridge, TN: Oak Ridge Associated Universities. Retrieved from https://orise.orau.gov/reacts/documents/medical-aspects-of-radiation-incidents.pdf

TABLE 34.6 Radiation Dose Producing Illness and/or Mortality

Condition	Whole-Body Dose—Sv (rem)
No observed effects	0.05 (5)
Chromosome damage	0.15 (15)
White cell depression	0.5 (50)
Radiation sickness begins	1 (100)
[a]LD$_{50}$ (assuming no medical treatment) LD$_{50}$ (with medical treatment)	4–5 (400–500) 7–8 (700–800)
[b]LD$_{100}$ (assuming no medical treatment)	8–10 (800–1,000)

[a]LD$_{50}$ equals dose at which 50% of the population exposed will die.
[b]LD$_{100}$ equals dose as which 100% of the population exposed will die.

Sources: Reprinted with permission from Linnemann, R. E. (2001). *Managing radiation medical emergencies*. Philadelphia, PA: Radiation Management Consultants and American College of Radiology. (2002). *Radiation disasters: Preparedness and responses for radiology*. Reston, VA: Author.

helpful information—he or she may recall recent radiology or radiation oncology procedures or may mention that he or she works in a facility with radiation-generating equipment, for example. Medical staff should also know that radiation injury is seldom, if ever, associated with charring, so charred tissue is typically a sign of thermal injury. However, patients near the site of a dirty bomb explosion may suffer thermal burns from the chemical explosion *and* be radioactively contaminated. Remember that exposure to radiation does not cause a person to become radioactive and that radiation burns do not manifest immediately. If you survey a burned patient and find positive counts with a radiation instrument, the wound is likely contaminated, but the burns themselves are likely *thermal* burns, *not* radiation burns.

There is no health risk to medical or emergency personnel from working with patients exposed to high levels of radiation. Irradiated patients do *not* become radioactive.

Clinical Signs of Radiation Exposure (See Table 34.6)

1. Nausea and vomiting (prodromal syndrome—if experienced shortly after exposure, the patient has probably received a lethal radiation dose)
2. Possible erythema when patient denies thermal or chemical exposure (may be localized, depending on source of radiation)
3. Blistering, ulcerated tissue, possible necrosis (following exposure to very high, localized exposure to radiation)
4. Depression in red and white blood cell counts (usually occurs a few to several weeks after exposure)
5. Elevated levels of chromosomal aberrations

Treatment for Patients Exposed to High Levels of Whole-Body Radiation (Table 34.7)

- Patients exhibiting signs of radiation sickness immediately after an accident have likely received a fatal dose of radiation. Treating their symptoms will help to make them comfortable until a physician specializing in such cases can be contacted for the most recent medical advice. Such advice is available from the REAC/TS center at the Oak Ridge National Laboratory (orise.orau.gov/reacts/).
- Patients receiving several sieverts (several hundred rem) of exposure will exhibit reduced immune system function. Such patients require medical support until their immune systems can recover.

Patient Management—Doses Greater Than 200 rad (Berger et al., 2007)

1. Use selective blocking of serotonin 5-HT$_3$ receptors or use 5-HT$_3$ receptor antagonists to treat vomiting.
2. Consider initiating viral prophylaxis.
3. Consider tissue and blood typing in anticipation of possible blood transfusions and/or bone marrow transplant.
4. Treat trauma as necessary and appropriate.
5. Consider consultation with hematologist and radiation experts to determine dosimetry, prognosis, use of colony-stimulating factors, stem cell transfusion, and so forth.
6. Draw blood for chromosome analysis (possible biodosimetry); use heparinized tube.
7. Note and record areas of erythema on body chart; take photographs if possible.
8. Begin supportive care in clean environment (reverse isolation).
9. Prevent and/or treat infections.
10. Use growth factors (e.g., GCSF, GMCSF, interleukin) to stimulate hematopoiesis.

11. Provide psychological support to patient and family.
12. Consider transfusions of stem cells via umbilical cord blood, peripheral blood, or bone marrow.
13. Consider platelet transfusions if platelet count is low or in case of bleeding.
14. Observe for erythema, hair loss, skin injury, mucositis, parotitis, weight loss, fever.

Caring for Radioactively Contaminated Patients (Table 34.8)

In the aftermath of the earthquake, tsunami, and nuclear reactor accident in Fukushima, local hospitals began receiving patients from the reactor plant and from the areas affected by the earthquake and tsunami. After the nuclear reactors began releasing

TABLE 34.7 Guidelines for Radiologically Exposed Patients at General Hospitals

Exposure Type	Possible Effects	Initial Treatment
External Whole-Body Exposure		
Localized exposure—usually to hands.	Localized erythema; possible blistering, ulceration, and necrosis.	Clinical observation and treatment of symptoms.
Total or partial whole-body exposure, minimal or delayed clinical signs.	No clinical signs in 3 plus hours after exposure, not life-threatening. Minor blood changes.	Clinical observation and treatment of symptoms. Sequential blood samples.
Total or partial whole-body exposure with early prodromal syndrome.	Acute radiation syndrome with severity depending on dose.	Treatment as noted earlier, possible specialized care. Full blood count and HLA typing prior to transfer to specialized center.
Total or partial whole-body exposure with thermal, chemical, or radiation burns.	Severe injuries, life-threatening.	Treat life-threatening conditions. Treat as above and early transfer to specialized facility.
External Contamination		
Low-level contamination, intact skin, cleaning possible.	No likely consequences, possible mild radiation burns.	Decontaminate skin, monitor medical condition.
Low-level contamination, skin intact, cleaning delayed.	Possible radiation burns. Possible percutaneous intake.	Consult with specialist if possible.
Low-level contamination with thermal, chemical, radiation burns, and/or trauma.	Internal contamination possible.	Consult with specialist if possible.
Extensive contamination and associated wounds.	Internal contamination probable.	Consult with specialist if possible.
Extensive contamination with thermal, chemical, radiation burns, and/or trauma.	Severe combined injuries and probable internal contamination.	First aid and treatment of life-threatening injuries, early transfer to specialized center.
Internal Contamination		
Inhalation and ingestion of minor quantities of radionuclides.	No immediate effects.	Consult with specialist if possible.
Inhalation and ingestion of large quantities of radionuclides.	No immediate effects.	Nasopharyngeal lavage. Early transfer to specialized center to increase excretion.
Absorption through damaged skin.	No immediate effects.	Consult with specialist if possible.
Major incorporation, with/without external irradiation, serious wounds, and/or burns.	Severe combined radiation injury.	Treat life-threatening conditions and transfer to specialized center.

HLA, human leukocyte antigen.

Source: Reprinted with permission from Armed Forces Radiobiology Research Institute. (1999). *Medical management of radiological casualties.* Bethesda, MD: Author.

TABLE 34.8 Some Radiation Accidents and Their Effects

Year	Place	Source	Activity	Origin	Dose (rad)	Effects
1962	Mexico	Co-60	Unknown	Industrial source	990–5,200	4 deaths
1965	U.S.A.	Accelerator	N/A	Industrial device	2,900–240,000 rad to partial body	One patient—leg and arm amputated
1967	U.S.A.	Accelerator	N/A	Industrial device	100–600 rad whole body; 600 rad to hands	3 persons irradiated, 1 person required amputation of hands
1968	Japan	Ir-192	5.26 Ci	Industrial source	15–130	3 cases of radiation sickness among 6 exposed
1974–1976	U.S.A.	Co-60	Various	Medical therapy	Various	426 patients overexposed
1987	Brazil	Cs-137	1,400 Ci	Abandoned source	100–800	4 deaths
1990	Spain	Therapy accelerator	N/A	Medical therapy	Various	27 patients overexposed, 18 fatally
1991	Vietnam	Accelerator	N/A	Industrial device	~1,000	One hand and several fingers amputated
1996	Costa Rica	Co-60	Unknown	Medical therapy	60% overdose	115 patients overexposed, 17 deaths
1999	Japan	U-235	N/A	Reactor fuel	300–1,700	3 workers exposed, 2 workers died
2001	Georgia	Sr-90	40,000 Ci	Radioisotopic thermal generator (RTG)	Unknown	Severe radiation burns, 1 death, amputations

radioactivity into the environment, there were concerns that these patients might be radioactively contaminated. It is important to note that only the two patients mentioned earlier—both nuclear power plant workers—were exposed to enough radiation to cause radiation injury. No medical workers were exposed to harmful levels of radiation or contamination from any of their patients.

Patients contaminated, even at very high levels, pose no threat to emergency response or medical personnel. Simple precautions, such as wearing latex gloves and a nuisance mask, changing outer clothing, and washing or showering after patient contact will suffice to protect medical staff. Even if such measures are not immediately possible, however, radioactive contamination does not pose a health risk to emergency responders or medical staff. *It is imperative that medical staff treat significant medical problems with whatever degree of urgency is required.* If a patient is only slightly injured, it may be appropriate to attempt decontamination before treating the patient, just as a physician will clean a laceration prior to suturing. However, serious injury requires immediate medical care that must be provided by the medical staff—the decontamination of staff, equipment, or facilities (including ambulances) can be performed by health physics personnel after the incident is resolved.

Potassium iodide (KI) is useful *only* for incidents involving the release of radioactive iodine, such as a nuclear power plant accident or a nuclear explosion. The use of KI will be recommended by the state or federal government if it is appropriate. KI is usually recommended only for children and young adults and only when the projected radiation dose to be averted is in excess of 50 mSv (5 rem) to the thyroid. It must be recognized that administering KI carries a slight risk of allergic reaction—it should be administered only when the risk from the radiation exposure is greater than the risk of administering KI.

Caring for Patients With Internal Radioactivity

Patients might receive internal contamination through accidental ingestion, inhalation, implantation of radioactive debris from an explosion, or absorption through open cuts and wounds. Internal contamination can cause high radiation exposures to internal organs and it is important to recognize and to administer medical countermeasures when appropriate.

The NCRP developed the Clinical Decision Guideline (CDG) to help medical practitioners identify levels of internal radioactivity that can produce a radiation dose of 0.25 Sv (25 rem) over a period of 50 years postexposure. An uptake of less than 1 CDG is not expected to have clinical significance for the patient (although even sub-CDG levels of exposure may warrant treatment if circumstances permit), while higher levels of exposure should be factored into clinical decision making. NCRP Reports #161 and #166 provide detailed information on how to determine whether or not a patient has had an uptake of 1 CDG. These reports also provide a great deal of information on medical countermeasures that are available for treating patients with a substantial uptake of RAMs—there is not sufficient room in this chapter to provide such details here.

Patients can be assessed for internal radioactivity via any of the following methods:

External counting using radiation detectors can be used to detect internal gamma-emitting radionuclides only. Detectors that can be used include Geiger counters, sodium iodide detectors, and nuclear medicine gamma cameras. External counting cannot detect internal alpha or beta emitters.

Nasal and oral swabs can be used to detect possible inhalation or ingestion of RAM. Such swabs can detect alpha, beta, and gamma radioactivity if counted with appropriate instruments. The presence of positive radioactivity on a swab indicates the likelihood of internal contamination but the absence of contamination cannot be used to rule out an uptake.

Urine samples can be used to detect RAM that has entered the bloodstream and been excreted. Urine samples can detect alpha, beta, or gamma emitters. Urine samples obtained too soon after exposure may not be representative of uptake because of the time needed (24 hours or more) for radioactivity to enter the blood and to pass into the urine.

Contamination of the face or head can indicate the potential for a patient to have been exposed to elevated levels of radioactivity. Patients with high levels of contamination are at greater risk of having had a significant uptake of radioactivity.

Radiological Control Methods

Patient Decontamination

1. Remove patient's clothing; dress in hospital scrubs or patient gown.
2. Rinse contaminated areas with saline solution or deionized water.
3. Gently wash contaminated areas with mild soap and cool to warm water.
4. Shower or bathe patient, using mild soap and cool to warm water.
5. Give sponge bath; discard sponge or washcloth as radioactive waste.
6. Flush open wounds with saline solution or deionized water.
7. Use standard sterilization practices prior to administering injections, suturing, or other practices that puncture or break the skin.

Emergency Department Contamination Control

1. Wrap patient in blankets to contain contamination and reduce contamination of facilities.
2. Establish dedicated routes for transporting contaminated patients.
3. Establish dedicated rooms for decontamination and care of contaminated patients.
4. Line dedicated routes and rooms with plastic to reduce contamination of fixed surfaces.

5. If possible, a hospital should consider establishing a trauma bay designed for use with contaminated patients. If possible, there should be a dedicated entrance for this room to minimize the risk of contaminating other parts of the hospital. Figure 34.13, adapted from NCRP Report #161, shows how such a trauma bay can be set up while Figure 34.14 shows a trauma bay that was used to receive contaminated patients in the aftermath of the nuclear reactor accident at the Fukushima Daiichi nuclear reactors.
6. Do not use rooms for noncontaminated patients until checked and released by radiation safety personnel.

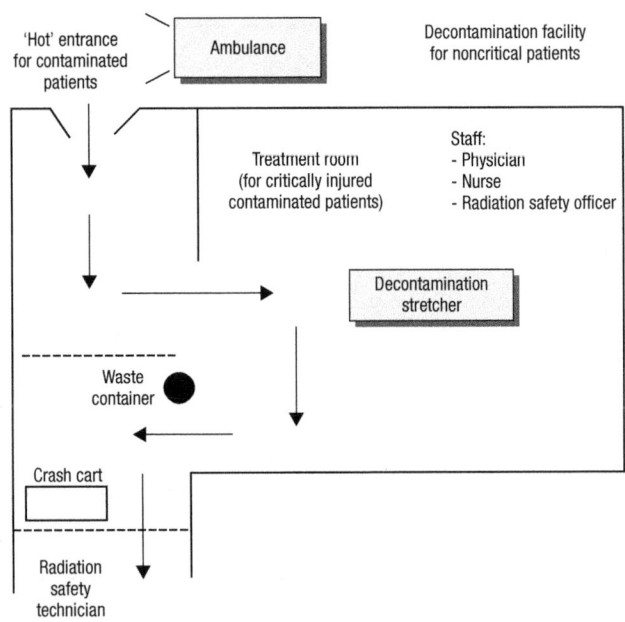

FIGURE 34.13 Stylized diagram of an emergency department and treatment room complex to receive radioactively contaminated patients. Dashed lines indicate radiological boundaries.

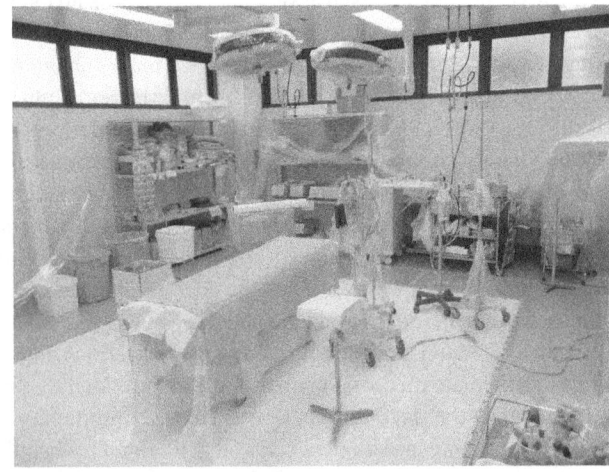

FIGURE 34.14 Contaminated patients' trauma bay at the Fukushima Medical University Hospital.

Medical Staff Contamination Control

1. Follow standard precautions—wear gloves, lab coats, shoe covers, and so forth, to reduce personnel contamination and to cover all exposed skin to the maximum extent possible.
2. Wear surgical masks or N95 masks to reduce the chance of contamination inhalation.
3. Securely bandage or cover all open cuts, scrapes, and other wounds.
4. Change gloves after treating each patient.
5. Remove shoe covers prior to leaving any contaminated area.
6. Wash hands and exposed skin thoroughly after treating each patient.
7. Change clothes and shower at the end of the shift or when leaving patient decontamination or treatment areas.
8. Medical personnel working with highly contaminated patients should consider performing a urine bioassay 24 to 72 hours after exposure to check for evidence of radionuclide uptake. About 20 mL of urine is required, of which 1 mL will be counted in a liquid scintillation counter.

Emergency Care for Badly Injured, Contaminated Patients

1. If the patient requires immediate attention, treat the patient first and worry about radiological controls when the patient's condition has stabilized. Rooms and medical staff can be decontaminated later.
2. Even badly contaminated patients pose no health risk to medical or emergency personnel.

Responsibilities of Radiation Safety Personnel, If Present

1. Survey all patients for contamination prior to their entry into uncontrolled areas in medical facilities.
2. Assist with patient decontamination when practical.
3. Assist with establishing controlled areas for patient transport and treatment.
4. Survey controlled areas periodically to determine necessity for replacing or renewing coverings.
5. Establish and perform confirmation surveys of boundaries delineating controlled areas.
6. Survey medical and emergency personnel prior to exiting controlled areas.
7. Perform bioassay measurements as necessary (probably at the end of the shift or the following day) to determine uptake of radionuclides by medical and emergency response personnel.
8. Perform bioassay measurements as necessary for patients thought to have been exposed to radioactive contamination.
9. Identify contaminating isotope(s).

MEDICAL RESPONSE TO NUCLEAR AND RADIOLOGICAL TERRORISM

In the event of a terrorist attack, people will suffer physical and psychological trauma. Physical effects will include those following the exposure to any explosion—broken bones, burns, shock, lacerations, blast lung, and so forth. These may be compounded by the presence of radioactive contamination and, in some cases, radiation sickness or injury. In addition, any terrorist attack will inflict psychological trauma, and medical personnel must be prepared to receive many patients who are worried, panicked, or suffering psychosomatically in spite of being physically well. In this light, even a simple headache or anxiety attack may be seen as evidence of radiation sickness.

It may be prudent to develop a plan for addressing the psychological effects of a radiological attack. Medical staff must be able to differentiate between real and perceived illness, and hospitals should have personnel and literature on hand to help people understand why they were sent home instead of being treated or admitted, and to address the other psychological needs of patients and their families.

To help determine the likelihood of whether a particular person might be suffering from radiation effects or contamination, medical personnel should make every effort to communicate with emergency response personnel at the scene of the attack, so that area hospitals are aware of the nature of the attack (i.e., nuclear weapon, RDD, exposure to a high-activity radioactive source), the highest radiation dose rates and contamination levels measured, and approximate extent of radiation or contamination. With this information, medical staff will have a rough idea, based on a patient's location at the time of the attack, as to whether the patient was likely exposed to sufficient radiation to cause various syndromes (Figure 34.15). For example, a person who is vomiting may have prodromal or gastrointestinal syndrome. If this person was a mile downwind of an RDD attack, however, this diagnosis makes no sense because he or she would not have been exposed to enough radiation to induce these syndromes. Before sending such patients home, though, they should be radiologically surveyed to make sure they are not contaminated—a precaution that would not be necessary for a patient who was *upwind* at the time of the attack.

Medical personnel should also be aware of the possibility of secondary attacks in any terrorist event. In the aftermath of the 9/11 terrorist attacks, emergency room staff at St. Vincent's Hospital in Manhattan performed some triage activities in the street outside their hospital—staff acknowledged (in conversations with me) that they did not realize until later that this left them vulnerable to secondary terrorist attack. If the demands of a mass casualty situation call for establishing medical triage outside a hospital, it may be prudent to first request law enforcement screening for secondary explosives and other threats.

Medical Response to RDD (Dirty Bomb)

An RDD ("dirty bomb") is a chemical explosive laced with radioactivity. *An RDD attack will probably lead to widespread contamination, contaminated patients and emergency responders, and victims of the blast itself, but will likely **not** result in widespread radiation injury or illness. Those close to the RDD may have radioactive shrapnel embedded in their bodies, contaminated wounds, and may have inhaled radioactive dust*

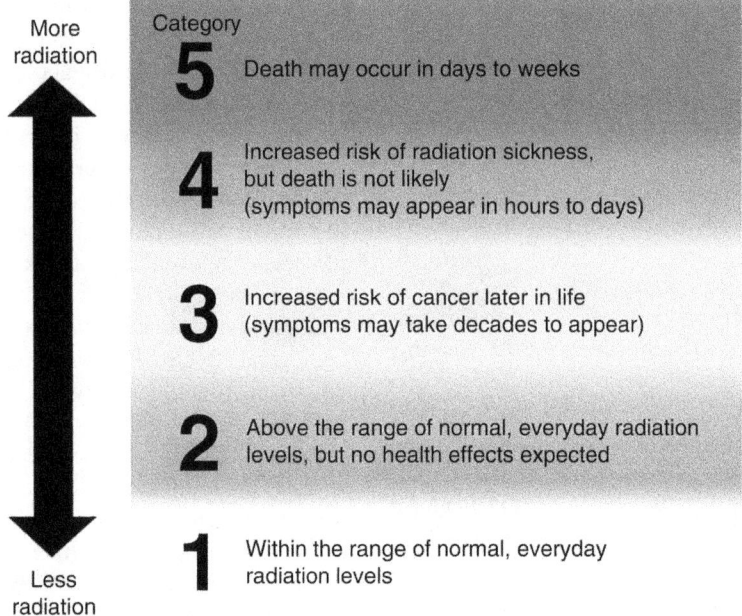

FIGURE 34.15 Radiation Hazard Scale developed by the Centers for Disease Control and Prevention.

Source: Centers for Disease Control and Prevention. Radiation Hazard Scale. Retrieved from emergency.cdc.gov/radiation/radiationhazardscale.asp

or smoke. In the case of an RDD attack, medical personnel will probably be confronted with large numbers of patients who are contaminated with radioactivity, some of whom may have very high contamination levels. Many more people may appear who are anxious or panicked, but are not likely to be ill from radiation exposure.

One caveat is that radioactive sources may be incorporated into an RDD, and they may survive the explosion essentially intact or might break apart into larger fragments. Such source fragments could give very high radiation doses to personnel handling them and could lead to localized radiation burns if handled with bare hands. In most cases, however, patients are expected to exhibit injuries typical of an explosion itself, with the presence of radioactive contamination as a complicating factor.

The medical response to RDD use should focus on injuries from the blast—thermal burns, broken bones, shock, lacerations, internal injury, crushing, and so forth. Lightly injured patients may be decontaminated prior to arrival at the hospital, and may simply be decontaminated, treated, and released at the scene. Patients who are sent home should be instructed to change their clothes, shower, and wash their hair (although conditioners should not be used as these can actually trap contamination on the hair) when they get home. More seriously injured patients may be decontaminated prior to treatment if their injuries permit—these may include patients with lacerations requiring suturing, but that are not life-threatening, or patients with sprains, contusions, or noncompound broken bones. Medical personnel must use their professional judgment in deciding how much, if any, radiological controls to take. Patients with life-threatening injuries must be treated immediately, without regard to contamination levels. An alternative to decontaminating a patient is to wrap the patient in sheets, blankets, or anticontamination clothing during transportation to the treatment room. This will help keep the patient from contaminating "clean" areas, although

the treatment room will require decontamination prior to use by uncontaminated patients.

Although medical personnel may need to treat patients who are still contaminated, these patients pose no health risk to nurses or physicians. Standard precautions will serve to further reduce an already low radiation dose. Medical caregivers should remember, too, that the typical nuclear medicine patient emits radioactivity and in many cases will have skin contamination from the nuclides that have been administered.

It may be helpful, weather permitting, to set up a triage and decontamination station outside the emergency room. After the nuclear reactor accident at Three Mile Island, the local hospital established a decontamination station in its parking garage, which was better able to handle large numbers of patients. This also kept patients with imagined radiation sickness from interfering with the smooth functioning of the emergency room. In a radiological attack, this will also help to minimize contamination levels in the emergency room when the immediate crisis has passed.

Medical staff working with contaminated patients should wear gloves, masks, shoe covers, and lab coats or other anticontamination clothing. They should change their clothing after treating each patient to reduce the chance of having skin contamination themselves, and they should change all clothes and shower after each shift. Shoe covers, gloves, masks, and anticontamination clothing must be removed before leaving a "hot" room (a room in which a contaminated patient has been treated).

The Centers for Disease Control and Prevention (CDC, 2016) advocates establishing Community Reception Centers (CRCs) in the aftermath of a sufficiently large radiological event. The purpose of a CRC is to provide radiological screening for uninjured or lightly injured people, to provide decontamination when necessary, and to refer those with likely internal contamination for radiological assessment and (if appropriate) medical countermeasures. Information on establishing and operating CRCs is available on the CDC website, the URL of which is provided in the references to this chapter. Medical personnel may be asked to provide medical screening and first aid in CRCs (if established). In addition, if CRCs are *not* established in the aftermath of a radiological or nuclear event, members of the public might appear at hospitals requesting radiological screening.

Medical Response to a Radiation-Emitting Device Attack

Instead of setting off an RDD, terrorists may simply set a high-activity radioactive source in a public place—this is referred to as a radiation-emitting device (RED). In such an attack, a relatively small number of people may suffer from radiation illness or injury (including the various syndromes or localized radiation burns if they handled the source). A larger number of people may appear at medical centers, suffering from anxiety rather than radiation sickness. Unfortunately, nausea and vomiting can result from either radiation sickness or extreme anxiety, and many patients may be unable to distinguish between the two. Although such an attack will likely injure fewer people than either an RDD or a nuclear weapon, there may still be hundreds of patients, depending on how the attack was planned and orchestrated. Because an attack of this type will likely not be associated with an explosion, it is prudent to assume that skin burns are radiation burns and to treat them accordingly. This may include skin grafts and removal of necrotic tissue, as well as pain relief.

All patients from the site of an irradiator attack should be evaluated for radiation sickness (including obtaining a baseline blood sample and complete blood count [CBC] analysis), and a health physicist or medical physicist should be consulted to attempt to determine the radiation dose to each patient. If the patient is conscious, it is essential to get as much information as possible about his or her exact location, travel paths, and the amount of time he or she spent in each place near the site of the radioactive source. For example, if a source is placed in an elevator, persons working on the 50th floor of a high-rise will generally receive more radiation dose than patients on lower levels (who likely do not need to use the elevator or can take the stairs). On the other hand, a person who has a nonstop ride to an upper level may receive a lower dose than one whose trip to the 10th floor was interrupted by frequent stops. Similarly, a person walking briskly by a large source may receive a far smaller dose than someone working at a distance of several meters for a prolonged period of time.

Regardless of the severity of a patient's injuries, patients pose absolutely no threat to medical personnel. Radiation burns from exposure to high levels of radiation are not radioactive, and there will be no radiation dose to medical personnel from treating such patients. The patients will likely be frightened, anxious, and in pain; this should not be exacerbated by medical staff taking unnecessary and elaborate precautions.

Finally, remember that the immune system is unusually sensitive to the effects of radiation exposure. Patients who have received enough radiation to cause burns or radiation sickness may suffer from suppression of their immune systems and may require medical follow-up and antibiotic support. Because there is sometimes an asymptomatic period following the prodromal period, it may be prudent to keep patients under observation for several days after treatment. It should also be remembered that patients who have received a fatal radiation dose might not succumb for several weeks or even months. These patients must be cared for during this time, even though those who have received doses in excess of 8 Sv (800 rem) are not likely to survive their exposure.

Medical Response to Nuclear Attack

Unlike the previous two scenarios, a nuclear attack will be truly devastating and many people will be killed and injured, many more will be traumatized, and a city's infrastructure may be severely damaged. Radioactive fallout can be present in dangerous concentrations over many tens of square miles and up to 10 miles downwind, and people can suffer from thermal and radiation burns as well as inhalation of fallout.

In addition to these effects, a nuclear explosion can cause broken glass to a distance of a few miles from the scene of the attack and can cause flash blindness to a distance of over 10 miles during the day and even further at night. Thus, medical personnel should be prepared to also treat injuries from flying (or falling) glass, temporary or permanent blindness, as well as injuries from traffic accidents when drivers are suddenly and unexpectedly unable to see. There will also be thermal damage—prompt burns from the thermal radiation emitted by the explosion itself as well as burns from the mass fires ignited by the blast's thermal pulse. In the aftermath of the explosion at Hiroshima, fires and thermal effects were deadly at distances greater than those at which the prompt radiation was fatal. Accordingly, medical personnel should also expect to see a very large number of burn victims, and for these victims to continue arriving for days after the attack as they are rescued or make their way to safety.

All other factors being equal, a larger weapon will produce more damage and will affect a larger area than will a smaller one. A weapon set off at ground level will produce more fallout (be "dirtier") than a high altitude burst because soil and building debris that are swept into the fireball will sweep up the radioactivity from the explosion itself and will produce intensely radioactive fallout. Rain will wash fallout from the air, giving higher radiation doses to people near the explosion, but lower doses to people at a distance. Other factors will influence the severity of any attack as well and are likely to vary considerably from site to site. Even under ideal circumstances, however, any nuclear attack will have a horrific impact on the city attacked.

That said, it must be noted that the area directly affected by the explosion, fires, and fallout—while large—will be only a portion of any large city and the rest of the city will still need to be taken care of. For example, a 10 kiloton (kT) explosion will utterly destroy an area about 0.5 mile or so in radius and extensive damage will extend to a distance of up to 1 mile in all directions. In addition, the radioactive plume might be dangerously radioactive to a distance of several miles and can be up to 0.5 mile or so across. This is not a trivial area—but such an attack in most major cities would still leave more than 75% of the city relatively undamaged and nonradioactive, but still potentially lacking food, drinking water, heat, and electrical power. The city, too, might suffer from civil unrest until order can be restored; emergency rooms might see patients with injuries from this unrest as well as those injured by the attack itself.

Even a single nuclear weapon will stress an area's emergency and medical response resources to the breaking point. If utilities are affected, medical personnel may be required to care for patients without reliable electrical power, heat, or water. Unlike many Cold War scenarios, though, it is not likely that any terrorist group will possess enough nuclear weapons to attack a city with more than a single device. This means that large parts of a city will likely remain intact and people from those parts of the city will be able to provide assistance at the site of an attack, and the national response infrastructure will remain intact.

In spite of these effects, medical personnel can play an important role in saving lives and treating the injured, as was shown in Hiroshima and Nagasaki after their respective nuclear attacks. Today, with the advantage of more than half a century of research and planning, medical personnel can be even more effective at mitigating the health effects of a nuclear terrorist attack.

A nuclear attack will combine all of the elements noted earlier on a large scale. People closest to the weapon will be killed immediately and those somewhat further away might receive a fatal dose of radiation. Depending on the yield of the device, local geography, weather, and other factors, however, people as close as several hundred meters may survive the explosion and its aftereffects. Radioactive fallout will lead to many patients being highly contaminated, some to the point of receiving a lethal radiation dose from their contamination if not promptly decontaminated. Complicating everything will be the presence of physical trauma—broken bones, thermal burns, crushing, lacerations, and so forth.

It is impossible to provide guidance in a book such as this one that will apply to any situation that may arise in a nuclear attack. Rather, it may be more appropriate to provide general guidance with the knowledge that medical personnel will have to react as appropriate, based on their own blend of experience, training, and knowledge. The general rules are the following:

1. Part of the triage process should include an assessment of radiation exposure received. For example, if a patient is vomiting or has diarrhea on arrival, there is a good chance the patient was exposed to a lethal dose of radiation, if the vomiting is due to radiation exposure and not due to stress or illness.

2. Accept that the emergency room will become contaminated and will require decontamination after the crisis has passed. Instead of trying to limit contamination to a few areas, it may make more sense to designate a few areas as "cold" areas and to use those areas for treating nonradiological patients. Alternately, it may be necessary to designate the entire emergency room as "hot" and to treat nonradiological patients in other parts of the hospital.

3. Contingency plans should include the loss of potable water, electricity, and/or heat. Medical staff should consider how they would continue to provide medical care to existing and incoming patients if utilities are lost.

4. Radioactive fallout can include "hot" particles. These particles can burn very localized parts of the skin, not affecting areas only a few centimeters away.

5. The distribution of fallout can be very patchy, depending on peculiarities of terrain, weather, weapon characteristics, and other factors. People close to the site of the explosion may have lower radiation doses than those further away.

6. Patients from near the site of the explosion may look frightening and may have injuries that are simply impossible to imagine in advance. For example, some patients in the aftermath of the Hiroshima and Nagasaki nuclear attacks were described as having skin hanging off of their bodies in addition to both thermal and radiation burns. Medical personnel must expect to be confronted with situations for which their experience and training give them no appropriate tools—technical or emotional.

7. Even patients receiving a lethal radiation dose can be helped. Painkillers and antibiotics can help to make patients comfortable and to help them survive until their family can be found. Remember that some patients who have received a fatal dose of radiation might not succumb for weeks or even months and they must be cared for during that time.

Lastly, you should be aware of how to protect yourself, your family, your colleagues, and your patients in the aftermath of a nuclear attack. Most important is to go inside as quickly as possible and to take shelter toward the center of the building on a lower level or basement (Figure 34.16). Once there, you should prepare to remain for up to 2 or 3 days to allow radioactivity to decay to levels permitting evacuation. During that time, the local, state, and/or federal government will be assessing radiation levels to determine the location of the fallout plume so that appropriate evacuation instructions can be provided; thus, you should monitor the media and/or Internet to remain aware and informed.

Regardless of the severity of a nuclear attack and its consequences, medical personnel must do their best to respond. There will be many patients who cannot be saved, but they can be made more comfortable and it may be possible to save them from indignity. There will be many more patients for whom medical care will mean the difference between life and death, and still others who may be able to assist with recovery once their injuries are treated.

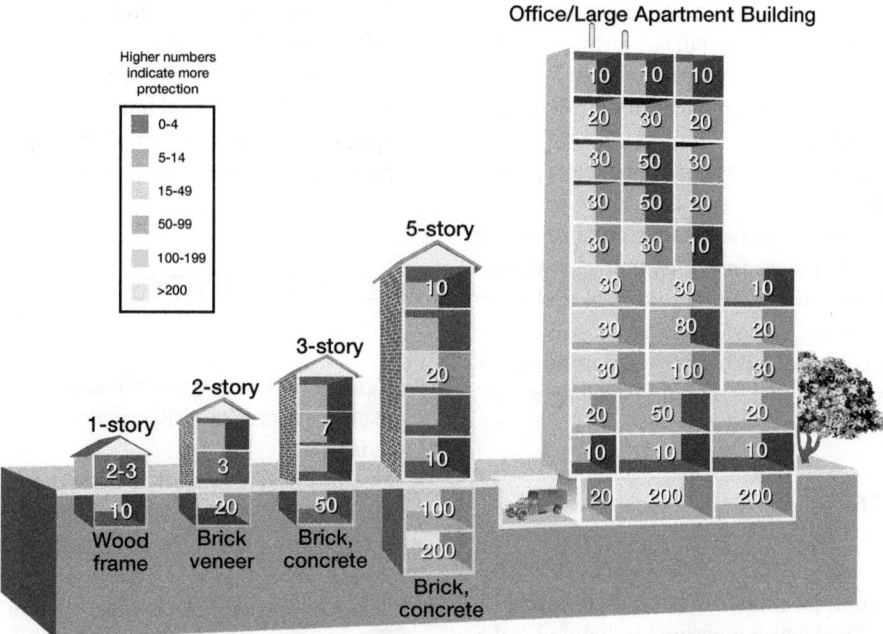

FIGURE 34.16 Protection factors for various locations inside of several types of structures.

Source: Federal Emergency Management Agency. (2010). Planning Guidance for a Response to a Nuclear Detonation. Retrieved from www.fema.gov/media-library/assets/documents/24879

QUESTIONS TO ASK WHEN RECEIVING AND CARING FOR RADIOLOGICAL PATIENTS (AMERICAN COLLEGE OF RADIOLOGY, 2002)

About the Incident

1. When did it occur?
2. What was the nature of the incident?
3. What other medical problems might we see?
4. What isotopes are involved and at what levels?
5. What on-site measurements have been made and what were the results?
6. Are other contaminants (biological, chemical) expected?

About the Patient

1. Was the patient contaminated? Is the patient now decontaminated?
2. Were contamination/radiation levels measured on the patient's skin? If so, what were the results?
3. Was the patient exposed to radiation or radioactive contamination?
4. Is the patient still emitting radiation following decontamination? If so, the patient might have internal contamination from inhalation, ingestion, or contamination of open wounds.
5. Are there any dosimetric measurements or estimates?
6. Have any therapeutic methods been attempted (blocking agents, isotopic dilution, chelation, etc.)?
7. What are the chemical and radiological properties of the contaminants?

Follow-Up

1. Has the patient's clothing been saved (if removed at the site)?
2. Have any physical samples (blood, urine, feces) been collected? If so, where are they?
3. What further laboratory work is planned or recommended?

For further information, see Figures 34.12 and 34.13.

CONTENTS OF A CONTAMINATION CONTROL KIT

- Pens and pencils
- Blank paper
- Survey maps for human body (outline of front and back to note location of injuries and contamination levels)
- Cotton swabs (for obtaining nasal or oral wipes)
- Filter paper for smear wipes
- Small Geiger counter (e.g., a Ludlum Model 2401P) for measuring contamination from medium- to high-energy beta- and gamma-emitting isotopes
- Mild soap
- Alcohol swabs
- Paper towels
- Shoe covers
- Latex gloves (or equivalent)
- Lab coats or other outer contamination control garments for medical staff

- Hospital gowns, scrubs, blankets, sheets, or coveralls (for dressing either patient or medical staff)
- Boundary tape (to delineate contamination zones)
- Small envelopes (for holding smear wipes prior to counting)
- Nuisance mask or surgical mask
- Plastic sheeting (to cover floor, examination tables, patient transportation routes)
- Stethoscopes, thermometers, blood pressure cuffs, and other "sacrificial" equipment for use on contaminated patients
- Small plastic bags (to cover stethoscope end and other objects that might become contaminated)
- Sample containers and zippered bags (to seal urine, feces, blood, dressings, wound exudates, clothing, bandages, etc.)

STUDY QUESTIONS

An RDD explodes, contaminating 10 city blocks with radioactive cobalt (Co-60). The highest measured radiation level is about 10 m from the site of the explosion and it reads about 150 mrem/hr. The average radiation dose through the affected area is 5 mrem/hr, and about 500,000 people live and work in this area. The device itself consisted of 1,000 pounds of explosive, set off near City Hall.

1. A firefighter is brought to the emergency room with extensive burns on his face and hands. Do you expect these to be radiation burns? Explain your reasoning.

2. A passerby is brought to the emergency room with severe lacerations and burns. She was about 100 m downwind of the explosion. List the radiological precautions you should take prior to treating her injuries. List radiological precautions to take after she is treated.

3. The next day, a policeman is brought to the emergency room. He was one of the first people at the scene and spent 10 hours helping evacuate and recover victims. He has a severe headache and is vomiting. Is this due to radiation exposure? Explain your reasoning.

4. When the immediate emergency has ended, what actions should you take to recover from this incident and return to normal operations?

5. How many additional cancer deaths do you expect to see as a result of the radiation exposure from this attack? List your assumptions and explain your reasoning.

   Answer the following questions individually.

6. What are four sources of natural background radiation? What is the average annual background radiation dose to people living in the United States and Canada?

7. List three kinds of radiation. Which is most penetrating? Which does the most damage to living cells?

8. A young woman comes into the emergency room, unconscious, following a motor vehicle accident. Following a series of x-rays, the attending physician orders a pelvic CT because of concerns about internal injury. The patient is of childbearing age and has a little "tummy," leading to questions about her pregnancy status. What actions should be taken?

INTERNET ACTIVITIES

- Centers for Disease Control and Prevention (includes information on Community Reception Centers). emergency.cdc.gov/radiation
- Health Physics Society. www.hps.org
- International Atomic Energy Agency. www.iaea.org
- International Council on Radiation Protection. www.icrp.org
- National Council on Radiation Protection and Measurements. www.ncrp.com
- Nuclear Regulatory Commission. www.nrc.gov
- Radiation Emergency Assistance Center/Training Site (REAC/TS) includes class schedule for "Medical Care and Planning in Radiation Accidents." orise.orau.gov/reacts/index.htm

REFERENCES

American College of Radiology. (2002). *Radiation disasters: Preparedness and response for radiology.* Reston, VA: Author.

Berger, M. E., Hurtado, R., Dunlap, J., Mutchinick, O., Valasco, M. G., Tostado, R. A., …, Ricks, R. C. (1997). Accidental radiation injury to the hand: Anatomical and physiological consideration. *Health Physics, 72*(3), 343–348.

Berger, M. E., Leonard, R. B., Ricks, R. C., Wiley, A. L., Lowry, P. C., & Flynn, D. F. (2007). Hospital triage in the first 24 hours after a nuclear or radiological disaster. Retrieved from https://www.yumpu.com/en/document/view/40196819/hospital-triage-in-the-first-24-hours-after-a-nuclear-or-radiological-

Centers for Disease Control and Prevention. (2016). Radiation hazard scale. Retrieved from https://emergency.cdc.gov/radiation/radiationhazardscale.asp

Linnemann, R. E. (2001). *Managing radiation medical emergencies.* Philadelphia, PA: Radiation Management Consultants.

National Council on Radiation Protection and Measurements. (2009). *Report #161—Management of persons contaminated with radionuclides: Handbook* (Vol. 1). Bethesda MD: Author.

Oliveira, A. R., Brandão-Mello, C. E., Valverde, N. J., Farina, R., & Curado, M. P. (1991). Localized lesions induced by Cs-137 during the Goiania accident. *Health Physics, 60*(1), 25–29.

Schauer, D. A., Coursey, B. M., Dick, C. E., McLaughlin, W. L., Puhl, J. M., Desrosiers, M. F., & Jacobson, A. D. (1993). Radiation accident at an industrial accelerator facility. *Health Physics, 65*(2), 131–140.

Wagner, L. K., Lester, R. G., & Saldana, L. R. (1997). *Exposure of the pregnant patient to diagnostic radiations: A guide to medical management* (2nd ed.). Milwaukee, WI: Medical Physics Publishing.

35

DECONTAMINATION AND PERSONAL PROTECTIVE EQUIPMENT

Tener Goodwin Veenema

LEARNING OBJECTIVES

When this chapter is completed, readers will be able to:

1. Define a hazardous materials (HAZMAT) incident.
2. Distinguish between first responders and first receivers and understand the implications for nurses' personal safety.
3. Describe the process for special conditions triage and decontamination during a chemical or radiological incident.
4. Describe the four levels of personal protective equipment (PPE) and when it is appropriate to use them.
5. List the Joint Commission and Occupational Safety and Health Administration (OSHA) requirements for emergency department (ED) preparedness for chemical incidents.
6. Describe the procedure for chemical decontamination in the hospital setting.
7. Describe the decontamination process for infants and small children.

KEY MESSAGES

A large-scale chemical or radiological release with mass casualties will create a significant burden and may quickly overwhelm the existing healthcare system.

Timely identification of the hazardous substances involved ensures safer and rational response efforts.

Decontamination must be available and provided quickly to patients involved in chemical and other HAZMAT incidents.

Decontamination of victims must be timely and thorough.

Decontamination must reduce or remove the chemical agent or radiation, while protecting the safety of the staff and preventing further contamination of the environment.

In treating patients with chemical and radiological exposures, decontamination is of primary importance *provided* the patient does not require immediate lifesaving interventions.

Before decontamination, only the most urgent first aid measures are provided: clearing the airways, protection of the cervical spine, and control of bleeding by applying compression.

The responders' safety always has to come first (using the appropriate PPE and determining a suitable treatment area).

EDs have a unique role in mass casualty decontamination and should employ evidence-based disaster planning.

During decontamination, nurses must use the appropriate level of PPE and know how to use it correctly to keep themselves safe and avoid becoming victims.

CHAPTER OVERVIEW

Disaster events may create a sudden influx of patients who have been exposed to a chemical agent, radiation, or other hazard that requires decontamination. Protecting nurses and other healthcare workers who respond to chemical or radiological HAZMAT mass casualty incidents is critical. Patient decontamination is an organized method of removing residual contaminants from the victim's hair, skin, and clothing and should be performed whenever known or suspected contamination has occurred with a hazardous substance through contact with aerosols, solids, liquids, or residual radiation. The degree of decontamination performed will depend on the situation. Nurses dealing with these types of emergencies may be exposed to hazards, either in the field or in the hospital setting. Ideally, only HAZMAT experts and other highly trained professionals should be responding to victims of chemical and radiation exposure at the site of the event. Nurse responders must approach contaminated sites with great caution and be prepared to self-decontaminate. Nurse receivers need to have a solid understanding of how to keep themselves and their patients safe while participating in decontamination procedures and patient care at the hospital.

HAZMATs come in the form of explosives, flammable and combustible substances, poisons, and radioactive materials. HAZMAT incidents can occur during production, storage, transportation, use, or disposal. Nurses and communities are at risk if a chemical is used unsafely or released in harmful amounts into the environment where individuals live, work, or play. Chemical emergencies may result from industrial explosions, transportation or agricultural accidents, police actions involving tear gas, or the intentional use of chemicals as agents of war by terrorists. The release of a chemical into the environment creates a HAZMAT incident that poses unique challenges for the healthcare system and for those individuals who participate in the response. "Contamination" or the "state of being contaminated" occurs when a person or persons inhale, ingest, inject, or absorb harmful substances as the result of exposure to chemical or biological agents and/or radiological materials (*American Heritage Dictionary of the English Language*, 2009). Victims who are chemically or radiation contaminated must be decontaminated as soon as possible, preferably before being brought to the hospital or into a clean treatment area. "Decontamination" is the removal or reduction of contaminants through the use of water, cleansers, or neutralizers. Emergency medical services (EMS) has specific procedures for triage during HAZMAT events, and in most communities, decontamination of victims is done before transport to a hospital. *EMS may transport nondecontaminated victims directly to the hospital,* however, and it is expected that many ambulatory victims will leave the scene before being triaged and decontaminated (Levitin & Siegelson, 1996; Sarc, 2012). Research supports that many casualties are likely to bypass on-site triage, first aid, and decontamination stations and go directly to hospitals (Auf der Heide, 2006). Hospital personnel should assume that individuals presenting to the hospital have *not* undergone adequate field decontamination until proven otherwise. Therefore, each hospital must have an evidence-based system in place to employ *special conditions triage* and decontaminate these arrivals, while ensuring the safety of staff and existing patients (Auf der Heide, 2006; Levitin et al., 2003).

A first receiver is defined by the OSHA as a healthcare worker at a hospital (away from the contaminated incident site) receiving contaminated victims. In contrast, first responders are people such as firefighters, law enforcement, and HAZMAT teams typically working at the site of the incident. The assumption in defining first receivers is that the hospital is not the primary incident site, but rather removed from the location of the incident (OSHA, 1997, 2005). OHSA's regulations (29 CFR 1910.120q) require that organizations involved in emergency response provide appropriate training to their workers; utilize an incident command system; have a written response plan detailing lines of authority, communication, site security, and control; possess medical and emergency alert procedures; and provide workers with appropriate protective equipment. *Nurses attempting to act as first responders without the proper training and equipment and without an organizational affiliation that provides them with OSHA protections place themselves at great risk.* The potential exists for nurses functioning in the roles of first responder or first receiver to become victims themselves, either from actual primary exposure (direct exposure to the contaminant) or secondary exposure (exposure to a person or object that has been contaminated by the primary source) to the toxins or from the inappropriate use and/or stressful physiological effects of wearing and working in personal protective gear. Emergency nurses have a high likelihood of participating in disaster response and as such should be adequately prepared (Hammond, Arbon, Gebbie, & Hutton, 2017).

EDs and EMS are responsible for managing chemical and radiation disasters, whether they result from industrial accidents or terrorist activities, and continue to be the primary providers of care to contaminated individuals (Auf der Heide, 2006; Levitin & Siegelson, 1996). In recognition of this responsibility, the Joint Commission, the Environmental Protection Agency (EPA), and OSHA require EDs to prepare for and have a written plan for potential HAZMAT incidents (Emergency Planning and Community Right-to-Know Act, 1986; Joint Commission, 1996; OSHA, 2005). The OSHA *Best Practices for Hospital-Based First Receivers of Victims From Mass Casualty Incidents Involving the Release of Hazardous Substances* document discusses elements of decontamination planning that should be included in the decontamination plan as an annex to the hospital's overall emergency operations plan. The determination of a workable HAZMAT plan requires careful thought and often professional input from ED physicians and nurses, medical toxicologists, HAZMAT teams, and industrial hygiene and safety officers. It also demands a careful investigation of the assumptions upon which these plans are based versus the scientific evidence regarding how people will actually behave during these types of events (Auf der Heide, 2006). Understandably, for most hospital staffs, treatment of chemical and radiation casualties presents an obscure and frightening situation. Chemical, biological, radiological, and nuclear (CBRN) agents are not usual hazards. Chemical agents are inherently complex materials because they can result in chain reactions, generating additional toxic substances. Medical personnel are seldom familiar with the health effects of such agents and this inevitably caps their effectiveness in responding to CBRN emergencies (Djalali et al., 2017). Hospitals must attend to ensuring that they have adequate amounts of antidotes available for the treatment of casualties, adequate showers and decontamination tents, the appropriate level and supply of protective gear and equipment for worker safety, and enough staff trained to decontaminate patients. Concern exists that hospital preparedness in major U.S. and international metropolitan areas is severely lacking for chemical and radiological terrorism (Keim, Pesik, & Twum-Danso, 2003; Kolleck, 2003; Wang, Huei-Tsair, & Chang, 2004). Finally, using a patient decontamination plan implemented without specific adaptation to the hospital and without practice can result in undesirable outcomes. The level of preparedness for a chemical or radiation mass casualty scenario should be established according to the existing threat and the available resources, and the plan should be tested to the full extent possible in regular full-scale hospital drills (Cox, 1994; Tur-Kaspa et al., 1999).

TRIAGE OF CONTAMINATED PATIENTS IN THE FIELD

Special conditions triage for chemical incidents will occur in specific places referred to as the "Zones of Operation" (Alibek et al., 2005).

Triage in the Zones of Operation

In setting up a site diagram for triage in the field, it is important to remember that three zones need to be identified (hot, warm, and cold); each is ideally upwind from the previous zone and not situated in a low-lying area. Note that all distances for each zone are estimates and will be incident-dependent based on the existing environmental conditions.

- *Hot zone*: The hot zone is the innermost zone and the area immediately adjacent to the location of the incident. Minimal triage and medical care activities take place and are limited to airway and hemorrhage control, administration of antidotes, and identification of expectant cases (dead or nonsalvageable). All staff are in protective gear in this area. In the hot zone, victims are located, given basic lifesaving measures, and then transported to the warm zone for decontamination.
- *Warm zone*: A distance of at least 300 ft from the outer perimeter of the hot zone, and upwind and uphill from the contaminated area. Rapid triage takes place to sort victims into critical, urgent, delayed, or, if they have deteriorated, expectant categories. As in the hot zone, only a minimal amount of treatment is rendered to provide essential stabilization. The priority is to commence decontamination. Nonambulatory victims go through litter decontamination, whereas ambulatory patients and any personnel wishing to leave the warm zone go through ambulatory decontamination before entering the cold zone. Those victims with the most severe signs/symptoms of contamination are given priority for decontamination. *All staff* in this area must wear the appropriate PPE.
- *Cold zone*: The area that is adjacent (and uphill and upwind) from the warm zone, into which decontaminated victims enter. As the victims enter this area, a more thorough triage is performed (including evaluation for secondary injuries), and victims are directed to treatment areas based on the severity and nature of illness or injury. PPE is maintained in this area in case the wind changes or victims arrive who have been improperly decontaminated (for further discussion, see Chapter 22). The purpose of this zone is to provide medical care and to transport victims to higher care facilities.

Triage in the Hospital Setting

Decontamination zones located at the hospital are established using barricades to clearly designate the perimeter of each zone. Victims are directed to the decontamination zone as a single point of entry to the hospital with all other means of entry in lockdown. Security personnel should assist with maintaining the integrity of the established zones and with moving traffic and personnel.

- *Warm zone*: This is an area that is adjacent to the hospital (usually the ED) that has a source of water (in cold climates it must be a warm water source) for decontamination, and barriers to control entrance and exit from the area. The triage station is at the entrance to the warm zone decontamination area. All ambulance and walk-in cases must enter the facility after going through this triage station. Cases that are clearly not contaminated enter the ED, and those that require decontamination go through the warm zone decontamination area before exiting into the clean zone in the ED (or noncontaminated area).
- *Clean zone*: This is the treatment area inside the ED or hospital where newly arriving patients and victims are sent after having been triaged and decontaminated. This area is considered clean or noncontaminated. Any staff or patients who have entered the warm zone must be decontaminated before entering the clean zone. Another more thorough triage is performed in the clean zone area.

In the hospital or at the scene of a mass chemical contamination, nurses may be asked to accurately decide which patients need care, in what order should they receive care, and in situations of severely constrained resources, who should not receive care at all. This is an extremely difficult scenario for the nurse and will create personal emotional distress. This type of disaster triage is best practiced in field exercises and drills prior to participation in a real event (Veenema, 2003).

DECONTAMINATION FOR CHEMICAL WARFARE AGENTS

Chemical warfare agents (CWAs) are a diverse group of extreme HAZMATs. There are five major classes of CWAs (CDC, 2013):

- *Nerve agents*: tabun, sarin, soman, GF, and VX
- *Tissue (blood) agents*: cyanide
- *Vesicants*: sulfur mustard and lewisite
- *Pulmonary agents*: phosgene and chlorine
- *Riot control agents (tear gas)*: mace (CN), pepper spray, and CS

Because of their toxic, explosive, and flammable properties, chemicals continue to be the weapons of choice for terrorist attacks and civilians may be exposed to them (Brennan, Waeckerle, Sharp, & Lillibridge, 1999). As potential weapons of mass destruction with the capability of causing a catastrophic medical disaster, CWAs easily may overwhelm any healthcare system. Because victims exposed to CWAs are likely to flee to the nearest hospital, nurses should be familiar with the various clinical presentations produced by CWAs (see Table 35.1) and the principles and practices of appropriate care (see Table 35.2). The onset of symptoms may not always be immediate; sometimes they may be delayed by several hours, as is the case with certain vesicants and pulmonary agents. Exposure to these agents can cause serious injury and death (for further discussion, see Chapter 29). Thus, rapid detection of the chemical is critical to the protection of first responders and emergency medical personnel, as well as to the effective treatment of victims (Brennan et al., 1999).

Personal Protective Equipment

The first consideration for decontamination should always be staff safety. EDs that are part of an emergency response plan for HAZMAT incidents must meet OSHA (2005) requirements for both staff training and response to HAZMATs, because they likely will be presented with a chemically exposed patient who has not been decontaminated at the scene. Under these regulations, emergency personnel who may decontaminate victims exposed to a hazardous substance should be trained at a minimum to the first-responder operational level. Staff require the appropriate level of PPE, and must know how to properly use it. PPE is the clothing and respiratory gear designed specifically to protect the healthcare provider while he or she is caring for a contaminated patient. To ensure the greatest possible protection for nurses in the workplace, hospital, and other healthcare facility, employers are responsible for:

TABLE 35.1 Chemical Warfare Agents and Descriptions and Examples

Agent Category	Brief Description	Example
Nerve agents	The most toxic of the known chemical warfare agents, nerve agents inhibit the body's normal functions.	Sarin
Vesicants	Chemical agents that cause blisters or sores.	Mustard gas
Tissue (blood) agents	Tissue (blood) agents that cause chemical asphyxiation by preventing body tissues from utilizing oxygen.	Cyanide
Pulmonary agents	Chemicals that cause severe irritation or swelling of the respiratory tract.	Chlorine
Riot control agents	Chemical compounds that temporarily inhibit a person's ability to function by causing irritation to the eyes, mouth, throat, lungs, and skin (i.e., tear gas).	Chlorobenzylidene malononitrile

Source: Centers for Disease Control and Prevention. (2017). Stockpiled chemical warfare agents. Retrieved from http://www.cdc.gov/nceh/demil/chemical_agent.htm

TABLE 35.2 Chemical Warfare Agents, Physiological Effects, and Antidotes or First Treatments

Type of Agent	Physiological Effect	Antidotes
Nerve agents	Inhibit the activation of acetylcholinesterase (AChE), which results in accumulation of neurotransmitters, and results in overstimulation of exocrine glands, skeletal and smooth muscles, and the central nervous system.	Atropine, Protopam (2-PAMCl), diazepam (for prolonged convulsions), *MARK I* Kit (contains two spring-loaded auto-injectors that contain atropine and 2-PAMCl).
Tissue (blood) agents (cyanide)	Binds with cytochrome oxidase at the cellular level, inhibiting aerobic metabolism. Results in tissue hypoxia.	Amyl nitrite (perles), sodium nitrite, sodium thiosulfate (*Pasadena Cyanide* Kit contains both sodium nitrite and sodium thiosulfate).
Vesicants	Tissue damage from alkylation of DNA or modification of other cellular macromolecules. Results in vesicles and blisters.	Decontamination with soap and water or 5% solution of bleach and water. British anti-Lewisite (BAL) for Lewisite.
Pulmonary agents	Cellular damage to the pulmonary capillaries and alveoli causing leakage of fluids into the alveolus and resulting in pulmonary edema.	No known antidote. Must provide oxygen and absolute rest.
Riot control agents	Local irritants.	Decontaminate with soap and water (which may initially increase burning sensation) or a solution of 6% sodium bicarbonate, 3% sodium carbonate, and 1% benzalkonium chloride.

Source: Stokes, E., Gilbert-Palmer, D., Skorga, P., Young, C., & Persell, D. (2004). Chemical agents of terrorism: Preparing nurse practitioners. *Nurse Practitioner, 29*(5), 30–39.

- Performing a "hazard assessment" of the workplace to identify and control physical and health hazards
- Identifying and providing appropriate PPE for employees
- Training employees in the use and care of the PPE
- Maintaining PPE, including replacing worn or damaged PPE
- Periodically reviewing, updating, and evaluating the effectiveness of the PPE program

In general, nurses should:

- Properly wear PPE
- Attend training sessions on PPE
- Care for, clean, and maintain PPE
- Inform a supervisor of the need to repair or replace PPE

Research following the Ebola virus disease outbreak in 2014 demonstrated that hospital staff may not be aware of the appropriate type or level of PPE needed or that they may deviate from the proper protocols for donning and doffing PPE and self-contaminate (Casanova et al., 2017; Kwon et al., 2016, 2017). In a simulation study where healthcare workers were videotaped donning and doffing PPE, 79% self-contaminated (Kang et al., 2017).

OSHA (2017) has identified the following four classes of personal protective clothing:

- *Level A* provides the highest level of skin, respiratory, eye, and mucus membrane protection. Equipment includes a fully encapsulated water- and vapor-proof suit, boots, gloves, and hardhat, which contains a self-contained breathing apparatus (SCBA). The suit should contain a cooling and communication system. Level A PPE is required by HAZMAT teams for use in the field.

- *Level B* is used when the highest level of respiratory protection is required, but skin and eye protection will suffice with splash-resistant gear. The equipment includes SCBA and splash-resistant clothing, hood, gloves, hardhat, boots, booties, and two-way communication and cooling system.
- *Level C* provides the same skin and eye protection as Level B, but uses an air-purifying respirator (APR; rather than a SCBA). The APR filters the air rather than providing oxygen from an outside source. The APR uses a hood rather than a mask, which reduces the risk of contamination around the edges of the mask and avoids the need for fit testing to ensure a proper fit. Level C gear is to be used only when the chemical contaminant is known and the criteria for use of an APR are met (Dickens, 2002).
- *Level D* provides standard work protection from splashes; no respiratory and minimal skin protection are required. The gear includes cover or standard work clothing, safety glasses, gloves, and face shield.

The higher the level of PPE, the higher the degree of protection for the healthcare provider; however, there is a higher level of burden that is due to weight, bulk, and the heat factor. Wearing PPE may present various problems for the nurse depending on the environment, the level of PPE that is required, and the duration that the PPE will be worn. Nurses should be prepared to expect any of the following conditions while wearing PPE:

- Extreme heat
- Poor ventilation
- Lack of peripheral vision because of the goggles or head gear

- Inhibited sense of touch because of the gloves
- Claustrophobia
- Heavy weight
- Fatigue
- Difficulty in communications

In the hospital setting, the safety officer will determine the level of PPE to be used. It is important to select the correct level of PPE. The minimum protective equipment required by OSHA regulations for nurses caring for patients contaminated with an unknown substance include chemical-resistant suits that guard against splash exposures and positive-pressure full-faced respirators (OSHA, 2002a, 2002b). Using this equipment requires specialized training; therefore, nurses must have appropriate training *prior* to being asked to participate in a response effort (Centers for Disease Control and Prevention [CDC]/National Institute for Occupational Safety and Health [NIOSH], 2013). Nursing skills may have to be adapted while wearing PPE. Participating in classroom instruction taught by HAZMAT experts and practice exercises involving donning and working in PPE will allow the nurse to become comfortable with the decontamination process.

The following cautions should be used when wearing PPE:

- Ensure proper fit of PPE. If PPE does not fit properly, it will not be effective.
- Do not use respirators in a flammable or explosive atmosphere.
- Keep batteries/battery packs away from heat and flame.
- Know the proper procedure for donning and removing PPE.

It is important to determine if your hospital or agency has *enough* PPE in the event of a disaster for *all its nurses* and if any mitigation plans are in place in the event of an equipment shortage. Ensuring that hospitals have adequate resources and training to mount an effective decontamination response in a rapid manner is essential (Levitin et al., 2003). Nurses need to know that there is enough PPE, where it is located, how to put it on, and what their role is during decontamination. It is critically important that *nurses know they are safe* to function effectively during decontamination procedures. This also affects their *willingness to come to work*. A process to notify decontamination personnel needs to be in place to allow members to assemble and don proper PPE when the hospital is notified of an impending arrival of contaminated patients.

Respirators

In the event of deployment of chemical weapons, emergency care providers will be at serious risk of exposure, and special respirators may be needed for additional protection. There are several types of respirators, each providing a different level of protection.

- Full facepiece APR
- Full facepiece APR retrofit
- Powered APR (PAPR)

- SCBA
- Closed-circuit SCBA
- Reusable elastomeric respirators[1]

Respirators protect the user in two basic ways. The first is by the removal of contaminants from the air. Respirators of this type include particulate respirators that filter out airborne particles and gas masks that filter out chemicals and gases. Other respirators protect by supplying clean respirable air from another source. Respirators that fall into this category include airline respirators that use compressed air from a remote source and SCBA that include their own air supply.

In U.S. workplaces requiring the use of respiratory protective devices, the OSHA requires the use of respirators approved by NIOSH. Industrial type approvals are in accordance with the federal respiratory regulations (Title 42, Code of Federal Regulations Part 84). The National Personal Protective Technology Laboratory (NPPTL), a Division of NIOSH, tests and approves respirators, and the Food and Drug Administration (FDA) regulates medical devices including N95 respirators (CDC, 2017). Development of respirator standards is in concert with various partners from government and industry. NIOSH states that respirators should be used only as a last line of defense when engineering control systems are not feasible. Engineering control systems, such as adequate ventilation or scrubbing of contaminants, should be used to avoid the need for respirators. The reader is cautioned that the science in this field is rapidly evolving, and it is essential that nursing professionals refer to reliable, established sources frequently to stay abreast of current changes. Up-to-date information may be obtained from the CDC at www.cdc.gov/niosh/npptl/respstdpg.html.

PATIENT DECONTAMINATION

Decontamination is the process of removing or neutralizing a hazard from the environment, property, or life form (Farmer, Jiminez, Rubinson, & Talmor, 2004). The goals of decontamination are to reduce or remove the hazardous agent while maintaining staff safety and to prevent further contamination of the environment. For victims, the goal is to prevent further harm and to enhance the potential for a full clinical recovery from the exposure. Decontamination needs to be accomplished as quickly as possible. For most chemical agents, there is a direct relationship between contact time and effect; therefore, physical removal is of the highest priority. Optimal decontamination requires identification and knowledge of the HAZMAT, but decontamination can occur without this exact knowledge.

The four basic methods for decontamination are (Hurst, 1997):

- *Physical removal*—Flushing with water or aqueous solutions. This method is highly effective and significantly dilutes or

---

[1] Elastomeric respirators are NIOSH-approved, half-facepiece, tight-fitting respirators that are made of synthetic or rubber material permitting them to be repeatedly disinfected, cleaned, and reused. They are equipped with exchangeable filter cartridges and may have disposable components. These elastomeric respirators are assigned the same protection classification (APF) as N95s. They are also available as full facepieces, which have a clear lens that covers the eyes as well as the nose and mouth.

reduces the amount of chemical agent on the skin or mucus membrane. For absorbent materials: Rub with flour followed by wet tissues. This is suggested for emergency situations where water flushing is not available. M291 resin: Used by the military; wallet-sized packets with resin-impregnated pads used for individual decontamination.

- *Chemical methods*—Water/soap wash: This is the most likely method to be used in the hospital setting. The chemical agent is removed via mechanical force as well as hydrolysis.
- *Oxidation*—Hypochlorite solutions are considered to be universally effective for removing organophosphates and mustard agents.
- *Hydrolysis*—Hydrolyzing agents: Alkaline hypochlorite is effective for hydrolyzing VX and G agents (for further information, see Table 35.3).

Patient Decontamination in the Field

Ideally, a HAZMAT team at the scene will be able to provide assistance regarding the specifics of the exposure and the potential treatment. A local poison control center also may be able to provide assistance. The Chemical Manufacturers Association provides 24-hour assistance in the specifics of treating a particular chemical exposure; it can be reached at (800) 424-9300. The Domestic Preparedness Chem/Bio Helpline can be reached at 800-368-6498. Online information is available at the CDC website at www.cdc.gov or the CDC hotline at 770-488-7100 (24 hours).

Patient Decontamination in the ED

When a patient presents to the ED, the nurse must ascertain that an exposure has taken place. Nurses should suspect chemical exposures for any mass casualty incident in which multiple ill persons with similar clinical complaints (point-source exposure) seek treatment at about the same time, or in persons who are exposed to common ventilation systems or unusual patterns of death or illness. The ED may or may not receive notification in advance that a chemical explosion or leak has occurred. In either case, ED healthcare providers have the following three primary goals in treating a patient who has been exposed to a HAZMAT and may be contaminated or who has not undergone adequate decontamination before arrival at the hospital:

1. Isolate the chemical contamination.
2. Appropriately decontaminate and treat the patient(s) while protecting hospital staff, other patients, and visitors.
3. Reestablish normal service as quickly as possible.

Healthcare providers caring for the patient should put on the appropriate PPE prior to coming into contact with contaminated patients. In most instances, this is Level B PPE.

Ideally, decontamination occurs outside the hospital by specially trained EMS providers. If this does not occur, prepare a decontamination area for the patient. If possible, the ideal location is outdoors (see Table 35.4). If indoor decontamination is necessary, a decontamination room is the next ideal location. Indoor decontamination should occur only in cases in which a controlled indoor environment may be maintained safely.

Control volatilization of the chemical to prevent displacement of ambient room oxygen, to prevent combustion, and to prevent levels of the chemical from reaching air concentrations deemed immediately dangerous to life or health for that specific hazard. To monitor this hazard effectively, the hospital requires testing equipment capable of identifying the chemical, its ambient air concentration, and ambient room oxygen concentrations. If such a room is not available, try to isolate the patient in a single large room after removing nonessential and nondisposable equipment. Ideally, this

TABLE 35.3 Decontamination Methods

Method	Description
Physical removal	• *Remove clothing—Clothing removal is decontamination*—encourage victims to remove clothing at least to their undergarments. • *Flush* with water or aqueous solutions. • *Absorb* contaminating agent with absorbent materials (e.g., rub with flour followed by wet tissues or use military M291 resin kits for spot decontamination of skin only). • *Scrape* bulk agent with a wooden stick (e.g., tongue depressor/popsicle stick). *Note:* Follow all of these actions with full decontamination at a medical treatment facility.
Chemical deactivation	• *Water/soap wash:* Chemical warfare agents have a generally low solubility and slow rate of diffusion in both fresh water and seawater. Therefore, the major effect of water and water combined with soap (especially alkaline soaps) is via a slow breakdown of the compound (i.e., hydrolysis) or through dilution of the agent and the mechanical force of the wash. When other chemical deactivation means are not available, washing with water or soap and water is a good alternative. • *Chemical solutions:* In the event of an emergency, you may be directed to perform decontamination with other chemical deactivation agents. These vary depending on the chemical warfare agent and may include alkaline solutions of hypochlorite.
Hydrolyzing agents	• Alkaline hypochlorite is effective for hydrolyzing VX and G agents.

TABLE 35.4 Hospital Decontamination Work Zones

Zone	Location	Description
Hot	Contamination site (prehospital)	Contaminated area where the release occurred. See earlier discussion of on-scene decontamination.
Warm/dirty	Adjacent to the hospital, usually near the emergency department (remote to the release site)	*Hospital decontamination area*: This area needs a source of water (cold climates require a warm water source) for decontamination and barriers to control entrance and exit from the area, which must be tightly controlled. Personnel working in this area (first receivers) have potential to be exposed to the contaminant(s) and, therefore, must wear the appropriate level of PPE (Level C minimum). At the entrance to the warm zone is the initial triage station. All ambulance and walk-in cases must enter the facility after going through this triage station. Victims who are clearly not contaminated skip the warm zone and enter the cold (clean) zone directly. All others proceed into the warm zone for decontamination.
Cold/clean	Hospital treatment area, often the emergency department	*Uncontaminated hospital treatment area (postdecontamination)*: Because no agent exposure is expected in this area, in most cases only standard (universal) precautions are needed for healthcare workers. This area needs to be tightly controlled so that only patients who have been triaged and decontaminated are allowed entry. Any potentially contaminated victims, clothing, PPE, and/or equipment should not be permitted entrance to this zone. Another more thorough triage is performed in the cold (clean) zone before treatment is begun based on the nature and acuity of signs and symptoms.

PPE, personal protective equipment.

room should be away from other patient care areas. Maintain ventilation to the area in which the patient is located, but be wary of further contamination of the hospital with recycled ventilation.

Establish a secure zone with yellow tape and permit only appropriately protected individuals to enter as needed. Include in the secure zone any area the patient may have contaminated while entering the ED.

On arrival of the patient, determine whether the patient requires any immediate lifesaving interventions. If these are required, stabilize the patient before or during decontamination.

Decontamination Procedures

The basic preparation steps in patient decontamination include the following:

- Get information. Identify the agent (if possible).
- Determine the level of PPE required.
- Mobilize security personnel and trained triage and decontamination staff.
- Control access to the decontamination site as well as to the hospital.
- Prepare decontamination area (warm zone should be outside the facility).
- Gather decontamination supplies and equipment (see Box 35.1).
  - Downwind of clean area, not located near facility air intake.
  - Area for decontamination triage: those with most severe signs or symptoms are triaged first.
  - Receptacles for contaminated clothing, valuables, and contaminated supplies.
  - Source of water (warm in cold climate areas), soap, and towels.

- Tape to demarcate dirty and clean sides.
- Screens for privacy or segregation by gender (if possible).
- Collection system for runoff water.
- Chemical agent monitor supplies (CAM).

Victim Decontamination

- Having the patient perform as much of the decontamination as possible is preferable to decrease the amount of cross-contamination.
- Remove all clothing (this will remove 80% to 90% of the contaminants).
- Place all clothing and valuables in a bag. Place these individual bags in a larger collection container, taking care to not touch the outside of the container.
- Wet skin and wash down with soap and water. Attention needs to be given to hair, face, hands, and other areas that were exposed and not covered by clothing. Avoid vigorous scrubbing to prevent skin breakdown. Wash for 5 to 10 minutes and rinse.
- Decontaminate open wounds by irrigation with saline or water for an additional 5 to 10 minutes.
- Try to avoid contaminating unexposed skin on the patient. Use surgical drapes if necessary.
- Flush exposed areas with soap and water for 10 to 15 minutes with gentle sponging.
- Irrigate exposed eyes with saline for 10 to 15 minutes, except in alkali exposures, which require 30 to 60 minutes of irrigation.
- Clean under fingernails with a scrub brush.
- Check for presence of agent using CAM or M-8 paper, and if positive, decontaminate again.
- Relocate to clean area, don dry clothing.
- Ideally, collect runoff water in steel drums if possible.

- IV setups and solutions can be left in during decontamination, but should be replaced as soon as possible with new, clean setups.
- Endotracheal tubes can remain in place during decontamination, but should be replaced as soon as possible with new, clean tubes.

For more detailed information, see Boxes 35.2 and 35.3. During the decontamination procedure, the victims must be monitored for signs of decompensation, and staff must be monitored for signs of exhaustion. Antidotes may need to be administered during decontamination procedures, and previous ambulatory individuals may have to have their decontamination on a gurney (see Box 35.4).

BOX 35.1 Baseline Decontamination Supplies and Equipment

- Containment equipment
- Pool or tank
- Tarps
- 6-mil construction plastic
- Fiberglass backboard
- Supports for ambulatory patients
- Sawhorses to support backboards
- Water supply
- Scissors for clothing removal
- Mild detergent (dishwashing liquid)
- 5-gallon buckets
- Sponges and soft brushes
- Towels and blankets/sheets
- Triage tags
- Disposable clothes and shoes for ambulatory patients
- Large plastic bags for contaminated clothing with predetermined unique ID tags to go on the bag and patient's wrist/neck
- Small plastic bags for patients' valuables
- Waterproof pens to mark bags
- Clear, zip-front body suits or large water-repellent blankets to minimize contamination to transport personnel and ambulances
- Duct tape (4 in.)

BOX 35.2 Procedures for Gross Individual Patient Decontamination

- Direct patient to the decontamination area (warm zone).
- Separate male and female patients if possible, and keep children with parents or older siblings, if possible.
- Instruct patients to wipe feet before entering decontamination area—use mat or remove shoes directly into plastic bag.
- Instruct patient to remove clothing.
- Place clothing in plastic bag with shoes, label the bag, and hold it during decontamination.
- Instruct patient to place valuables in a small plastic bag, label the bag, and hold it during decontamination.
- Brush or wipe off particulate matter.
- Instruct patient to step into shower, close eyes and mouth, and raise arms above head.
- Instruct patient to rotate twice, slowly.
- Instruct patient to walk out of shower into secondary (definitive) decontamination area.

BOX 35.3 Procedures for Secondary (Definitive) Individual Patient Decontamination

- If possible, keep male and female patients separate.
- Make sure all clothing is removed, bagged, and labeled.
- Brush or vacuum any remaining particulate matter off of skin.
- Decontaminate systematically from the head down with water.
- Water-wash contaminated area gently under a stream of water and scrub gently using a soft brush with soap.
- Use warm, never hot, water.
- Decontaminate exposed wounds and eyes before intact skin areas; do not introduce contaminants into wounds.
- Cover wounds with a waterproof dressing.
- Remember the back, under skin folds, axilla, ears, and genitalia.
- Remove contaminants to the level that they are no longer a threat to the patient or response personnel.
- Allow ambulatory patients to decontaminate themselves.
- Provide instructions in multiple languages to ensure that patients understand the problem and follow instructions.
- Administer medicines or ventilation support to seriously ill patients while undergoing decontamination.
- Administer invasive procedures in the contamination reduction zone (on-scene) or warm zone (hospital setting) only when it is absolutely necessary.
- Isolate the patient from the environment by wrapping in blanket/sheet to prevent the spread of any remaining contaminants.
- Direct men and women to segregated treatment areas, if possible.
- Soap, brushes, sponges, and other equipment used for decontamination should be placed in a trashcan and not carried into the support zone (on-scene) or the cold (clean) zone (hospital setting).

BOX 35.4 Procedures for Individual Nonambulatory Patient Decontamination

- Apply C-collar immediately if a cervical spine injury is suspected.
- Place plastic sheet on cart, cover with sheet, place victim on sheet.
- Remove all clothing and place in plastic bag and label the bag.
- Place valuables in a small plastic bag and label properly.
- Brush or wipe off particulate matter.
- Rinse patient gently using handheld sprayer; begin with face and airway, then open wounds (cover patient's mouth and pinch nose when washing face).
- Ensure axilla, genitalia, and the back are rinsed.
- Use nonrebreather mask or bag-valve-mask to protect airway.

(continued)

> **BOX 35.4** Procedures for Individual Nonambulatory Patient Decontamination (*continued*)
>
> - Wash from head to toe using tepid, not hot, water and soap 5 minutes when agent is nonpersistent and 8 minutes when a persistent or unknown agent.
> - Wash and rinse creases such as ears, eyes, axilla, groin; rinse for about 1 minute; roll patient to side if needed.
> - Wash around IV site(s) and IV setup. Replace IV once out of decontamination.
> - Thoroughly dry patient and cover with a blanket.
> - Soap, brushes, sponges, and other equipment used for decontamination should be placed in a trashcan and not carried into the support zone (on-scene) or the cold (clean) zone (hospital setting).
> - Open wounds should be covered with dressings after decontamination is complete.
> - Transfer patient to clean backboard and exit into cold zone for rapid assessment, triage, and assignment to a treatment area.

PEDIATRIC CONSIDERATIONS

Children presenting to the ED needing decontamination require special consideration. When dealing with children in a disaster situation, nurses must not only work to identify, triage, and decontaminate a potentially large number of children, they also must take special precautions to ensure that the emotional and psychological trauma experienced by the children is minimized (Mueller, 2006). Children lack the cognitive ability to make clear and rational decisions and are likely to refuse to follow directions. Children are unpredictable and are unable to fully understand the event as it is occurring. They will become distressed when separated from their parents, and healthcare providers dressed in PPE will appear threatening to young victims. Adolescents may be reluctant to undress for decontamination. Infants and small children will need to be held throughout the decontamination process and will be extremely fearful. Special considerations should include the following:

- Allow children and parents (or other adults known to them) to remain together.
- Constantly reassure and offer compassion to a child if the child is separated from his or her parent(s)—children will be fearful.
- Attempt to reunite children with their parents if they were separated during the course of the disaster.
- Take time to inform and reassure older children of the current situation.
- Prevent children from developing hypothermia.
- Use a water temperature of 100°F.
- Wash/shower for 5 minutes.
- Use great caution—*wet infants are slippery.*

The Children's Hospital of Boston, in conjunction with Dr. Michael Shannon, Chief, Division of Emergency Medicine, has developed an instructional video entitled "The Decontamination of Children" to teach individuals who will need to care for children contaminated with chemicals. This valuable teaching and learning resource can be obtained by contacting: AHRQ Publications Clearinghouse; (800) 358–9295; ahrqpubs@ahrq.gov.

EVACUATION OF THE ED

Decontamination helps protect nurses and other healthcare providers and maintains the viability of the ED as a treatment center. Mismanagement of the process may result in illness in healthcare providers and contamination of the ED; and severe ED contamination may necessitate departmental closure, which is potentially catastrophic in a mass casualty incident. Evacuation of the ED rarely is indicated; however, it remains a possibility. In most situations, isolation of the contamination is all that is required.

Nurses should contact the chief nurse executive or hospital administrator-on-call and consider evacuation of the ED in the following situations:

- Toxic materials are spilled in the ED.
- Nearby HAZMATs are threatening the hospital.
- A patient is contaminated with a volatile toxic or flammable chemical and is decontaminated insufficiently prior to entering the ED.

If symptoms start to occur outside the isolation area or the situation requires urgent decision making without time to identify the contaminant, consider evacuation. Odor does not predict toxicity reliably.

SUPPORTIVE MEDICAL AND NURSING CARE

Saving lives always depends on ensuring the ABCs: adequate airway, breathing, and circulation. The care of patients who have experienced chemical contamination is nursing intensive. These patients may require one-to-one staffing ratios, an impossibility during a mass casualty event. Greater contamination or exposure more likely results in victims who require early intubation and ventilation (having an adequate supply of ventilators and respiratory therapists available in the ED is an important component of planning). Conversely, adequate ventilation may be impossible because of the intense muscarinic effects of certain nerve gas exposures (copious airway secretions, bronchoconstriction). In this situation, administer atropine before initiating other measures. In some patients, large quantities of atropine may be required, rapidly depleting hospital supplies. Administering succinylcholine to assist intubation is relatively contraindicated because nerve agents prolong the drug's paralytic effects.

SEIZURES

Victims of certain chemical exposures will experience seizure activity. Patients must be protected from harm. Benzodiazepines are the mainstays in seizure treatment. Liberal doses are required;

titrate to effect. Termination of seizure activity may reflect onset of flaccid paralysis from the nerve agent rather than adequacy of anticonvulsant therapy. A bedside electroencephalogram (EEG) may be required to assess ongoing seizure activity.

SUMMARY

Hazardous chemical incidents create unique challenges for first responders and first receivers, including nurses. A large-scale chemical or radiation release with mass casualties will create a significant burden and may quickly overwhelm the existing healthcare system. Special conditions triage must be employed to appropriately sort victims of the exposure. Decontamination must be available and provided quickly to patients involved in chemical and other HAZMAT incidents. Decontamination must reduce or remove the chemical agent while protecting the safety of the staff and preventing further contamination of the environment. Hospitals in the United States and across the world must be prepared to handle a sudden influx of large numbers of casualties requiring triage and decontamination. Above all, *safety is of the utmost priority during disaster response.* Proper antidotes and equipment, a clearly written emergency response plan articulating policies and procedures, leadership and lines of communication, and adequate staff training and evaluation drills are required to ensure the provision of a safe environment for staff as well as patients during disaster triage and decontamination. All nurses should be (at a minimum) aware of the basic processes regarding mass triage models for HAZMAT events and decontamination procedures.

STUDY QUESTIONS

1. During triage for mass casualty chemical incidents, what are the differences in the triage activities in the hot, warm, and cold zones?

2. What are the five major classes of CWAs? Can you describe their basic physiological effects?

3. Describe the primary goals of decontamination.

4. A 32-year-old worker at a large photochemical plant presents to the ED following a massive explosion. He was exposed to large volumes of an unknown chemical, both in liquid and gaseous states. He presents unconscious and with slow respiratory rate and stridor. What are the priorities for care?

5. Why is staff safety such an important factor for the disaster manager during response to a chemical incident?

6. You are the triage nurse in the ED on a cold and windy Saturday afternoon. Two women present to the ED with complaints of cough, runny eyes, headache, and report smelling a foul odor. Ten minutes later, three more people arrive with the same complaint. Five minutes later, eight more patients present to the ED with a similar story. Identify how you would manage this situation.

7. What level of PPE is needed by the nurse caring for a victim of a chemical contamination of an unknown agent?

HOTLINES/HELPLINES

Centers for Disease Control and Prevention
Phone: 770-488-7100 (24 hours)

Domestic Preparedness Chemical/Biological HelpLine
Phone: 800-368-6498
Provides technical assistance during business hours to eligible state and local emergency responders and their organizations.

FEMA
Chem/Bio Hotline 800-424-8802 (24 hours)
Radiological Hotline 202-586-8100 (24 hours)
Report a Chemical, Biological, or Radiological emergency incident.
FEMA, Office of National Preparedness: Preparedness News and Information)

National Response Center Hotline
Phone: 800-424-8802 (24 hours)
Receives reports of oil, chemical, biological, and radiological releases and actual or potential domestic terrorism; provides technical assistance to emergency responders; and connects callers with appropriate federal resources.

Nuclear Regulatory Commission Operations Center
Phone: 301-816-5100 (collect calls accepted)
Accepts reports of accidents involving radiological materials.

REFERENCES

Alibek, K., Dashiell, T., Dwyer, A., Lane, S., Patrick, W., Ponikvar, D., ..., Sidell, F. (2005). *Jane's chem-bio handbook* (3rd ed.). Alexandria, VA: Jane's Information Group.

American Heritage Dictionary of the English Language (4th ed., 2009). Boston, MA: Houghton Mifflin Harcourt.

Auf der Heide, E. (2006). The importance of evidence-based disaster planning. *Annals of Emergency Medicine, 47*(1), 34–49. doi:10.1016/j.annemergmed.2005.05.009

Brennan, R. J., Waeckerle, J. F., Sharp, T. W., & Lillibridge, S. R. (1999). Chemical warfare agents: Emergency medical and emergency public health issues. *Annals of Emergency Medicine, 34*(2), 191–204. doi:10.1016/S0196-0644(99)70229-5

Casanova, L. M., Erukunuakpor, K., Walsh, V. L., Kraft, C., Shane, A., Ray, S., ..., Jacob, J. T. (2017). Multicenter evaluation of viral self-contamination during doffing of Ebola-level personal protective equipment. *American Journal of Infection Control, 45*(6), S17. doi:10.1016/j.ajic.2017.04.276

Centers for Disease Control and Prevention, National Center for Environmental Health. (2013, June 25). Chemical agent information. Retrieved from https://www.cdc.gov/nceh/demil/chemical_agent.htm

Centers for Disease Control and Prevention, National Institute for Occupational Safety and Health. (2013, September). What's special about chemical, biological, radiological, and nuclear (CBRN) air-purifying respirators

(APR)? NIOSH fact sheet. Retrieved from https://www.cdc.gov/niosh/docs/2013-157/pdfs/2013-157.pdf

Centers for Disease Control and Prevention, Department of Health and Human Services. (2017, September 5). Elastomeric and powered-air purifying respirators in U.S. healthcare. Retrieved from https://www.cdc.gov/niosh/npptl/pdfs/ElastomericPAPR-Healthcare.pdf

Cox, R. D. (1994). Decontamination and management of hazardous materials exposure victims in the emergency department. *Annals of Emergency Medicine, 23*(4), 761–770. doi:10.1016/S0196-0644(94)70312-4

Dickens, G. (2002). A basic review of personal protection equipment (PPE). In P. Maniscalco & H. Christen (Eds.), *Understanding terrorism and managing consequences* (pp. 301–311). Upper Saddle River, NJ: Prentice Hall.

Djalali, A., Della Corte, F., Segond, F., Metzger, M. H., Gabilly, L., Grieger, F., …, Ingrassia, P. L. (2017). TIER competency-based training course for the first receivers of CBRN casualties: A European perspective. *European Journal of Emergency Medicine, 24*(5), 371-376. doi:10.1097/MEJ.0000000000000383

Emergency Planning and Community Right-to-Know Act, 42 U.S.C. §11001-§11050 (1986). Retrieved from https://www.govinfo.gov/content/pkg/USCODE-2011-title42/html/USCODE-2011-title42-chap116.htm

Farmer, J. C., Jiminez, E. J., Rubinson, L., & Talmor, D. S. (2004). *Fundamentals of disaster management: A handbook for medical professionals* (2nd ed.). Des Plaines, IL: Society for Critical Care Medicine.

Hammond, K., Arbon, P., Gebbie, K., & Hutton, A. (2017). Why a disaster is not just normal business ramped up: Disaster response among ED nurses. *Australasian Emergency Nursing Journal.* Retrieved from http://www.aenj.com.au/article/S1574-6267(17)30064-2/fulltext

Hurst, C. (1997). Decontamination. In Brig. Gen. R. Zajtchuck (Ed.), *Textbook of military medicine: Medical aspects of chemical and biological warfare* (pp. 351–360). Falls Church, VA: Office of the Surgeon General, Department of the Army.

Joint Commission. (1996). *1996 comprehensive accreditation manual for hospitals.* Oakbrook Terrace, IL: Author.

Kang, J., O'Donnell, J. M., Colaianne, B., Bircher, N., Ren, D., & Smith, K. J. (2017). Use of personal protective equipment among health care personnel: Results of clinical observations and simulations. *American Journal of Infection Control, 45*(1), 17–23. doi:10.1016/j.ajic.2016.08.011

Keim, M. E., Pesik, N., & Twum-Danso, N. A. (2003). Lack of hospital preparedness for chemical terrorism in a major U.S. city: 1996–2000. *Prehospital and Disaster Medicine, (18)*3, 193–199. doi:10.1017/S1049023X00001059

Kolleck, D. (2003). Canadian emergency department preparedness for a nuclear, biological or chemical event. *Canadian Journal of Emergency Medicine,* (1), 18–26. doi:10.1017/S148180350000806X

Kwon, J. H., Burnham, C. A. D., Reske, K., Liang, S., Hink, T., Wallace, M., …, Dubberke, E. R. (2016, October). Healthcare worker self-contamination during standard and Ebola virus disease personal protective equipment doffing. *Open Forum Infectious Diseases, 3*, Suppl 1, p. 1387. Oxford University Press. doi:10.1093/ofid/ofw172.1090

Kwon, J. H., Burnham, C. A. D., Reske, K. A., Liang, S. Y., Hink, T., Wallace, M. A., …, Dubberke, E. R. (2017). Assessment of healthcare worker protocol deviations and self-contamination during personal protective equipment donning and doffing. *Infection Control and Hospital Epidemiology, 38*(9), 1–7. doi:10.1017/ice.2017.121

Levitin, H. W., & Siegelson, H. J. (1996). Hazardous materials. Disaster medical planning and response. *Emergency Medicine Clinics of North America, 14*(2), 327–348.

Levitin, H. W., Siegelson, H. J., Dickinson, S., Halpern, P., Haraguchi, Y., Nocera, A., & Turineck, D. (2003). Decontamination of mass casualties: Re-evaluating existing dogma. *Prehospital and Disaster Medicine, 18*(3), 200–207. doi:10.1017/S1049023X00001060

Mueller, C. (2006). The effects of weapons of mass destruction on children. *Journal for Specialists in Pediatric Nursing, 11*(2), 114–128. doi:10.1111/j.1744-6155.2006.00053.x

Occupational Safety and Health Administration. (1997). *Hospitals and community emergency response: What you need to know. Emergency Response Safety Series.* Washington, DC: U.S. Department of Labor.

Occupational Safety and Health Administration. (2002a). *Fact sheet: What is personal protective equipment?* Retrieved from http://www.osha.gov/OshDoc/data_General_Facts/ppe-factsheet.pdf

Occupational Safety and Health Administration. (2002b). *Personal protective equipment guidelines.* Retrieved from http://www.osha.gov/SLTC/personalprotectiveequipment/index.html

Occupational Safety and Health Administration. (2005). *OSHA best practices for hospital-based first receivers of victims.* Retrieved from http://www.osha.gov/dts/osta/bestpractices/html/hospital_firstreceivers.html

Occupational Safety and Health Administration. (2017). Section VIII: Chapter 1. Chemical protective clothing. In *OSHA technical manual.* Retrieved from https://www.osha.gov/dts/osta/otm/otm_viii/otm_viii_1.html

Sarc, L. (2012). Incidents caused by hazardous material. In S. Lennquist (Ed.), *Medical response to major incidents and disasters.* Berlin, Germany: Springer.

Stokes, E., Gilbert-Palmer, D., Skorga, P., Young, C., & Persell, D. (2004). Chemical agents of terrorism: Preparing nurse practitioners. *Nurse Practitioner, 29*(5), 30–39.

Tur-Kaspa, I., Lev, E., Handler, I., Siebner, R., Shapira, Y., & Shemer, J. (1999). Preparing hospitals for toxicological mass casualties events. *Critical Care Medicine, 27*(5), 873–874. doi:10.1097/00003246-199905000-00045

Veenema, T. (2003). Chemical and biological terrorism preparedness for staff development specialists. *Journal for Nurses in Staff Development, 19*(5), 215–222.

Wang, T.-L., Huei-Tsair, C., and Chang, H. (2004). Hospital preparedness for weapons of mass destruction incidents: An initial assessment. *Annals of Disaster Medicine, 2*(2), 74–78. doi:10.1067/mem.2001.118009

SPECIAL TOPICS IN DISASTERS

36

U.S. NATIONAL DISASTER NURSE READINESS: PRACTICE AND EDUCATION FOR A PREPARED WORKFORCE

Joanne C. Langan, Anne Griffin, Alicia R. Gable, and Aram Dobalian

LEARNING OBJECTIVES

When this chapter is completed, readers will be able to:

1. Discuss the rationale for a prepared nursing workforce.
2. Discuss disaster nursing roles and responsibilities.
3. Identify key disaster-nursing competencies and expectations for new graduate nurses and licensed nurses according to role.
4. Describe disaster-related education and training opportunities for nurses.
5. Define the types of disaster drills in which nurses may participate and the advantages and disadvantages of each type of drill.

KEY MESSAGES

In the United States, nurses will be expected to respond to disaster situations regardless of workplace setting, type of clinical practice, or skill set.

All nurses are expected to have basic foundational disaster preparedness and response skills; disaster nurses or those in advanced practice will be expected to lead nurses with less disaster skills and training.

Basic disaster preparedness education is available in courses on college campuses, online through formal educational institutions, and online through approved governmental and nongovernmental agencies.

Nurses are more likely to retain knowledge and be most effective if they are active participants in regularly scheduled disaster drills and exercises.

Nurses can access online learning opportunities for disaster preparedness and response and become contributors to strategies to improve survivor outcomes for communities, groups, and individuals.

CHAPTER OVERVIEW

This chapter provides the reader with a broad overview of the importance of national nurse readiness for disasters and large-scale public health emergencies. This means ensuring that every nurse is prepared for disaster planning, response, mitigation, and recovery. Because nurses provide care at all levels and during each phase of a disaster, they are essential in helping to prepare communities, groups, families, and individuals for disasters, reduction of vulnerabilities, and appropriate and effective response. This chapter discusses disaster and public health emergency education and training for nurses at all levels of clinical and administrative practice. The chapter also describes the recently established U.S. Society for the Advancement of Disaster Nursing, an ongoing national initiative to create, practice, and disseminate evidence-based disaster preparedness and response strategies.

RATIONALE FOR A PREPARED NURSING WORKFORCE

Disasters are largely unpredictable; with the potential to happen anywhere, at any time, with little or no notice. The potential is there for any practicing nurse to be called upon to respond. Nurses may need to respond to a wide variety of disasters or public health emergencies with the expectation of minimizing both morbidity and mortality, despite chaotic and suboptimal conditions. Nurses will be expected to recognize and respond to triggering events that would force them to transition from providing care as usual to responding to an unanticipated "surge" of patients with requisite crisis standards of care. Such a significant shift requires preparation well in advance of the event. The Bureau of Labor Statistics (BLS) reports that registered nurses held 2.95 million jobs in 2016 and have a growth projection of 15% through 2024 (BLS, 2017). Nurses are the largest segment of the healthcare workforce (BLS, 2017). This number of healthcare providers is significant as the effectiveness of the healthcare system's response to disasters depends heavily on the surge capacity of the nursing workforce (U.S. Department of Health and Human Services [HHS], 2013; National Advisory Council on Nursing Education and Practice [NACNEP], 2009). Registered nurses are well positioned to improve population health outcomes during times of disaster

given their broad scope of practice and collaboration with a diverse range of healthcare professionals.

Consistently ranked by the public as trusted sources of health information (American Nurses Association [ANA], 2016), nurses have far-reaching influence. Key organizations have highlighted the nursing profession's broad scope and available potential during disasters. The Institute of Medicine (IOM, 2011) report, *The Future of Nursing: Leading Change, Advancing Health*, endorsed the nursing profession's breadth and untapped potential as the frequency and intensity of major disasters have increased (Hay & Mimura, 2010; U.S. Agency for International Development, 2015).

The American Red Cross (ARC, 2012) report, *The Future of American Red Cross Nursing: A Blueprint for Action*, aligned three of the eight IOM Report recommendations with its strategic and business priorities and outlined how nurses can and should be actively engaged. Mobilization of the nursing workforce can enhance surge capacity, strengthen disaster readiness, and build community resiliency. Disaster experts endorse and support efforts to adequately prepare the nursing workforce with the required knowledge and skills (Stanley & Wolanski, 2015). While many nurses may complete their careers without ever having to respond to a major disaster, a lack of preparation could contribute to devastating morbidity and mortality outcomes.

The next section outlines unique disaster-nursing knowledge required for nurses to respond to disaster situations.

PRACTICES OF A PREPARED NURSING WORKFORCE

Nurses will continue to rely heavily on the general nursing skills they use every day (Box 36.1) during a disaster response. Nurses routinely assess patient needs, provide and coordinate clinical care. As patient advocates, they are integral members of the healthcare team. Registered nurses oversee the work of licensed practical nurses (LPNs), nurse assistants, and other nonlicensed personnel. They may also need to be competent in rendering a broad scope and spectrum of care specific to stages of the disaster life cycle. In the predisaster or nondisaster stage, nurses with experience and expertise will educate other nurses, patients, and the public in disaster preparedness and the mitigation of disaster trauma.

Nurses prepare patients for discharge from the healthcare facility by considering the condition of the patient, anticipated

BOX 36.1 Twenty-First-Century Professional Activities Associated with Registered Nurses

- Perform physical exams and record health histories
- Triage patients according to established acuity levels
- Administer pharmaceuticals (medications, vaccines, chemotherapeutic agents, etc.)
- Interpret patient's vital signs and laboratory data
- Monitor patient's physical, mental, and emotional status
- Use critical thinking and clinical decision making to inform care plans
- Administer evidence-based nursing interventions
- Collaboration with other healthcare professionals to coordinate care
- Direct and supervise care delivered by ancillary health-care personnel
- Provide counseling and education to patients, families, and communities
- Provide leadership across all healthcare settings
- Promote standards for quality and safety
- Advance ethical and equitable access to high-quality care for all
- Support the essentials of public health
- Advocate for health policies that improve population health
- Prepare for and respond to disasters and public health emergencies
- Conduct research to advance practice and improve patient outcomes

Source: © Tener Goodwin Veenema 2018

BOX 36.2 Examples of Unique Disaster-Nursing Activities

- Allocation of scarce resources (e.g., staff, equipment, supplies, power)
- Operate under altered standards of care that affect delivery of care as usual
- Triage
- Large-scale event management
- Communicate using Incident Command System (ICS)
- Clinical management and correct use of PPE for conditions rarely encountered (e.g., Ebola or SARS; chemical, biological, radiological and nuclear exposures)
- Implement decontamination
- Crisis leadership
- Medical service planning and coordination
- Rapid needs assessment to determine healthcare and critical resource capacity
- Mass prophylaxis and immunization
- Isolation and quarantine

PPE, personal protective equipment; SARS, severe acute respiratory syndrome.

healthcare needs, and placement requirements. They recommend modifications that must be made either to the placement, the environment, or possible hazards. They build safety measures into the discharge plan to accommodate limitations that may be new to the patient. They use the principle of mitigation to reduce or eliminate hazards. For example, how will the patient evacuate the building/house in the event of a fire? Are there steps or elevators to use or to avoid?

In other aspects of the disaster life cycle, the pre- and postdisaster stages, public policy can be impacted by nurse input on lessons learned from previous disaster experiences, and recommendations can be proposed for evidence-based strategies to minimize the effects of disasters. Much can be learned by the evaluation of these past disaster and public health emergencies and this information should be incorporated into developing future disaster preparedness and response plans. Nurses who have prior disaster response experience can have a profound effect on leaders in public policy in offering advice for keeping the public safe in future events.

When a disaster occurs, and through all stages of the disaster life cycle, nurses continue to assess patient needs and provide and coordinate clinical care despite a suboptimal environment. For nurses based in prehospital or acute care settings, they may serve as first responders, hospital-based receivers, or assist with meeting the demand for patient surge and triage. Public health

nurses may be called upon to assist with surge capacity, but also may have more population-based roles, such as providing mass prophylaxis or immunizations in the community, conducting rapid needs assessments, undertaking surveillance or contact tracking, or preparing risk communication and educational resources.

Some nurses play a more indirect role by covering shifts of those nurses who are deployed to respond or by assisting with documentation and administrative responsibilities. Nurses have multiple opportunities to volunteer with disaster relief groups, such as the American Red Cross, the Medical Reserve Corps, and the National Disaster Medical System. Although nurses do not need to be prepared for all potential roles, a minimum set of skills for disaster response is considered a professional duty. As an integral part of the healthcare team, nurses are responsible for a variety of essential response activities (McHugh, 2010). Some examples are identified within Box 36.2.

Nurses should be considering their own self-protection in their workplace settings, school environments, homes they visit, and so forth. Nurses need to be aware of potential risks in the environment such as biological, chemical, radiological risks, as well as weapons and fire. While safety professionals (e.g., fire, police, HAZMAT) will secure the area, nurses will respond to an area after it is deemed safe by these professionals and enter only after they have donned the appropriate respective personal protective equipment (PPE). This recommendation is no different than the policies and procedures for nurses who wear PPE before entering patient rooms on isolation precautions. Additionally, nurses who are prepared in their own homes and have prepared family members will be more willing and likely to respond in disaster situations. They will be reassured that they can answer the call for their nursing expertise knowing their family members know what to do in their absence to be safe and secure.

EDUCATING A PREPARED NURSING WORKFORCE

Ideally, clinical competencies should drive professional clinical nursing practice and serve as criteria for evaluating nurses. Competencies are most useful when they are research-driven or have gone through either an evidence-based review or a rigorous consensus process. Because disasters are unpredictable and emergent in nature, collecting data during disasters presents a logistical challenge. Therefore, most disaster competencies lean heavily on lessons learned and retrospective evaluation of disaster response (Daily, Padjen, & Birnbaum, 2010; Hsu et al., 2006; International Council of Nurses [ICN], 2009; Loke & Fung, 2014; Schultz, Koenig, Whiteside, & Murray, 2012; Walsh et al., 2012).

Historically, attempts have been made to methodically define disaster competencies for nurses, midwives, clinical nurse specialists, certified registered nurse anesthetists, emergency department nurses, community/public health nurse educators, nurse faculty, and those who deploy through organized response such as the American Red Cross, the National Disaster Medical System, or the Medical Reserve Corp (see Daily, 2010; Al Thobaity, Plummer, & Williams, 2017 for a review of competencies).

While there are common content domains across all nursing competencies (e.g., communication, planning, decontamination and safety, incident command structure and ethics) (Al Thobaity et al. 2017), Table 36.1 illustrates some of the unique and varied competencies required by specialty. It is important to note that "competency requirements are inconsistent across

TABLE 36.1 Examples of Disaster-Nursing Competencies

Competency	Author	Targeted Professional(s)	Sample of Competency Statements Unique to Targeted Professional(s)
Emergency and Disaster Preparedness: Core Competencies for Nurses	Gebbie and Qureshi (2002)	All Nurses	• Identify and locate the agency's emergency response plan • Describe emergency response functions or roles and demonstrate them in regularly performed drills • Demonstrate the use of equipment (including PPE) and the skills required in emergency response during regular drills • Describe communication roles in emergency response • Recognize deviations from the norm that might indicate an emergency and describe appropriate action • Participate in continuing education to maintain up-to-date knowledge in relevant areas • Participate in evaluating every drill or response and identify necessary changes to the plan
Public Health Nurse Competencies for Surge	Polivka et al. (2008)	Public Health Nurses (PHN)	Conduct a rapid assessment of the event to determine: • Nature and extent of the event • Population affected • Indicators of mass exposure • Safety concerns Demonstrate PHN technical skills, for example: • Administer medication/vaccination at mass dispensing sites • Organize mass dispensing sites • Conduct case investigation • Assure population-based infection control • Apply personal protection and safety measures, including the use of PPE • Preserve possible evidence and chain of custody • Deliver health education regarding infectious diseases
Disaster Core Competencies for Acute Care Medical Personnel	Schultz et al. (2012)	ED Nurses, Physicians and Out-of-Hospital EMS	• Identify need for decontamination • Explain the need for PPE and protection of staff performing decontamination • Describe environmental and privacy factors that affect decontamination • List necessary equipment for decontamination • List the necessary requirements and specifications for a patient-holding area for use before decontamination • Sort patients according to those capable of self-decontamination versus those needing assistance • Describe the method for containing and tracking personal/contaminated items • Identify and perform all steps necessary for decontamination, including rewarming, reclothing, and retriage

EMS, emergency medical services; PPE, personal protective equipment.

groups. [There is] little attempt to validate if those competencies are accurate or address the full spectrum of required skill sets" (Littleton-Kearney & Slepski, 2008, p. 105).

Competencies are most valuable when they are maintained, updated, and accompanied by the parallel educational materials. As a first step, established professional organization(s) along with qualified disaster nursing experts could coordinate a review of all existing published competencies to determine a limited set that would be beneficial to all nurses. Formal dissemination of a refined set of disaster-nursing competencies for both pre- and postlicensure nurses could be accomplished with the endorsement of accrediting bodies, licensing organizations, academia, and private sector healthcare.

Pre-Licensure Disaster Education

To assure consistent delivery of disaster education to all nurses, it is important to understand the factors that influence how and what nurses are taught and tested on so that disaster preparedness education can be methodically and consistently integrated into the academic programs leading to multiple pathways to licensure.

Several organizations provide accreditation for nursing schools within the United States (see Table 36.2). Each accrediting body covers various types of programs (e.g., baccalaureate, diploma, associate) and each describes a unique set of curriculum standards for schools of nursing to meet. The content and the number of academic hours to cover all material is left to each individual school to select and, therefore, educational programs vary by nature. For example, the American Association of Colleges of Nursing (AACN) added requirements to the 2008 edition of the *Essentials of Baccalaureate Education* requiring schools to provide disaster education (e.g., on risk communication, emergency preparedness and disaster response including self-protection), but each school of nursing is given the flexibility to determine the content to use and the amount of time to be devoted to it. Similarly, the National League for Nursing (NLN) does not itemize specific requirements for disaster education within its stated competencies for graduates of nursing programs but, following the 2014 Ebola outbreak (ICN, 2009), issued a recommendation to incorporate Ebola-type disaster preparedness training into nursing curricula addressing standard infection control measures.

To assure consistent delivery of disaster education for all nurses, regardless of program type, accrediting bodies could endorse the dissemination of standard disaster-nursing competencies within curriculum guidelines.

Content for curriculum development is also driven by licensing requirements. Upon completion of an accredited nursing education program, nurses are required to successfully pass a professional licensing exam, known as the National Council Licensure Examination, or NCLEX-RN, before they can practice as registered nurses. The NCLEX-RN is developed by the National Council of State Boards of Nursing. Every 3 years, new subject areas can be added based on the relevance and frequency of needed skills (National Council of State Boards of Nursing [NCSBN], 2016). Even though disasters are becoming more frequent (Hay & Mimura, 2010; U.S. Agency for International Development, 2015), they do not occur at the same rate as other pressing changes in healthcare (e.g., hospital-acquired infections, new treatment modalities). This may account for the paucity of disaster preparedness test items on this very important licensing test. The NCSBN-RN test plan includes those items that are deemed essential for new graduate nurses to know. These items are selected based on surveys completed by practicing nurses. The section of the test plan related to safety and infection control lists some key areas related to disaster preparedness and response (see Box 36.3).

Disasters impacting healthcare settings can have devastating consequences for both patients and staff. Incorporating substantial disaster-nursing content into the NCLEX exam would help drive the inclusion of more consistent disaster-nursing content into nursing school curricula.

Post-Licensure Disaster Education

To assure disaster nursing educational programming is refreshed and updated as nurses integrate into the workforce, it is important to understand some of the key stakeholders influencing continuing education requirements for the licensed nurse. See Table 36.3 for several examples of key stakeholders influencing continuing education for nurses.

Because nurses need to react quickly during an escalating situation (Newton, 2017, p. 107), just-in-time education and

TABLE 36.2 Accrediting Bodies for Schools of Nursing

Accrediting Organization	Program Type
Accreditation Commission for Education in Nursing (ACEN), previously NLNAC and wholly owned subsidiary of the National League for Nursing (NLN).	Accredits all types of nursing education programs: clinical doctorate/DNP specialist certificate, master's/post-master's certificate, baccalaureate, associate, diploma, and practical nursing programs in the United States and internationally.
Commission on Collegiate Nursing Education (CCNE), affiliated with the American Association of Colleges of Nurses (AACN).	Accredits baccalaureate and master's nursing education programs.
National League for Nursing Commission for Nursing Education Accreditation (NLN-CNEA), an autonomous accreditation division of the National League for Nursing (NLN).	Petitioning to accredit LPN/LVN, diploma, associate, bachelor, master's, and clinical doctorate degree programs.

BOX 36.3 Section of NCLEX-RN Test Blueprint

Safety and Infection Control—protecting clients and healthcare personnel from health and environmental hazards.

Related content includes but is not limited to:

- Accident/Error/Injury Prevention
- Emergency Response Plan
- Safe Use of Equipment
- Security Plan
- Ergonomic Principles
- Standard Precautions/Transmission-Based Precautions/ Surgical Asepsis
- Handling Hazardous and Infectious Materials
- Home Safety
- Reporting of Incident/Event/Irregular Occurrence/ Variance
- Use of Restraints/Safety Devices

Source: National Council of State Boards of Nursing. (2016). 2016 NCLEX-RN test plan. Retrieved from https://www.ncsbn.org/RN_Test _Plan_2016_Final.pdf

training is typically provided in response to specific disasters. The use of PPE for nurses and other healthcare providers during the "Ebola scare" (HHS, 2014) serves as an example.

Another approach would be to provide ongoing disaster and public health emergency education and training per expected response in conjunction with the Centers for Medicare and Medicaid Services regulations or accreditation standards. Consistent, required content can be made available to key stakeholders who have a vested interest in assuring what licensed nurses know and that they are meeting expectations.

While many institutions have published a variety of educational and training competencies in emergency and disaster preparedness, a common core of nursing competencies includes a personal preparedness plan and knowledge in the nurse's specific role in emergencies and disasters regardless of setting and the nurse's basic nursing preparation. Those who desire to become members of disaster response teams will require more extensive, formal training and preparation (Speraw & Persell, 2013). For example, Sigma Theta Tau International (STTI, 2017) offers an online program of study titled, "Emergency Nursing: Understanding the Profession." This course is offered for a fee and provides continuing

TABLE 36.3 Key Stakeholders Influencing Continuing Education of the Licensed Registered Nurse

Education Domain	Stakeholder	Continuing Education Requirement
License Renewal	Nevada State Board of Nursing	Beginning January 1, 2005, all nurses renewing their licenses must have completed a 4-hour bioterrorism course as part of the CE renewal requirement.
Fire	2015 Edition of NFPA 101: Life Safety Code	19.7.1.1: The administration of every healthcare occupancy shall have, in effect and available to all supervisory personnel, written copies of a plan for the protection of all persons in the event of a fire, for their evacuation to areas of refuge, and for their evacuation from the building when necessary. 19.7.1.2: All employees shall be periodically instructed and kept informed with respect to their duties under the plan required by 19.7.1.1. 19.7.1.6: Drills shall be conducted quarterly on each shift to familiarize facility personnel (nurses, interns, maintenance engineers, and administrative staff) with signals and emergency action required under varied conditions.
	The Joint Commission EC.02.03.03	The hospital conducts fire drills once per shift per quarter in each building defined as a healthcare occupancy by the Life Safe Code
Emergency Response Role	The Joint Commission EM.03.01.03 EP's 1–12	The hospital trains staff for their assigned emergency response roles.
Respiratory Protection	Occupational Safety and Health Administration (OSHA) 29 CFR 1910.134	Train, at least annually, all employees required to use a respirator on how to use the respirator effectively in emergency situations, including situations in which the respirator malfunctions. This includes education to employees about hazardous potential exposures, proper PPE donning (placing) and doffing (removing).
Bloodborne Pathogens	Occupational Safety and Health Administration (OSHA) 29 CFR 1910.1030	Provide initial and annual bloodborne pathogens training to employees with occupational exposure. Provide information on the appropriate actions to take and persons to contact in the event of an emergency involving contact with blood or other potentially infectious materials.

CE, continuing education; NFPA, National Fire Protection Associaton; PPE, personal protective equipment.

education for nurses. The American Nurses Credentialing Center (ANCC, 2017) has developed a National Healthcare Disaster Certificate. The test is a competency-based, entry-level exam. Registered nurses may apply to take the exam with 3 years of disaster experience. Competencies tested are based on response to a wide range of situations in a team-based approach (ANA, 2017).

Educational Strategies

Experiential Learning—Simulation Drills and Exercises

A basic teaching method is to practice what is learned in a more active way to retain knowledge. Drills or exercises are those active methods to help learners retain knowledge about disaster preparedness and response. Disaster simulations, conducted through drills and exercises, educate individuals about disaster preparedness and train them to respond appropriately to a variety of disaster scenarios. While some healthcare organizations have not experienced a disaster, they still need to plan and practice potential disaster scenarios to be prepared. These simulations or practice drills may involve healthcare professionals and community citizens. Healthcare professionals should also be aware of Community Emergency Response Team (CERT) drills and exercises (Federal Emergency Management Agency [FEMA], 2015). This program educates citizens about disaster preparedness and trains them in basic disaster response skills. Following this training, CERT members can assist others in the community with fire safety, light search and rescue and disaster medical operations (FEMA, 2015). Box 36.4 describes three types of simulated disaster drills or exercises. Regardless of drill type, it is critical to prepare postdrill summaries and evaluations that identify opportunities for improvement. Nurses should be represented on the committees that plan, execute, and review each type of drill or simulation. In this way, nurses from various practice settings and varying skill levels will be better prepared to help themselves and others in a real disaster.

BOX 36.4 Types of Drills and Exercises

TABLETOP EXERCISES

Tabletop exercises are activities that are held in an informal setting, around a table through the use of a facilitator. The purpose of this type of exercise is to generate discussion regarding a simulated emergency. It is most helpful if drills and exercises address a real or perceivable threat to the organization. Tabletops are a means of testing policies and procedures as well as to evaluate disaster preparedness plans and processes. A variety of personnel, including general staff and leadership, should be present to explore the response to a real situation. Nurses are integral members of the participating team. The facilitator presents the objectives of the exercise and guides the scenario and discussion. This type of exercise, like all drills and exercises, should be discussed in a no-blame environment; all are there to learn, not to be criticized. The exercise concludes with a review or "hot wash" when the objectives have been met or when time is called (FEMA, 2015).

FUNCTIONAL DRILLS

A functional drill is a verbal drill; there is no actual fieldwork. It focuses on reviewing and "running through" plans, policies, and procedures. Those in leadership and management, direction, command and control typically "staff" this kind of drill. While a tabletop exercise asks participants to discuss what they might do, a functional exercise asks the command team to "take actions" in making decisions. A functional exercise simulates movement of personnel and equipment. The functional exercise is a bit more realistic in the simulation of a disaster than a tabletop as it is conducted in real time in a classroom-type setting (FEMA, 2015).

FULL-SCALE EXERCISES

Full-scale exercises are the most realistic type of drill. This is because they are executed in a field environment that mimics a real disaster. Many persons are involved including mock victims who wear moulage, a variety of response agencies, as well as observers and evaluators. A description of the scenario is shared among participants and an incident commander (IC) is typically in the incident command center, leading the exercise. Functional teams are used to evaluate the situation and begin working immediately. Additional personnel and resources may be mobilized and actually triage, treat, and transport mock victims. This type of exercise requires rapid problem solving, critical thinking, and effective responses to complex and realistic situations (FEMA, 2015). Problem solving and critical thinking are familiar skills and competencies for nurses at all levels; it is important that they be actively involved and practice these skills in an interdisciplinary exercise.

Full-scale exercises may be the most complex and resource-intensive of all exercises because of the staging in large indoor or outdoor spaces and the large numbers of volunteers and trained personnel who are necessary for realistic effect of the exercise. Many activities occur simultaneously and additional events may be inserted throughout the drill. Safety officers, facilitators, and observers/evaluators are all used and add to the number of personnel required for a successful full-scale exercise. While it is complex and resource-intensive, this type of exercise offers great participant learning and identifies opportunities for improvement for all (FEMA, 2015).

SUPPORTING EVIDENCE-BASED DISASTER-NURSING PRACTICE

Each disaster or public health emergency presents an important opportunity to inform future preparedness, response and recovery efforts, and ensure evidence-based practice among nurses and other healthcare workers. Lurie, Manolio, Patterson, Collins, and Frieden (2013) underscore the importance of conducting rigorous research in disaster settings: "The knowledge that is generated through well-designed, effectively executed research in anticipation of, in the midst of, and after an emergency is critical to our future capacity to better achieve the overarching goals of preparedness and response: preventing injury, illness, disability, and death and supporting recovery" (p. 1251).

Ensuring the proper research infrastructure is in place to conduct research during or shortly after disasters is essential. Conducting research in the context of disaster response poses significant challenges in terms of research design, implementation, and human participants' protection given the inherently unpredictable and chaotic nature of disasters. Common barriers include institutional review board (IRB) delays or restrictions, lack of a rapid or sustainable research funding, and uncertainty about how to best integrate research into response frameworks (IOM, 2014; Lurie et al., 2013), among others. Important data from disasters are often missed due to these barriers. HHS has significant efforts underway to develop a more integrated system to address these barriers such as: identifying experts in research design and topical areas of concern, utilizing prefunded research networks, instituting a centralized IRB to facilitate rapid and appropriate review, identifying and prioritizing research needs, developing and pre-approving generic protocols and instruments that can be easily adapted to different disaster scenarios, and addressing community concerns (Lurie et al., 2013). These investments in "scientific preparedness" should facilitate disaster research.

In terms of research priorities for disaster nursing, some topic areas, such as nurses' willingness to respond to disasters, have been studied and provide an evidence base for organizational policies (e.g., offering family and pet care for staff), and personal actions (e.g., personal and family preparedness) that promote willingness to respond (Connor, 2014). An international Delphi panel study (Ranse et al., 2014) highlighted the need to study the role nurses can play in providing psychosocial support during disasters and the psychosocial well-being of nurses who assist in disasters. However, the literature on nursing's unique role in disasters is lacking (Veenema et al., 2016, 2017). As a result, Veenema et al. (2016) recommended "establishing a focused research agenda based on a needs assessment that documents gaps in the literature, nursing knowledge and skills, and available resources" (p. 9). To that end, a Delphi panel study is underway that will identify research priorities for disaster nursing in the United States and researchable questions (Couig et al., 2017).

As each unfortunate disaster or tragedy occurs, we continue to discover better means of improving survivor outcomes. It is imperative that we engage experienced nurses and healthcare providers in research related to knowledge gained and lessons learned about disasters. In addition, nurses have many opportunities to become more knowledgeable and actively involved in disaster nursing. The following section describes a nursing society that is improving the practice of disaster nursing on a national level.

SOCIETY FOR THE ADVANCEMENT OF DISASTER NURSING

The Society for the Advancement of Disaster Nursing (SADN) stemmed from Disaster Nursing Call to Action launched by the Veterans Emergency Management Evaluation Center (VEMEC). This 2014 foundational work was under the auspices of the Office of Patient Care Services, Veterans Health Administration (VHA), U.S. Department of Veterans Affairs (VA), with the support of the VA Office of Nursing Services and VHA Office of Emergency Management.

VEMEC initiated the Disaster Nursing Call to Action to identify the first action steps toward improving the practice of disaster nursing in the United States. Building on the 2011 IOM/Robert W. Johnson Foundation [RWJF] report, *The Future of Nursing: Leading Change, Advancing Health*, and the coalitions developed as part of the RWJF/American Association of Retired Persons (AARP) *Future of Nursing: Campaign to Action*, VEMEC convened nursing leaders from government, academia, and the private sector to develop an agenda to expand the pivotal role nurses can play as patient educators, responders, and leaders in disaster preparedness.

Panelists and participants collaborated to define a vision for the future of disaster nursing (Box 36.5), along with

---

BOX 36.5 Vision for the Future of Disaster Nursing in the United States

VISION

"To create a national nursing workforce with the knowledge, skills, and abilities to respond to disasters and public health emergencies in a timely and effective manner.

Ideally, nurses would:

- Possess the minimum knowledge base, skills, and abilities regarding disaster response and public health emergency preparedness;
- Respond directly or provide indirect support (e.g., shift coverage for those deploying or critical data collection) during a disaster event or public health emergency;
- Promote preparedness amongst individuals in their care, families, communities, and within the organizations they represent; and
- Demonstrate a commitment to professional preparedness by participating in disaster planning, drills, and exercises within and beyond their specialty environment."

Source: Veenema, T. G., Griffin, A., Gable A. R., MacIntyre, L., Simons, R. N., Couig, M. P., ... Larson, E. (2016). Nurses as leaders in disaster preparedness and response: A call to action. *Journal of Nursing Scholarship, 48*, 5. doi:10.1111/jnu.12198

BOX 36.6 Recommendations: Practice, Education, Policy, and Research

Practice

- Healthcare and related organizations support clinical nursing practice during disasters to reflect crisis standards of care and address common barriers to willingness of nurses to respond to a disaster.
- Establish a collective effort among nurse leaders to advance the practice of disaster nursing and public health emergency preparedness and response.

Education

- Develop a national set of disaster-nursing competencies to be integrated into the AACN Essentials of Nursing and NLN Guidelines for Nursing.
- Establish coalitions of schools of nursing to develop evidence-based and competency-driven didactic and clinical learning opportunities using multiple delivery platforms that can be integrated into the undergraduate and/or graduate nursing curricula.
- Broaden lifelong, continuing educational opportunities in disaster nursing and public health emergency preparedness and response for nurses through healthcare and related organizations across all healthcare settings.
- Establish a national clearinghouse of information to provide guidance and resources on disaster nursing.

Policy

- Conduct review of national policies and planning documents addressing disasters and public health emergencies to ensure that they elevate, prioritize, and address the practice of disaster nursing in federal, state, and local emergency management operations.
- Encourage a culture of volunteerism through national nursing professional organizations by engaging their members to align with volunteer agencies and participate in disaster response.
- Facilitate timely and efficient deployment of nurses and other healthcare workers to disaster areas by expanding liability protections for volunteers and providing coverage for volunteers harmed while responding.

Research

- Establish a research agenda based on a thorough needs assessment to document gaps in literature, nursing knowledge and skills, and available resources.
- Expand research methods to include interventional studies and use both quantitative and qualitative designs.
- Increase the number of doctoral-level nurse scientists serving as principal investigators on disaster research projects.

AACN, American Association of Colleges of Nursing; NLN, National League for Nursing.

12 recommendations to support the vision within nursing practice, education, policy, and research (Box 36.6; see Veenema et al., 2016 for a summary). This work serves as a roadmap for creating a national nursing workforce with the knowledge, skills, and abilities to respond, either directly or indirectly (e.g., through supportive roles), to disasters and public health emergencies in a timely and effective manner (Veenema et al., 2016). Since then, a growing number of nurses from across the country have volunteered their time and expertise to work toward the proposed vision for the U.S. nursing workforce.

Building on this earlier work, the Johns Hopkins School of Nursing hosted a meeting in December 2016 that marked the formation of the SADN. The group identified its mission and vision (Box 36.7) and initiated its strategic planning process. In addition to the mission of preparing every nurse, the organization plans to advance professionalism within disaster nursing and designate it as a nursing specialty (Veenema et al., 2017). Furthermore, four national workgroups have been formed in the areas of disaster-nursing practice, education, policy, and research. An update on workgroup activities was recently published (Couig et al., 2017). By enhancing nurses' roles as leaders, educators, responders, policy makers, and researchers in disaster preparedness and response, SADN represents an important step toward the goal of strengthening the resiliency of the national nursing workforce.

It is important that nurse leaders consider placing the disaster preparedness and response materials, content, and expectations of nurses at varying levels of practice. For example, educators should consider expanding educational opportunities in disaster response and emergency preparedness to enhance nurse interest in learning and greater likelihood of a timely and appropriate response if a disaster occurs (Langan, Lavin, Wolgast, & Veenema, 2017). Prelicensure students, new nurse graduates, nurse administrators, and advanced practice registered nurses have vastly different disaster preparedness and response duties that will dictate their learning needs.

BOX 36.7 SADN Mission and Vision

SOCIETY FOR THE ADVANCEMENT OF DISASTER NURSING (SADN)

Mission: Every nurse a prepared nurse
Vision: Create a national nursing workforce with the knowledge, skills, and abilities to respond to disasters and public health emergencies in a timely and effective manner.

Source: See disasternursing.org for more information.

The SADN recommends that a national workgroup review existing published competencies. From this review, specific leveled nursing competencies would be discussed with key organizations to endorse them and recommend adoption into the educational process.

SUMMARY

The nation's nurses and healthcare providers need access to evidence-based disaster education and training. Competency-driven education will ensure that our nursing workforce is prepared with the knowledge, skills, and abilities to respond to any kind of disaster in an appropriate manner. While many nurses may complete their careers without ever having to respond to a major disaster, a lack of preparation could contribute to increased negative outcomes during disasters. Academic and service nurse leaders likewise need to be prepared, acknowledge the necessity of disaster nursing education, and advocate for programs of study. Nurses are obligated to remain current educationally and aware of trends and rapidly changing demands of healthcare delivery. When nurses are educated, practiced, and prepared for all kinds of disasters and emergencies, they will be better able to protect themselves, their patients, families, and communities.

STUDY QUESTIONS

1. Why should all nurses be prepared for disasters?

2. List three basic disaster competencies that all nurses should be prepared to perform in disaster preparedness and response.

3. How might disaster preparedness/response competencies and expectations differ for newly licensed nurses compared with more experienced nurses?

4. How does personal preparedness equipment (PPE) during disaster response vary from PPE worn in usual (non-emergency) patient care settings?

5. What are the advantages and disadvantages of tabletop, functional, and full-scale exercises?

6. Describe learning opportunities that nurses may engage in to become competent and confident in disaster preparedness and response.

7. Describe how key stakeholders can influence or require curricular content regarding emergency preparedness for pre- and post-licensure nurses?

REFERENCES

Al Thobaity, A., Plummer, V., & Williams, B. (2017). What are the most common domains of the core competencies of disaster nursing? A scoping review. *International Emergency Nursing, 31*, 64–71.

American Nurses Association. (2016). Nurses rank #1 most trusted profession for 15th year in a row. Retrieved from https://www.nursingworld.org/news/news-releases/2016/nurses-rank-1-most-trusted-profession-for-15th-year-in-a-row/

American Nurses Association. (2017). Who will be there? Ethics, the law and a nurse's duty to respond in a disaster. Retrieved from https://www.nursingworld.org/~4af058/globalassets/docs/ana/ethics/who-will-be-there_disaster-preparedness_2017.pdf

American Nurses Credentialing Center. (2017). National Healthcare Disaster Certification. Retrieved from https://www.nursingworld.org/our-certifications/national-healthcare-disaster

American Red Cross. (2012). *The future of American Red Cross nursing: A blueprint for action*. Washington, DC: Author.

Bureau of Labor Statistics, U.S. Department of Labor. (2017). *Occupational outlook handbook, 2016–2017 edition: Registered nurses*. Retrieved from https://www.bls.gov/ooh/healthcare/registered-nurses.htm

Connor, S. B. (2014). When and why health care personnel respond to a disaster: the state of the science. *Prehospital and Disaster Medicine, 29*(3), 270–274.

Couig, M. P., Gable, A., Griffin, A., Langan, J. C., Katzburg, J. R., Wolgast, K. A., ... Veenema, T. G. (2017). Progress on a call to action: Nurses as leaders in disaster preparedness and response. *Nursing Administration Quarterly, 41*(2), 112–117. doi:10.1097/NAQ.0000000000000226

Daily, E., Padjen, P., & Birnbaum, M. (2010). A review of competencies developed for disaster healthcare providers: Limitations of current processes and applicability. *Prehospital and Disaster Medicine, 25*, 387–395. doi:10.1017/S1049023X00008438

Federal Emergency Management Agency. (2015). CERT drills and exercises. Retrieved from https://www.fema.gov/media-library/assets/documents/27997

Gebbie, K. M., & Qureshi, K. (2002). Emergency and disaster preparedness: Core competencies for nurses: What every nurse should but may not know. *AJN The American Journal of Nursing, 102*(1), 46–51.

Hay, J., & Mimura, N. (2010). The changing nature of extreme weather and climate events: Risks to sustainable development. *Geomatics, Natural Hazards and Risk, 1*(1), 3–18. doi:10.1080/19475701003643433

Hsu, E. B, Thomas, T. L., Bass, E. B., Whyne, D., Kelen, G. D., & Green, G. B. (2006). Healthcare worker competencies for disaster training. *BMC Medical Education, 6*, 19. doi:10.1186/1472-6920-6-19

Institute of Medicine. (2011). *The future of nursing: Leading change, advancing health*. Washington, DC: National Academies Press.

Institute of Medicine. (2014). *Enabling rapid and sustainable public health research during disasters*. Washington, DC: National Academies Press.

International Council of Nurses. (2009). *ICN framework of disaster nursing competencies*. Geneva, Switzerland: World Health Organization and International Council of Nurses.

Langan, J. C., Lavin, R., Wolgast, K. A., & Veenema, T. G. (2017). Education for developing and sustaining a health care workforce for disaster readiness. *Nursing Administration Quarterly, 41*(2), 118–127. doi:10.1097/NAQ.0000000000000225

Littleton-Kearney, M. T., & Slepski, L. A. (2008). Directions for disaster nursing education in the United States. *Critical Care Nursing Clinics of North America, 20*, 103–109, viii. doi:10.1016/j.ccell.2007.10.008

Loke, A. Y., & Fung, O. W. (2014). Nurses' competencies in disaster nursing: Implications for curriculum development and public health. *International Journal of Environmental Research and Public Health, 11*, 3289–3303. doi:10.3390/ijerph110303289

Lurie, N., Manolio, T., Patterson, A. P., Collins, F., & Frieden, T. (2013). Research as a part of public health emergency response. *New England Journal of Medicine, 368*, 1251–1255. doi:10.1056/NEJMsb1209510

McHugh, M. D. (2010). Hospital nurse staffing and public health emergency preparedness: Implications for policy. *Public Health Nursing, 27*(5), 442–449.

National Advisory Council on Nursing Education and Practice. (2009). *Challenges facing the nurse workforce in a changing environment. Part I: Surge capacity: Educating the nursing workforce for emergency and disaster preparedness*. Rockville, MD: Health Resources and Services Administration.

National Council of State Boards of Nursing. (2016). 2016 NCLEX-RN test plan. Retrieved from https://www.ncsbn.org/RN_Test_Plan_2016 _Final.pdf

Newton, E. E. (2017). Preparing for the big one: Emergency preparedness for nursing leaders. *Nursing Administration Quarterly, 41*, 101–111. doi:10.1097/NAQ.0000000000000215

Polivka, B. J., Stanley, S. A., Gordon, D., Taulbee, K., Kieffer, G., & McCorkle, S. M. (2008). Public health nursing competencies for public health surge events. *Public Health Nursing, 25*(2), 159–165.

Schultz, C. H., Koenig, K. L., Whiteside, M., & Murray, R. (2012). Development of national standardized all-hazard disaster core competencies for acute care physicians, nurses, and EMS professionals. *Annals of Emergency Medicine, 59*, 196–208. e1. doi:10.1016/j.annemergmed.2011.09.003

Sigma Theta Tau International. (2017). Emergency nursing: Understanding the profession. Retrieved from http://www.nursingsociety.org

Speraw, S., & Persell, D. F. (2013). National nurse preparedness: Achieving competency-based practice. In T. G. Veenema (Ed.), *Disaster nursing and emergency preparedness* (3rd ed., pp. 669–685). New York, NY: Springer Publishing.

Stanley, S., & Wolanski, T. A. B. (2015). *Designing and Integrating a Disaster Preparedness Curriculum*. Indianapolis, IN: Sigma Theta Tau.

United States Agency for International Development. (2015). Emerging pandemic threats. Retrieved from http://www.usaid.gov/what-we-do/ global-health/pandemic-influenza-and-other-emerging-threats

U.S. Department of Health and Human Services. (2013). The *US nursing workforce: Trends in supply and education*. Washington, DC: Health Resources and Services Administration.

U.S. Department of Health and Human Services. (2014). 35 hospitals designated as Ebola treatment centers. Retrieved from http://wayback.archive-it. org/3926/20170127184726/https://www.hhs.gov/about/news/2014/12/02/35- us-hospitals-designated-as-ebola-treatment-centers.html

Veenema, T. G., Griffin, A., Gable A. R., MacIntyre, L., Simons, R. N., Couig, M. P., … Larson, E. (2016). Nurses as leaders in disaster preparedness and response: A call to action. *Journal of Nursing Scholarship, 48*, 187–200. doi:10.1111/jnu.12198

Veenema, T., Lavin, R. P., Griffin, A., Gable, A. R., Couig, M. P., Dobalian, A. (2017). Call to action: Advancing disaster nursing education in the United States. *Journal of Nursing Scholarship, 49*(6):688–696.

Walsh, L., Subbarao, I., Gebbie, K., Schor, K. W., Lyznicki, J., Strauss-Riggs, K., … James, J. J. (2012). Core competencies for disaster medicine and public health. *Disaster Medicine and Public Health Preparedness, 6*, 44–52. doi:10.1001/dmp.2012.4

37

AMERICAN RED CROSS DISASTER HEALTH SERVICES AND DISASTER NURSING: NATIONAL CAPABILITY — LOCAL COMMUNITY IMPACT

Mary Casey-Lockyer, Linda M. MacIntyre, J. Christie Rodgers, and Valerie Cole

LEARNING OBJECTIVES

When this chapter is completed, readers will be able to:

1. Describe the foundations for the work of the American Red Cross, including its Congressional Charter, and the fundamental principles of the International Red Cross and Red Crescent Movement.
2. Describe the role of the American Red Cross as a colead with the Federal Emergency Management Agency (FEMA) for Emergency Support Function #6 Mass Care and support agency for Emergency Support Function #8: Public Health and Medical Services as identified in the National Response Framework.
3. Discuss nurse roles in disaster preparedness, response, and recovery phases.
4. Discuss operational and strategic roles of Red Cross partners in promoting health before, during, and after disasters.

KEY MESSAGES

The American Red Cross responds to nearly 64,000 disasters annually, most of them at the local community level, and has the ability to deploy volunteers nationally (American Red Cross, 2017a).

The American Red Cross prevents and alleviates human suffering in the face of emergencies by mobilizing the power of volunteers and the generosity of donors (American Red Cross, 2017b).

The American Red Cross is part of the International Federation of Red Cross and Red Crescent Movement (IFRC), one of the 190 national societies throughout the world movement (IFRC, 2017a).

The American Red Cross is the only nongovernmental organization (NGO) with colead responsibility in the National Response Framework (NRF): Emergency Support Function (ESF) #6 (Mass Care).

The American Red Cross has the capacity to engage thousands of volunteer nurses and other health professionals in disaster preparedness, response and recovery activities, as well as participating in community resilience efforts.

CHAPTER OVERVIEW

The American Red Cross (Red Cross) has played an integral role in disaster response in communities across the United States since 1881. This chapter provides an overview of the structure and governance of the Red Cross, its conceptual foundation, fundamental principles and Congressional Charter, working with partners, and a detailed description of how nursing fits into that mission. The role of the Red Cross nurse, shelter nursing, and the core components of disaster response practice in the Red Cross are presented.

The American Red Cross responds to nearly 64,000 disasters annually, most of them at the local community level, and has the ability to deploy volunteers nationally (American Red Cross, 2017a). The Red Cross is a humanitarian nongovernmental organization (NGO) that is recognized for providing relief to survivors of disasters and assisting people to prepare for, respond to, and recover from emergencies (American Red Cross, 2017b). The Red Cross responds to all types of disasters, both natural and man-made, to include hurricanes, floods, earthquakes, fires, wildfires, and other events. Specifically, the Red Cross is ready to assist and support disaster survivors to meet disaster-caused needs. The Red Cross works closely with federal partners such as FEMA and the Department of Health and Human Services (HHS) in disasters. Its workers, both volunteers and employees, also participate in National Voluntary Organizations Active in Disaster (NVOAD), an association of organizations that mitigates and alleviates the impact of disasters; provides a forum promoting cooperation, communication, coordination, and collaboration; and fosters more effective delivery of services to communities affected by disaster (NVOAD, 2017).

Today, in addition to domestic disaster relief, the Red Cross offers humanitarian services in five other areas: community services that help individuals in need; support and comfort for military members, veterans, and their families; the collection, processing, and distribution of lifesaving blood and blood products; educational programs that promote health and safety; and

international relief and development programs. The Red Cross provides wraparound community and international services through its Congressional Charter and the fundamental principles of the International Red Cross and Red Crescent Movement, all the while maintaining a neutral and impartial stance in assisting individuals, families, and communities (see Boxes 37.1 and 37.2).

CONGRESSIONAL CHARTER

The Congressional Charter of 1905 includes the statement that the American Red Cross will "carry on a system of national and international relief in time of peace and apply the same in mitigating the sufferings caused by pestilence, famine, fire, floods, and other great national calamities, and to devise and carry on measures for preventing the same" (American Red Cross, 2007). This charter not only grants authority but also specifies the agency's duties and obligations to the nation, disaster survivors, and the donors who support its work.

The 1905 Congressional Charter also granted to the Red Cross to act "in accord with the military authorities as a medium of communication between the people of the United States and their armed forces" (American Red Cross, 2017c). The Red Cross continues to provide communications, training, and other humanitarian services to members of the U.S. military and their families around the world. Red Cross field staff, who frequently live and work in the same locations as deployed U.S. troops, also give comfort to military members thousands of miles from home by providing emergency messages regarding deaths and births, distributing comfort kits and blank cards for troops to send home to loved ones.

INTERNATIONAL RED CROSS AND RED CRESCENT MOVEMENT

In 1919, Red Cross national societies (led by the American Red Cross) established what would become the International Federation of Red Cross and Red Crescent Societies (IFRC, 2017b). The International Federation provides a forum for national societies to discuss common objectives, and its secretariat

Humanity: The International Red Cross and Red Crescent Movement, born of a desire to bring assistance without discrimination to the wounded on the battlefield, endeavors, in its international and national capacity, to prevent and alleviate human suffering wherever it may be found. Its purpose is to protect life and health and to ensure respect for the human being. It promotes mutual understanding, friendship, cooperation, and lasting peace among all peoples.

Impartiality: It makes **no discrimination as to nationality, race, religious beliefs, class, or political opinions.** It endeavors to relieve the suffering of individuals, being guided solely by their needs, and to give priority to the most urgent cases of distress.

Neutrality: In order to continue to enjoy the confidence of all, the Movement may **not take sides in hostilities or engage at any time in controversies** of a political, racial, religious, or ideological nature.

Independence: The Movement is independent. The **National Societies,** while auxiliaries in the humanitarian services of their governments and subject to the laws of their respective countries, **must always maintain their autonomy** so that they may be able at all times to act in accordance with the principles of the Movement.

Voluntary Service: It is a voluntary relief movement **not prompted** in any manner **by desire for gain.**

Unity: There can be **only one Red Cross or one Red Crescent Society in any one country.** It must be open to all. It must carry on its humanitarian work throughout its territory.

Universality: The **International Red Cross and Red Crescent Movement,** in which all societies have equal status and share equal responsibilities and duties in helping each other, **is worldwide.**

Source: American Red Cross. (2017d). American Red Cross: Who we are. Retrieved from http://www.redcross.org/about-us/who-we-are/mission-and-values

helps coordinate international relief provided outside of conflict areas. Today, the International Federation comprises 190 Red Cross and Red Crescent societies, a secretariat based in Geneva, and regional delegations strategically located around the world to support global coordination and response (IFRC, 2017c). The International Federation works to alleviate suffering through a range of activities, such as:

- Organizing and coordinating international disaster relief operations.
- Providing assistance to refugees outside conflict areas;

- The American Red Cross is a $2.7 billion humanitarian services organization.
- An average of 91 cents of every dollar the American Red Cross spends is invested in humanitarian services and programs.
- There are 36 American Red Cross blood services regions. In 2017, the American Red Cross collected more than 4.8 million units of blood from nearly 2.8 million volunteer donors.
- Each year the Red Cross provides 369,000 services to military members, veterans, and civilians.
- Approximately 820,000 people a year attend Red Cross disaster education presentations.
- Nearly 5.9 million people a year receive Red Cross training and information in first aid, water safety, and other skills that help save lives.
- Each year, the American Red Cross helps reconnect, on average, more than 5,000 families separated by war and disaster around the world.
- Nearly 314,000 people a year proudly call themselves American Red Cross volunteers.

Source: American Red Cross. (2017e). American Red Cross: Our history. Retrieved from http://www.redcross.org/about-us/our-work/disaster-relief

- Promoting national disaster preparedness programs;
- Helping national societies improve the services they deliver to individuals in need in their local communities.

Please refer to Figure 37.1 for an illustration of how the American Red Cross fits within the International Red Cross and Red Crescent Movement.

AMERICAN RED CROSS HISTORICAL BACKGROUND

The concept of the Red Cross originated in 1859 when Henry Dunant, a Swiss businessman, traveled to Solferino (now Italy) to petition Napoleon III on a matter of land rights. He came on the aftermath of a bloody battle between the armies of imperial Austria and the Franco-Sardinian alliance, with 40,000 men dead or dying on the battlefield and the wounded without any medical attention. Dunant, a lifelong humanitarian, organized the local community to gather needed materials and provide care to the injured of both armies. On his return to Geneva, he called for the creation of national relief societies to assist those wounded in war, and pointed the way to the future Geneva Conventions (Gumpert, 1938).

In October 1863, the International Red Cross Movement was created in Geneva, Switzerland, to provide nonpartisan care to the wounded and sick in times of war. The Red Cross emblem, the Geneva cross, was adopted at this first international conference as a symbol of neutrality and was to be used by

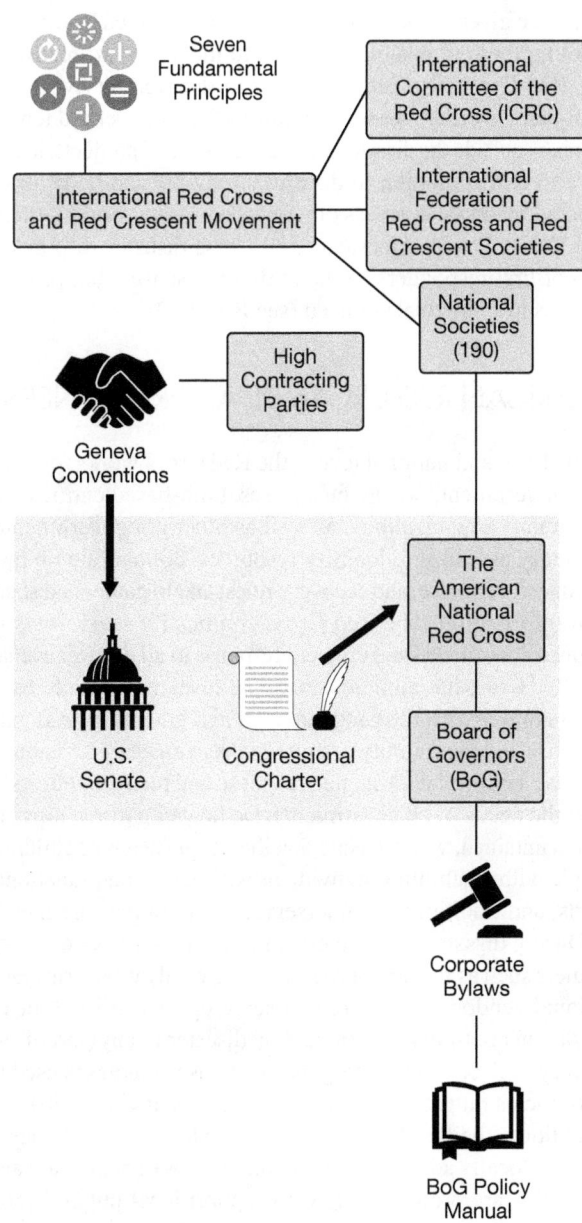

FIGURE 37.1 International Red Cross and Red Crescent Movement with American Red Cross.

national relief societies. In August 1864, the representatives of 12 governments signed the Geneva Convention Treaty and, eventually, the extraordinary efforts of Henry Dunant led to the establishment of the International Red Cross. Today, the Red Cross Movement includes the Geneva-based International Committee of the Red Cross and the International Federation of Red Cross and Red Crescent Societies (www .ifrc.org), including the American Red Cross (American Red Cross, 2017f). Modeled after the International Red Cross, the American Red Cross was founded in the late 19th century by Clara Barton (1821–1912). While Barton did not originate the concept of the Red Cross, she established the Red Cross Society in America that continues to this day. She successfully organized the American Association of the Red Cross in Washington, DC on May 21, 1881, created to serve America in peace and in war, during times of disaster and national calamity. Barton's organization added a new focus to the International Red Cross

Movement by adding disaster relief to battlefield assistance. She served as the organization's volunteer president until 1904.

American Red Cross nurses have been a vital force since 1909, supporting communities with compassion and professional skills and strengthening the Red Cross with innovative support. Jane Delano, a leading pioneer in the nursing profession, created the Red Cross nursing division. Through her efforts as the first chairman of the National Committee on Red Cross Nursing, the image of the Red Cross nurse became a national symbol. More than 370,000 Red Cross nurses have enrolled in the Nursing Service since its inception. These nurses volunteered for service in times of war and disaster and created programs for emergency response and the advancement of healthcare in peacetime. A woman of incredible energy, Delano (Figure 37.2) served as superintendent of the Army Nurse Corps from 1909 to 1912. During the same time, she became chairperson of the new National Committee on Red Cross Nursing Service and created the plan for the first volunteer nursing unit of the American Red Cross (Dock et al., 1922). She emphasized the importance of having a ready supply of nurses in case of military conflict. Under her skillful leadership, the American Red Cross Nursing Service became the recognized nursing reserve for the Army, Navy, and Public Health Service.

In 1912, Delano resigned from the Army Nurse Corps to volunteer full time with the Red Cross. She wanted to increase the enrollment of Red Cross nurses. As a result, when the United States entered World War I in 1917, there were over 8,000 registered nurses (RNs) immediately available for duty. By the Armistice in November 1918, over 20,000 Red Cross nurses had volunteered to serve at home and overseas (Dock et al., 1922). While she was organizing Red Cross Nursing for service to the military, Delano developed Red Cross courses for the training of nurses' aides and coauthored a textbook: *Elementary Hygiene and Home Care of the Sick* (Dock et al., 1922). Delano also established the Red Cross Town and Country Nursing Service for delivering healthcare to rural areas of the country, renamed in 1918 as the American National Red Cross Public Health Nursing Service.

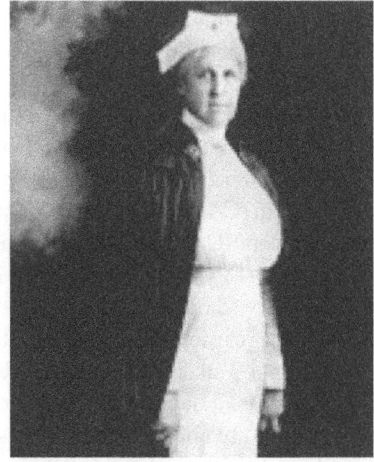

FIGURE 37.2 Jane Delano (1862–1919), Founder of the American Red Cross Nursing Service.

Source: American Red Cross. (2011). Retrieved from https://intranet.redcross .org/content/redcross/categories/our_services/vol-services/onboard-engage/ nursing-health.html retrieved 06_20_2018.

OVERVIEW OF AMERICAN RED CROSS DISASTER CYCLE SERVICES

The Red Cross responds to all types of natural and human-created disasters. Red Cross disaster relief focuses on meeting an individual's immediate disaster-caused needs to include assistance at the community level. When a disaster threatens or strikes, the Red Cross provides shelter, food, distribution of emergency supplies, disaster health and mental health services to address basic human needs. The core of Red Cross disaster relief involves

---

BOX 37.3 American Red Cross Disaster Response Capabilities at a Glance

- **Staff Resources**: More than 35,000 trained workers in Disaster Human Resources System (94% volunteers). Approximately 38% can be deployed across the country; the remainder can be mobilized within their local community.
- **Disaster Health Services**: A nationwide network of thousands of Red Cross disaster health services workers trained to provide health assessments, illness and injury surveillance, and casework, replacement of medication, medical equipment, and general health services.
- **Disability Integration**: A network of disaster responders who work closely with national headquarters, division and regional staff to promote best practices and ensure there is a consistent and dedicated focus on providing services to persons with access and functional needs, including persons with disabilities.
- **Disaster Mental Health**: A nationwide network of thousands of Red Cross disaster mental health workers trained to provide approved Disaster Mental Health interventions (including psychological first aid, crisis intervention, and referral) that focus on basic care, support, and comfort of individuals experiencing disaster-related stress.
- **Sheltering**: The National Shelter system contains more than 61,000 potential shelter locations with supplies to support 350,000 people.
- **Emergency Assistance**: Thousands of Red Cross caseworkers are trained to help after disasters of all sizes with the support of tools including the Red Cross Client Assistance System (CAS) and the multiagency Client Assistance Network (CAN) to provide families with the items, means, or services to promote their recovery.
- **Reunification**: Loved ones can search for the status of those who have registered on the online Red Cross system of Safe and Well during a disaster. Red Cross disaster apps feature a one touch "I'm Safe" button that helps people use social media outlets to alert family and friends of their status.

Source: American Red Cross. (2017h). American Red Cross: Core and pillar processes. Retrieved from https://intranet.redcross.org/content/redcross/categories/our_services/disaster-cycle-services/core-and-pillar-processes/respond/respond-toolkit.html

---

assistance given to individuals and families affected by disaster, enabling them to resume activities to move toward recovery. The Red Cross also provides food to disaster survivors and emergency workers, handles inquiries from concerned family members outside the disaster area, provides blood products, health and safety information to disaster survivors, and helps those affected by disaster access other needed resources (American Red Cross, 2015). American Red Cross disaster responders are not first responders in the traditional sense—but provide services to individuals in need (see Box 37.3).

AMERICAN RED CROSS DISASTER PARTNERS

At the local and national levels, the Red Cross works together with government, private businesses, faith-based entities and community organizations, as well as other nongovernmental voluntary agencies to identify resources; collaborate on preparedness, response, and recovery roles; and to gather and share vital information. The Red Cross continually seeks ways to ensure a coordinated and efficient response to all disaster events. The Red Cross has numerous national-level memorandums of understanding (MOUs) and letters of agreement (LOAs) with response and community organizations to ensure provision of effective and well-coordinated response and recovery efforts to meet the needs of all constituents. Dedicated partnerships are also maintained, which ensure that the unique needs of children, people with disabilities, individuals with access and functional needs, and traditionally underserved communities are met.

During disasters, the American Red Cross works with key partners such as the Southern Baptists, the Salvation Army, and national vendors to prepare and serve up to 1 million meals per day in communities affected by disaster in any part of the country. A fleet of 342 emergency response vehicles is used to serve meals on mobile routes (American Red Cross, 2017g). In addition, the Red Cross partners with the Medical Reserve Corps, a locally administered volunteer corps of healthcare and nonhealthcare professionals who support local public health entities and provide support during local disaster events.

The National Response Framework (NRF) and the Red Cross

The American Red Cross is the only NGO with colead responsibility for an ESF in the National Disaster Response Framework (FEMA, 2014). The purpose of ESF #6—*Mass Care, Emergency Assistance, Temporary Housing, and Human Services* coordinates and provides life-sustaining resources, essential services, and statutory programs when the needs of disaster survivors exceed local, state, tribal, territorial, and insular area government capabilities (FEMA, 2017). FEMA is lead federal agency and with Red Cross as colead, the agencies work together to help state governments and NGOs plan, coordinate, and provide a breadth of mass care services for people affected by disasters. Some of the mass care services that are the focus of these joint efforts include sheltering, feeding, distribution of emergency supplies, and reunification services.

In addition to sharing a lead role in the ESF #6, the American Red Cross is named as a support agency in several other ESFs, including ESF #8: Public Health and Medical Services Annex. This support could involve activities such as providing support for vaccine administration or providing both physical and mental healthcare for individuals and families in general population shelters (American Red Cross, 2017i). At the request of HHS, the American Red Cross coordinates with the American Association of Blood Banks (AABB) Interorganizational Task Force on Domestic Disasters and Acts of Terrorism to provide blood products and services through regional blood centers as needed (AABB, 2011).

The National Emergency Repatriation Plan and the Red Cross

The National Emergency Repatriation Plan (NERP) is implemented when international conditions require return of U.S. citizens and dependents from a foreign country under emergency conditions. The U.S. Department of State and HHS jointly coordinate the implementation of NERP. HHS notifies Disaster Services at National Headquarters of the implementation of the plan and may also contact local chapters of the point of entry. Under the NERP, the Red Cross has agreed to provide congregate shelters, mass feeding, first aid, triage assistance, and repatriation of human remains post event, should it be necessary.

For example, less than a week after the 2010 Haiti earthquake, the Department of Defense and U.S. Customs converted a gymnasium into a processing center for repatriated Haitians returning to the United States. In making plans for the processing center operations, the government called on two organizations for help: The Florida Department of Children and Families, and the American Red Cross (2010a). Chapter volunteers provided support to thousands arriving at Homestead Air Force Base under Operation Unified Response, the U.S. military's Haitian relief effort. People arrived from Haiti disoriented, thirsty, hungry, and injured. There were many infants, most without diapers, wipes, baby bottles, formula, or baby food. Red Cross volunteers brought a human touch to the repatriation process. The Red Cross also provided volunteer translators to greet people and offer comfort when they arrived (Figure 37.3).

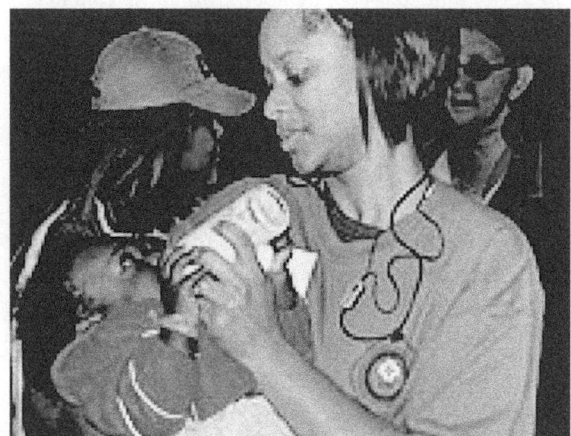

FIGURE 37.3 A Miami chapter Red Cross volunteer comforts a baby who had just arrived on a flight from Haiti.
Source: Photo, by Peter Macias for the American Red Cross (2010).

The Aviation Disaster Family Assistance Act and the Red Cross

In 1996, the National Transportation Safety Board (NTSB; www .ntsb.gov) was assigned the role of integrating the resources of the federal government with those of local and state authorities and the airlines to meet the needs of aviation disaster survivors and their families. As a result, the Federal Family Assistance Plan for Aviation Disasters was developed and implemented. The plan describes the airline and federal responsibilities in response to an aviation crash involving a significant number of passenger fatalities or injuries (NTSB, 2017).

In addition, the Aviation Disaster Family Assistance Act (ADFAA) of 1996 mandated that the NTSB identify a human service organization to coordinate childcare, spiritual care, family assistance, and mental health services for survivors and the families of the deceased, including the coordination of a nondenominational memorial service. The NTSB named the American Red Cross as the coordinating agency for these services. When ADFAA is enacted and certain disaster incident criteria are met, the American Red Cross chapter in the affected area deploys a team of disaster responders who work with local, state, and federal resources to meet the crisis support needs of those involved (NTSB, 2017).

In 2008, similar legislation was passed, focusing on rail passenger accidents. The Rail Passenger Disaster Family Assistance Act sets out comparable requirements for Amtrak and future intra- and interstate high-speed passenger rail operators and the NTSB (NTSB, 2017). In rail transportation disaster and certain other types of transportation disasters (e.g., marine, highway, or pipeline incidents), the Red Cross also provides services for families under the coordination of the NTSB. Specifically, the role of the Red Cross disaster mental health (DMH) teams involved in this type of response fulfills the required U.S. and U.S. commonwealth provision of:

■ Establishing a liaison at the NTSB Joint Family Support Operations Center
■ Providing psychosocial and emotional support services in coordination with the disaster response team of air carriers involved in accidents
■ Ensuring an environment where families can grieve in private
■ Coordinating childcare and spiritual care services
■ Providing emotional and physical support of families during their memorial service planning

AMERICAN RED CROSS AT THE LOCAL, REGIONAL, AND NATIONAL LEVELS

Local communities are served by Red Cross chapters that meet the day-to-day needs of individuals affected by local emergencies, such as single-family house fires (the most common type of disaster) or floods, tornadoes and other disasters affecting small, localized areas. These needs typically include short-term shelter, food, and the provision of mental health and physical health services (American Red Cross, 2008).

When a disaster exceeds the human and material resources of a given Red Cross chapter, the affected chapter joins with other chapters in their regional area for assistance. In situations where the demands of a given incident exceed what the local and regional chapters can provide, the Red Cross deploys resources by using proximity deployment (i.e., the nearest available resources to achieve speed to scale) from across the nation.

RED CROSS NURSING

There are significant roles for nurses in Red Cross Disaster Cycle Services, including the care and support for individuals with functional and access needs who have been displaced from their usual support systems post disaster. FEMA defines functional needs support services (FNSS) as the following: services that enable individuals with access and functional needs to maintain their independence in a general population shelter. Examples of support services include durable medical equipment (DME), consumable medical supplies (CMS), and personal assistance services (PAS). Individuals requiring FNSS may have physical, sensory, mental health, and cognitive and/or intellectual disabilities affecting their ability to function independently without assistance. Others who may benefit from FNSS include women in the late stages of pregnancy, seniors, and people whose body mass requires special equipment (FEMA, 2017).

Nurses who volunteer for the Red Cross need excellent critical thinking, assessment and referral skills; they need to be able to remain calm, flexible, and creative while working effectively with people under stress in unusual environments. Red Cross nurses work with disaster survivors as well as Red Cross volunteers serving those survivors. Red Cross nurses need to understand public health nursing practice (nursing care delivered in community settings) to best deliver nursing assessment, care, and referrals to clients in a general population shelter, as well as to ensure a safe and healthy physical environment in the "new neighborhood" created by the incident. Other disaster practice attributes required include good communication skills, an ability to quickly understand and apply reference materials, and good personal health accompanied by physical stamina.

Disaster Health Services nurses comprise more than 3,000 of the approximately 20,000 health professional volunteers involved at all levels and service areas of the American Red Cross. Disaster nurses usually have affiliation in one or more of three Disaster Service areas: disaster health services, DMH, disability integration and staff wellness. The Creed of the Red Cross Nurse was written by Lona Trott in 1953 (see Box 37.4). The specific nursing role in disaster response is addressed following an overview of nursing roles across the Red Cross organization.

Nurses' activities in the American Red Cross include, but are not limited to (American Red Cross, 2011):

- *Direct service provision*: examples include: local response on Disaster Action Teams (DATs), support to DATs when health and mental health needs are identified, supporting the Home Fire Campaign (a program to reduce morbidity and mortality due to home fires by 25% over 5 years), deployment to national incidents, review of chapter health status records for volunteers, DMH response and/or referrals, volunteering in military clinics and hospitals, client casework in Disaster Cycle Services, Service to the Armed Forces or International Services, blood collection teams, supporting first aid stations, and emergency communications for military service members and their families.
- *Teaching and developing courses*: for example: disaster health services, staff wellness, mental health workshops, blood donor education, education about the measles & rubella initiative, psychological first aid, cardiopulmonary resuscitation/automated external defibrillator (CPR/AED), first aid–nurse assistant training, and babysitting.
- *Leading in management and supervisory roles*: for example: project leads; chapter, regional or division-level executives; blood services regional leadership; and Nursing Network Division, Associate and Regional Nurse Leader positions that work across the organization.
- *Serving in consultant, subject-matter expert, or capacity development roles*: for example: Disaster Health Services Advisors and DMH Advisors at both the regional and divisional levels; Service Line and Staff Wellness Advisors; Nursing Network Biomedical, International Services; and Service to the Armed Forces Nurse Consultants, national workgroup and committee members.
- *Functioning in governance and advisory roles*: for example: Red Cross local board or committee member; Nursing Network Senior Nurse Consultants; National Nursing Committee; National Board of Governors.

Office of the Chief Nurse and Red Cross Nursing

The Office of the Chief Nurse is responsible for health professional recruitment and engagement throughout the Red Cross to help meet the organization's mission and goals to serve communities.

BOX 37.4 Creed of the Red Cross Nurse

I believe in the ideals of democracy and the concept of universal brotherhood. I acknowledge no barriers of country, race, class, or creed.

I believe it is my privilege and my duty to teach others some of the knowledge and skill that I possess so that they too may know the satisfaction of competence in dealing with illness and pain.

To bring comfort to those who are in trouble, to alleviate suffering, and to conserve life is my mission. Wherever disaster calls there I shall go. I ask not for whom, but only where I am needed.

Under the banner of the Red Cross, symbolic of the finest instincts of man, I find fulfillment in helping to animate the spirit of kindness and mercy that embraces the world.

Lona L. Trott, R. N., 1953

In addition, the Office of the Chief Nurse represents Red Cross nursing with external health-related professional organizations, educational institutions, the Federal Nursing Service Council, and federal committees. The office is led by the chief nurse, supported by the volunteer national chairperson of nursing who leads the National Nursing Committee (NNC), and the nursing network director. This work is supported by thousands of nurse volunteers and nursing students (American Red Cross Office of Nursing, 2011).

The NNC provides a strategic and collaborative forum to advise the Red Cross and its nursing leadership. The annual Chief Nurse Initiatives provide prioritized roles for health professionals in each line of service (biomedical services, disaster cycle services, international services, preparedness, health & safety services, and service to the Armed Forces).

All Red Cross nurses belong to the Red Cross Nursing Network. Nursing Network leaders are committed to helping the Red Cross recruit and retain nurses and other health professionals in all business lines of service. The Nursing Network receives guidance from the NNC and the chief nurse. Nursing Network activities are aligned with the Chief Nurse Initiatives and current organizational goals to build Red Cross health professional capacity and effective service delivery.

ROLE OF THE AMERICAN RED CROSS NURSE DURING A DISASTER

Nurses are involved at all levels of the Red Cross: supporting individuals impacted by disaster; providing case management; supporting members of the military, veterans, and their families; educating communities about health and prevention; assisting to ensure that lifesaving blood is available when needed; leveraging Academic Service Learning to meet community needs; working to eradicate measles and rubella; serving in local and national leadership positions; serving on boards; and more. Because nurse involvement is such an essential part of American Red Cross disaster services, nurses participate in various components of the readiness, mitigation, response, and recovery phases of a disaster. The Red Cross nursing function in disasters involves caring for clients, both disaster survivors and volunteer responders.

In December 2014, the Veterans Emergency Management and Evaluation Center in the Department of Veterans Affairs convened a panel of subject matter experts in disaster health nursing to discuss disaster nursing recommendations to increase nurse disaster readiness to better serve individuals, families, and communities (Veenema et al., 2016). Recommendations specifically addressed each of four core areas: nurse practice, education, policy, and research. The experts were in consensus that nurses need to be personally prepared for disasters—having a disaster kit, a plan for their family members and pets who rely on them, and to take training as needed. This belief was consistent with previously published literature. In a survey of 6,428 healthcare workers, Qureshi et al. (2005)

documented that barriers to healthcare worker ability to report to duty during a disaster included transportation, childcare, eldercare, and pet responsibilities. Barriers in willingness to report to duty during a disaster included fear and concern for personal/family safety and health concerns (Qureshi et al., 2005). Veenema, Walden, Feinstein, and William (2008) documented that knowledge base, sense of clinical competence, and perception of personal safety were all critical factors associated with a nurse's willingness to respond. The Red Cross provides information on disaster kits and making disaster plans. The Red Cross, FEMA, and many other organizations offer disaster training that can help nurses become competent in all phases of the disaster cycle: supporting communities with disaster mitigation and preparedness, disaster response, and recovery.

The three primary Red Cross Disaster Cycle Services available to healthcare professionals include *disaster health services, DMH,* and *staff wellness.* All three areas require that the Red Cross volunteer complete a background check, enroll in general disaster orientation training as well as specific function training, and meet the specific functions eligibility requirements (American Red Cross, 2017i).

In larger disasters, "just-in-time" training may be provided to address surge capacity needs for volunteer responders. On a disaster response operation, one individual may be assigned responsibility for multiple health professional activities.

Functional Needs Support Services in Shelters

In November 2010, the FEMA published a new set of guidelines in order to "... provide planning guidance that can be incorporated into existing shelter plans to State emergency managers and shelter planners to meet access and functional needs in general population shelters ... [and] identify methods of achieving a lawful and equitable program through the delivery of functional needs support services (FNSS) for children and adults" (FEMA, 2010). This guidance was developed in consultation with the Red Cross and other key stakeholders, and reflects an inclusive approach to sheltering that parallels the Red Cross commitment. It provides guidance to local emergency managers and shelter operators on how to develop plans to serve people with disabilities and people with access and/or functional needs during disasters. It also promotes our shared goal of integrating people with access and/or functional needs including those with disabilities into general population shelters.

The Red Cross carries out its commitment to inclusiveness by assisting each client to identify his or her needs and assisting the client to find resources to meet those needs. In some cases, Red Cross shelter workers, including Disaster Health Services workers, will provide the needed services directly; in other cases, they will coordinate with a governmental or nongovernmental partner to offer the required assistance. There are key planning and readiness steps that Red Cross chapters take to prepare to meet the functional and/or access needs of general population shelter clients, to include the following (American Red Cross, 2010b):

- Work with the local disability community and governmental partners to identify the types of disability-related and/or functional or access needs people are likely to have in an emergency.
- Determine which tasks and responsibilities related to functional and/or access needs will be performed by the Red Cross and put systems in place to achieve them, using local and/or national Red Cross resources.
- Work with local community partners and federal, state, tribal, and local governments, including public health departments, to identify the resources these partners can bring and the tasks and responsibilities they will perform.
- Establish relationships with DME companies, CMS companies, pharmacies, home healthcare agencies, and the public health department and identify how they can help meet client needs in a general population sheltering operation.

Disaster health professionals in collaboration with Red Cross Disability Integration responders are a key player in meeting the FNSS goal and continue to provide wraparound services and care for disaster-affected communities in close collaboration with other disaster response agency partners.

Disaster Health Services

Disaster Health Services provides essential health and preventive services to ensure the highest quality of care to clients affected by disaster. This activity may supplement the existing service delivery system for community healthcare and may coordinate its effort with the local public health system and medical/nursing communities (Figure 37.4).

Red Cross Disaster Health Services allows licensure scope of practice for nurses. This means that nurses within Disaster Cycle Services can provide care according to their level of education and licensure.

The Red Cross uses a RN-led model in disaster shelters. The overall goal is to increase the capability of the health response team to better serve clients and communities.

Red Cross Disaster Health Services

- Conduct health assessments of disaster-affected individuals and communities to determine appropriate response and care needs.
- Provide hands-on care if necessary.
- Refer individuals/families to appropriate healthcare resources and services to maintain client independence and expedite recovery.
- Provide initial emergency first aid to the injured.
    - Provide assistance to clients who may need replacement medications, consumable health supplies, and medical equipment to disaster clients.
- Assign disaster health services personnel to various sites such as shelters, emergency aid stations, integrated care condolence teams, hospital and healthcare facility visits, outreach teams and multiagency resource centers, assigning resources and partnering with others as appropriate.
- Provide healthcare appropriate to the community setting.
- Collect, record, and provide morbidity and mortality surveillance data to public health partners to include the Centers for Disease Control and Prevention (CDC).
- Collaborate with local public health authorities for environmental concerns, health hazards, disease and infection prevention, and surveillance.
- Follow up with clients as appropriate in the recovery phase (usually through the local chapter).

Disaster Health Services Team

- Registered Nurses (RNs)
- Nurse Practitioners (NPs)
- Licensed Practical and Vocational Nurses (LPNs/LVNs)
- Emergency Medical Technicians—All Levels (EMTs)
- Physicians (MDs and DOs)
- Certified Nurses' Aides (CNAs) (Local deployment only)
- Student Caregiver (any of the above categories in training with local deployment only)

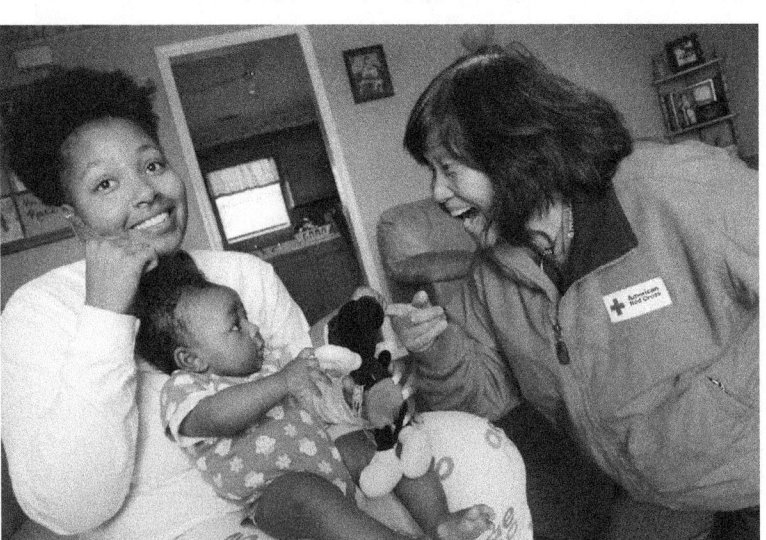

FIGURE 37.4 Three-month-old Kyinda receives a Red Cross Mickey Mouse from Carmen Young, Red Cross nurse who supports Kyinda and her mother Courtney in the 2017 southern tornadoes and storms.

Source: Photo by Daniel Cima for the American Red Cross.

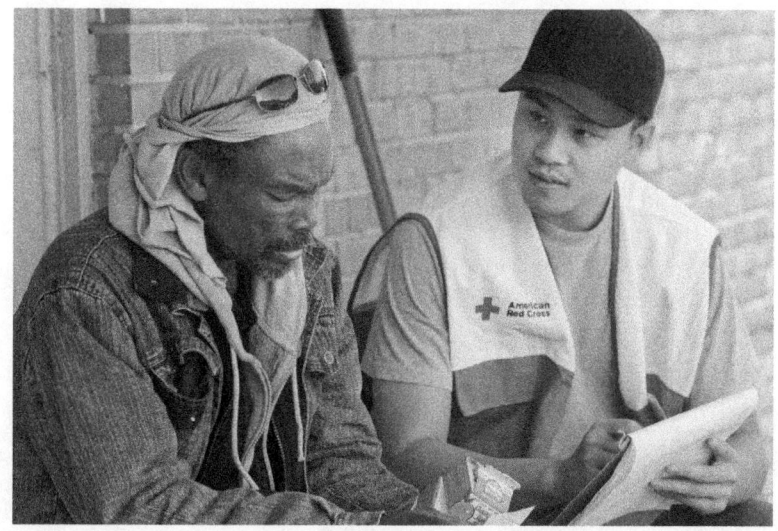

October 2017, Fair Bluff, NC. Shelter resident Earl Edge meets with Nam Ngo, Red Cross Nurse after Hurricane Matthew.
Source: Photo by Daniel Cima for the American Red Cross.

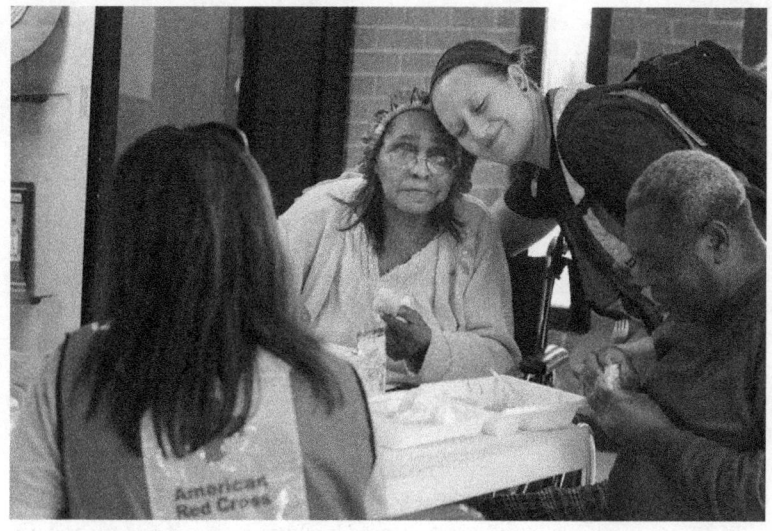

FIGURE 37.5 Red Cross nurse Sarah Adkin with Dorothy Peterson in Kinston, NC, October 2017.
Source: Photo by Daniel Cima for the American Red Cross.

Assignment Settings

Disaster health services personnel will work in three categories of settings, depending on their expertise and experience:

- *Red Cross Shelters*—where disaster survivors take temporary shelter to meet their basic needs for daily living (Figure 37.5)
- *Red Cross Multiagency Resource Centers*—where disaster clients interview with caseworkers and support agencies such as the Lion's Club, United Way, Salvation Army, and organizations assembled during disasters
- *Outreach*—to include home visits, integrated care condolence teams, staging areas, feeding kitchens or mobile feeding sites, warehouses and emergency aid stations (early field sites where the survivor's immediate needs are met; American Red Cross, 2017j).

Disaster Mental Health

The DMH function provides for, and responds to, the psychosocial and emotional needs of people affected by disaster, both survivors as well as paid and volunteer Red Cross staff, across the continuum of disaster preparedness, response, and recovery. DMH volunteers work throughout the relief operation alongside other disaster response workers in any disaster setting.

The American Red Cross DMH team is the largest DMH response force in the nation. Approximately 3,500 volunteers respond to over 60,000 disasters per year, from single-family fires to catastrophic disasters affecting thousands of individuals. The DMH services they provide are intended to augment the community's mental health services when a disaster challenges the existing capacity to respond to increased service demand. This increase in demand for mental health services is caused by both disaster-*aggravated* and disaster-*caused* mental health needs among individuals directly and indirectly affected by the disaster (American Red Cross, 2017m).

Disaster Mental Health Volunteer Eligibility

The DMH team consists of volunteers who are currently or previously licensed mental health professionals. There is no distinction made among types of mental health educational degrees and DMH workers are not generally addressed by professional titles. A DMH volunteer could be a social worker; licensed professional counselor; marriage and family therapist; psychiatric nurse; psychiatrist; psychologist; school counselor; or school psychologist.

Psychiatric nurses must be currently state licensed as a RN (or previously licensed within 5 years of joining the Red Cross DMH team) and have a minimum of 2 years of experience working in a psychiatric setting. New DMH volunteers are required to take Red Cross DMH-specific trainings to familiarize them with Red Cross policy and procedure and appropriate DMH intervention strategies (American Red Cross, 2017m).

Assumptions of Disaster Mental Health Services

DMH services are provided based on the assumption that many people are resilient. A significant minority will develop postdisaster psychological distress and DMH services are intended to alleviate immediate emotional distress and mitigate long-term consequences. Most individuals and families function adequately during and after disaster; however, their effectiveness in daily activities may be diminished.

DMH interventions are short term and can range from as little as 10 minutes of support to a much longer period of time. A worker will have limited contact with each client, generally no more than three instances. The most effective interaction will often involve problem solving and task-centered activities to address basic needs and the reduction of stress (American Red Cross, 2017m).

Disaster Mental Health Response

Using professional knowledge and skills, DMH workers focus on basic care, comfort, and support to those experiencing disaster-related stress by applying the three elements of DMH intervention.

The elements of the DMH response form a continuum of services from environmental and individual assessment using the 3Rs—Reactions, Risk Factors, Resilience—to targeted interventions appropriate to clients and workers in the disaster setting. In practice, these elements are fluid. In a single encounter, one might practice several elements at the same time or move from one element to another without intermediate steps.

Element 1: Environmental assessment and individual assessment using the 3Rs
Element 2: Promotion of resilience and coping including enhanced psychological first aid and psychoeducation

Element 3: Targeted interventions including: secondary assessment, referrals, crisis intervention, casualty support, and advocacy

More About the 3Rs

Individual assessment is accomplished using the 3Rs:

- Reactions to the stress of the event
- Risk factors of the individual
- Resilience of the individual

When assessing the mental health needs of disaster-affected individuals and families, it is important to take each of the Rs into consideration. While exposure-based risk factors are important to listen for, the client's current presentation and the factors associated with his or her resilience all contribute to understanding a person's emotional needs and likelihood for needing future services.

Reactions can manifest in any or all of the following categories: emotions/feelings; cognitive impacts/thoughts; physical effects; behaviors; spiritual beliefs.

Risk factors, including an individual's experiences and impacts from a disaster, can be predictors for long-term consequences. Risk factors can fall into the following categories: relational losses; physical/economic losses and transitions; threats to life; and loss of community/lifestyle.

Resilience refers to an individual's ability to cope effectively and adapt well to difficult challenges such as tragedy, adversity, or significant stressful experiences. Resilience is influenced by an individual's environment. It involves thoughts, behaviors, and ways of reacting that can be learned and developed. The more resilient an individual is, the less risk he or she has of having long-term mental health challenges.

Individual resilience is shaped by three key aspects of each person's life. These are: the factors of birth—personality, ethnicity, economic and cultural background; past history and life experiences that influence how he or she handles stressors; and perceived social support systems that include family, friends, school, work, and community. These aspects can have a positive or negative influence on an individual's resilience depending on the specific experience and the person's reaction to that experience (American Red Cross, 2017m).

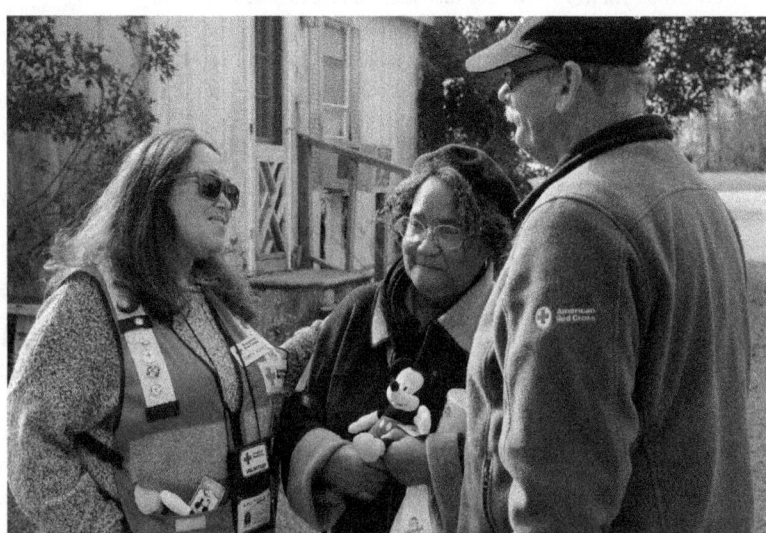

January 2017, Thomasville, GA. Carrie Abram shares her story about her family and the storms with Red Cross Disaster Mental Health Volunteer Elizabeth Woods.

Source: Photo by Daniel Cima for the American Red Cross.

Staff Mental Health

The DMH function is also responsible for providing psychosocial and emotional support for American Red Cross workers and other responders when requested. During a disaster response, DMH workers promote worker self-care on the individual level by distributing brochures containing resilience-building strategies to workers before and after deployment. These strategies are designed to help disaster workers manage stress reactions while working on the disaster response and returning home. DMH workers also contact Red Cross workers who have recently returned home from deployment to give them an opportunity to talk about their experience and any stressors still impacting them. The Red Cross Force Health Protection training for disaster leaders provides guidance and recommendations for promoting workforce resilience and psychological well-being (American Red Cross, 2017m).

Staff Wellness

The staff wellness activity supports the mission of the American Red Cross in providing relief to the survivors of disaster by promoting a healthy workforce available to serve on disaster relief operations.

The staff wellness activity on disaster relief operations is usually assisted by nurses from disaster health services, either through collaborative or formal assignments.

What They Do

- Provide worker education on pertinent disaster health issues during orientation and throughout the disaster relief operation
- Conduct prescreening health evaluations of potential Red Cross disaster responders
- Discuss with disaster responders the requirements of the role that the disaster responder wishes to fill and assist the disaster responder to decide if that is the role that he or she can fulfill
- Provide preventive, episodic, and emergency care and follow-up for Red Cross workers through direct care and/or referral
- Consult regarding health and safety issues associated with the work site or living quarters locations
- Make appropriate worker referrals, which may include accompanying staff to the treatment facility or to the home of residence
- Document worker illnesses and injuries for epidemiological review and insurance review
- Advise regarding maintenance of a safe and healthy work environment

SHELTER NURSING—THE ART OF DISASTER CARE

Shelters are unique, dynamic environments and health professionals working in shelter environments must draw on a variety of skill sets. General population shelters house people of all ages and present intersections for demographic, health, behavioral, cultural, and ethnic diversity. Diverse populations seek safety in shelters and an awareness of the community demographics is essential to starting, maintaining, and closing a shelter. The Red Cross uses a team approach with several units operating simultaneously within a shelter. This includes mass care, disaster health service, staff wellness, mass feeding, mental health, casework, community services, disaster public affairs, and facility management, as well as both governmental and nongovernmental liaisons. Red Cross nurses receive extensive training on how to set up, maintain, and close a shelter operation.

Disaster Health Services Competencies

To work effectively within a disaster environment, Red Cross nurses and volunteers are expected to develop and maintain certain competencies to ensure quality service. Competencies are applied to practice in differing ways, depending on the situation and the environment.

- *Critical thinking*—Use clinical judgment and decision-making skills in assessing the client for appropriate, timely individual, family, and community care.
- *Assessment*—Assess the safety issues for clients, other volunteers, and self in any disaster situation.
- *Technical skills*—Use the appropriate skill level based on client assessment and training/education.
- *Illness and disease management*—Provide population-based surveillance and take appropriate reporting action as necessary, partnering with the local and state public health department and CDC as indicated.
- *Information and healthcare technologies*—Use computer technology competently to communicate health information.
- *Ethics*—Maintain professional behavior in the practice of health services delivery and maintain the confidentiality of clients in all settings.

Red Cross Disaster Health Services in Shelter Operations

Red Cross Disaster Health Services provides an essential service to disaster survivors in a shelter environment. The following statement is an excerpt from the Disaster Health Services support to Clients Job Tool that assists the Disaster Health Services disaster responder to understand their work in a shelter environment. This outlines the multiple tasks needed to support clients in a shelter (American Red Cross, 2017k).

Providing Disaster Health Services in the Shelter Environment Toolkit

- Procure the Disaster Health Services kit that has been established by the chapter or region and bring to the shelter location.
- Obtain over-the-counter medications through pre-event chapter or regional procedures from local resources.
- Introduce yourself to the shelter manager.
- Coordinate with the shelter manager to accomplish the following:

- Identify and set up a Disaster Health Services area for confidential client interviews and request items needed for secure storage of records and supplies (e.g., drawer, file cabinet, cooler, room with a lock).
- Confirm that the shelter registration staff is completing the Registration Intake tool for each family unit at the time of registration. Although the Registration Intake tool is designed for the entire family, there could be a need to use more than one form if the family has several individuals with needs. In addition, the Registration Intake tool may be laminated and placed at the Shelter registration table with a log generated with the family or individual.
- Establish a Disaster Health Services–designated area to be staffed by one Disaster Health Services worker for confidential communication.
- Move actively about the shelter throughout the waking shelter hours leaving one Disaster Health Services worker in the designated Disaster Health Services area.
- Assist clients to identify their disaster-related health needs by moving about the shelter and interacting with clients through the Cot-to-Cot© method to assist clients to identify their health-related needs.
- Assist clients, including individuals with access and functional needs, to identify their needs.
- Prioritize the health needs of incoming shelter residents and residents who may already be present in the shelter using professional knowledge, skills, and orientation.
- Address critical health needs by activating the Emergency Medical system of 911. Urgent health needs will be addressed as quickly as possible.
- Prioritize providing personal care of clients, including hands-on care for assistance with activities of daily living, such as incontinence care or wound care.
- Understand that clients with access and functional needs, including those with disabilities, may readily identify their needs.
- Stop and listen to the clients and follow the clients' leads on meeting their needs.
- Move about the shelter to assist clients with their needs every 2 to 4 hours or more frequently as needed.
- Provide care to clients as needed, including but not limited to hands-on assistance with activities of daily living, wound care, assistance with monitoring of glucose levels, blood pressure checks, assistance with minor illnesses or injuries, and health education.
- Assist other Red Cross Disaster workers to maintain their health while responding.
- Perform Disaster Health Services casework by making contacts for the clients for medical needs and/or provide financial assistance to replace medically related items.
  - Connect clients to existing and intact caregivers, primary care providers, DME providers, CMS providers, PAS providers.
  - Determine if caregivers used before the disaster are currently available to meet the clients' health needs. (Did the disaster also affect providers?)
  - Contact alternate caregivers who have been mutually agreed on by the client and/or guardian.

- Network with local resources for goods and services that can be donated, loaned, or rented instead of purchased.
- Provide financial assistance to replace medications, DME, and/or CMSs as well as meet other disaster-related health needs to the limit of $500 and record in CAS.
- Determine if there is a valid prescription and/or if a new prescription is needed. A 3- to 7-day supply may be appropriate, but a 30-day supply is acceptable.
- Ask the client if DME or CMS is needed (e.g., canes, walkers, wheelchairs, O2 concentrators, colostomy supplies).
- Identify options for obtaining these needs.
- Enlist the assistance of the Disaster Relief Operations Disability Coordinator in obtaining the above resources.
- Ask vendors whether discounts are available.

Document all actions on the confidential Client Health Record to maintain client confidentiality (American Red Cross, 2017l).

SUMMARY

As a donor-funded, volunteer-driven NGO, the American Red Cross has provided disaster relief across the nation and around the globe for over 130 years. This NGO, with its unique Congressional Charter for disaster response and relief in times of national emergency, relies on the donations of time, money, and blood that the U.S. population so freely gives to accomplish its mission. Responding to over 64,000 disasters each year, Red Cross nurses and other volunteers fill a vital role in community resilience nationwide. Establishing shelters and emergency aid stations, providing meals, health assessment and care, emotional support and mental healthcare, the Red Cross remains a constant in the fabric of American lives.

The authors gratefully acknowledge Dianne Yeater and Sharon A. R. Stanley for their work on this chapter.

REFERENCES

American Association of Blood Banks. (2011). Disaster response. Retrieved from http://www.aabb.org/programs/disasterresponse/Pages/default.aspx#1

American Red Cross. (2007). Congressional charter of the National American Red Cross. Retrieved http://www.redcross.org/images/MEDIA_CustomProductCatalog/m4240124_charter.pdf

American Red Cross. (2008). About us. Retrieved from http://www.redcross.org/about-us

American Red Cross. (2010a). Touch of humanity for repatriates arriving from Haiti. Retrieved from http://www.redcross.org/portal/site/en/menuitem.1a019a978f421296e81ec89e43181aa0/?vgnextoid=06f4416215d46210VgnVCM10000089f0870aRCRD

American Red Cross. (2010b). *Serving people with disabilities and others with functional and/or access needs in Red Cross shelters*, 2010–009. Washington,

DC: American Red Cross Disaster Services. Retrieved from http://www.redcross.org/portal/site/en/menuitem.d229a5f06620c6052b1ecfbf43181aa0/?vgnextoid=f5195032f953e110VgnVCM10000089f0870aRCRD&vgnextchannel=d18859f392ce8110VgnVCM10000030f3870aRCRD

American Red Cross. (2011). Retrieved from https://intranet.redcross.org/content/redcross/categories/our_services/vol-services/onboard-engage/nursing-health.html retrieved 06_20_2018

American Red Cross. (2015). Retrieved from https://intranet.redcross.org/content/dam/redcross/documents/our_services/DisasterCycleServices/core-and-pillar-processes/respond/RespondProgramEssentials.pdf

American Red Cross. (2017a). American Red Cross: Our work in disaster relief. Retrieved from http://www.redcross.org/about-us/our-work/disaster-relief

American Red Cross. (2017b). American Red Cross: Mission and values. Retrieved from http://www.redcross.org/about-us/who-we-are/mission-and-values

American Red Cross. (2017c). American Red Cross federal charter. Retrieved from http://embed.widencdn.net/pdf/plus/americanredcross/e5mfayep2z/history-federal-charter.pdf?u

American Red Cross. (2017d). American Red Cross: Who we are. Retrieved from http://www.redcross.org/about-us/who-we-are/mission-and-values

American Red Cross. (2017e). American Red Cross: Our history. Retrieved from http://www.redcross.org/about-us/our-work/disaster-relief

American Red Cross. (2017f). American Red Cross: Our history, Part II. Retrieved from http://www.redcross.org/about-us/who-we-are/history

American Red Cross. (2017g). American Red Cross: Disaster cycle services. Retrieved from https://intranet.redcross.org/content/redcross/categories/our_services/disaster-cycle-services/dcs-capabilities/logistics/transportation/disaster-vehicles.html

American Red Cross. (2017h). American Red Cross: Core and pillar processes. Retrieved from https://intranet.redcross.org/content/redcross/categories/our_services/disaster-cycle-services/core-and-pillar-processes/respond/respond-toolkit.html

American Red Cross. (2017i). American Red Cross: Government operations toolkit. Retrieved from https://intranet.redcross.org/content/redcross/categories/our_services/disaster-cycle-services/dcs-capabilities/government_partnerships/government-operations-toolkit/national-response-framework.html

American Red Cross. (2017j). American Red Cross: Standards and procedures. Retrieved from https://intranet.redcross.org/content/dam/redcross/documents/our_services/DisasterCycleServices/dcscapabilities/individual_clientservices/health_services/DisasterHealthServicesStandardsAndProcedures.pdf

American Red Cross. (2017k). American Red Cross: Disaster health services support to clients. Retrieved from https://intranet.redcross.org/content/dam/redcross/documents/our_services/DisasterCycleServices/dcs-capabilities/individual_clientservices/health_services/DHSSupportToClientsJT.pdf

American Red Cross. (2017l). Disaster health services standards and procedures. Retrieved from https://intranet.redcross.org/content/dam/redcross/documents/our_services/DisasterCycleServices/dcs-capabilities/individual_clientservices/health_services/DisasterHealthServicesStandardsAndProcedures.pdf

American Red Cross. (2017m). Disaster mental health standards and procedures. Retrieved from https://intranet.redcross.org/content/dam/redcross/documents/our_services/DisasterCycleServices/dcs-capabilities/individual_clientservices/disaster_mental_health/DisasterMentalHealthStandardsAndProcedures.pdf

American Red Cross Office of Nursing. (2011). https://intranet.redcross.org/content/redcross/categories/our_services/vol-services/onboard-engage/nursing-health.html. Retrieved 06_10_2018

Dock, L., Pickett, S. E., Noyes, C. D., Clement, F. F., Fox, E. G., & Van Meter, A. R. (1922). *History of Red Cross nursing*. New York, NY: MacMillan.

Federal Emergency Management Agency. (2010). Guidance on planning for integration of functional needs support services in general population shelters. Washington, DC: Department of Homeland Security. Retrieved from https://www.fema.gov/pdf/about/odic/fnss_guidance.pdf

Federal Emergency Management Agency. (2014). NRF (National Response Framework) Resource Center. Retrieved from https://www.fema.gov/media-library/assets/documents/32230

Federal Emergency Management Agency. (2017). Emergency Support Function #6—Mass care, emergency assistance, temporary housing, and human services annex. Retrieved from https://www.fema.gov/media-library-data/1470149820826-7bcf80b5dbabe158953058a6b5108e98/ESF_6_MassCare_20160705_508.pdf

Gumpert, M. (1938). *Dunant: The story of the Red Cross*. New York, NY: Oxford University Press.

International Federation of Red Cross and Red Crescent Services. (2017a). International Federation of Red Crescent: Who we are. Retrieved from http://www.ifrc.org/en/who-we-are/the-movement/national-societies

International Federation of Red Cross and Red Crescent Services. (2017b). International Federation of Red Crescent: Who we are: History. Retrieved from http://www.ifrc.org/en/who-we-are/history

International Federation of Red Cross and Red Crescent Services. (2017c). International Federation of Red Crescent: Who we are: The movement. Retrieved from http://www.ifrc.org/en/who-we-are/the-movement

National Transport Safety Board. (2017). Family assistance operations: Planning and policy. Retrieved from https://www.ntsb.gov/tda/Pages/default.aspx

National Volunteer Organizations Active in Disaster. (2017). Retrieved from https://www.nvoad.org

Qureshi, K., Gershon, R. R., Sherman, M. F. Straub, T., Gebbie, E., McCollum, M., …, Morse, S. S. (2005). Health care workers' ability and willingness to report to duty during catastrophic disasters. *Journal of Urban Health: Bulletin of the New York Academy of Medicine, 82*(3), 378–388. doi:10.1093/jurban/jti086

Veenema, T. G., Griffin, A., Gable, A. R., MacIntyre, L., Simons, N, Couig, M. P., …, Larson, E. (2016). Nurses as leaders in disaster preparedness and response: —A call to action. *Journal of Nursing Scholarship, 48*(2), 1–4. doi:10.1111/jnu.12198

Veenema, T. G., Walden, B., Feinstein, N., & Williams, J. P. (2008). Factors affecting hospital-based nurses' willingness to respond to a radiation emergency. *Disaster Medicine and Public Health Preparedness, 2*(4), 224–229. doi:10.1097/DMP.0b013e31818a2b7a

38

DIRECTIONS FOR DISASTER NURSING RESEARCH AND DEVELOPMENT

Janice B. Griffin Agazio, Lynn A. Slepski, Roberta Proffitt Lavin, Mary Pat Couig, Kandra Strauss-Riggs, and Richard Ricciardi

LEARNING OBJECTIVES

When this chapter is completed, readers will be able to:

1. Describe the purpose of research in disaster prevention, preparedness, response, and recovery.
2. Describe the challenges frequently encountered when conducting clinical research following disasters and public health emergencies.
3. Explore ethical, legal, and logistical issues related to conducting disaster research.
4. Appreciate the importance of protecting human subjects in disaster research.
5. Assess the Haddon matrix and Crisis Conceptual Nursing Model as potential frameworks for disaster nursing research.
6. Determine the value of both qualitative and quantitative methods to the conduct of research in disaster situations.
7. Identify gaps in current disaster nursing research.

KEY MESSAGES

Research during disasters is complex and challenging.

The goal of disaster nursing research is to advance knowledge in the field to maximize the quality of healthcare provided throughout the event.

Research design must be matched to the study question.

Because of the nature of the research problem(s), significant challenges may be encountered regarding access to subjects, research design, and data collection.

Protection of human subjects participating in research is of paramount importance.

Nurses can contribute to research addressing all phases of disaster prevention, preparedness, response, and recovery.

CHAPTER OVERVIEW

The potential for natural or human-caused disasters will always exist. Enhancing our capacity to prevent, mitigate, prepare for, respond to, and recover from disasters, however, will increase disaster resilience and improve our capacity to confront disasters. Conducting disaster nursing research has significant scientific, ethical, legal, and practical complexities, making it difficult. Unlike clinical research, where the emphasis is on the individual and protecting individual rights, in disasters the focus is on whole populations of affected persons. This chapter provides a conceptual framework for disaster research. The framework upon which research is based will impact both the design of the research and the broader applicability to the emergency health services community, including nurses. In 1972, Haddon introduced a conceptual framework that utilized three epidemiologic principles: "(a) an external agent, (b) a susceptible host, and (c) an environment that brings the host and agent together ..." (Institute of Medicine [IOM], 2003, p. 27). By applying these principles to public health concepts, he believed it was possible to introduce a pathway to systematically analyze strategies for loss reduction and resource allocation (Haddon, 1973). When combined with the Crisis Conceptual Nursing Model (CCNM)—which address the concepts of dynamic equilibrium, hazardous events, and crises within the traditional concepts of a nursing conceptual framework—the conceptual model is ideally suited for disaster-related research in nursing. Attention to the legal and ethical issues surrounding disaster research is paramount, and researchers must be sensitive to the challenges in addressing these issues.

Conducting research during disasters is complex and challenging. In 2015, the IOM, renamed the National Academy of Medicine (NAM, 2015), published proceedings from its Disaster Research Response Workshop. The report, "Enabling Rapid and Sustainable Public Health Research During Disasters: Summary of a Joint Workshop by the Institute of Medicine and the U.S. Department of Health," describes recommendations for defining and conducting research during disasters. In 2017, the NAM published a second report, "Integrating Clinical Research into Epidemic Response: The Ebola Experience" (NAM, 2017), that analyzed the clinical trials that were conducted during the 2014 epidemic and considered the many scientific, ethical, and practical issues related to the conduct of research in similar contexts. These reports highlight the challenges frequently encountered when conducting clinical research following disasters and public health emergencies.

Conducting research focused on disasters is a legitimate and appropriate task for the nursing profession. Several strengths of the nursing profession are key to conducting research to improve the management of disasters: (a) nurses are team players and work effectively in interdisciplinary teams needed in disaster situations; (b) nurses can play key roles at the forefront in disaster prevention, preparedness, response, recovery, and evaluation; (c) nurses historically integrate the psychological, social support, spiritual, and family-oriented aspects of care with physiological needs of patients/clients; and (d) nurses are available and practicing across the spectrum of healthcare delivery system settings and can be mobilized rapidly if necessary. To capitalize upon the strengths of the profession to make a difference in disaster situations, research must be conducted related to the nursing role and the impact of nursing on both the client (individual and community) and the environment, and the healthcare delivery system. The research must be purposeful and outcomes driven, that is, conducted with the intent to change or to improve the outcomes of care in disaster situations and the recovery of the community. Ideally, this would involve collaboration among nurse researchers with differing strengths in research design, focus, and disaster response, to achieve improved outcomes at the client level, the provider level, and the systems level at all stages of a disaster. A disaster nursing research agenda would include the following: research related to education and intervention at the individual and community levels; educational research targeted toward the nurse as a provider; and health services research targeted toward maximizing the potential of the appropriate use of nurses by systems with health policy implications highlighted for the future. This agenda would explore the possible roles for nurses in all phases of a disaster response and recovery, evaluate the education and preparation for these roles, and analyze how nurses have been used by health systems and communities in actual disaster situations.

CONCEPTUAL FRAMEWORKS FOR DISASTER NURSING RESEARCH

The purpose of nursing research is to improve quality of care received in disasters and public health emergencies. Donabedian's (1982) structure, process, and outcome approach to quality management provides a suggested framework. However, Holzemer and Reilly (1995) expanded the original approach to develop an Outcomes Model for Health Care Research, which provides a comprehensive framework for the development of a nursing research agenda for disaster management related to quality of care. By extending the work of Donabedian, Holzemer and Reilly's attention is focused on the interactions and linkages among structure, process, and outcomes at the levels of the client, the provider, and the setting. Because the disaster research agenda needs to address outcomes at the client level, the provider level, and the systems level, this framework is useful in analyzing the research that has been accomplished and in identifying gaps that would inform future research, as well as serving as a model for designing comprehensive research.

William Haddon (1972) introduced a conceptual framework for categorizing highway safety phenomena that came to be known as the Haddon matrix. His approach drew strongly from his background in epidemiology by utilizing the epidemiological principles of: "1) an external agent, 2) a susceptible host, and 3) an environment that brings the host and agent together ..." (IOM, 2003, p. 27). By applying these principles to public health concepts, he believed it was possible to introduce a pathway to systematically analyze strategies for loss reduction and resource allocation (Haddon, 1973).

Haddon (1973) introduced 10 countermeasure strategies to reduce losses from the phenomena of the transfer of energy to animate and inanimate objects in manners that cause damage. The 10 strategies that in some ways mirror primary, secondary, and tertiary health promotion, include:

1. Prevent the production of the form of energy (e.g., kinetic, thermal, electric, ionizing radiation).
2. Reduce the amount of energy produced.
3. Prevent release of the energy.
4. Modify the rate of release of the energy from the source.
5. Separate people from release of the energy in time and/or distance.
6. Separate people in time/distance and also by use of barriers or shielding.
7. Modify the contact surface and points at which people may come in contact with the energy.
8. Reduce losses in people by strengthening the structure that might be damaged by the energy release.
9. Move rapidly to detect and evaluate damage that occurred or is occurring to counter continuation and extension.
10. Restore the infrastructure by encompassing all the preceding measures and stabilize for repair and rehabilitation (Haddon, 1995).

The 10 aforementioned strategies are helpful guides in applying the Haddon matrix to a problem. It can also be easily applied to healthcare research that focuses more broadly on the disaster and prevention as well as the healthcare response and there are examples of its use across aspects of disaster research, including violence, burns and fire safety, defense, and emergency medical response (Scott-Parker & MacKay, 2015). In fact, it was identified as one of the six most influential articles in *Injury Prevention* (Runyan, 1998, 2015).

Assumptions of the Haddon Matrix

Haddon (1973) identified assumptions and limitations that must be taken into consideration when utilizing the Haddon matrix. First, "there is no logical reason why the rank order (or priority) of loss-reduction countermeasures generally considered must

parallel the sequence, or rank order, of causes contributing to the result ..." (p. 359). Second, once a person is injured, there may not always be a possibility to completely eliminate an undesirable result. Third, if the energy release is of a magnitude that cannot possibly be countered by existing measures, then the more essential contention is to eliminate the threat. Expanding upon the third assumption, if nuclear power plants are highly likely to fail and release large quantities of ionizing radiation, then the only countermeasure is to eliminate nuclear power plants. Obviously, this is not a foreseeable case as the world is currently too dependent on power.

The fourth assumption deserves greater attention; it contends that for each strategy there is an opposite strategy for those who desire to cause damage. A terrorist may seek ways to intentionally alter one of the 10 strategies. For example, he or she may choose to damage the normal alerting systems that inform the public of an imminent release of ionizing radiation, thus preventing affected individuals from taking appropriate action. However, Haddon (1973) offers a more positive example of a physician correcting the function of the anterior pituitary through the use of ionizing radiation.

Two final assumptions are critical to adequately utilize the framework. First, despite all possible pre-event countermeasures, accidents will happen. The final and most important assumption is that, when considering all possible loss reduction countermeasures, the emphasis must be on the countermeasure that has the greatest effect on reducing the damage (Haddon, 1972).

Concepts

The design of the Haddon matrix has four basic concepts distributed over three phases. The phases form rows representing the potential points of intervention in an injury, pre-event, event, and postevent. The concepts initially formed three columns representing the influencing factors of human, vehicle or equipment, and environment. Over time the Haddon matrix was expanded to encompass more public health problems and is now represented as four concepts in columns, which are host, agent or vehicle, physical environment, and social environment (Barnett et al., 2005).

Runyan (1998) introduced a third dimension of value criteria to the Haddon matrix to facilitate decision making regarding countermeasures by adding policy analysis principles. In essence, the value criteria included the addition of a cost-benefit analysis. If considering, for example, the distribution of potassium iodide (KI) in a nuclear power plant meltdown like the one in Japan, then one might add a set of value criteria that includes feasibility, preferences, equity, cost, and effectiveness. For example, one might use the thyroid cancer literature on children, regarding the effectiveness of KI following the Chernobyl accident, to assess the effectiveness of the intervention. Cost may include not only the amount of the KI tablets, but also the cost of public education on when and how to use the tablets—as opposed to informing the public of the likelihood of the event and the cost of treatment of thyroid cancer if the KI is not available.

Whether or not one chooses to include the third dimension, the first two sides of the matrix have remained relatively consistent over the last two decades and the concepts are well defined to allow for evidence-based decision making

(Scott-Parker & MacKay, 2015). Host is the person or object at risk of injury. The agent is whatever causes the injury or damage. The vector is the delivery mechanism. Physical environment is where the injury occurs. Social environment is the social, cultural, or legal norms in the community where the injury occurs (Barnett et al., 2005; Runyan, 1998). Pre-event is before the event occurs; event is the occurrence of the event or crisis phase; and postevent is after the event or consequences phase. The definitions are consistent with preparedness, response and mitigation, and recovery in the current all-hazards approach to disaster preparedness.

Relationships Among the Concepts

Using the Haddon matrix to focus on loss reduction, rather than prevention alone, allows the observer to analyze the information using a structured approach that helps to clarify the interrelationships among concepts in the three phases (Haddon, 1972). The columns represent the interacting factors that influence injury prevention (Runyan, 1998). By examining the phases (pre-event, event, and postevent) with the concepts of host, agent, physical environment, and social environment, there is a possibility to analyze the interaction as a means to identify possible population-based interventions (Runyan, 1998). For example, in the pre-event phase of a nuclear power plant accident, the functions should include actions to ensure public safety, including distribution of KI. Table 38.1 provides examples of functions that can be included in a Haddon matrix for preventing injuries related to an ionizing radiation release. Additionally, the cells of the matrix identify risk factors and interventions as they would occur across all phases of an event (IOM, 2004). For research, the matrix provides foci for structuring studies toward, for example, prevention in the pre-event phase or most effective care of injuries in the event and postevent phases.

Sandifer et al. (2017) recently developed the Disaster-Pressure-State-Ecosystem Service-Response-Health (DPSERH) model. This conceptual model was specifically developed to address ecological disasters and the related health effects. The DPSERH model is an important addition as the number of ecological and climate-related disasters has significantly increased since 1960 with floods and severe storms being the greatest percentage of disasters (Federal Emergency Management Agency [FEMA], 2017). The model, like the Haddon

matrix, considers both environmental and health outcomes, but is more complex in its approach. Importantly it makes the link between the pressure exerted by the disaster and the health outcomes. Thus, it is not just what is directly caused by a disaster that impacts health, but what moderates the impact and what is exacerbated by a disaster that is essential to consider. There are many aspects of DPSERH that are consistent with the Haddon matrix, but it is more limited in that it addresses primarily environmental issues such as water quality, habitat structure and function, biodiversity, nonharvested biota, and fishery (harvested) species (Sandifer et al., 2017).

CRISIS CONCEPTUAL NURSING MODEL

The CCNM is a nursing developmental model, which was derived from the crisis theory created by Lindemann and Caplan, and was adapted for use by the University of Connecticut faculty members. Lindemann was a psychiatrist who had firsthand experience with the Coconut Grove fire of 1942. Lindemann drew upon the fields of public health and social science in an attempt to escape the medical model, which he viewed as a major contributing factor that resulted in the institutionalization of the mentally ill, in part because he ascribed that the medical model inadequately addressed the bereavement process (Fawcett & Murphy, 1983). If a person experienced a disaster, which overwhelmed his or her ability to cope effectively, then a crisis ensued. Fawcett and Murphy (1983) viewed crisis as an opportunity flowing from "any event that challenges the assumed state and forces the individual to change his view of, or readapt to, the world, himself, or both" (p. 47).

Caplan brought to crisis theory the perspective of public health and a belief in prevention. He believed that individuals in crisis are more accommodative to the intervention and the intervention is important to achieve a positive outcome. Caplan identified three stages of a crisis: (a) a perceived change in a person's state of mental equilibrium, (b) the inability to solve the problem through one's normal problem-solving techniques, and (c) a person's mentality returns to a state of equilibrium if the crisis is successfully resolved (as cited in Fawcett & Murphy, 1983). Because Lindemann and Caplan did not address the whole person, the faculty of the University of Connecticut added a biophysical component to the theory. The faculty members

TABLE 38.1 The Haddon Matrix

Phases	Host	Agent/Vector	Physical Environment	Social Environment
Pre-event				
Event				
Postevent				
(Optional) Cost-cutting value criteria	**Feasibility**	**Cost**	**Effectiveness**	**Preferences**

Source: Adapted from Barnett, D. J., Balicer, R. D., Blodgett, D., Fews, A. L., Parker, C. L., & Links, J. M. (2005). The application of the Haddon matrix to public health readiness and response planning. *Environmental Health Perspectives, 113*(5), 553. doi:10.1289/ehp.7491

recognized that a person could have an altered physical status while continuing to function on a higher level after a crisis was resolved. For example, Christopher Reeve suffered an injury that left him a quadriplegic, but most of the country witnessed his growth and contributions to society that resulted from his crisis, despite eventually dying from complications of his condition.

Assumptions

The first and most important assumption of the CCNM is that a person can achieve a higher level of functioning through the nursing process. The nursing process passes through the pre-crisis, crisis, and postcrisis stages, which are viewed as a continuum. Because individuals are in a state of dynamic equilibrium within the environment, there is a possibility to prevent a state of disequilibrium by reducing risk factors and enhancing coping (Thibodeau, 1983). For example, there is a possibility to reduce the risk of thyroid cancer in children from ionizing radiation by providing KI to vulnerable populations and teaching them how to respond if there is a release of ionizing radiation.

Concepts

The crisis model addresses the concepts of dynamic equilibrium, hazardous events, and crisis within the traditional concepts of a nursing conceptual framework. People are physiological, psychological, and social beings who function dynamically within the environment (Hawkins, 1983). Individuals are vulnerable to crisis, but have the problem-solving ability to address the crisis. People live within a larger environment that is inclusive of the internal and external environment. The external environment includes everything outside the person, such as friends, family, and the air one breathes (Fawcett & Murphy, 1983). A hazardous event can result from disequilibrium within either the internal or external environment, which can lead to a crisis if there is an inadequate coping mechanism (Hawkins, 1983).

Health is measured on a continuum that is in a state of flux between wellness–illness–wellness where illness is a "state of disequilibrium or maladaption," and wellness is "physical, emotional, and social well-being" (Hawkins, 1983, p. 78). An important point to note is that crisis does not necessarily indicate illness; rather, a crisis offers the opportunity for growth.

The concept of nursing is considered to be the facilitator for effective coping and resource identification during certain crises. When a person is not able to meet his or her own needs, then the nurse intervenes and assists that individual with those needs to "prevent crisis and restore wellness" (Hawkins, 1983, p. 79).

Life is divided into stages of pre-crisis, crisis, and postcrisis. Pre-crisis is considered a state of dynamic equilibrium between people and the environment. When a hazardous event occurs and a problem is perceived or identified, then the result may be adequate problem solving leading to recovery or inadequate problem solving leading to a crisis. The crisis stage occurs when a nurse would assist in identifying additional internal and external resources to either reduce the effect of the crisis or return the person to a state of equilibrium. Postcrisis is the period of time after the crisis has occurred that leads to dysfunction via a chronic condition from which the person cannot recover to a higher level of wellness under the circumstances.

Relationships Among the Concepts

The concepts of nursing, person, environment, and health are in a state of dynamic equilibrium. The nurse functions at two levels: as a stage manager who helps to identify resources—guiding an individual through crisis—and as a human being who is also a system in dynamic equilibrium with the environment. When a hazardous event occurs, there is the potential to disrupt the state of equilibrium, thus resulting in a change in the state of wellness. The person's perception of the event and his or her coping mechanisms will determine whether he or she interprets the event as a crisis. Nurses work to assist the person with event interpretation as well as the identification and utilization of coping mechanisms, which the nurse does in an effort to maintain the highest level of wellness. If pre-crisis efforts are unsuccessful in maintaining the state of equilibrium, then a crisis occurs and the nurse will work to lessen or cure disequilibrium. Successful identification of resources assists the person in a state of crisis to return to a state of equilibrium; an unsuccessful resolution may result in the continued possibility of death (Fawcett & Murphy, 1983).

MERITS OF MODELS

Haddon Matrix

Evaluation of the Haddon matrix reveals a biased approach toward problem solving and crisis prevention. The concepts of host, agent or vector, physical environment, and social environment are well defined and linked—leaving no apparent gaps. Like the crisis nursing model, the concepts are linked in each of three phases of a crisis that results in a logically consistent framework socially congruent and focused on a multidisciplinary approach to injury prevention. Through the knowledge of hazardous events, this prevention-oriented model is ideal for a multidisciplinary approach.

Because the focus of the Haddon matrix is based on reducing the effects of a hazardous event rather than merely prevention, the model is particularly appropriate for use in public health preparedness issues. The Haddon matrix breaks down problems into manageable components and facilitates decision making, planning, understanding of potential threats, and allocation of resources (Barnett et al., 2005).

Crisis Conceptual Nursing Model

Evaluation of the CCNM reveals a distinct bias toward a holistic and wellness-based approach where a crisis is viewed as an opportunity for growth. The concepts of person, environment, health, and nursing are well defined and linked to crisis intervention, leaving no apparent gaps (Figure 38.1). Furthermore, each concept is linked in each of three phases of a crisis resulting in a logically consistent framework that is socially congruent with the focus of nursing being the patient and not the problem (Fawcett & Murphy, 1983). Through the knowledge of hazardous events, the goal-directed approach can readily produce nursing protocols that guide practice. The utility of the CCNM is evident in health promotion prior to a hazardous event and has shown to be useful in practice (Hawkins, 1983).

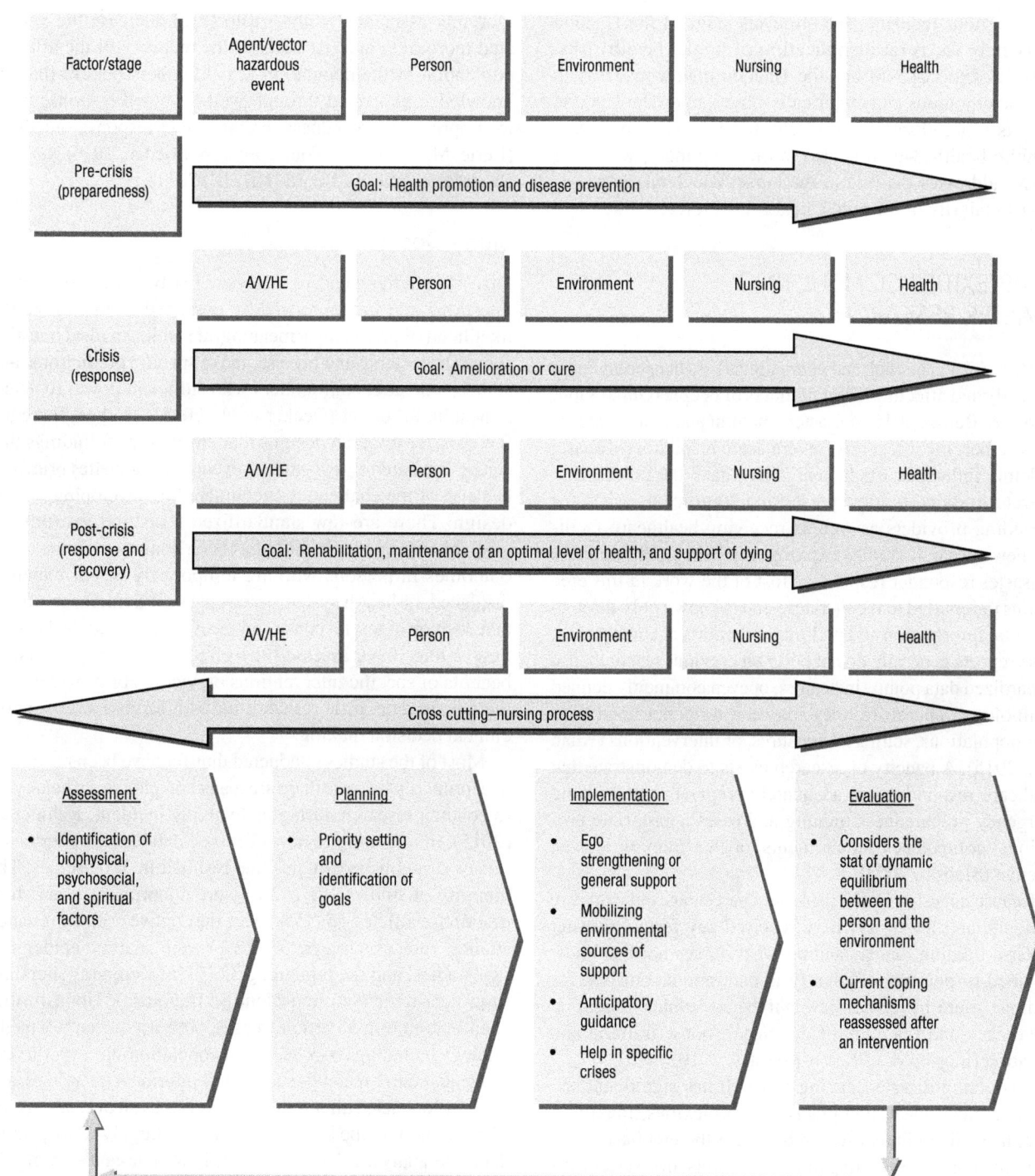

FIGURE 38.1 Crisis conceptual nursing model with Haddon elements (A/V/HE).

A, agent; HE, hazardous event; V, vector.

IMPLICATIONS FOR USING MODELS FOR DISASTER NURSING RESEARCH

Research is undertaken to systematically address questions related to specific phenomena. The use of a conceptual framework helps to structure the observations of the researcher. By utilizing different frameworks, researchers are likely to have unique perspectives from which to approach observed phenomena.

The CCNM is well designed to generate research questions related to nursing interventions at each stage of a crisis. One

method for accomplishing the intervention is through the design of research to determine problem-solving mechanisms of the client to hazardous events in the precrisis stage.

The Haddon matrix is also well designed for research approaches in all stages of crisis. In some ways, the approaches are likely to be similar to those in the CCNM. The goal of research using the CCNM is to address questions that arise from providing direct patient care (Hawkins, Thibodeau, Utley-Smity, Igou, & Johnson, 1993), whereas the goal of research utilizing the Haddon matrix is related to the reduction of adverse effects of a hazardous incident. The pre-event stage of the Haddon matrix may focus on identification of public health risks. Analysis of the CCNM and the Haddon matrix reveal both to be parsimonious and empirically observable. The Haddon matrix is a multidisciplinary approach that is most applicable to public health, which is also multidisciplinary, while the CCNM addresses the role of the nurse, which encompasses the vast majority of the public health workforce.

COMPLEXITIES CONDUCTING DISASTER RESEARCH

Disasters (local, national, and international) are happening more frequently and affecting larger numbers of people (Guha-Sapir, Hoyois, & Below, 2016). Disasters, natural and man-made, as well as emerging infections (severe acute respiratory disease, pandemic influenza, Ebola, and Zika), have the potential to generate mass casualties, presenting significant issues for responding providers as well as receiving healthcare facilities. Few research studies explore emergency preparedness or disaster responder response. Most of the work in this area remains unreported in the literature and is known only through anecdotal information and preliminary reports at conferences. These reports generally do not build on previous research, use standardized data points, indicators, or even commonly defined terminology. Therefore, they may not be generalizable to other populations, settings, exposures, or interventions (Khan et al., 2015). A paucity of research exists to demonstrate that healthcare responders are adequately prepared, that existing emergency preparedness training addresses appropriate professional competency requirements, or that training is even effective (Slepski, 2007).

Because nurses comprise the largest percentage of healthcare providers, and few if any have received any formal disaster response training, understanding what nurses need to know and need to perform efficiently is paramount. Further, for example, there have been few published studies validating the efficacy and retention of disaster response training and education (Slepski & Littleton-Kearney, 2010).

Conducting disaster nursing research has significant scientific, ethical, legal, and practical complexities, making it difficult. Unlike clinical research, where the emphasis is on the individual and protecting individual rights, in disasters, the focus is on whole populations of affected persons. As a result, there are difficulties in obtaining subjects, designing a realistic research design, collecting data, as well as the timing of the research in relation to an evolving incident. While prospective designs have the potential to identify and correct problems in the immediate moment, doing so has the potential to divert scarce resources, like food, shelter, water, and transportation, from the response. There are also significant sensitivities associated with surveying disaster victims and their significant others, the community and responders, and the potential development of posttraumatic stress (Walker, Garmon, & Ellerson, 2005). According to Birnbaum, Daily, and O'Rourke (2015), there are four ultimate goals in conducting disaster research entailing the use of epidemiological or interventional studies: (a) decrease the risk that a hazard will produce a disaster; (b) decrease the

mortality associated with disasters; (c) decrease the associated morbidity; and (d) enhance the recovery of the affected population or the population at risk. Others believe that the knowledge generated through well-designed response studies improves preparedness, practice, and response outcomes (Lurie, Manolio, Patterson, Collins, & Frieden, 2013; National Biodefense Science Board [NBSB], 2011).

Study Design

Disaster studies need to address clearly stated, important questions and be appropriately designed to maximize the likelihood of producing a meaningful result. An ideal question should be testable and precise, make specific predictions, and address potential confounders with sufficient power to detect a meaningful effect (Decker et al., 2013). To date, there are few disaster research designs that ensure robust findings that can be compared across studies, events, and societies primarily because of the challenges encountered in developing a good design. There are few standardized tools and instruments available. For example, little has been done to examine client outcomes in persons who are temporarily or permanently displaced, or health systems recovery postincident, or studies that develop or test response and recovery concepts or theories. Few studies have assessed the effects, efficiency, costs, or benefits of specific interventions on victims or providers and there is, to date, little research-based information to support clinical decision making.

Most of the studies conducted thus far have been retrospective, primarily because there are many complexities when trying to conduct research during an evolving incident. Kahn et al. (2015), in a scoping review of mixed databases, undertook a review of published studies that resulted in 300 articles. The majority of studies 186 (62%) were nonprimary research or descriptive articles, 45 (15%) were descriptive primary research studies, such as surveys, 37 (12%) were analytic epidemiology studies, and the remaining 32 (11%) were gray literature (non-peer-reviewed, nonscientific literature). Upon further examination of a 58 article subset, 60% used a survey methodology including cross-sectional population surveys, surveys using qualitative methods such as key informant interviews, and surveys conducted after training exercises as an evaluation tool. They found that the cohort studies were largely retrospective database analyses. Norris (2006), in a meta-analysis of 225 disaster studies conducted over 20 years, found: 31% used convenience sampling; 27% were based on census information; 19% were probability-based; 17% were purposive; and only 6% were clinical studies. She noted that "certain desirable characteristics (longitudinal designs, representative samples) have been decreasing in prevalence over time whereas others (early assessment) have been increasing" (p. 173).

Why Disaster Research Is So Difficult

RESEARCH DESIGNS MUST BE MATCHED TO THE QUESTION AND PROTECT STUDY SUBJECTS

Generally, studies can be grouped according to the type of information they are generating: short term to guide decision making or longer term to explicate the effects of the incident on the affected communities or the environment (NBSB, 2011). Each requires different approaches. High-quality research can produce knowledge about the health impacts of an event or quantify the benefit of types of interventions if an appropriate design is implemented. While many types of disasters may occur, important research questions can be anticipated and protocols, including data collection tool templates, can be developed nationally in advance, especially for types of incidents described in the FEMA's 15 National Planning Scenarios (NBSB, 2011). Giarratano, Savage, Barcelona-deMendoza, and Haville (2014) also suggest that a study already in progress before a disaster occurs can be transformed by adding new measures, such as mental health assessments, to make use of baseline data that are already collected. Study designs should be matched to best answer the research question, taking into account potential problems of obtaining informed consent, autonomy, independent versus participant observation, and the testing of new interventions.

SIGNIFICANCE AND FEASIBILITY

Decker et al. (2013) looked at a number of important factors to consider when undertaking a disaster study. Under public health significance and scientific importance, they highlighted the need to determine if the proposed study: had the potential to provide new knowledge or information; could be generalized to other situations or populations; confirmed or refuted a preliminary or preexisting hypothesis; answered questions that needed to be answered; or contributed to or improved the public health response. As part of the significance consideration, they looked at the size of the affected population and the estimated risk. When evaluating feasibility, they included as factors to consider: access to the area; ability to collect reliable data, especially if data could be lost if not collected immediately; study size and statistical power; ability to identify and locate subjects and an appropriate control or comparison population (if needed); and adequacy of resources to support, conduct, and complete the study among others. Of note, maintaining necessary confidentiality and addressing other potential ethical issues and obtaining timely Institutional Review Board (IRB) approval were called out.

IDENTIFYING AND RECRUITING SUBJECTS

Following established human research guidelines (National Institutes of Health [NIH], 2007), disaster research must be conducted in an ethical manner. Selections should be fair and impartial and align with the goals of the study.

Sampling Size

Recruiting sufficient numbers of subjects is difficult. Norris (2006) found that sample sizes in the 225 disaster studies that she reviewed were small (median 150) and resulted in studies that lacked power.

Identifying Healthcare Responders Is Difficult

Often many different organizations deploy responders or, as history as demonstrated, volunteers just show up without any previous training or affiliation with an organization. Responder rosters with names and contact information is often not obtainable. As a result, many researchers turn to convenience samples accessed

during conferences where responders are likely to attend, resulting in persons with "self-selected" roles (Slepski, 2007).

Accessing Sufficient Numbers of Responder Types

Many times, responders come with different backgrounds, training, experience, and expectations. When small numbers of responder types (e.g., emergency medical technicians or respiratory technicians) are combined, skill sets and roles are different, making comparisons difficult (Slepski, 2007).

Identifying and Recruiting Disaster Victims at the Individual, Family, or Community Level

Disaster victims are vulnerable, especially children, the elderly, persons with mobility limitations, persons with English as a second language, as well as the economically and educationally disadvantaged (Ferreira, Buttell, & Ferreira, 2015; Flanagan, Gregory, Hallisey, Heitgerd, & Lewis, 2011; NIH, 2007). They may suffer the most severe consequences from disaster. Giarratano et al. (2014) believe that persons with chronic physical or mental health conditions or who lack social or material resources before a disaster are at greater risk of developing disaster-related health issues. Early in a response, survivors often confuse research with response operations (Hunt et al., 2016). As a result, they may be more easily subjected to coercion and as a result of their trauma, may have difficulty providing informed consent. Haney and Elliot (2012) found that participants were initially hesitant to participate, expressing worry that researchers were exploiting their pain for personal or professional gain. When evacuation is not needed, subjects can be recruited where they gather—in emergency shelters, community centers, health clinics, or where disaster management workers enroll survivors for benefits. Finding subjects for follow-on data collection can be challenging. When evacuation takes place, however, there are few mechanisms to identify where victims evacuate and when they leave to return to their homes. For example, there are no publicly available lists and disaster workers are compelled to protect victim contact information (Browne & Peek, 2014). Further, the purpose of a disaster study may not be intended to benefit persons experiencing the disaster. As such, subjects bear the burden and risks of participating, including inconvenience, emotional distress, psychological discomfort, loss of dignity, breach of confidentiality, unwanted media attention, or pressure to consent to research to avoid appearing unpatriotic or unhelpful (Collogan, Farris, Donal-Sewell, Borja, & Fleischman, 2004). The NIH (2007) identified four critical ethical considerations when identifying subjects for disaster studies: the decisional capacity of potential participants who have been affected; their vulnerability; the risks and benefits of participation; and their ability to give informed consent. Ferreira et al. (2015) consider these recommendations too broad and provide more practical approaches to operationalizing the considerations. For example, as part of mitigating potential risks, they recommend deidentification and the avoidance of photography of participants.

Data Collection

TIMELY DATA COLLECTION IN THE CONTEXT OF ETHICAL AND LEGAL CONSIDERATIONS

Disasters evolve over time. Their scale, timing, and unpredictability often overwhelm local capabilities and resources (Khan et al., 2015; Nelson, Lurie, Wasserman, & Zakowski, 2007). Data collection must have appropriate privacy protections and ethical safeguards in place. While there is often a desire to collect baseline data as early as possible, doing so may divert limited resources, cause distraction from saving lives and speeding recovery, and interrupt survivors as they attempt to regain stability (Hunt et al., 2016). In many instances, data collection could be delayed and still achieve the same results. North and Pfefferbaum (2002) recommend that data collection should be timed to allow survivors to: bury their dead; obtain housing if lost during the event; seek assistance from relief organizations; and report losses to their insurance companies.

THREATENING AND DIFFICULT ENVIRONMENTS

Accessing a disaster site to collect reliable data may be difficult. The environment is often hazardous, constantly changing, and highly charged, and is often subject to the conflicting agendas of the local population, politicians, and scientists. In many instances, perimeters are established requiring credentials, generated by the disaster response lead, to pass through. The disaster zone is often chaotic. There may be environmental impediments such as fire, smoke, damaged buildings, or flood waters. In the case of communicable disease, personal protective equipment may be required to prevent disease transmission. Contaminated objects, such as signed consent documents as well as electronic devices such as tablets and phones used for data collection, may need to be disinfected before leaving the area, which may not be possible. Nurse researchers who deploy to the field must address the potential for language barriers, the logistics of reliable transportation and living accommodations, issues surrounding position (gender or ethnicity), and research team stress (Mukherji, Ganapati, &Rahill, 2014) as well as safety concerns (Cox, 2008). The University of California, Berkley has safety guidelines consisting of general field safety guidelines, physical and environmental hazards, animals and pests (which includes snakes) and diseases (www.ehs.berkeley.edu/pubs/fieldresearchsfty.pdf). If access to the disaster is limited or if local infrastructure is not severely impacted, telephone or Internet surveys can be implemented quickly, often through the use of social media, and more efficiently than in-person interviews (Cox, 2008; Hugelius, Adolfsson, Gifford, & Örtenwall, 2017; Schlenger & Silver, 2006). Researchers need to be prepared for the recounting of trauma and distress when interviewing participants who live through a disaster's impact and loss (Giarratano et al., 2014).

FUNDING

Obtaining external funding for disaster research is limited. Whereas in the past, many agencies had "preapproval" mechanisms, most no longer offer this. The NBSB (2011) recommended the establishment of funding mechanisms to support a rapid and robust scientific response to disasters, within hours or days, suggesting contracts or funded research centers. This recommendation has not been enacted. In the meantime, several funding organizations exist. For example, the Natural Hazards Center Quick Response Grant Program provides funds for researchers to quickly travel to disaster-affected areas to capture perishable data. The Center has preferred topics especially for quick-response grants (hazards.colorado.edu/research/quick-response/guidelines). Similarly, the National Science Foundation, through its Rapid Research Response mechanism, can award up to $200,000 for up to 1 year.

WORKING WITH IRBs

IRBs must evaluate the soundness of disaster protocols, balancing the risks and benefits to the subject, and the need to collect data as soon as possible. A key challenge is obtaining a timely review that is also rigorous and holds to core ethical principles. Few IRBs have opportunities to develop expertise specific to disaster research and its review or have the requisite understanding of current cultural and societal realties being experienced where the research will be carried out, especially if the study will be conducted in another nation, during an expedited review (Hunt et al., 2016). In their study of international IRBs, IRB members sought information on gender norms, decision-making structures, and cultural values in the disaster-affected community. For large-scale, international events often involving nongovernmental organizations, efforts are underway to develop guidance and ethical frameworks by the World Health Organization and Doctors Without Borders, among others (Hunt et al., 2016).

Haney and Elliot (2012) found that when researchers sought approval from their local IRB after Hurricane Katrina, the university had closed and the IRB members had dispersed. While the NBSB (2011) "Call to Action" recommended the establishment of a Public Health Emergency Research Review Board within the Department of Health and Human Services (HHS) to expedite the review of research protocols before, during, and after a disaster, creation of such a new body for this purpose seems duplicative. The National Center for Disaster Medicine and Research (the National Center) was developed as a result of the 2006 Pandemic and All Hazards Preparedness Act and its reauthorization (113-5; 2013) and the 2007 Homeland Security Presidential Directive-21, Public Health and Medical Preparedness. The initial legislation identified the Departments of Defense, HHS, Homeland Security (DHS), and Transportation and the Veterans Administration as members. According to its Charter, the National Center develops and propagates disaster medicine core competencies, standardized education and training curricula, and research. Specifically, the report communicates how the National Center serves as a clearinghouse and converts translation of research findings into disaster-related medical and public health programs and best practice guidelines available to federal, state, local, and tribal governments; academia; and the private sector (National Center, 2017). The National Center has all of the prerequisites for assembling a national-level IRB, in that it has experienced subject matter experts in the areas of disaster medicine, disaster public health, occupational medicine, industrial hygiene, toxicology, epidemiology, psychology, and emergency response, as well as awareness of specific subject matter experts who could supplement the organic elements of the National Center depending on the type of disaster and could be rapidly convened to review, refine, prioritize, and approve any previously developed generic research plans without the bias associated with required funding. While so chartered, neither HHS or the DHS, whose secretary, according to the DHS (2016), has been delegated authority from the president for Stafford Act responses, have provided any significant financial support to the National Center. Until such a national

IRB is established, nurse researchers should consider seeking preapproval of generic research studies that can later be tailored, perhaps using nationally developed templates, based on the likelihood of disasters and their areas of expertise, rather than waiting for an incident to occur (Hunt et al., 2016).

Nurse researchers have much to learn both from the work done historically and more recently by nurses, as well as from interdisciplinary researchers in disaster medicine. Although both highlight the approach and value of retrospective research, by defining the target population as those impacted by the disaster situation, more research can be accomplished with potential for a greater impact in phases of prevention, preparedness, response, and recovery. From a systems evaluation perspective, it is also critical that nurses be at the forefront in developing the science and planning to be appropriately used in disaster situations. This can start with an active involvement in the process to evaluate the lessons learned from recent disasters such as the terrorist acts of September 11, 2001 (9/11) and Hurricane Katrina.

FUTURE NURSING RESEARCH AGENDA AND POLICY IMPLICATIONS

Disaster nursing research has produced important lessons for education and practice (Gebbie & Qureshi, 2002; Kako, Mitani, & Arbon, 2012). While critical research continues to inform policy and practice, the field faces the same challenges that all disaster-related specialties confront when attempting to make evidence-based decisions during the preparedness, response, and recovery phases of a disaster. There is not enough high-quality research that can inform disaster health activities (Gebbie & Qureshi, 2002). Disaster health research varies significantly based on the research question(s) being pursued. It can include a variety of methods: surveillance and epidemiology, surveys, key informant interviews, mixed methods (Koenig & Schultz, 2010). First-person accounts from healthcare professionals who played a role in a disaster, whether a natural or man-made event, are a common method for disseminating information about the medical and public health impacts of particular disasters. While these are valuable for identifying the gaps and challenges confronted by individual providers, they do not follow standard metrics that can be compared across events to build a consistent evidence base.

After Action Reports are the traditional emergency management tool used to assess the operational activities immediately following an event. These documents are rarely published or shared with the disaster response community. They typically focus on the successful aspects of a particular response with some suggestions for future changes that are often relevant only for a particular community or facility (Lurie et al., 2013).

The challenges of conducting research during, or in the immediate aftermath of, disasters are myriad. Events can move quickly and health professionals are, of course, focused on saving lives and treating injuries—not on data collection. There is also the issue of trust in the impacted community and the need to involve the community by following principles of community-based participatory research.

Leaders in the field of public health emergency response have proposed ways to incorporate research into the Incident Command System and other disaster response and recovery activities (Gebbie & Qureshi, 2002; Lurie et al., 2013). The efforts of the National Institutes of Health Disaster Research Response program are focused on developing standards and open access tools for standardized data collection, protocols, regulatory documents, and other materials (Strauss-Riggs, Yeskey, Miller, Arnesen, & Goolsby, 2017).

As noted, the disaster health community would do well to move toward developing a learning health system to systematically collect and rapidly share data. The uniform Utstein-style of data collection and reporting has been utilized in a variety of medical settings to inform providers' rapid, evidence-based decision making (Cummins et al., 1991; Miller et al., 2016). The field of disaster medicine has adapted the style for what has been termed, "disaster medical response (DMR)" (Ringdal, Coats, & Lefering, 2008). A variety of DMR data elements and indicators have been defined by expert consensus panels and a medical operation coordination scale was developed for use in the acute phase of a medical response (Debacker et al., 2012; Ringdal et al., 2008). The disaster health community can adopt these indicators and tools to better align the research questions and outcomes necessary to advance the science and build the critically needed disaster health evidence base.

Any future nursing research agenda must focus on not only provider outcomes that include preparation, readiness, protection, resilience, and recovery, but also increasingly on both client and healthcare system outcomes. With the use of technology (particularly the Internet) and advances in computer and communication systems, the challenge is to use both to the fullest extent in all phases of disaster management. To improve outcomes as described in Haddon's and the CCNM frameworks, there are ample opportunities for a new research agenda that must involve nurse researchers. Nurses have traditionally focused on patient or client advocacy and education for health promotion and prevention. One of the clearest needs for the future is the research that must be focused on the client's needs at both the individual and community levels, as well as considering the environment in which disasters occur. To explicate this aspect of the research, however, nurses will need to think creatively about how to adapt some of the research that has been conducted related to provider preparation and readiness. With the continued threat of terrorism, natural disasters, or man-made events complicated by technology such as nuclear power, healthcare consumers' awareness and need for preparation and education are heightened. Nurses providing for patients/clients across healthcare settings have a unique opportunity to respond to interest and concerns. Consequently, there is an opportunity for practice-based research initiatives in public health departments, primary care clinics, and acute care settings.

Much has been done to identify areas where there are gaps in the literature as well as best practices. The Katrina Report (White House, 2008), commissioned by the White House, identified inadequate preparation and response. It found knowledge, skills, and abilities that differed from previously developed disaster response capabilities and best practices, including the following:

- Knowledge, skills, and abilities needed for immediate public health and medical support
- Identification, triage of acutely sick and injured persons
- Management of chronic medical issues in large numbers of evacuees, especially those with special needs

- Assessment, communication, and mitigation of public health risks
- Management of mortuary needs
- Re-establishment of impacted healthcare delivery systems and public health infrastructures
- Effectiveness of existing emergency preparedness and disaster response educational programs

Khan et al. (2015) surveyed stakeholders to identify gaps in disaster literature. They identified 12 themes for future research:

1. Attitudes and beliefs of responders, including willingness to respond and equity
2. Capacity assessment and capacity building at the community, multisectoral levels, including gender considerations, high-risk or at-risk populations
3. Collaboration and system integration, especially organizational capacity including acute, long-term, community, and primary care, and emergency medical services
4. Communicable disease control
5. Communication with the public, health, or governmental systems, and social media
6. Education, training, and exercises for clinicians, leadership, and public health practitioners
7. Ethical considerations
8. Planning
9. Psychosocial impacts of emergencies on communities and health workers
10. Public health considerations for sheltering and evacuation, including functional needs assessments
11. Quality improvement and performance standards, including measure and metrics
12. Surveillance, epidemiology, and public health information, including rapid needs assessments and risk assessments

Finally, Ranse, Hutton, Jeeawody, and Wilson (2014) conducted the first international study to develop consensus on nursing research priorities using a three-round Delphi technique of nurses who were members of the World Association for Disaster and Emergency Medicine and World Society of Disaster Nursing. Participants prioritized research addressing the psychosocial aspects of disaster nursing as having the greatest need. The areas of clinical practice, disaster education and training, and curriculum development were ranked as a lower priority. Ranked as lowest priority by the group were studies surrounding strategy, relationship, and networking.

Policy Considerations

As Tip O'Neill is historically credited with the phrase, "all politics are local," so too it can be said that *all policy is local* as well. With nursing being the largest healthcare workforce and consistently rated in Gallup polls as the most ethical and honest profession in healthcare (Gallup Poll, n.d.), nurses are well positioned to advocate for disaster preparedness policy development, implementation, and evaluation. Although the field of disaster preparedness and response has acknowledged specific professional competencies, the complexity of the science necessitates an interprofessional approach to conducting research and translating research into evidence-based policy.

Future disaster research is needed in many areas to address gaps in evidence to inform policy. Some of these would include:

- Support of vulnerable populations (children, elderly, frail elderly, pregnant women, disabled, and seriously mentally ill)
- Workforce models
- Role of artificial intelligence and information technology
- Coordination of aid and scarce resources
- Methods to deliver psychological first aid
- State and local community use of TeleHealth
- Command, control, and communication—organizational barriers preventing effective communication and decision making
- Processes and procedures to provide care for the volunteer's families while deployed during disaster response
- Scope of practice and regulatory policies that identify competencies currently performed by physicians and nurses that can be performed by other members of the health workforce team
- Human capacity asset tracking
- Collaboration among multisector disaster response networks
- Response to cyberattacks
- Strengthening capacity to detect, prevent, respond to, and recover from biologic pathogens
- Methods to distribute biological countermeasures
- Triage and ethics of decision making during mass casualty events
- Promotion of health and wellness to optimize personal and community readiness and personal safety—sustainment of a culture of prevention
- Enhancing resilience

SUMMARY

While the number and scale of disasters is increasing, disaster research is in its infancy, with few studies reported in the literature. More research is needed to make planning and response evidence-based. Conducting research in the midst of an evolving incident is difficult, primarily because of the unique and unpredictable nature of the events. Designing disaster research that helps to expand the state of the science as well as identify best practices is at best difficult. Nurses should be leaders in conducting disaster research that can inform practice, education, health systems delivery, as well as health policy. More attention should be given to rigorous, scientific evaluation of these areas before, during, and after a disaster.

STUDY QUESTIONS

1. What is the purpose and value of nursing research in disaster situations?

2. How would the agenda for nursing research be shaped for the future to address client needs, provider needs, and issues for and effect on healthcare delivery systems?

3. What are some of the challenges for researchers trying to conduct both retrospective and prospective research related to disaster care?

4. Is there research related to preparedness and to the development of provider competencies that can serve as a building block for future research?

5. Where are the most pressing gaps in the disaster nursing literature?

6. How can the lessons learned in the field from nurses be captured and translated into future research?

7. What are some of the key interdisciplinary research questions surrounding the use of advancing technologies by local communities and on a national scale during disaster prevention, preparedness, response, and recovery?

INTERNET ACTIVITIES

Several Internet sites are available for nurse researchers to obtain information related to current research and opportunities for future funding of research related to disaster situations. These include but are not limited to:

Federal grants: www.grants.gov (Search preparedness or by federal agency.)

U.S. Department of Health and Human Services:

1. Office of the Assistant Secretary for Preparedness and Response; www.phe.gov/Preparedness/planning/hpp/Pages/funding.aspx

2. The Centers for Disease Control and Prevention; www.cdc .gov/funding/resources/index.html

3. The Division of Nursing; bhw.hrsa.gov/grants/nursing

4. The National Institute for Nursing Research: www.ninr .nih.gov/researchandfunding/dea/desp/oep/fundingopportunities

Department of Defense:

1. The TriService Nursing Research Program, www.usuhs.edu/ tsnrp/ (Eligible TSNRP applicants are limited to active duty, reserve, or retired military nurses from the U.S. Army, Navy, or Air Force, or National Guard Nurse Corps Officers.)

Additional sites that might be helpful to nurse researchers and students attempting to locate research and other content related to disaster nursing include:
Department of Health and Human Services: www.hhs.gov

1. Office of the Assistant Secretary for Preparedness and Response (ASPR), Public Health Emergency; www.phe .gov/preparedness/Pages/default.aspx

   a. National Disaster Medical System; www.phe.gov/ preparedness/responders/ndms/Pages/default.aspx
   b. Technical Resources, Assistance Center, Information Exchange (TRACIE) asprtracie.hhs.gov/assistance-center

2. Centers for Disease Control and Prevention; www.cdc.gov

   a. Office of Public Health Preparedness and Response; www .cdc.gov/phpr/index.htm
   b. Preparedness and Emergency Response Learning Centers (PERLC); www.cdc.gov/phpr/perlc.htm (Alabama, Arizona, Florida, Illinois, Iowa, Maryland, Massachusetts, Minnesota, New York, North Carolina, Oklahoma, Texas, Washington)
   c. CDC Emergency Preparedness; emergency.cdc.gov

3. National institutes of Health, National Library of Medicine; Disaster Information Management Research Center: disasterlit.nlm.nih.gov

Department of Homeland Security: www.dhs.gov

1. Federal Emergency Management Agency; www.fema.gov

Department of Defense

1. The Uniformed Services University of the Health Sciences; www.usuhs.mil

   a. National Center for Disaster Medicine and Public Health; www.usuhs.edu/ncdmph

2. U.S. Army Medical Research Institute of Chemical Defense, https://usamricd.apgea.army.mil

3. Center for Global Health Engagement; www.usuhs.edu/cghe

Other:

1. Association of State and Territorial Health Officials, Preparedness, www.astho.org/Programs/Preparedness/News-Updates

2. Center for Excellence in Disaster Management & Humanitarian Assistance; www.cfe-dmha.org

3. Emory University, Rollins School of Public Health, Center for Public Health Preparedness and Research; cphpr.emory.edu

4. Evidence Aid; www.evidenceaid.org

5. Public Health Learning Network; nnphi.org/phln

6. Saint Louis University, College for Public Health and Social Justice, Institute for Biosecurity; www.slu.edu/ public-health-social-justice/research/centers_institutes/ institute_bsdp.php

REFERENCES

Barnett, D. J., Balicer, R. D., Blodgett, D., Fews, A. L., Parker, C. L., & Links, J. M. (2005). The application of the Haddon matrix to public health readiness and response planning. *Environmental health Perspectives*, *113*(5), 561–566. doi:10.1289/ehp.7491

Birnbaum, M. L., Daily, E. K., & O'Rourke, A. P. (2015). Research and evaluations of the health aspects of disasters, Part I: An overview. *Prehospital and Disaster Medicine*, *30*(5), 512–522. doi:10.1017/ S1049023X15005129

Browne, K. E., & Peek, L. (2014). Beyond the IRB: An ethical toolkit for long-term disaster research. *International Journal of Mass Emergencies and Disasters, 32*(1). Retrieved from http://www.ijmed.org/articles/651

Collogan, L. K., Farris, T., Donal-Sewell, R., Borja, S., & Fleischman, A. R. (2004). Ethical issues pertaining to research in the aftermath of disaster. *Journal of Traumatic Stress, 17*(5), 363–372. doi:10.1023/B:JOTS.0000048949.43570.6a

Cox, C. W. (2008). Research considerations when studying disasters. *Critical Care Nursing Clinics of North America, 20*(1), 111–119. doi:10.1016/j.ccell.2007.10.003

Cummins, R. O., Chamberlain, D. A., Abramson, N. S., Allen, M., Baskett, P. J., Becker, L., … Eisenberg, M. S. (1991). Recommended guidelines for uniform reporting of data from out-of-hospital cardiac arrest: the Utstein Style. A statement for health professionals from a task force of the American Heart Association, the European Resuscitation Council, the Heart and Stroke Foundation of Canada, and the Australian Resuscitation Council. *Circulation, 84*(2), 960–975. doi:10.1161/01.cir.84.2.960

Debacker, M., Hubloue, I., Dhondt, E., Rockenschaub, G., Rüter, A., Codreanu, T., … Castrèn M. (2012). Ustein-style template for uniform data reporting of acute medical response in disasters. *PLOS Currents Disasters, 4*, e4f6cf3e8df15a. doi:10.1371/4f6cf3e8df15a

Decker, J. A., Kiefer, M., Reissman, D. B., Funk, R., Halpin, J., Bernard, B., … Howard, J. (2013). A decision process for determining whether to conduct responder research following disasters. *American Journal of Disaster Medicine, 8*(1), 25–33. doi:10.5055/ajdm.2013.0108

Department of Homeland Security. (2016). *National response framework* (3rd ed.). Retrieved from https://www.fema.gov/media-library-data/1466014682982-9bcf8245ba4c60c120aa915abe74e15d/National_Response_Framework3rd.pdf

Donabedian, A. (1982). *Explorations in quality assessment and monitoring: The criteria and standards of quality.* Ann Arbor, MI: Health Administration Press.

Fawcett, J., & Murphy, E. (1983). Evaluation of the crisis theory conceptual framework. In M. B. White (Ed.), *Curriculum development from a nursing model: The crisis theory framework* (pp. 213–223). New York, NY: Springer Publishing.

Federal Emergency Management Agency. (2017). Disaster declaration by year. Retrieved from https://www.fema.gov/disasters/grid/year

Ferreira, R. J., Buttell, F., & Ferreira, S. B. (2015). Ethical considerations for conducting disaster research with vulnerable populations. *Journal of Social Work Values and Ethics, 12*(1), 29–140.

Flanagan, B. E., Gregory, E. W., Hallisey, E. J., Heitgerd, J. L., & Lewis, B. (2011). A social vulnerability index for disaster management. *Journal of Homeland Security and Emergency Management.* Retrieved from https://www.researchgate.net/profile/Barry_Flanagan/publication/274439003_A_Social_Vulnerability_Index_for_Disaster_Management/links/569e582d08ae192a92a4a2fd.pdf

Gallup Poll. (n.d.). Americans rate healthcare providers high on honesty, ethics. Retrieved from http://www.gallup.com/poll/200057/americans-rate-healthcare-providers-high-honesty-ethics.aspx

Gebbie, K., & Qureshi, K. (2002). Emergency and disaster preparedness: Core competencies for nurses: What every nurse should but may not know. *American Journal of Nursing, 102*(1), 46–51. doi:10.1097/00000446-200201000-00023

Giarratano, G., Savage, J., Barcelona-deMendoza, V., & Harville, E. W. (2014). Disaster research: A nursing opportunity. *Nursing Inquiry, 21*(3), 259–268. doi:10.1111/nin.12049

Guha-Sapir, B., Hoyois, P., & Below, R. (2016). Annual disaster statistical review 2015: The numbers and trends. Centre for Research on the Epidemiology of Disasters. Retrieved from http://www.emdat.be/publications

Haddon, W. (1972). A logical framework for categorizing highway safety phenomena and activity. *Journal of Trauma, 12*(3), 193–207. doi:10.1097/00005373-197203000-00002

Haddon, W. (1973). Energy damage and the ten countermeasure strategies. *Human Factors, 15*(4), 355–366. doi:10.1177/001872087301500407

Haddon, W. (1995). Energy damage and the 10 countermeasure strategies. *Injury Prevention, 1*, 40–44. doi:10.1136/ip.1.1.40

Haney, T. J., & Elliot, J. R. (2012). The sociological determination: A reflexive look at conducting local disaster research after Hurricane Katrina. *Sociology Mind, 3*(1), 7–15. doi:10.4236/sm.2013.31002

Hawkins, J. W. (1983). A developmental model: The crisis model. In J. A. Thibodeau (Ed.), *Nursing models: Analysis and evaluation* (pp. 77–88). Monterey, CA: Wadsworth.

Hawkins, J. W., Thibodeau, J. A., Utley-Smity, Q. E., Igou, J. F., & Johnson, E. E. (1993). Using a conceptual model for practice in a nursing wellness centre for seniors. *Perspectives, 17*(4), 11–16.

Holzemer, W. L., & Reilly, C. A. (1995). Variables, variability and variations research: Implications for medical informatics. *Journal of American Medical Informatics Association, 2*, 183–190. doi:10.1136/jamia.1995.95338871

Hugelius, K., Adolfsson, A., Gifford, M., & Ortenwall, P. (2017). Facebook enables disaster research studies: The use of social media to recruit participants in a post-disaster setting. Retrieved from https://www.ncbi.nlm.nih.gov/pmc/articles/PMC5300848/?report=printable

Hunt, M., Tansey, C. M., Anderson, J., Boulanger, R. F., Eckenwiler, L., Pringle, J., & Schwartz, L. (2016). The challenge of timely, responsive and rigorous ethics review of disaster research: Views of research ethics committee members. Retrieved from http://journals.plos.org/plosone/article?id=10.1371/journal.pone.0157142

Institute of Medicine. (2003). *Preparing for the psychological consequences of terrorism: A public health strategy.* Washington, DC: National Academies Press.

Institute of Medicine. (2004). *Preparing for the psychological consequences of terrorism: A public health strategy.* Washington, DC: National Academies Press.

Kako, M., Mitani, S., & Arbon, P. (2012). Literature review of disaster health research in Japan: Focusing on disaster nursing education. *Prehospital and Disaster Medicine, 27*(2), 178–183. doi:10.1017/S1049023X12000520

Khan, Y., Fazli, G., Henry, B., de Villa, E., Tsamis, C., Grant, M., & Schwartz, B. (2015). The evidence base of primary research in public health emergency preparedness: A scoping review and stakeholder consultations. *BioMed Central Public Health.* Retrieved from https://bmcpublichealth.biomedcentral.com/articles/10.1186/s12889-015-1750-1

Koenig, K., & Schultz, C. (2010). *Disaster medicine: Comprehensive principles and practices.* New York, NY: Cambridge University Press.

Lurie, N., Manolio, T., Patterson, A. P., Collins, F., & Frieden, T. (2013). Research as a part of public health emergency response. *The New England Journal of Medicine, 368*(13), 1251–1255. doi:10.1056/NEJMsb1209510

Miller, A., Yeskey, K., Garantziotis, S., Arnesen, S., Bennett, A., O'Fallon, L., … Hughes, J. (2016). Integrating health research into disaster response: The new NIH Disaster Research Response Program. *International Journal of Environmental Research and Public Health, 13*(7), 676. doi:10.3390/ijerph13070676

Mukherji, A., Ganapati, N. E., & Rahill, G. (2014). Expecting the unexpected: Field research in post-disaster settings. Retrieved from https://www.researchgate.net/profile/Guitele_Rahill/publication/271740520_Expecting_the_unexpected_Field_research_in_post-disaster_settings/links/56322d3208ae0530378fb6c1.pdf

National Academy of Medicine. (2015). *Enabling rapid and sustainable public health research during disasters: Summary of a Joint workshop by the Institute of Medicine and the U.S. Department of Health and Human Services.* Washington, DC: National Academies Press. doi:10.17226/18967

National Academy of Medicine. (2017). Integrating clinical research into epidemic response: Ebola experience. Retrieved from http://nationalacademies.org/hmd/~/media/Files/Report%20Files/2017/epidemicclinicaltrials-report-highlights.pdf

National Biodefense Science Board. (2011). Call to action: Include scientific investigations as an integral component of disaster planning and response. Retrieved from https://www.phe.gov/Preparedness/legal/boards/nprsb/Documents/nbsbrec14.pdf

National Center for Disaster Medicine and Public Health. (2017). 2017 Annual report. Retrieved from https://www.usuhs.edu/sites/default/files/media/ncdmph/pdf/ncdmph_2017_ar_5082.pdf

National Institutes of Health. (2007). Ethical issues to consider in developing, evaluating, and conducting research post-disaster. Retrieved from https://www.nimh.nih.gov/funding/grant-writing-and-application-process/ethical-issues-to-consider-in-developing-evaluating-and-conducting-research-post-disaster.shtml

Nelson, C., Lurie, N., Wasserman, J., & Zakowski, S. (2007). Conceptualizing and defining public health emergency preparedness. *American Journal of Public Health, 97*(S1), S9–11. doi:10.2105/AJPH.2007.114496

Norris, F. H. (2006). Disaster research methods: Past progress and future directions. *Journal of Traumatic Stress, 19*(2), 173–184. doi:10.1002/jts.20109

North, C. S., & Pfefferbaum, B. (2002). Research on the mental health effects of terrorism. *Journal of the American Medical Association, 228*(5), 633–636. doi:10.1001/jama.288.5.633

Ranse, J., Hutton, A., Jeeawody, B., & Wilson, R. (2014). What are the research needs for the field of disaster nursing? An international Delphi study. *Prehospital and Disaster Medicine, 29*(5), 448–454. doi:10.1017/S1049023X14000946

Ringdal, K. G., Coats, T. J., & Lefering, R. (2008). The Utstein template for uniform reporting of data following major trauma: A joint revision by SCANTEM, TARN, DGU-TR and RITG. *Scandinavian Journal of Trauma, Resuscitation and Emergency Medicine, 16*(1):7. doi:10.1186/1757-7241-16-7

Runyan, C. W. (1998). Using the Haddon matrix: Introducing a third dimension. *Injury Prevention, 4*, 302–307. doi:10.1136/ip.4.4.302

Runyan C. W. (2015). Using the Haddon matrix: Introducing the third dimension. *Injury Prevention, 21*, 126–130. doi:10.1136/ip.4.4.302rep

Sandifer, P. A., Knapp, L. C., Collier, T. K., Jones, A. L., Juster, R., Kelble, C. R., ... Sutton-Grier, A. E. (2017). A conceptual model to assess stress-associated health effects of multiple ecosystem services degraded by disaster events in the Gulf of Mexico and elsewhere. *Geohealth, 1*(1), 17–36. doi:10.1002/2016GH000038

Schlenger, W. E., & Silver, R. C. (2006). Web-based methods in terrorism and disaster research. *Journal of Traumatic Stress, 19*(2), 185–193. doi:10.1002/jts.20110

Scott-Parker, B., & MacKay, J. M. (2015). Research and practice in a multidimensional world: A commentary on the contribution of the third dimension of the Haddon matrix to injury prevention. *Injury Prevention, 21*, 131–132. doi:10.1136/injuryprev-2015-041568

Slepski, L. A. (2007). Emergency preparedness and professional competency among health care providers during hurricanes Katrina and Rita: Pilot study results. *Disaster Management and Response, 5*(4), 99–110. doi:10.1016/j.dmr.2007.08.001

Slepski, L. A., & Littleton-Kearney, M. T. (2010). Disaster nursing educational competencies. In R. Powers & E. Daley (Eds.), *International disaster nursing* (pp. 549–560). New York, NY: Cambridge University Press.

Strauss-Riggs, K., Yeskey, K., Miller, A., Arnesen, S., & Goolsby, C. (2017). Translating battlefield practices to disaster health. *Disaster Medicine and Public Health Preparedness, 11*(4), 1–2. doi:10.1017/dmp.2016.196

Thibodeau, J. A. (1983). Types of conceptual model. In J. A. Thibodeau (Ed.), *Nursing models: Analysis and evaluation* (pp. 43–65). Monterey, CA: Wadsworth.

Walker, P., Garmon, S., & Ellerson, K. (2005). Research issues in preparedness for mass casualty events, disaster, war and terrorism. *Nursing Clinics of North America, 40*(3), 551–564. doi:10.1016/j.cnur.2005.04.008

White House Katrina Report. (2008). A failure of initiative: Final Report of the Select Bipartisan Committee to investigate the preparation for and response to hurricane Katrina. Retrieved from https://www.gpo.gov/fdsys/pkg/CRPT-109hrpt377/pdf/CRPT-109hrpt377.pdf

---

CASE STUDY 38.1

Public Health Service and Military Disaster Nursing Research

The U.S. Public Health Service and U.S. military have a long history of involvement in humanitarian and disaster relief missions. According to Walker et al. (2011), hundreds of civilians received humanitarian assistance following the Korean War. This assistance was repeated during the Vietnam War between 1963 and 1975 as part of Medical Civic Action Projects (MEDCAPS) as healthcare was provided by U.S. military physicians and nurses. Through the involvement of the U.S. Navy ships, the *Comfort* and the *Mercy,* many military members have had the opportunity to assist with international disasters through humanitarian missions such as posttsunami in Indonesia (Yates, 2005). During this mission, personnel aboard the *USNS Mercy* provided care to 9,500 patients and performed over 20,000 procedures that included 285 surgical cases during the first 2 months at its offshore location. The *USNS Mercy,* traditionally stationed on the West Coast, has responded to humanitarian crises in the Pacific islands, the Philippines, and invasion of Iraq, while the *USNS Comfort,* berthed on the east U.S. coast, responded to the terrorist attacks in New York, Hurricane Katrina, and the Haiti earthquake (Drayton, 2013). Rivers, Gordon, Speraw, and Reese (2013) and River et al. (2017) directly studied military nurses who served as first caregivers as members of local reserve and National Guard units. Comparably, Elliott (2015) used narrative inquiry to extract themes from interviews of 10 military nurses postdeployment to identify issues in fitting back into their home stateside environment.

Following 9/11 and the start of Operations Iraqi Freedom and Enduring Freedom in Afghanistan, military nursing research focused on wartime operations; patient care delivery and transport; and nursing skills, readiness, and competencies. Multiple descriptive studies provided information on nursing practice in humanitarian missions or operations other than war (Agazio, 2010; Agazio, Goodman, & Padden, 2014), the shipboard practice environment (Cox, 2005; Gehring, 2005; King, 2015), advanced practice nurses (Aberle, Bethards, Orsega, & Ricciardi, 2003), and flight–nursing skill sets for critical care transport (Dremsa-Brewer, 2003; McNeill, 2006; Mortimer, 2005). McNeill, Pierce, Dukes, and Bridges (2014) detail the issues encountered during en route care to increase patient safety during transport. Agazio (2010) completed a 3-year project to compare nursing competencies and patient care challenges in humanitarian missions or operations other than war missions such as in Bosnia, Hungary, and Somalia from those skills needed in wartime operations. Agazio, Goodman, Opanubi, and McMullen (2016) further extended the findings from this study to focus upon the management of ethical issues that emerged in nursing practice during the war time environment.

The Commissioned Corps of the U.S. Public Health Service (USPHS), one of the seven U.S. uniformed services, and the civilian component of HHS, have responded to humanitarian emergencies and disasters both in the United States and around the world. After 9/11, the numbers of deployed PHS commissioned officers increased to respond to natural and man-made disasters including major deployments to Hurricanes Katrina and Rita. PHS officers were deployed to Liberia to care for healthcare workers infected with the

(continued)

CASE STUDY 38.1 (*continued*)

Ebola virus (Mosquera, Braun, Hulett, & Ryszka, 2015), and most recently to Texas, Florida, Puerto Rico, and the U.S. Virgin Islands following the devastating hurricane season of 2017. PHS Commissioned Corps nurses reflected on their deployment to Ground Zero (Knebel et al., 2010) and described the psychological impact of working at the disaster scene and care provided to the rescuers, both psychological and physical. Tyree-Debisette, Brown, and Chamberlain (2006) described the lived experience of those affected by Hurricane Katrina, including evacuation issues, a lack of safe shelters, environmental and climate challenges, and access to care. Nursing issues included long hours delivering care, physiological and psychological needs, as well as leadership responsibilities and the ability to conduct assessments on the shelter's ability to provide health services.

REFERENCES

Aberle, C. J., Bethards, K. J., Orsega, S. M., & Ricciardi, R. (2003). Designing a medical humanitarian assistance course for advanced practice nurses in the uniformed services. *Military Medicine, 168*(9), 729–732. doi:10.1093/milmed/168.9.729

Agazio, J. (2010). Army nursing practice challenges in Humanitarian and Wartime Missions. *International Journal of Nursing Practice, 16*(2), 166–175. doi:10.1111/j.1440-172X.2010.01826.x

Agazio, J., Goodman, P., Opanubi, O., & McMullen, P. (2016). Ethical issues encountered by military nurses during wartime. *Annual Review of Nursing Research, 34*(1), 227–246. doi:10.1891/0739-6686.34.227

Agazio, J., Goodman, P., & Padden, D. (2014). Impact of deployment on military families. *Annual Review of Nursing Research, 32*, 109–133. doi:10.1891/0739-6686.32.109

Cox, C. W. (2005). Shipboard nursing on aircraft carriers: The perceptions of twelve Navy nurses. *Nursing Outlook, 53*(5), 247–252. doi:10.1016/j.outlook.2005.02.007

Drayton, A. (2013). Nursing onboard mercy class naval hospital ships. *Journal of Emergency Nursing, 39*(6), 581–590. doi:10.1016/j.jen.2013.08.006

Dremsa-Brewer, T. (2003). CCATT nurses' deployed experience. TSNRP funded study abstract. Retrieved from https://www.usuhs.edu/node/3488

Elliott, B. (2015). Military nurses' experiences returning from war. *Journal of Advanced Nursing, 71*(5), 1066–1075. doi:10.1111/jan.12588

Gehring, J. (2005). Nursing, core values, and caring during Operation Iraqi Freedom. Retrieved from https://www.usuhs.edu/node/3424

King, H. (2015). Global Health Engagement Missions: Lessons learned aboard US naval hospital ships. TSNRP funded study abstract. Retrieved from https://www.usuhs.edu/tsnrp/funded-study/global-health-engagement-missions-lessons-learned-aboard-us-naval-hospital-ships

Knebel, A. R., Martinelli, A. M., Orsega, S., Doss, T. L., Balingit-Wines, A. M., & Konchan, C. L. (2010). Ground zero recollections of US Public Health Service nurses deployed to New York City in September 2001. *Nursing Clinics of North America, 45*(2), 137–152. doi:10.1016/j.cnur.2010.02.010

McNeill, P. (2006). Critical care performance in a simulated military aircraft cabin environment. TSNRP funded study abstract. Retrieved from https://www.usuhs.edu/node/3534

McNeill, M. M., Pierce, P., Dukes, S., & Bridges, E. J. (2014). En route care patient safety: Thoughts from the field. *Military Medicine, 179*(8), 11–18. doi:10.7205/MILMED-D-13-00522

Mortimer, D. (2005). Wartime critical care ground transport problems. Retrieved from http://131.158.7.207/cgi-bin/tsnrp/search_studies.cgi?id=268

Mosquera, A., Braun, M., Hulett, M., & Ryszka, L. (2015). U.S. Public Health Service Response to the 2014–2015 Ebola Epidemic in West Africa: A Nursing Perspective. *Public Health Nursing, 32*(5), 550–554. doi:10.1111/phn.12217

Rivers, F. M., Dukes, S., Hatzfeld, J., Yoder, L. H., Gordon, S., & Simmons, A. (2017). Understanding post-deployment reintegration concerns among en route care nurses: A mixed-methods approach. *Military Medicine, 182*, 243–250. doi:10.7205/MILMED-D-16-00209

Rivers, F. M., Gordon, S., Speraw, S., & Reese, S. (2013). U.S. Army nurses' reintegration and homecoming experiences after Iraq and Afghanistan. *Military Medicine, 178*(2), 166–173. doi:10.7205/MILMED-D-12-00279

Tyree-Debisette, A., Riley Brown, C., & Chamberlain, N. (2006). A nursing perspective from United States Public Health Service nurses. *Journal of Professional Nursing, 22*(5), 270–272. doi:10.1016/j.profnurs.2006.07.011

Walker, S. G., Ward, J. B., Montalvo, M., Cunliffe, C., Beadling, C., & Riley, K. (2011). A new paradigm for military humanitarian medical operations: Mission-generic metrics. *Military Medicine, 176*(8), 845–851.

Yates, M. (2005). Medical-surgical nurses volunteer to aid tsunami victims. *MEDSURG Nursing, 14*(5), 331–334.

CASE STUDY 38.2

Department of Veterans Affairs

The mission of the U.S. Department of Veterans Affairs (VA) is to provide care for and honor our nation's veterans. A "Fourth Mission" is to "ensure care and continuity of operations during emergencies and disasters and to support local, state, and national all-hazards planning and response under the National Response Framework" (VA, 2014, 2015). The Veterans Emergency Management Evaluation Center (VEMEC) was established in 2010 to support VA's "Fourth Mission" with a focus on establishing a scientific evidence base and on researching best practices (VA,

2017a). Recent work includes research and practice in the areas of nursing leadership roles, home-based primary care and veterans' level of preparedness, VA communications during disasters, veterans' disaster resiliency, and nonprofit organizations' ability to serve veterans during disasters (VA, 2017b). Dobalian, Claver, Riopelle, Wyte-Lake, & Canelo (2017) recently published a comprehensive research agenda that proposed research questions for behavioral health, workforce, resiliency, continuity of operations, and communications.

(*continued*)

CASE STUDY 38.2 (*continued*)

REFERENCES

Dobalian, A., Claver, M., Riopelle, D., Wyte-Lake, T., & Canelo, I. (2017). The development of a Veterans Health Administration emergency management research agenda. *PLOS Currents Disasters*, Edition 1. doi:0.1371/currents.dis.c0c84b1b680388649227be71823e6adf

United States Department of Veterans Affairs. (2014). FY 2014-2020 strategic plan. Washington, DC: Author. Retrieved from https://www.data.va.gov/dataset/department-veterans-affairs-fy-2014-2020-strategic-plan

United States Department of Veterans Affairs. (2015). VHA Office of Emergency Management. Retrieved from https://www.va.gov/VHAEMERGENCYMANAGEMENT/OEM_About.asp

United States Department of Veterans Affairs. (2017a). Community preparedness & response. Retrieved from https://www.publichealth.va.gov/about/vemec/projects/

United States Department of Veterans Affairs. (2017b). VEMEC: About us. Retrieved from https://www.publichealth.va.gov/about/vemec/index.asp

39

IMPROVING CHILDREN'S HEALTH OUTCOMES THROUGH PEDIATRIC DISASTER RESEARCH AND POLICY

Janice B. Griffin Agazio

LEARNING OBJECTIVES

When this chapter is completed, readers will be able to:

1. Discuss the impact of disasters on children since the September 11 (9/11) terrorist attacks.
2. Discuss findings from research detailing the impact of disasters on children.
3. Identify the challenges of designing and conducting research with children during the phases of disaster prevention, preparedness, response, and recovery.
4. Determine the value of both qualitative and quantitative methods to the conduct of research in disaster situations.
5. Discuss the challenges of identifying evidence-based intervention strategies.
6. Identify gaps in the research in studying the effects of disasters on children.
7. Articulate lessons learned in preparing for the next disaster and best practices in preparing responders for pediatric care.

KEY MESSAGES

Children may be more susceptible to the mental health effects of disasters due to exposure to death and destruction, but many symptoms resolve over time.

Cross-culturally, and across different types of disasters, commonalities exist in the response and
duration of children's symptomatology in the short and long term.

Environmental and protective factors may mitigate posttraumatic symptoms (PTS) in children by
1 year postdisaster.

Most strategies developed to date for short- and long-term intervention have limited research support.

Challenges exist to conducting research into the impact of disasters on children and adolescents.

CHAPTER OVERVIEW

*Disasters are increasing in their frequency and intensity with
some more devastating than ever before. The magnitude may
appear more impactful due to the immediacy of media coverage and the Internet. In the years since the 9/11 tragedy,
children have been exposed to the devastation of hurricanes,
tsunamis, earthquakes, floods, and other natural disasters
and human-made disasters of genocide, war, terrorism, and
epidemics. In 2017 alone, the world witnessed multiple disaster
events including the devastation of Hurricanes Harvey, Irma,
and Maria in Texas, Florida, across the Caribbean and Puerto
Rico and the Virgin Islands, a 7.1 magnitude earthquake in
Mexico, a mass shooting in Las Vegas, and massive landslides
and flooding in Sri Lanka, Southeast Asia, and Sierra Leone
with significant loss of life.*

*Disasters are defined as "a calamitous event that generally
involves an injury of loss of life and destruction of property . . .
[affecting] both small and large populations" (Hagan, the
Committee on Psychosocial Aspects of Child and Family Health,
& the Task Force on Terrorism, 2005, p. 787). Research on
children following these events has resulted in findings that
increase awareness of healthcare professionals for resultant
symptomology and effects, plus provide an impetus and direction
for interventions. The sentinel events of September 11, 2001,
as noted by Lengua, Long, Smith, and Meltzoff (2005), had
"a dramatic effect on most U.S. citizens and on individuals
worldwide" and many studies have considered the immediate
and lasting effects of this disaster on both adults and children
in subsequent research.*

*Since 2001, the wars in Afghanistan and Iraq have affected
millions of families and children as parents have been deployed,
many repeatedly, for varying amounts of time separating them
from their children at various points in their development to
unclear long-term effects. In addition, many children have lost
a parent or greeted one parent returning home with posttraumatic stress disorder (PTSD), amputations, or recovering from
other physical or psychological injuries. Research addressing
children's adjustments to parental deployments and separations
as well as addressing military member and spousal readjust-
ment document the impact as these conflicts conclude (Agazio,
Goodman, & Padden, 2014; Padden & Agazio, 2013). Osofsky
and Chartrand (2013) note that while the stress of military
deployment cannot "be equated with the experience of disaster, certain similarities exist—for example, heightened family
distress, disruption of family support systems and schedules,
and an impact on parenting" (pp. 68–69).*

*Children are traumatized beyond witnessing disasters in
person. Lengua et al. (2005) demonstrated that effects may
occur and persist even when children are geographically
removed from the disaster itself. These researchers were
already conducting a study on child, family, and contextual
influences on children's development prior to the 9/11 attacks.
Following up with the same instrumentation 6 months afterward, children in Seattle, exposed at a distance to the 9/11
events, demonstrated persistent PTSD symptoms and worries
while controlling for any preattack symptomology. In 2013,
many children watched the Boston Marathon bombing unfold
in real time on news channels, where three people were killed
including a school-aged child, and 264 others were injured,
16 of whom later required amputations (Comer et al., 2014).
Children were exposed to the intensive media coverage of the
manhunt that followed and then could relive the event in a
popular 2017 movie Patriot's Day, Similarly, multiple movies
and documentaries made about other disasters such as 9/11,
for example, Fahrenheit 9/11, World Trade Center, and United
93, or the Phuket tsunami, The Impossible, make these distant
events appear real and immediate. Saylor, Cowart, Lipovsky,
Jackson, and Finch (2003) surveyed 179 Grade K–5 students
and their parents at four Southwestern schools 1 month after
9/11 using the Pediatric Emotional Distress scale, the Parent
Response of Post-Traumatic Symptoms, and the children's
report of PTS to assess effects of media exposure via the
Internet, TV, and print media. Interestingly, as expected,
higher levels of PTSD symptoms were detected with increased
exposure to negative images. What was not expected was that
a comparable level of symptoms occurred in conjunction with
exposure to positive images as well. The authors concluded
that "greater amounts of exposure, both positive and negative,
correspond with more PTSD symptoms" (p. 1636). While not
necessarily a direct link of causation, other factors could have
been influential, such as distressed parents may have watched
more about the event, thus the child could have picked up
the parental response in conjunction with the media images.
They noted that more research is needed in this area, especially in guiding parents and teachers regarding children's
media exposure. These results mirrored that of Mijanovich
and Weitzman (2010) who also analyzed data collected post
9/11 that included 10- to 18-year-old youths, distant to the
actual events, who displayed symptoms of emotional distress
following the disaster. Man-made disasters such as these not
only traumatize those in the immediate area, but there may
also be a distance effect for children through media exposure
(Sharlin, Moin, & Yahav, 2006).*

WHY ARE CHILDREN'S RESPONSES DIFFERENT FROM ADULTS IN DISASTERS?

In children, physiological, cognitive, and developmental differences may provide a dissimilar picture of effects than that of adults and need to be accounted for in terms of intervention, prevention, and education. Physical injuries may occur that may also affect children differently than adults. Burke, Iverson, Goodhue, Neches, and Upperman (2010) point out the obvious that children are smaller than adults meaning that what treatments work, and what equipment is needed in adults, do not necessarily translate into appropriateness for children. A different skill set is also needed for the providers to scale down for appropriate interventions, doses, and procedures to treat children's needs.

Physically, children are at different stages in their maturation and abilities. Fendya (2006) provides a description of physiological differences that may impact on pediatric care during a disaster. Depending on the age of the child, head size may predispose a child to more susceptibility to head or neck trauma. Explosive events such as the Boston bombing may expose a child to more head and neck trauma due to falling, or the amount of debris dispersed. Their weaker neck muscles, as well as a proportionally larger tongue, can also be risk factors in ventilation as positioning can cause compression of the airway. Children may respond differently if exposed to toxic agents and, mechanically, production of mucus and other secretions may more easily block their airways. Children have more immature ventilatory structures, such as fewer alveoli for gas exchange; higher oxygen demands; and faster respiratory rates so that hypoxemia may occur more quickly with fewer compensatory mechanisms as would be found in an adult. Their normally faster respiration rate will contribute to quicker absorption of hazardous materials, for example, in a chemical or aerosolized event. Children have a smaller total circulating blood flow, so are at more risk of hypovolemia in situations of blood loss. However, in cases of hemorrhage, increased heart rate and peripheral constriction may act to compensate for blood loss and perhaps "effectively mask impending shock" (p. 164). Abdominal organs are more at risk for injury due to a more cartilaginous rib cage providing less protection for a proportionately larger liver and spleen. While the skin provides an effective barrier to infection and thermoregulation, the skin of a child comparably covers a larger area than that of an adult putting them at higher risk to heat and fluid loss when injured, especially by cold, burns, or chemical agents.

Developmentally and emotionally, children are also at risk. Fendya (2006, p. 164) notes that a child's response to disaster is dependent upon "psychological maturity, prior experiences of the child, coping skills, the emotional well-being of the parent or caretaker, and supportive resources." Age, cognitive level, and ego strength also factor in developmentally to how much children will comprehend about the circumstances of a disaster and their survival and coping abilities. Burke et al. (2010) also point out that younger children may not have the motor skills to be able to remove themselves from hazardous situations and the cognitive ability to recognize dangerous circumstances, and in fact may move toward the danger if looking for a parent or familiar environment. Coping skills are also less well developed that may lead to psychological reactions following the event that can have long-lasting implications such as PTSD, anxiety, or other issues.

The American Association of Pediatrics Workgroup on Disasters has detailed stages of children's emotional responses to disasters. First, in the immediate occurrence, children may react with "fright, disbelief, denial, grief, and feelings of relief if loved ones have not been harmed" (Hagan et al., 2005, p. 791). A few days to several weeks after the event, the second stage begins where children may display regressive behaviors and continued signs of emotional distress to include depression, fear, anxiety, apathy, hostility, sleep disturbances, and aggressive behaviors. These symptoms may persist and professional intervention such as counseling is appropriate, especially for extreme distress or persistent symptoms. Research has shown that symptomology more than 1 month after the event may lead to development of PTSD or other persistent behavioral disorders such as acting out, violence, and depression.

In general, developmentally, children react differently depending on their age. For infants, the loss of their routine activities and consistent care provider may lead to "regression and detachment" (Hagan et al., 2005). Being too young to understand what is happening and not being able to understand, nor verbalize, infants and toddlers exhibit their distress through crying, sleep disturbances, irritability, separation anxiety, and an exaggerated startle response (Hagan et al., 2005). Toddlers and preschoolers may regress to earlier stages of dependence with bedwetting, separation anxiety, nightmares, and night terrors. Younger school-aged children, while old enough to understand explanations, tend to focus on specific details of the event and personal safety concerns. Older school-aged children are able to grasp more ramifications regarding the scope of injuries and loss of life and display more "empathy for families who were affected by the crisis, have a greater willingness to analyze how or why a tragedy occurred, and focus more on the safety of the society as a whole" (Hagan et al., 2005, p. 791). Reactions may include both internalizing and externalizing behaviors as they respond to the event.

In addition to age and developmental differences, Hagan et al. (2005) also note that there may be gender, cultural, and other risk factors for how children react to disasters. Boys tend to display more externalizing behavioral symptoms and take longer to recover emotionally. Cultural aspects may influence reaction such as, after 9/11, individuals of Middle Eastern origin felt a negative reaction of racism and bigotry directed toward them and were targeted for violent attacks despite being U.S. citizens. Those who have experienced previous violence, such as through abuse, war, or disasters, are at risk for more adverse reactions, such as those who had survived Hurricane Katrina (2005) only to then face further risk and evacuation during the oil spill, or those families in Sri Lanka whose country was in turmoil for years before the earthquake and tsunami. Children who have less stable home environments, lower social support, or have experienced other losses are also at particular increased risk for long-term emotional consequences, such as those involved in Hurricane Katrina already struggling with poverty in New Orleans. Evacuation became particularly traumatic for these families with no means of leaving the city ahead of the storm and fewer opportunities once the streets were flooded and escape routes clogged.

RESEARCHING CHILDREN EXPERIENCING DISASTERS

Challenges exist to conducting research regarding the impact of disasters on children and adolescents. As noted by Masten and Osofsky (2010), disasters occur without warning and with such devastation that trying to conduct research in the midst of those circumstances poses ethical dilemmas as well as logistical challenges. They also point out that research under these conditions can pose danger to the researcher as well as further harm to those affected in the disaster. In an ideal situation, predisaster conditions would be measured to compare to postdisaster responses. That naturally is difficult when most disasters are not predictable. Although, serendipitously, as previously mentioned, the Seattle study of children and families was concurrent with the disaster and had comparative data for school-aged children's reactions pre- and post-9/11 as part of a larger study started before the attacks (Lengua et al., 2005). Similarly, an early study of Kenyan children was started prior to the eruption of violence in that country that provided baseline data for preschoolers (Kithakye, Morris, Terranova, & Myers, 2010).

Pfefferbaum et al. (2013) conducted a comprehensive review of methods used to research children's disaster responses across 165 reports that included 83 publications from the 9/11 attacks, 29 regarding the 2004 Indian Ocean tsunami; and 53 on Hurricane Katrina. Predominantly, cross-sectional studies were the most frequent design used to study the effects of disasters on children. They note that some researchers were able to pull pre-event data for comparison either through archival sources or from nondisaster studies. Studies were noted to use qualitative designs, either through individual interviews or focus groups with children or adolescents. In their review, Pfefferbaum et al. noted that most of the research was conducted within 12 months of the event with a few studies being longitudinal.

Pfefferbaum et al. (2013) emphasized that determining the time between measurements needs to be carefully planned so that reactions occurring across the trajectory are not lost due to too much time between intervals. They also noted that baseline information may also be available if data were collected prior to, or predisaster, as part of another study. Access to children who have directly experienced the disaster should be limited. Sampling across the studies examined in the Pfefferbaum and others' review was obtained through convenience-, purposive-, random-, and census-sampling methods. Some of the research targeted specific ethnic groups, geographical location, type or severity of disaster exposure, or age groups. They also noted that most of the research considered individual, family, and social factors that could be linked to children's reactions and adjustments. Due to sampling constraints, most often they found that the studies were predictive or correlational in nature and not able to determine cause and effect determinations, a weakness inherent in most disaster research. The team further compared the studies for themes among the variables of interest. Some were focused upon children's direct exposure to the event versus others that were from indirect through media coverage and content. Studies were broken down between those with interpersonal exposure such as through a caregiver that could include loss or injury to someone close or known to the child. Outcomes included in the studies were directed primarily toward negative reactions and concerns although a small body of research is developing to include posttraumatic growth and how children overcome trauma. Some of these studies have focused upon the results of interventional research and programs directed toward mitigating disaster effects.

CHILDREN'S REACTIONS TO DISASTER

Sharlin et al. (2006) focused on the short- and long-term symptoms of fear in 747 Israeli students in their study to determine the effects of the threat of prolonged terrorist attacks. None of the children had previously experienced or witnessed a terror attack directly; however, living in Haifa, the threat of an attack was ever present. Data were collected following three attacks occurring over the course of the study in Israel. Using instruments to measure children's reaction to terror and the Child Behavioral Checklist, the study found that "prolonged terror" did not lead to pathological behavioral problems detected in the children's self-reports. The rate of fear overall was relatively low and, as noted by the authors, "most children understood the dangers to terror, yet they were not overly preoccupied by this" (p. 102). In addition, new terror attacks were not noted to increase fears within the repeated measures over time. The authors attributed the findings to perhaps some habituation to living under this threat, or to perhaps some adaptation as a defense mechanism. They recommended further research to discern individual internal responses, possible internal consequences, or projections of fear onto the parents as a coping mechanism.

Following Hurricane Katrina, Kronenberg et al. (2010) assessed the trauma symptoms, recovery patterns, and life stresses of 387 children between the ages of 9 and 18 using the National Child Traumatic Stress Network Hurricane Assessment and Referral tool for children and adolescents. The study focused on the reactions of children from a severely impacted area 2 to 3 years after the hurricane and hypothesized that PTS recovery would vary based on demographic factors such as age, gender, and life stresses. Participants were assessed each school year over a 3-year period beginning immediately after the hurricane. The authors demonstrated that PTSD and depression symptoms decreased over time and that the experience was related to gender and age. Younger children and women scored higher on depression and PTSD scales. Life stressor variables were not significant predictors for PTSD or depression. Consultation with a mental health professional and endorsement of family and school support were identified as positive influences upon recovery from the trauma. The findings of this study provided a hopeful picture for children exposed to the devastation of Katrina and the stress resistance demonstrated in the decreasing symptomology over time.

Following up on the effects of Katrina, Lai, Kelley, Harrison, Thompson, and Self-Brown (2015) used latent profile analysis to identify typologies of distress for 353 children aged 8 to 15 who were living in southern Louisiana during Katrina and were assessed at 3 to 7 months and 14 to 17 months after the storm. Arguing that many studies have considered only one diagnostic symptom, this study examined co-occurrence of posttraumatic stress, anxiety and depression, school problems, life threat and loss/disruption, and mitigating variables of social support and exposure to community and family violence. This study was particularly interesting for the typology of symptoms the researchers identified indicating perhaps a group of children at particular risk who may need early and continued interventions. Like many postdisaster research studies, the largest group of children experienced only a minimal number of symptoms. Twenty percent of the children fell into a group with PTS only; that percentage was also comparable to other research in the literature. However, unique to this study, a third group of children were identified who displayed moderate PTS along with high anxiety and depression. This third group was displaying symptoms a year after the hurricane with similar school and behavioral difficulties as those who fell initially into the high PTS group. The children in both of these high-risk groups had similar risk factors to include "perceived life threat, immediate loss and disruption, and community violence exposure," (p. 1266) that, according to the researchers, support the need to assess for these risk factors as these may be predictive of continued difficulties in postdisaster symptomology. Another interesting finding was that children who had strong parental support were less likely to fall into the mixed category and were more often in the PTS-only group if there were symptoms postdisaster. This would indicate that there is a protective, or mitigating, factor in developing internalizing symptoms when social support is present.

Not all children escaped unscathed despite the hopeful findings from these reported studies. McLaughlin et al. (2009) administered a telephone survey to 797 parents of children 4 to 17 years of age who were contacted in the Federal Emergency Management Administration–defined disaster area affected by Hurricane Katrina. Data were collected in three waves: first, 5 to 7 months after the disaster; at 7 to 10 months; and finally, 15 to 19 months afterward. Surveys employed included the Strength and Difficulties Questionnaire for identifying serious emotional disturbances; a hurricane-related stressors questionnaire; and sociodemographic factors. Serious emotional disturbances were identified in almost 15% of the sample. As in other studies, 80% of this sample was stressed by the loss of housing as well as housing adversity and loss of a loved one. According to the study, "virtually all" of the serious emotional disturbance occurred in the youth with multiple hurricane-related stressors that were exacerbated by low income levels. The prevalence remained high at the final measurement time point suggesting a need for intensive mental health services and that distress can persist, at least for these participants, up to 2 years after the event. Osofsky, Kronenberg, Bocknek, and Hansel (2015) identified similar risk factors for persistence of symptomology in their study of 914 younger children, aged 3 to 5 years at the time of Hurricane Katrina. Focusing primarily upon effects from attachment, like older children in the previous study, those with additional family and environmental risk factors found that symptomology could persist over a longer time, but for the most part, the younger children symptomology would decrease over time and, as they commented, may speak to the child's resilience and ability to "rebound following disaster" (p. 506).

Reviewing the literature, multiple studies were located for post-Katrina assessments for its effects on children. Madrid, Grant, Reilly, and Redlener (2006), who were staff in the National Center for Disaster Preparedness at Columbia's Mailman School of Public Health, launched Operation Assist to coordinate and organize medical, mental, and public health efforts during the immediate and long-term recovery and dispatched mobile medical units to the more hard-hit areas. Reporting on the experiences and findings from their work with families, their paper offers a 10-week overview of the needs and care provided during this period. From their experiences, they developed several recommendations to mitigate and promote resilient child outcomes. In the immediate period following the disaster, these recommendations included "rapid family reunification; helping families recognize strengths and resources; assisting evacuee integration to the community; … proactive measures to cope with losses and changes; … ready access to basic human needs; [and] treating individuals with respect and dignity …" (p. S452).

Dolan and Krug (2006) reiterated many of these same recommendations in describing lessons learned during Katrina. They described the situation in New Orleans in the days after the hurricane where many children were found alone looking for family members. During their journeys to find their loved ones, the children would pass dead bodies of humans and animals floating in the water to add to their mental distress. Evacuation buses separated families who assumed when they placed members in the seats that they would end up at the same evacuation point. Difficulties were especially evident in locating parents for younger children who could not share their names or verbalize descriptions of their parents and previous address. The authors described scenarios of rescue personnel circulating digital photographs taken of children at evacuation points to try to match children with parents. Dolan and Krug cited a case in Sri Lanka as an example of an infant boy who was claimed by nine sets of parents following the tsunami. DNA testing eventually had to be used to establish accurate parentage. Similarly, Jemtrud, Rhoades, and Gabbai (2010) noted that the average age of the Katrina-separated child was 5.7 years of age and had been relocated multiple times in the evacuation process before there was time to start reunification efforts. By that time, the child may have been the only informant and too young to provide reliable details. Sadly by January 2006, months after the disaster, there were still several hundred children who had not been reunited (Dolan & Krug, 2006). Multiple researchers and responders have urged development of strategies that would improve early and accurate reunification in planning for future disasters (Dolan & Krug, 2006; Jemtrud et al., 2010). In addition, they urged improved strategies as well for non–English-speaking children, developmentally and culturally appropriate mental health interventions, and considerations for evacuation of community-based and hospitalized children with special needs and technology dependence. Osofsky, Osofsky, Weems, King, and Hansel (2015) add to these recommendations with a focus upon preparation in communities prior to disaster.

Pfefferbaum, Tucker, and Nitiema (2015) focused upon adolescents in their comparison pilot study between 14

African Americans who had relocated to Oklahoma after direct exposure to Hurricane Katrina and nine African American youth who were from a local urban community with no direct exposure. This study combined psychometric assessment of PTSD symptomology, depression, and externalizing behaviors with physiological measures of cortisol and dexamethasone suppression 19 to 29 months after the event. Compared to community participants, the survivors demonstrated higher PTSD and depressive symptoms and lower morning levels of cortisol. Perhaps due to the small sample size, the study failed to detect differences in cortisol suppression between the two groups, even though it was hypothesized that the stress experienced by the Katrina survivors and resultant symptoms would show an effect on the hypothalamic–pituitary–adrenal (HPA) axis. Since the HPA axis is a major part of the body's response to stress, exploring the physiological correlates of stress response has previously indicated some dysregulation, but with limited research to date, this relationship has not been conclusively established. Weems (2015) cites further studies exploring physiological responses to disaster and long-term consequences. Work in this area is ongoing with links being tracked in central nervous systems effects hormonal responses, and psychophysiology such as changes in vagal tone related to disaster reactions.

In a qualitative approach using phenomenology, 15 adolescents, between 12 and 17 years of age, who had been exposed to Hurricane Katrina and were all relocated to the Baton Rouge area, participated in face-to-face interviews to describe the lived experiences and behavioral changes experienced as a result of the disaster (Mearidy-Bell, 2013). After the disaster, the participants identified isolation and withdrawal, increased arguments, avoidance of relationships, and overprotectiveness as behavioral changes they experienced. Some also noted using excessive eating and sleeping as behaviors that changed after the hurricane. The participants described the lived experiences of the hurricane as changes they had to make in their lives such as changing homes, schools, and communities. Some noted that parents lost their jobs in many cases due to the relocation and others had lost loved ones or friends in the disaster. These stresses led to more arguments with family members and pulling back emotionally from making new friends and being more watchful over family members to protect from any harm. Studies such as this can lend insight into the quantitative findings as these adolescents shared stories and thoughts behind some of the behaviors described in other studies.

Super Storm Sandy struck the east coast, Canada, and the Caribbean in 2012. Quinn et al. (2016) recruited a convenience sample of 141 children in New Jersey to complete the National Child Traumatic Stress Network (NCTSN) Hurricane Stressor assessment tool for children and adolescents in an online study 15 to 20 months after the storm. Younger children completed the scale with parental assistance. The research was concerned that these particular results could have reflected parental influence on the findings as at least 35% of the preschoolers were reported to have significant behavioral changes after the storm such as increased worry and clinginess. Additional results were grouped by age category and reflected findings similar to those previously discussed for older children. These participants were heavily affected as 82.5% reported

homes that were damaged or destroyed in the storm. Many of the school-aged and adolescent participants reported struggles in classroom behaviors such as difficulty concentrating, falling grades, and not being able to complete their work. As well, the school-aged and adolescent children expressed increased anxiety regarding the possibility of another super storm coming, especially when hearing weather reports.

After the Boston bombing, Comer et al. (2014) surveyed 460 Boston area parents regarding their children's functioning in the 6 months after the attack regarding the amount and type of exposure and effects upon resultant psychosocial functioning. Outreach was made through schools, community advertisement, and local pediatrician offices to reach families living within a 25-mile radius of the bombing to ask parents to complete an online survey. The sample included 15% who attended the marathon; 47% who saw an increased presence of heavy police presence in their neighborhood; and 100% who experienced the shelter-in-place order. Several who attended the marathon had seen some of the injured and dead and all were part of the mass evacuation from the scene. Approximately 11% of those attending displayed PTS that was at a rate about six times more than those not in attendance. One interesting aspect of this study was the inclusion of how much media exposure the children experienced during the newscast of the bombing and subsequent manhunt. Most parents did not limit TV exposure and reported up to 3 hours of coverage during the day of the bombing. Despite being distant from the actual events, children in both groups displayed PTS. The conclusion of the study was to provide a caution to broaden clinical efforts of assessment and intervention to those who may indirectly be affected by the disaster itself, especially those exposed to in-the-moment coverage that may appear to imply a threat in the immediate environs of these children.

Findings in disaster research with children seem to be consistent cross-culturally. Children who were exposed to a 1998 hurricane in Puerto Rico were compared to those who were not. These children displayed internalizing symptoms postdisaster exposure that persisted even at 18 months, although most had diminished by 30 months after the event (Felix et al., 2011). McDermott, Cobham, Berry, and Kim (2014) screened 71 children and 191 adolescents after a category 5 cyclone disaster in Australia at approximately 3 months (T1) and then at 18 months (T2) following exposure. As in previous studies, a majority (81.2%) of children and adolescents displayed no to mild symptoms at time 1 and time 2. For those identified as having moderate to severe PTS at time 1, the majority had resolved these symptoms at the 18-month time period (55%). These authors had completed a previous study with children following the tsunami in 2004 with similar findings. Implications from studies demonstrating these findings include a hopeful outcome for children. They note that most children, even if demonstrating PTS 3 months after a disaster, have a high possibility of resolving symptoms unless exposed to another trauma or disaster. In contrast, children who remain symptomatic at 3 months have a 30% to 45% chance of remaining symptomatic long term, especially if not treated effectively at the time of the trauma. Based on their findings, McDermott et al. (2014) recommend that, if severe to very severe symptoms are detected at the time of the event, a formal mental health assessment should be triggered postevent to intervene early to prevent chronicity. Lieber (2017) described the effects of the 2011 Japan combined disaster of earthquake, tsunami, and radiation meltdown for 3,650 elementary and middle school children. Interestingly in Japan, most mental healthcare has been provided in private facilities focused upon more long-term care. Their systems failed as a result of the need to intervene in a more community-based response. In contrast to other studies, this study found that younger children were more at risk for higher distress symptoms that suggested a greater need for increased intervention for the aged child as well. Yonekura, Ueno, and Iwanaka (2013) provided further lessons learned from the unusual triple disaster that stressed existing medical systems and emergency response on so many fronts with a variety of injuries from radiation exposure, earthquake injuries, and tsunami devastation.

Jia et al. (2010) explored the effects of the 2008 Sichuan earthquake upon 596 children between the ages of 8 and 16 years who were in the severely affected areas of the quake. Their findings mirror those from other studies in terms of the amount, type, and duration of the PTS following the disaster. Interestingly in this study, the authors addressed findings in previous research that found ethnic minorities to be disproportionally affected by disasters such as in Hurricane Katrina where the ethnic makeup of New Orleans was around 60% African American at the time. They specifically examined differences in Han versus other ethnic groups in the affected area of China and found that the minorities "possessed possibly stronger resilience" than the Han, or dominant cultural group (p. 1387), which could possibly be a finding requiring further study. Navarro et al. (2016) also noted cross-cultural similarities in their study when comparing psychological symptoms between 494 Louisiana children experiencing Hurricane Katrina and 333 Chilean children who experienced the 2010 earthquake and tsunami. The authors noted that findings, even though occurring in different parts of the world, emphasize the importance of having supportive behavioral health services available (p. 552).

PARENTAL INFLUENCES ON CHILDREN'S REACTIONS TO DISASTERS

A separate body of research literature has considered how parental reactions affect children experiencing a disaster and several examples will be discussed here. Proctor et al. (2007) included 117 two-parent families with a child aged 4 to 5 at the time of the Northridge earthquake in Los Angeles in 1994. As is usual in studies that possess pre-event data, this study was ongoing at the time of the quake with the focus upon family conflict using behavioral observations of parental interactions. Approximately 8 months after the quake, parents were mailed surveys that assessed quake exposure and individual and family functioning and were asked to respond to each item twice, once for reactions within the first month after the event and the second to reflect up to 8 months afterward. The majority of the families had been affected by the earthquake (85%) with 59% experiencing home damage, loss of possessions (50%), and financial impacts (39%). Children demonstrated distress both

at the first month reflection (90.7%) and at the eighth month (71.8%) to include fear, difficulty in sleeping, and recurrent worries and thoughts about the quake. In using parental distress as a moderator variable in a regression equation, the mother's distress was found to be a significant predictor of persistent distress in the girls whereas for boys, neither father nor mother distress predicted their distress. Earthquake impact significantly predicted both parental and child distress for both genders. What was most interesting about the study were the mediating effects noted between pre-earthquake parenting behaviors related to the earthquake impact and children's persistent distress. These authors caution that more work is needed in this area to discern how parental reactions and parenting behaviors can affect children's responses to disaster. They pointed out that many studies usually include just an individual focus and the effects are most likely more multidimensional and should involve family context as an important variable. In contrast, Kilic, Ozguven, and Sayil (2003) found more influence from father behavior such as detachment and irritability related to more significant impact on children's symptoms.

Comparably, Kelley et al. (2010) examined the effect of parental distress and parenting practices on children following Hurricane Katrina including 381 parent–child dyads from New Orleans and neighboring parishes during the storm. Using a combination of instruments, measures were completed twice: at 3 to 7 months and 14 to 17 months post-Katrina. Using path analysis, beyond detailing effects upon the children that were comparable to other studies, a path "emerged indicating that children who reported more hurricane loss had parents who reported more maladaptive coping and, in turn, these parents were more likely to use corporal punishment, which increased their children's risk for PTSD symptoms in T1 and T2" (p. 588). This finding supported previous work in the area that suggests that poor parenting behaviors may exacerbate children's PTS postdisasters perhaps due to less positive social support. The use of corporal punishment, used as a proxy for harsher parenting styles, can "elevate child anxiety" and thus not provide a mediating or moderating presence to offset the effects of the disaster (p. 588). Endo (2007) and others had analogous findings in their study of 288 children following the 2004 Japan earthquake in relating adverse parental mental health related to the children's behavioral problems postdisaster. Another factor found to predict higher PTSD in adolescents were parents who displayed overprotectiveness and excessive control postdisaster in their own coping (Bokszczanin, 2008). In contrast, Sriskandarajah, Neuner, and Catani (2015) found protective factors provided by parents that promoted recovery in the children whereby the overprotective behavior of the parents was perceived as caring behavior. The difference could perhaps have a cultural overlay as this latter study was conducted in Sri Lanka and the former in Poland. The findings from this battery of research studies suggest that parental coping has an impact on child recovery and resolution of symptoms and needs more research to discern the multiple factors of parental influence.

Sadly, many children lose one or both parents in a disaster. Kalantari and Vostanis (2010) reached out to 86 children 7 to 13 years of age who experienced such a loss in the 2004 Bam earthquake in Iran. Using the Strengths and Difficulties questionnaire and self-report questionnaire, children who had lost either a father (48.8%), mother (25.6%), or both parents were compared to a control group that had not experienced such a loss. For those who had a surviving parent, there was a significant correlation between the surviving parent's mental health problems and the degree of the children's behavioral and emotional problems. For the remaining parent, mental health issues were predicted from variables of governmental support and house rebuilding, indicating that these were highly stressed families due to loss coupled with economic difficulties. While not surprising that loss of a parent would be related to symptomology in the children, the findings provided a clear research implication for early and continued intervention for these children at particular risk.

RESEARCH-BASED INTERVENTIONS WITH CHILDREN EXPOSED TO DISASTERS

Pfefferbaum, Newman, and Nitiema (2016) recently published a review of intervention strategies and their comparative effectiveness. They noted that these interventions have focused on enhancing pre-event resilience and skill building as well as coping strategies useful during and after the crisis. Some interventions are effective in disaster preparation, such as in school-based programs, while others are more individually focused. Postdisaster programs have been studied with some limited findings on effectiveness. For example, psychosocial first aid (PFA) was shown to decrease psychological symptoms slightly in a school-based program following diverse traumatic events. Debriefing has also been used postdisaster, but only a few studies have been conducted with children using this strategy. Methodological differences in how debriefing has been used in children have prevented any definitive recommendations for how and when to use this strategy. The same is true for inconclusive studies of using psychoeducation, a technique where "information about an event or situation, potential reactions, coping and available services and resources" are part of an informational package (p. 194). Cognitive behavioral interventions have been the mainstay of most child disaster treatment. Two manualized interventions, Cognitive Behavioral Intervention for Trauma in Schools and Trauma-Focused Cognitive Behavioral Therapy have been used successfully for children with severe to moderate PTSD symptoms, although children with at-risk levels of PTSD months out from the event may need additional services and individualized therapies. This modality seems particularly useful in the first year following the disaster, as La Greca and Silverman (2009) determined that most children recover within that period. Other interventions they included as possible strategies are stress management and stress reduction practices, grief and traumatic grief interventions, and psychopharmacological medications with some promising results. A Cochrane Review meta-analysis of child PTSD from disaster exposures did not identify one treatment as superior to any other and found the evidence amassed to date to be "fair," indicating that much work still needs to be done to find efficacious and effective interventions to help children experiencing disasters (Gillies, Taylor, Gray, O'Brien, & D'Abrew, 2013).

La Greca and Silverman (2009) offered a helpful typology in their review of treatment options. They advised conceptualizing the interventions as those designed for the immediate aftermath; for short-term recovery; or focused upon the long term. In the immediacy of the disaster, besides focusing upon physical safety, according to these authors, the most effective interventions are those that are "brief and present focused ... [with a goal to] reduce or prevent long-term psychological difficulties" (p. 4). Strategies in this period would include critical incident debriefing, psychological first aid, and use of psychoeducational materials. For the most part, research-based evidence on the effectiveness of these interventions is unfortunately limited to scant, although PFA and the educational focus are promising (Gillies et al., 2013; La Greca & Silverman, 2009; Newman et al., 2014). Short-term recovery modalities are aimed toward the usual 15% to 18% of children who will report severe to very severe PTS and could go on to have persistent symptomology, and, as has been seen in the previously reported studies, most will resolve during the first year after the disaster.

As for the other interventions, evidence for the effectiveness of the approaches in the short-term recovery period is limited. Psychoeducation, in combination with other approaches like cognitive behavioral therapy, is typically provided in this period. Long-term recovery interventions most often incorporate cognitive behavioral therapy, but this modality needs more research validation. Results of studies are promising, however, in that "reductions in youth PTS have been significantly greater for cognitive behavioral therapy (CBT) than for other comparison control conditions" (p. 6). Like other reviews, La Greca and Silverman described additional possible interventions such as multimodality trauma treatments that appear to have resulted in significant improvements in PTSD symptoms that were sustained on follow-up. Other potentially successful interventions are emerging to include the comprehensive multimodal combination of education, a strengths model of child intervention, and promotion of child resilience. This approach was used with children in Haiti and, with the training of local providers to administer the intervention, promoted sustainability and partnership between a Haitian-based nongovernmental organization (NGO) and the U.S. Playmakers organization and team.

PEDIATRIC PERSPECTIVES ON DISASTER PREPARATIONS

Many of the papers detailing necessary preparations for being able to address pediatric needs after a disaster have emerged as "lessons learned" from previous events. Farfel et al. (2011), who responded to the Haiti earthquake, found that children were treated most frequently for orthopedic injuries and infectious diseases. Consequently, efforts in improving sanitary conditions were paramount as gastrointestinal infectious diseases such as cholera were particularly prevalent in that disaster and were also observed after the 2004 earthquake/tsunami in Indonesia. Medically, the providers were also challenged in managing concurrent chronic illnesses on top of the demand for acute care interventions. Sanitation concerns were also worrisome for open wound treatment as tetanus infections are a major health issue in Haiti as only 53% of the population was appropriately vaccinated at the time of the disaster. Due to this concern, pediatric patients were routinely vaccinated as a preventive measure. Medical facilities were challenged by the number of individuals needing surgical intervention, so many procedures were performed under conscious or deep sedation, for example, in debridement procedures. Similarly, facilities could be overwhelmed by the influx of patients and were not sufficiently supplied for pediatric patients. Farfel et al. (2011) noted that prescored adult medications needed to be adapted to pediatric dosages or capsules opened and sprinkled on food for those unable to swallow pills. Language was an issue in the French-speaking culture and interpreters were challenged by the need to inquire about medical history or communicate treatment details. Logistically, medical facilities were confronted with the breakdown of normal infrastructure in obtaining electricity, clean water, and maintaining clean environments for patient care. The challenges of working in this environment highlighted the need for efficient triage to manage patients; adequate supplies, patient capacity, and surgical capabilities; and consideration of pediatric physiological and psychological needs.

Most experts advise planning ahead for these types of events even if the likelihood of occurrence is low. The American Academy of Pediatrics published a guide for pediatricians (Hagan et al., 2005) advising all to be aware of the potential for disasters in their communities and recommends reaching out to schools, other professionals, and community agencies to discuss potential disaster scenarios; how an evacuation would proceed; where to shelter in place; as well as identifying resources that would be available to families in the area. Burke et al. (2010) provide a framework organizing disaster planning to include steps to: plan, practice, prepare, partner, and develop a process for family reunification. Within each of these steps they suggest specific activities to accomplish a comprehensive approach to planning pre-event.

A key component of disaster preparedness stems from adequate education and training of those who will respond to the disaster. The American Academy of Pediatrics has issued several policy statements that include rich resources from that organization as well as links to governmental agencies involved in disaster response. Nursing specialty organizations such as the National Association of Pediatric Nurse Practitioners; Society of Pediatric Nurses (Sterling, 2011); and colleges of nursing have been meeting at a national level to develop educational materials for pediatric disaster preparedness for personal readiness and for specific types of care needed in different disaster situations. Fox and Timm (2008) described efforts to focus educational preparation on "specific agents (ie chemical, biological, and radiological)" man-made disasters with the associated equipment and supplies needed for large-scale exposures and community and environmental effects (p. 146), while others detail specific care needs in these types of disasters (Committee on Environmental Health, 2003; Endom, 2013; Mulligan, Levy, & Rokusek, 2009; Ratnapalan et al., 2013; Ryan et al., 2011; Siegel, Strauss-Riggs, & Needle, 2014). Gaps remain in not only developing materials to use in education, but also in efforts to train and reach personnel to insure readiness (Dolan & Krug, 2006; Fox & Timm, 2008). As well, research is needed to determine best modalities for

education and preparation of healthcare providers and personnel for immediate mobilization.

SUMMARY

In summary, the research on children's reactions to disasters has indicated that while children may be more susceptible to mental health effects due to exposure to death and destruction, many symptoms resolve over time. Reactions to disasters may include symptoms of PTSD, depression, and anxiety manifesting as clinginess, crying, sleep disturbances, withdrawal, or outbursts of temper. Their reactions may be exacerbated and recovery lengthened if the child concurrently has risk factors present such as previous disaster experiences; loss of a loved one; exposure to violence; family instability; low income; impaired parental mental health; or multiple symptomology in response to the disaster (Lieber, 2017). Cross-culturally, and across ethnic groups, commonalities exist in the response and duration of symptomatologies. Children may be affected even by being indirectly exposed to the disaster event through media sources and parental reactions to the disaster. Several protective factors have also been identified: male gender, younger age, parental support, and early reunification. Prominent among the findings, most studies and anecdotal accounts have detailed recommendations for preparing for future disasters involving children and lessons learned from providing care in previous disaster situations. Despite challenges in conducting research during and in the aftermath of disasters, it is only by doing so that healthcare providers, emergency personnel, and community agents will determine best practices and research-based approaches for effective interventions and preventive services.

REFERENCES

Agazio, J., Goodman, P., & Padden, D. (2014). Impact of deployment on military families. *Annual Review of Nursing Research, 32*, 109–133. doi:10.1891/0739-6686.32.109

Bokszczanin, A. (2008). Parental support, family conflict, and overprotectiveness: Predicting PTSD symptom levels of adolescents 28 months after a natural disaster. *Anxiety, Stress & Coping, 21*(4), 325–335. doi:10.1080/10615800801950584

Burke, R. V., Iverson, E., Goodhue, C. J., Neches, R., & Upperman, J. S. (2010). Disaster and mass casualty events in the pediatric population. *Seminars in Pediatric Surgery, 19*(4), 265–270. doi:10.1053/j.sempedsurg.2010.06.003

Comer, J., Dantowitz, A., Chou, T., Edson, A., Elkins, R., Kerns, C., ... Green, J. (2014). Adjustment among area youth after the Boston marathon bombing and subsequent manhunt. *Pediatrics, 134*(1), 7–14. doi:10.1542/peds.2013-4115

Committee on Environmental Health. (2003). Radiation disasters and children. *Pediatrics, 111*(6), 1455. doi:10.1542/peds.111.6.1455

Dolan, M. A., & Krug, S. E. (2006). Pediatric disaster preparedness in the wake of Katrina: Lessons to be learned. *Clinical Pediatric Emergency Medicine, 7*(1), 59–66. doi:10.1016/j.cpem.2006.01.004

Endo, T. (2007). Parental mental health affects behavioral changes in children following a devastating disaster: A community survey after the 2004 Niigata-Chuetsu earthquake. *General Hospital Psychiatry, 29*(2), 175–176. doi:10.1016/j.genhosppsych.2006.09.006

Endom, E. E. (2013). Bioterrorism and the pediatric patient: An update. *Clinical Pediatric Emergency Medicine, 14*(2), 102. doi:10.1016/j.cpem.2013.04.001

Farfel, A., Assa, A., Amir, I., Bader, T., Bartal, C., Kreiss, Y., & Sagi, R. (2011). Haiti earthquake 2010: A field hospital pediatric perspective. *European Journal of Pediatrics, 170*(4), 519–525. doi:10.1007/s00431-011-1423-8

Felix, E., Hernández, L. A., Bravo, M., Ramirez, R., Cabiya, J., & Canino, G. (2011). Natural disaster and risk of psychiatric disorders in Puerto Rican children. *Journal of Abnormal Child Psychology, 39*(4), 589–600. doi:10.1007/s10802-010-9483-1

Fendya, D. G. (2006). When disaster strikes: Care considerations for pediatric patients. *Journal of Trauma Nursing: The Official Journal of the Society of Trauma Nurses, 13*(4), 161–165. doi:10.1097/00043860-200610000-00005

Fox, L., & Timm, N. (2008). Pediatric issues in disaster preparedness: Meeting the educational needs of nurses: Are we there yet? *Journal of Pediatric Nursing, 23*(2), 145–152. doi:10.1016/j.pedn.2007.12.008

Gillies, D., Taylor, E., Gray, C., O'Brien, L., & D'Abrew, N. (2013). Psychological therapies for the treatment of post-traumatic stress disorder in children and adolescents. *Cochrane Review Journal, 8*(3), 1004–1116. doi:10.1002/ebch.1916

Hagan, J. F., Jr., The Committee on Psychosocial Aspects of Child and Family Health, & The Task Force on Terrorism. (2005). Psychosocial implications of disaster or terrorism on children: A guide for the pediatrician. *Pediatrics, 116*(3), 787–795. doi:10.1542/peds.2005-1498

Jemtrud, S. M., Rhoades, R. D., & Gabbai, N. (2010). Reunification of the child and caregiver in the aftermath of disaster. *Journal of Emergency Nursing, 36*(6), 534–537. doi:10.1016/j.jen.2009.04.020

Jia, Z., Tian, W., He, X., Liu, W., Jin, C., & Ding, H. (2010). Mental health and quality of life survey among child survivors of the 2008 Sichuan earthquake. *Quality of Life Research, 19*(9), 1381–1391. Retrieved from http://www.jstor.org/stable/40927186

Kalantari, M., & Vostanis, P. (2010). Behavioural and emotional problems in Iranian children four years after parental death in an earthquake. *International Journal of Social Psychiatry, 56*(2), 158–167. doi:10.1177/0020764008101854

Kelley, M. L., Self-Brown, S., Le, B., Bosson, J. V., Hernandez, B. C., & Gordon, A. T. (2010). Predicting posttraumatic stress symptoms in children following Hurricane Katrina: A prospective analysis of the effect of parental distress and parenting practices. *Journal of Traumatic Stress, 23*(5), 582–590. doi:10.1002/jts.20573

Kilic, E. Z., Ozguven, H. D., & Sayil, I. (2003). The psychological effects of parental mental health on children experiencing disaster: The experience of Bolu earthquake in Turkey. *Family Process, 42*(4), 485–495. doi:10.1111/j.1545-5300.2003.00485.x

Kithakye, M., Morris, A. S., Terranova, A. M., & Myers, S. (2010). The Kenyan political conflict and children's adjustment. *Child Development, 81*, 114–1128. doi:10.1111/j.1467-8624.2010.01457.x

Kronenberg, M. E., Hansel, T. C., Brennan, A. M., Osofsky, H. J., Osofsky, J. D., & Lawrason, B. (2010). Children of Katrina: Lessons learned about post disaster symptoms and recovery patterns. *Child Development, 81*(4), 1241–1259. doi:10.1111/j.1467-8624.2010.01465.x

La Greca, A. M., & Silverman, W. K. (2009). Treatment and prevention of posttraumatic stress reactions in children and adolescents exposed to disasters and terrorism: What is the evidence? *Child Development Perspectives, 3*(1), 4–10. doi:10.1111/j.1750-8606.2008.00069.x

Lai, B. S., Kelley, M. L., Harrison, K. M., Thompson, J. E., & Self-Brown, S. (2015). Posttraumatic stress, anxiety, and depression symptoms among children after Hurricane Katrina: A latent profile analysis. *Journal of Child and Family Studies, 24*(5), 1262–1270. doi:10.1007/s10826-014-9934-3

Lengua, L. J., Long, A. C., Smith, K. I., & Meltzoff, A. N. (2005). Pre-attack symptomatology and temperament as predictors of children's responses to the September 11 terrorist attacks. *Journal of Child Psychology & Psychiatry, 46*(6), 631–645. doi:10.1111/j.1469-7610.2004.00378.x

Lieber, M. (2017). Assessing the mental health impact of the 2011 Great Japan earthquake, tsunami, and radiation disaster on elementary and middle school children in the Fukushima prefecture of Japan. *PLOS ONE, 12*(1). doi:10.1371/journal.pone.0170402

Madrid, P. A., Grant, R., Reilly, M. J., & Redlener, N. B. (2006). Short-term impact of a major disaster on children's mental health: Building resiliency in the aftermath of Hurricane Katrina. *Pediatrics, 117*(5), S448. doi:10.1542/peds.2006-0099U

Masten, A., & Osofsky, J. (2010). Disasters and their impact on child development: Introduction to the special section. *Child Development, 81*(4), 1029–1039. Retrieved from http://www.jstor.org/stable/40801458

McDermott, B., Cobham, V., Berry, H., & Kim, B. (2014). Correlates of persisting posttraumatic symptoms in children and adolescents 18 months after a cyclone disaster. *Australian & New Zealand Journal of Psychiatry, 48*(1), 80–86. doi:10.1177/0004867413500349

McLaughlin, K., Fairbank, J. A., Gruber, M. J., Jones, R. T., Lakoma, M. D., Pfefferbaum, B., ... Kessler, R. C. (2009). Serious emotional disturbance among youths exposed to Hurricane Katrina 2 years postdisaster. *Journal of the American Academy of Child and Adolescent Psychiatry, 48*(11), 1069–1078. doi:10.1097/CHI.0b013e3181b76697

Mearidy-Bell, L. (2013). Adolescent victims of natural disasters: A phenomenological study on lived experiences and behaviors displayed after a crisis. *Journal of Human Behavior in the Social Environment, 23*(4), 536–551. doi:10.1080/10911359.2013.765818

Mijanovich, T., & Weitzman, B. C. (2010). Disaster in context: The effects of 9/11 on youth distant from the attacks. *Community Mental Health Journal, 46*(6), 601–611. doi:10.1007/s10597-009-9240-5

Mulligan, D. A., Levy, L., & Rokusek, C. F. (2009). Preparation for terrorist threats: Explosive devices. *Clinical Pediatric Emergency Medicine, 10*(3), 140–143. doi:10.1016/j.cpem.2009.07.008

Navarro, J., Pulido, R., Berger, C., Arteaga, M., Osofsky, H., Martinez, M., ... Hansel, T. (2016). Children's disaster experiences and psychological symptoms: An international comparison between the Chilean earthquake and tsunami and Hurricane Katrina. *International Journal of Social Work, 59*(4), 545–558. doi:10.1177/0020872814537850

Newman, E., Pfefferbaum, B., Kirlic, N., Tett, R., Nelson, S., & Liles, B. (2014). Meta-analytic review of psychological interventions for children survivors of natural and man-made disasters. *Current Psychiatry Reports, 16*(9), 1–10. doi:10.1007/s11920-014-0462-z

Osofsky, J. D., & Chartrand, M. M. (2013). Military children from birth to five years. *The Future of Children, 23*(2), 61–77. doi:10.1353/foc.2013.0011

Osofsky, J., Kronenberg, M., Bocknek, E., & Hansel, T. C. (2015). Longitudinal impact of attachment-related risk and exposure to trauma among young children after hurricane Katrina. *Child & Youth Care Forum, 44*(4), 493–510. doi:10.1007/s10566-015-9300-7

Osofsky, J. D., Osofsky, H. J., Weems, C. F., King, L. S., & Hansel, T. C. (2015). Trajectories of post-traumatic stress disorder symptoms among youth exposed to both natural and technological disasters. *Journal of Child Psychology and Psychiatry, 56*(12), 1347–1355. doi:10.1111/jcpp.12420

Padden, D., & Agazio, J. (2013). Caring for military families across the deployment cycle. *Journal of Emergency Nursing, 39*(6), 562–569. doi:10.1016/j.jen.2013.08.004

Pfefferbaum, B., Newman, E., & Nitiéma, P. (2016). Current evidence for selecting disaster interventions for children and adolescents. *Current Treatment Options in Psychiatry, 3*(2), 192–205. doi:10.1007/s40501-016-0079-4

Pfefferbaum, B., Tucker, P., & Nitiéma, P. (2015). Adolescent survivors of Hurricane Katrina: A pilot study of hypothalamic–pituitary–adrenal axis functioning. *Child & Youth Care Forum, 44*(4), 527–547. doi:10.1007/s10566-014-9297-3

Pfefferbaum, B., Weems, C., Scott, B., Nitima, P., Noffsinger, M., Pfefferbaum, R., ... Chakraburtty, A. (2013). Research methods in child disaster studies: A review of studies generated by the September 11, 2001, terrorist attacks; the 2004 Indian Ocean tsunami; and Hurricane Katrina. *Child & Youth Care Forum, 42*(4), 285–337. doi:10.1007/s10566-013-9211-4

Proctor, L. J., Fauchier, A., Oliver, P. H., Ramos, M. C., Rios, M. A., & Margolin, G. (2007). Family context and young children's responses to earthquake. *Journal of Child Psychology and Psychiatry, 48*(9), 941–949. doi:10.1111/j.1469-7610.2007.01771.x

Quinn, M., Gillooly, D., Kelly, S., Kolassa, J., Davis, E., & Jankowski, S. (2016). Evaluation of identified stressors in children and adolescents after super storm Sandy. *Pediatric Nursing, 42*(5), 235–241.

Ratnapalan, S., Martimianakis, M. A., Cohen-Silver, J. H., Minnes, B., MacGregor, D., Allen, U., … Daneman, D. (2013). Pandemic management in a pediatric hospital. *Clinical Pediatrics, 52*(4), 322–328. doi:10.1177/0009922812474890

Ryan, C., Antoon, A., Fagan, S., Goverman, J., Lawlor, D., Sheridan, R., & Tompkins, R. (2011). Considerations for preparedness for a pediatric burn disaster. *Journal of Burn Care & Research, 32*(5), E165–E166. doi:10.1097/BCR.0b013e31822ac9a4

Saylor, C. F., Cowart, B. L., Lipovsky, J. A., Jackson, C., & Finch, A. J., Jr. (2003). Media exposure to September 11: Elementary school students' experiences and posttraumatic symptoms. *The American Behavioral Scientist, 46*(12), 1622–1642. doi:10.1177/0002764203254619

Sharlin, S. A., Moin, V., & Yahav, R. (2006). When disaster becomes commonplace reaction of children and adolescents to prolonged terrorist attacks in Israel. *Social Work in Health Care, 43*(2), 95–114. doi:10.1300/J010v43n02_07

Siegel, D., Strauss-Riggs, K., & Needle, S. (2014). Prioritization of pediatric chemical, biological, radiologic, nuclear, and explosive disaster preparedness education and training needs. *Clinical Pediatric Emergency Medicine, 15*(4), 309–317. doi:10.1016/j.cpem.2014.10.002

Sriskandarajah, V., Neuner, F., & Catani, C. (2015). Parental care protects traumatized Sri Lankan children from internalizing behavior problems. *BMC Psychiatry, 15*(1), 1–11. doi:10.1186/s12888-015-0583-x

Sterling, Y. M. (2011). Society of pediatric nurses public policy committee position statement on disaster management for children and families. *Journal of Pediatric Nursing, 26*(1), 97–100. doi:10.1016/j.pedn.2010.10.004

Weems, C. F. (2015). Biological correlates of child and adolescent responses to disaster exposure: A bio-ecological model. *Current Psychiatry Reports, 17*(7), 1–7. doi:10.1007/s11920-015-0588-7

Yonekura, T., Ueno, S., & Iwanaka, T. (2013). Care of children in a natural disaster: Lessons learned from the great east Japan earthquake and tsunami. *Pediatric Surgery International, 29*(10), 1047–1051. doi:10.1007/s00383-013-3405-6

40

INFORMATION TECHNOLOGY IN DISASTER MANAGEMENT

Adam B. Rains

LEARNING OBJECTIVES

When this chapter is completed, readers will be able to:

1. Characterize the difference between information technology (IT) and information systems (IS).
2. Identify and describe key examples and roles for information and communication technologies in disaster management.
3. Identify and describe the technological and human components of key disaster IS.
4. Describe the specific roles of information and communication technologies in logistics, early warning, decision support, and telemedical systems.
5. Formulate strategies to encourage adoption of available information technologies into disaster response plans.
6. Define the role of telemedicine in extending the provision of clinical care during a disaster.
7. Discuss the potential role of social media in disaster risk reduction and emergency management.

KEY MESSAGES

Advances in information and communication technology (ICT) are changing the way we prepare for and respond to disasters.

In disasters, information can be as valuable a resource as food, water, or shelter. Disaster management requires timely information for effective planning and decision making.

Informatics and information management are concerned with the process by which data become information, knowledge, and, eventually, wisdom.

ICT are tools, whereas IS describe how these tools are integrated with human activity and protocols to further a goal.

Disaster management is reliant on a variety of key technologies and systems including: telecommunications, direct and remote sensing, information processing, logistics, decision support, early warning systems (EWS), telemedicine, and the Internet.

Involving nurses and first responders in developing and implementing IS is a critical means to ensure system suitability, usability, and effectiveness.

Nurses, as early adopters of IT, can drive improvements in disaster response.

CHAPTER OVERVIEW

The hallmark of modern disaster management is the effective and efficient use of IT. Disaster management is now reliant upon a broad variety of key technologies and systems including: telecommunications, direct and remote sensing, information processing, logistics, decision support, EWS, telemedicine, and the Internet. Early adoption of these technologies by nurses will enhance preparedness and mitigation strategies, expand clinical capacity, facilitate decision making, and ultimately drive improvements in population-based outcomes.

Information and communication are critical resources across all phases of the disaster management life cycle (International Federation of the Red Cross and Red Crescent Societies, 2005; Reddick, 2011; Sagun, 2010). In many ways information is as essential a resource in disasters as food or water. The demand for accurate, timely, and appropriately targeted information is a recurrent theme of this book and indeed much of the emergency management literature.

This chapter thus surveys existing and emergent ICT and IS across the disaster management life cycle. Although, in common parlance, these terms are sometimes used synonymously, there exists an important functional distinction that is especially important for disaster management.

ICT—or sometimes more narrowly IT—is the acquisition, storage, processing, and dissemination of data or information through a combination of computing and telecommunications. This is typically understood to include computers, embedded systems, network infrastructure, software, telephony, broadcast technology (radio, TV, etc.), Internet, wireless communications, scanners, and sensors as well as all manner of digital audio, video, and imaging equipment. In essence, ICT encompasses all technological means of capturing, handling, or exchanging information in any form.

In contrast, the term IS refers to a combination of ICT, human activity, and organizational policies/processes intended to make practical use of information. While the term can have quite different meanings depending on context, here we use it to emphasize the confluence of technology and human actions in pursuit of a defined goal or function (e.g., determining when to evacuate, selecting the number of vaccines doses needed in a specific area, finding the epicenter of an earthquake).

INFORMATION AND DISASTER MANAGEMENT

Modern disaster management relies on a number of important forms of ICT. While various typologies have been suggested (Pine, 2007; Sagun, 2010), here we discuss several key forms of supporting technology and progress to an exploration of archetypal information systems for disaster management. In doing so, we loosely follow the path from data collection to storage, interpretation, and contextualization and, finally, to the various ways in which this information informs decision making.

Despite the growing recognition of the mitigating impact of ICT in disaster response (Toya & Skidmore, 2015), there exists considerable unrealized potential for promoting rapid and large-scale collaboration in disaster management. The National Research Council's Committee on Using Information Technology to Enhance Disaster Management highlights six IT-enabled capabilities with the potential for significant benefit (Box 40.1).

Telecommunications

Few developments have had as profound or wide-ranging impact on humanity as the growth of global telecommunications and networking. Most aspects of modern life are in some way dependent on the ability to rapidly convey

---

BOX 40.1 Key IT-Enabled Capabilities

1. More robust, interoperable, priority-sensitive communications
2. Better situational awareness and a common operating picture
3. Improved decision support, resource tracking, and allocation
4. Greater organizational agility for disaster management
5. Better engagement of the public
6. Enhanced infrastructure survivability and continuity of societal functions

Source: Adapted From National Research Council, Committee on Using Information Technology to Enhance Disaster Management. (2007). In R. R. Rao, J. Eisenberg, & T. Schmitt (Eds.), *Improving disaster management: The role of IT in mitigation, preparedness, response, and recovery* (pp. 5–9). Washington, DC: National Academies Press.

information over a distance; even short-term disruptions can have severe social and economic consequences (Marchetti, 2010). Communication is a critical need at all stages of disaster management. Breakdown in communications—through physical damage, network disruption, or congestion—is a hallmark of many disasters and a primary focus of recovery efforts (National Research Council [NRC], 2007; Wrobel & Wrobel, 2009).

The telecommunications infrastructure is typically understood to include fixed cable networks (copper, fiber optic), wired and wireless (global system for mobiles [GSM], cellular, universal mobile telecommunications system [UMTS], WiFi, Bluetooth) communication protocols and equipment as well as the numerous devices that make use of these networks (wired and mobile phones, computers, two-way radios, etc.). While a detailed discussion of telecommunications technology and standards is beyond the scope of this text, in the sections that follow we touch frequently on the role of technology in supporting information exchange. Indeed, so significant is the availability of communications to information management processes that any discussion of IT should be understood to include some aspect of telecommunications.

Alerting and Warning Technology

Alerting technology is a general label for ICT and systems (warning systems) intended to widely disseminate critical information or send targeted notifications relating to an impending disaster. In practice, this can include a variety of telecommunications and broadcast media as well as conventional signaling systems such as sirens, alarms, or public address systems. Meissen and Voisard (2010) suggest a valuable typology as well as strengths and weaknesses for available alerting and warning technologies:

1. *Classical Alert Systems (sirens, claxons, alarms, PA systems, etc.):* These tend to be short-range, susceptible to utilities disruptions, and capable of only limited message nuance. In addition, they require that individuals have a preexisting understanding of the alert's meaning and appropriate action to take.
2. *Radio and TV Broadcasts:* Manual and automated broadcast of warning messages using analog or digital television and radio broadcast channels is a common alerting methodology. A familiar example is the Emergency Alert System (EAS) maintained by the Federal Emergency Management Agency (FEMA), National Weather Service (NWS), and the Federal Communications Commission (FCC). EAS and similar systems can reach a wide audience and deliver detailed response information, and provide the ability to regionally target alert messages.
3. *Mobile Radio Networks:* The proliferation of mobile phones, pagers, and other devices with wireless network (cellular, pagers, WiFi, GSM, UTMS) access provides a means of delivering targeted messages to a wide and geographically distributed audience.
4. *Fixed Cable Networks (Copper Wire, Fiber Optic):* Fixed cable (wired) networks provide access through standard and digital telephony, cable television, and Internet access.

While susceptible to physical disruptions, wireline systems provide high bandwidth and targeted, always-on access suitable for alerting.
5. *Satellite Communications:* Satellite systems, particularly those employing low earth orbit communications satellites, provide an ideal and robust, if resource-intensive, means of providing alerting during the response phase. Despite increasing availability and decreasing cost, the number of satellite communications receivers remains quite limited.
6. *Telecontrol Systems:* A number of modern devices such as GPS (global positioning systems) units, weather radios, and onboard navigation systems support external control and push notification. U.S. National Oceanic and Atmospheric Administration (NOAA) systems such as the NOAA Weather Radio All Hazards (NWR) network provide the ability to disseminate regionally targeted and detailed warnings even when the receiving unit (weather radio) is in standby mode. Other examples include the proposed transmission of alerts via the traffic notification service present on most modern satellite navigation units.

Direct and Remote Sensing

Sensors—devices that measure or detect some physical property (e.g., temperature, vibration, presence of a chemical)—represent one of the primary data sources for modern disaster management. In addition to providing individual-level information for clinicians and first responders (e.g., patient monitors, portable detectors), data obtained from sensor networks or through remote sensing play a pivotal role in early warning, situational awareness, and decision making. Furthermore, developments supporting the storage, integration, and representation of sensor data increasingly underpin a range of functions across the disaster management life cycle (prediction, trending, and evaluation).

Direct sensing is characterized by the need for physical contact between the sensor and the entity being measured. Examples include familiar diagnostic (e.g., thermometers, immunoassays) tools and environmental monitoring devices (e.g., seismometers, rain gauges, particulate profilers) as well as chemical and biological "point detectors" introduced in previous chapters.

In contrast, *remote sensing* involves collecting data "at a distance" through the interpretation of propagated signals (e.g., light, sound, radio waves). This can be accomplished by interpreting existing environmental signals (e.g., reflected sunlight in satellite imagery) or using actively generated emissions (e.g., microwave radiation in Doppler radar). While the term has become virtually synonymous with longer distance and satellite-based sensing methods, remote sensing includes a variety of shorter range applications such as medical imaging, crowd scanning, asset tracking, and standoff detection for potential biochemical threats (Kosal, 2003).

Fostered by progressive improvements in supporting technology (communications, miniaturization, energy efficiency, detection capability) and economies of scale, the last 30 years have seen massive growth in the number and diversity of prepositioned, mobile, and postincident deployable sensors (NRC, 2007). This has included the introduction of novel sensing methods (see Box 40.2), the use of sensors in new contexts (oil spills, forest

BOX 40.2 Selected Sensing Methods for Disaster Management

Infrared Detectors and Thermal Cameras: A form of passive remote sensing that can be used to determine the amount of heat emitted by an object or individual. Aside from diagnostic and fire detection applications, thermal imagery has been used with moderate success to scan crowds for individuals with febrile illness (severe acute respiratory syndrome [SARS], influenza, dengue; Bitar, Goubar, & Desenclos, 2009; McBride, Buikstra, & FitzGerald, 2010; Shu et al., 2005).

Pulsed-Doppler Radar: An active remote sensing method that can be used to monitor the movement, position, size, shape, and speed of nonsolid objects (clouds, precipitation, chemical plumes). Sometimes referred to as weather surveillance radar (WSR), this method involves directing pulses of microwave radiation at a target and interpreting changes in the returned reflection to gather information.

LiDAR (Light Detection and Ranging, "Laser Radar"): Conceptually similar to other forms of radar but uses more energetic, shorter wavelength emissions (light) in the ultraviolet, visible, and near-infrared spectrum. In addition to detection and ranging, this method permits the visualization of finer detail (down to single molecules), three-dimensional imaging, and temperature sensing. Often used in meteorological and mapping applications, light detection and ranging (LiDAR) and laser spectroscopy are seeing increased use in biological and chemical agent identification such as the U.S. Army's Long Range Biological Standoff Detection System (LR-BSDS), Short Range Biological Standoff Detection System (SR-BSDS), and Laser Induced Breakdown Spectroscopy (LIBS) system (Kosal, 2003; Munson, Gottfried, De Lucia, & Miziolek, 2008).

Surface Acoustic Wave (SAW): Technology provides an electromechanical means of augmenting and miniaturizing direct sensing methods for the identification of chemical and biological agents (i.e., point detectors). In simple terms, SAW-based sensors generate a tiny amount of electrical current in response to contact with an agent-specific substrate (e.g., antibody, selectively absorbent polymer). This technology permits the construction of compact sensor arrays with the ability to detect numerous specific agents.

fires, air quality, biosurveillance), and the increasing availability of timely satellite-based remote sensing data. Advances in wireless communications and data processing have facilitated remote monitoring of sensor inputs (telemetry), greater use of mobile sensor platforms (aircraft/unmanned aerial vehicles [UAVs], ships and sensor buoys, air-dropped sacrificial sensors), and the creation of more robust, efficient sensor networks.

Multiple individual sensors can be combined to form networks of varying formality, threat specificity, and geographic scale (Sagun, 2010). In addition to providing improved coverage,

the availability of multiple heterogeneous sensor inputs permits cross-validation (minimizing false positives), allows spatial and temporal tracking, and provides a contingency against the failure of one or more parts of the network (Toya & Skidmore, 2015). As an example, data from a widespread series of seismic, sea level, orbital, and deep-sea pressure sensors are used by the Japanese Meteorological Agency (JMA) to detect, verify, and track the development and progression of potential tsunamis (Joseph, 2011). The NOAA, U.S. Geological Survey (USGS), and NWS integrate data from similarly diverse sources (weather spotters, weather stations, remote sensing, sensor buoys, satellite imagery) in detecting and tracking natural disasters and extreme weather. While sensor network data are increasingly central to this process, it will likely never fully supplant eyewitness observations from first responders, emergency management personnel, radio operators, and citizen volunteers (Coleman, Knupp, Spann, Elliott, & Peters, 2011; Doswell, Moller, & Brooks, 1999).

Since the 1960s, the U.S. NWS's Skywarn⁻ program (www.weather.gov/skywarn) has assembled a federated network of more than 300,000 trained, volunteer weather spotters. Technological improvements (GPS, mobile Internet) and the development of allied programs (e.g., Spotter Network) have enhanced coverage, timeliness, and accessibility of spotter data and have improved the ability to train, track, and coordinate volunteer spotters (Jans & Keen, 2012). Skywarn spotters gather key details on emergent weather (description, location, wind speed, direction, hail size, etc.) and relay the data through a variety of communication channels (radio, telephone, Internet) to their regional NWS office for processing and redistribution. The success of such volunteer-based, participatory sensing programs has been extended to other regions (NWS Illinois' Significant Weather Observing Program [SWOP]; Citizen Weather Observer Program [CWOP]; Skywarn Europe) and common threats (e.g., Community Collaborative Rain, Hail and Snow Network [CoCoRaHS]; Tornado and Storm Research Organisation [TORRO]; Alfonso, Chacon, & Peña-Castellanos, 2015; Reges et al., 2016).

Historically, cost considerations associated with the deployment, monitoring, and maintenance of large-scale sensor networks limited their application to high-impact military and environmental threats (e.g., nuclear attack, earthquake, tsunami). The confluence of collective action coordinated through the Internet (i.e., citizen science, participatory sensing), economies of scale borne of the mobile tech boom, and the massive growth in wired and wireless connectivity have supported the creation of novel, inexpensive sensor networks (Cranswick, Gardner, Hammond, & Banfill, 1993). Since it is often impossible or impractical to ensure that dedicated sensors are positioned in all potential areas of risk, new efforts increasingly seek to incorporate inputs from the myriad sensor-enabled devices (e.g., mobile phones, computers, smart home devices, building systems, vehicles, appliances) that populate modern life (NRC, 2007).

An interesting illustration of this trend can be seen in efforts over the past 20 years to develop sustainable, volunteer-based seismic sensing networks. The Personal Seismic Network—a series of volunteer-purchased seismometers deployed in private buildings and connected via dial-up modem—was one early attempt to address urban gaps in existing, sensing networks (Cranswick et al., 1993). More recent programs, such as the USGS NetQuakes, Community Seismic Network, and Home

Seismic Network have capitalized on the decreasing cost of micro-electromechanical system (MEMS) sensors and increased connectivity to build out low-cost, high-density sensing networks (Kohler, Heaton, & Cheng, 2013; Luetgert, Oppenheimer, & Hamilton, 2010).

Started in 2008, the Quake-Catcher Network (QCN) aims for even greater coverage and mobility by incorporating data from Internet-connected computers and mobile devices with internal MEMS accelerometers (e.g., shake/drop/orientation sensors; Cochran, Lawrence, Christensen, & Jakka, 2009). Using the provided software, enrolled computers monitor built-in or externally connected sensors and transmit notifications (measurement, time, location) to the QCN servers whenever a strong motion is detected. Server software analyzes the strength, timing, and geographical distribution of these notifications to separate cultural noise (e.g., traffic, doors slamming) from relevant seismic activity (Quake-Catcher, 2017). QCN's detection of earthquakes using multiple, inexpensive sensors compares favorably with existing systems (Chung et al., 2011; Cochran et al., 2012) and provides a good model for the future of web-based participatory sensing.

The growing use of smart devices means more potential sensing data but the heterogeneity and diversity of devices present a problem of making sense of the resulting data. Given the widespread impact of disasters, there is increasing focus on improving interagency and international collaboration through the standardization and sharing of sensor data. This hinges on the development and implementation of standards for interoperability, networking, and data exchange such as the CCSI (Common CBRN Sensor Interface), ORCHESTRA (Open Architecture and Spatial Data Infrastructure for Risk Management), and SANY (Sensors ANYwhere) project architectures.

The future holds much promise for the role of individual sensors and sensor networks in disaster management. As we move toward ubiquitous sensing and continuous real-time monitoring, greater emphasis must be placed on what we do with the data collected. Increased sensor density and diversification must be associated with improvements in interoperability, processing, management, and presentation necessary for turning these data streams into usable information for situational awareness and decision making (NRC, 2007; Sagun, 2010; Zdravkovic, Noran, Panetto, & Trajanović, 2015).

INFORMATION MANAGEMENT AND PROCESSING

Effective disaster management requires timely information for effective planning and decision making (Subedi, 2010). New technologies have gone a long way toward addressing concerns of data availability and shifted the focus to efficient organization, processing, storage, analysis, modeling, and representation (NRC, 2007). The rubric "information management" is used here to loosely group a variety of the means by which data (unorganized facts) become information, knowledge, and eventually wisdom. As most examples are dependent on local or distributed computing, they might alternately be classed "computer-based" technologies (Sagun, 2010).

In addition to abundant direct and remote sensing data streams, disaster management information systems draw on data gathered from user input, historical records, surveillance, and communication with other systems. In practice, these might include patient vital signs and medical records, damage reports, geospatial imagery, incident action plans, and environmental data as well as logistics and inventory information at varying levels of granularity (Aung & Whittaker, 2013; Hristidis, Chen, Li, Luis, & Deng, 2010; Naumann & Raschid, 2006).

New methods and technologies—such as artificial intelligence, machine learning, data mining, natural language processing, and semantic web—are opening up the possibility of systems collecting and processing their own data. An intriguing example is Google's aggregation and surveillance of influenza-related search queries to provide short-term prediction of regional physician visits (Dugas et al., 2013; Ginsberg et al., 2008; www.google.org/flutrends). While, at present, the sustainability and reliability of such methods is currently highly dependent on human oversight, they nonetheless provide a potentially sensitive form of early warning (Lazer, Kennedy, King, & Vespignani, 2014).

As storage and analysis capabilities have increased, so too has the need to extract patterns and useable information from every larger pool data. Traditional modeling techniques have been supplemented by semiautomated, procedural analysis and hypothesis generation. Data mining at its core is an effort to elucidate implicit, previously unknown/unsuspected and potentially useful information from large data structures. In brief, this method entails management and integration of data sources, preprocessing of data in preparation for mining, application of the data mining algorithms and tasks, and post-processing evaluation of information rendered by the overall process. Analytic methods in data mining as well as general modeling include association mining, exploratory data analyses, classification, clustering, principal component analyses, regression, natural language processing, and content retrieval (Hristidis et al., 2010).

The demands of data processing and information management in the context of disaster response present unique challenges including the existence of numerous data producers and information consumers, varying levels of data trustworthiness and completeness, heterogeneous terminology and formats, time sensitivity, as well as highly dynamic and user-specific information requirements (Hristidis et al., 2010). Outside the response phase, time constraints are lessened but the overall data space is no less complex. Systems must contend with diverse spatial and temporal data covering a wide range of media (NRC, 2007).

Drawing on a fusion of cartography, demography, statistics, and database technology, geographical information systems (GIS) is a broad term for the methods and technological means used to gather, manipulate, manage, analyze, and represent geographically referenced data. This includes explicitly geospatial data such as maps, satellite imagery, and geolocation data (e.g., GPS coordinates) as well as a wide variety of data sources for which a geographical position may be inferred (e.g., disease incidence in a ZIP code, number of free beds at a location). In addition to providing an intuitive means of connecting disparate data streams, GIS facilitates novel pattern identification, analytic exploration, and modeling.

Over the past decade, GIS has proven to be a useful tool in disaster management. While principally employed during response (impact assessment, resource allocation), a spatial perspective is needed to draw meaning from a growing volume of real-time sensing data (Tomaszewski, Szarzynski, Radestock, & Wirkus, 2015). Since 1993, FEMA has made the use of GIS technology a central part of disaster response efforts. Among many functions, the agency's E-GIS team is responsible for pre- and postincident mapping, geographical modeling, and damage assessment as well as specific requests from disaster managers and other agencies (gis.fema.gov).

LOGISTICS AND RESOURCE MANAGEMENT

Logistical problems in disasters often result from a failure to coordinate resource distribution rather than from resource shortages (Auf der Heide, 1996). While information systems to address the management of personnel, supply chain, and materials have long been used in business and industry (enterprise resource planning [ERP]; content management system [CMS]), supply chain systems, only more recently has such an approach become the norm in emergency management (NRC, 2007). As experience has shown, manual methods for managing this type of information are fraught with inefficiency and potential risk. As a resource-driven discipline, logistics and inventory control systems have numerous potential uses in disaster management. These include systems for preregistration and certification of personnel, spatial asset and people tracking, inventory control, shelter and site registration, and interagency resource coordination (Christopher & Tatham, 2014).

From a technological perspective, the design of such systems is dependent on the scale of information exchange (e.g., single agency, local, nationwide), anticipated transaction volume, and means used to update resource status and inventory (e.g., manual entry, bar code scanner, radio frequency identification device (RFID) tags, wireless transponders). Thus a smaller, manual, entry-based inventory system might require a single computer with an isolated database instance, whereas larger systems depend on a scalable distributed architecture capable of contending with multiple simultaneous and geographically disparate inputs and requests for information. Such a system would require a robust distributed relational database, user interfaces for data input and reporting, and a means of keeping system data up to date (sensor data, manual inputs, etc.).

A key lesson from the tragedy of September 11, 2001 is that, during a crisis, coordination and certification of medical and other specialized personnel can itself become a burden on response efforts (Weiner, 2006). A variety of governmental, professional, and private groups (Community Emergency Response Team, American Red Cross, American Nurses Association, Médecins Sans Frontières) have sought to address this concern through the creation of web-based credentialing and precertification programs. Such systems serve not only to create a repository of trained personnel but, when coordinated effectively, will ensure that specific volunteers are not counted twice as an available resource. Similar civilian volunteer matching and management systems include the HandsOn Network

(www.handsonnetwork.org) and National Voluntary Organizations Active in Disaster (www.nvoad.org).

In recognition of the importance of resource management for interagency coordination, FEMA's National Preparedness Directorate (NPD) has developed, through the auspices of the Preparedness Technology Analysis and Coordination (P-TAC) center, a local inventory management tool (preptoolkit.fema.gov/web/nims-tools). The Incident Resource Inventory System (IRIS) allows users to document and share resource information with other agencies. Users can define and select resources based on mission requirements, capabilities, availability, and desired response time (FEMA, 2011).

A variety of commercial systems, such as WebEOC (www.esi911.com) and E-Teams, are in use by emergency management departments for information management, coordination, and decision support. The Free Open Source Software (FOSS) community also has a significant role to play in developing technology and systems for disaster management logistics (NRC, 2007). The Sahana Software Foundation has launched a progression of local and web-based tools (Mayon, Eden, Vesuvius, Krakatoa, Sahana) addressing humanitarian needs management, shelter registry, community preparedness and response, triage, missing persons location and family reunification, and personnel coordination (sahanafoundation.org).

As the possibilities for real-time spatial tracking of patients, responders, materials, and resources increase, the line between resource management, logistics, and decision support system becomes ever more fuzzy. As the examples presented suggest, a detailed resource inventory is not a goal in and of itself; it is how the data is used that is critical to disaster management and response.

DECISION SUPPORT SYSTEMS

Decision support systems (DSS) are a special class of information system intended to support or guide the activity of decision makers situated at different levels on a chain of command. In effect, a DSS is a means of guiding individuals through a complex decision-making process by bringing together their judgment, normative processes (protocols, models, rules), and situational information. While the term has a long history and may be broadly understood to include various nontechnical decision-making guidance tools (nomograms, diagnostic decision trees, etc.), for the purposes of this discussion we focus on computer and ICT-based systems.

Formal definitions of DSS vary greatly; however, they are typically understood to include certain key domain-specific characteristics and goals (Parker & Al-Utabi, 1986). These are summarized by Cioca and Cioca (2010) as endeavoring to do the following:

- Support and improve, and not supplant, human reasoning
- Assist individuals in decision making for unstructured and semistructured problems which cannot be solved through reasoning, judgment, or using other types of information systems
- Adapt to changes in the decision-making and support context

- Provide ease-of-use for nontechnical users (managers, decision makers, et al.) including support for novel individual decision processes and decision-making styles
- Augment existing real-world methods (and not merely computerize existing processes)
- Integrate use of analytic models, techniques, and data access
- Incorporate multiple data and knowledge source
- Improve the efficiency, but not necessarily the effectiveness, of decision making
- Contribute to productivity increases through improved quality, suitability, and appropriateness of decisions

From a systems architecture standpoint, DSS include certain key elements:

1. **A data repository, database, or means of storing information relating to the domain of interest.** This might include sensor and user inputs, data on past events, clinical records, logistics data, inventory, or any number of raw or processed data streams relevant to the decision-making context.
2. **A model representing the decision-making context.** This model is a manifestation or articulation of organizational rules and processes relating to the decision domain. The model may itself be entirely prescriptive, the product of a priori modeling and prediction, or may draw on various forms of machine learning and artificial intelligence to generate an emergent or malleable structure.
3. **A user interface to permit decision makers to interact with the system in an efficient manner.** This might take the form of a software dashboard, web-based client, or proprietary control system and include a means of both entering data and representing guidance or other system outputs.
4. **A system user.** Depending on the context, in disaster DSS, the system user may be a clinician, first responder, incident commander, administrator, governmental planner, or other decision maker.

DSS have numerous applications related to disaster management. Historically rooted in management and business information systems, DSS have been applied to logistics, supply chain management, environmental regulation, sustainable development, and, notably, in guiding clinical decision making (clinical DSS; Chan, Killeen, Griswold, & Lenert, 2004; Cioca & Cioca, 2010; Kondaveti & Ganz, 2009; Wallace & Balogh, 1985).

Since providing guidance and support in decision making is an important functionality of many disaster ICT applications, DSS are often a key component of situational awareness, logistics, telemedicine, and EWS. The National Research Council's Committee on Using Information Technology to Enhance Disaster Management (NRC) characterizes decision support in disasters as follows:

> … decision support focuses on assisting them [users, decision-makers] in formulating prospective actions, primarily by helping them understand and assess characteristics and consequences of alternative courses of action. Decision support is about explicitly recording candidate course(s) of action and generating, analyzing, and evaluating those alternatives. (2007, p. 48)

Definitions of decision support have grown to encompass elements such as artificial intelligence, data mining, online analysis, and knowledge management. Functionally, disaster decision support systems (DDSS) may include dynamic decision evaluation, triggering and "nagging" at key junctures to ensure action is taken, organizational authority structures to identify the next in a chain of command, data tracking, analysis, simulation, warning generation, and maintenance of a traceable log of system actions (NRC, 2007).

Recent years have seen a proliferation of DSS for various disaster scenarios. In their survey of the topic, Hristidis et al. (2010) cite a range of systems for specific disasters including: forest fires (Kohyu, Weiguo, & Yang, 2004), oil spills (Pourvakhshouri & Mansor, 2003), hurricanes (Lindell & Prater, 2007; Tufekci, 1995), floods (Wang, Qin, & Wang, 2004), evacuation (Pidd, de Silva, & Eglese, 1996; Silva, 2001), and rescue operations (Farinelli, Grisetti, Iocchi, & Lo Cascio, 2003). Other examples include systems for detecting, predicting damage, assessing loss, and selection of response measures for earthquakes such as the web-based WaveLet system (Yong et al., 2001), and E-DECIDER (Emergency Data Enhanced Cyber Infrastructure for Disaster Evaluation and Response; e-decider.org).

Another prominent example is the Department of Homeland Security's (DHS's) Unified Incident Command and Decision Support (UICDS) framework (www.uicds.us). The system's primary goal is to "enable information sharing and decision support among commercial, academic, volunteer, and government incident management technologies used across the country to prevent, protect, respond, and recover from natural, technological, and terrorist events" (Morentz, 2008; Pottebaum et al., 2016). While users do not interface with the UICDS system directly, it provides a backbone intended to support the National Response Framework (NRF), National Incident Management System (NIMS), and Incident Command System (ICS).

The Open Advanced System for Disaster and Emergency Preparedness (OASIS) project is a European Commission–backed initiative to develop a framework, standards, and user interfaces tailored to the needs of the emergency response community. This flexible, open architecture was developed to facilitate cooperation of systems across organizations and provide a basis for a unified European disaster and emergency management system. OASIS supports a variety of extrinsic decision support options as well as in-system guidance in the selection of event scenarios and recovery actions (Andrienko & Andrienko, 2005).

While a great number of DDSS focus on high-level administrative, logistic, and incident command decision making, new tools are being developed to guide field teams, clinicians, and first responders (Garshnek & Burkle, 1999). One example is the ReadyRN Clinical Decision Support Software (CDSS) which provides clinical, diagnostic, preventive, systemic, and shelter management guidance to nurses and clinicians. Using an adaptive hierarchical presentation structure (model), the ReadyRN CDSS tool allows rapid access to background materials, diagnostic guidelines, GIS data, geospatial imagery, and real-time situational data using a computer or smartphone (Figure 40.1).

By weighting information sources depending on user preferences, inputs, and data aggregated from other users

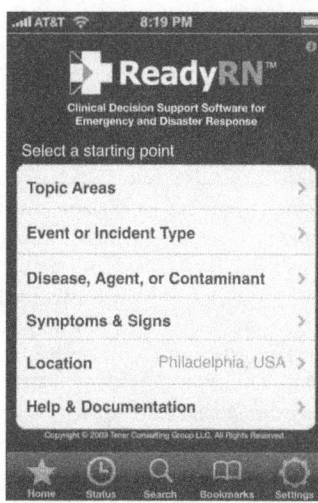

FIGURE 40.1 ReadyRN smartphone app for disaster nursing (2017).

Source: Tener Consulting Group, LLC. Copyright 2011. All rights reserved.

(currently and for past-related incidents), this tool aims to simplify navigation of the vast range of data relevant to nurses and first responders (Veenema & Rains, 2009).

EARLY WARNING SYSTEMS

In the context of disaster response, the term EWS describes an integrated collection of technology and human activities intended to provide advance notice and actionable information regarding some impending threat. In their review, Meissen and Voisard (2010) indicate that the definitions of EWS are quite variable and dependent on interpretation of what constitutes "early warning." While providing early warning is the ultimate goal of many mitigation and preparedness activities, an EWS is usually understood to include certain key features (monitoring, forecasting, alerting).

The UN International Strategy for Disaster Reduction (UN/ISDR) has defined a complete, effective EWS as comprising four interrelated elements: risk knowledge, monitoring and warning service, dissemination and communication, and response capability (Table 40.1).

From an organizational perspective, this view places appropriate focus on the role of human activity in EWS development, implementation, maintenance, and response. It also suggests some of the ways in which ICT directly (e.g., remote sensing, warning generation, communications) and indirectly (e.g., risk modeling, training, response simulation, decision support) supports warning systems. In terms of system architecture, Meissen and Voisard (2010) suggest a series of four key EWS components: monitoring and data collection, information processing, warning generation, and alert dissemination.

A commonly cited example of a highly integrated and effective EWS is the Japanese Meteorological Association's Earthquake Early Warning (EEW) system. Drawing on sensor network data (seismographs, deep-sea pressure sensors, sea level monitors, sensor buoys, weather stations), this system seeks to identify dangerous seismic events and provide early warning regarding the development and landfall of tsunamis (Joseph, 2011). Data are aggregated at a series of monitoring centers, processed, used to assess risk, and, when warranted, generate and disseminate targeted warnings through a variety of communications and alerting channels (radio, sirens, mobile messaging, etc.). Technology aside, a significant part of the success of the EEW system lies in well-established and practiced public response plans and evacuation routes.

TELEMEDICINE

Telemedicine can be loosely described as the use of ICT to deliver healthcare services at a distance. Definitions of telemedicine have evolved along with supporting technology (wireless communications, digital patient records) and may broadly include a range of medical services and delivery modalities (Sood et al., 2007; Whitten & Sypher, 2006). These include store-and-forward (i.e., asynchronous) systems employing email or text messaging as well as real-time (synchronous) systems using voice, two-way video, diagnostic sensor data, augmented reality, or telepresence (e.g., remote control of surgical robots).

TABLE 40.1 The Four Elements of Effective Early Warning Systems

Risk Knowledge	Monitoring and Warning Service
Systematically collect data and undertake risk assessments	*Develop hazard monitoring and early warning services*
Are the hazards and the vulnerabilities well known? What are the patterns and trends in these factors? Are risk maps and data widely available?	Are the right parameters being monitored? Is there a sound, scientific basis for making forecasts? Can accurate and timely warnings be generated?
Dissemination and Communication	Response Capability
Communicate risk information and early warnings	*Build national and community response capabilities*
Do warnings reach all of those at risk? Are the risks and the warnings understood? Is the warning information clear and useable?	Are response plans up to date and tested? Are local capacities and knowledge made use of? Are people prepared and ready to react to warnings?

Source: Adapted from United Nations, International Strategy for Disaster Reduction. (2006). *Global survey of early warning systems.* Retrieved from https://www.unisdr.org/files/3612_GlobalSurveyofEarlyWarningSystems.pdf

TABLE 40.2 Telemedical Functions in Disaster Management

Stage	Phase One: Predisaster Preparedness	Phase Two: Disaster Relief Operations	Phase Three: Postdisaster Rehabilitation
Activities	• Hazard assessments • Planning and development • Evaluation of technological and administrative infrastructure • Training and drills of clinicians, responders, and those at risk	• Robot-assisted medical care • Patient tracking and telemetry • Mobile prehospital management • Telediagnostics • Clinical decision support systems • Telesurgery and teleconsultation	• Telepsychiatric intervention • Early warning systems • Disaster medicine • Epidemiology • Telerehabilitation

Source: Adapted from Patoli, A. Q. (2006). Role of telemedicine in disaster management. *EHealth International Journal, 2*(2), 34.

Telemedicine has shown considerable success in care delivery to outlying regions and holds considerable promise as a means of addressing stresses on the U.S. healthcare system.

Patoli (2006) classifies telemedicine's roles in disaster management into three distinct phases, each with its own technological needs and requirements (Table 40.2). At the level of supporting technology, telemedical activities in the response phase are likely to demand: satellite communications or other long-range uplink, ICT-enabled clinical and environmental sensors, local area wireless networking and communications equipment, on-scene video monitoring, and independent power source (batteries, generator; Haynes & Saleem, 2008; Simmons et al., 2003).

Due to the dependence of telemedical systems on a functional communications infrastructure, their application in extreme or disaster conditions has traditionally been limited to large governments, corporations, and military humanitarian missions (Doarn, Barrigan, & Poropatich, 2011; Garshnek & Burkle, 1999). Trends toward greater availability of satellite-based communications channels, improved resilience of ground-based networking, and the decreased cost and power demands of field equipment (e.g., portable medical devices, patient monitors) have all contributed to more widespread application of disaster telemedicine (Chan et al., 2004; Garshnek & Burkle, 1999; Figure 40.2).

Architectures such as Wireless Internet Information System for Medical Response in Disasters (WIISARD) and WISTA provide a means of creating a wireless, incident area network (802.11b, Bluetooth) that permits communications and data exchange at the disaster site. A more powerful communications link (e.g., satellite connection) can then be used to relay data between this incident area network and a remotely situated control center (Buono, Chan, & Griswold, 2008; Chu & Ganz, 2007).

The availability of wireless networking at the disaster site opens up a range of telemedical options including decision support, expert guidance, remote patient monitoring, access to remotely held patient records, and care prioritization. As an example, one component of the WIISARD architecture is an intelligent triage tag (iTag/ITT) that stores patient and transport details, permits spatial tracking, and provides a real-time stream of data for offsite planning (Lenert, Palmer, Chan, & Rao, 2005).

While telemedical systems have moved toward increasing complexity, it is important to recognize that much can be accomplished with little (Garshnek & Burkle, 1999; Whitten & Sypher, 2006). Often, once basic communication and power infrastructure have been restored, a wide variety of telemedical recovery functions may be accomplished through telephone, email, text chats, informational websites and support groups, and social media (Crowe, 2011; Wootton & Bonnardot, 2010).

As with other IT, successful development, implementation, and use of telemedical systems hinges on human factors. Effective delivery of telemedical care in a disaster requires that frontline staff (nurses, physicians, first responders) become conversant with systems and protocols through regular training and simulations/drills (Garshnek & Burkle, 1999; Patoli, 2006; Whitten & Sypher, 2006).

THE INTERNET AS A DISASTER MANAGEMENT RESOURCE

Growth and expanding access to the Internet has had a transformative influence on a wide spectrum of human activities, not least of which is disaster management. The emergence of a globally interconnected network of computing systems

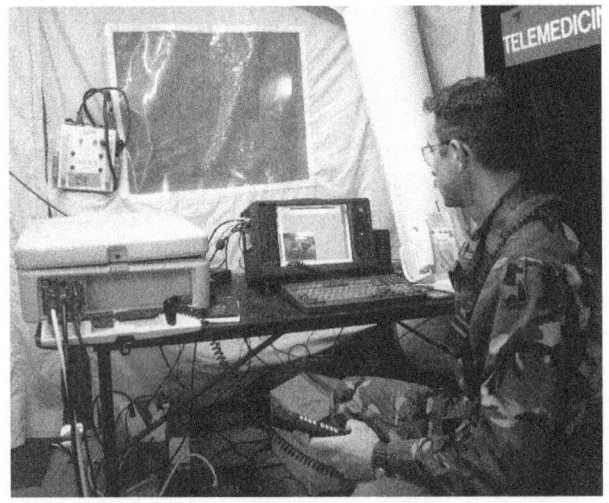

FIGURE 40.2 U.S. Army Mobile MedCam for telemedicine.
Source: SPC Gary A. Bryant, U.S. Army (970424-A-AF423–002).

(network of networks) capable of multimodal communications, data storage, and processing provides a low-cost backbone critical to a wide variety of disaster management functions. Furthermore, the existence of common standards for interoperability and communication as well as broad and increasingly robust access resulting from the proliferation of wireless, Internet-connected devices makes the Internet an ideal platform for a range of disaster management applications.

Beyond enabling novel forms of data collection, dissemination, training, and risk communication through static or interactive websites, the Internet provides a number of modalities for asynchronous (email, site comments) and synchronous communications (text/voice/video, web conferencing, voice over internet protocol [VOIP]) and data exchange (file transfer protocol [FTP], web-connected databases). Interactivity allows users to explore, customize, and contextualize information in new ways and can enable the elucidation of hidden patterns and relationships. Projects such as GapMinder (www.gapminder.org) and Emergency and Disaster Information Service (EDIS; hisz .rsoe.hu/alertmap/index2.php) demonstrate some of the ways in which the web can serve as an aggregation and exploration point for seemingly disparate data streams. In addition, the ability to deliver content dependent on known or collected user parameters (user type, knowledge level, location, interest area) permits more tailored and nuanced warning and alerting capabilities (Meissen & Voisard, 2010). Given considerations of increasing bandwidth and the value of asynchronous communications, the Internet is also a key channel for many forms of telemedicine (Garshnek & Burkle, 1999).

Social media is a blanket term for websites, services, and applications enabling user-mediated discussion, content creation and sharing, and the formation of social networks (Boyd & Ellison, 2007). Examples include microblogs (Twitter, Sina Weibo), meeting and messaging services (WhatsApp, Skype), social networking sites (Facebook, Google+, LinkedIn), as well as a variety of content sharing and discussion platforms (Instagram, Reddit, YouTube, Flickr). Globally distributed and collectively boasting daily visit counts in the tens to hundreds of millions, these sites and services have, to many, become a de facto news source (Alexa, 2017; Beaujohn, 2012), especially during a crisis (Thomas, Schrock, & Friedman, 2016), emergency management (Wukich & Steinberg, 2016), or in circumstances of restrictive or absent governmental structures (Al-Saggaf & Simmons, 2015; Dandoulaki & Halakia, 2010; Murthy & Longwell, 2013).

Growth in the diversity, popularity, and constant availability of social media has amplified the value of the Internet as a disaster management resource (Alexander, 2014; Crowe, 2011). Houston et al. (2015) highlight 15 key functions across the disaster lifecycle including information sharing, crisis communication, threat detection, social support, and response coordination. As projects such as Google Flu and the USGS "Did You Feel It?" program illustrate, much can be gleaned from even the simplest data streams (Dugas et al., 2013). Frequently updated, accompanied by contextualizing geographical and temporal metadata, and often accessible through documented application program interfaces (APIs), social media content provides a rich data source for individual users and in aggregate.

As social media companies derive value from the size of their user base, the volume of user-contributed content, frequency of return visits, and diversity of data they amass, these services have a distinct profit motive for ensuring they remain engaging. Beyond the many capabilities and technological synergies made possible by the growth of social media, it is perhaps the level of user engagement they engender that is the greatest boon to disaster management.

SUMMARY

Effective disaster management requires sharing information, resources, and decision making among stakeholders to improve coordination, reduce uncertainty, and help to evaluate strategic costs and benefits. As we have seen, IT plays a considerable and growing role in the management and mitigation of disasters through facilitated communications, more accurate and timely data collection, improved information processing and contextualization, and support for collaboration and key decision-making functions. However, to realize the potential of ICT to disaster management, a number of technical, institutional, and organizational challenges must be addressed (NRC, 2007; Sagun, 2010).

IT and systems for disaster response must contend with complex, time-sensitive, and geographically distributed data streams as well as potential damage, component aging and failure, power and communications disruptions, interference, and crowding. Potential barriers to IT adoption and sustainability include costs of implementation, maintenance, and training; heterogeneous or nonstandard organizational processes; integration with existing and potentially outdated institutional systems; and individual and institutional resistance to change. Effective application of ICT and information systems to disaster management requires continued focus on improved interoperability through the creation of common standards and data interchange formats. Careful consideration must be given to system robustness and necessary redundancy in key components (e.g., communications, power) to ensure fail-safe operation. Furthermore, contingency and system recovery plans are needed to ensure continuity of operations in the event of a partial or complete system failure.

A final, pivotal consideration is that systems should be suitable to the task and closely reflect real-world organizational and individual user requirements. Considerations of usability, flexibility, and appropriateness will ultimately determine the nature of user interactions and the utility of ICT tools. As such, the creation of effective systems must extend from the involvement of nurses, first responders, and decision makers in all phases of system design, development, implementation, maintenance, and evaluation.

REFERENCES

Alexa. (2017). Alexa ranking and site information for selected top social media sites. Retrieved from https://www.alexa.com/topsites/category/Computers/Internet/On_the_Web/Online_Communities/Social_Networking

Alexander, D. E. (2014). Social media in disaster risk reduction and crisis management. *Science and Engineering Ethics, 20*(3), 717–733. doi:10.1007/s11948-013-9502-z

Alfonso, L., Chacon, J., & Peña-Castellanos, G. (2015). Allowing citizens to effortlessly become rainfall sensors. In *36th IAHR World Congress*, The Hague, The Netherlands (pp. 1520–0477).

Al-Saggaf, Y., & Simmons, P. (2015). Social media in Saudi Arabia: Exploring its use during two natural disasters. *Technological Forecasting and Social Change, 95*, 3–15.

Andrienko, N., & Andrienko, G. (2005). A concept of an intelligent decision support for crisis management in the OASIS project. In P. van Oosterom, S. Zlatanova, & E. M. Fendel (Eds.), *Geo-information for disaster management* (pp. 669–682). Berlin, Germany: Springer.

Auf der Heide, E. (1996). Disaster planning, Part II. Disaster problems, issues, and challenges identified in the research literature. *Emergency Medicine Clinics of North America, 14*(2), 453–480. doi:10.1016/S0733-8627(05)70262-5

Aung, E., & Whittaker, M. (2013). Preparing routine health information systems for immediate health responses to disasters. *Health Policy and Planning, 28*(5), 495–507. doi:10.1093/heapol/czs081

Beaujohn, A. (2012). Pew: Half of Americans get news digitally, topping newspapers, radio. Retrieved from https://www.poynter.org/news/pew-half-americans-get-news-digitally-topping-newspapers-radio

Bitar, D., Goubar, A., & Desenclos, J. C. (2009). International travels and fever screening during epidemics: A literature review on the effectiveness and potential use of non-contact infrared thermometers. *Euro Surveillance, 14*(6), ii.

Boyd, D. M., & Ellison, N. B. (2007). Social network sites: Definition, history, and scholarship. *Journal of Computer-Mediated Communication, 13*, 210–230. doi:10.1111/j.1083-6101.2007.00393.x

Buono, C., Chan, T., & Griswold, W. (2008, May). WIISARD: Wireless internet information system for medical response to disasters. In *Proceedings of the 5th International ISCRAM Conference*, Washington, DC.

Chan, T., Killeen, J., Griswold, W., & Lenert, L. (2004). Information technology and emergency medical care during disasters. *Academic Emergency Medicine, 11*(11), 1229–1236. doi:10.1197/j.aem.2004.08.018

Christopher, M., & Tatham, P. (Eds.). (2014). *Humanitarian logistics: Meeting the challenge of preparing for and responding to disasters*. London, UK: Kogan Page.

Chu, Y., & Ganz, A. (2007). WISTA: A wireless telemedicine system for disaster patient care. *Mobile Networks and Applications, 12*, 201–214. doi:10.1007/s11036-007-0012-6

Chung, A. I., Neighbors, C., Belmonte, A., Miller, M., Sepulveda, H. H., Christensen, C., ... Lawrence, J. F. (2011). The Quake-Catcher Network Rapid Aftershock Mobilization Program following the 2010 M 8.8 Maule, Chile Earthquake. *Seismological Research Letters, 82*(4), 526–532. doi:10.1785/gssrl.82.4.526

Cioca, M., & Cioca, L. I. (2010). Decision support systems used in disaster management. In S. J. Chiang (Ed.), *Decision support systems* (pp. 371–390). Rijeka, Croatia: InTech.

Cochran, E. S., Lawrence, J. F., Christensen, C., & Jakka, R. S. (2009). The Quake-Catcher Network: Citizen science expanding seismic horizons. *Seismological Research Letters, 80*(1), 26–30. doi:10.1785/gssrl.80.1.26

Cochran, E. S., Lawrence, J. F., Kaiser, A., Fry, B., Chung, A., & Christensen, C. (2012). Comparison between low-cost and traditional MEMS accelerometers: A case study from the M7.1 Darfield, New Zealand, aftershock deployment. *Annals of Geophysics, 54*(6). doi:10.4401/ag-5268

Coleman, T. A., Knupp, K. R., Spann, J., Elliott, J. B., & Peters, B. E. (2011). The history (and future) of tornado warning dissemination in the United States. *Bulletin of the American Meteorological Society, 92*(5), 567–582. doi:10.1175/2010BAMS3062.1

Cranswick, E., Gardner, B., Hammond, S., & Banfill, R. (1993). Recording ground motions where people live. *Eos, Transactions American Geophysical Union, 74*(21), 243–244. doi:10.1029/93EO00393

Crowe, A. (2011). The social media manifesto: A comprehensive review of the impact of social media on emergency management. *Journal of Business Continuity & Emergency Planning, 5*(1), 409–420.

Dandoulaki, M., & Halakia, M. (2010). Social media (Web 2.0) and crisis information: Case Study Gaza 2008–09. In E. Asimakopoulou & N. Bessis (Eds.), *Advanced ICTs for disaster management and threat detection: Collaborative and distributed frameworks*. Hershey, PA: IGI Global.

Doarn, C. R., Barrigan, C. R., & Poropatich, R. K. (2011). Application of health technology in humanitarian response: U.S. military deployed health technology summit: A summary. *Telemedicine Journal and E-Health, 17*(6), 501–506. doi:10.1089/tmj.2011.0088

Doswell III, C. A., Moller, A. R., & Brooks, H. E. (1999). Storm spotting and public awareness since the first tornado forecasts of 1948. *Weather and Forecasting, 14*(4), 544–557. doi:10.1175/1520-0434(1999)014<0544:SSAPAS>2.0.CO;2

Dugas, A. F., Jalalpour, M., Gel, Y., Levin, S., Torcaso, F., Igusa, T., & Rothman, R. E. (2013). Influenza forecasting with Google flu trends. *PLOS ONE, 8*(2): e56176. doi:10.1371/journal.pone.0056176

Farinelli, A., Grisetti, G., Iocchi, L., & Lo Cascio, S. (2003). Design and evaluation of multiagent systems for rescue operations. In *Proceedings of 2003 IEEE/RSJ International Conference on Intelligent Robots and Systems*, Las Vegas, NV.

Federal Emergency Management Agency. (2011). Incident Resource Inventory System (IRIS) user's guide v4. Retrieved from http://www.fema.gov/library

Garshnek, V., & Burkle, F. M. (1999). Applications of telemedicine and telecommunications to disaster medicine: Historical and future perspectives. *Journal of the American Medical Informatics Association, 6*(1), 26–37. doi:10.1136/jamia.1999.0060026

Ginsberg, J., Mohebbi, M. H., Patel, R. S., Brammer, L., Smolinski, M. S., & Brilliant, L. (2008). Detecting influenza epidemics using search engine query data. *Nature, 457*(7232), 1012–1014. doi:10.1038/nature07634

Haynes, J. D., Saleem, M., & Kanwal, M. (2008). Telemedicine and Information Technology for Disaster Medical Scenarios. In *Encyclopedia of Healthcare Information Systems* (pp. 1303–1310). Hershey, PA: IGI Global.

Houston, J. B., Hawthorne, J., Perreault, M. F., Park, E. H., Goldstein Hode, M., Halliwell, M. R., ... Griffith, S. A. (2015). Social media and disasters: a functional framework for social media use in disaster planning, response, and research. *Disasters, 39*(1), 1–22.

Hristidis, V., Chen, S.-C., Li, T., Luis, S., & Deng, Y. (2010). Survey of data management and analysis in disaster situations. *Journal of Systems and Software, 83*(10), 1701–1714. doi:10.1016/j.jss.2010.04.065

International Federation of the Red Cross and Red Crescent Societies. (2005). *World disasters report 2005: Focus on information in disasters*. Bloomfield, CT: Kumarian Press.

Jans, J. J., & Keen, C. (2012). Enriching the modern day storm spotter through technology & education enhancements. In *92nd American Meteorological Society Annual Meeting*, New Orleans LA.

Joseph, A. (2011). *Tsunamis: Detection, monitoring, and early-warning technologies*. Amsterdam, The Netherlands: Elsevier Science.

Kohler, M. D., Heaton, T. H., & Cheng, M. H. (2013, April). The Community Seismic Network and Quake-Catcher Network: Enabling structural health monitoring through instrumentation by community participants. In *Proceedings of the SPIE*, International Society for Optical Engineering, Bellingham, WA.

Kohyu, S., Weiguo, S., & Yang, K. T. (2004). A study of forest fire danger prediction system in Japan. In *Proceedings of the 15th International Workshop on Database and Expert Systems Applications (DEXA'04)*, IEEE Computer Society, Washington, DC.

Kondaveti, R., & Ganz, A. (2009). Decision support system for resource allocation in disaster management. In *Proceedings of the Annual International Conference of the IEEE Engineering in Medicine and Biology Society. IEEE Engineering in Medicine and Biology Society Conference*, Minneapolis, MN (pp. 3425–3428).

Kosal, M. E. (2003). *The basics of chemical and biological weapons detectors*. Monterey, CA: Center for Nonproliferation Studies, Monterey Institute of International Studies.

Lazer, D., Kennedy, R., King, G., & Vespignani, A. (2014). The parable of Google flu: Traps in big data analysis. *Science, 343*, 1203–1205. doi:10.1126/science.1248506

Lenert, L. A., Palmer, D. A., Chan, T. C., & Rao, R. (2005). An Intelligent 802.11 Triage Tag for medical response to disasters. In *AMIA Annual Symposium Proceedings* (p. 440). Washington, DC: American Medical Informatics Association.

Lindell, M. K., & Prater, C. S. (2007). A hurricane evacuation management decision support system (EMDSS). *Natural Hazards, 40*(3), 627–634. doi:10.1007/s11069-006-9013-1

Luetgert, J. H., Oppenheimer, D. H., & Hamilton, J. (2010, December). The NetQuakes Project; Research-quality Seismic Data Transmitted via the Internet from Citizen-hosted Instruments. In *American Geophysical Union Fall Meeting Abstracts*.

Marchetti, N. (2010). *Telecommunications in disaster areas*. River Publishers Series in Communications. Aalborg, Denmark: River Publishers.

McBride, W. J. H., Buikstra, E., & FitzGerald, M. (2010). Investigation of febrile passengers detected by infrared thermal scanning at an international airport. *Australian and New Zealand Journal of Public Health, 34*, 5–10. doi:10.1111/j.1753-6405.2010.00466.x

Meissen, U., & Voisard, A. (2010). Current state and solutions for future challenges in early warning systems and alerting technologies. In E. Asimakopoulou & N. Bessis (Eds.), *Advanced ICTs for disaster management and threat detection: Collaborative and distributed frameworks*. Hershey, PA: IGI Global.

Morentz, J. W. (2008, May). Unified incident command and decision support (UICDS): a Department of Homeland Security initiative in information sharing. In *2008 IEEE conference on technologies for homeland security* (pp. 321–326). Piscataway, NJ: IEEE.

Munson, C. A., Gottfried, J. L., De Lucia, F. C., & Miziolek, A. (2008). Detection of indoor chemical and biological hazards using the man-portable laser-induced breakdown spectrometer (MP-LIBS). *Applied Optics, 47*, G48. doi:10.1364/AO.47.000G48

Murthy, D., & Longwell, S. A. (2013). Twitter and disasters: The uses of Twitter during the 2010 Pakistan floods. *Information, Communication & Society, 16*(6), 837–855.

National Research Council, Committee on Using Information Technology to Enhance Disaster Management. (2007). In R. R. Rao, J. Eisenberg, & T. Schmitt (Eds.), *Improving disaster management: The role of IT in mitigation, preparedness, response, and recovery*. Washington, DC: National Academies Press.

Naumann, F., & Raschid, L. (2006, October 25–27). Information Integration and Disaster Data Management (DisDM) Workshop on Information Integration, Philadelphia, PA.

Parker, B. J., & Al-Utabi, G. A. (1986). Decision support systems: The reality that seems to be too hard to accept? *International Journal of Management Science, 14*(2), 135–143.

Patoli, A. Q. (2006). Role of telemedicine in disaster management. *EHealth International Journal, 2*(2), 34.

Pidd, M., de Silva, F. N., & Eglese, R. W. (1996). A simulation model for emergency evacuation. *European Journal of Operational Research, 90*(3), 413–419. doi:10.1016/0377-2217(95)00112-3

Pine, J. C. (2007). *Technology in emergency management*. Wiley Pathways Series. Hoboken, NJ: Wiley.

Pottebaum, J., Schäfer, C., Kuhnert, M., Behnke, D., Wietfeld, C., Büscher, M., & Petersen, K. (2016, May). Common information space for collaborative emergency management. In *2016 IEEE symposium on technologies for homeland security (HST)* (pp. 1–6). Piscataway, NJ: IEEE.

Pourvakhshouri, S., & Mansor, S. (2003). Decision support system in oil spill cases. *Disaster Prevention and Management, 12*(3), 217–221. doi:10.1108/09653560310480695

Quake-Catcher. (2017). The Quake-Catcher Network. Retrieved from http://quakecatcher.net

Reddick, C. (2011). Information technology and emergency management: Preparedness and planning in US states. *Disasters, 35*(1), 45–61. doi:10.1111/j.1467-7717.2010.01192.x

Reges, H. W., Doesken, N., Turner, J., Newman, N., Bergantino, A., & Schwalbe, Z. (2016). COCORAHS: The evolution and accomplishments of a volunteer rain gauge network. *Bulletin of the American Meteorological Society, 97*(10), 1831–1846. doi:10.1175/BAMS-D-14-00213.1

Sagun, A. (2010). Efficient deployment of ICT tools in disaster management process. In E. Asimakopoulou & N. Bessis (Eds.), *Advanced ICTs for disaster management and threat detection: Collaborative and distributed frameworks*. Hershey, PA: IGI Global.

Shu, P. Y., Chien, L. J., Chang, S. F., Su, C. L., Kuo, Y. C., Liao, T. L., … Huang, J. H. (2005). Fever screening at airports and imported dengue. *Emerging Infectious Diseases, 11*(3), 460–462. doi:10.3201/eid1103.040420

Silva, F. N. (2001). Providing decision support for evacuation planning: A challenge in integrating technologies. *Disaster Prevention and Management, 10*(1), 11–20. doi:10.1108/09653560110381787

Simmons, S. C., Murphy, T. A., Blanarovicii, A., Workman, F., Rosenthal, D. A., & Carbone, M. (2003). Telehealth technologies and applications for terrorism response: A report of the 2002 Coastal North Carolina domestic preparedness training exercise. *Journal of the American Medical Informatics Association, 10*, 166–176. doi:10.1197/jamia.M1205

Sood, S., Mbarika, V., Jugoo, S., Dookhy, R., Doarn, C. R., Prakash, N., & Merrell, R. C. (2007). What is telemedicine? A collection of 104 peer-reviewed perspectives and theoretical underpinnings. *Telemedicine Journal and E-Health: The Official Journal of the American Telemedicine Association, 13*(5), 573–590. doi:10.1089/tmj.2006.0073

Subedi, J. (2010). Disaster informatics: Information management as a tool for effective disaster risk reduction. In E. Asimakopoulou & N. Bessis (Eds.), *Advanced ICTs for disaster management and threat detection: Collaborative and distributed frameworks* (pp. 80–94). Hershey, PA: IGI Global.

Thomas, T. L., Schrock, C., & Friedman, D. B. (2016). Providing health consumers with emergency information: A systematic review of research examining social media use during public crises. *Journal of Consumer Health on the Internet, 20*(1–2), 19–40. doi:10.1080/15398285.2016.1142927

Tomaszewski, B., Judex, M., Szarzynski, J., Radestock, C., & Wirkus, L. (2015). Geographic information systems for disaster response: A review. *Journal of Homeland Security and Emergency Management, 12*(3), 571–602. doi:10.1515/jhsem-2014-0082

Toya, H., & Skidmore, M. (2015). Information/communication technology and natural disaster vulnerability. *Economics Letters, 137*, 143–145. doi:10.1016/j.econlet.2015.10.018

Tufekci, S. (1995). An integrated emergency management decision support system for hurricane emergencies. *Safety Science, 20*, 39–48. doi:10.1016/0925-7535(94)00065-B

United Nations, International Strategy for Disaster Reduction. (2006). *Global survey of early warning systems*. Retrieved from https://www.unisdr.org/files/3612_GlobalSurveyofEarlyWarningSystems.pdf

Veenema, T. G., & Rains, A. B. (2009, November). Clinical decision support for nurses: Restoring public health following a disaster. *Presentation given at the American Public Health Association (APHA) Annual Conference*, Philadelphia, PA.

Wallace, W. A., & Balogh, F. (1985). Decision support systems for disaster management. *Public Administration Review, 45*(SI), 134–146. doi:10.2307/3135008

Wang, L., Qin, Q., & Wang, D. (2004, September 20–24). Decision support system of flood disaster for property insurance: Theory and practice. In *Proceedings 2004 IEEE International Geoscience and Remote Sensing Symposium* (Vol. 7, pp. 4693–4695).

Weiner, E. (2006). Informatics can play a key role in emergency preparedness and response. *Nursing Outlook, 54*(1), 55–57. doi:10.1016/j.outlook.2005.11.005

Whitten, P., & Sypher, B. D. (2006). Evolution of telemedicine from an applied communication perspective in the United States. *Telemedicine Journal and E-Health: The Official Journal of the American Telemedicine Association, 12*(5), 590–600. doi:10.1089/tmj.2006.12.590

Wootton, R., & Bonnardot, L. (2010). In what circumstances is telemedicine appropriate in the developing world? *Journal of the Royal Society of Medicine, Short Reports, 1*(5), 37. doi:10.1258/shorts.2010.010045

Wrobel, L. A., & Wrobel, S. M. (2009). *Disaster recovery planning for communications and critical infrastructure*. London, UK: Artech House Telecommunications Library, Artech House.

Wukich, C., & Steinberg, A. (2016). 11 Social media for emergency management. In S. M. Zavattaro & T. A. Bryer (Eds.), *Social Media for Government: Theory and Practice* (p. 140). New York, NY: Routledge.

Yong, C., Chen, Q. F., Frolova, N., Larionov, V., Nikolaev, A., Pejcoch, J., … Ugarov, A. N. (2001). Web based decision support tool in order to respond to strong earth-quakes. In *Proceedings of TIEMS 2001*, Oslo, Norway.

Zdravkovic, M., Noran, O., Panetto, H., & Trajanović, M. (2015). Enabling interoperability as a property of ubiquitous systems for disaster management. *Computer Science and Information Systems, 12*(3), 1009–1031. doi:10.2298/CSIS141031011Z

Epilogue

DISASTER RECOVERY: CREATING HEALTHY, RESILIENT, AND SUSTAINABLE COMMUNITIES AFTER DISASTERS

Tener Goodwin Veenema

In the aftermath of a disaster, the evidence of death, injury, and devastation can overwhelm both victims and responders. The effects on healthcare range from situations that immediately burden the system with large numbers of patients to catastrophes that strain the effective functioning and long-term fiscal sustainability of services. The evidence of destruction and the inevitable life changes that the disaster has caused become rapidly apparent. The social fabric of the community may have unwoven and the geography may appear representative of a war zone. Chaos and ambiguity may reign. The disaster continuum plays out—leaving its victims and responders in its wake. Yet the disaster response is not over—in fact, the final recovery and evaluative phases of the disaster continuum are just beginning. And in all probability, the role of the nurse is never more important than during the recovery.

In the almost 20 years that have passed since the first edition of this book was released, we have witnessed a significant increase in the number of devastating disasters and large-scale public health emergencies. Across the globe, we have witnessed nurses quick to respond. At the heart of our profession, we bring care and compassion to all victims of these horrific events. We bring highly refined assessment skills and evidence-based strategies to optimize disaster-impacted population health outcomes. In the aftermath of response, our focus shifts to recovery. Nursing, with roots firmly planted in health promotion and wellness and the provision of holistic healthcare and human services, now must address *holistic disaster recovery* with the goals being to assist individuals and communities to move forward and create a more sustainable future. Healthy, resilient, and sustainable communities develop, maintain, and leverage collaborative relationships among government, corporations, community organizations, and individual households that enable them to more effectively respond to and recover from disasters and emergencies.

A healthy community is defined as one in which a diverse group of stakeholders collaborate to use their expertise and local knowledge to create a community that is socially and physically conducive to health. Community members are empowered and civically engaged, assuring that all local policies consider health. The community has the capacity to identify, address, and evaluate its own health concerns on an ongoing basis, using data to guide and benchmark efforts. As a result, a healthy community is safe, economically secure and environmentally sound, as all residents have equal access to high quality educational and employment opportunities, transportation and housing options, prevention and healthcare services, and healthy food and physical activity opportunities (Health Resources in Action, 2013). Disasters, inarguably destructive, can however provide communities access to previously unavailable resources and opportunities for transformation to advance a vision of a healthier and more resilient and sustainable community. However, leveraging the disaster recovery process to this end necessitates an understanding of the diverse determinants that influence health and healthy communities (Institute of Medicine [IOM], 2015). It requires an appreciation of what resiliency truly is (Burkle, 2012). It is increasingly understood that health is influenced largely by the natural and locally built social environments within communities—the social determinants of health, defined by the World Health Organization (WHO) as "the conditions in which people are born, grow, live, work and age. These circumstances are shaped by the distribution of money, power and resources at global, national and local levels" (WHO, 2014).

In April 2015, the Institute of Medicine ([IOM]; now National Academy of Medicine) published a report, *Healthy, Resilient and Sustainable Communities After Disasters*, in response to concerns that disaster recovery efforts tended to focus upon rebuilding and hardening infrastructure rather than on strengthening the resiliency of individuals and communities. The report proposed that disaster recovery initiatives should be forward thinking and used to enhance the health of communities and individuals. It articulated 12 recommendations using a framework of vision, assessment, planning, and implementation to integrate health considerations into recovery decision making (IOM, 2015).

RECOMMENDATIONS FOR DISASTER RECOVERY IN THE UNITED STATES

Recommendation 1: Develop a Healthy Community Vision for Disaster Recovery
Recommendation 2: Integrate Health Considerations Into Recovery Decision Making Through the National Disaster Recovery Framework
Recommendation 3: Facilitate the Engagement of the Whole Community in Disaster Recovery Through Simplified and Accessible Information and Training
Recommendation 4: Enhance and Leverage Social Networks in Community Health Improvement and Recovery Planning

Recommendation 5: Establish Pathways by Which Health Information Can Inform Recovery Decision Making
Recommendation 6: Leverage Recovery Resources in a Coordinated Manner to Achieve Healthier Post-Disaster Communities
Recommendation 7: Ensure a Ready Health Information Technology Infrastructure
Recommendation 8: Develop a National Disaster Behavioral Health Policy
Recommendation 9: Develop an Integrated Social Services Recovery Framework
Recommendation 10: Design for Healthy Post-Disaster Communities
Recommendation 11: Mitigate Against Future Health Hazards
Recommendation 12: Ensure Healthy and Affordable Post-Disaster Housing (IOM, 2015).

At the time of publication of this book, progress toward achieving these recommendations has been mixed. The delayed recovery status of Puerto Rico, more than 100 days post Hurricane Maria, suggests that much work remains to be done.

SOCIAL DETERMINANTS OF HEALTH & DISASTER RECOVERY

Physical Rebuilding

"The social determinants of health are the circumstances in which people are born, grow up, live, work, and age, and the systems put in place to deal with illness. These circumstances are in turn shaped by a wider set of forces: economics, social policies, and politics" (WHO, 2014). How do we address the impact disasters have on the social determinants of health? How do we restore healthy neighborhoods and help communities that have been impacted by disasters to rebuild? Attention must focus upon the built, natural, and social environments. In postdisaster situations, the physical rebuilding–reconstruction planning, assistance, funding, and responsibility for recovery and rebuilding is often centralized and comes from the top down. This type of reconstruction approach is often managed by city, state, or federal governments and, depending on the location of the disaster, by an international agency, such as the United Nations. Centralized management and support are vital to effective and efficient reconstruction that follows best practices. Emergency funding can be appropriated and distributed to areas affected by the disaster, and myriad governmental and nongovernmental organizations (NGOs) are coordinated to move reconstruction forward.

Despite this centralized approach, postdisaster rebuilding is a local task. Rebuilding is a task undertaken by individual homeowners and business owners and healthcare systems at the local level. While centralized authorities can support and stimulate this effort, the actual work of rebuilding a community (other than public infrastructure) is a bottom-up decentralized process. The decisions made by tens of thousands of individuals determine the outcome. These decisions are made by individuals with the knowledge they possess in response to the specific context of their situation. They may take their cues from their neighbors and from what other *local* individuals are deciding. Decision making will be reflective of the social and cultural norms in place in the predisaster community. Individuals will need support for their ideas and decisions. Understanding that each community will have its own unique perspectives, priorities, and timelines will allow for the implementation of a meaningful recovery plan that is both pragmatic and respectful of the citizens it is designed to help.

Restoration of Livelihoods

Individuals, families, and localities need a source of income to survive. Restoration of the economic security of a disaster-affected region is critical to its survival. Yet the restoration of livelihoods is often the largest and most difficult hurdle for long-term recovery. In communities with high rates of poverty before the disaster, the impact of the event may destroy any remaining economic fabric for years to come. Efforts to restore the economic integrity of the community must be swift and include a plan for sustainability. Rebuilding the economy means the restoration of businesses and trade and the establishment of new sources of local employment. International aid and governmental funding will need to be administered in a manner that supports employment opportunities and reflects a long-term vision for the affected community. Returning people to work not only provides income but gives a sense of purpose and hope for the future.

Shelter

Efforts to establish safe, secure housing is a major challenge in recovery planning. Frequently, it is poorly constructed housing that may have contributed to the community's vulnerability prior to the event. Shelter may need to occur as an evolving process starting with temporary shelter and moving to intermediate housing to permanent housing or relocation. Meaningful recovery planning will incorporate multiple options and a degree of redundancy to ensure adequate shelter for all affected individuals and families. Environmental impact and the potential for future disasters should also be taken into account in identifying locations for shelter.

The Role of the Nurse

How can nurses contribute to holistic disaster recovery and create a healthier and more sustainable future for communities? Communities need nurses who are prepared and willing to respond. *We must all accept our professional mandate as a global profession to be prepared.* We share our knowledge and experiences with each other through professional conferences, the establishment of disaster nursing task forces, and in the literature. We write and speak of the lessons that we have learned and identify strategies for avoiding future mistakes. We applaud the efforts of those valiant nurses who have responded to their communities in times of need. We band together to advocate on behalf of those populations which are vulnerable and at higher risk for poor outcomes from the effects of a disaster. We acknowledge the looming threat of global climate change and its potential impact on the frequency

and intensity of disasters. We partner with our colleagues in medicine, public health, and emergency management, and work to focus on improving community outcomes and fostering environmental stability.

We as nurses need to continually seek and accept leadership positions in disaster planning, response, and recovery initiatives. We need to clearly understand the concept of *sustainability* and what that means in terms of community planning and building codes, environmental health and safety, and promoting a sense of harmony and togetherness. We bring our respect for cultural differences and our value for the uniqueness of each individual to each response. The disaster recovery process is multifaceted and involves numerous steps and the inclusion of many individuals and organizations. The disaster recovery process is long, cumbersome, and often painful. It encompasses adaptive responses to unexpected and untoward events, advocacy planning to ensure the future safety of populations, and policy and legislative adjustments. It mandates extensive investigation and exploration of what went right and what went wrong. It demands an evaluation of every agency's response.

Disaster recovery is a social process that encompasses planning for future events, public policy development, and social awareness/learning. This mandates the establishment of organizational relationships and intergovernmental linkages—and the processes for collaboration and coordination that enhance recovery efforts. We must understand how the disaster recovery process can be used to maintain and enhance the quality of life. We need to design recovery strategies for enhancing quality of life, pursue new strategies for improving the quality of life, and institute systems for the ongoing monitoring of the quality of life. In doing so, we can work to correct preexisting social and economic disparities and reduce vulnerability to future disaster events.

Nurses need to understand and become active in policy making at both their federal and state levels. Familiarity with existing disaster policies; the concepts of negotiation, regionalism, and paternalism on the part of the federal government with regard to disaster recovery; and the role of leadership and charisma are important components of policy making. The importance of using strategies that protect the quality of the environment, address rebuilding economic vitality in a community, and include protections for social and intergenerational equity are critical to achieving sustainable improvements.

Nurses need to understand how the *funding* of the disaster recovery process is supposed to occur and what national and international disaster recovery programs exist (and how they are evolving). Debate surrounds many recovery issues related to funding, such as whether or not at-risk families should be relocated, and what the government's role (in terms of long-term commitment) to the disaster recovery process should be. Who should pay for what and for how long? In the United States, what is the role of the federal government versus that of the states? When should disaster areas seek congressional aid? Is FEMA disaster funding realistically sustainable? What are the "hard" decisions that need to be made? What areas should be rebuilt and what areas should not? What is the risk if the hazard persists? What are individuals' understanding of risk? What are the expectations of the public and of the media? What type of social learning needs to take place for communities to better position themselves for mitigation and recovery? How do we create a less vulnerable society? How do we protect the quality of our environment to sustain life on our planet? What is the role for academia in disaster response and recovery?

These are difficult questions at best, yet the foundation for successful disaster recovery and the creation of disaster-resistant sustainable communities lies within them. As a nation, we must not succumb to apathy but force ourselves to plan for the unexpected, prepare for the unlikely, and establish *sustainable community partnerships with effective avenues of communication.* These discussions will most likely take place at the highest levels of our government—and no one is better prepared to contribute to this discussion than a nurse.

REFERENCES

Burkle, F. M., Jr. (2012). The limits to our capacity: Reflections on resiliency, community engagement and recovery in 21st century crises. *Disaster Medicine and Public Health Preparedness*, 5(Suppl. 2), 176–181. doi:10.1001/dmp.2011.52

Health Resources in Action. (2013). Defining healthy communities. Retrieved from https://hria.org/wp-content/uploads/2016/10/defininghealthycommunities.original.pdf

Institute of Medicine. (2015). *Healthy, resilient, and sustainable communities after disasters: Strategies, opportunities, and planning for recovery.* Washington, DC: National Academies Press.

World Health Organization. (2014). Health impact assessment. Retrieved from http://www.who.int/hia/en

Appendix I

AT-A-GLANCE: CAPABILITY DEFINITIONS, FUNCTIONS, AND ASSOCIATED PERFORMANCE MEASURES

CAPABILITY 1: COMMUNITY PREPAREDNESS

Definition: Community preparedness is the ability of communities to prepare for, withstand, and recover—in both the short and long terms—from public health incidents. By engaging and coordinating with emergency management, healthcare organizations (private and community-based), mental/behavioral health providers, community and faith-based partners, state, local, and territorial, public health's role in community preparedness is to do the following:

- Support the development of public health, medical, and mental/behavioral health systems that support recovery
- Participate in awareness training with community and faith-based partners on how to prevent, respond to, and recover from public health incidents
- Promote awareness of and access to medical and mental/behavioral health resources that help protect the community's health and address the functional needs (i.e., communication, medical care, independence, supervision, transportation) of at-risk individuals
- Engage public and private organizations in preparedness activities that represent the functional needs of at-risk individuals as well as the cultural and socioeconomic, demographic components of the community
- Identify those populations that may be at higher risk for adverse health outcomes
- Receive and/or integrate the health needs of populations that have been displaced due to incidents that have occurred in their own or distant communities (e.g., improvised nuclear device or hurricane)

Functions and Associated Performance Measures: This capability consists of the ability to perform the functions listed below. At present there are no Centers for Disease Control and Prevention (CDC)-defined performance measures for these functions.

Function 1: Determine risks to the health of the jurisdiction

Function 2: Build community partnerships to support health preparedness

Function 3: Engage with community organizations to foster public health, medical, and mental/behavioral health social networks

Function 4: Coordinate training or guidance to ensure community engagement in preparedness efforts

CAPABILITY 2: COMMUNITY RECOVERY

Definition: Community recovery is the ability to collaborate with community partners, (e.g., healthcare organizations, business, education, and emergency management) to plan and advocate for the rebuilding of public health, medical, and mental/behavioral health systems to at least a level of functioning comparable to preincident levels, and improved levels where possible.

This capability supports National Health Security Strategy Objective 8: Incorporate Post-Incident Health Recovery Into Planning and Response. Postincident recovery of the public health, medical, and mental/behavioral health services and systems within a jurisdiction is critical for health security and requires collaboration with and advocacy by the public health agency for the restoration of services, providers, facilities, and infrastructure within the public health, medical, and human services sectors. Monitoring the public health, medical, and mental/behavioral health infrastructure is an essential public health service.

Functions and Associated Performance Measures: This capability consists of the ability to perform the following functions. At present there are no CDC-defined performance measures for these functions.

Function 1: Identify and monitor public health, medical, and mental/behavioral health system recovery needs

Function 2: Coordinate community public health, medical, and mental/behavioral health system recovery operations

Function 3: Implement corrective actions to mitigate damages from future incidents

CAPABILITY 3: EMERGENCY OPERATIONS COORDINATION

Definition: Emergency operations coordination is the ability to direct and support an event or incident with public health or medical implications by establishing a standardized, scalable system of oversight, organization, and supervision consistent with jurisdictional standards and practices and with the National Incident Management System.

Functions and Associated Performance Measures: This capability consists of the ability to perform the following functions. Associated CDC-defined performance measures are also listed.

Function 1: Conduct preliminary assessment to determine need for public activation

Function 2: Activate public health emergency operations
Measure 1: Time for preidentified staff covering activated public health agency incident management lead roles (or equivalent lead roles) to report for immediate duty; Performance Target: 60 minutes or less

Function 3: Develop incident response strategy
Measure 1: Production of the approved Incident Action Plan before the start of the second operational period

Function 4: Manage and sustain the public health response

Function 5: Demobilize and evaluate public health emergency operations
Measure 1: Time to complete a draft of an After Action Report and Improvement Plan

CAPABILITY 4: EMERGENCY PUBLIC INFORMATION AND WARNING

Definition: Emergency public information and warning is the ability to develop, coordinate, and disseminate information, alerts, warnings, and notifications to the public and incident management responders.

Functions and Associated Performance Measures: This capability consists of the ability to perform the following functions. Associated CDC-defined performance measures are also listed.

Function 1: Activate the emergency public information system

Function 2: Determine the need for a joint public information system

Function 3: Establish and participate in information system operations

Function 4: Establish avenues for public interaction and information exchange

Function 5: Issue public information, alerts, warnings, and notifications
Measure 1: Time to issue a risk communication message for dissemination to the public

CAPABILITY 5: FATALITY MANAGEMENT

Definition: Fatality management is the ability to coordinate with other organizations (e.g., law enforcement, healthcare, emergency management, and medical examiner/coroner) to ensure the proper recovery, handling, identification, transportation, tracking, storage, and disposal of human remains and personal effects; certify cause of death; and facilitate access to mental/behavioral health services to the family members, responders, and survivors of an incident.

Functions and Associated Performance Measures: This capability consists of the ability to perform the following functions. At present there are no CDC-defined performance measures for these functions.

> Function 1: Determine role for public health in fatality management
> Function 2: Activate public health fatality management operations
> Function 3: Assist in the collection and dissemination of antemortem data
> Function 4: Participate in survivor mental/behavioral health services
> Function 5: Participate in fatality processing and storage operations

CAPABILITY 6: INFORMATION SHARING

Definition: Information sharing is the ability to conduct multijurisdictional, multidisciplinary exchange of health-related information and situational awareness data among federal, state, local, territorial, and tribal levels of government, and the private sector. This capability includes the routine sharing of information as well as issuing of public health alerts to federal, state, local, territorial, and tribal levels of government and the private sector in preparation for, and in response to, events or incidents of public health significance.

Functions and Associated Performance Measures: This capability consists of the ability to perform the following functions. At present there are no CDC-defined performance measures for these functions.

> Function 1: Identify stakeholders to be incorporated into information flow
> Function 2: Identify and develop rules and data elements for sharing
> Function 3: Exchange information to determine a common operating picture

CAPABILITY 7: MASS CARE

Definition: Mass care is the ability to coordinate with partner agencies to address the public health, medical, and mental/behavioral health needs of those impacted by an incident at a congregate location. This capability includes the coordination of ongoing surveillance and assessment to ensure that health needs continue to be met as the incident evolves.

Functions and Associated Performance Measures: This capability consists of the ability to perform the following functions. At present there are no CDC-defined performance measures for these functions.

> Function 1: Determine public health role in mass care operations
> Function 2: Determine mass care needs of the impacted population

> Function 3: Coordinate public health, medical, and mental/behavioral health services
> Function 4: Monitor mass care population health

CAPABILITY 8: MEDICAL COUNTERMEASURE DISPENSING

Definition: Medical countermeasure dispensing is the ability to provide medical countermeasures (including vaccines, antiviral drugs, antibiotics, antitoxins, etc.) in support of treatment or prophylaxis (oral or vaccination) to the identified population in accordance with public health guidelines and/or recommendations.

Functions and Associated Performance Measures: This capability consists of the ability to perform the following functions. Associated CDC-defined performance measures are also listed.

> Function 1: Identify and initiate medical countermeasure dispensing strategies
> Function 2: Receive medical countermeasures
> Function 3: Activate dispensing modalities
>> Measure 1: Composite performance indicator from the Division of Strategic National Stockpile in CDC's Office of Public Health Preparedness and Response
> Function 4: Dispense medical countermeasures to identified population
>> Measure 1: Composite performance indicator from the Division of Strategic National Stockpile in CDC's Office of Public Health Preparedness and Response
> Function 5: Report adverse events

CAPABILITY 9: MEDICAL MATERIAL MANAGEMENT AND DISTRIBUTION

Definition: Medical material management and distribution is the ability to acquire, maintain (e.g., cold chain storage or other storage protocol), transport, distribute, and track medical material (e.g., pharmaceuticals, gloves, masks, and ventilators) during an incident and to recover and account for unused medical material, as necessary, after an incident.

Functions and Associated Performance Measures: This capability consists of the ability to perform the following functions. Associated CDC-defined performance measures are also listed.

> Function 1: Direct and activate medical material management and distribution
>> Measure 1: Composite performance indicator from the Division of Strategic National Stockpile in CDC's Office of Public Health Preparedness and Response

Function 2:   Acquire medical material
        Measure 1:   Composite performance indicator from the Division of Strategic National Stockpile in CDC's Office of Public Health Preparedness and Response

Function 3:   Maintain updated inventory management and reporting system
        Measure 1:   Composite performance indicator from the Division of Strategic National Stockpile in CDC's Office of Public Health Preparedness and Response

Function 4:   Establish and maintain security
        Measure 1:   Composite performance indicator from the Division of Strategic National Stockpile in CDC's Office of Public Health Preparedness and Response

Function 5:   Distribute medical material
        Measure 1:   Composite performance indicator from the Division of Strategic National Stockpile in CDC's Office of Public Health Preparedness and Response

Function 6:   Recover medical material and demobilize distribution operations
        Measure 1:   Composite performance indicator from the Division of Strategic National Stockpile in CDC's Office of Public Health Preparedness and Response

CAPABILITY 10: MEDICAL SURGE

Definition: Medical surge is the ability to provide adequate medical evaluation and care during events that exceed the limits of the normal medical infrastructure of an affected community. It encompasses the ability of the healthcare system to survive a hazard impact and maintain or rapidly recover operations that were compromised.

Functions and Associated Performance Measures: This capability consists of the ability to perform the following functions. At present there are no CDC-defined performance measures for these functions.

Function 1:   Assess the nature and scope of the incident
Function 2:   Support activation of medical surge
Function 3:   Support jurisdictional medical surge operations
Function 4:   Support demobilization of medical surge operations

CAPABILITY 11: NONPHARMACEUTICAL INTERVENTIONS

Definition: Nonpharmaceutical interventions are the ability to recommend to the applicable lead agency (if not public health)

and implement, if applicable, strategies for disease, injury, and exposure control. Strategies include the following:

- Isolation and quarantine
- Restrictions on movement and travel advisory/warnings
- Social distancing
- External decontamination
- Hygiene
- Precautionary protective behaviors

Functions and Associated Performance Measures: This capability consists of the ability to perform the following functions. At present there are no CDC-defined performance measures for these functions.

Function 1:   Engage partners and identify factors that impact nonpharmaceutical interventions
Function 2:   Determine nonpharmaceutical interventions
Function 3:   Implement nonpharmaceutical interventions
Function 4:   Monitor nonpharmaceutical interventions

CAPABILITY 12: PUBLIC HEALTH LABORATORY TESTING

Definition: Public health laboratory testing is the ability to conduct rapid and conventional detection, characterization, confirmatory testing, data reporting, investigative support, and laboratory networking to address actual or potential exposure to all hazards. Hazards include chemical, radiological, and biological agents in multiple matrices that may include clinical samples, food, and environmental samples (e.g., water, air, and soil). This capability supports routine surveillance, including pre-event or preincident and post-exposure activities.

Functions and Associated Performance Measures: This capability consists of the ability to perform the following functions. Associated CDC-defined performance measures are also listed.

Function 1:   Manage laboratory activities
        Measure 1:   Time for sentinel clinical laboratories to acknowledge receipt of an urgent message from the CDC Public Health Emergency Preparedness (PHEP)-funded Laboratory Response Network biological (LRN-B) laboratory
        Measure 2:   Time for initial laboratorian to report for duty at the CDC PHEP-funded laboratory

Function 2:   Perform sample management
        Measure 1:   Percentage of Laboratory Response Network (LRN) clinical specimens without any adverse quality assurance events received at the CDC

PHEP-funded LRN-B laboratory for confirmation or rule-out testing from sentinel clinical laboratories

Measure 2:   Percentage of LRN nonclinical samples without any adverse quality assurance events received at the CDC PHEP-funded LRN-B laboratory for confirmation or rule-out testing from first responders

Measure 3:   Ability of the CDC PHEP-funded Laboratory Response Network chemical (LRN-C) laboratories to collect relevant samples for clinical chemical analysis, package, and ship those samples

Function 3:   Conduct testing and analysis for routine and surge capacity

Measure 1:   Proportion of LRN-C proficiency tests (core methods) successfully passed by CDC PHEP-funded laboratories

Measure 2:   Proportion of LRN-C proficiency tests (additional methods) successfully passed by CDC PHEP-funded laboratories

Measure 3:   Proportion of LRN-B proficiency tests successfully passed by CDC PHEP-funded laboratories

Function 4:   Support public health investigations

Measure 1:   Time to complete notification between CDC, on-call laboratorian, and on-call epidemiologist

Measure 2:   Time to complete notification between CDC, on-call epidemiologist, and on-call laboratorian

Function 5:   Report results

Measure 1:   Percentage of pulsed field gel electrophoresis (PFGE) subtyping data results for *Escherichia coli* O157:H7 submitted to the PulseNet national database within 4 working days of receiving an isolate at the PFGE laboratory

Measure 2:   Percentage of PFGE subtyping data results for *Listeria monocytogenes* submitted to the PulseNet national database within 4 working days of receiving an isolate at the PFGE laboratory

Measure 3:   Time to submit PFGE subtyping data results for *Salmonella* to the PulseNet national database upon receipt of an isolate at the PFGE laboratory

Measure 4:   Time for CDC PHEP-funded laboratory to notify public health partners of significant laboratory results

CAPABILITY 13: PUBLIC HEALTH SURVEILLANCE AND EPIDEMIOLOGICAL INVESTIGATION

Definition: Public health surveillance and epidemiological investigation is the ability to create, maintain, support, and strengthen routine surveillance and detection systems and epidemiological investigation processes, as well as to expand these systems and processes in response to incidents of public health significance.

Functions and Associated Performance Measures: This capability consists of the ability to perform the following functions. Associated CDC-defined performance measures are also listed.

Function 1:   Conduct public health surveillance and detection

Measure 1:   Proportion of reports of selected reportable diseases received by a public health agency within the jurisdiction-required time frame

Function 2:   Conduct public health and epidemiological investigations

Measure 1:   Percentage of infectious disease outbreak investigations that generate reports

Measure 2:   Percentage of infectious disease outbreak investigation reports that contain all minimal elements

Measure 3:   Percentage of acute environmental exposure investigations that generate reports

Measure 4:   Percentage of acute environmental exposure reports that contain all minimal elements

Function 3:   Recommend, monitor, and analyze mitigation actions

Measure 1:   Proportion of reports of selected reportable diseases for which initial public health control measure(s) were initiated within the appropriate time frame

Function 4:   Improve public health surveillance and epidemiological investigation systems

CAPABILITY 14: RESPONDER SAFETY AND HEALTH

Definition: The responder safety and health capability describes the ability to protect public health agency staff responding to an incident and the ability to support the health and safety needs of hospital and medical facility personnel, if requested.

Functions and Associated Performance Measures: This capability consists of the ability to perform the following functions. At present there are no CDC-defined performance measures for these functions.

Function 1: Identify responder safety and health risks
Function 2: Identify safety and personal protective needs
Function 3: Coordinate with partners to facilitate risk-specific safety and health training
Function 4: Monitor responder safety and health actions

CAPABILITY 15: VOLUNTEER MANAGEMENT

Definition: Volunteer management is the ability to coordinate the identification, recruitment, registration, credential verification, training, and engagement of volunteers to support the jurisdictional public health agency's response to incidents of public health significance.

Functions and Associated Performance Measures: This capability consists of the ability to perform the following functions. At present there are no CDC-defined performance measures for these functions.

Function 1: Coordinate volunteers
Function 2: Notify volunteers
Function 3: Organize, assemble, and dispatch volunteers
Function 4: Demobilize volunteers

Source: Centers for Disease Control and Prevention. (2011, March). Public Health Preparedness Capabilities: National standards for state and local planning. Retrieved from https://www.cdc.gov/phpr/readiness/00_docs/DSLR_capabilities_July.pdf

Note: Updated Centers for Disease Control and Prevention (CDC) Public Health Preparedness and Response Capabilities will be released in 2018 by the CDC. These updated capabilities address a shift from planning to execution and will include cross-cutting topics, including pandemic influenza/immunization, public health informatics, tribal populations, and populations at risk for being disproportionately impacted (vulnerable populations and environmental health). See https://www.cdc.gov/phpr/readiness/capabilities.htm.

Appendix II

SEQUENCE FOR PUTTING ON PERSONAL PROTECTIVE EQUIPMENT

CENTERS FOR DISEASE CONTROL AND PREVENTION SEQUENCE FOR PUTTING ON PERSONAL PROTECTIVE EQUIPMENT (PPE)

The type of PPE used will vary based on the level of precautions required, such as standard and contact, droplet or airborne infection isolation precautions. The procedure for putting on and removing PPE should be tailored to the specific type of PPE.

1. GOWN
- Fully cover torso from neck to knees, arms to end of wrists, and wrap around the back
- Fasten in back of neck and waist

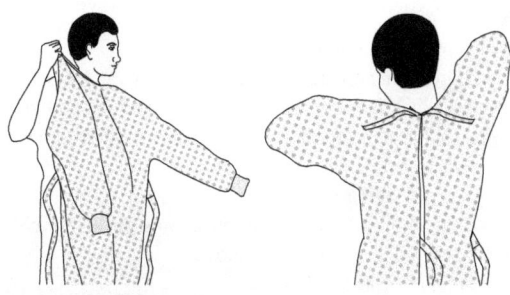

2. MASK OR RESPIRATOR
- Secure ties or elastic bands at middle of head and neck
- Fit flexible band to nose bridge
- Fit snug to face and below chin
- Fit-check respirator

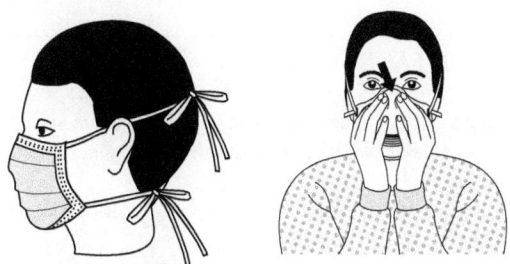

3. GOGGLES OR FACE SHIELD
- Place over face and eyes and adjust to fit

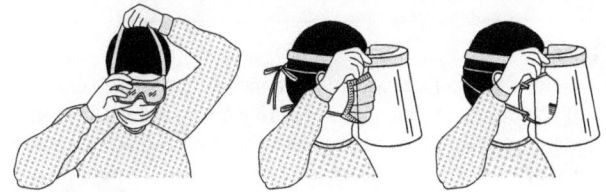

4. GLOVES
- Extend to cover wrist of isolation gown

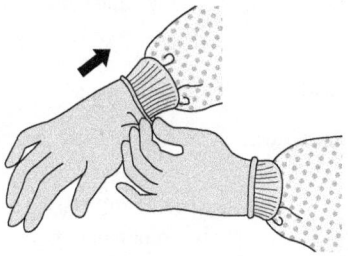

USE SAFE WORK PRACTICES TO PROTECT YOURSELF AND LIMIT THE SPREAD OF CONTAMINATION

- Keep hands away from face
- Limit surfaces touched
- Change gloves when torn or heavily contaminated
- Perform hand hygiene

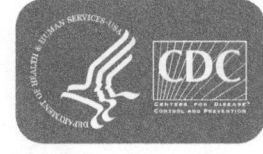

HOW TO SAFELY REMOVE PPE EXAMPLE 1

There are a variety of ways to safely remove PPE without contaminating your clothing, skin, or mucous membranes with potentially infectious materials. Here is one example. **Remove all PPE before exiting the patient room** except a respirator, if worn. Remove the respirator **after** leaving the patient room and closing the door. Remove PPE in the following sequence:

1. GLOVES

- Outside of gloves are contaminated!
- If your hands get contaminated during glove removal, immediately wash your hands or use an alcohol-based hand sanitizer
- Using a gloved hand, grasp the palm area of the other gloved hand and peel off first glove
- Hold removed glove in gloved hand
- Slide fingers of ungloved hand under remaining glove at wrist and peel off second glove over first glove
- Discard gloves in a waste container

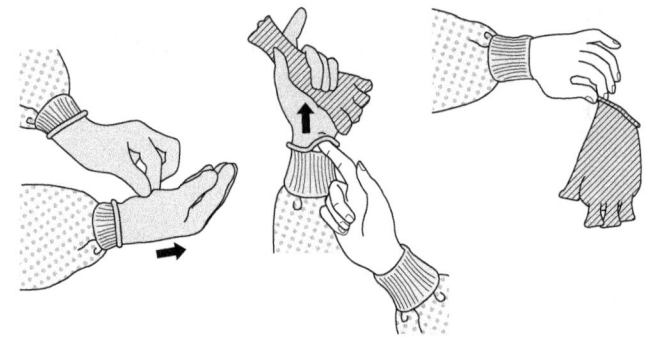

2. GOGGLES OR FACE SHIELD

- Outside of goggles or face shield are contaminated!
- If your hands get contaminated during goggle or face shield removal, immediately wash your hands or use an alcohol-based hand sanitizer
- Remove goggles or face shield from the back by lifting head band or ear pieces
- If the item is reusable, place in designated receptacle for reprocessing; otherwise, discard in a waste container

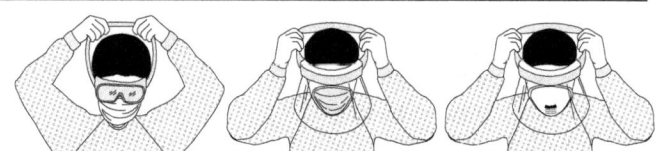

3. GOWN

- Gown front and sleeves are contaminated!
- If your hands get contaminated during gown removal, immediately wash your hands or use an alcohol-based hand sanitizer
- Unfasten gown ties, taking care that sleeves do not contact your body when reaching for ties
- Pull gown away from neck and shoulders, touching inside of gown only
- Turn gown inside out
- Fold or roll into a bundle and discard in a waste container

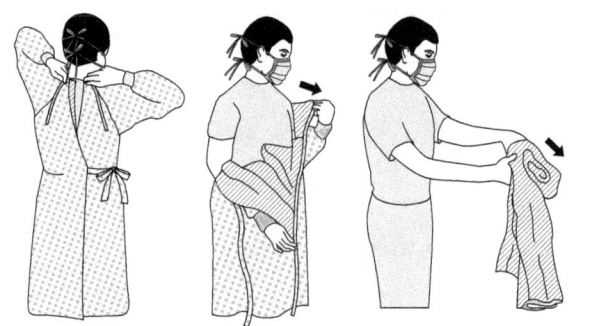

4. MASK OR RESPIRATOR

- Front of mask/respirator is contaminated—DO NOT TOUCH!
- If your hands get contaminated during mask/respirator removal, immediately wash your hands or use an alcohol-based hand sanitizer
- Grasp bottom ties or elastics of the mask/respirator, then the ones at the top, and remove without touching the front
- Discard in a waste container

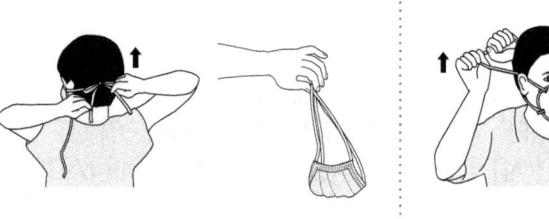

5. WASH HANDS OR USE AN ALCOHOL-BASED HAND SANITIZER IMMEDIATELY AFTER REMOVING ALL PPE

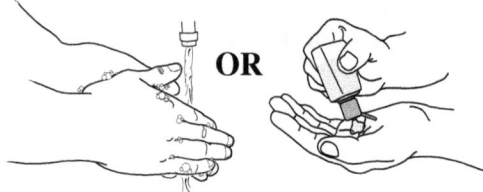

PERFORM HAND HYGIENE BETWEEN STEPS IF HANDS BECOME CONTAMINATED AND IMMEDIATELY AFTER REMOVING ALL PPE

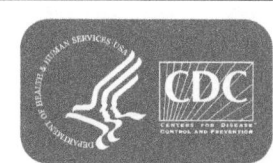

HOW TO SAFELY REMOVE PPE EXAMPLE 2

Here is another way to safely remove PPE without contaminating your clothing, skin, or mucous membranes with potentially infectious materials. **Remove all PPE before exiting the patient room** except a respirator, if worn. Remove the respirator **after** leaving the patient room and closing the door. Remove PPE in the following sequence:

1. **GOWN AND GLOVES**
   - Gown front and sleeves and the outside of gloves are contaminated!
   - If your hands get contaminated during gown or glove removal, immediately wash your hands or use an alcohol-based hand sanitizer
   - Grasp the gown in the front and pull away from your body so that the ties break, touching outside of gown only with gloved hands
   - While removing the gown, fold or roll the gown inside-out into a bundle
   - As you are removing the gown, peel off your gloves at the same time, only touching the inside of the gloves and gown with your bare hands; place the gown and gloves into a waste container

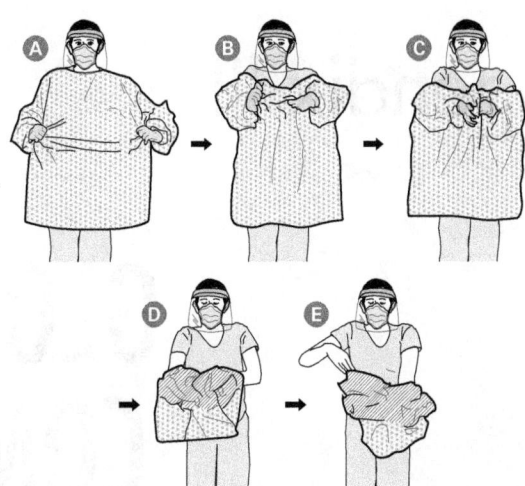

2. **GOGGLES OR FACE SHIELD**
   - Outside of goggles or face shield are contaminated!
   - If your hands get contaminated during goggle or face shield removal, immediately wash your hands or use an alcohol-based hand sanitizer
   - Remove goggles or face shield from the back by lifting head band and without touching the front of the goggles or face shield
   - If the item is reusable, place in designated receptacle for reprocessing; otherwise, discard in a waste container

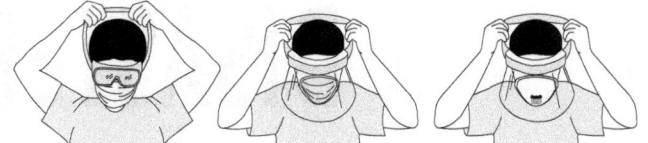

3. **MASK OR RESPIRATOR**
   - Front of mask/respirator is contaminated—DO NOT TOUCH!
   - If your hands get contaminated during mask/respirator removal, immediately wash your hands or use an alcohol-based hand sanitizer
   - Grasp bottom ties or elastics of the mask/respirator, then the ones at the top, and remove without touching the front
   - Discard in a waste container

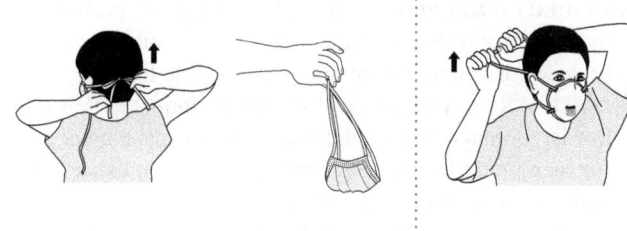

4. **WASH HANDS OR USE AN ALCOHOL-BASED HAND SANITIZER IMMEDIATELY AFTER REMOVING ALL PPE**

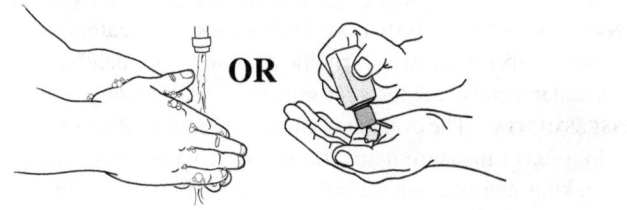

PERFORM HAND HYGIENE BETWEEN STEPS IF HANDS BECOME CONTAMINATED AND IMMEDIATELY AFTER REMOVING ALL PPE

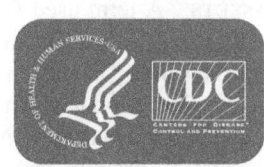

Source: Centers for Disease Control and Prevention. (n.d.). Sequence for putting on personal protective equipment (PPE). Retrieved from https://www.cdc .gov/hai/pdfs/ppe/PPE-Sequence.pdf

Appendix III

GLOSSARY OF TERMS COMMONLY USED IN DISASTER PREPAREDNESS AND RESPONSE

ADVANCED LIFE SUPPORT A medical procedure performed by paramedics that includes the advanced diagnosis and protocol-driven treatment of a patient in the field.

AFTERSHOCKS A sequence of smaller earthquakes that follow larger magnitude earthquakes; aftershocks may be felt for many months after an earthquake and can exacerbate damage; also a type of ground failure.

ALARM PROCEDURE A means of alerting concerned parties to a disaster; various optical and acoustical means of alarm are possible including flags, lights, sirens, radio, and telephone.

ANALYSIS-EPIDEMIOLOGICAL MEASURES Indicators such as descriptive statistics, specific disease and/or death rates, secular trends, and tests for sensitivity and validity.

ASSESSMENTS The evaluation and interpretation of short- and long-term measurements to provide a basis for decision making and to enhance public health officials' ability to monitor disaster situations.

ASSETS A term used for all resources required, including human, to adequately respond to a disaster.

AVALANCHE The sudden slide of a huge mass of snow and ice, usually carrying with it earth, rocks, trees, and other debris.

BASIC LIFE SUPPORT Noninvasive measures used to treat unstable patients, such as extraction of airway obstructions, cardiopulmonary resuscitation, care of wounds and hemorrhages, and immobilization of fractures.

BECQUEREL (BQ) A unit of nuclear activity (e.g., 1 Bq represents the amount of radioactive substance that disintegrates in 1 sec); this unit replaces the curie.

BIOTERRORISM The unlawful release of biological agents or toxins with the intent to intimidate or coerce a government or civilian population to further political or social objectives; humans, animals, and plants are often targets.

BRANCH An organizational level that has functional or geographical responsibility for major parts of the incident command system (ICS) or incident operations (the incident commander may establish geographical branches to resolve span-of-control issues, or functional branches to manage specific functions [e.g., law enforcement, fire, and emergency medical]; a branch is managed by the Branch Director).

CASE One (unit) documented incidence of disease.

CASE DEFINITION Standardized criteria for deciding whether a person has a particular disease or health-related condition; often used in investigations and for comparing potential cases; case definitions help decide which disaster-specific conditions should be monitored with emergency information surveillance systems.

CASE MANAGEMENT The collaborative process that assesses, plans, implements, coordinates, monitors, and evaluates the options and services required to meet an individual's health needs.

CASUALTY Any person suffering physical and/or psychological damage that leads to death, injury, or material loss.

CASUALTY CLEARING STATION A collecting point for victims that is located in the immediate vicinity of a disaster site where triage and medical treatment can be provided.

CENTRAL HOLDING AREA A location from which ambulances leave to pick up patients from the casualty clearing station, or deliver patients to neighboring hospitals according to a victim distribution plan.

COMMUNITY EMERGENCY RESPONSE TEAM (CERT) The CERT program supports local response capability by training volunteers to organize themselves and spontaneous volunteers at the disaster site, to provide immediate assistance to victims and to collect disaster intelligence to support responders' efforts when they arrive.

COMMUNITY PROFILE The characteristics of the local environment that are prone to a chemical or nuclear accident (these characteristics can include population density; age distribution; number of roadways, railways, and waterways; type of buildings; and local relief agencies).

COMPREHENSIVE EMERGENCY MANAGEMENT A broad style of emergency management, encompassing prevention, preparedness, response, and recovery.

CONCEPT A view or idea persons hold about something, ranging from something highly concrete to something highly abstract.

CONSEQUENCE MANAGEMENT An emergency management function that includes measures to protect public health and safety, restore essential government services, and provide emergency relief to governments in the event of terrorism. (Consequence management responses are managed by the Federal Emergency Management Agency [FEMA] and use protocols established under the National Response Plan. Consequence management efforts can also include support missions as described in other federal operations plans, such as predictive modeling, protective action recommendations, and mass decontamination.)

CONTAMINATION An accidental release of hazardous chemicals or nuclear materials that pollute the environment and place humans at risk.

CONTINGENCY PLAN An emergency plan developed in expectation of a disaster; often based on risk assessments, the availability of human and material resources, community preparedness, and local and international response capabilities.

COORDINATION A systematic exchange of information among principal participants to carry out a unified response in the event of an emergency.

COVERT RELEASES (of a biological agent) An unannounced release of a biological agent that causes illness (detection of a biological agent is dependent on traditional surveillance methods; if undetected, a covert release of a contagion has the potential to spread widely before it is detected).

CRISIS MANAGEMENT Administrative measures that identify, acquire, and plan the use of resources needed to anticipate, prevent, and/or resolve a threat to public health and safety (e.g., terrorism).

DATA COLLECTION Gathering, assembling, and delivering data to a centralized collection point.

DECONTAMINATION The removal of hazardous chemicals or nuclear substances from the skin and/or mucus membranes by showering or washing the affected area with water or by rinsing with a sterile solution.

DISASTER Any event, typically occurring suddenly, that causes damage, ecological disruption, loss of human life, deterioration of health and health services, *and* which exceeds the capacity of the affected community on a scale sufficient to require outside assistance. These events can be caused by nature, equipment malfunction, human error, or biological hazards and disease (e.g., earthquake, flood, fire, hurricane, cyclone, typhoon, significant storms, volcanic eruptions, spills, air crashes, drought, epidemic, food shortages, and civil strife).

DISASTER CASE MANAGEMENT The formal process of organizing and providing a timely, coordinated approach to assess disaster-related needs including healthcare, mental health, and human services needs that were caused or exacerbated by the event and may adversely impact an individual's recovery if not addressed.

DISASTER CONTINUUM OR EMERGENCY MANAGEMENT CYCLE The life cycle of a disaster or emergency.

DISASTER EPIDEMIOLOGY The study of disaster-related deaths, illnesses, and injuries in humans; also includes the study of the factors and determinants that affect death, illness, and injury following a disaster. (Methodology involves identifying and comparing risk factors among disaster victims to those who were left unharmed. Epidemiological investigations provide public health professionals with information on the probable public health consequences of disasters.)

DISASTER FIELD OFFICE (DFO) The office established in or near the disaster area that supports federal and state response as well as recovery operations. The DFO houses the Federal Coordinating Officer (FCO), the Emergency Response Team (ERT), the State Coordinating Officer (SCO), and support staff. Often referred to as the Joint Field Office (JFO/JOC) when shared by multiple agencies.

DISASTER INFORMATICS The theoretical and practical operation of processing information and communicating in a disaster situation.

DISASTER SEVERITY SCALE A scale that classifies disasters by the following parameters: the radius of the disaster site, the number of dead, the number of wounded, the average severity of the injuries sustained, the impact time, and the rescue time.

DISASTER VULNERABILITY A measure of the ability of a community to absorb the effects of a severe disaster and to recover; vulnerability varies with each disaster, depending on the disaster's impact on the affected population or group.

DISASTER-PRONE The level of risk that is related to the hazard or the immediate cause of a disaster, which is determined by analyzing the history of past events as well as new conditions that may increase the risk of a disaster taking place.

DISPATCH COMMUNICATIONS SYSTEM A system used to assign ambulance personnel and other first responders.

DIVISION The organizational level that has responsibility for operations within a defined geographical area (the division level is the organizational level between single resources, task forces, or strike teams and the branch level).

EMERGENCY Any natural or man-made situation that results in severe injury, harm, or loss of humans or property.

EMERGENCY MANAGEMENT AGENCY (EMA) Also referred to as the Office of Emergency Preparedness (OEP); the EMA, under the authority of the governor's office, coordinates the efforts of the state's health department, housing and social service agencies, and public safety agencies (e.g., state police) during an emergency or disaster; the EMA also coordinates federal resources made available to the states, such as the National Guard, the Centers for Disease Control and Prevention (e.g., Epidemic Intelligence Service officers), and the Public Health Service (e.g., Agency for Toxic Substances Disease Registry [ATSDR]).

EMERGENCY MEDICAL SERVICES (EMS) SYSTEM   The coordination of the prehospital system (e.g., public access, dispatch, emergency medical technicians and medics, ambulance services) and the inhospital system (e.g., emergency departments, hospitals, and other definitive care facilities and personnel) to provide emergency medical care.

EMERGENCY MEDICAL TECHNICIANS (EMTS) AND PARAMEDICS (EMT-PS)   Trained emergency medical respondents (both paramedics and EMTs are trained to diagnose and treat most common medical emergencies in the field and to provide medical treatment while en route to the hospital; paramedics are more highly trained than EMTs).

EMERGENCY OPERATIONS CENTER (EOC)   The location where departmental heads, governmental officials, and volunteer agencies coordinate the response to an emergency.

EMERGENCY PUBLIC INFORMATION   Information disseminated to the public in anticipation of an emergency that continues for the duration of the emergency; emergency public information directs actions and gives instructions.

EMERGENCY RESPONSE TEAM   A team of federal personnel and support staff that is deployed by FEMA during a major disaster or emergency; the duty of the team is to assist the FCO in carrying out his or her responsibilities under the Stafford Act; team members consist of representatives from each federal department or agency that has been assigned primary responsibility for an emergency support function (ESF) as well as key members of the FCO's staff.

EMERGENCY SUPPORT FUNCTION (ESF)   A functional area of response activity established to coordinate the delivery of federal assistance during the response phase of an emergency. (ESF's mission is to save lives, protect property, preserve public health, and maintain public safety; ESF represents the type of federal assistance most needed by states overwhelmed by the impact of a catastrophic event on local and state resources.)

ENHANCED FUJITA SCALE   Updated scale using a set of wind estimates (not measurements) based on damage occurring from a tornado.

EPIDEMIC   The occurrence of any known or suspected contagion that occurs in clear excess of normal expectancy (a threatened epidemic occurs when the circumstances are such that a disease may reasonably be anticipated to occur in excess of normal expectancy).

ESF-6 MASS CARE   Mass Care includes sheltering and feeding victims of disaster, emergency first aid, family reunification, and the distribution of emergency relief supplies; the American Red Cross (ARC) is designated by the National Response Plan (NRP) as the primary agency responsible for ESF Mass Care.

ESF-8 HEALTH AND MEDICAL   Led by the U.S. Public Health Service's OEP, ESF-8 Health and Medical serves as the basis for federal response to the health needs of disaster victims.

EVACUATION   An organized removal of civilians from a dangerous or potentially dangerous area.

EVALUATION   A detailed review of a disaster relief program designed to determine whether program objectives were met, to assess the program's impact on the community, and to generate lessons learned for the design of future projects (evaluations are most often conducted at the completion of important milestones, or at the end of a specified period).

EVALUATION RESEARCH   The application of scientific methods to assess the effectiveness of programs, services, or organizations established to improve a patient's health or prevent illness.

EXPOSURE SURVEILLANCE   To look for exposure to risk (in a disaster setting, exposure may be based on the physical or environmental properties of the disaster event; also known as a "risk factor variable," "predictor variable," or "independent variable").

EXPOSURE VARIABLE   A characteristic of interest; also known as "risk factor" or "predictor variable."

FAMINE EARLY WARNING SYSTEM   A system established by the U.S. Agency for International Development to monitor a number of factors that are predictive of famine including climate, availability of food, and nutrition-related morbidity.

FEDERAL COORDINATING OFFICER (FCO)   The person appointed by FEMA following a presidential declaration of a severe disaster or of an emergency to coordinate federal assistance. (The FCO initiates immediate action to ensure that federal assistance is provided in accordance with the disaster declaration, any applicable laws or regulations, and the FEMA–state agreement. The FCO is also the senior federal official appointed in accordance with the provisions of Public Law No. 93–288, as amended [the Stafford Act], to coordinate the overall consequence management response and recovery activities. The FCO represents the president as provided by Section 303 of the Stafford Act by coordinating the administration of federal relief activities in the designated disaster area. Additionally, the FCO is delegated responsibilities and performs those for the FEMA director as outlined in Executive Order 12148 and those responsibilities delegated to the FEMA regional director in the Code of Federal Regulations, Title 44, Part 205.)

FEDERAL ON-SCENE COMMANDER (OSC)   The official designated upon the activation of the Joint Operations Center who ensures appropriate coordination of the U.S. government's overall response with federal, state, and local authorities; the OSC maintains this role until the U.S. Attorney General transfers the Lead Federal Agency (LFA) role to FEMA.

FIRST RESPONDER   Local police, fire, and emergency medical personnel who arrive first on the scene of an incident and take action to save lives, protect property, and meet basic human needs.

FUJITA SCALE   A scale used to measure the strength of tornadoes.

FUNCTIONAL MODEL OF PUBLIC HEALTH RESPONSE IN DISASTERS   A model for identifying what disaster-related activities are the responsibility of public health officials; this model also identifies the interface between the core components of professional public health training and emergency management functions, as well as the relationship between the framework of activities typically conducted by the emergency management community and public health practice.

GOLDEN HOUR   A principle that states that unstable victims must be stabilized within 1 hour following injury to reduce the risk of death.

GROUP   The organizational level that has responsibility for a specified functional assignment in an emergency or disaster (e.g., perimeter control, evacuation, fire suppression; a group is managed by a group supervisor).

HAZARD   The probability that a disaster will occur (hazards can be caused by a natural phenomenon [e.g., earthquake, tropical cyclone], by failure of man-made energy sources [e.g., nuclear reactor, industrial explosion], or by an uncontrolled human activity [e.g., conflict, overgrazing]).

HAZARD IDENTIFICATION/ANALYSIS   The process of determining what events are likely to occur in a specified region or environment (e.g., earthquakes, floods, industrial accidents).

HAZARD SURVEILLANCE   An assessment of the occurrence, distribution, and secular trends relating to different levels of hazards (e.g., toxic chemical agents, physical agents, biomechanical stressors, and biological agents) that are responsible for disease and injury.

IMPACT PHASE   A phase during a disaster when emergency management activities focus on warning and preparedness.

INCIDENT ACTION PLAN (IAP)   A written document, developed by the incident commander or the planning section of the ICS, that details which actions will be conducted by the ICS in response to an incident. (IAPs are developed for a specific time period, often referred to as "operational periods," and are based on the specific needs of an incident. The incident commander is responsible for the oversight and implementation of the IAP.)

INCIDENT COMMAND SYSTEM (ICS)   The model for the command, control, and coordination of a response to an emergency; provides the means to coordinate the efforts of individual agencies.

INTEGRATED COMMUNICATIONS   A system that uses a common communications plan, standard operating procedures, clear text, common frequencies, and common terminology.

INTEGRATED RECOVERY PROGRAMS (IRPS)   Versatile recovery programs that respond to a variety of community needs. (IRPs often coordinate recovery activities and stimulate economic rehabilitation by working with various sectors of the community. For example, IRPs may include work schemes to repair community facilities that enable disaster victims to access cash and replace their lost possessions.)

INTENSITY   A roman numerical index from I to XII that describes the physical effects of an earthquake to a specific area. (These values are subjective. Intensity is a measurement of the nature and spatial extent of the distribution of damage. The most commonly used scale is the 12-point Modified Mercalli Intensity [MMI]. An earthquake has many intensities [perceived effects], but only one magnitude [force]. The MMI does not indicate an earthquake's magnitude.)

INTERNATIONAL ASSISTANCE   Assistance provided by one or more governments or voluntary organizations to a country in need, usually for development or for an emergency.

JOINT INFORMATION CENTER (JIC)   A center located at the scene of an emergency established to coordinate federal public information; it is also the central point of contact for all news media; public information officials from participating state and local agencies often collocate here.

JOINT OPERATIONS CENTER (JOC)   The JOC acts as the focal point for the management and direction of on-site activities, coordination and establishment of state requirements and priorities, as well as the coordination of the federal response; JOCs are established by the LFA and are under the operational control of the federal on-scene coordinator.

LANDSLIDE   A massive or rapid descent of damage-causing soil and rock (landslides are the most common and widespread type of ground failure and may include falls, topples, slides, spreads, and flows of soil and/or rock on unstable slopes).

LATRINES   A pit designed to capture and contain excreta; most often trenches with multiple platforms across them, or solitary pits surrounded by a structure.

LD50   The amount of a substance (the lethal dose) that results in the death of 50% of the subjects who are exposed to it.

LEAD AGENCY   The federal department or agency that is assigned the lead responsibility under U.S. law for the management and coordination of the federal response in a specific functional area (lead agencies support the LFA during all phases of the response).

LEAD FEDERAL AGENCY (LFA)   The agency designed by the president to lead and coordinate the federal response. (The type of emergency determines which agency becomes the LFA. In general, the LFA establishes operational procedures to assemble and work with the cooperating agencies to provide the LFA with support. These agencies support the LFA in carrying out the president's policy by furnishing the LFA with an initial assessment of the situation, developing action plans, monitoring and updating operational priorities, and ensuring that each agency exercises its authority within the boundaries of the law. Specific responsibilities of an LFA vary according to each agency's statutory authority.)

LIAISON   An agency official who works with individual agencies or agency officials to coordinate interagency communications.

LIQUEFACTION   Occurs primarily in young, shallow, loosely compacted, water-saturated sand and gravel deposits that are subjected to ground shaking; it results in a temporary loss of load-bearing strength.

LOCAL GOVERNMENT   Any county, city, village, town, district, political subdivision of any state, Indian tribe or authorized tribal organization, or Alaskan native village or organization, including rural communities, unincorporated towns and villages, or any other public entity.

LOSS   A range of adverse consequences that can impact communities and individuals (e.g., damage, loss of economic value, loss of function, loss of natural resources, loss of ecological systems, environmental impact, health deterioration, mortality, morbidity).

MAGNITUDE   A numerical quantity invented by Charles F. Richter that determines the size and scope of an earthquake by using a measure called a Richter. (The magnitude of an earthquake is the total amount of energy released after adjusting for differences in epicentral distance and focal depth. Magnitude is determined on the basis of instrumental records, whereas intensity is determined by subjective observations of an earthquake's damage. Moderate earthquakes have magnitudes of 5.5 to 6.9; larger earthquakes have magnitudes of 7.0 to 7.9; and strong earthquakes have magnitudes of 8.0 and greater. The energy of an earthquake increases exponentially with magnitude. For example, a magnitude 6.0 earthquake releases 31.5 times more energy than a magnitude 5.0 earthquake or approximately 1,000 times more energy than a magnitude 4.0 earthquake.)

MAN-MADE OR HUMAN-GENERATED DISASTERS; COMPLEX EMERGENCIES   Technological events that are caused by humans and occur in human settlements (e.g., fire, chemical spills and explosions, and armed conflict).

MASLOW'S THEORY OF HUMAN MOTIVATION AND HIERARCHY OF BASIC NEEDS   Proposes a hierarchical structure for human needs, from physiological drives to needs for safety, belonging, love, esteem, and self-actualization at the top of the pyramid.

MAXIMUM CONTAMINANT LEVEL (MCL)   The maximum permissible level of a contaminant in water in a public water system. The MCL is established by the Environmental Protection Agency (EPA). MCLs are defined in the Safe Drinking Water Act as the level that may be achieved with the use of the best available technology, treatment techniques (TTs), and other means that the EPA finds are available after taking cost into consideration.

MEASURES OF BIOLOGICAL EFFECTS   A gauge of health in humans that indicates the impact of a disaster (examples include laboratory typing of organisms where infectious disease outbreaks occur, biochemical testing of exposures to toxic chemicals to assess exposure levels, and anthropometric measurements [e.g., height-to-weight ratio] that indicate the type and degree of malnutrition in famine situations).

MEASURES OF PHYSICAL EFFECTS TO INDICATE MAGNITUDE   An assessment of environmental conditions whose levels are negatively impacted because of a disaster (e.g., the height of river above flood stage, the level of pollutants in air after a forest fire, and the level of toxic chemicals in drinking water or sediment).

MEASURING ENVIRONMENTAL HAZARDS   Assessing the occurrence, distribution, and the secular trends that affect the level of hazards (e.g., toxic culture agents, physical agents, biomechanical stressors, biological agents) responsible for disease and injury.

MEDICAL COORDINATION   The coordination between healthcare providers during the transition from the prehospital to the hospital phase of patient care; simplification and standardization of materials and methods are a prerequisite.

MITIGATION   Measures taken to reduce the harmful effects of a disaster by attempting to limit the disaster's impact on human health and economic infrastructure.

MODIFIED MERCALLI SCALE   A scale that indicates the intensity of an earthquake by assessing the degree of damage on a particular location.

MONITORING   A process of evaluating the performance of response and recovery programs by measuring a program's outcomes against stated objectives (monitoring is used to identify bottlenecks and obstacles that cause delays or programmatic shortfalls that require assessment).

MORTALITY DATA   Information about the number of deaths used to assess the magnitude of a disaster, evaluate the effectiveness of disaster preparedness, evaluate the adequacy of warning systems, and aid contingency planning by identifying high-risk groups.

NATIONAL HEALTH SECURITY STRATEGY (NHSS) 2018   The purpose of the NHSS was to refocus the patchwork of disparate public health and medical preparedness, response, and recovery strategies to ensure that the nation is prepared for, protected from, and resilient in the face of health threats or incidents with potentially negative health consequences. It is the first comprehensive strategy focusing specifically on protecting people's health in the case of a large-scale incident that puts health and well-being at risk. It contains two goals: build community resilience; and strengthen and sustain health and emergency response systems. These overarching goals are supported by 10 detailed strategic objectives, such as developing and maintaining the workforce needed for national health security; and ensuring timely and effective communication.

NATIONAL INCIDENT MANAGEMENT SYSTEM   Provides a template for incident management regardless of size, scope, or cause. The template includes a core set of concepts, doctrines, principles, organizational processes, and terminology. It standardizes emergency management, personnel and resource management procedures, promoting coordination during planning and response. There are five interrelated components: preparedness, communications and information management, resource management; command and control; and ongoing management and maintenance.

NATIONAL PREPAREDNESS GOAL   Describes the core capabilities required for each of the five mission areas: prevention, protection, mitigation, response, and recovery.

NATIONAL RESPONSE FRAMEWORK (NRF)   Enacted in January 2008, supersedes the National Response Plan and serves as a guide to how the nation conducts comprehensive incident response using an all-hazards approach to respond to natural and man-made disasters. Built on its predecessor, it includes guiding principles that detail how federal, state, local, tribal, and private sector partners, including the healthcare sector, prepare for and provide a unified domestic response through improved coordination and integration. (The NRF is designed to address the consequences of any disaster or emergency situation in which there is need for federal assistance under the authorities of the Robert T. Stafford Disaster Relief and Emergency Assistance Act, 42 U.S.C. 5121 et seq. The NRF includes 15 ESFs, each of which has a designated coordinator and primary agency and supporting agencies. The NRF works hand in hand with the National Incident Management System and incorporates the tenets of the ICS.

NATURAL DISASTERS   Natural phenomena with acute onset and profound effects (e.g., earthquakes, floods, cyclones, tornadoes).

NATURAL-TECHNOLOGICAL (NA-TECH) DISASTERS   Natural disasters that create technological emergencies, such as urban fires that result from seismic motion, or chemical spills that result from floods.

ON-SCENE COORDINATOR (OSC)   The federal official predesignated by the EPA and U.S. Coast Guard to coordinate and direct the response and removals of oil or hazardous materials under the National Oil and Hazardous Substances Pollution Contingency Plan.

OUTCOME SURVEILLANCE   To look for a health outcome or health event of interest, usually illness, injury, or death; also known as the "response variable," "dependent variable," or "effect variable" (e.g., the ARC/Centers for Disease Control and Prevention's Health Impact Surveillance System records mortality in disaster events in which the ARC has served).

OUTCOME VARIABLE   A health event, usually encompassing illness, injury, or death; also known as a "response variable."

OVERT RELEASE   An announced release of a biological agent, by terrorists or others; this type of release allows for treatment before the onset of disease.

PANDEMIC AND ALL-HAZARDS PREPAREDNESS ACT   Originally passed in 2006, this law amended the Public Health Service Act to require the secretary of Health and Human Services (HHS) to lead all federal public health and medical responses to public health emergencies. Included in this legislation were many requirements to improve the ability of the nation to respond to a public health or medical disaster or emergency, such as the creation of the office of the assistant secretary for Preparedness and Response (ASPR) and the requirement to establish a near–real-time electronic nationwide public health situational awareness capability to enhance early detection of, rapid response to, and management of potentially catastrophic infectious disease outbreaks and other public health emergencies.

PHASES OF THE EMERGENCY PLANNING MODEL   The model is composed of five phases, each corresponding to a type of activity involved in preparing for and responding to a disaster; the phases include planning (preparedness), mitigation, response, recovery, and evaluation.

PLANNING   To work cooperatively with others in advance of a disaster to initiate prevention and preparedness activities.

POSTDISASTER SURVEILLANCE   Observations conducted by health authorities after a disaster to monitor health events, detect sudden changes in disease occurrence, follow long-term trends of specific diseases, identify changes in agents and host factors for the diseases of interest, and detect changes in health practices for treating disease.

POSTIMPACT PHASE   The period of time after a disaster event; often associated with the activities of response and recovery.

PREIMPACT PHASE   The period of time before a disaster strikes; often associated with mitigation and prevention activities.

PREPAREDNESS   All measures and policies taken before an event occurs that allow for prevention, mitigation, and readiness. (Preparedness includes designing warning systems, planning for evacuation and relocation, storing food and water, building temporary shelter, devising management strategies, and holding disaster drills and exercises. Contingency planning is also included in preparedness as well as planning for postimpact response and recovery.)

PRESIDENTIAL POLICY DIRECTIVE 8 (PPD-8)   Issued in March 2011, this directed the development of a national preparedness goal that identifies core capabilities as well as a national preparedness system to guide preparedness for the threats that pose the greatest risk to the security of the nation (Department of Homeland Security). These threats include both natural and man-made incidents such as terrorism, cyberattacks, pandemics, and catastrophic natural disasters.

PREVENTION   Primary, secondary, and tertiary efforts that help avert an emergency; these activities are commonly referred to as "mitigation" in the emergency management model (e.g., prevention activities include cloud seeding to stimulate rain in a fire; in public health terms, prevention refers to actions that prevent the onset or deterioration of disease, disability, and injury).

PRIMARY PREVENTION   Preventing the occurrence of death, injury, or illness in a disaster (e.g., evacuation of a community in a flood-prone area, sensitizing warning systems for tornadoes and severe storms).

PUBLIC ACCESS SYSTEM   An emergency telephone system by which the public notifies authorities of a medical emergency; accessed by dialing 911.

PUBLIC HEALTH SURVEILLANCE   The systematic collection, analysis, and interpretation of the health data that are used to plan, implement, and evaluate public health programs; also used to determine the need for public health action.

PUBLIC INFORMATION OFFICER   The official at headquarters or in the field responsible for preparing, coordinating, and disseminating public information; he/she relies on the cooperation of federal, state, and local agencies.

RADIATION   Energy emitted by atoms that are unstable radiation with enough energy to create ion pairs in matter.

RADIO BANDS   A collection of neighboring radio frequencies; frequencies are allocated on different bands; each two-way radio is designed for a specific band (a radio designed to work on one band will not work on another band).

RADIOACTIVE CONTAMINATION   The presence of radiation-emitting substances (radioactive materials) in a place where it is not desired.

RAPID NEEDS ASSESSMENT   A collection of techniques (i.e., epidemiological, statistical, anthropological) designed to provide information about an affected community's needs following a disaster.

READINESS   Links preparedness to relief; an assessment of readiness reflects the current capacity and capabilities of the organizations involved in relief activities.

RECOVERY   Actions of responders, government, and the victims that help return an affected community to normal by stimulating community cohesiveness and governmental involvement. (One type of recovery involves repairing infrastructure, damaged buildings, and critical facilities. The recovery period falls between the onset of the emergency and the reconstruction period.)

RECOVERY PLAN   A plan to restore areas affected by disaster; developed on a state-by-state basis with assistance from responding federal agencies.

RED CROSS   (also known as the "American Red Cross" or the "International Red Cross") A comprehensive designation used for all or one of the components of the International Red Cross and Red Crescent Movement, a worldwide organization active in humanitarian work. (This organization has three components: The International Committee of the Red Cross [ICRC], which acts primarily as a neutral intermediary during armed conflict and includes the Guardian of the Geneva Conventions, an advocate for the protection of war victims; the League of the Red Cross and Red Crescent Societies [LRCS]; an international federation of the National Societies, active in nonconflict disasters and natural calamities; and the National Red Cross or Red Crescent Society, a worldwide relief organization specific to individual countries.)

REGIONAL OPERATIONS CENTER (ROC)   Temporary operations facility used in the coordination of federal response and recovery activities; located at the FEMA Regional Office (or at the Federal Regional Center) and led by the FEMA regional director or deputy regional director until the Disaster Field Office becomes operational.

REHABILITATION OR RECONSTRUCTION   A long-term developmental project that follows a disaster or emergency that reconstructs a community's infrastructure to preexisting levels; is often associated with an opportunity to improve a community rather than to simply "reconstruct" a preexisting system.

RELIEF   Action focused on saving lives. (Relief activities often include search and rescue missions, first aid, and restoration of emergency communications and transportation systems. Relief also includes attention to the immediate care of survivors by providing food, clothing, medical treatment, and emotional care.)

REPORT FORMAT   The instrument on which surveillance data are reported.

REPORTING UNIT FOR SURVEILLANCE   The data source that provides information for the surveillance system. (Reporting units often include hospitals, clinics, health posts, and mobile health units. Epidemiologists select reporting units after they define "what a case is" because the source of data is dependent on that definition.)

REPRESENTATIVENESS   The accuracy of the data when measuring the occurrence of a health event over time and its distribution by person and place.

RESOURCE MANAGEMENT   A management style that maximizes the use of and control over assets; this management style reduces the need for unnecessary communications, provides for strict accountability, and ensures the safety of personnel.

RESPONSE   The phase in a disaster when relief, recovery, and rehabilitation occur; also includes the delivery of services, the management of activities and programs designed to address the immediate and short-term effects of an emergency or disaster.

RICHTER SCALE   A scale that indicates the magnitude of an earthquake by providing a measure of the total energy released from the source of the quake; the source of an earthquake is the segment of the fault that has slipped.

RISK AS A FUNCTION OF HAZARD AND VULNERABILITY   A relationship that is frequently illustrated with the following formula, although the association is not strictly arithmetic: Risk equals Hazard times Vulnerability.

RISK ASSESSMENT   A systematic process that determines the likelihood of adverse health effects to a population after exposure to a hazard; health consequences may depend on the type of hazard and damage to infrastructure, loss of economic value, loss of function, loss of natural resources, loss of ecological systems, environmental impacts, deterioration of health, mortality, and morbidity. (The major components of a risk assessment include a hazard identification analysis and a vulnerability analysis that answer the following questions: What are the hazards that could affect a community? What can happen as a result of those hazards? How likely is each of the possible outcomes? When the possible outcomes occur, what are the likely consequences and losses? Risk assessment is a fundamental planning tool for disaster management, especially during prevention and mitigation activities.)

RISK INDICATOR   Descriptor that denotes risks that may cause a disaster.

RISK MANAGEMENT   The process of deciding which action to take when a risk assessment indicates that a danger of loss exists. (Risk management includes a range of actions [e.g., prevention, mitigation, preparedness, recovery] that are designed to mitigate an increasing risk of natural and technological hazards, decrease a risk to existing levels, and plan ways to respond to natural and technological hazards as well as catastrophic events.)

SAFFIR–SIMPSON WIND SCALE   A scale used to measure strength of hurricanes; now revised and updated to establish a more accurate measurement and basis for comparison of hurricane wind.

SECONDARY PREVENTION   Mitigates the health consequences of disasters. (Examples include the use of carbon monoxide detectors when operating gasoline-powered generators after the loss of electric power, employing appropriate occupant behavior in multistory structures during earthquakes, and building "safe rooms" in dwellings located in tornado-prone areas. Secondary prevention may be instituted when disasters are imminent.)

SIZE-UP/ASSESSMENT   To identify a problem and assess the potential consequences. (Initially, a size-up is the responsibility of the first officer to arrive at the scene of an emergency. Size-ups continue throughout the response phase and continuously update the status of the incident, evaluate the hazards present, and determine the size of the affected area as well as whether the area can be isolated. A size-up also determines if a staging area will be needed and where it should be located to allow for the best flow of personnel and equipment.)

SPAN OF CONTROL   The number of individuals managed by a single supervisor (the manageable span of control for one supervisor ranges from three to seven individuals, with five as optimum).

STAGING AREA   An area where resources are kept while awaiting assignment.

STATE COORDINATING OFFICER   An official designated by the governor of an affected state upon the declaration of a major disaster or emergency to coordinate state and local disaster assistance efforts with those of the federal government and to act in cooperation with the FCO to administer disaster recovery efforts.

STOCKPILE   An area or storehouse where medicine and other supplies are kept in the event of an emergency.

STRESS   Physical, mental, or emotional strain or tension.

STRIKE TEAM   A group of resources of the same size and type (e.g., five patrol units, three drug K-9 teams).

SUPPLY MANAGEMENT PROGRAM (SUMA)   A computer system that sorts and classifies supplies to prepare inventories of relief supplies that are sent to disaster-stricken countries (developed by the Pan American Health Organization).

SURVEILLANCE   The ongoing and systematic collection, analysis, and interpretation of health data essential to the planning, implementation, and evaluation of public health practice; systems are designed to disseminate data in a timely manner and often include both data collection and disease monitoring.

TABLE-TOP EXERCISE   Method of evaluation of a disaster preparedness plan.

TASK FORCE   A combination of single resources that is assembled for a particular operational need with common communications and one leader.

TECHNOLOGICAL HAZARD   A potential threat to human welfare caused by technological factors (e.g., chemical release, nuclear accident, dam failure; earthquakes and other natural hazards can trigger technological hazards as well).

TERTIARY PREVENTION   The minimization of the effects of disease and disability among those with preexisting health conditions. (Tertiary prevention shields persons with health conditions from negative health effects relating to a disaster. Examples of tertiary prevention include protecting persons with respiratory illnesses and those prone to respiratory conditions from the haze and smoke that originates from forest fires, and sheltering elderly who are prone to heat illnesses during episodes of extreme ambient temperatures.)

THEORY   A set of interrelated constructs (concepts), definitions, and propositions that present a systematic view of phenomena by specifying relations among variables, with the purpose of explaining and predicting the phenomena.

TIMELINESS   How quickly information or surveillance data can be made available.

TOP–DOWN   A command function that is established by the first officer to arrive on the scene, who then becomes the incident commander.

TOXICOLOGICAL DISASTER   A serious environmental pollutant that causes illness by a massive, accidental escape of toxic substances into the air, soil, or water; these disasters affect humans, animals, and plants.

TOXIN   A substance capable of causing a harmful effect.

TREATMENT TECHNIQUE (TT)   An enforceable procedure or level of technological performance that public water systems must follow to ensure control of a water contaminant. (When there is no reliable method that is economically and technically feasible to measure contaminants at particularly low concentrations, a TT is set rather than a MCL. An example of a TT rule is the surface water treatment rule, which includes disinfection and filtration.)

UNITY OF COMMAND   A hierarchical methodology that states that each person within an organization should report to only one superior.

VICTIM DISTRIBUTION   A victim distribution plan defines the transport distribution of victims among neighboring hospitals according to their hospital treatment capacity; these plans often avoid taking victims to the nearest hospital because walking victims will overcrowd hospitals closest to the disaster site.

VOLUNTARY AGENCY (VOLAG)   A nonprofit, nongovernmental, private association maintained and supported by voluntary contributions that provides assistance in emergencies and disasters.

VULNERABILITY   The susceptibility of a population to a specific type of event; it is also associated with the degree of possible or potential loss from a risk that results from a hazard at a given intensity. (The factors that influence vulnerability include demographics, the age and resilience of the environment, technology, social differentiation, and diversity as well as regional and global economics politics.)

VULNERABILITY ANALYSIS   The assessment of an exposed population's susceptibility to the adverse health effects of a particular hazard.

WARNING AND FORECASTING   Monitoring events to determine the time, location, and severity of a disaster.

WEAPONS OF MASS DESTRUCTION (WMD)   Any device, material, or substance used in a manner, in a quantity or type, or under circumstances evidencing an intent to cause death or serious injury to persons or significant damage to property.

Appendix IV

CREATING A PERSONAL DISASTER PLAN

One of the most important steps you can take in preparing for emergencies is to develop a household disaster plan.

1. Learn about the natural disasters that could occur in your community from your local emergency management office or American Red Cross chapter. Learn whether hazardous materials are produced, stored, or transported near your area. Learn about possible consequences of deliberate acts of terror. Ask how to prepare for each potential emergency and how to respond.
2. Consider becoming an American Red Cross disaster nurse.
3. Talk with employers and school officials about their emergency response plans.
4. Talk with each member of your household about potential emergencies and how to respond to each. Talk about what you would need to do in an evacuation.
5. Plan how your household would stay in contact if you were separated. Identify two meeting places: the first should be near your home—in case of fire, perhaps a tree or a telephone pole; the second should be away from your neighborhood in case you cannot return home.
6. Pick a friend or relative who lives out of the area for household members to call to say they are okay.
7. Draw a floor plan of your home. Mark two escape routes from each room.
8. Post emergency telephone numbers by telephones. Teach children how and when to call 911.
9. Make sure everyone in your household knows how and when to shut off water, gas, and electricity at the main switches. Consult with your local utilities if you have questions.
10. Stay up to date with all of your certifications (e.g., CPR, ACLS, PALS, TNCC).
11. Reduce the economic impact of disaster on your property and your household's health and financial well-being.

- Review property insurance policies before disaster strikes—make sure policies are current and be certain they meet your needs (type of coverage, amount of coverage, and hazard covered—flood, earthquake).
- Protect your household's financial well-being before a disaster strikes—review life insurance policies and consider saving money in an "emergency" savings account that could be used in any crisis. It is advisable to keep a small amount of cash or traveler's checks at home in a safe place where you can quickly gain access to them in case of an evacuation.
- Be certain that health insurance policies are current and meet the needs of your household.

12. Consider ways to help neighbors who may need special assistance, such as the hearing impaired, elderly, or the disabled.
13. Make arrangements for pets. Pets are not allowed in public shelters. Service animals for those who depend on them are allowed.
14. Do not rely on the Internet or cell phone for communication. Both may be unavailable during a disaster. Have a personal communications backup plan.

EMERGENCY PLANNING FOR PEOPLE WITH SPECIAL NEEDS

If you or someone in your family has a disability or special need, you may have to take additional steps to protect yourself and your household in an emergency. If you know of friends or neighbors with special needs, help them with these extra precautions. Examples include:

- Hearing impaired may need to make special arrangements to receive a warning.
- Mobility impaired may need assistance in getting to a shelter.

- Households with a single, working parent may need help from others both in planning for disasters and during an emergency.
- Non–English-speaking people may need assistance planning for and responding to emergencies. Community and cultural groups may be able to help keep these populations informed.
- People without vehicles may need to make arrangements for transportation.
- People with special dietary needs should have an adequate emergency food supply.

1. Find out about special assistance that may be available in your community. Register with the office of emergency services or fire department for assistance, so needed help can be provided quickly in an emergency.
2. Create a network of neighbors, relatives, friends, and coworkers to aid you in an emergency. Discuss your needs and make sure they know how to operate necessary equipment.
3. Discuss your needs with your employer.
4. If you are mobility impaired and live or work in a high-rise building, have an escape chair.
5. If you live in an apartment building, ask the management to mark accessible exits clearly and to make arrangements to help you evacuate the building.
6. Keep extra wheelchair batteries, oxygen, catheters, medication, food for guide or hearing-ear dogs, or other items you might need. Also, keep a list of the types and serial numbers of medical devices you need.
7. Those who are not disabled should learn who in their neighborhood or building is disabled so that they may assist them during emergencies.
8. If you are a caregiver for a person with special needs, make sure you have a plan to communicate if an emergency occurs.

DISASTER SUPPLY KITS

You and your family may need to survive on your own for 3 days or more. This means having your own water, food, and emergency supplies. Try using backpacks or duffel bags to keep the supplies together.

Assembling the supplies you might need following a disaster is an important part of your disaster plan. You should prepare emergency supplies for the following situations:

- A disaster supply kit with essential food, water, and supplies for at least 3 days—this kit should be kept in a designated place and be ready to "grab and go" in case you have to leave your home quickly because of a disaster, such as a flash flood or major chemical emergency. Make sure all household members know where the kit is kept.
- Consider having additional supplies for sheltering or home confinement for up to 2 weeks.
- You should also have a disaster supply kit where you work. This should be in one container, ready to "grab and go" in case you have to evacuate the building.
- A car kit of emergency supplies, including food and water, to keep stored in your car at all times. This kit would also include flares, jumper cables, and seasonal supplies.

The following checklists will help you assemble disaster supply kits that meet the needs of your household. The basic items that should be in a disaster supply kit are water, food, first-aid supplies, tools and emergency supplies, clothing and bedding, and specialty items. You will need to change the stored water and food supplies every 6 months, so be sure to write the date when you store it on all containers. You should also rethink your needs every year and update your kit as your household changes. Keep items in airtight plastic bags and put your entire disaster supply kit in one or two easy-to-carry containers such as an unused trash can, camping backpack, or duffel bag.

Water: The Absolute Necessity

1. Stocking water reserves should be a top priority. Drinking water in emergency situations should not be rationed. Therefore, it is critical to store adequate amounts of water for your household.
   - Individual needs vary, depending on age, physical condition, activity, diet, and climate. A normally active person needs at least 2 quarts of water daily just for drinking. Children, nursing mothers, and ill people need more. Very hot temperatures can double the amount of water needed.
   - Because you will also need water for sanitary purposes and, possibly, for cooking, you should store at least 1 gallon of water per person per day.
2. Store water in thoroughly washed plastic, fiberglass, or enamel-lined metal containers. Do not use containers that can break, such as glass bottles. Never use a container that has held toxic substances. Sound plastic containers, such as soft drink bottles, are best. You can also purchase food-grade plastic buckets or drums.
   - Containers for water should be rinsed with a diluted bleach solution (1 part bleach to 10 parts water) before use. Previously used bottles or other containers may be contaminated with microbes or chemicals. Do not rely on untested devices for decontaminating water.
   - If your water is treated commercially by a water utility, you do not need to treat water before storing it. Additional treatments of treated public water will not increase storage life.
   - If you have a well or public water that has not been treated, follow the treatment instructions provided by your public health service or water provider.
   - If you suspect that your well may be contaminated, contact your local or state health department or agriculture extension agent for specific advice.
   - Seal your water containers tightly, label them, and store them in a cool, dark place.
   - It is important to change stored water every 6 months.

Food: Preparing an Emergency Supply

1. If activity is reduced, healthy people can survive on half their usual food intake for an extended period or without any food for many days. Food, unlike water, may be rationed safely, except for children and pregnant women.

2. You do not need to go out and buy unfamiliar foods to prepare an emergency food supply. You can use the canned foods, dry mixes, and other staples on your cupboard shelves. Canned foods do not require cooking, water, or special preparation. Be sure to include a manual can opener.

3. Keep canned foods in a dry place where the temperature is fairly cool. To protect boxed foods from pests and to extend their shelf life, store the food in tightly closed plastic or metal containers.

4. Replace items in your food supply every 6 months. Throw out any canned food that becomes swollen, dented, or corroded. Use foods before they go bad, and replace them with fresh supplies. Date each food item with a marker. Place new items at the back of the storage area and older ones in front.

5. Food items that you might consider including in your disaster supply kit are: ready-to-eat meats, fruits, and vegetables; canned or boxed juices, milk, and soup; high-energy foods like peanut butter, jelly, low-sodium crackers, granola bars, and trail mix; vitamins; foods for infants or persons on special diets; cookies, hard candy; instant coffee, cereals, and powdered milk.

First-Aid Supplies

Assemble a first-aid kit for your home and for each vehicle:

- The basics for your first-aid kit should include:
  - First-aid manual
  - Sterile adhesive bandages in assorted sizes
  - Assorted sizes of safety pins
  - Cleansing agents (isopropyl alcohol, hydrogen peroxide)/soap/germicide
  - Antibiotic ointment
  - Latex gloves (two pairs)
  - Petroleum jelly
  - 2-in. and 4-in. sterile gauze pads (4 to 6 each size)
  - Triangular bandages (three)
  - 2-in. and 3-in. sterile roller bandages (three rolls each)
  - Cotton balls
  - Scissors
  - Tweezers
  - Needle
  - Moistened towelettes
  - Antiseptic
  - Thermometer
  - Tongue depressor blades (two)
  - Tube of petroleum jelly or other lubricant
  - Sunscreen
- It may be difficult to obtain prescription medications during a disaster because stores may be closed or supplies may be limited. Ask your physician or pharmacist about storing prescription medications. Be sure they are stored to meet instructions on the label and be mindful of expiration dates—be sure to keep your stored medication up to date.
- Have an extra pair of prescription glasses or contact lenses.
- Have the following nonprescription drugs in your disaster supply kit:
  - Aspirin and nonaspirin pain reliever
  - Antidiarrhea medication
  - Antacid (for stomach upset)

- Syrup of ipecac (use to induce vomiting if advised by the poison control center)
- Laxative
- Vitamins

Tools and Emergency Supplies

It will be important to assemble these items in a disaster supply kit in case you have to leave your home quickly. Even if you do not have to leave your home, if you lose power it will be easier to have these items already assembled and in one place.

- *Tools and other items*:
  - A portable, battery-powered radio or television and extra batteries (also have a NOAA weather radio, if appropriate for your area)
  - Flashlight and extra batteries
  - Signal flare
  - Matches in a waterproof container (or waterproof matches)
  - Shut-off wrench, pliers, shovel, and other tools
  - Duct tape and scissors
  - Plastic sheeting
  - Whistle
  - Small canister, A-B-C-type fire extinguisher
  - Tube tent
  - Compass
  - Work gloves
  - Paper, pens, and pencils
  - Needles and thread
  - Battery-operated travel alarm clock
- *Kitchen items*:
  - Manual can opener
  - Mess kits or paper cups, plates, and plastic utensils
  - All-purpose knife
  - Household liquid bleach to treat drinking water
  - Sugar, salt, pepper
  - Aluminum foil and plastic wrap
  - Resealing plastic bags
  - If food must be cooked, small cooking stove and a can of cooking fuel
- *Sanitation and hygiene items*:
  - Washcloth and towel
  - Towelettes, soap, hand sanitizer, liquid detergent
  - Toothpaste, toothbrushes, shampoo, deodorants, comb and brush, razor, shaving cream, lip balm, sunscreen, insect repellent, contact lens solutions, mirror, feminine supplies
  - Heavy-duty plastic garbage bags and ties—for personal sanitation uses—and toilet paper
  - Medium-sized plastic bucket with tight lid, small shovel for digging a latrine
  - Disinfectant and household chlorine bleach
- *Household documents and contact numbers*:
  - Personal identification, cash (including change) or traveler's checks, and a credit card
  - Copies of important documents: birth certificate, marriage certificate, driver's license, social security cards, passport, wills, deeds, inventory of household goods, insurance papers, immunization records, blank and credit card

account numbers, stocks, and bonds. Be sure to store these in a watertight container.

- Emergency contact list and phone numbers
- Map of the area and phone numbers of places you could go
- An extra set of car keys and house keys

Clothes and Bedding

- One complete change of clothing and footwear for each household member. Shoes should be sturdy work shoes or boots. Rain gear, hat and gloves, extra socks, extra underwear, thermal underwear, sunglasses.
- Blankets or a sleeping bag for each household member, pillows

Specialty Items

Remember to consider the needs of infants, elderly persons, disabled persons, and pets and to include entertainment and comfort items for children.

- For baby
- For the elderly
- For pets
- Entertainment: books, games, quiet toys, and stuffed animals

It is important for you to be ready, wherever you may be when disaster strikes. With the checklists above, you can now put together an appropriate disaster supply kit for your household:

- A disaster supply kit kept in the home with supplies for at least 3 days.
- Although it is unlikely that food supplies would be cut off for as long as 2 weeks, consider storing additional water, food, clothing, bedding, and other supplies to expand your supply kit to last up to 2 weeks.
- A workplace disaster supply kit. It is important to store a personal supply of water and food where you work; you will not be able to rely on water fountains or coolers. Women who wear high heels should be sure to have comfortable flat shoes at their workplace in case an evacuation requires walking long distances.
- A car disaster supply kit. Keep a smaller disaster supply kit in the trunk of your car. If you become stranded or are not able to return home, having these items will help you be more comfortable until help arrives. Add items for severe winter weather during months when heavy snow or icy roads are possible—salt, sand, shovels, and extra winter clothing, including hats and gloves.

Source: Modified from Federal Emergency Management Agency. (2011). *Are you Ready? A guide to citizen preparedness* (H-34). Retrieved from https://www.fema.gov/pdf/areyouready/areyouready_full.pdf

CDC'S PUBLIC HEALTH EMERGENCY PREPAREDNESS PROGRAM: EVERY RESPONSE IS LOCAL

CDC'S PUBLIC HEALTH EMERGENCY PREPAREDNESS PROGRAM:
EVERY RESPONSE IS LOCAL

State and local health departments must stand ready to handle many different types of emergencies that threaten the health and safety of families, communities, and the nation.

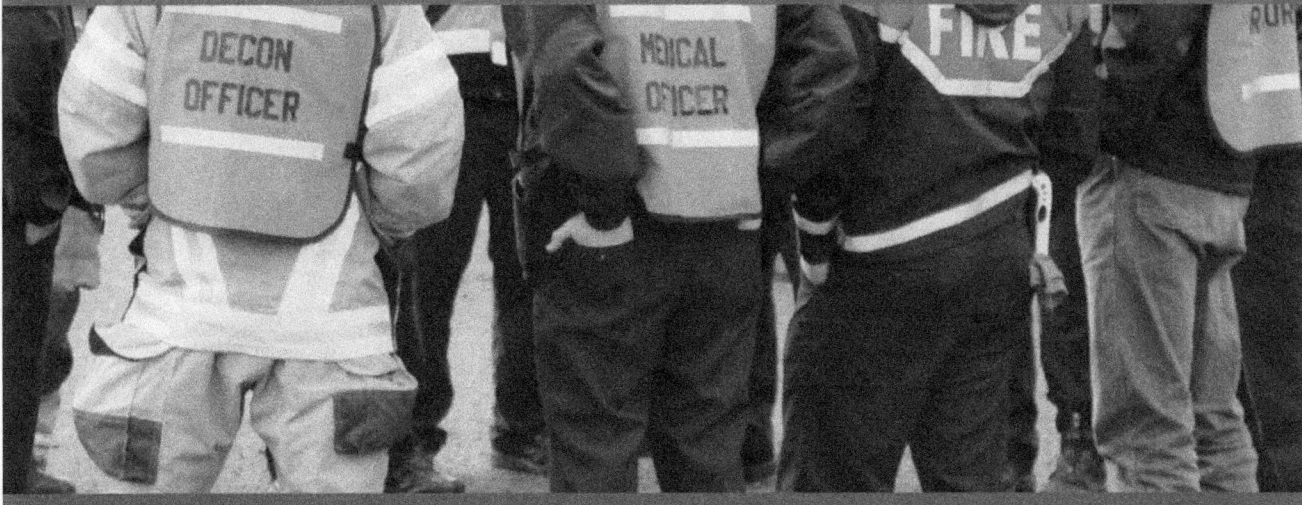

WHY IT MATTERS

Communities must be ready to respond to emergencies – both those they expect and those that come without warning. The terrorist and anthrax attacks of 2001 clearly demonstrated that states need expertise and resources in place before disaster strikes. Since 9/11, CDC's Public Health Emergency Preparedness (PHEP) program has partnered with states to prepare and plan for emergencies, resulting in measurable improvement.

IMPROVEMENTS IN PUBLIC HEALTH EMERGENCY PREPAREDNESS SINCE 9/11

PHEP JURISDICTIONS WHO:	THEN	NOW
Can mobilize staff during an emergency	20%	98%
Have an Incident Command System with pre-assigned roles in place	5%	100%
Have identified point-of-dispensing (POD) sites	0%	100%
Have sufficient storage and distribution capacity for critical medicines and supplies	0%	98%

WHY CDC?

CDC's experience and expertise helps U.S. communities prepare for, withstand, and recover from emergencies. We remain committed to training and growing a strong public health workforce by providing resources, funding, and partnerships to rapidly identify and respond to public health threats.

The Public Health Emergency Preparedness program provides:

Guidance: Annual evidence-based guidance to ensure state and local jurisdictions have the most current information to better protect their communities

Technical Assistance: Operational know-how to ensure state and local public health departments are ready to respond

Evaluation: Measurement and evaluation of states' capabilities to prepare for any public health emergency

PREPAREDNESS IN ACTION

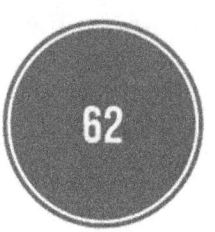

62

Since 2002, the PHEP program has provided support to 62 state, local, and territorial public health departments across the nation to protect Americans and save lives

487

In 2016, CDC and the 50 state health departments conducted 487 operational readiness reviews nationwide, including in the 72 largest metropolitan areas, to make sure life-saving medicines and supplies can reach the right people at the right time

SIX DOMAINS OF PREPAREDNESS:

CDC's PHEP program works to advance six main areas of preparedness so state and local public health systems are better prepared for emergencies that impact the public's health.

COMMUNITY RESILIENCE
Preparing for and recovering from emergencies

INCIDENT MANAGEMENT
Coordinating an effective response

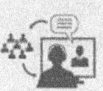

INFORMATION MANAGEMENT
Making sure people have information to take action

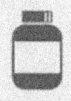

COUNTERMEASURES AND MITIGATION
Getting medicines and supplies where they are needed

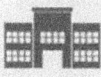

SURGE MANAGEMENT
Expanding medical services to handle large events

BIOSURVEILLANCE
Investigating and identifying health threats

PUBLIC HEALTH PREPAREDNESS AND RESPONSE
READY FOR EMERGENCIES

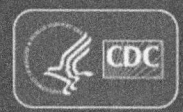

U.S. Department of
Health and Human Services
Centers for Disease
Control and Prevention

Source: CDC (2018). CDC Public Health Emergency Preparedness Program. Retrieved from https://www.cdc.gov/phpr/whatwedo/phep.htm

Appendix VI

RADIATION INFOGRAPHICS

RADIATION CONTAMINATION VERSUS EXPOSURE

EXTERNAL CONTAMINATION

External contamination occurs when radioactive material comes into contact with a person's skin, hair, or clothing.

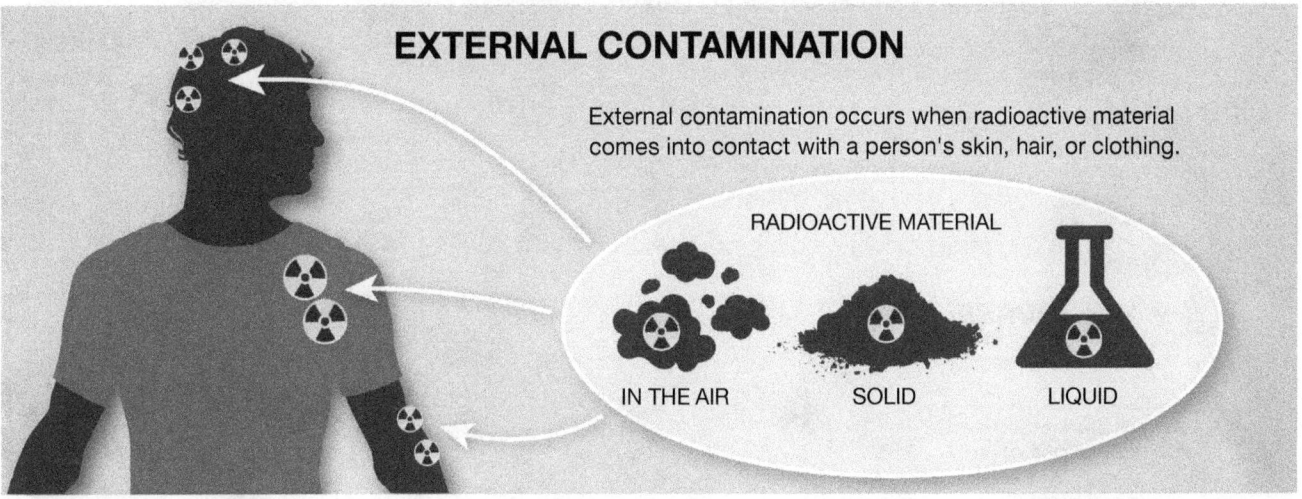

RADIOACTIVE MATERIAL

IN THE AIR   SOLID   LIQUID

INTERNAL CONTAMINATION

Internal contamination can occur when radioactive material is swallowed or breathed in.

Internal contamination can also occur when radioactive material enters the body through an open wound.

Different radioactive materials can accumulate in different body organs.

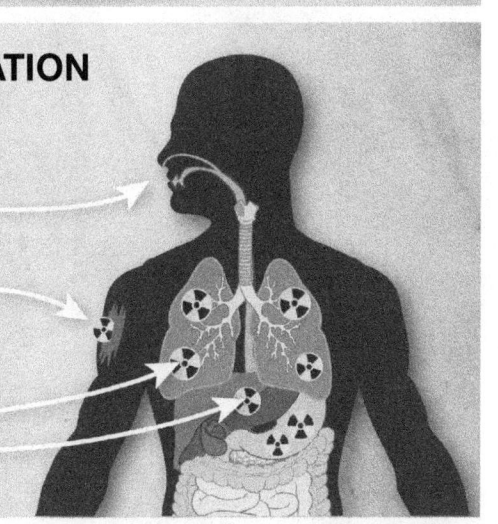

RADIATION EXPOSURE

Another word for radiation exposure is irradiation.

Radioactive materials give off a form of energy that travels in waves or particles.

A person exposed to radiation is not necessarily contaminated with radioactive material.

For a person to be contaminated, radioactive material must be on or inside of his or her body.

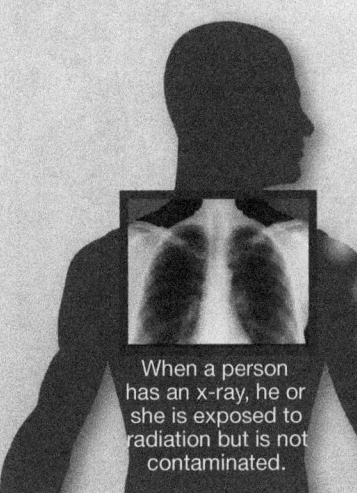

When a person has an x-ray, he or she is exposed to radiation but is not contaminated.

When a person is exposed to certain types of radiation, the energy may penetrate the body.

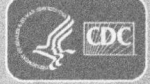

U.S. Department of Health and Human Services
Centers for Disease Control and Prevention

http://emergency.cdc.gov/radiation

DECONTAMINATION FOR YOURSELF AND OTHERS

① TAKE OFF OUTER LAYER OF CLOTHING

Taking off your outer layer of clothing can remove up to 90% of radioactive material.

Put the clothing in a plastic bag or other sealable container.

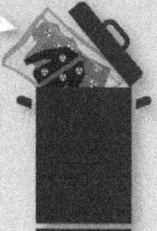

Be very careful in removing your clothing to prevent radioactive dust from shaking loose.

Put the bag in an out-of-the-way place, away from other people and pets.

② WASH YOURSELF OFF

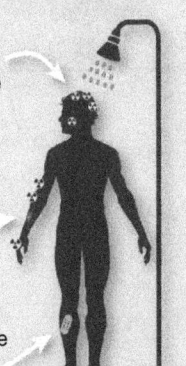

If you can take a shower:

Use soap and shampoo. Do not use conditioner because it will cause radioactive material to stick to your hair.

Do not scald, scrub, or scratch your skin.

Keep cuts and scrapes covered when washing to keep from getting radioactive material in open wounds.

If you cannot take a shower:

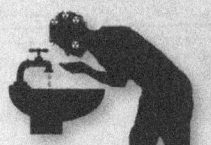

Wash your hands, face, and parts of your body that were uncovered at a sink or faucet. Use soap and plenty of water.

If you cannot use a sink or faucet:

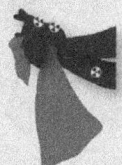

Use a moist wipe, clean wet cloth, or damp paper towel to wipe the parts of your body that were uncovered. Pay special attention to your hands and face.

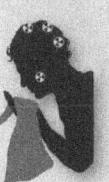

Blow your nose and wipe your eyelids, eyelashes, and ears with a moist wipe, clean wet cloth, or damp paper towel.

③ PUT ON CLEAN CLOTHES

If you have clean clothes:

Clothes stored in a closet or drawer away from radioactive material are safe to wear.

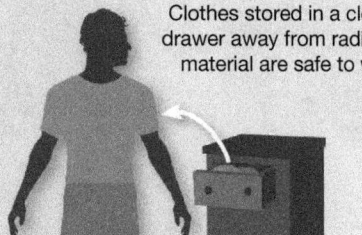

If you do not have clean clothes:

Take off your outer layer of clothing, shake or brush off your clothes, and put your clothes back on.

Rewash your hands, face, and exposed skin at a sink or faucet.

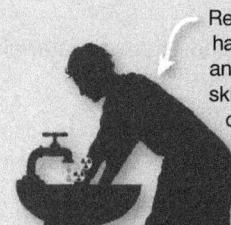

④ HELP OTHERS AND PETS

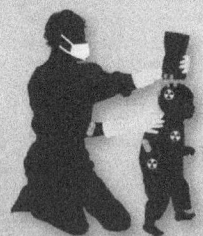

Wear waterproof gloves and a dust mask if you can.

Keep cuts and scrapes covered when washing to keep radioactive material out of the wound.

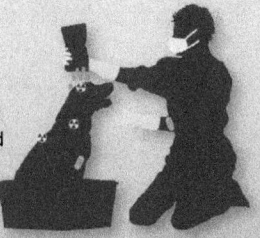

Rewash your hands, face, and parts of your body that were uncovered at a sink or faucet.

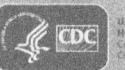

U.S. Department of Health and Human Services Centers for Disease Control and Prevention

STAY TUNED FOR UPDATED INFORMATION FROM PUBLIC HEALTH OFFICIALS.

http://emergency.cdc.gov/radiation

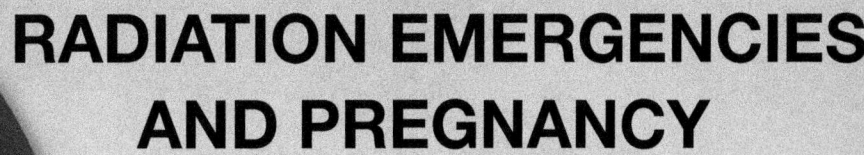

RADIATION EMERGENCIES AND PREGNANCY

After a radiation emergency, pregnant women should follow instructions from emergency officials and seek medical attention as soon as emergency officials say it is safe to do so.

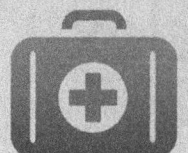

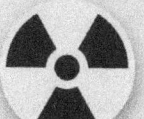

Prenatal radiation exposure occurs when a pregnant woman's abdomen is exposed to radiation.

For most radiation exposures, the radiation dose to the fetus is lower than the dose to the woman. A pregnant woman's abdomen partially protects the fetus from radiation sources that are outside her body.

If a pregnant woman swallows or breathes in radioactive materials, these may be absorbed into her bloodstream. From the woman's blood, radioactive materials may pass through the umbilical cord to the fetus or concentrate in areas of the mother's body near the womb and expose the fetus to radiation.

Health effects to the fetus from radiation exposure can be severe, even at radiation doses too low to make the mother sick. These health effects can include miscarriage, stunted growth, deformities, abnormal brain function, and cancer.

A fetus is most sensitive to radiation between weeks 2 and 18 of pregnancy. A fetus will become less sensitive to radiation during later stages of pregnancy.

In the rare event of a radiation emergency, radiation experts can answer questions from pregnant women and their healthcare providers about radiation exposure and pregnancy.

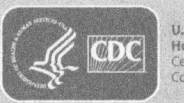

U.S. Department of
Health and Human Services
Centers for Disease
Control and Prevention

http://emergency.cdc.gov/radiation

Index

CPSIA information can be obtained
at www.ICGtesting.com
Printed in the USA
BVHW012321270721
613074BV00002B/8